# POTTER AND PERRY'S
# FOUNDATIONS IN NURSING THEORY AND PRACTICE

**Edited by**

## Hazel B M Heath

MSc, BA(Hons), RN, RCNT, RNT, DipN(Lond), CertEd, FETC, ITEC

*Senior Teacher and Subject Leader in Nursing Theory and Practice,*
*St Bartholomew & Princess Alexandra & Newham College of Nursing and Midwifery, London.*
*Adviser on Nursing and Older People to the Royal College of Nursing of the United Kingdom.*
*Freelance Consultant, Lecturer and Writer.*

 Mosby

## *Dedication*

*To Stanley Raymond Sims and Phyllis Margaret Sims*
*Thank you*

MOSBY
An imprint of Harcourt Publishers Limited

**M** is a registered trademark of Harcourt Publishers Limited
Mosby

© Times Mirror International Publishers Limited 1995
© Harcourt Publishers Limited 1999
© Harcourt Publishers Limited 2000

First published in 1995
    Reprinted 1999
    Reprinted 2000

ISBN 0 7234 2005 X

British Library Cataloguing in Publication Data
A catalogue record for this book is available from the British
Library.

Printed in China

| | |
|---|---|
| **Project Manager:** | Louise Crowe |
| **Developmental Editor:** | Amy Salter |
| **Designer:** | Lara Last |
| **Production:** | Joseph Lynch |
| **Cover Illustration:** | Ian Hands |
| **Cover Photograph:** | Cover photograph © 1994 Bruce Bailey/Select Photos, London |
| **Index:** | Nina Boyd |
| **Publisher:** | Griselda Campbell |

# Contents

# Clinical Skills

# Contributors

The following people edited, reviewed, and contributed new chapters to this book:

**Marion Allison**, BA(Hons), RGN, RNT, DipNEd(Lond), DipN(Lond)
CliniMed Lecturer in Stoma Care Nursing
St Bartholomew & Princess Alexandra & Newham College of Nursing and Midwifery
*Chapters 20, 23*

**Elizabeth Atchison**, MSc, RN, RNT, CertEd
MacMillan Senior Lecturer
Faculty of Health Care and Social Studies
University of Luton
*Chapter 11*

**Loretta Bellman**, MPhil, BSc(Hons), RGN, RCNT, RNT, CertEd
Adviser/Lecturer in Nursing
Institute of Advanced Nursing Education
Royal College of Nursing of the United Kingdom
*Chapter 29*

**Carmel Blackie**, BEd(Hons), RN, RNT, HVL, SCM, HV
Lecturer in Primary Health Care Nursing
St Bartholomew & Princess Alexandra & Newham College of Nursing and Midwifery
and
the Joint Academic Department of General Practice
The Medical College of St. Bartholomew's Hospital and the Royal London Hospital
Specialist reviewer for Community Nursing

**Diane Bosley**, BA(Hons), RCNT, SRN, OND, DipN(Lond)
Formerly Lecturer
St Bartholomew & Princess Alexandra & Newham College of Nursing and Midwifery
*Chapter 3*

**Helen Caulfield**, LLB, MA
Solicitor
Royal College of Nursing of the United Kingdom
*Chapter 13*

**Mary Cooke**, MSc(Econs), BSc(Hons), RGN, CM, DipArom, PGCE(A), CertHypnosis, CertReflex, FRSH, RCN
Senior Lecturer in Professional Studies, Health Economics & Complementary Medicine
Practising Nurse
University of East London
*Chapter 32*

**Alison Coutts**, MSc, BSc, RGN, PGCEA
Lecturer in Biological Sciences
St Bartholomew & Princess Alexandra & Newham College of Nursing and Midwifery
*Chapter 21*

**Michelle Cowen**, BEd(Hons), RGN, DipN(Lond), RCNT, ENB 100, RNT
Formerly Lecturer in Intensive Care Nursing

St Bartholomew & Princess Alexandra & Newham College of Nursing and Midwifery
*Chapter 25*

**Carol L. Cox**,  PhD, MSc, BSc, MAEd, RN, RNT, PG DipEd, CCRN, CNA
Head of Department of Nursing
St Bartholomew & Princess Alexandra & Newham College of Nursing and Midwifery
*Chapters 1, 2, 7, 9*

**Stuart J. Darby**, BA(Hons), RGN, RMN, RHV, DPSN
Head of Community Nursing Development Team
Camden and Islington Community Health Services NHS Trust
*Chapter 19*

**Andrea Fox-Hiley**, BSc(Hons), RN, RCNT, RNT, DipN(Lond), CertEd, ITEC
Lecturer in Continuing Care
St Bartholomew & Princess Alexandra & Newham College of Nursing and Midwifery
*Chapter 3*

**Barbara Hancock**, RNMH, ENB 870, 936
Head of Learning Disabilities Services
Guild Community Health Care NHS Trust
Specialist reviewer for Learning Disabilities Nursing

**Judith Handyside**, RGN, RSCN, RCNT, RNT, DipNEd(Lond), AdDipChildDev(Lond)
Lecturer in Children's Nursing
St Bartholomew & Princess Alexandra & Newham College of Nursing and Midwifery
*Chapter 26*

**Haoli James**, BSc(Hons), RGN, ENB 998, 100
Independent Nurse Consultant in Tissue Viability
London
*Chapter 30*

**Abigail Masterson**, BSc, MN, RGN, PGCEA
Institute of Advanced Nursing Education
Royal College of Nursing of the United Kingdom
*Chapter 24*

**Lyn Meehan**, BSc, RGN, DipN, DNCert, CertEd,
Director of Community Nursing Studies
Bloomsbury and Islington College of Nursing and Midwifery
*Chapter 19*

**Angela Monaghan**, MA, RGN, RM, RNT
Senior Lecturer in Adult Continuing Care, Primary Care Nursing
St Bartholomew & Princess Alexandra & Newham College of Nursing and Midwifery
*Chapter 15*

**Pam Parker**, MA(Ed), BA(Hons), RGN
Senior Lecturer for Education/Examinations and Assessment
St Bartholomew & Princess Alexandra & Newham College of Nursing and Midwifery
London
*Chapters 14, 16*

**Irene Schofield**, MSc, RGN, RNT, CertEd, CertGerontology, CertOncolN
Lecturer in Care of the Older Adult
St Bartholomew & Princess Alexandra & Newham College of Nursing and Midwifery
*Chapter 6* (Older Adult)

**Lesley Sheldon**, BSc(Hons), RN, RSCN, DipN, DipNEd, CertPublicPol
Lecturer in Children's Nursing
St Bartholomew & Princess Alexandra & Newham College of Nursing and Midwifery
*Chapter 6* and Specialist reviewer for Children's Nursing

**Rosemary H. Sheng**, BA(Hons), RMN, RCNT, DipN(Lond), RNT, DipNEd(Lond)
Senior Lecturer in Mental Health Nursing & Learning Disabilities/Mental Handicap Nursing
St Bartholomew & Princess Alexandra & Newham College of Nursing and Midwifery
*Chapters 6, 10* and Specialist reviewer for Mental Health Nursing

**Dorothy Stables**, MSc, BA(Hons), RN, RM, MTD, DipN(Lond)
Midwife/Lecturer in Biological Sciences
St Bartholomew & Princess Alexandra & Newham College of Nursing and Midwifery
*Chapter 6* and Specialist reviewer for Mother & Child Nursing

**David Taylor**, RN, RCNT, RNT, CertEd, FETC, ENB 249, ENB 934
Lecturer Cardiothoracic Nursing
St Bartholomew & Princess Alexandra & Newham College of Nursing and Midwifery
*Chapters 5, 28*

**Nicola Thomas**, BSc(Hons), RGN, PGDip(Ed), ENB 136,
Lecturer in Renal Nursing
St Bartholomew & Princess Alexandra & Newham College of Nursing and Midwifery
*Chapter 18*

**Verena Tschudin**, BSc(Hons), RN, RM, DipCouns
Senior Lecturer
University of East London
*Chapter 12*

**David Turner**, MSc, BA, RGN, ENB 870, 941, 998
Lecturer
Buckinghamshire College
Formerly Ward Manager, St Bartholomew's Hospital & Newham College of Nursing and Midwifery
*Chapter 22*

**Janet Vickers**, MSc, BSc(Hons), RN, RSCN, PGCE, DipHEd
Senior Lecturer, Applied Biological Sciences
St Bartholomew & Princess Alexandra & Newham College of Nursing and Midwifery
*Chapter 17*

**Neslyn Watson-Druee**, MSc, BA(Hons), RGN, RNT, DipHEd, RHV, RM, PGCE, MIPD
Management Consultant, London
*Chapter 8*

**Carole Webster**, BSc(Hons) (Pharmacology), RGN, RM, DipN, DipNEd, RNT, DipHE (Biol), ENB 100
Formerly Lecturer
St Bartholomew & Princess Alexandra & Newham College of Nursing and Midwifery
*Chapters 4, 18, 22, 31*

**Isabel White**, BEd(Hons), RGN, RNT, RSCN, DipLScNurs
Lecturer, Practitioner in Clinical Oncology
Thames Valley University & Hammersmith Hospitals NHS Trust
*Chapter 27*

# Acknowledgements

The editor and publisher gratefully acknowledge the following people for their assistance with this book:

Patricia A. Potter, RN, MSN and Anne G. Perry, RN, MSN, Ed D., Bruce Bailey, Carol Bavin, Ann Cowcher, Catherine Ebinezer, Debbie Fisher, Andrea Ford, Phyl MacKenzie, Georgina Massy, Paul Moorbath, The Royal London Hospitals Trust, Madeleine Sowden, Hannah Tudge, Christopher Walker

**Reviewers:** Elaine Andrews, Sue Atkins, Chris Brooker, Dr Philip Burnard, Eloise Carr, Steve Cavanagh, Glenda Cook, Mrs E Desira, Helena Gyory, Noel Knopp, Tom Lewis, Rose Maconaghie, Miss E A Matthew, James McAllister, Catherine A McEvoy, Donna Mead, Marian Moody, Janet Scammell, Dot Stables, Kevin Teasdale, Mrs L C M Toner,

**Contributors to the U.S. edition of this book:** Della Aridge, RN, MSN; Susan Cole, RN, MSN, CCRN; Dorothy McDonnell Cooke, RN, PhD; Sharon H. Cox, MSN, CNAA; Catherine Doerrer, RN, MSN; Sally M. Featherstone, RN, MN, CS: Lois K. Hess, RN, JD; Nancy C. Jackson, RN, BSN, MSN, CCRN; Sister Kathleen Krekeler, RN, PhD; Pamela A. Lesser, RN, MS; Gail B. Lewis, RN, MSN; Annette Lueckenotte, RN, MS CS; Mary Kay Knight Macheca, RN, MSN(R), CDE; Sharon L. Merritt, RN, EdD; Ann M. Popkess, RN, BSN; Susan A. Reed, RNCS, MSN; Janet Robuck, MS, RD; Judith A. Roos, RN, MSN; Janice Rumfelt, RNC, MSN(R), EdD; Rachel E. Spector, RN, PhD, CTN; Martha Spies, RN, MSN; Joetta A. Vernon, RN, MS; Mary Walker, RN, MA; Valerie Yancey, BA, AD, BSN, MSN.

# Foreword

Radical changes in the National Health Service are creating complex challenges for nurses, who must be able to function effectively in the new health care climate. The major overhaul of the National Health Service (NHS and Community Care Act 1990) has been a catalyst for major changes in health care, giving new shape and direction to the provision of health and social services. Health strategies are moving away steadily from the hospital dominated focus for the major provision of health care to the provision of local, accessible and relevant services.

Nursing curricula, preparing nurses to meet health care needs into the next century, should therefore be sensitive to the political, social and economic pressures which are directing health care strategies. The political emphasis on health promotion and disease prevention demands comprehensive primary health care within the community, rather than institutional settings, and as care becomes more community centred, acute hospital services will be rationalised and reduced.

There are clearly implications for nurse educationalists, to ensure that education programmes facilitate student nurses' learning towards:
"an emphasis on care in the community,
on care in the home,
on assessing health needs, and promoting self-care and independence"
(Project 2000 - A New Preparation for Practice 1986).

Nursing curricula should also be sensitive to the varied needs of a range of client groups: the adult, the older person, the child, those with disturbance of mental health and individuals with learning disabilities. Furthermore, the practitioners of the future will be required to contribute to the planning, assessment and development of services. It is imperative that the initial education programmes leading to qualification, should enable the development of relevant skills, knowledge and expertise to act as the bedrock for a lifelong progression of professional learning. This is essential when considering the changing pattern of needs for health care, and the subsequent changes to the delivery of care.

The education process preparing students for practice should move them forward through a foundation programme embedded in health, developing a body of knowledge and skills related to normal living, normal reactions to stress, and coping and supporting. Theory and practice must be interrelated and integrated, grounded in social, behavioural and biological sciences, enabling the students to achieve learning outcomes which are responsive to the stated goals of the National Health Service:
- to restore health
- to teach self-care
- to promote independent living as far as possible
- to respect the values and desires of the individual patient/client.

These goals must be placed in the social context, where there are many differing general and special needs. A significant number of people have limited access to health care: people who are homeless, unemployed or coping as a single parent, or as a consequence of changes in family structures.

For nurses to be prepared to function effectively in a constantly changing health service and to respond to the complex needs of society, education must be a liberating process, enabling them to grow in their capacity to make well informed decisions with confidence. Prior to the implementation of Project 2000 (A New Preparation for Practice) which commenced in September 1989, the emphasis lay with nurse training rather than with education. Now, in preparing the "knowledgeable doer", students are educated and trained establishing a process which will be continued throughout their working life. They will develop skills in reflection, critical thinking, seeing other possibilities, generating new ideas, assessing information and making appropriate decisions. Students need to be able to challenge preconceptions, calling on their knowledge and skills to bring about change and innovation.

In the Department of Health's *Nursing, Midwifery and Health Visiting Education: A Statement of Strategic Intent (1994)*, the fundamental principles for nursing education are stated, including the requirement that it be patient-focused, practice-led and student-centred:
"recognising the individuality of students....
.... and making programmes accessible, attractive
and challenging, in terms of both personal and professional development".
"Students must be placed at the centre of the learning experience, which is explicitly practice-led and research-based."

How can this education process be facilitated? In part, by learning resources which will challenge students, hold their interest and encourage them to develop skills in seeking out information for themselves, an essential prerequisite to becoming truly research minded.

This book will prove to be such a resource, as a research orientated source of knowledge, guiding and informing practice. It interrelates fundamental nursing principles with relevant skills, considering each situation logically and analytically. It will help nurses to have the skills, knowledge and attributes to make sound clinical judgements in assessing, planning, implementing and evaluating care, recognising the primacy of each patient's/client's interests. Above all, the outcome must be a nurse who is caring and conscious of each person's needs, capable of responding to these needs, in a highly skilled and sensitive manner.

It is a privilege to write this Foreword as Chairman of the Management Board of St Bartholomew and Princess Alexandra and Newham College of Nursing and Midwifery. As Chairman of the English National Board for Nursing, Midwifery and Health Visiting (1988-1993), I was committed totally to the reform of nurse education in the United Kingdom. I am confident that this textbook will make a major and significant contribution to the curricula for future students of nursing.

Professor Jean E Hooper CBE

# Foreword by Student Nurses

This book is exactly what students need in their Common Foundation Course. It is the only book we have found which comprehensively covers all the aspects of nursing practice linked to theory, and prepares students for all of the branches.

It clearly explains the biological, psychosocial and other theories on which nursing is based, and it also describes in detail all the relevant aspects of care such as nursing skills, caring for people undergoing particular investigations or treatments, and assisting in examinations. This is particularly helpful in clinical situations when we need to know how to deliver care appropriately. The book also contains immediately accessible information about the UK health care system, health targets and the development of nursing in the UK.

Most nursing books are adult-orientated, and we particularly like the highlights on mental health, learning disabilities, adult and children's nursing. Together with the further reading, these can help all of us to work towards our chosen branch programmes, but also to appreciate the scope of the other branches.

The chapter outlines, learning outcomes and key concepts sections are helpful in letting us quickly find a particular subject, and in using as a guide to read through the chapter. The key terms are useful for checking definitions and the critical thinking questions help us reflect on what we have read.

We found the book easy to read. Everything is clearly explained and well set out. The book is also good value for money.

Claire Bannister
Jacqueline Mary Binnie
Jacqueline Cox
Unesu Audrey Chindabata

(April 1993 Cohort, St Bartholomew & Princess Alexandra & Newham College of Nursing and Midwifery)

# Preface

Planning our new pre-registration programme, the nursing subject group at St Bartholomew's College became aware of the need for a comprehensive textbook which would support the students in developing their caring skills, alongside the building of their theory base.

Rather than totally reinvent the wheel, a committed team of lecturers, specialists and clinicians set about adapting the popular US text *Fundamentals of Nursing : Concepts, Process and Practice 3 ed* by Patricia A. Potter and Anne G. Perry. The selection of content to be revised was guided by the United Kingdom Central Council curriculum requirements, and the 1989 Statutory Instrument No 1456, which lists the outcomes to be achieved by students undertaking pre-registration programmes.

## THE CONTENT OF THE BOOK

New chapters written for the UK book include Culture, Ethnicity and Religion, Legal Issues and Complementary Therapies. The chapters based on the US text have been adapted to reflect UK populations, cultures, health care, nursing practice, terminology and research base. In particular, the chapters now consider the experience of UK pre-registration students caring for patients/clients of different ages and with varying care needs.

*Foundations in Nursing Theory and Practice* comprehensively introduces the concepts integral to nursing and health care, such as individuality, human needs, health, illness, culture, religion, development and loss. It works through the processes fundamental to nursing practice such as communication, assessment, research, planning, ethical decision-making, intervention, teaching and evaluation. In addition, specialists have contributed highlighted inserts and recommended reading which enable students to work towards their branch programmes.

The content focuses on individuals and individual experiences, and on health rather than ill health. It also discusses nursing practice in a variety of settings.

### Use of the terms patient/client
In most cases the terms individual, person or people have been used to denote the UK population, and those who receive health care. When discussing specific situations, the title patient/client has been adopted. Although more cumbersome than a single term, it more accurately reflects the terminology used by nurses in the diversity of settings in which they practice.

### Clinical practice guidelines, protocols and procedures
Nursing practice in the UK is currently guided by a variety of formats. Guidance for nurses may be presented as standards of care, clinical practice guidelines, management protocols, or nursing procedures.

There is currently much debate on which format will improve the quality of care, organisational information, and the implementation of research findings. In experiencing a variety of formats, students will develop their own views. A separate content's page has been included listing those clinical skills included in this book.

## THE STRUCTURE OF THE BOOK

**Unit 1: Foundations of Contemporary Nursing** introduces the student to the profession of nursing, the current health care context, and the process of nursing with particular emphasis on assessment and documentation.

**Unit 2: The Nurse and the Patient/Client** details the concepts and processes fundamental to the health of human beings, be they patients/clients or nurses. Content includes growth and development, human needs, culture, ethnicity and religion, health and illness, stress and adaptation, loss, death and grieving.

**Unit 3: Professional Nursing Concepts and Processes** discusses the concepts, principles and processes which underpin and guide nursing practice. These include values and ethics, legal issues, research communication, teaching and learning.

**Unit 4: Human Needs and Nursing Practice** details the theory and practice of how nurses assist patients and clients to meet fundamental needs for oxygen, fluids, sleep, nutrition, elimination, mobility and hygiene.

**Unit 5: Nursing Practice and Nursing Skills** details specific aspects of nursing practice such as controlling pain or infection, administering medications and using complementary therapies. It also considers nursing people who have sensory alterations, who are at risk of tissue viability problems, or who are undergoing surgery.

## THE FORMAT OF THE CHAPTERS

The chapters are designed to aid effective student learning and to assist readers in quickly finding particular subjects. Each chapter contains:

**Chapter outline** - the chapter content at a glance.

**Learning outcomes** - the main concepts which can be learned from the chapter.

**Special focus boxes** - to link the topics in the chapters to nursing practice with children, adults, people with mental health needs and those with a learning disability.

**Boxed highlights** - to emphasize important issues relevant to the chapter, such as cultural diversity, or varying priorities around the UK.

**Nursing process stages** - to present clearly the nurse's role in assessing, planning, implementing and evaluating care.

**Nursing skills procedures, principles and guidelines** - to give detailed guidance on the fundamental caring skills.

**Illustrations** - there are clear diagrams and photographs to illustrate the text.

**Chapter summary** - to provide an overview of the topics discussed in the chapter.

**Key terms** - to highlight new terminology, and to enable the terms to be found quickly in the chapter.

**Critical thinking exercises** - to encourage reflection on practical situations, and to assess critically understanding of the content.

**References** - to give full citations of the literature and research on which the chapter is based.

**Further reading** - recommendations for further resources on adult, children's, mental health and learning disabilities nursing, which assist in understanding the needs of particular patients/clients.

We hope you enjoy using *Foundations in Nursing Theory and Practice*. Should you have any comments about the book, please write to me care of the Publishers - we'll be pleased to hear from you.

Hazel B.M. Heath
February 1995

# unit 1

## Foundations of Contemporary Nursing

# The Profession of Nursing

## CHAPTER OUTLINE

## LEARNING OUTCOMES

After studying this chapter you should be able to:
- *Define the key terms listed.*
- *Discuss the historical development of professional nursing.*
- *Discuss the historical and modern definitions, philosophies, and theories of nursing practice.*
- *Describe the issues addressed in the UKCC position statement on scope of practice.*
- *Describe the aims of the UKCC Code of Professional Conduct.*
- *Describe the most common practice settings for nurses.*
- *Describe the roles and functions of a nurse.*
- *List the five characteristics of a profession and discuss how nursing demonstrates these characteristics.*
- *Discuss the influence of social and economic changes on nursing practice.*
- *Discuss the influence of political issues on nursing practice and health care policy.*
- *Identify current trends in nursing practice.*

Modern nursing involves many activities, concepts, and skills related to basic sciences, social sciences, growth and development, contemporary issues, and other areas. Nursing as a profession is unique because it addresses the responses of individuals and families to actual and potential health problems in a humanistic and holistic manner (Roper *et al*, 1983). Nurses have many roles, such as carers, decision makers, advocates, and teachers, and they must often assume several roles at the same time. Because of the diversity of nursing roles, nurses need a **philosophy of nursing** to guide their practice. Over the years, nurses have developed many philosophies and definitions of nursing. The following **definition of nursing**, written by Virginia Henderson and adopted by the **International Council of Nurses (ICN)** (1973), is a concise statement with which most nursing theorists would agree:

*The unique function of the nurse is to assist the individual, sick or well, in the performance of those activities contributing to health, its recovery, or to a peaceful death, that the client would perform unaided if he had the necessary strength, will, or knowledge. And to do this in such a way as to help the client gain independence as rapidly as possible.*

The profession of nursing is complex and multifaceted. Nurses practise in many settings that emphasize different aspects of nursing care and nursing roles. In addition, individuals can become registered nurses through a variety of educational programmes, and a variety of career opportunities become available as nurses gain experience and continue their education.

Expertise in nursing is the result of knowledge and clinical experience. The expertise required to interpret clinical situations and make complex decisions is the basis for the advancement of nursing practice and the development of nursing science (Benner, 1984; Benner and Tanner, 1987). To deliver nursing care, the nurse must be able to make relevant observations, recognize health problems, and develop appropriate plans to address those problems (Tanner et al, 1987). Expertise is gained through this continual process.

The profession of nursing evolves as society and health care needs and policies change. Nursing responds and adapts to changes, meeting new challenges as they arise.

## HISTORICAL PERSPECTIVE

Nursing was distinguished in its early history as a form of community service and was originally related to a strong instinct to preserve and protect the family (Donahue, 1985). Nursing began as the desire to keep people healthy and provide comfort, care, and assurance to the sick. Although the general goals of nursing have remained relatively the same over the centuries, the practice of nursing has been influenced by society's changing needs, and thus nursing has gradually evolved into a modern profession.

Nursing is as old as medicine. Throughout history, nursing and medicine have been interdependent. During the era of Hippocrates, medicine was practised without nursing, and during the Middle Ages, nursing was practised without medicine (Donahue, 1985).

In ancient cultures, religious beliefs and myths were the bases for health care and medical practice. Religious leaders assumed the responsibility for diagnosis and treatment, and many cultures believed that illness was caused by the gods' displeasure. In these cultures, nurses usually had a role subservient to religious leaders.

Many ancient societies did not value human life in the same way we do today, so the care takers of life were less respected. Nurses delivered custodial care and depended on physicians or priests for direction (Kelly, 1981). Under the direct supervision of a physician the nurse tended to the hygiene of clients in the home. Nurses did not participate in activities to promote health or teach families how to care for the sick.

One consistent role from early civilization is that of the midwife. Throughout history, the midwife has been accepted in the role of assisting women during childbirth and has been seen as separate from, but complementary to, the role of the nurse.

Under the influence of Christianity, nurses began to gain respect, and the practice of nursing expanded. One of the earliest records of Christian nursing detailed the formation of the Order of the Deaconesses, a group somewhat like today's Health Visitors and District Nurses. The Order's goals included to meet the following **basic needs** of the society (Dolan et al, 1983; Donahue, 1985), and to mirror Christian doctrine:

- to feed the hungry
- to give water to the thirsty
- to clothe the naked
- to visit the imprisoned
- to shelter the homeless
- to care for the sick
- to bury the dead.

Historically, both men and women have held the role of nurse. The entry of women into nursing can be traced to approximately AD 300 (Shryock, 1959; Donahue, 1985). Women entered nursing because the social position of Roman women improved (Shryock, 1959), Christians taught that men and women are equal before God (Shryock, 1959; Dolan et al, 1983), and Christians appealed to women "to carry on His work on behalf of all who were in distress" (Shryock, 1959).

The Benedictine order, founded in the sixth century, increased the number of men entering nursing. Although the Benedictines were scholars, librarians, teachers, and agriculturalists, nursing the sick eventually became the chief function and duty of their community life (Donahue, 1985).

During the Middle Ages, the Crusades became a stimulus for expanded nursing and health care. Military nursing orders for men were formed, and hospitals were established. After the Crusades, large cities began to develop and grow with the decline of feudalism. The extensive population growth in cities led to certain health problems and an increased need for health care. Some of these problems still exist in urban areas today (WHO, 1992), although the mortality rates associated with them have greatly declined.

Secular groups were also formed to meet specific health care needs during the Middle Ages. The Hospital Brothers of St Anthony cared for victims of the disease which became known as *St Anthony's fire*, the Brothers of Misericordia in Italy provided transportation services for the ill (Fig. 1-1), and the Alexian Brothers (a group still active today) cared for victims of bubonic plague.

The lack of hygiene and sanitation, and the increasing poverty in urban centres resulted in serious health problems in the fifteenth to seventeenth centuries. Societal factors, such as laws punishing the poor, and the Window Tax (which led to decreased ventilation because landlords bricked in windows to avoid paying the tax), created conditions and health needs to which nursing responded.

The Sisters of Charity was founded in 1633 by St Vincent de Paul. The sisters cared for people in hospitals, asylums, and poorhouses. In addition, the sisters became widely known as visiting nurses because they cared for sick people in their homes. The first supervisor of the Sisters of Charity was Louise de Gras, a widow of high social standing. de Gras, who entered the order and was later known as St Louise de Marillac, established perhaps the first educational programme to be associated with a nursing order. She recruited intelligent, refined, and compassionate women (Donahue,

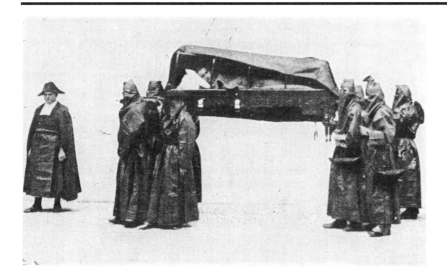

**Fig. 1-1** The Brothers of Misericordia taking a patient to the hospital in Florence.
From Dolan JA *et al: Nursing in society,* ed 15, Philadelphia, 1983, Saunders.

1985) and offered a programme that included experience in the care of the sick in the hospital, as well as home visits.

In the eighteenth century, the further growth of cities brought an increase in the number of hospitals and a larger role for nurses. Smallpox epidemics in the French colonies and during the Revolutionary War in the English colonies increased the need for nursing services. Nursing skills and knowledge were generally passed on by experienced nurses because there was still little formal education for them.

During the nineteenth century, the Deaconess Order was revived by Protestant churches. The Deaconess Institute at Kaiserswerth, Germany, was established in 1836 by Pastor Theodore Fliedner . The regeneration of this nursing order was stimulated by the recognition of the need for the services of nurses. In October 1846, Florence Nightingale received the *Yearbook of the Institution of Deaconesses at Kaiserswerth.* In 1847, she went to Kaiserswerth to work with the Deaconesses (Woodham-Smith, 1983; Donahue, 1985).

In 1853, Nightingale went to Paris to study with the Sisters of Charity and was later appointed superintendent of the British General Hospitals in the Crimea. During this period, she brought about major reforms in hygiene, sanitation, and nursing practice and reduced the mortality rate at the Barracks Hospital in Scutari, from 42.7% to 2.2% in 6 months (Cohen, 1984; Woodham-Smith, 1983; Donahue, 1985).

In 1860, Nightingale wrote *Notes on Nursing: What It Is and What It Is Not* for the lay person. Her philosophy of nursing practice reflected the changing needs of society. She saw the role of nursing as having "charge of somebody's health" based on the knowledge of "how to put the body in such a state to be free of disease or to recover from disease" (Nightingale, 1860). During the same year, she developed the first organized programme of training for nurses, the Nightingale Training School for Nurses at St Thomas' Hospital in London (Fig. 1-2).

Nurses and nurse educators are revising nursing practice and curricula to meet the ever-changing needs of society. Advances in high technology, rising acuity of clients, early discharge of clients from hospitals and the transfer of services from the acute to the community sector require nurses to have a strong and current knowledge base from which to practise.

## CONCEPTUAL AND THEORETICAL MODELS OF NURSING PRACTICE

The development of nursing science and theory is a scholarly activity. Developing this science involves generating knowledge; although this knowledge can be used with knowledge from other disciplines, it is designed to advance and support nursing practice and health care (Hinshaw, 1989). One method for creating nursing's scientific knowledge base is through the development and use of **nursing theory**.

Historically, nursing theories were studied in an isolated academic environment independent of nursing practice. There is, however, a contemporary move towards **theory-based practice**. Nurses now and in the future need to have models of care from which their practice is based (Parse, 1990).

As nursing continues to evolve, nurses theorize about the nature of nursing practice, the principles on which practice is based, and the proper goals and functions of nursing in society. Conceptual and theoretical nursing models are used to provide knowledge to improve practice, guide research and curricula, and identify the domain and goals of nursing practice. Nursing theories provide the nurse with goals for assessment, planning, implementation and evaluation; common ground for communication; and professional autonomy and accountability. They also guide future directions for nursing research, practice, education, and management (Marriner-Tomey, 1989; Chinn and Jacobs, 1987; Fawcett, 1989; Meleis, 1985; Torres, 1986; Parse, 1987; Chinn and Kramer, 1991).

A historical review of the last 120 years demonstrates that nursing has developed a growing body of knowledge. **Nursing concepts and theories** have evolved since Nightingale, who, in establishing the discipline of nursing, spoke with firm conviction about the "nature of nursing as a profession that required knowledge distinct from medical knowledge" (Nightingale, 1860). The overall goal of this knowledge has been to explain the practice of nursing as different and distinct from the practice of medicine, psychology, and social work (Torres, 1986; Chinn and Jacobs, 1987; Fawcett, 1989; Chinn and Kramer, 1991).

A significant milestone influencing the development of nursing concepts and theory was the establishment of the journal,

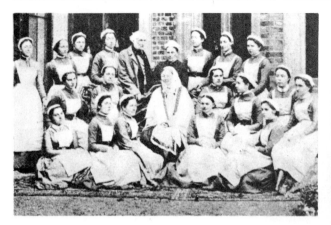

**Fig. 1-2** Florence Nightingale *(centre)* and students at St Thomas' Hospital in London in 1887. From Dolan JA *et al*: *Nursing in society*, ed 15, Philadelphia, 1983, Saunders.

### Children's Nursing
### Applying nursing models

Models for nursing can also be applied to children's nursing. The model needs to reflect the actual and/or potential health situation in which the nurse meets the child and family. The model must also reflect that the child is a unique, developing individual whose interests are paramount. The child has physical, psychological, social, cultural and spiritual needs which must be met. The child also has rights; therefore, information must be geared towards his/her developmental stage and ability to understand and provide informed participation regarding his/her care (RCN, 1992). The model must also reflect the partnership with the child's family and that children have a right to have a parent or guardian accompanying them during hospitalization and treatment.

*Nursing Research*, in 1952. Today, many journals report on the scientific investigations being conducted by nurses and other professionals. They have encouraged scientific productivity and have helped to provide the framework for a questioning attitude that has set the stage for further inquiries into theoretical nursing (Meleis, 1985).

In the mid-1950s, nursing leaders began to formulate theoretical views of nursing and concerns about subjects to include or exclude from nursing curricula. Teachers College Columbia University in the US offered masters and doctoral programmes in nursing education and administration (Meleis, 1985). Several prominent nurse theorists graduated from this institution; these include Peplau, Henderson, Hall, Abdellah, King, Wiedenbach, and Rogers.

During the 1960s, Yale University School of Nursing in the US defined nursing even further: "Nursing was considered a process rather than an end, an interaction rather than content, and a relationship between two human beings rather than an interaction between unrelated nurse and patient" (Meleis, 1985).

In 1961, Ida Jean Orlando discussed the process of nursing in her book *The Dynamic Nurse-Patient Relationship*. This led to the formulation of the nursing process by Yura and Walsh in 1967 as nurses know it today.

Macfarlane, in December of 1973, introduced the nursing process to the UK at a nursing conference in Manchester. Following its introduction, nurses in the UK began to incorporate the nursing process of assessment, planning, implementation and evaluation into their practice.

Theory development has been emphasized in the UK from the 1980s. For example, the four UK National Boards, the accrediting institutions for nursing education programmes, have emphasized a theory-based curriculum as a requirement for accreditation and validation of nursing programmes. Thus, colleges of nursing are expected to use a conceptual framework in the development and implementation of their curricula.

Definitions and theories of nursing can help the student nurse understand how the roles and actions of nurses fit together in nursing. The following sections describe, in chronological order, concepts basic to selected nursing theories.

### Nightingale's Theory

Contemporary authors are beginning to explore Florence Nightingale's work as a potential theoretical and conceptual model for nursing (Chinn and Jacobs, 1987; Marriner-Tomey, 1989; Meleis, 1985; Torres, 1986). Meleis (1985) notes that Nightingale's concept of environment as the focus of nursing care and her admonition that nurses need not know all about the disease process are early attempts to differentiate between nursing and medicine.

Nightingale did not view nursing as limited merely to the administration of medications and treatments but rather as orientated towards providing fresh air, light, warmth, cleanliness, quiet, and adequate nutrition (Nightingale, 1860; Torres, 1986). Through observation and data collection, she linked the client's health status with environmental factors and, as a result, initiated improved hygiene and sanitary conditions during the Crimean war.

Torres (1986) notes that Nightingale provided basic concepts and propositions that could be validated and used for practice in nursing. Nightingale's "descriptive theory" provides nurses with a way to think about nursing or a frame of reference that focuses on patients and the environment (Torres, 1986). Nightingale's letters and writings direct the nurse to act on behalf of the client. Her principles encompass the areas of practice, research, and education. Most importantly, her concepts and principles shaped and delineated nursing practice (Marriner-Tomey, 1994). Nightingale taught and used the nursing process, noting that "vital observation [assessment] . . . is not for the sake of piling up miscellaneous information or curious facts, but for the sake of saving life and increasing health and comfort."

### Peplau's Theory

Hildegard Peplau's theory (1952) focuses on the individual, nurse, and interactive process (Peplau, 1952); the result is the nurse-client relationship (Torres, 1986; Marriner-Tomey, 1994; Fawcett, 1993). According to this theory the client is an individual with a felt need, and nursing is an interpersonal and therapeutic process. Nursing's goal is to educate the client and family and to help the client reach mature personality development (Chinn and Jacobs, 1987). Therefore, the nurse strives to develop a nurse-client relationship in which the nurse serves as a resource person, counsellor, and surrogate.

When the client seeks help, the nurse first discusses the nature of the problem and explains the services available. As the nurse-client relationship develops, the nurse and client mutually define the problem and potential solutions. The client gains from this relationship by using available services to meet needs, and the nurse assists the client in reducing anxiety related to the health care problem. Peplau's theory is unique in that the collaborative nurse-client relationship creates a "maturing force" through which interpersonal effectiveness assists in meeting the client's needs (Beeber, Anderson and Sills, 1990). When the original needs have been resolved, new needs may emerge. The nurse-client interpersonal relationship is characterized by the following overlapping phases: orientation, identification, explanation, and resolution (Chinn and Jacobs, 1987; Fawcett, 1993).

Peplau's theory and ideas were developed to provide a design for the practice of mental health nursing. Nursing research on anxiety, empathy, behavioural tools, and tools to evaluate verbal responses resulted from Peplau's conceptual model (Marriner-Tomey, 1989).

## Henderson's Theory

Virginia Henderson's nursing theory (1955) involves basic needs of the whole person. The following needs, often called *Henderson's 14 basic needs,* provide a framework for nursing care (Henderson, 1966):
1. Breathe normally
2. Eat and drink adequately
3. Eliminate by all avenues of elimination
4. Move and maintain a desirable position
5. Sleep and rest
6. Select suitable clothing; dress and undress
7. Maintain body temperature within normal range
8. Keep the body clean and well groomed
9. Avoid dangers in the environment
10. Communicate with others
11. Worship according to faith
12. Work at something that provides a sense of accomplishment
13. Play or participate in various forms of recreation
14. Learn, discover, or satisfy the curiosity that leads to normal development and health.

## Abdellah's Theory

The nursing theory developed by Faye Abdellah *et al* (1960) emphasizes delivering nursing care for the whole person to meet the physical, emotional, intellectual, social, and spiritual needs of the client and family. When using this approach, the nurse needs knowledge and skills in interpersonal relations, psychology, growth and development, communication, and sociology, as well as a knowledge of the basic sciences and specific nursing skills. The nurse is a problem solver and decision maker. The nurse formulates an individualized view of the client's needs, which may occur in the following areas:

1. Comfort, hygiene, and safety
2. Physiological balance
3. Psychological and social factors
4. Sociological and community factors.

## Orlando's Theory

To Ida Orlando (1961), the client is an individual with a need that, when met, diminishes distress, increases adequacy, or enhances well-being (Chinn and Jacobs, 1987). Orlando's theory focuses on nurses' reactions to client behaviour in terms of the client's immediate need (Torres, 1986). Orlando's theory contains a conceptual framework for professional nursing. Three elements: client behaviour, nurse reaction, and nurse actions, compose the nursing situation (Marriner-Tomey, 1989). After nurses thoroughly assess the client's need, they recognize the impact of that need on the client's level of health and then act automatically or deliberately to meet the need, ultimately reducing the client's distress (Chinn and Jacobs, 1987, Orlando, 1990).

## Levine's Theory

Myra Levine's nursing theory, formulated in 1966 and published in 1973, views the client as an integrated being who interacts with and adapts to the environment. Levine believes that nursing intervention is a conservation activity, with conservation of energy as a primary concern (Fawcett, 1989). Health is viewed in terms of the conservation of energy in the following areas, which Levine calls the *four conservation principles of nursing:*
1. Conservation of patient energy
2. Conservation of structural integrity
3. Conservation of personal integrity
4. Conservation of social integrity.

With this approach, nursing care involves conservation activities aimed at the optimal use of the client's resources.

## Johnson's Theory

Dorothy Johnson's theory of nursing (1968) focuses on how the patient adapts to illness and how actual or potential stress can affect the ability to adapt. The goal of nursing is to reduce stress so that the patient can move more easily through recovery (Johnson, 1968). Johnson's theory focuses on basic needs in terms of the following categories of behaviour:
1. Security-seeking behaviour
2. Nurturance-seeking behaviour
3. Master of oneself and one's environment according to internalized standards of excellence
4. Taking in nourishment in socially and culturally acceptable ways
5. Ridding the body of waste in socially and culturally acceptable ways
6. Sexual and role-identity behaviour
7. Self-protective behaviour.

According to Johnson (1980), the nurse assesses the patient's needs in these categories of behaviour, called *behavioural subsystems.* Under normal conditions the patient functions effectively in the environment. When stress disrupts normal adaptation, behaviour becomes erratic and less purposeful. The nurse identifies this inability to adapt and provides nursing care to resolve problems in meeting the patient's needs.

## Rogers' Theory

In her theory, Martha Rogers (1970, 1986, 1989) considers the unitary human being as an energy field coexisting within the universe. The human being is in continuous interaction with the environment. In addition, the human being is a unified whole, possessing personal integrity and manifesting characteristics that are more than, and different from, the sum of the parts (Rogers, 1970). The unitary human being is a

*multi-dimensional energy field identified by pattern and manifesting characteristics that are specific to the whole and which cannot be predicted from the knowledge of parts* (Marriner-Tomey, 1989).

The four dimensions used in Rogers' theory energy fields, openness, pattern and organization, and multi-dimensionality, are used to derive principles about how human beings develop.

Rogers views nursing primarily as a science and is committed to nursing research. Nursing therefore incorporates knowledge of the basic sciences and physiology, as well as nursing knowledge.

## Orem's Theory

Dorothea Orem (1971) developed a definition of nursing that emphasizes the client's self-care needs. Orem describes her philosophy of nursing in this way:

*Nursing has as a special concern man's needs for self-care action and the provision and management of it on a continuous basis in order to sustain life and health, recover from disease or injury, and cope with their effects. Self-care is a requirement of every person: man, woman, and child. When self-care is not maintained, illness, disease, or death will occur. Nurses sometimes manage and maintain required self-care continually for persons who are totally incapacitated. In other instances, nurses help persons to maintain required self-care by performing some but not all care measures, by supervising others who assist patients, and by teaching and guiding individuals as they gradually move toward self-care.*

Thus the goal of Orem's theory is helping the patient perform self-care. According to Orem (1971), nursing care is necessary when the client is unable to fulfill biological, psychological, developmental, or social needs. The nurse determines why a client is unable to meet these needs, what must be done to enable the client to meet them, and how much self-care the client is able to perform (Orem, 1995).

Orem's universal self-care needs are:

1. Sufficient intake of air, water and nutrition
2. Satisfactory eliminative functions
3. Activity balanced with rest
4. Time spent alone balanced with time spent with others
5. Prevention of danger to the self
6. Being "normal".

## King's Theory

Imogene King's theory (1971) focuses on the interpersonal relationship between client and nurse. The nurse-patient/client relationship is the vehicle for the nursing process, which is a dynamic interpersonal process in which the nurse and client are affected by each other's behaviour, as well as by the health care system (King, 1971). The nurse's goal is to use communication to assist the client in re-establishing or maintaining a positive adaptation to the environment.

## Neuman's Theory

Betty Neuman (Neuman and Young, 1972) defines a total-person model incorporating the holistic concept and an open-systems approach (Marriner-Tomey, 1989). To Neuman, the person is a dynamic composite of physiological, sociocultural, and developmental variables that function as an open system. As an open system, the person interacts with, adjusts to, and is adjusted by the environment, which is viewed as a stressor (Chinn and Jacobs, 1987). Stressors disrupt the system. Neuman's model includes intrapersonal, interpersonal, and extrapersonal stressors. Intrapersonal stressors are forces occurring within the person; interpersonal stressors, such as role expectations which occur between people, and extrapersonal stressors, such as financial circumstances, occur outside the person (Neuman, 1982; Marriner-Tomey, 1994).

Neuman believes that nursing is concerned with the whole person. She uses the term "client" when discussing the patient. The goal of nursing is to assist individuals, families, and groups in attaining and maintaining a maximal level of total wellness (Neuman and Young, 1972). The nurse assesses, manages, and evaluates client systems. Nursing focuses on the variables affecting the client's response to the stressor (Chinn and Jacobs, 1987). Nursing actions are in the primary, secondary, and tertiary levels of prevention. Primary prevention focuses on strengthening a line of defence through the identification of actual or potential risk factors associated with stressors. Secondary prevention strengthens internal defences and resources by establishing priorities and treatment plans for identified symptoms, and tertiary prevention focuses on readaptation. The principal goal in tertiary prevention is to strengthen resistance to stressors through client education and to assist in preventing a recurrence of the stress response (Chinn and Jacobs, 1987; Marriner-Tomey, 1994; Torres, 1986; Neuman, 1982). However, client education is a component of primary, secondary and tertiary prevention.

## Roy's Theory

Sister Callista Roy's adaptation theory (Roy and Obloy, 1979; Roy, 1980) views the patient as an adaptive system. According to Roy's model, the goal of nursing is to help the person adapt to changes in physiological needs, self-concept, role function, and interdependent relations during health and illness (Marriner-Tomey, 1994). The need for nursing care arises when the patient cannot adapt to internal and external environmental demands. All individuals must adapt to the following demands:

1. Meeting basic physiological needs
2. Developing a positive self-concept
3. Performing social roles
4. Achieving a balance between dependence and independence.

The nurse determines what demands are causing problems for a patient and assesses how well the patient is adapting to them. Nursing care is then directed at helping the patient adapt.

## Watson's Theory

Watson's philosophy of caring (1979) attempts to define the outcome of nursing activity in regard to the humanistic aspects of life (Watson, 1979; Marriner-Tomey, 1994). The action of nursing is directed at understanding the interrelationship of health, illness, and human behaviour. Nursing is concerned with promoting and restoring health and preventing illness.

Watson's theory is designed around the caring process, which she defines as 10 "carative" factors. Each factor describes the caring process of how a patient attains or maintains health or dies peacefully. Caring represents all of the factors the nurse uses to deliver health care to the patient (Watson, 1987).

## Roper et al's Theory

Roper, Tierney and Logan (1980) designed a model for nursing based on 12 **activities of living**. This developmental model is based on the life-span of the person from infancy to old age, and is used extensively by nurses throughout the UK. Roper *et al* (1990) suggest the model can be used in a variety of settings and view the model as an essential aspect when documenting patient care. The model contains the idea that actual and potential problems can place a person anywhere along a continuum from total dependence to independence. The goal of nursing is to advance the patient from dependence to independence so that the patient can perform his or her own activities of living. The activities of living are:

1. Maintaining a safe environment
2. Communicating
3. Breathing
4. Eating and drinking
5. Eliminating
6. Personal cleansing and dressing
7. Controlling body temperature
8. Mobilising
9. Working and playing
10. Expressing sexuality
11. Sleeping
12. Dying.

## THE SCOPE OF PROFESSIONAL PRACTICE

Scope of practice is related to responsibilities which fall within the nurse's, midwife's and health visitor's educational background, experience and area of practice. *The Scope of Professional Practice*, a position statement published in 1992 by the United Kingdom Central Council for Nursing, Midwifery, and Health Visiting, addresses the application of knowledge and the simultaneous exercise of judgement and skill required by the nurse, midwife and health visitor in providing care. In this document, the UKCC acknowledges that practice takes place within the context of continual change. Change results from advances in research leading to improvements in care. As such, nurses, midwives and

### The Midwife

- provides sound family planning information and advice
- prescribes or advises on the examinations necessary for the earliest possible diagnosis of pregnancies at risk
- cares for and assists the mother during labour and monitors the condition of the fetus *in utero*
- conducts spontaneous deliveries
- examines and cares for the new-born infant; takes all initiatives necessary in case of need; carries out immediate resuscitation where necessary
- cares for and monitors the progress of the mother in the postnatal period
- gives all necessary advice to the mother on infant care to enable her to ensure the optimum progress for the new-born infant
- carries out the treatment prescribed by a doctor and maintains all necessary records
- is employed in a variety of settings, including hospital and community
- training includes 18-month post-registration course after completing RN (Registered Nurse) course; or three-year, full-time course for those entering midwifery with no previous nursing education

Portions adapted from the *European Community Midwives' Directives* (80/155/EEC Article 4).

health visitors must be sensitive, and responsive to the needs of individual patients/clients, and have the capacity to adjust in changing circumstances.

The UKCC further acknowledges that education and experience form the foundation upon which nurses, midwives and health visitors exercise judgement and skill. Within the *Scope of Professional Practice* (1992) document, the *Code of Professional Conduct* and the principles for adjusting the **scope of professional practice** are addressed.

## NURSING PRACTICE

Nurses practise in a variety of settings, in many roles within those settings, and with other health carers in the allied health professions. The practice of nursing is guided in part by managers in hospitals and other health care agencies and institutions. In the United Kingdom, standards of practice for the nurse, midwife and health visitor are guided primarily by the UKCC *Code of Professional Conduct* (1992).

### Standards of Nursing Practice (Code of Professional Conduct)

As nursing has gained independence as a profession, it has increasingly set its own **standards for practice**. Standards for practice are important as objective guidelines for nurses to provide care, and as criteria for evaluating care. When standards are clearly defined, patients/clients can be assured they are receiving high-quality care, nurses know exactly what is necessary to give nursing care, and managers can determine that care meets acceptable standards. Moreover, standards of practice are important if a legal dispute arises over whether a nurse practised appropriately in a particular case. The UKCC (1992) has published standards of nursing practice which are delineated in the *Code of Professional Conduct for the Nurse, Midwife and Health Visitor* (see box).

## Practice Settings

As nursing's role in the health care system has expanded, the settings in which nurses practise have also increased. There is currently a thrust for nurses, midwives and health visitors to expand their practice in primary health care as changes in health care delivery assume new dimensions in the community.

## Hospitals and Other Institutions

The largest group of practising nurses is found in NHS hospitals or other health care institutions. Due to changes in government policy regarding hospital stays, patients are being discharged from hospitals earlier, frequently requiring continued nursing care in the home. Today's hospital-based professional nurse is being educated to provide good nursing care and to be able, through early discharge planning, to meet the home care needs of patients. NHS reform and the shift from acute care to community care will further challenge and stretch nursing practice.

The increased older adult population and rising acuity rates have resulted in part from new disease entities and new forms of supportive therapy. Infections associated with acquired immunodeficiency syndrome (AIDS), organ transplantation, and technological equipment used in the critical care setting are a few factors contributing to a higher percentage of critically ill patients in hospitals.

In addition to the rising acuity rate, there has been a sharp upward spiralling of health care costs. The challenge to keep health spending within national budgets is affecting all of the health care systems of the developed world (Holliday, 1992). To adjust for this increase, hospitals are reducing the number of people on their staff without decreasing the workload. Professional nurses are caught in this dilemma (McClure, 1991). Today's professional nurses are challenged to meet the multiple health care needs of patients, with reduced resources.

In hospitals, nursing services operate 24 hours a day. Hospitals use different staffing patterns to meet the need for nursing care. Some hospitals have three 8-hour shifts, whereas other hospitals use two 12-hour shifts or three 10-hour shifts that overlap during the early morning, late afternoon, and night. The roles and responsibilities of nurses employed in hospitals vary because hospitals differ widely in size, organizational structure and in function.

Regardless of the practice environment, nurses are challenged to deliver quality care. Nursing research linking quality patient outcome studies with cost effectiveness provides documentation that nurses are meeting the challenge.

Patients in hospitals generally require 24-hour nursing care. Hospitals may be acute, long-term, or rehabilitation care facilities. Nurses employed in an acute-care setting care for patients with severe illnesses and complex problems. Today these patients are usually more dependent and more seriously ill than patients in the past, due to shorter periods of hospitalization. As a

## The Profession of Nursing Specialty Areas within the Registered Nurse Status

After completing the **Common Foundation Programme** within the Diploma of Higher Education, student nurses continue their education in a **branch programme** that leads to one of the following specialties:

### Adult General Nurse RN (Part 12)

- cares for adults who have, or are recovering from, a physical illness
- employed in general hospital or community settings
- workplace varies, from long-stay hospital wards, operating theatres or intensive care areas; to community areas such as patients'/clients' homes or health centres

[description also applies to RN (Part 1)]

### Mental Health Nurse RN (Part 13)

- cares for adults or children who have, or are recovering from, a mental illness
- employed in long- and short-term psychiatric hospital or community settings
- can specialize as a nurse therapist through post-registration training

[description also applies to RN (Part 3)]

### Mental Handicap Nurse RN (Part 14)

- cares for adults or children who have a mental handicap (learning disability)
- clients/patients vary, from those with profound mental and physical handicaps requiring continual care, to those learning to live in the community
- employed in hospitals; community, residential and day care settings; as well as in patients'/clients' homes

[description also applies to RNMH (Part 5)]

### Children's Nursing RN (Part 15)

- cares for sick children in a variety of settings, such as children with infectious diseases, chronic illnesses, or new-borns in intensive care units
- employed in general hospital or community settings
- role also involves working with parents and families of sick children

[description also applies to RSCN (Part 8)]

From Lowry M: *Becoming a nurse,* London, 1993, Mosby.

result, nursing practice in acute-care settings has become more specialized and complex. The skills and knowledge needed to practise in this setting are determined by the clinical area of practice.

The rapid rise in the number of older adults, patients with chronic illnesses, and those with functional impairments has resulted in the growth of long-term care facilities. Long-term care has been provided in NHS hospitals and nursing homes, but is now increasingly provided by the independent sector of health care.

Rehabilitation facilities generally employ many types of health care professionals. The goal of these organizations is to

## Code of Professional Conduct

The Code of Professional Conduct provides guidelines for practice in nursing, midwifery and health visiting.

*As a registered nurse, midwife or health visitor, you are personally accountable for your practice and, in the exercise of your professional accountability, must:*

1. *act always in such a manner as to promote and safeguard the interests and well-being of patients and clients;*
2. *ensure that no action or omission on your part, or within your sphere of responsibility, is detrimental to the interests, condition or safety of patients/clients;*
3. *maintain and improve your professional knowledge and competence;*
4. *acknowledge any limitations in your knowledge and competence and decline any duties or responsibilities unless able to perform them in a safe and skilled manner.*

From: *Code of Professional Conduct*, London, 1992, United Kingdom Central Council for Nursing, Midwifery and Health Visiting.

## Further Reading

*Code of Professional Conduct (1992)* — provides guidelines for standards of practice for every registered nurse, midwife and health visitor.

*The Scope of Professional Practice (1992)* — defines professional practice, the role of education in practice, and the scope of practice for the nurse, midwife, health visitor, and those practising in residential care and social services sectors.

*Guide for Students of Nursing and Midwifery (1992)* — addresses the Nurses, Midwives and Health Visitors Acts of 1979 and 1992, provides information about the professional register, and gives advice for students of nursing and midwifery.
Available from: United Kingdom Central Council for Nursing, Midwifery and Health Visiting, 23 Portland Place, London, W1N 3AF.

*Nursing: the Nature and Scope of Professional Practice (1992)* — provides a brief overview of the definition, nature and practice of nursing, and of the interaction between nurses and other health care workers.
Available from: Royal College of Nursing, 20 Cavendish Square, London, W1M 0AB.

teach disabled patients/clients to achieve a maximal level of function and to teach families to help them reach that level.

### Community Settings

The number of nurses employed in **community-based** practice settings is increasing. The rising costs of institutional care, coupled with changing demography, health trends, client expectation and a need to provide health care within budgetary limits, have created the need for community-based nursing services aimed at health promotion and disease prevention (NHS Executive, 1993).

Nursing in community-based settings is concerned primarily with health promotion and maintenance, education and management, and coordination and continuity of care within the community (see Chapter 2). Community-based nurses assess the health needs of individuals, families, and communities and help patients/clients cope with threats to health and problems of illness. Whereas institutional health care focuses on the individual and family, community-based nursing is directed towards the health of the community and the interaction of individuals within that community. A community can be a particular location such as an urban or rural area or a group of people related by occupation, school, or another common interest or characteristic. Thus, community-based nurses are employed in a variety of practice settings, including general practice surgeries, community and occupational health centres, schools, home health care agencies, and private practices.

### PRIMARY HEALTH CARE CENTRES

Primary health care centres offer comprehensive programmes for health maintenance and promotion, protection, education, treatment, and coordination of care within the community.

Primary health care centres provide ambulatory care (care sought by people able to come to the centres), as well as a variety of health services. People seeking health care at a primary health care centre usually live in the local community. Trends within the provision of health care are increasing the role and function of primary health care centres (WHO, 1992). Nurses are central to this development (Department of Health, 1990).

Nurses employed in these centres often work more independently than nurses working in institutional settings. Primary health care centres also employ other health professionals, but nurses generally provide most of the care. In some settings, doctors are called in only when specific needs arise. Some examples of primary health care services are planned parenthood clinics, child health and family care and mental health centres. Nurses within primary care have usually undergone a course of further study, after their initial education, for example, health visitors and district nurses. As nursing is evolving, other nurses, such as practice nurses, are developing their role within GP practices, and education for this group is increasing.

### SCHOOLS

Community-based health services are common in schools and on college and university campuses. Nursing services include health education in disease prevention, health promotion, and sex education. In addition, nurses working in schools may provide care for students with non-emergency acute illnesses such as upper respiratory tract infections, influenza, and viruses. School nurses also make referrals for students and their families when additional, more specialized health care is needed. School nurses work closely with health visitors in relation to child surveillance and child protection.

## OCCUPATIONAL HEALTH SETTINGS

Many companies in large office buildings and factories provide health services to employees in occupational health centres located on the premises. Nursing care in these settings involves five areas. The nurse may develop programmes aimed at increasing health and safety in the workplace by reducing the number of occupational accidents, the risk of occupational disease, or the transmission of a contagious disease among the workers. The nurse may provide programmes for health promotion, disease prevention, and health education. The nurse also treats non emergency acute illnesses and provides first aid. In emergency situations, such as heart attacks or trauma, the nurse may give emergency care. The nurse may also refer employees to additional health resources, such as their local general practitioner, when necessary.

## PUBLIC HEALTH

As assessment of health needs of individuals and communities becomes more central to purchasing targetted health services, so the role of the nurse within Public Health increases. This involves the search for health needs, and action to improve health by mobilization of community resources through partnership with clients and targetting services towards greatest need.

### Other Settings

The settings previously discussed are the most common areas in which nurses are employed, but there are a number of other settings in which nurses' roles and responsibilities vary widely. A practice nurse employed in a doctor's surgery, for example, may have little independent responsibility, but a nurse in joint practice with other nurses or other health care professionals may provide care with much independence. Nurses are also employed in educational and research positions.

## ROLES AND FUNCTIONS OF THE NURSE

Contemporary nursing requires that the nurse possess knowledge and skills in a variety of areas. In the past the principal role of nurses was to provide care and comfort as they carried out specific nursing functions, but changes in nursing have expanded the role to include increased emphasis on health promotion and illness prevention, as well as concern for the patient/client as a whole. The contemporary nurse functions in the interrelated roles of carer, decision maker, protector and client advocate, manager, rehabilitator, comforter, communicator, teacher, and empowerer.

### Carer

As carer, the nurse helps the patient/client regain health through the healing process. Healing is more than just curing a specific disease, although treatment skills that promote physical healing are important to carers. The nurse addresses the **holistic health care** needs of the patient/client, including measures to restore emotional and social well-being. The carer helps the person and family set goals and meet those goals with a minimal cost of time and energy.

### Decision Maker

To provide effective care, the nurse uses decision-making skills throughout the nursing process. Before undertaking any nursing action, whether it is assessing the patient's/client's condition, giving care, or evaluating the results of care, the nurse plans the action by deciding the best approach for each person. In some situations the nurse makes these decisions alone or with the patient/client and family, and in other cases the nurse works with other health care professionals.

### Protector and Patient Advocate

As protector the nurse helps maintain a safe environment for the patient/client and takes steps to prevent injury and protect the patient/client from possible adverse effects of diagnostic or treatment measures. Confirming that a patient/client does not have an allergy to a medication and providing immunization against disease in a primary health care setting are examples of the nurse's protective role.

In the role of patient/client advocate, the nurse protects the person's human and legal rights and provides assistance in asserting those rights if the need arises. For example, the nurse may provide additional information for a patient/client who is trying to decide whether to accept treatment. The nurse may also defend patients'/clients' rights in a general way by speaking out against policies or actions that might endanger individuals' well-being or conflict with their rights.

### Manager

Nurses coordinate the activities of other members of the health care team, such as health care support workers, when managing the patient's/client's total care. Nurses must also manage their own time and the resources of the practice setting when concurrently providing care to several patients/clients. Differentiated practice models offer nurses opportunities to make decisions about their career paths. In a differentiated practice setting, such as a nursing development unit, nurses can choose between roles as primary nurses (managers) of patient care or as associate nurses who carry out the care prescribed by primary nurses (Manthey, 1990). As managers, nurses coordinate and delegate care responsibilities and supervise other health care workers.

### Rehabilitator

Rehabilitation is the process by which individuals return to maximal levels of functioning after illness, accidents, or other disabling events. Frequently patients/clients experience physical or emotional impairments that change their lives, and the nurse helps them adapt as fully as possible. Rehabilitative activities range from teaching patients/clients to walk with crutches to helping patients/clients cope with lifestyle changes often associated with chronic illness.

### Comforter

The role of comforter, caring for the patient/client as a person, is a traditional and historical one in nursing and has continued to be important as nurses have assumed new roles. Because nursing care must be directed to the whole person rather than simply the body, comfort and emotional support often help give the patient/client strength to recover. While carrying out nursing activities, nurses can provide comfort by demonstrating care for the patient/client as an individual with unique feelings and needs. As comforter, nurses should help the patient/client reach therapeutic goals rather than encourage emotional or physical dependence.

## Communicator

The role of communicator is central to all other nursing roles. Nursing involves communication with patients/clients and families, other nurses and health care professionals, resource people, and the community. Without clear communication, it is impossible to give care effectively, make decisions with patients/clients and families, protect patients/clients from threats to well-being, coordinate and manage patient/client care, assist the client in rehabilitation, offer comfort, or teach. The quality of communication is a critical factor in meeting the needs of individuals, families, and communities.

## Teacher

As teacher, the nurse explains to patients/clients concepts and facts about health, demonstrates procedures such as self-care activities, determines that the patient/client fully understands, reinforces learning or patient/client behaviour, and evaluates progress in learning. Some teaching can be unplanned and informal, such as when a nurse responds to a question about a health issue in casual conversation. Other teaching activities may be planned and more formal, such as when the nurse teaches a person with diabetes mellitus to self-administer injections. The nurse uses teaching methods that match the person's capabilities and needs and incorporates other resources, such as the family, in teaching plans.

## Empowerer

The nurse works in partnership with patients/clients, their carers, and the community in order to help individuals and communities take charge of their lives and health, and to make informed choices.

## Career Roles

The preceding roles and functions apply to all nurses. Career roles, on the other hand, are specific employment positions. Because of increasing educational opportunities for nurses, the growth of nursing as a profession, and a greater concern for job enrichment, the nursing profession offers expanded roles and different kinds of career opportunities. Examples of career roles include nurse educators, clinical nurse specialists, nurse managers and nurse researchers.

## Nurse Educator

Nurse educators works primarily in a college or university, staff development department of a health care agency, or a client teaching centre. They have a background in clinical nursing, which provides them with practical skills and theoretical knowledge. Educators in a college of nursing prepares students to function as nurses. They are responsible for teaching current nursing practice theory and necessary skills in skills laboratories and clinical settings. They undertake specialized training in education and are registered with the UKCC as qualified teachers of nurses. They are usually required to have degrees in nursing, nursing education or a specialty related to nursing. In addition, they generally have a specific clinical specialty and advanced clinical experience.

Nurse educators in staff development departments of health care institutions provide educational programmes for nurses within their institution. These programmes vary and may include orientation of new nurses to wards or units, and in-service education such as teaching about new equipment or procedures.

The primary focus of the nurse educator in a client education centre is to teach ill or disabled patients and families to provide care in the home. In most health care agencies, however, the budget does not permit a separate patient education centre. Therefore, staff nurses usually incorporate education into a client's plan of care and do the teaching themselves. An example of a client education centre would be a cardiac rehabilitation centre in which teaching following open heart or transplant surgery is conducted by specialist nurses.

## Clinical Nurse Specialist

The clinical nurse specialist (CNS) has expertise in a specialized area of practice. A CNS works in a critical, acute, long-term, or primary health care setting. In addition, a CNS may specialize in the management of a disease such as cancer, diabetes mellitus, or cardiovascular or pulmonary disease or in a specific field such as paediatrics or nursing older people. The CNS functions as a clinician, educator, manager, consultant, and researcher within the area of practice to plan or improve the quality of nursing care for the patient/client and family.

## Nurse Manager

A nurse manager manages patient/client care and the delivery of specific nursing services within a health care agency. This manager may hold a middle management position, such as ward sister or senior nurse or supervisor, or an upper-level management position, such as director of nursing services or chief nurse. Since the early 1990s, with the NHS reforms, many Directors of Nursing Services are not active managers, but professional heads of nursing with an advisory role. Functions of managers include budgeting, staffing, strategic planning of programmes and services, employee evaluation, and employee development.

## Nurse Researcher

The nurse researcher investigates problems to improve nursing care and to further define and expand the scope of nursing practice. The nurse researcher may be employed in an academic setting, hospital, or independent professional or primary health care setting.

## NURSING AS A PROFESSION

### Professionalism

Nursing is not simply a collection of specific skills, and the nurse is not simply a person trained to perform specific tasks. Nursing is a **profession**.

No one factor absolutely differentiates a job from a profession, but the difference is important in terms of how nurses practise. When we say a person acts "professionally", for example, we imply that the person is conscientious in actions, knowledgeable in the subject, and responsible to self and others. Etzioni (1961) describes professions in terms of the following primary characteristics:

1. A profession requires an extended education of its members, as well as a basic liberal foundation
2. A profession has a theoretical body of knowledge leading to defined skills, abilities, and norms
3. A profession provides a specific service
4. Members of a profession have autonomy in decision making and practice
5. The profession as a whole has a code of ethics for practice.

Nursing clearly shares, to some extent, each of these characteristics. Nursing is still evolving as a profession, however, and faces controversial issues as nurses strive for greater professionalism.

### Education

As a profession, nursing requires that its members possess a significant amount of education. The issue of standardization of nursing education is a major controversy today. Most nurses agree that nursing education is important to practice and that it must respond to changes in health care created by scientific and technological advances.

### Theory

As nursing has emerged as a profession, nursing knowledge has been developed through nursing theories. Theoretical models serve as frameworks for nursing curricula and clinical practice. Nursing theories also lead to further research that increases the scientific basis of nursing practice.

A theory is a way of understanding a reality, and in this general sense, all practising nurses use the theories they have learned. Several of the approaches described in the section on definitions and philosophies are parts of fully developed nursing theories.

### Service

Nursing has always been a service profession, although in the past the service was usually viewed as a charitable one. Today, nursing is a vital and indispensable component of the health care delivery system.

### Autonomy

Autonomy means that a person is reasonably independent and self-governing in decision making and practice. It has been difficult for nurses to attain the degree of autonomy enjoyed by other professionals. In the past, doctors, hospital managers, and others in the health care delivery system have found nursing autonomy difficult to understand and support. Through clinical competence and greater educational preparation, however, nurses are increasingly taking on more independent roles.

With increased autonomy, comes greater responsibility and accountability. *Accountability* means the nurse is responsible, professionally and legally, for the type and quality of nursing care provided. The nurse is accountable for keeping abreast of technical skills and knowledge needed to perform nursing care (UKCC, 1992). The nursing profession itself regulates accountability through nursing audits and standards of practice.

---

### Children's Nursing
### Education for children's nurses

Project 2000 is the central route into children's nursing. Students undergo a Common Foundation Programme with other students studying the other disciplines of nursing and then, after 18 months of study, the student branches into studying the art and science of children's nursing.

There are other routes of entry — some colleges still provide the Post-Registration course in Sick Children's Nursing (RSCN). However, most of the colleges which provide the child branch of Project 2000 are either already providing a fast-track, modified branch for adult mental health/learning disability diplomats to become Registered in Children's Nursing, or have plans to do so. (There are also Bachelor and Masters degrees available in Children's Nursing.)

Some colleges offer many continuing educational programmes for children's nurses e.g. Nursing Care of the Acutely Ill Child, Health and Development, or Caring for Children with Special Needs. These are examples of courses presently offered; however, consumer demand will dictate which courses are available in the future.

### Nursing and Other Health Care Workers

The work of health care professionals often overlaps and the team is interdependent. The division of work should be based on mutual recognition of each profession's expertise and of what will most benefit the patient. The shared approach should not put at risk the care which only the nurse can provide. Nor should it limit the nurse's responsibility for deciding what nursing care is needed. It is an important part of nursing to refer a patient, where necessary, to other health care professionals and to carry out treatment initiated by others.

Nurses may also delegate work to other people, in particular to nursing auxiliaries and health care support workers. The nurse is responsible for the decision to delegate and must be sure that the assistant is competent.

From: Royal College of Nursing: *Nursing — the nature and scope of professional practice, Issues in nursing and health*, London, March 1992, RCN.

### Code of Conduct

Nursing has a code of conduct, which defines the principles by which nurses function (see p.11). In addition, nurses incorporate their own values and ethics into practice.

## Professional Organizations

A **professional organization** is created to deal with issues of concern to those practising in the profession. In the UK the major professional nursing organizations are the United Kingdom Central Council for Nursing, Midwifery and Health Visiting (UKCC), and the National Boards for Nursing, Midwifery and Health Visiting. The UKCC functions as the primary regulatory body for standards of practice and registration. **National Boards** delineate minimal course requirements and accredit educational programmes for nursing, midwifery and health visiting. The UKCC and the National Boards are concerned with the improvement of nursing education, nursing service, and health care delivery in the United Kingdom.

Some professional organizations for nurses focus on specific interests such as critical care, nursing management or research. The Royal College of Nursing (RCN) of the UK, for example, is the largest professional union of nurses in the world. The RCN works to develop the art and science of nursing, to improve standards of practice, and to foster the welfare of nurses in all areas. The RCN also offers advanced education, conferences and various publications. A variety of services are also offered by UNISON, the Health Service trade union.

Student nurses may become student members of some professional organizations, such as the RCN, and may then enjoy cost reductions in seminars and nursing conventions. The RCN considers issues of importance to student nurses and often cooperates in activities and programmes with other professional organizations.

## SOCIETY'S INFLUENCE ON NURSING

Throughout history, nursing has responded to society's needs. Contemporary nursing education, practice, and research are an outgrowth of economic, technological, demographic, sociological, and political issues.

### Technological Advances

In recent years, scientific and technological advances have affected almost every aspect of life. Health care has changed in many ways, including the use of new equipment, new diagnostic tests and treatment measures, and new drugs. Nursing has adapted and will continue to respond to these changes with continuing education, in-service programmes, and other educational approaches. Nursing is also uniquely concerned with the *human* side of technological advances. While society generally accepts technological advances in health care, individual patients/clients often experience problems related to them. For example, dialysis machines have been used for many years to treat people with kidney problems, but that fact does not lessen the emotional conflict a person may experience after learning that dialysis is needed. As health care technology becomes increasingly complex and sophisticated, nurses must help patients/clients adjust to the use of technology in care.

### Demographic Changes

Demographic changes affect the whole population. Changes that have influenced health care in recent decades include the population shift from rural areas to urban centres; increasing life spans; the higher incidence of chronic, long-term illness; and the increased incidence of diseases such as alcohol dependency and lung cancer. Nursing as a profession responds to such changes by exploring new methods for providing care, by changing educational emphases, and by establishing practice standards in new areas. To better meet the changing health care needs of people, the nurse also responds to demographic changes in the population served by the practice setting.

### Consumer Movement

The consumer movement is a heightened awareness of the value and costs of products and services available in the United Kingdom. Linked to this is the concept of self-determination and individualism. Health care is being influenced by the consumer movement in ways as diverse as the shift to primary health care in the community, to concern about the rising costs of health care in the NHS. Consumers are becoming more knowledgeable about health and illness and are becoming more vocal in their desire for high-quality care. Health care consumers are also becoming more aware of their rights as patients, and the nurse supports these rights in the role of patient/client advocate. Because nurses generally interact with patients more than other health care professionals, they must often answer questions about the quality of health care and, in some circumstances, the costs of health care. Quality assurance and audits are now central to nursing and other health care activity (Ellis, 1993).

### Health Promotion

Related to the consumer movement is a greater emphasis in society on health promotion and illness prevention. Exercise and nutrition are subjects that interest many people. Nursing has responded to this greater concern for health promotion in many ways, from programmes in the community to specific health promotion and teaching activities for patients/clients in hospitals and other health care settings. Health promotion activities are a part of many of the roles of a nurse, including carer, patient/client advocate, rehabilitator, communicator and teacher. Health promotion gains more emphasis in a health system striving to make best use of limited resources.

### Women's Movement

The women's movement has brought about many changes in society, as women have increasingly sought economic, political, occupational and educational equality. Nursing is responding in two ways. Because most nurses are women, they are increasingly asserting their equal rights as human beings, employees and health care professionals. The women's movement has encouraged nurses to seek greater autonomy and responsibility in providing care in an environment that has been and continues to be male dominated (Bunning and Campbell, 1990). The women's movement has caused female patients/clients to seek more responsibility for and control over their bodies, health, and lives in general. As women become more aware of their own needs and unique qualities, they seek health care that can help them meet those needs.

## Human Rights Movement

Like the women's movement, the human rights movement is changing the way society views the rights of *all* of its members, including minorities, patients with terminal illness, pregnant women, and older adults. Many groups have special health care needs, and nursing has responded by respecting all patients/clients as individuals with a right to good care and with basic human rights. Nurses advocate the rights of all patients and clients.

## TRENDS IN NURSING

This chapter has emphasized that nursing is not a static, unchanging profession but is continually growing and evolving as society changes, as health care emphases and methods change, as lifestyles change – and as nurses themselves change. To speak of nursing at all is to speak of nursing as it is at a given time, and in this sense, this chapter is about trends in nursing.

The current philosophies and definitions of nursing demonstrate the holistic trend in nursing to address the whole person in all dimensions, in health and illness, and in interaction with the family and community. Nursing continues to draw on the social sciences and other fields as the focus of nursing care expands.

Trends in nursing practice include a growing variety of settings in which nurses have greater independence. Nurses continue to gain autonomy and respect as members of the health care team. Nursing roles continue to expand with the broadening focus of nursing care.

Trends in nursing as a profession include the growing emphasis on the aspects of nursing that characterize it as a profession, including education, theory, service, autonomy, and ethical codes. The activities of professional organizations reflect all the trends in nurse education and practice. All the influences of society on nursing also reflect trends in contemporary nursing.

In summarising 'the challenges for nursing and midwifery in the 21st century', the Chief Nursing Officers of Wales, Scotland, England and Northern Ireland concluded that current changes 'offer great opportunities'. The concept for the future, they beleived, should be reflected in training and development, and produce 'caring, positive nurses who can face a turbulent and uncertain future with confidence in themselves and their values' (The Heathrow Debate, 1993).

## SUMMARY

Nursing is a complex and multifaceted profession. The nurse's role includes that of carer, teacher, counsellor, advocate, researcher and empowerer. The nurse needs theoretical or **conceptual models** from which to practise in a variety of settings. The professional growth and development of today's nurse requires information on research and on ways to perform a research study, as well as on the use of findings in a clinical practice setting. The standards of practice set forth by the UKCC (1992) provide guidelines for competent, safe, and professional practice. Historical origins of nursing have assisted today's health professionals in their development and future needs.

## Key Concepts

- Nursing is an essential part of society; it has grown out of society and has evolved with it.
- Nursing has responded to the health care needs of society, which were influenced by economic, social, and cultural variables of a specific era.
- Formalized education programmes for professional nursing were established in the nineteenth century by Florence Nightingale.
- Nursing definitions reflect changes in the practice of nursing and help bring about changes by identifying the domain of nursing practice and guiding research, practice, and education.
- Conceptual and theoretical nursing models provide knowledge to improve practice, guide research and nursing curricula, and identify the domain and goals of nursing practice.
- Nursing standards provide the guidelines for implementing and evaluating nursing care.
- The multiple roles and functions of the nurse include carer, decision maker, protector, client advocate, manager, rehabilitator, comforter, communicator, teacher and empowerer.
- Specific employment positions include nurse educator, clinical nurse specialist, manager and researcher.
- Nursing is a profession encompassing educational preparation for the nurse, nursing theory, a provided service, autonomy, and a code of conduct.
- Professional nursing organizations deal with issues of concern to nursing within the nursing profession.
- Changes in society, such as increased technology, new demographic patterns, consumerism, health promotion, and the women's and human rights movements, have led to changes in nursing.

## CRITICAL THINKING EXERCISES

1. You are assigned to care for a patient who needs to learn how to manage cardiac drugs. Describe the criteria you would use to select a nursing theory for a basis for clinical practice.
2. You are assigned to interview a nurse in an expanded role. What information would you need about the role before conducting your interview?
3. Part of your education includes experiences in different types of health care settings. What differences would you expect between nurses who practise in hospitals, long-term care facilities, and primary health care settings? Would you expect any commonalities?
4. Consider a nursing model which might be appropriate to use in a mental health care setting, whether this be institutional or community care.

## Key Terms

## REFERENCES

Abdellah FG et al: *Patient-centered approaches to nursing,* New York, 1960, Macmillan.

Beeber L, Anderson CA, Sills GM: Peplau's theory in practice, *Nurs Sci Q* 3(1):6, 1990.

Benner P: *From novice to expert: excellence and power in clinical nursing practice, Menlo Park,* Calif, 1984, Addison-Wesley.

Benner P, Tanner C: How expert nurses use intuition, *Am J Nurs* 87(1):23, 1987.

Bunning S, Campbell JC: Feminism and nursing: historical perspectives, *ANS* 12(4):11, 1990.

Chinn PL, Jacobs MK: *Theory and nursing: a systematic approach,* ed 4, St Louis, 1994, Mosby.

Cohen IB: Florence Nightingale, *Sci Am* 250(128):137, 1984.

Department of Health: *The Heathrow Debate, The Challenges for nursing and midwifery in the 21st century,* London, 1993, DOH.

Department of Health: *The NHS and Community Care Act 1990,* London, 1990, HMSO.

Dolan JA et al: *Nursing in society: a historical perspective,* ed 15, Philadelphia, 1983, Saunders.

Donahue MP: *Nursing: the finest art, an illustrated history,* St Louis, 1985, Mosby.

Ellis R, Whittington D: *Quality assurance in health care,* Sevenoaks, kent, 1993, Edward Arnold.

Etzioni A: *The semi-professionals and their organizations,* New York, 1961, Free Press.

Fawcett J: *Analysis and evaluation of conceptual models of nursing,* ed 2, Philadelphia, 1989, Davis.

Fawcett J: *Analysis and evaluation of nursing theories,* Philadelphia, 1993, Davis.

Henderson V: *The nature of nursing, Am J Nurs* 64:62, 1964.

Henderson V: *The nature of nursing,* New York, 1966, Macmillan.

Hinshaw AS: Nursing science: the challenge to develop knowledge, *Nurs Sci Q* 2(4):162, 1989.

Holliday I: *The NHS transformed,* London, 1992, Baseline Books.

International Council of Nurses: *Code for nurses,* Geneva, 1973, The Council.

Johnson DE: Theory in nursing: borrowed and unique, *Nurs Res* 11:206, 1968.

Johnson DE: The behavioral system for nursing. In Riehl JP, Roy C, editors: *Conceptual models for nursing practice,* ed 2, New York, 1980, Appleton-Century-Crofts.

Kelly LY: *Dimensions of professional nursing,* New York, 1981, Macmillan.

King IM: *Toward a theory for nursing,* New York, 1971, John Wiley & Sons.

Levine MC: *An introduction to clinical nursing,* ed 2, Philadelphia, 1973, Davis.

Manthey M: 1990 nursing: a profession of choice, *Nurs Manage* 21(9):17, 1990.

Marriner-Tomey A: *Nursing theorists and their work,* ed 3, St Louis, 1994, Mosby.

McClure ML: Nursing and hospital cost containment, *J Prof Nurs* 7(1):4, 1991.

Meleis AI: *Theoretical nursing: development and progress,* Philadelphia, 1985, Lippincott.

Neuman B: *The Neuman systems model: application to nursing education and practice,* New York, 1982, Appleton-Century-Crofts.

Neuman BM, Young RJ: A model for teaching total person approach to patient problems, *Nurs Res* 21:264, 1972.

NHS Executive: *New world new opportunites: nursing in primary health care,* London, March 1993, HMSO.

Nightingale F: *Notes on nursing: what it is and what it is not,* London, 1860, Harrison & Sons.

Orlando IJ: *The dynamic nurse-patient relationship: function, process, and principles,* New York, 1961, Putnam.

Orlando IJ: *The dynamic nurse-patient relationship: function, process, and principles,* New York, 1990, National League for Nursing.

Orem DE: *Nursing: concepts of practice,* New York, 1971, McGraw- Hill.

Orem DE: *Nursing: concepts of practice,* ed 5, St Louis, 1995, Mosby.

Parse RR: *Nursing science: major paradigms, theories, and critiques,* Philadelphia, 1987, Saunders.

Parse RR: Nursing theory-based practice: a challenge for the 90s, *Nurs Sci Q* 3(2):53, 1990.

Peplau HE: *Interpersonal relations in nursing,* New York, 1952, Putnam.

Rogers ME: *An introduction to the theoretical basis of nursing,* Philadelphia, 1970, Davis.

Rogers ME: The science of unitary human beings. In Malinski VM: *Explorations on Martha Roger's science of unitary human beings,* Norwalk, 1986, Appleton-Century-Crofts.

Rogers ME: Nursing, a science of unitary human beings. In Riehl-Sisca JP, *Conceptual models for nursing practice,* ed 3, Norwalk, 1989, Appleton-Century-Crofts.

Roy C, Obloy SM: *The practitioner movement: toward a science of nursing, Am J Nurs* 79:1698, 1979.

Roy C: The Roy adaptation model. In Riehl JP, Roy C, editors: *Conceptual models for nursing practice,* New York, 1980, Appleton- Century-Crofts.

Royal College of Nursing: *Paediatric nursing, a philosophy of care,* London 1992, RCN.

Roper N, Tierney A, Logan W: *The elements of nursing,* ed 3, London, 1990, Churchill Livingstone.

Roper N, Tierney A, Logan W: *Using a model for nursing,* London, 1983, Churchill Livingstone.

Shryock RH: *The history of nursing: an interpretation of the social and medical factors involved,* Philadelphia, 1959, Saunders.

Tanner CA et al: Diagnostic reasoning strategies of nursing and nursing students, *Nurs Res* 36(6):358, 1987.

Torres G: *Theoretical foundations of nursing,* Norwalk, 1986, Appleton-Century-Crofts.

United Kingdom Central Council for Nursing, Midwifery and Health Visiting: *The scope of professional practice,* London, 1992, UKCC.

United Kingdom Central Council for Nursing, Midwifery and Health Visiting: *Code of professional conduct,* London, 1992, UKCC.

Watson J: *Nursing: the philosophy and science of caring,* Boston, 1979, Little, Brown & Co.

Watson J: Nursing on the caring edge: metaphorical vignettes, *ANS* 10(1):10, 1987.

Woodham-Smith C: *Florence Nightingale,* New York, 1983, McGraw-Hill.

World Health Organization: *The role of health centres in the development of urban systems: report of a WHO study group on primary health care in urban areas,* Geneva, 1992, WHO.

Yura H, Walsh M: *The nursing process: assessing, planning, implementing, evaluating,* ed 3, New York, 1978, Appleton-Century-Crofts.

## FURTHER READING
### Adult Nursing

Aggleton P, Chalmers H: Models and theories (series), *Nurs Times* 80(36):24-28,1984.

Aggleton P, Chalmers H: *Nursing models and the nursing process,* London, 1986, Macmillan.

Cavanagh S: Orem's model in action, in *Nursing models in action series,* London, 1991, Macmillan.

Dickoff J, James P: A theory of theories: a position paper, *Nurs Res* 17(3):197, 1968.

Easterbrook J, editor: *Elderly care — towards holistic nursing (using a model series),* London, 1987, Hodder & Stoughton.

Fairman JA: Sources and references for research in nursing history, *Nurs Res* 36(1):56, 1987.

Leininger MM: *Transcultural care, diversity and universality: a theory of nursing,* Thorofore, 1985, Slack.

Newton C: The Roper–Logan–Tierney model in action, in *Nursing models in action series,* London, 1991, Macmillan.

Pearson A, Vaughan B: *Nursing models for practice,* London, 1986, Heinemann.

Savage J, Kershaw B: *Models for nursing,* London, 1990, Scutari.

Silva MC, Rothbart D: An analysis of changing trends in philosophies of science on nursing theory development and testing, *ANS* 6(2):1, 1984.

Stevens BJ: *Nursing theory: analysis, application, evaluation,* ed 2, Boston, 1984, Little, Brown & Co.

Walker LO: Toward a clearer understanding of the concept of nursing theory, *Nurs Res* 20(5):428, 1971.

### Children's Nursing

British Paediatric Association: *Care of critically ill children.* Report of the multidisciplinary working party, London, 1993, BPA.

Burr S: Paediatric nursing: past, present and future, *JRSH* 4:155, 1987.

RCN, 1988. Paediatric nursing — a philosophy of care, *Nurs Standard* 6(48):32, 1992.

Chalmers B: Annotation: care of children in hospital, *Child Care Health Devel* 19:119, 1993.

Miles I: The emergency of sick children nursing - part 1 and 2, *Nurs Education Today* **vol**:133, 1986.

NHS Executive: *A vision for the future,* London, 1993, Department of Health.

Report of the Platt Committee, London, 1989, HMSO.

Webb N et al: Care by parent in hospital, *BMJ* 291:176, 1985.

Welch L: Orem of roly; two concepts of nursing, *Paediatr Nurs* 5: 24, 1993.

Welch L: Applying Orem's model, *Paediatr Nurs* 6:14, 1993.

While A, editor: *Caring for children using nursing models,* London, 1991, Edward Arnold.

### Learning Disabilities Nursing

Blunden R, Allen D, editors: *Facing the challenge: an ordinary life for people with learning difficuliteis and challenging behaviour,* London, 1987, King's Fund Centre.

RCN :*The role and function of the domiciliary community nurse for people with learning disability,* London, 1992, RCN.

Shanley E & Starrs TA: *Learning disabilities: a handbook of care,* Edinburgh, 1993, Churchill Livingstone.

Sines D: The specialist nurse in mental handicap, *Nursing Standard* 15 (52): 36-39, 1991.

Sines D & Bicknell JC: *Caring for mentally handicapped people in the community,* London, 1985, Harper & Row.

Thompson T & Mathias P: *New approaches to competence: examples from nursing and social work,* In Thompson T and Mathias P: Standards and mental handicap: keys to competence. London, 1992, Bailliere Tindall.

### Mental Health Nursing

Chapman G E: *Politics, power and psychiatric nursing,* In Brooking, J et al. A textbook of psychiatric and mental health nursing. Edinburgh, 1992, Churchill Livingstone.

Collister B: *Psychiatric nursing : person to person,* London, 1988, Edward Arnold.

Cormack D: *Psychiatric nursing described,* London, 1983, Royal College of Nursing.

Giddey M : Mental health care in a changing society. In Giddey M, Wright H, editors: *Mental health nursing,* London, 1993, Chapman & Hall.

Kesey K: *One flew over the cuckoo's nest,* London, 1962, Picador.

Nolan P: *A History of mental health nursing,* London, 1994, Chapman and Hall.

CHAPTER 2

# The Health Care System

## CHAPTER OUTLINE

**Evolution of the National Health Service**

**Types of Health Care Services**
*Health promotion*
*Illness prevention*
*Diagnosis and treatment*
*Rehabilitation*

**Types of Agencies**
*Outpatient agencies*
*Institutions*
*Primary health care — community-based agencies*
*Support groups, self-help groups and voluntary agencies*
*Hospices*

**Factors Influencing Health Care Delivery**
*Society and the consumer's movement*
*New knowledge and technology*
*Legal and ethical issues*
*Economics*
*Politics*

**The Patient/Client and the Health Care System**
*Right to health care*
*Rights within the system*
*Entry into the system*

**Issues Affecting Health Care in the Next Decade**

**The Role of Information Technology**

## LEARNING OUTCOMES

After studying this chapter, you should be able to:
■ *Define the key terms listed.*
■ *Discuss major events in the evolution of the health care system.*
■ *Describe the various health care services available.*
■ *Discuss the types of agencies within the health care system.*
■ *Discuss the influence of social factors on health care delivery.*
■ *Suggest ways in which information technology affects care provision.*
■ *Differentiate between the legal and ethical rights of the patient/client and describe the impact of these on standards of care.*
■ *Discuss the patient's/client's right to health care and describe the patient's/client's rights within the health care delivery system.*
■ *Describe some issues related to the health care delivery system.*
■ *Explain solutions for some of these issues.*

The National Health Service (NHS) is undergoing change. National Health Service institutions are not thriving economically. The NHS is centrally funded through a universal contributory framework and is free at the point of delivery. However the cost of health care is rising. Because of central funding, and rising costs, there is a demand for greater control, effective regulation, and evidence that quality health care is being received by patients/clients. Control and effective regulation are viewed as essential to ensure the best use of available resources whilst costs are contained. The National Health Service is working through the NHS reforms to find better ways to provide effective health care at a lower cost. At the same time, it is being evaluated closely by **regulatory agencies**, such as the Audit Commission, the NHS Executive and the Department of Health. These regulatory agencies focus on the outcomes of health care and whether patients/clients benefit from intervention by an improved state of health and/or with the capacity to manage their continued health care needs.

Rising costs and restricted health care services lower the frequency and quality of care for people from varying socio-economic backgrounds. Many individuals wait months or years before they may gain access to health care in the NHS. Those who use private health insurance may have immediate access to health care in the private sector. Income, employment, social class, and geographic location frequently dictate accessibility to private health insurance and the type of health care received.

NHS reforms have introduced **market concepts** into the

NHS and have created a split between health care purchasers and providers. General practitioners are central to the reorganized NHS and are the 'gate-keepers' of access to hospital and other NHS services. General practitioners are currently either 'fundholders', responsible for their practice budget and purchasing health care services for their practice population, or are 'non-fundholders'. Non-fundholder patient/client care is purchased by the district health authority. It has been suggested that this has created a two-tier system and gross inequality (Holliday, 1992).

Nursing is a major component of the health care system. Nurses make up the largest employment group within the system. The average nursing population in an acute care facility can be as high as sixty percent. Nursing services are necessary for virtually every patient/client seeking care of any type, including health promotion, diagnosis and treatment, and rehabilitation. Because nursing is such an important part of the health care delivery system and because the delivery of nursing services is tied to other components of the health care delivery system, nurses need to understand the system to effectively deliver quality care within it. Every nurse practising today needs to appreciate that health care now operates within a business ethos. The success of this business depends on nursing's participation in changing the systems for delivering cost-effective care and creating strategies to ensure that patients/clients receive quality care and equal access to care.

## EVOLUTION OF THE NATIONAL HEALTH SERVICE

The NHS began giving universal health care for the first time in the UK on 5 July, 1948, as the result of passing the National Health Service Act of 1946. This initiative was a result of an increasing awareness of social inequality, and was commenced by the wartime coalition government and was enacted and developed by the post-war Labour government.

The concept of the NHS was built on the belief that health care is the right of every person regardless of his or her ability to pay. Funding for this National Health Service (NHS) would be provided largely from general taxation.

It is generally believed that the NHS was the first innovation in the UK health care system. Before 1948, there was considerable state provision. In 1911 the National Insurance Act allowed free care from general practitioners for manual workers and others receiving limited incomes. Medicines and various forms of health care were also provided free. The service was funded by contributions from employees, employers and the State. All general practitioners were entitled to be on the panel of those who provided care under the National Insurance Act, and general practitioners were often known as 'Panel Doctors'.

The NHS was legislated by the government, based upon the Beveridge Report of 1942. Beveridge postulated that living conditions could be improved through a comprehensive approach to health care and proposed extensive reforms of the social security system as well as an extension of the National Insurance Programme. The report assumed State-provided health care services would be comprehensive. The government accepted the concept and published a White Paper outlining its plans in 1944. In 1945 the task of creating the NHS fell to the newly elected Labour government and its health minister, Aneurin Bevan (Connah and Pearson, 1991).

The NHS unified various health care provisions into a national structure. It inherited a variety of health resources that had evolved over the years. Workhouses, built to house the destitute under the Poor Law, became hospitals and were passed on to the NHS. The Poor Law measures were discarded when the NHS was instituted.

When the NHS was established, the distribution of beds and staff between different parts of the country was not equal. This was true in relation to health care as a whole. It was evident there was little coordination of health care services. Thus, hospitals were organized through the NHS on a regional basis.

A tripartite system was created under the NHS, in which each hospital, family practitioner and local health authority were involved in contributing to the system. Primary health care services as we know them today were provided in the NHS by independent contractors. General practitioners and community nurses were governed by the local authorities. Community nurses remained outside the NHS structure until 1974. Executive Councils assumed the role previously provided by insurance committees. Dental and ophthalmic services were included as independent contractors.

As an entirely new regional structure was created for hospitals, regional boards were appointed by the Health Minister to oversee the management of the hospitals. The boards in turn appointed committees for the hospitals. The hospital management committees primarily followed the administrative pattern of voluntary hospitals, with the chief officer being the Hospital Secretary. These committees oversaw either a local group of hospitals, or one large teaching hospital. The Medical Officer of Health for the local authority had substantial powers and responsibilities regarding public health issues.

Aneurin Bevan insisted on a first-class health service (Connah and Pearson, 1991). This was in part to ensure the participation of the doctors, but also to command the confidence of the population and ensure quality across the UK. However, Treasury and Health Department officials miscalculated the original cost of the NHS and it was under-resourced. Therefore there was little capital development and modernization before the 1960s. Some small changes were made with the introduction of Churchill's incoming Conservative government. Prescription charges were initiated.

Beveridge envisaged a **decentralized health system**. Bevan and the government introduced a centralized and unitary structure based on a nationalized hospital sector. The present reform programme of **decentralization** is a major change in the philosophy of health care in the UK (Holliday, 1992).

In 1966 the General Practitioner's Charter introduced a number of reforms concerning general practitioner remuneration and incentives for practice. It replaced a per capita payments system with one that compensated for heavier work-loads. The purpose of the Charter was to encourage improvements in practice premises and employment of ancillary staff.

The Cogwheel Report of 1967 brought about additional changes in the NHS system. Hospital doctors became organized into speciality groupings so that clinical and administrative medical work could be undertaken more sensibly. In addition, as a result of the Salmon Report in 1966, nursing services were reorganized. The reorganization abolished the hospital matron and introduced the senior nurse staffing structure. Career progression emerged within the health care system for nurses.

February 1974 bought further changes, designed by Sir Keith Joseph, to the NHS structure. At this time, staff were having difficulty working in the tripartite structure and the service was not considered to be unified. In addition, regional hospital boards were replaced by regional health authorities. Hospital management committees were disbanded. Executive councils were abolished and replaced by family practitioner committees which were appointed by the health authorities. In addition, community health and school health services were moved from government control to that of the health authority. This brought community nursing into the tripartite health structure of the NHS. The new structure facilitated strategic planning which is critical to effective and efficient health care.

This new structure was not considered satisfactory by the medical organizations (Ham, 1990). A new layer of management had been added which appeared to take decision-making away from the front line and move it to the district level. Medical organizations linked this to the allegation that the NHS was seriously under financed. The new management system was less efficient and thus more costly.

To address these problems, an NHS planning system was introduced, and by 1976 a Resource Allocation Working Party had been established. It recommended a formula for redistributing funds out of the Thames regions to other parts of the country where funding was badly needed. The long-term intention was to increase the strategic capacity of the NHS. However, dissatisfaction with the structural reforms persisted. In 1982, further reorganization abolished area health authorities. District health authorities were created to oversee particular aspects of health care, such as acute care services and community services.

In 1983 the Health Secretary, Norman Fowler, commissioned Sir Roy Griffiths to appraise the NHS management style and to suggest improvements. The Griffiths Report highlighted the absence of identifiable leaders within management. It recommended the appointment of a general manager at every level, from national to individual unit. Proposals within the report were accepted by the government. One major proposal was the establishment of an NHS Supervisory Board and NHS Management Boards at a national level. Two boards were established which have now become respectively the Policy Board and the NHS Executive (NHSE).

Due to financial crisis in the Public Sector, Prime Minister Margaret Thatcher requested a further review of the NHS in 1988. Kenneth Clarke, the Secretary of State, finalized the details of plans to revise the health care system. Two White Papers, Working for Patients (DOH, 1989a), and Caring for People (DOH, 1989b), formed the basis of the National Health Service and Community Care Act of 1990 (Connah and Pearson, 1991).

This is the biggest reform of UK health care since the introduction of the NHS. This Act fundamentally altered the NHS structure by:

- injecting more competition into the system creating an internal market within the NHS
- introducing a purchaser/provider split focusing on health gain and outcomes of care
- re-routing funding to follow the patients/clients.

Health authorities began to purchase health care on behalf of their resident populations via contracts and the referral patterns of local general practitioners. Hospitals and community health units became NHS Trusts; those who chose not to, or who were not allowed to, remained as Directly Managed Units. Trusts have direct control over their own resources and operations. As fundholders, some general practitioners began to purchase hospital and community health services for their patients from a 'mixed economy' of care.

Health care is a business; as a result, central issues are escalating costs and the availability of quality health care services. Financial pressures have forced hospitals and other health care institutions to shift organizational priorities. There is concern that institutions will make financial incentives a priority over quality, humane care.

In today's health care economy, nursing professionals are in a position to restructure care delivery systems while maintaining a level of excellence in health care. More than ever, the role of nursing in patient advocacy will be critical to ensure that the health care needs of all populations are served.

## TYPES OF HEALTH CARE SERVICES

A variety of health care services are available to patients/clients and families, depending on the nature and extent of a health problem. The types of services offered often depend on the site in which patients/clients seek health care (for example, a hospital or mental health facility). Nurses play an active role in all forms of the health care service. The types of services can best be categorized as health promotion, illness prevention, diagnosis and treatment, and rehabilitation (Table 2-1).

### Health Promotion

**Health promotion** services have developed rapidly within the health care delivery system. Health promotion activities, including specific health education programmes, are designed to help patients/clients reduce the risk of illness, maintain maximal function, and promote habits related to good health. Health promotion activities take place in many settings, but the majority are offered within **primary health care**. For example, some hospitals and clinics offer programmes such as prenatal nutrition classes in which the essentials of good nutrition during pregnancy, after childbirth, and for the infant are taught. These classes promote the general health of the woman, the fetus, and the infant. The four regions of the UK have developed strategies, set out health promotion targets and are the basis of health promotion activity.

## Illness Prevention

**Illness prevention** is another type of service provided by the health care delivery system. The nurse helps prevent illness by assisting the patient/client and family in reducing risk factors and avoiding the need for primary, secondary, or tertiary health care. Usually, prevention activities involve the patient/client directly and include measures such as periodical physical examinations and identification of familial risk factors for illnesses such as cardiovascular disease. After risk factors are identified, the patient/client can engage in positive health practices such as changing the diet to prevent illness.

Illness prevention activities also include environmental programmes to reduce the threat of illness or disability. For example, sanitation and water treatment programmes to prevent the spread of disease.

Occupational safety measures in the workplace and educational programmes are also illness-prevention activities. In the painting and construction industry, for example, the use of respirators by employees exposed to dust and paint fumes reduces the risk of lung disease.

Public education programmes and legislation are also involved in illness and injury prevention. Laws requiring the use of approved infant or toddler restraint seats and safety belts in cars, for example, are directed at preventing severe injury or death.

Preventive health education and practices are generally effective in reducing the risk of disease and disability, and prevention activities help improve the individual's and community's level of health. It is also becoming evident that preventive measures can reduce the costs of health care. The strategies are intended to build upon the preventative aspect of health care services.

## Diagnosis and Treatment

The diagnosis and treatment of illness have traditionally been the most commonly used services of the health care delivery system. Advances in technology and computers have resulted in more sophisticated diagnostic procedures and greater chances for early

### Examples of Health Promotion Targets throughout the UK

**England** - By 2000, infant mortality should be less than 15 per 100,000 live births.
**Northern Ireland** - By 1997 the proportion of energy derived from saturated fat in the diet should be reduced to less than 15% (from 17.5%) and from total fats to less than 35% (from 40%).
**Scotland** - By the year 2000, there will be a 30% reduction in smokers aged 12-24, and a 20% reduction in smokers aged 25-65.
**Wales** - By 2002 there will be a 30% reduction in deaths from circulatory diseases, at least a 15% reduction in deaths from lung cancer among people aged 45-64 and at least a 15% reduction in suicides.

The Health of the Nation (*HMSO*, 1992b)
A Regional Strategy for Northern Ireland (*Northern Ireland Office*, 1991)
Scotland's Health (*Scottish Office*, 1992)
Caring for the Future (*NHS Cymru Wales*, 1992)

## TABLE 2-1 The Three Levels of Prevention

| Primary Prevention | | Secondary Prevention | | Tertiary Prevention |
|---|---|---|---|---|
| **Health Promotion** | **Specific Protection** | **Early Diagnosis and Prompt Treatment** | **Disability Limitations** | **Restoration and Rehabilitation** |
| Health education | Use of specific immunizations | Case-finding measures: individual and mass | Adequate treatment to arrest disease process and prevent further complications | Provision of hospital and community facilities for retraining and education to maximize use of remaining capacities |
| Good standard of nutrition adjusted to developmental phases of life | Attention to personal hygiene | Screening surveys | Provision of facilities to limit disability and prevent death | Education of the public and industries to use rehabilitated persons to the fullest possible extent |
| Attention to personal development | Use of environmental sanitation | Selective examinations | | |
| Provision of adequate housing and recreation and agreeable working conditions | Protection against environmental hazards | Cure and prevention of disease process to prevent spread of communicable disease, prevent complications, and shorten period of disability | | |
| Marriage counselling and sex education | Protection from accidents | | | Selective placement |
| Genetic screening | Use of specific nutrients | | | Work therapy in hospitals |
| Periodic selective examinations | Protection from carcinogens | | | Use of sheltered colony |
| | Avoidance of allergens | | | |

Modified from Leavell H, Clark AE: Preventive medicine for doctors in the community, New York, 1965, McGraw-Hill.

diagnosis. Many new diagnostic tests are noninvasive and painless. Furthermore, diagnostic services can now be brought to a patient/client; some health authorities have equipped motorized vans with diagnostic x-ray equipment and offer services at sites, such as public libraries.

Nurses' activities in the community can be directed at early diagnosis and education. For example, nurses can teach women about breast self-examination, enabling them to discover a breast mass at an early stage and to seek early treatment. In other community settings, such as schools, special programmes have been organized to detect health problems, such as hypertension, elevated cholesterol, or visual or hearing impairments, at an early stage.

Treatment methods have also expanded because of advances in technology and knowledge. Patients/clients are receiving newer, more innovative health care treatments based on the most recent research. Treatment of illnesses has also expanded outside hospitals and other institutions, even to the home. When treatment is initiated within an institution, nurses teach the patient/client and family to complete the treatment plan at home.

## Rehabilitation

**Rehabilitation** is the restoration of a person to normal or near-normal function after a physical or mental illness, injury, or chemical addiction. Rehabilitation was once available primarily for patients/clients with illnesses or injury to the nervous system, but the health care system has expanded its scope of such services. Today, specialized rehabilitation services, such as cardiovascular rehabilitation programmes, help individuals and their families adjust to necessary changes in lifestyle after heart attacks. Pulmonary rehabilitation programmes aim to increase the exercise tolerance of people with chronic pulmonary diseases.

Rehabilitation services begin the moment a patient/client enters the health care system with an illness or injury. Initially, rehabilitation may focus on the prevention of complications related to the illness or injury. As the condition stabilizes, rehabilitation is directed at maximizing the person's functioning and level of independence.

These programmes take place in many health care settings, including specific rehabilitation institutions, outpatient settings, and the home. Frequently, people needing long-term rehabilitation have severe disabilities affecting their ability to carry out activities of living. When rehabilitation services are provided in outpatient settings, patients/clients receive treatment at specified times during the week, but remain at home the rest of the time. Specific rehabilitation strategies are applied to the home environment so that maximal levels of function and independence can be achieved. District nurses and other members of the health care team visit people in their homes and provide nursing care. They also help individuals and families learn to adapt to illness or injury.

## TYPES OF AGENCIES

As a result of the expansion of the health care system and increasing specialization, the variety and number of health care agencies have increased. Services once delivered primarily by hospitals are now provided in many other types of settings through agencies that include outpatient, institutional (e.g. day care surgery), community-based, volunteer, hospice, and government programmes.

## Outpatient Agencies

People who do not require hospitalization can receive health care in an alternative site such as a doctor's general practice surgery, clinic, or other ambulatory care facility. Outpatient services are generally directed at the diagnosis and treatment of acute and chronic illnesses. An outpatient setting is designed to be convenient and easily accessible to patients/clients.

## General Practice Surgeries

General practice surgeries provide primary care for a large segment of the population (around 99%), but 1 in 7 people of some populations in inner cities are not registered (Tomlinson, 1992). These people, for example the homeless, are the most 'at risk' and are a challenge to health care professionals. Doctors have tended to focus on the diagnosis and treatment of specific illnesses rather than on health promotion and other services. With the changes in health care due to NHS reforms, general practice surgeries now offer a wider range of diagnostic and therapeutic services. The nature and scope of general practice is changing radically. Practices are being encouraged to extend their services, leading to new roles for doctors and nurses.

Nurses employed in general practice surgeries can assume many roles. Some practice nurses register patients/clients, take observations, prepare the patient/client for examination or laboratory studies, and provide basic information. Other practice nurses working with doctors have the expanded role of conducting physical examinations and histories, offering health education, and recommending therapies for patients/clients in stable health. This aspect of nursing in general practice is evolving into the controversial 'nurse practitioner'. Currently, practice nurses are employed by the general practitioner. Health visitors and district nurses are employed by the District Health Authority (DHA) Community Services (Trust or Directly Managed Unit), and are increasingly working with patient/client groups from aligned or attached general practitioner practices.

## Clinics

Clinics have traditionally involved a department in a hospital where patients/clients not requiring hospitalization receive medical care. General practice surgeries or community clinics deliver aspects of primary health care, such as immunizations. The roles of nurses in a clinic are very similar to those of nurses in a general practice surgery.

## Minor Injury Units/Satellite Centres

Minor Injury Units or Satellite Centres, like clinics, provide health services on an **outpatient** basis. The centres may be affiliated with hospital trusts or may function independently in a health authority or special district. Although the centre may be located within an **inpatient** facility, most are located away from major inpatient institutions. A satellite centre is an example of an ambulatory care centre that provides services to patients/clients for minor injuries or illnesses such as lacerations and influenza. The centre offers an alternative to a hospital accident and emergency department.

## Institutions

Institutional agencies include hospitals, long-term care facilities, continuing care facilities, nursing, residential and dual registered homes, and psychiatric/mental health facilities. Rehabilitation centres offering health care services to patients/clients are also considered to be health care institutions.

## Hospitals

Hospitals traditionally have been the major agency of the health care system. Care which has traditionally been provided in hospital is shifting to the community. Typically a patient/client would come to a hospital for diagnosis and treatment. The individual would remain hospitalized until almost fully recovered. However, increasing costs are changing how people are cared for in hospitals. A person may be given initial treatment in hospital and then be expected to recover at home. When the person is not fully recovered, alternative care sites are found, including extended care facilities, nursing homes, and home care.

Today, people who enter hospitals are usually acutely ill and need comprehensive and specialized health care. The services provided by hospitals vary considerably. Small rural hospitals may offer limited accident and emergency, and diagnostic services, as well as general inpatient services. In comparison, large urban teaching hospitals offer comprehensive, state-of-the-art diagnostic services, accident and emergency care, surgical intervention, intensive treatment units, inpatient services, and rehabilitation facilities. Larger hospitals also offer professional staff from a variety of specialities such as social service, physical and occupational therapy, and speech therapy. The focus in hospitals is to provide the highest quality of care possible so that patients/clients can be discharged early but safely to the home or to a facility that can adequately manage remaining health care needs.

Nurses who work in hospitals have opportunities to work in a variety of roles and departments. The care of patients/clients on a nursing ward or within an intensive treatment unit requires the nurse to have the knowledge and skills for applying the nursing process, providing patient/client education, coordinating health care services and discharge planning, and delivering a variety of therapies. As the depth of nursing knowledge increases, many nurses specialize in their practice. This allows them to become expert in the care of select patient/client populations. Many hospitals have, for example, specialized wards for the care of people with oncological, orthopaedic, pulmonary, or cardiac problems. Other opportunities within a hospital setting may include the role of patient/client educator, nurse manager, clinical nurse specialist, and infection control nurse.

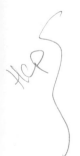

## Long-term Care

**Long-term care** embraces all forms of continuing personal or nursing care and associated domestic services for people who are unable to look after themselves without some degree of support. Within this definition, these services can be provided in patients'/clients' own homes, at a day centre, or in a NHS or private nursing home setting (Laing, 1993).

Long-term care most often describes the institutional care of people who have chronic illness or disability (Ebrahim *et al*, 1993). The residents within long-term care institutions were historically those who lived within the Victorian workhouses, particularly older people with physical or mental frailty and adults of all ages who had chronic disability. The stigma of the workhouses has influenced the way these long-term care units have been viewed by many people, and particularly the low levels of funding they have traditionally received (Ebrahim *et al*, 1993).

## Continuing Care Units

Continuous health care for physically and mentally frail people, particularly older people, has traditionally been funded by the National Health Service and provided mainly within hospitals and nursing homes. In recent years the number of NHS continuing care beds for both physically and mentally ill older people has reduced markedly (Rickford, 1993; Alzheimers Disease Society, 1993), whereas the numbers of beds provided in private sector nursing homes is gradually increasing.

## Nursing Homes

A **Nursing Home** is defined as a facility that provides, or intends to provide, nursing and clinical care for people suffering from any sickness, injury or infirmity. These homes are registered under part II of the Registered Homes Act 1984 and are inspected by the Health Authority's Nursing Homes Inspectors. Private hospitals can also be included within this definition and are therefore subject to the same regulatory mechanisms.

## Residential Care Homes

A Residential Care Home is defined as a facility that provides, or intends to provide, personal care in a residential setting. These facilities are registered under part I of the Registered Homes Act 1984 and are inspected by the Local Authority's Residential Care Home Inspectors.

People who live in residential care homes should be sufficiently independent to need assistance with personal care only. Health care is organized and given by the community nursing team and resident's general practitioner.

## Dual Registered Homes

Dual Registered Homes provide differing levels of support including both personal and nursing care. They are registered under both parts I and II of the Registered Homes Act 1984, and are inspected by both Local Authorities and Health Authorities. Dual Registered Homes pay dual registration fees.

The provisions of the 1984 Registered Homes Act and its amendments are highly complex and are currently the subject of debate. The debate has increased since the implementation of the NHS and Community Care Act and the Government's deregulation initiatives.

## Psychiatric/Mental Health Facilities

People who have emotional or behavioural problems, for example depression or eating disorders, often require specific counselling and therapy in a variety of mental health care settings. These services may be offered within the National Health Service or within the independent health sector. Inpatient, day patient and outpatient facilities are available depending on the nature of the problem and the needs of the individual.

A person may seek mental health care services voluntarily, or involuntarily under one of the provisions of the Mental Health Act (1983), if there is danger of the patient/client harming others or harming himself or herself.

People requiring mental health services are usually referred to as 'clients' in order to emphasize their citizenship and choice. A multidisciplinary approach is usually adopted when considering the mental health needs of the individual client. A comprehensive nursing assessment is carried out involving the client, and his or her family and significant others. At times, a social work assessment and occupational therapy assessment will also be conducted.

A range of interventions is available to help meet specific needs of the client. These could include occupational therapy, cognitive or behavioural therapy, or client-centred counselling, stress management programmes and drug therapy. The nurse facilitates the ability of the client to take an active part in the programme of care.

When a client is considered suitable for discharge, the multidisciplinary team discusses the discharge plan with the individual, his or her family and other care agencies. Clients may be discharged home with follow-up by community psychiatric nurses. Alternatively, the client may be referred onto **day care** within either health or social services. Clients may also wish to seek additional support from a range of self-help groups organized by people who have experienced similar mental health problems.

Having a psychiatric diagnosis or treatment in a mental health care setting can be a stigmatizing experience. After treatment, many people are reluctant to remain associated with professional mental health organizations. Therefore, discharge planning is essential to the treatment programme in order to safeguard the wellbeing of the client and the community to which he or she is returning.

With the closure of large mental institutions small units have been set up to focus particularly on the specific needs of people with long-term mental illness so that they can be rehabilitated in the community.

## Rehabilitation Centres

A **rehabilitation centre** is a residential institution providing therapy and training to restore individuals to optimal levels of functioning and independence. Rehabilitation centres actively involve patients/clients and families in providing health care. The goal of rehabilitation is to decrease the person's dependence on the care provided so that he or she assumes responsibility for personal care.

Rehabilitation centres employ people from nursing, medicine, and professions allied to health, such as occupational therapy and physiotherapy. Many rehabilitation centres focus on physical rehabilitation programmes to teach the patient/client and family to achieve maximal physical function after a stroke, head or spinal cord injury, or other physical impairment. Drug rehabilitation centres help the person become free from drug dependence and return to the community. Nurses employed in rehabilitation centres are committed to long-term continuity of nursing services and must be knowledgeable in their specialized area.

## Primary Health Care Agencies — Community-Based Agencies

Primary Health Care agencies focus on providing health care to people within their neighbourhoods. The strategies developed by the four regions of the UK include aims and objectives to provide increased community care services. Examples of such agencies are day care hospitals/centres, crisis intervention centres, support groups, self-help groups and volunteer agencies. Nurses may have a variety of roles within these settings.

## Day Care Hospitals/Centres

Day hospitals are used for the assessment, treatment, rehabilitation and maintenance of the physical and mental health of people (National Audit Office, 1994). The majority of day hospitals cater primarily for older people. The range of services offered include nursing, medicine, physiotherapy, occupational therapy, speech therapy, dietetics, chiropody and hearing therapy. Day hospitals aim to meet local needs and priorities and thus fulfil different functions in different areas throughout the UK.

Day centres may be organized by Local Authorities, voluntary bodies or organizations within the private sector. They provide social care and recreational activities, particularly aimed at relieving isolation and loneliness.

## Crisis Intervention Centres

**Crisis intervention centres** and their teams provide 24-hour emergency psychiatric care and counselling to people experiencing extreme stress or conflict, often involving suicide attempts or drug or alcohol abuse. The services may be delivered directly on the premises, or counselling may be provided over the telephone. The primary objectives of crisis intervention centres are to help the person cope with the immediate problem and to offer guidance and support for long-term therapy.

Some voluntary organizations and charities offer help and support in crisis situations. For example, the Samaritans offer a 24-hour telephone helpline for people who are suicidal or disparing. Some Samaritan centres also offer a drop-in service during specified hours.

Many different organizations offer telephone helplines. Lists of these organizations are given in local telephone directories.

## Support Groups, Self-Help Groups and Voluntary Agencies

**Support groups**, **self-help groups**, and **voluntary agencies** are usually non profit-making and may be established nationally or within a community to meet a specific need. The groups or agencies may be run by charities, voluntary groups or individuals who have experienced similar problems to those they aim to help. These organizations provide information, advice, support, advocacy and practical help. They may also have programmes for the prevention and detection of specific illnesses. Some charity and voluntary agencies provide financial support for the training of doctors and nurses, as well as for research directed at the prevention, detection, and treatment of certain diseases. Many health professionals donate time and resources to agencies within their specialty. Multi-agency cooperation is vital to ensure the effectiveness of services provided.

### Hospices

The trend of seeking care outside of institutions has led to the development of hospices to meet the holistic needs of the terminally ill. A **hospice** is a system of family-centred care designed to make the terminally ill person comfortable and ensure a satisfactory lifestyle through the terminal phase of illness. Hospice care can benefit people in the terminal phases of any disease, such as cardiomyopathy, multiple sclerosis, acquired immunodeficiency syndrome (AIDS), cancer, emphysema, or renal disease.

A patient/client entering a hospice has reached the terminal phase of illness, and the individual, family, and doctor have agreed that no further treatment could reverse the disease process. The individual and family must accept the fact that the hospice will not use emergency measures, such as cardiopulmonary resuscitation, to prolong life. Instead, the hospice provides pain control and comfort measures to maintain the quality of life. Hospices do not have rigid visiting policies or other prescribed limits, and the environment for the patient/client and health care workers is very relaxed.

Hospices are operated in many settings. Independent hospices provide only hospice care and are not affiliated with a hospital, but have good medical and nursing backup, for example, the International St Joseph's Hospice, or 'Jospice'. Other hospices operate within a hospital setting, and many hospitals are now developing hospice units in a separate area of the institution.

Hospice nurses are committed to the philosophy and objectives of the facilities for which they work. They provide care and support for the patient/client and family during the terminal phase and continue to give the family emotional support throughout the grieving period.

Some organizations affiliated with hospices also offer respite care. Caring for a terminally ill spouse or relative can be emotionally and physically draining. **Respite care** provides a primary care provider such as a spouse or family member the opportunity to have some time alone. A nurse or specially trained volunteer comes to the home so that the primary care provider can run errands or have a break from the responsibility of direct care. The respite care service is important in maintaining the health of the care giver and family.

## FACTORS INFLUENCING HEALTH CARE DELIVERY

Changes in the health care delivery system have increased rapidly during the last decade. The present system is the result of changes associated with social and consumer influences, new knowledge and technology, legal and ethical trends, and economic and political factors. An understanding of the factors influencing the health care system will enable nurses to adjust to changes, create better ways of providing nursing care, and develop new nursing roles.

### Society and the Consumer's Movement

Consumers of health care delivery services have increased their knowledge and awareness of health promotion, illness prevention, and treatment practices (Downie *et al*, 1991). As a result, these consumers are exerting pressure on the government to influence health care and its delivery. No longer do consumers simply accept a health care professional's recommendations. Consumers expect information to be provided so they can gain an understanding of health problems and their implications.

As consumers have become more knowledgeable about health in general, they have gained a greater awareness of the

---

### Some Aims/Objectives for Health and Social Provision throughout the United Kingdom

**Wales** - In order to promote *maternal and early child health,* family planning strategies are developing. These will ensure that family planning is available to all who need it and particularly through young people's advisory services. The strategy will also target high risk pregnancies.

**Northern Ireland** - There should be further development of community care services in order to facilitate the discharge from hospital of people with a learning disability. This should reduce the numbers of people in learning disability hospitals from just under 1000 in 1991 to less than 700 by 1997.

**England** - The Department of Health aims to reduce the level of disability caused by *mental illness* by improving significantly the treatment and care of mentally disordered people.

**Scotland** - Health Boards are meeting the challenges of HIV and AIDS by setting up special AIDS units in Dundee, Edinburgh and Glasgow, needle and syringe exchange schemes in many areas and targeting over £73 million to national public education campaigns.

Caring for the Future (*NHS Cymru Wales*, 1992)
A Regional Strategy for Northern Ireland (*Northern Ireland Office*, 1991)
The Health of the Nation (*HMSO*, 1992b)
Scotland's Health (*Scottish Office*, 1992)

impact of lifestyle on health. As a result, consumers have expressed a greater need for knowledge and services related to illness prevention and health promotion. Similarly, businesses and corporations have instituted programmes to promote wellness and fitness. The cost of health care has a direct impact on businesses. Increased sick time and disability of employees cause significant financial loss. The interest society holds for more information about health care is growing. Consumers seek diagnosis and treatment of illness, but this is no longer the exclusive or even primary focus of health care. More people wish to learn about self-care, so they may remain as independent as possible (Downie et al, 1991).

Another major influence on societal trends has been people born during the decade after World War II. This segment of the population is now middle-aged and is beginning to express concerns about the availability and quality of health care. As this group approaches old age, significant changes will probably occur in health care delivery systems. For example, primary health care services which help people with chronic disease to achieve a high level of wellness and functioning, are becoming more important.

The health care beliefs and practices of society are as complex as those of an individual, depending on continuously evolving values, ethics, concepts of health, and other factors. In general, however, consumers' desire for health promotion, health protection, and new cures and treatments has led to changes in the health care delivery system. Many institutions and community-based agencies provide a wide range of outpatient health promotion and health protection programmes on a regular basis. Volunteer agencies have been formed to meet specific needs in health protection and promotion, and consumers have become more active in fund raising to support research in these areas.

## New Knowledge and Technology

Scientific knowledge continues to increase rapidly. Research has led to new treatments and cures for life-threatening conditions such as cancer, cardiovascular diseases, and diabetes mellitus. People have the opportunity to receive the most advanced treatment in the form of organ transplantation, laser surgery, and even gene-alteration therapies.

The challenges of this knowledge explosion are related to three factors. First, it is increasingly difficult for health care professionals to remain well informed about advances in their field. With the volume of knowledge available, it is difficult to remain a generalist. For example, a practising nurse has trouble remaining competent in all areas of general nursing practice. More care givers are becoming specialized, so they can focus on exclusive areas of knowledge and skills (such as oncology or critical care). Institutions must bear the costs of keeping professional staff educated and updated on advances in health care.

A second factor is the cost related to technology. New third-generation antibiotics, diagnostic imaging equipment, and specialized beds are just a few examples of technologies that are introduced daily into health care settings. Consumers must ask about whether these new technologies improve the quality of care and are cost effective. Nurses play a key role in evaluating new products and determining whether they help improve nursing practice. The costs of technologies are eventually transferred to patients/clients. The ultimate factors in the use of technologies may be the economic resources available and the wants and needs of society as a whole.

The third factor of advanced technology relates to its impact on health care delivery. Because technology causes greater specialization in health care, there is a risk of more fragmentation in care. It is important to have a single care giver who coordinates a patient's/client's health management. For example, one doctor directs the course of therapy, using advice from radiologists, surgeons, and perhaps rehabilitation experts. However, diverse specialization usually introduces multiple carers who do not always communicate clearly to ensure well coordinated patient/client care. Increased fragmentation of care also adds to health care costs.

## Legal and Ethical Issues

As people become more aware of their rights to health care and humane treatment, legal and ethical issues arise when care becomes compromised (see Chapter 13). Health care providers are under increased scrutiny as consumers gain a better understanding of their health problems. Safe, efficacious, and humane health care is an expectation of society (Seedhouse, 1986; Seedhouse and Cribb, 1989). When this expectation is unmet, legal actions can be taken against care givers, and the ethical dilemmas that arise are enormous.

A **legal right** is that to which a person is entitled by law. For example, a person has a legal right to competent registered professionals and safe practices within a medical treatment centre. In contrast, an ethical right, such as a person's desire to refuse life-saving therapies, has no legal guarantees. Ethics defines the principles or standards governing proper conduct (see Chapter 12). The legal and ethical concerns raised by consumers are changing the health care system. Standards are being implemented to ensure that health care staff are competently educated. Policies within an institution dictate proper procedures for obtaining patient/client consent to treatment. Institutions have created **ethics committees** to review professional practices and offer guidance when patient/client rights are threatened. More attention is being given to patient/client advocacy. Health care institutions are more intent on keeping patients/clients and families informed and ensuring that staff members are responsible for their practice. The Patient's Charter (DOH, 1992a) and Working in Partnership (DOH, 1994) are two examples of recommended changes in the way in which health services should be organized and care is approached to protect the rights of patients/clients.

## Economics

Ultimately, someone must pay for all health care services. People with private resources or health insurance policies are generally able to seek health promotion and health protection services from the private sector. Those without private insurance seek health services through the NHS.

As the National Health Service and Community Care Act (DOH, 1990) reforms have been instituted, doctors have begun to avoid hospitalization for their patients/clients whenever possible. There is an increasing focus on primary health care, and with this more people are being treated in the community. Health care which is provided locally, with a focus on health promotion, is viewed as cost effective in the long term.

Due to the large number of people treated in NHS hospitals, planning for their discharge has a high priority and should be implemented the first day of hospital admission. The NHS and Community Care Act (DOH, 1990) requires health authorities and Social Services to develop adequate joint discharge planning arrangements. In some hospitals and other institutions, a high ratio of nurses to patients/clients is viewed as too expensive, so there has been a re-analysis of the appropriate methods for delivering care with fewer nurses. In an attempt to further reduce nursing costs, lower-salaried, non-professional health care workers may be employed.

Rising costs and changing demographics have caused some hospitals to close and others to consolidate their services into large hospitals. Some smaller, rural hospitals have been unable to diversify their services in order to compete with larger hospitals.

### Politics

The health care delivery system is influenced by political decisions and factors. Through health care legislation, government affects how health care is provided. The NHS and Community Care Act (DOH, 1990) is an example of legislation that is reshaping how health care is provided. For example, a government that makes health care a high priority can benefit the health care delivery system by increasing funding for health education and research.

## THE PATIENT/CLIENT AND THE HEALTH CARE SYSTEM

People usually have little or no interaction with the health care system while experiencing good health. An exception to this is families with children under 5 years of age who are regularly visited by a health visitor. If people become ill, or are motivated for other reasons to seek health care, they must enter the health care system. This is usually via a general practitioner, however some patients/clients enter the system by walking into a clinic or hospital accident and emergency department.

Patients/clients entering the system have specific rights. Society generally believes that all people have a right to health care. However, after people enter the health care system, they become patients or clients and thus have certain rights within the system. As health care consumers, people have a general right to determine what kind of health care should be available for present and future needs. Each of these rights affects how health care is delivered, but practices ensured by

these rights are also influenced by society's attitudes and the system itself. The Patient's Charter (DOH, 1992a) was developed as a result of the belief that all people have specific rights in relation to their health care.

### Right to Health Care

Society has generally come to believe that all people have a right to health care, regardless of cultural, economic, or other factors. This belief has led to the development of the National Health Service, which seeks to meet the health care needs of all people, regardless of their ability to pay.

### Rights within the System

Patients/clients have the right to information about their diagnosis and treatment, fees for services, and continuity of care. Patients/clients have the right to refuse any diagnostic or treatment procedures. Above all, patients/clients have the right to information about their health and privacy while receiving health care. Not all users of the health care service are aware of their rights or have the power to demand those rights; for example, older people and those with mental health problems.

One of the patient's/client's specific legal rights in any health care facility is informed consent, which is obtaining permission from the patient/client to perform certain kinds of actions. Informed consent must be obtained before beginning any invasive procedure, administering an experimental drug, or placing a patient/client in a research study (see Chapter 13).

Patient's/client's rights and informed consent affect the way the health care system delivers care. Most agencies have committees to evaluate patient/client suggestions and complaints about the delivery of health care. Nurses advocate for patients/clients. The need to protect patient's/client's rights sometimes results in increased work and/or paperwork, however this protection is necessary to ensure that all patients/clients maintain their rights within the health care system.

### Entry into the System

The most common ways that individuals enter the health care system are entry by referral from a health team member, such as a doctor or health visitor, or entry when the patient/client has a specific health need. Other methods of entry are self-referral, employer referral, and social referral. For people with mental health needs, these pathways are often inadequate and many of these individuals are brought to health care via the police, the courts and prison services.

A patient/client may enter the system by referral from a health team member in the case of an acute, potentially life-threatening problem, such as severe chest pain, or in the case of a less threatening problem such as a rash of unknown cause. In an emergency situation a patient/client typically contacts his or her general practitioner who refers that person directly to the accident and emergency department. In less acute situations the nurse often refers the patient/client to the system. Such referrals may be given to a neighbour seeking advice, a child and family at a school where the nurse practices, or to the family of a person to whom the nurse has previously provided care.

People also enter the system on their own because of a specific need. For example, a college student may seek health care for treatment of a sore throat or gastrointestinal upset and thus may enter the health care system at the primary care level through the health service centre at the university. Another student may be involved in a severe automobile accident and enter the health care system through a hospital accident and emergency department.

Regardless of the manner of entry into the system, all patients/clients encounter nurses and nursing services. The first impression the patient/client has of the care delivered by a nurse may form a significant and lasting impression about nursing and health care in general. Nurses therefore have the opportunity to increase patient/client awareness of such services and the types of quality care they can, and should, expect.

## ISSUES AFFECTING HEALTH CARE IN THE NEXT DECADE

### Issue: Fragmented Care

Advanced scientific knowledge and technology have resulted in the increasing specialization of health care in areas such as cardiac disease, kidney disease, and cancer. Although specialization allows each professional to provide patients/clients with highly advanced care, the delivery of total care may be fragmented if it is not managed well. The number of doctors in general practice is declining in some areas of the United Kingdom, and due to the increasing practice of referral many people may have a different doctor for each specific problem. As a result, care is not provided for the individual as a whole person. This fragmentation of care inhibits comprehensive assessment of personal dynamics and its impact on the level of health of the person. When many specialists are involved, there is an increased chance of losing the patient/client to follow-up, over-medicating or under-medicating the patient/client, and decreasing his or her quality of life because of the time involved in obtaining care.

Nurses are taught to care for the patient/client holistically. Generally, within the health care delivery system, it is the nurse who assumes the responsibility of coordinating the patient's/client's care, so that care is not fragmented.

### Solution: Managed Care and Case Management

In the past, care givers from all disciplines, such as nursing, medicine and social work, managed a patient's/client's care within a hospital by contributing their own plans of care. There has always been an objective to coordinate the work of all care givers so that a single plan is followed with favourable outcomes. This is not always easy to accomplish, and depends upon the nursing delivery-of-care model used and the collaboration of all care givers. For example, team nursing may be focused on the tasks of nursing care. When this occurs, there is a danger that little effort may be given to ensure continuity of discharge planning and

participation by all care givers. Managed-care and case-management systems are improving collaboration of care givers and the ability to deliver quality services. The product of most health care agencies is the provision of services by health care professionals in an efficient and effective manner with expected outcomes (Pierog, 1991). With managed care and case management, one care giver coordinates care, from admission through to discharge, from an acute-care setting into the primary health care environment. A multidisciplinary plan is implemented so that all care givers work with one plan to achieve the same patient/client outcomes.

A popular tool used in managed care and case management is the critical pathway. These are multidisciplinary treatment plans that sequence interventions over a projected length of stay for specific case types. Initially developed by Zander (1988) at the New England Medical Center in Boston, a critical path tells care givers what care needs to be given and when so that a patient/client is discharged on time and in as healthy a condition as possible. Ideally, critical pathways incorporate expected outcomes throughout hospitalization and at the time of discharge. A primary nurse, often called a care manager, coordinates a patient's/client's progress through a pathway. The nurse is responsible for communicating with other care givers so that the individual's progress is uninterrupted. In some settings, the nurse care manager may continue to coordinate care on a pathway after the patient/client has been transferred to a different ward.

If pathways are developed correctly, fewer resources (for example, laboratory or radiological tests) are used and the clinical outcomes of care (for example, avoidance of complications or successful achievement of rehabilitation) are realized in a desired time frame. By reducing costs and ensuring quality outcomes, critical pathways are a solution to major health care delivery problems. Critical pathways may also be developed for extended care facilities.

Nursing has always supported a holistic model for health care, integrating the person, care givers, society, environment, and health. However, the present health care system continues to emphasize curing rather than caring for an individual. Nursing can make a significant contribution by becoming more involved in all levels of health care. Nurses can provide services at a more cost-effective and qualitative level than other providers (Maraldo, 1989). Consumers must learn what nurses can offer in preventive and in primary care services. In addition, nurses should take an active lead in re-organizing and coordinating health care systems.

### Issue: Ill Health and Disability in the Older Adult Population

Older adults comprise a significant portion of patients/clients within the health care system. Chronic illnesses affect older adults more often than children or young adults. Because people live longer, the number of individuals with chronic disease grows. Quality of life versus increased longevity also becomes an issue as doctors develop treatments that prolong life. The health care system must address the special care requirements of the chronically ill by providing proper health care facilities and ensuring that professionals are appropriately prepared to care for the needs of older adults.

## Solution: Specialist Care for Older People

As the population of older adults increases, it becomes critical for nursing and other professions to understand the unique science of gerontology. For a long time, doctors and nurses have accepted paediatrics as a branch of medicine concerned with the development and care of children. Only during the past few decades has a specific body of knowledge been established pertaining to the physiological characteristics of ageing, diseases of ageing, and the psychological, economical, and sociological problems of older adults.

An older adult has different health concerns from a middle-aged adult. Gunter (1987) defines gerontological nursing as a health service that incorporates gerontological nursing methods and specialized knowledge about the aged to establish conditions within the patient/client and/or environment that will increase health-conducive behaviours, minimize health losses and disability, provide comfort and sustenance, and facilitate diagnosis, palliation, and treatment of disease in the aged.

The rapidly growing speciality of gerontological nursing prepares nurses to design strategies aimed at helping older adults (including those who are chronically ill or disabled) maintain functioning and independence. The collaboration of all health care disciplines is needed for improved care. More services designed to provide high quality care for older adults are needed.

## Issue: Quality of Care

As public awareness about health care improves and as the statistics for performance of the health care system become available, quality of care will become a serious issue. To determine the quality of health care, a person must ask about the outcomes of care. Outcomes are the result (desirable or undesirable) of care delivered (Williams, 1991). For example, nosocomial (hospital-acquired) infection rates, surgical wound healing, and ability to perform self-care, are all outcomes.

## Solution: Quality Improvement

Efforts to ensure and improve the quality of health care have never been as important as they are today. The health care agencies that survive in the next decade will be able to guarantee a superior level of quality of care.

Quality management is less well developed in health care than in industry. The terms most frequently discussed in the health care literature are quality assurance and quality improvement. **Quality assurance** (QA) is the ongoing systematic monitoring or evaluation of nursing practice, medical practice, or practice of other disciplines. Traditionally, QA has focused on clinical practice, providing information on the appropriateness of nursing care processes and activities. QA programmes direct staff to inspect and repair rather than prevent, innovate, and develop personnel

(Schroeder, 1988). Quality improvement (QI) has become the new focus in health care. Quality improvement programmes are identified as total quality management (TQM) or continuous quality improvement (CQI). These are integrated, coordinated approaches to improving practices and services. A focus is the elimination of barriers that impede patients'/clients' use of the health care system at a nursing unit or agency. The King's Fund accrediting agenda is to encourage active collaboration among health care disciplines in order to identify the best possible clinical practice that can guarantee repeated favourable outcomes for patients/clients.

## THE ROLE OF INFORMATION TECHNOLOGY IN HEALTH CARE DELIVERY

As the profession of nursing develops, it continues to embrace new technology. Perhaps the most important type of technology to influence nursing practice in recent years is the **computer and information technology (IT)**. Consider the following examples:

- The NHS Executive's Information Management and Technology Strategies project that by the year 2000 all large hospitals and 90% of general practices will have IT systems. These systems will be networked (connected to one another) locally and nationally, and GPs will be linked to their local hospital. Family health services authorities and purchasers of local health services will be able to access data collected by these systems in order to estimate local health needs and to plan services (DOH, 1992b).

---

**Information Technology and Nursing**

**Useful Resources**

British Computer Society
Nursing Specialist Group
Doddinghurst Road
Doddinghurst
Essex CM15 0QP
0127 7824366

Strategic Advisory Group on Nursing Information Systems (SAGNIS)
NHSE
Nursing Division, Room 7E11
Quarry House
Quarry Hill
Leeds LS2 7UE
0532 546065

NHS Executive Information Management Group (IMG)/NHS Register of Computer Applications
IMG Information Point
c/o Anglia & Oxford Regional Health Authority
Union Lane
Cambridge CB4 1RF
0223-62274

- The Strategic Advisory Group on Nursing Information Systems (SAGNIS) is overseeing the Nursing Terms Project, which is developing a 'nursing thesaurus' in order to integrate nursing terminology uniformly into information systems throughout Europe (RCN, 1993).
- European Action — Information Requirements for Nursing Practice is a project led by the Danish Institute for Health and Nursing Research focussing on the information requirements for nursing practice and the European classification of nursing interventions and patient outcomes. The project is funded by Advanced Informatics in Medicine (AIM), a research and development programme of the Directorate General XIII (RCN, 1993).
- Increasingly, nursing care plans and patient records are becoming computerized (see Chapter 5). The single patient-based electronic record is a key element of the NHS Information Management and Technology strategy, and of Information Systems for Nurses, Midwives and Health Visitors, the strategic statement of the NHSE Information Management Group (DOH, 1992b).

With these and other developments occurring, it is clear that today's student nurses must become familiar with (and comfortable with) computer technology. Computers are changing the way in which health care is delivered and managed — a trend that will certainly affect the management and delivery of nursing care.

## SUMMARY

The National Health Service in the United Kingdom is undergoing significant changes. Change is due to government policy, the NHS reforms and health care provision shifting to the community. Therefore patterns and use of health care by patients/clients is changing. New emphases are emerging for primary health care. Health care consumers are demanding accessible high quality health promotion and health protection services. The increasing population of older adults in the United Kingdom requires solutions to improve the quality and availability of health care for this population segment.

Although today's health care delivery system is improved over previous systems, financing it has placed a burden on government resources. Technological advances have resulted in high quality specialized care, but specialization has led to fragmentation of care when care is not managed well. Additionally, health care services are still unevenly distributed.

Nurses are in a position to influence the future of health care. The traditional medical model for health care is not viewed as responsive to the holistic needs of patients/clients. Cost-effectiveness, expansion of nursing services, and quality improvement are just some examples of nursing activities that will help solve some of the issues within our health care system.

## CHAPTER 2 REVIEW

### Key Concepts

- Health care services are provided in a large number of settings, across all age groups, and for the chronically and acutely ill.
- Consumers are requesting more information, especially on services related to illness prevention and health promotion.
- Increased technology and new biomedical equipment increase the range of available treatments.
- A nation's economy directly affects the fiscal resources of the health care delivery system.
- Health promotion activities are designed to help people reduce the risk of illness, maintain maximal function, and promote lifestyle habits related to good health.
- Illness prevention activities are directed at helping the person and family reduce risk factors.
- Diagnosis and treatment activities are usually disease-specific, with the goal of curing the patient/client.
- Rehabilitation allows an individual to return to a level of normal or near-normal function after a physical or mental illness, injury, or chemical dependency.
- Primary health care (community-based) agencies focus on providing health care to people within their neighbourhoods.
- Crisis intervention centres provide emergency psychiatric treatment and counselling to patients/clients experiencing extreme stress or conflict.
- Mental health agencies provide inpatient and outpatient counselling services to patients/clients with behavioural or emotional illnesses.
- A hospice provides family-centred care to help patients/clients maintain satisfactory levels of comfort and lifestyles through the terminal phases of illness.
- Patients/clients may enter the health care system through referral and because of specific health needs.
- Nursing is able to reduce health care costs by implementing cost- containment measures such as primary care, and case management.

### CRITICAL THINKING EXERCISES

1. Discuss the advantages and disadvantages of market forces in the quality, delivery and accessibility of health care services.

2. Describe the community services available to a person who has schizophrenia and is living in the community. What are the advantages and disadvantages of care in the community for this person?

3. Consider Mr Matthews, a 68-year-old man who will have surgery to replace the joint in his hip. Afterwards, extensive therapy will be needed for him to again walk normally. Describe the type of health care services that will be available for Mr Matthews.

## Key Terms

## REFERENCES

Alzheimers Disease Society: *NHS psychogeriatric continuing care*, December, 1993.

Beveridge W: *Report on social insurance and allied services: Cmd 6404* (The Beveridge Report), London, 1992, HMSO.

Connah B, Peerson R: The NHS story. In National Association of Health Authorities and Trusts: *NHS Handbook*. London, 1991, HMSO.

Department of Health: *The mental health act,*. London, 1983, HMSO.

Department of Health: *Working for patients*, London, 1989a, HMSO.

Department of Health: *Caring for people,* London, 1989b, HMSO.

Department of Health: *National health service and community care act*, London, 1990, HMSO.

Department of Health: *The patient's charter*, London, 1992a, HMSO.

Department of Health: *The health of the nation*, London, 1992b, HMSO.

Department of Health: *Working in partnership: a collaborative approach to care*, London, 1994, HMSO.

Downie R, Fyfe C, Tannahill A: *Health promotion models and values*. Oxford, 1991, Oxford University Press.

Ebrahim S, Wallis C, Brittis S, et al: Long-term care for elderly people, *Quality in Health Care*, 2:198, 1993.

Godber G: *First report of a joint working party on the organisation of medical work in hospitals (The Cogwheel Report )*, London, 1967, HMSO.

Griffiths, Sir R: *NHS management inquiry report*, London 1983, Department of Health.

Gunter L M: Nomenclature: what is in the name "gerontic nursing"? *J Gerontol Nurs* 13:7, 1987 (editorial).

Ham C: *The new national health service*. Oxford, 1990, Radcliffe.

Holliday I: *The NHS transformed*. London, 1992, Baseline Books.

HMSO: *The health of the nation: a consultation document for health in England.* London, 1991, HMSO.

Laing W: *Financing long-term care*. London, 1993, Age Concern.

Maraldo PJ: The nursing solution, *Health Manage Q* 11(4):18, 1989.

National Audit Office: *National health service day hospitals for elderly people in England*. London, 1994, HMSO.

NHS Cymru Wales: *Caring for the future, 1992,* Cardiff, 1992, Central Office of Information, the Welsh Office.

NHS Executive: *IM&T infrastructure overview,* London, 1992, HMSO.

Northern Ireland Office: *A regional strategy for the Northern Ireland Health and Personal Social Services 1992–1997*, Belfast, 1991, Northern Ireland Office.

Pierog LJ: Case management: a product line, *Nurs Adm Q* 15(2):16, 1991.

Rickford F: Long-stay beds for elderly cut by 40%, *The Guardian*, 5th August, 1993.

Royal College of Nursing: *Euroforum,* no. 2, London, 1993, RCN.

Salmon B: *The senior nursing structure (The Salmon Report)*, London, 1966, HMSO.

Schroeder P: Directions and dilemmas in nursing quality assurance, *Nurs Clin North Am* 23(3):657, 1988.

Scottish Office: *Scotland's Health: a challenge to you*, Edinburgh, 1992, Scottish Office.

Seedhouse D: *Health: the foundations for achievement*, Chichester, 1986, John Wiley & Sons.

Seedhouse D, Cribb A: *Changing ideas in health care*, Chichester, 1989, John Wiley & Sons.

Tomlinson, B: *Report of the inquiry into London's health service: medical education and research*, London, 1992, HMSO.

Williams A D: Development and application of clinical indicators for nursing, *J Nurs Care Qual* 6(1):1, 1991

Zander K: Managed care within acute care settings: design and implementation via nursing care management, *Health Care Superv* 6(2):27, 1988.

## FURTHER READING

### Adult Nursing

Chaplin N: *Health care in the United Kingdom*, Brentford, Middlesex, 1982, Kluwer Medical.

Harrison S et al: *The dynamics of British health policy*, London, 1990, Unwin Hyman.

Townsend P, Davidson N, Whitehead M: *Inequalities in health: the Black report, the health divide*, London, 1988, Penguin Books.

Wertheimer A, editor: *A chance to speak out: consulting service users and carers about community care*, London, 1991, King's Fund Centre.

### Children's Nursing

Audit Commission: *Children first: a study of hospital services*, London, 1993, HMSO.

Department of Health: *Welfare of children and young people in hospital*, London, 1991, HMSO.

DOH: *An introduction to the children act*, London, HMSO, 1989.

Leenders, F: Children first, *Community Outlook*, July 90:4, 1990.

Report of the Committee on Child Health Services: *Fit for the future*, London, 1976, HMSO.

Richardson, J: Integrating services in community child care, *Nurs Standard* 3(8):32, 1993.

While A, Barriball L: School nursing: history, present practice and possibilities reviewed, *J Adv Nurs*, 18:1202, 1993.

### Learning Disabilities Nursing

Allen D et al, editors: *Meeting the challenge*, London, 1991, King's Fund Centre.

Emerson E et al, editors: *Evaluating the challenge: a guide to evaluating services for people with learning difficulties and challenging behaviour*, London, 1991, King's Fund Centre.

House of Commons: *National Health Service and Community Care Act 1990 Chapter 19*, London, 1990, HMSO.

Hubert J: *Home-bound—crisis in the care of young people with severe learning difficulties: a story of twenty families,* London, 1991, King's Fund Centre.

NHS Executive HSG: *Health services for people with learning disability (mental handicap),* London, 1992, DoH.

Sine SD (ed): *Towards integration: comprehensive services for people with mental handicaps,* London, 1988, Harper & Row.

Sines D: *Service provision: developments in the National Health Service,* In Thompson T & Mathias P: Standards and mental handicap: keys to competence, London, 1992, Bailliere Tindall.

Ward L, editor: *Getting better all the time? Issues and strategies for ensuring quality in community services for people with mental handicap,* London, 1987, King's Fund Centre.

Wertheimer A, editor: *Making it happen: employment opportunities for people with severe learning difficulties.* London, 1991, King's Fund Centre.

## Mental Health Nursing

Bean P, Mounser P: *Discharge from mental hospitals (Issues in mental health series),* London, 1993, Mind Publications in association with MacMillan Publishers.

Braisby D et al: *Changing futures: housing and support services for people discharged from psychiatric hospitals,* London, 1988, King's Fund Centre.

Brown H, Smith H , editors: *Normalisation—the reader for the 90s,* London, 1992, Tavistock/Routledge.

Butler T: *Changing mental health services: the politics and the policy,* London, 1993, Chapman & Hall.

McIver S: *Obtaining the views of users of mental health services,* London, 1991, King's Fund Centre.

Tomlinson, D: *Utopia, community care and the retreat from the asylums,* Milton Keynes, 1991, Oxford University Press.

Turner-Crowson J: *Reshaping mental health services: implications for Britain of US experience,* London, 1993, King's Fund Centre.

# The Process of Nursing

## CHAPTER OUTLINE

## LEARNING OUTCOMES

After studying this chapter, you should be able to:

■ *Define the key terms listed.*
■ *Describe the advantages and disadvantages of task allocation, team nursing, patient/client allocation, primary nursing, and the named nurse.*
■ *Describe and discuss the varying definitions of the nursing process.*
■ *Describe the relationship between the nursing process and models of care.*
■ *Differentiate between objective and subjective data.*
■ *State the possible sources of data for a nursing assessment.*
■ *Describe interpersonal skills involved in assessment and suggest how they might affect the assessment process.*
■ *List the components of a nursing care plan and describe its uses.*
■ *Describe the differences between care plans used in hospital and community health settings, and care plans used in different speciality areas.*
■ *Develop a care plan from a nursing assessment.*
■ *Discuss the process of priority setting.*

■ *Describe goal setting.*
■ *Discuss the process of selecting nursing interventions.*
■ *Define the implementation process.*
■ *Give examples of evaluation measures used to determine progress towards outcomes.*
■ *List the four steps involved in goal evaluation.*
■ *Describe the benefits of quality assurance programmes in a health care setting.*

Nursing practice in the UK has undergone a steady period of change and development since the 1960s. Chapter 1 describes the development of nursing as a profession, and the concepts, theories and models of nursing.

Alongside the development of nursing theory and the health care system the practice of nursing has developed. This development has been particularly marked during the past two decades. The nursing process has been implemented as the major framework for delivering care, and systems for the organization of nursing have changed and evolved.

In order to better understand the process of contemporary nursing and to place the nursing process into context, it is helpful to discuss the various systems of care delivery and how these have developed.

## THE DEVELOPMENT OF SYSTEMS FOR CARE DELIVERY

### Task Allocation

For many decades, nursing was organized within a system of 'caring by task'. One nurse performed the same task for each patient/client. For example, the same nurse would record the temperatures of all the patients/clients. The overall responsibility for care rested with the ward sister, who delegated the tasks to nurses with appropriate skills. Communication channels were hierarchical; the doctor spoke to the sister, who spoke to the staff nurse, who spoke to the nurse delivering care.

Junior nurses learned each task by constant repetition. Indeed, they often became quick and skillful. Unfortunately, this system of care did not always help the students to understand the consequences of their actions. Active thinking and questioning about the tasks had traditionally been discouraged.

The patients/clients were usually passive recipients of care. Their needs were often seen as interrupting the routine of work. Patient/client contact was fragmented, and this may have prevented the nurse and patient/client from developing an effective relationship. Menzies (1960) suggested that, by focusing their work on tasks rather than on patients/clients, nurses could protect themselves from the emotional burden which could result from developing a caring relationship.

This method of organizing care, though useful in areas where the workforce frequently changed, often resulted in care which was fragmented and offered little continuity (Proctor, 1989).

During the 1960s there were significant pressures on nursing and a growing dissatisfaction with task allocation. In 1972 the Briggs Committee documented nurses' frustration with this method. There began a growing trend to move towards more patient-orientated approaches to organizing nursing care. These included **team nursing, patient/client allocation** and, more recently, **primary nursing**.

### Team Nursing

Team nursing is a method of allocating a group of nurses to a group of patients/clients (Waters, 1985). Within teams, care could be task-centred, patient/client-centred, or a combination of both.

Team leaders are responsible to the charge nurse/sister or nurse manager for the care given. Channels of communication function through the team leader.

Team nursing varies in its effectiveness. The team can build relationships with patients/clients and continuity can be maintained if team members work closely together. Alternatively, the care can become disjointed, particularly if the team is disrupted or if the team leader is unable to give adequate support and supervision to team members (Roper *et al*, 1985).

### Patient/Client Allocation

Within this system an individual nurse takes responsibility, within his or her level of competence, for the care of an identified group of patients/clients. This responsibility may extend for a period of time or may change from day to day.

Patient/client allocation can facilitate the development of caring relationships between the patient/client and nurse. The system can work well in wards or specialized areas, such as Intensive Therapy Units, and may be combined with team nursing. It can also be a helpful introduction for students into planning and implementing care, although it is essential that a named, qualified nurse supervises students or nursing assistants delivering care.

Within this system care can become fragmented, particularly if allocations change on a day-to-day basis (Pearson, 1988). Communication channels can become complex if one nurse plans care while another implements it.

### Primary Nursing

A **primary nurse** is responsible for planning patient/client care and is accountable for that care 24 hours a day, seven days a week. This ensures both individualized care and continuity. The primary nurse is usually the main care giver, although there is some variation in this (Manthey, 1980). Due to the responsibility and accountability demanded by this autonomous method of nursing, only experienced qualified nursing staff should undertake this role (Manthey *et al*, 1970).

The supporting role is that of an **associate nurse**, who continues the care prescribed in the primary nurse's absence. Local protocols are usually established for this responsibility. In some cases, students may work as associate nurses.

There are many advantages for people being nursed within this system. Increased security and a satisfying relationship between patient/client and care giver are two examples. Communication channels are straightforward; the primary nurse liaises directly with the patient/client, family, doctors, ward sister, therapists, and other nurses.

The increased responsibility for care and improved job satisfaction are commonly cited advantages for staff undertaking the primary nurse role. However, the demands of caring so intensively can be stressful for the care giver, and a supportive, knowledgeable management structure is a prerequisite for primary nursing to succeed (Pearson, 1983).

### Named Nurse

In 1992, the Patient's Charter stated that each patient should have a **named nurse** responsible for his/her care. This is implemented in various settings through a named nurse or midwife, key worker, or case manager system (DOH, 1992).

## THE DEVELOPMENT OF THE NURSING PROCESS

The nursing process first came into nursing in the UK in the 1970s. At this time there was a feeling that a system was needed to unify the study of nursing with nursing practice, and to develop nursing as a *process* rather than a *series of actions.*

The nursing process was originally derived from business management systems as an organizational or problem-solving framework. It was first described in a nursing context in the early 1950s and was implemented into nursing in the US in the early 1960s.

In 1977 the General Nursing Council recommended that the nursing process be used in the UK in order to "provide a unifying thread for the study of patient care, and a helpful framework for nursing practice" (GNC, 1977). The nursing process was included in the syllabus for general nurse training.

The nursing process as used in the UK is not an exact copy of that used in the US. It was adapted to accommodate the nursing care setting of the UK. In the US, the literature described the process as a mechanism to achieve professional status and thus improve patient/client care. In the UK, it was seen initially in terms of improving the quality of care and enhancing nurses' job satisfaction (De La Cuesta, 1983).

By 1983 the process became embodied into a statute which required that first-level nursing practitioners be able to assess, plan, implement, and evaluate care (Rule 18 of the Nurses, Midwives and Health Visitors Act).

## THE STRUCTURE OF THE NURSING PROCESS

The nursing process is usually described as having four main components (Table 3-1):

* assessment
* planning
* implementation
* evaluation.

## Definitions of the Nursing Process

Since the nursing process first came to the United Kingdom, the ways in which it has been used, and thus defined, have evolved. In 1979, Kratz defined the nursing process as:

*Basically a problem-solving approach to nursing that involves interaction with the patient, making decisions, and carrying out nursing actions based on an assessment of an individual patient's situation.*

In 1988, Yura and Walsh gave a broader definition. They described the nursing process as:

*... the core and essence of nursing; it is central to all nursing actions; it is applicable in any setting and within any theoretical conceptual reference. It is flexible and adaptable, adjustable to a number of variables, yet sufficiently structured so as to provide a base from which all systematic nursing actions can proceed.*

In reviewing the literature, Walton (1986) suggests that there are four main ways in which the nursing process has been interpreted:

* as an ideology associated with professional aims, status, autonomy and aspirations for identity
* as a system of work organization, often equated with Primary Nursing, Team Nursing and Patient Allocation
* as a system of recording
* as a tool for education and practice, aimed at bringing ideals of individualized care closer to reality.

### TABLE 3-1 Summary of Nursing Process

| Component | Purpose | Steps |
|---|---|---|
| Assessment | To gather, verify, and communicate data about the patient/client so data base is established. To identify health care needs of the patient/client | 1. Collecting nursing health history<br>2. Assessing physical, psychological, social, and spiritual needs/desires<br>3. Assisting with physical examination<br>4. Collecting all relevant data |
| Planning | To identify the patient's/client's goals; to determine priorities of care, to determine expected outcomes, to design nursing strategies to achieve goals of care | 1. Identifying patient/client goals<br>2. Establishing expected outcomes<br>3. Selecting nursing actions<br>4. Delegating actions<br>5. Writing nursing care plan<br>6. Consulting |
| Implementation | To complete nursing actions necessary for accomplishing plan | 1. Reassessing patient/client<br>2. Reviewing and modifying existing care plan<br>3. Performing nursing actions |
| Evaluation | To determine the extent to which goals of care have been achieved | 1. Comparing patient/client response to criteria<br>2. Analysing reasons for results and conclusions<br>3. Modifying care plan |

In 1992, Marks-Maran suggested that some confusion had arisen because of the varying ways in which the nursing process has been viewed. Specifically, that there is often little distinction made between the process and the documentation used. Marks-Maran also suggested that the nursing process could be used as a vehicle for bringing into practice humanistic value systems, philosophies of care, models of nursing, quality assurance and the concept of caring (Marks-Maran, 1992).

## The Relationship of the Nursing Process to Nursing Models

The nursing process can be viewed as a delivery system for the concepts, values and models of nursing (see Chapter 1 for an explanation of models of nursing).

Walsh (1989) suggests that:

*A model tells us what the nursing care should be like, the nursing process describes how it should be organized.*

Roper *et al* (1985) describe the use of process with their model of nursing and emphasize that the model is the framework of concepts and thus provides guidelines for using the process of nursing.

When implementing the **Roper *et al* Model of Living**, the nursing process would focus on the following aspects:

- **Assessing** – helps to establish previous routines, levels of independence, and problems, both actual and potential, related to each activity of living. (The model emphasizes partnership with the patient/client and mutual assessment of an individual activity of daily living.)
- **Planning** – sets goals related to the place of the patient/client on the dependence-independence continuum in any one activity of living and identifies movement to be made.
- **Implementing** – aims to promote the patient's/client's normality and independence in activities of living or to re-educate. The role of the nurse is described in terms of preventing, solving, alleviating, and coping activities.

- **Evaluating** – determines the extent to which the goals have been achieved in the movement of the activity of living towards independence. Evaluating is also a stepping stone for **reassessment**, re-examination, and modification of problem statements, goals, goal dates and care given.

Thus, the activities of living are used as the criteria for which assessment data are collected. Goals for care and expected outcomes are prioritized. Nursing intervention is planned and a day-to-day record kept. Outcomes are evaluated and problems reassessed with the patient/client.

Using **Henderson's Model of Nursing** (1966) the focus of the stages of the nursing process would be different:

- **Assessing** – helps to establish which of the 14 basic needs (see Chapter 7) the patient/client requires assistance with and what has caused the lack of independence in the fulfilment of these needs.
- **Planning** – negotiates patient/client-centred goals to help individuals meet their basic needs, return to independence, or to die a peaceful death.
- **Implementing** – aims to help patients/clients meet their 14 basic needs, to perform activities to maintain health, to recover from illness, or to aid in a peaceful death.
- **Evaluating** – determines the degree to which the patient/client is able to meet fundamental needs without nursing assistance and the extent to which the model has been successful in directing nursing intervention.

Thus, the fundamental needs are used as the basic components on which assessment data are collected and care is planned. Henderson emphasizes the involvement of family members and the role of the health care team in planning. Nursing intervention addresses the relationship between nurse and patient/client in implementing measures to meet the patient's/client's needs. Evaluation provides data about the patient's/client's functional abilities pre- and post-nursing care, and the person's response to that care.

**Information Sources**

**Information from patient**
Verbal history
Visible signs
Observable behaviour

**Other professionals**
Community staff
District nurse
Health visitor
Community
psychiatric nurse
G.P.
Physiotherapist
Social worker

**DATA**

**Additional information**

from family/significant
other friends and
acquaintances,
employer, neighbours,
colleagues, home help

**Other documents as
information sources**
Previous medical records
Letter of referral/discharge summaries
Pathology reports
X-ray reports, scans, etc.
Patient symptom diaries
School or employer's letters

**Fig 3-1** Possible sources of patient/client information (data).

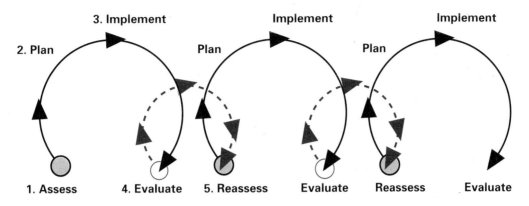

**Fig 3-2** The dynamic, continuous nature of the nursing process.

## THE NURSING PROCESS IN PRACTICE

The nursing process can be used in all care delivery settings. It can be used flexibly to facilitate creative nursing practice.

The importance of the patient/client as an individual is paramount. Each individual has his or her own particular needs and problems to be discovered and incorporated into the delivery of nursing care. The care offered should be **holistic**; that is, encompassing the whole person including the physical, psychological, social and spiritual aspects of their beings.

In practice, the purposes of the nursing process are:
- to help the nurse identify the patient's/client's health care needs from a holistic perspective
- to determine priorities of care by setting goals or expected outcomes
- to establish a nursing care plan to meet those needs
- to evaluate the effectiveness of nursing care in achieving the stated goals.

Throughout the process, the nurse collects and analyses data from a variety of sources (Fig. 3-1). Using this information the nurse, in association with the patient/client, identifies actual and potential health care needs and problems, and determines priorities of care by setting goals.

The nurse then develops and implements an individualized care plan and evaluates the patient's/client's responses to the plans, determining whether or not the goals have been achieved. If the goals have not been met, the nurse modifies the original plan of care. Evaluation and modification continue the creativity of this process.

It is essential that the patient/client is consulted throughout the process whenever possible. This dynamic process can develop and change in response to alterations in the patient's/client's condition. In this way, the cycle of care is continuous (Fig. 3-2).

### Documenting the Nursing Process

Each health care setting and each professional group will have documents which have been adapted to their own and their patient's/client's needs. The documents may also reflect the underlying philosophy or model of the area.

**Nursing documentation** is used not only to record the care of a particular person, but also to communicate between members of the care team. It is essential that documentation is legible, accurate and factual. In some cases documents may be used in a court of law and their importance cannot be overemphasized. When care is prescribed, it is necessary for the order to be signed by a qualified nurse.

Student nurses writing in nursing documentation are usually required to obtain counter-signatures from the trained nurse supervising them (for more detail about nursing documentation, see Chapter 5).

## NURSING ASSESSMENT

Yura and Walsh (1988) describe assessment as:

*... the act of reviewing a human situation from a data base in order to affirm the wellness state and diagnose potential client problems; to affirm an illness state diagnosing the client's particular problems; determining the potential for problems and identifying the wellness aspects of the ill client.*

**Assessment** is the process of gathering information about a patient/client. It consists of a variety of activities which are carried out simultaneously.

Assessment can also take place during the course of other activities. For example, when discussing with an individual how he or she is feeling, the nurse can simultaneously assess posture, breathing, mood and skin colour (see Chapter 4).

Assessment is not a once-only activity, but needs to be repeated frequently as the patient's/client's condition changes. Every interaction with an individual can offer valuable information on the person's changing health status or the effectiveness of the nursing care.

Information can be gathered from a variety of sources and is often referred to as **data** (see Fig. 3-1). The types of data collected vary according to the purpose of the assessment. For example, data gathered on admission will differ from that required when mobility is being considered, and it will differ again if discharge is being contemplated.

The consideration and interpretation of the data collected will enable the nurse to identify any problems, actual or potential, and to plan appropriate care in conjunction with the patient/client.

**TABLE 3-2 Assessment of Functional Health Patterns**

| | |
|---|---|
| 1. Health perception/health management | Assessment of general health, ways patients/clients keep healthy, past experience of treatments, hospital, fears/worries, current perception of health, smoking/drinking habits. |
| 2. Nutrition | Daily food and fluid intake. Likes and dislikes. Appetite, weight, dental history. |
| 3. Elimination | Bowel and urinary elimination pattern. Any excess sweating. |
| 4. Activity and exercise | Perception of energy, ability and desire to exercise – type and frequency, leisure activities/play activities. Perceived ability for: (code level – see Functional Level Code below) feeding, dressing, home maintenance, bathing, grooming, toileting, mobility, bed mobility, cooking. Functional Level Code: Level 0: Full self-care Level I: Requires use of equipment or device Level II: Requires assistance/supervision from another person Level III: Requires assistance/supervision from another person; requires equipment or advice Level IV: is dependent and does not participate |
| 5. Sleep and rest | Sleep and rest pattern, effects of sleep, factors influencing rest and sleep. |
| 6. Cognitive - perceptual ability | Hearing, sight, change in memory. Learning ability, whether information is needed. Pain, discomfort, site/nature of pain, frequency, what helps. |
| 7. Self-perception | Self-image, self-esteem in relation to health state, what may be causing anger, fear, anxiety. |
| 8. Roles and relationships | Home situation which may influence health. Next of kin, partner, sources of support. People who need contacting able to visit. Family commitments and dependants. |
| 9. Sexuality and reproduction | Sexual needs, changes relating to health state and effects on partner. Females - menstrual cycles. Contraceptive requirements. Questions, anxieties, fears about sexuality relating to health care and current health state. |
| 10. Coping - stress - tolerance pattern | Effects of life events in recent past. Coping abilities - what helps when anxieties arise. What and who is helping in this situation. |
| 11. Values and beliefs | Spiritual needs, religious persuasion and practices. Cultural factors and their current influence. |
| 12. Other | Any other factors or issues relevant to the individual. |

Adapted from: Gordon M: *Manual of nursing diagnosis* 1993-1994, St Louis, 1993, Mosby.

In 1982, Marjory Gordon introduced a typology (analysis based on types) of functional health patterns (see Table 3-2). This framework is not conceptually linked to one nursing theoretical model. Thus, it is adaptable to all models (Gordon, 1994). The **functional health pattern model** can be used with individuals, families, or communities, and it evolves from the relationship between the patient/client and the environment.

For each of the 11 patterns, the nurse assesses patients/clients by organizing patterns of behaviour and physiological responses that pertain to a functional health category. The nurse then compares assessment data with the patient's/client's baseline (for example, usual blood pressure, weight, and nutritional intake); with

established norms based on age, gender, height, and weight; and with cultural, social, or other norms, such as religious practices, ethnic dietary guidelines, and health care practices (Gordon, 1994).

The assessment of each of the 11 patterns represents the interaction of the patient/client and the environment, which Gordon calls 'biopsychosocial integration'. No one health pattern can be understood without knowledge of the other patterns (Gordon, 1994). Description and evaluation of health patterns assist the nurse in identifying functional patterns (patient/client strengths) and dysfunctional patterns, which assist in developing the nursing care plan (Gordon, 1994). For example, the sleep-rest pattern focuses the nursing assessment on the patterns of sleep,

### Learning Disabilities Nursing
### Assessing people with learning disabilities

Many of the problems and behaviours exhibited by people with learning disabilities are situation-specific; therefore, when assessing these patients/clients, it is important to involve everyone who can usefully contribute to the process. It is also important to remember that a person admitted to an assessment unit for a behavioural assessment will not necessarily behave in the same way he or she behaved at home. For this reason, all staff should reserve their opinions and judgements until the patient/client adapts to the assessment unit. Ideally, assessment should be performed in the place where the problems arise.

Assessment of self-help skills is an essential and valuable component of an assessment. However, the patient's/client's carer(s) may not have given him or her the opportunity to develop such skills. Giving the person a chance to rehearse a self-help activity, therefore, may reveal that the person is more able to perform the skills than is apparent initially.

The language used in the assessment process should be simple and straightforward. It is important to ensure that the patient/client understands what he or she is being asked to do. If English is not the patient's/client's first language, then arrange for a translator. Also take into account sensory impairments, such as hearing or sight disorders. Ensure the assessment is conducted in a 'natural' setting; for example, conduct a dressing assessment when the patient/client is getting dressed — not in an artificially contrived test situation where the patient/client may be anxious about failure.

Ideally, physical assessment should be a continuous process, and staff should be skilled in recognizing and understanding the importance of small changes in the patient's/client's physical condition. Changes in appetite and sleep patterns, skin condition, and bladder and bowel habit, for example, can indicate the onset of a physical disorder that requires intervention.

rest, and relaxation. It includes patterns of sleep and rest-relaxation periods during the 24-hour day, as well as the individual's perception of the quality and quantity of sleep and rest, and perception of energy level. Also included are aids to sleep (for example, medications, meditation, night-time routines) (Gordon, 1994). For example, the assessment of Mr Roberts' sleep-rest pattern reveals that he has difficulty falling and remaining asleep. He describes the quality of his sleep as "poor" and states that he averages about '3 hours of sleep per night'. He reports that, at times, he feels he is awake throughout the whole night. Further assessment reveals that the patient/client uses over-the-counter sleeping aids, drinks caffeinated beverages, exercises vigorously, and snacks heavily before retiring. The assessment data support a dysfunctional sleep-rest pattern, that results in identification of the problem of sleep disturbance.

## Data Collecting

Data collected during assessment should be descriptive, concise, and complete, and should not include interpretative statements. The patient's/client's perception of a symptom, the perceptions and observations of the family, or the observation of a member of the health care team, may all contribute to descriptive data. For example, a patient/client may describe his pain as, 'a sharp, throbbing pain in the abdomen.' The nurse's observation would be, 'The patient lies on his side holding the right side of his abdomen. Facial grimacing was present throughout the assessment.' The nurse has recorded only her observations. If the nurse had said 'the patient tolerates pain poorly,' this would be her interpretation or opinion and it is inappropriate to record these in a nursing assessment.

Frequently, using the patient's own words can be helpful. Use of correct medical terms can help summarize information, for example, 'Patient described a constant, sharp, throbbing pain in the upper right quadrant of the abdomen. Pain began 48 hours before admission, 2 hours after a high-fat meal. Pain was not relieved by antacids.' In order to confirm that all the relevant data have been collected the nurse should consider, "Do I have the information to answer the questions, 'When?' and 'Where?'", and 'What is the duration and influencing factors?'

Collecting inaccurate, incomplete, or inappropriate data can lead to the incorrect identification of the patient's/client's needs. Inaccurate and incomplete data result if the nurse fails to collect all the data relevant to a specific area, or if the nurse is disorganized, unskilled, jumps to conclusions or makes unsupported assumptions.

## Types of Data

During assessment, the nurse obtains two types of data, subjective and objective. Subjective data is the patient's/client's perception about his or her health problem, for example, the presence of pain is a subjective finding. Only the patient/client can provide information about its frequency, location, and intensity. Subjective data usually include feelings of anxiety, physical discomfort or mental stress. Although only the patient/client can provide the subjective data relevant to these feelings, the nurse must be aware that these problems can result in physiological changes, which can be measured. For example, a patient/client may say that he feels anxious (subjective feeling), and the nurse may observe that he has facial flushing and an elevated pulse rate (objective observation and measurement).

Objective data are observations or measurements made by the data collector. The measurement of objective data is based on an accepted standard, such as centigrade scale, or some other unit of measurement. Within the changing health care market, there is an increasing need for nurses and other care providers to be able to evaluate the effectiveness, or outcomes, of their work. This has led to increased use of scales, profiles, indicators and other tools which can assist nurses to offer more objective measurements of the effectiveness of their work.

For example, Linear Analogue Self-Assessment Scales (LASA Scales) can be completed by patients/clients to measure the effects of a disease (such as pain; these are called pain scales or pain thermometers), the side-effects of treatment (such as nausea), psychological responses (such as anxiety) or abilities to perform daily activities (such as to make a cup of tea). Taken over the course of time, these scales can provide a more objective measurement of change than subjective assessments by a health care worker.

## Sources of Data
### PATIENT/CLIENT
In most situations the patient/client is the best source of information. By assessing and observing the physical status of the person, the nurse gains valuable **baseline data**. In conversation, the patient/client who is mentally orientated and able to answer questions appropriately can provide the most relevant and accurate information about his or her own health, lifestyle, previous medical history, and changes in activities of living. Even patients/clients who appear to be disorientated can offer the nurse valuable and relevant information towards the overall assessment.

### FAMILY
Family members, and sometimes friends and neighbours, can be interviewed as the primary sources of information for those patients/clients unable to speak for themselves. In emergency situations, families may be the only source of information about

the onset of the illness, past medical history, current medication, allergies, and other useful information of help to the health care team.

### HEALTH CARE TEAM MEMBERS
The team consists of medical staff, nurses, physiotherapists, dietitians, speech therapists, occupational therapists, social workers, and many other professional and nonprofessional workers. It is important that the nurse remembers that these individuals may have additional information about the patient/client that he or she is currently assessing, and that they will need access to the documents that he or she is preparing. Maintaining effective communication within the team makes a positive contribution towards patient/client care.

### MEDICAL RECORDS
The present and past medical records of the patient/client can be a useful source of information about past illness, treatment, and the individual response of the patient/client to these experiences.

### OTHER RECORDS
Other records, such as educational or employment records, may contain pertinent health data. Community, day-care or clinic records can also be of value. It may be necessary to obtain the patient's/client's permission in order to obtain these records.

### CONFIDENTIALITY
All patient information is potentially sensitive, and confidentiality must be maintained at all times. It is worth noting that if any information is stored on a computer, the Data Protection Act may apply. Patients/clients have limited access to their medical records granted under the Access to Health Records (see Chapter 13).

### LITERATURE REVIEW
Reviewing the medical and nursing literature about an illness and it's treatment will help you to complete the data base. The review will increase your knowledge and help you to understand the cause of the symptoms, and the relevance of the treatment.

## Communicating
Only a skilled communicator will be able to assess a patient/client adequately. Students will develop communication skills if allowed to observe their senior colleagues communicating with patients/clients. It is essential for the student to practice his or her skills under the supervision of a senior colleague. The main communication skills and techniques used in assessing are listed here; these are offered as an *aide-mémoire* rather than a comprehensive list (see Chapter 15 for full explanations):

- nonverbal communication
- use of questions
- use of language
- listening
- silence
- encouraging the person to continue talking

**Mental Health Nursing**
**Issues in mental health assessment**

Intra- and interpersonal skills lie at the heart of mental health nursing assessment. Nurses must be aware of their own values, beliefs, and biases in relation to people with mental health needs and/or mental illnesses. As professional carers, nurses can make decisions about people's lives which may have profound implications. Thus, nurses must be acutely aware of their impact on patients/clients and should realize their understanding of another individual can only be partial at best.

Increasingly, nursing assessment in mental health nursing is underpinned by nursing models. For example, if the philosophy of care is derived from Peplau and a psychodynamic basis, then the nursing assessment will focus on the discovery of met and unmet needs. The nurse-patient/client relationship will be expected to develop through phases of orientation and identification during the nursing assessment.

In mental health care, the issue of patient/client safety is of paramount importance. The nursing assessment must satisfy nurses that the patient's/client's safety is not compromised in any way. Where the patient/client is not in the position to make decisions about his or her safety, nurses must take steps to assess the individual's safety needs, so that appropriate steps can be taken to safeguard his or her well-being.

• paraphrasing
• clarifying
• information giving
• summarizing.

## Assessment Interview

Ideally, the first assessment interview should be conducted as soon as possible after the patient's/client's admission. The patient's/client's condition and need for immediate treatment will often delay this first assessment. As observation is an important assessment skill, data can be gathered while helping the patient/client undress, or get comfortable in bed. For example, any changes in the skin's physical appearance, the presence of scars, bruising, or swelling can be noted while assisting the admitting doctor.

## Purpose

Patterns of health and illness are identified by collecting data about the physical, developmental, intellectual, emotional, social and spiritual dimensions (Fig. 3-3). A clear understanding of exactly what data is required and why it is being gathered will help you plan and conduct the interview.

### Adult Nursing
### Assessing mental health needs in older age

### What is 'normal'?

Making sense of what is called 'normality' and what is happening now in older age is dependent upon understanding the balance between a number of factors that may also be superimposed on pre-existing conditions. These factors include the following:
• physical state in relation to illness and disease
• mental state
• behaviour
• social factors
• biographical factors
• professional perspectives, expectations and viewpoints

A number of mental health assessment tools have also been developed. The following is a simplified guide to areas that need to be considered and included as part of the nursing contribution to assessment:
• physical state in relation to health and disease
• illness and disease
• vision and hearing
• side-effects from drugs and/or medication
• sudden change in environment
• changes to self care and independent living
• health threats to long established routine
• health belief models and how much in control a person feels.

From Royal College of Nursing: *Assessing mental health needs in old age*, London, 1993, RCN. Used with permission.

## Self-awareness

Be aware of the influences of secondary socialization, because you will have taken on the norms and values common to other nurses (see Chapter 12). It is necessary for any health professional to consider his or her own values, attitudes, and beliefs, to facilitate effective decision making, and contribute to his or her self-knowledge (Steele and Harmon, 1983). Displaying any form of discrimination or prejudice is unacceptable in dealing with patients/clients.

Contrary to commonly held opinion, nurses do not always consider the rights and fears of their patients/clients, even to the extent of 'labelling' some as 'difficult' or 'unpopular' (Stockwell, 1972).

## Conducting an Interview

There are some general guidelines that are appropriate for all interviews:
•   the nurse must remember that his or her interviewee is unwell, is possibly anxious, and may be in pain.
•   timing is important; ensure the patient/client is as comfortable as his or her condition allows. Several short interviews with breaks may suit the person better than trying to get everything finished in one go..The information gained in this way will probably be more comprehensive.
•   most nursing interviews will involve discussion of personal or intimate information; try to provide privacy if possible.
•   good manners dictate that you should introduce yourself.
•   as soon as is practical, tell the patient/client what you hope to achieve by this meeting, and how long you expect it to take.
•   guidelines for effective interviews have been described in Argyle (1978). At the very least, the nurse and patient/client should be at the same eye level and easily able to achieve eye contact when desired.

### Children's Nursing
### Techniques for assessing children

Assessing a child's response to illness and hospitalization is very complex and is a priority to any intervention of care. Assessment needs to be dynamic and flexible, and should include areas such as physical, social, emotional and spiritual development; nutritional status; peer and sibling relationships; and speech and language development.

When assessing children, do not 'talk at' them with a battery of questions, rather, talk 'with' them to gain constructive information. Remember also to assess each child as an individual.

It is also important to assess parent's responses to their child's illness and coping strategies parents have developed. Observe nonverbal cues and ask questions, such as, "Does it worry you when Sarah cries?" to yield more valuable information than just noting that Sarah cries. Also assess how much parents would like to be involved in their child's care in hospital and plan the care accordingly.

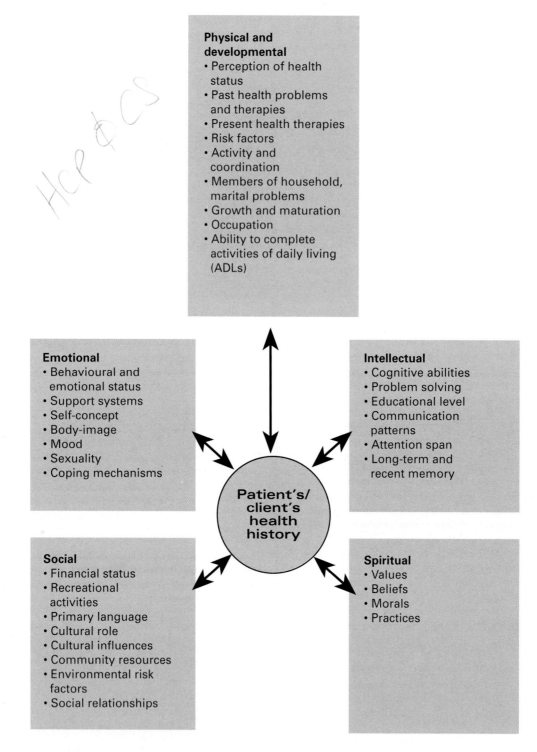

**Physical and developmental**
• Perception of health status
• Past health problems and therapies
• Present health therapies
• Risk factors
• Activity and coordination
• Members of household, marital problems
• Growth and maturation
• Occupation
• Ability to complete activities of daily living (ADLs)

**Emotional**
• Behavioural and emotional status
• Support systems
• Self-concept
• Body-image
• Mood
• Sexuality
• Coping mechanisms

**Intellectual**
• Cognitive abilities
• Problem solving
• Educational level
• Communication patterns
• Attention span
• Long-term and recent memory

**Patient's/client's health history**

**Social**
• Financial status
• Recreational activities
• Primary language
• Cultural role
• Cultural influences
• Community resources
• Environmental risk factors
• Social relationships

**Spiritual**
• Values
• Beliefs
• Morals
• Practices

**Fig 3-3** Dimensions for gathering data for health history.

## Data Collected During an Assessment
### BIOGRAPHICAL DATA

It is important to check the accuracy of the patient's/client's current address and telephone number (see Fig. 3-4). Verify the spelling of names, and ensure that you have the forename and surname in the correct order. This is not always as easy as it sounds! In these days of rapid discharge from the hospital it is also extremely important to have the right 'significant other'

named, with both and day and night telephone numbers where possible. In addition, it is important to be able to contact family members at any time, especially if the patient's/client's condition deteriorates rapidly.

Unexpected deteriorations and deaths are difficult for everyone, but if the person's family or partner cannot be contacted it can add to the emotional distress experienced by the loved ones.

## PATIENT'S DETAILS

**Surname** BROWNE **Title** Mrs

**Other names** ELIZABETH **Age** 84 yrs

**Date of birth** 12/2/10

**Address** 117 The Cottages, South Norwood. SE25 6SH.

**Telephone number** 0181-689-2627

**Religion** Church of England

**Religious/Cultural needs**
Regular attendee of Sunday services

**Present/Previous occupation**
Housewife and retired Schoolteacher.

**Effect of illness on occupation**
Unable to cook, shop, or do housework.

**Hobbies/Interests**
Member of Townswomen's Guild - enjoys needlepoint and reading fiction.

**Person to be contacted**
John Browne, RAF, Wildenrath, Germany.

**Relationship** Son

**Inform at night** Neighbour Mr Hatch

**Address** 115 The Cottages, South Norwood. SE25 6SH.

**Telephone number(s)** 0181-689 2243

## MEDICAL DETAILS

**Provisional diagnosis** Chest infection

**Actual diagnosis**

**Operation(s)** None

**Allergies** None known

**Relevant medical history and drug therapy**
Arthritis for last 20 yrs, takes aspirin/codeine for pain. Never been in hospital before.

**Patient's reason for admission**
Chest infection

**Patient's understanding of illness and treatment**
"Admitted as I can't cope whilst my breathing is so bad."

**Family's understanding of illness/treatment**
Alone on admission

## ADMISSION/DISCHARGE DETAILS

**Hospital number** 100123

**Date(s) of admission** 12/12/94 09.30 hrs

**CARE AT HOME**

**Housing conditions**
2 bedroom terraced cottage - own property

**Community services received** None

**Social problems due to admission of illness**
Worried about cat 'Smokey' (who is with neighbour going on holiday tomorrow).

**DISCHARGE PLANNING**

**Predicted date of discharge**

**Money with administrator**

**Outpatient appointment(s)**

**Community services requested**

| Name | Age | Religion | Consultant | C.R. no. |
|---|---|---|---|---|
| Elizabeth Browne | 84 yrs | C/E | Dr James | 100123 |

Fig 3-4  Assessment sheet with biographical detail.

## PAST HEALTH HISTORY

There is sometimes an obvious link between the patient's/client's past and present illness; for example, a past myocardial infarction, and a current congestive cardiac failure. Even if the relevance of past health history is not immediately apparent, encouraging the patient/client to talk about his or her health can consolidate the nurse-patient/client relationship.

## PRESENT ILLNESS

The effects of the current illness on the patient/client, his or her daily life, and his or her family should be systematically recorded (see Chapter 5).

## RELEVANT SOCIAL HISTORY

The type of home and support available to the patient/client may influence not only the course of his or her illness, but also how easily he or she can be rehabilitated. For example, living on a fixed, inadequate income may contribute to insufficient heating and a diet lacking in essential nutrients. A fourth storey bedsit may no longer be a viable home for a person with residual paralysis after a cerebral-vascular accident. All this information will enable other members of the multidisciplinary team to plan the best possible discharge for each patient/client.

The patient's/client's family is obviously also important for several reasons. The medical history of family members may be relevant to the patient's/client's illness, because some conditions, such as diabetes mellitus and hypertension, are familial.

A supportive and caring family is of value to the individual at all stages of an illness. For some people, friends or neighbours provide the emotional and practical help needed, and may have a closer relationship to the patient/client than his or her immediate family.

## HEALTH BEHAVIOURS

Any behaviours which are likely to influence the individual's health, either negatively or positively, are worth noting. Regular exercise, a low fat diet, a moderate alcohol intake with the avoidance of tobacco and other drugs, are all positive health-promoting behaviours. Alcohol in large amounts, and a lack of exercise, combined with a high fat diet, smoking or drug use, are behaviours which are likely to have adverse health effects.

## EMPLOYMENT HISTORY

The individual's employment history may indicate exposure to dangerous substances, such as coal dust or asbestos, or to a stressful working environment. Any job which constantly demands the meeting of unrealistic deadlines, taking work home, and missing time off should be regarded as a potential health risk.

## PHYSICAL FUNCTION

The nurse is required to assess each system of the body, noting any variation from the patient's/client's usual performance.

Any artificial aid in use should also be noted, for example, spectacles, contact lenses, hearing aids and walking aids. Careful observation of the patient/client, and painstaking attention to accuracy in recording all data obtained will yield the information needed to identify the individual's problems. Working with the patient/client, the nurse will then plan how these problems can be resolved.

## Assessment Conclusions

The end stage of assessment results in a conclusion about problems or needs, and is derived from a comparison between the patient's/client's normal functioning and changes brought about by present health status and needs. This is usually in the form of a problem or needs statement which facilitates the setting of goals for care. A problem statement should have three elements:

- What the problem is.
- What it is caused by.
- How it affects the patient/client.

## NURSING CARE PLANS

One product of the assessment component is the nursing care plan, which is based on assessment data and the patient's/client's identified problems or needs.

### Nursing Diagnosis

In the US the second major component of the nursing process is **Nursing Diagnosis**. A nursing diagnosis describes the patient's/client's actual or potential response to a health problem. In the US the North American Nursing Diagnosis Association (NANDA) meets to develop, refine and promote a taxonomy of nursing diagnostic terminology for use by professional nurses. Lists of NANDA-approved diagnoses are common in US nursing textbooks.

The potential use of nursing diagnosis in the UK has been debated in UK nursing literature (Mason and Webb, 1993) but nursing diagnosis has not been widely adopted outside the US. Various reasons have been proposed for this. Mason and Webb suggest that the role of the nurse as a diagnostician has been a contentious issue and hence the term diagnosis may be problematic. Other writers suggest that most nurses do, in fact, 'diagnose' people's nursing needs, but that they use different terminology. For example, the nursing diagnosis could be the conclusions drawn from assessment information.

There are both advantages and disadvantages to adopting nursing diagnoses in the UK. For example, diagnoses may assist in providing frames of reference for reasoning and decision-making skills, but wholesale adoption of the American system might create hostility (Webb, 1992).

Whatever terminology is used, the conclusion that nurses and patients/clients reach about problems, care needs and common goals are a vital part of the process of nursing, if values about partnerships in decision making are to be made a reality (Marks-Maran, 1992).

## Purpose of Care Plans

The **nursing care plan** is a written guideline for patient/client care. The purpose of written care plans is to:

- document the patient's/client's health care needs
- determine, by assessment, the patient's/client's problem, and the priorities and goals formulated during planning
- coordinate nursing care
- promote continuity of care
- list goals to be used in the evaluation of nursing care
- communicate pertinent assessment data, a list of problems, and therapies to other nurses and health care professionals
- decrease the risk of incomplete, incorrect, or inaccurate care

The advantages of care plans include:

- coordinated nursing care, specialty consultations, and scheduling of diagnostic tests so that nursing actions to be delivered can be quickly identified. In hospitals, and outpatient and community-based settings, the patient/client often receives care from more than one nurse, doctor, allied health professional, and health worker.
- coordinated resources used to deliver nursing care. If all equipment and supplies are included in the care plan, the nurse's time is used more effectively in providing care as opposed to locating supplies.
- enhanced continuity of nursing care by listing specific nursing actions necessary to achieve the goals of care. These nursing activities can be carried out throughout the day and from day to day. A correctly formulated nursing care plan facilitates the continuity of care from one nurse to another. As a result, all nurses have the opportunity to deliver the same quality of care.
- organized information exchanged by nurses in change-of-shift reports. Nurses focus these reports on nursing care and treatments delineated in care plans. At the end of shifts, nurses discuss care plans with the next care givers. Thus, all nurses are able to discuss current and pertinent information about the patient's/client's care plan.
- planned discharged needs of the patient/client. Incorporating the goals of the care plan into discharge planning is particularly important for a patient/client who will be undergoing long-term rehabilitation in the community. The adaptation of the care plan enhances the continuity of nursing care between nurses in the hospital and community.

Day-case surgery and earlier discharges from hospitals require the nurse to plan discharge needs on the care plan the moment the patient/client enters a health care setting. Mortensen and McMullin (1986) note that incomplete assessments and the absence of measurable outcome criteria extend patient/client stays in short-term, one-day surgical centres. Patient/client stays were lengthened because there were no documented, measurable criteria for discharge readiness on the postoperative nursing care plan, resulting in confusion among all the health care professionals as to when the patient/client could safely be discharged from the setting.

## Involving the Patient's/Client's Family

When developing an individualized care plan, the nurse involves the family and patient/client. The family can help the individual meet health goals. In addition, meeting some of the *family's* needs can improve the patient's/client's level of wellness.

A complete care plan is the blueprint for nursing action. It provides direction for implementation of the plan and a framework for evaluation of the patient's/client's response to nursing actions.

## Care Plans in Various Settings

The structure of the nursing care plan varies from one health care setting to another. For example, a care plan used in a hospital is different from one used in a community health setting. The nursing care plan developed for the patient/client returning home may focus on long-term health needs. In addition, the patient/client and family may assume more responsibility for care because the individual is receiving nursing care in the home. Although the structure of the care plan varies depending on the setting, its overall purpose is to provide a written guideline for care so that the health care needs of the patient/client and subsequent therapies are communicated among the health care team. Figures 3-5–3-9 illustrate care plans that have been adapted for different areas of care – an adult in the community, a child in hospital, an adult with mental health needs, and an adult with a learning disability, and an adult in hospital. Different models have been used in structuring the care provision required.

## Institutional Care Plans

Hospital care plans are concise documents that become part of the patient's/client's records. Traditionally, many hospitals used the 'Kardex' system. Kardex is a trade name for a card-filing system that allows quick reference to the particular needs of the patient/client for certain aspects of nursing care. Information about medications, activity levels, level of self-care, diet, treatments, and care is usually included in this system. Each institution has its own format for **nursing documentation**, but the basic information contained in it is universal. The care plan section of the nursing documentation also has variations. For example, one institution might use a three-column nursing care plan, which includes the problem, goal, and nursing action. Another institution may incorporate a four-column nursing care plan, which includes the nursing problem, goal, nursing action, and evaluation. Many nursing units are developing documentation reflecting particular nursing models. (For details on the legal, professional and accountability issues of care plan writing, see Chapter 5.)

## CORE CARE PLANS

The need to efficiently organize the nurse's time has resulted in **core care plans**, some of which are preprinted (see Chapter 29 for an example of a care plan). Formats are created for a specific clinical area (for example, coronary care, abdominal surgery, postpartum, and day-case surgery units). Each care plan lists patient/client problems, goals, and interventions.

After completing a nursing assessment, the nurse will

**The City and Hackney Authority**
**Community Nursing Division**

**TO BE RETAINED IN PATIENT'S HOME AND COMPLETED AT EACH VISIT**
Date commenced 6/12/94

Name    Hilda Flood

Address    16 Normanton Road

Tel No.    0171 - 634349

Religion    R/C                    Date of birth    15/2/1934

Person to be contacted    Mr John Flood

Relationship    Husband

Address    As above

Tel No.    As above

District Nurse    Sister James

GP    Dr. Gordon                    Tel No.    0171 - 342894

Nursing base    Stepney Health Centre

Social Worker    —

| Services | Sun | Mon | Tue | Wed | Thrs | Fri | Sat |
|---|---|---|---|---|---|---|---|
| Home Help | | | | | | | |
| Meals on Wheels | | | | | | | |
| Laundry a) House-bound b) Incontinent | | | | | | | |
| Day Centre | | | | | | | |
| Day Hospital | | | | | | | |
| Twilight Service | | | | | | | |
| Chiropody | | | | ✓ | | | |
| Others | | | | | | | |

Date completed 6/12/94

| Date | No. | Nursing Action | Signture |
|---|---|---|---|
| 6/12/94 | 1 | Clean and redress leg ulcer - ulcer clean. granulating. See wound chart for size reduction. | D. Bosley |
| | | | |

Name    Hilda Flood

Address    16 Normanton Road    Centre    Stepney

**Fig 3-5** A sample of a care plan for an adult used in the community setting.

## CITY AND HACKNEY PROVIDER UNIT NURSING CARE PLAN

| STICK ADDRESSOGRAPH HERE | PROBLEM/NEED |
| --- | --- |
| | LINK WORD *Bronchitis* |
| | WARD: *Salter* |

| DATE | PATIENT PROBLEM/NEED | RGN SIGNATURE | REVIEW DATE |
| --- | --- | --- | --- |
| 6/1/95 | Ranjit is experiencing difficulty with his breathing due to broncholitis | L.Sheldon | |
| | | | |
| | **GOAL** | | |
| 6/1/95 | Ranjit's respiratory rate will be reduced to 40 breaths per minute within 24 hours and pulse rate will be reduced to 100 bpm within 24 hours. | L.Sheldon | |
| | **NURSING ACTION/INSTRUCTION** | | |
| 1. | Nurse Ranjit with head elevated if possible. | L.Sheldon | |
| 2. | Record $O_2$ saturation levels hourly, report if these fall below 97%. | L.Sheldon | |
| 3. | Administer $O_2$ via headbox if prescribed. | L.Sheldon | |
| 4. | Record $O_2$ levels hourly | L.Sheldon | |
| 5. | Administer nebulisers if prescribed. | L.Sheldon | |
| 6. | Monitor apex and respiratory rate hourly noting signs of difficulty in breathing i.e. sternal recession, nasal flaring. | L.Sheldon | |
| 7. | Observe Ranjit's colour for signs of pallor and/or cyanosis. | L.Sheldon | |
| | **EVALUATION** | | |
| | Ranjit's observations have returned within normal limits. $O_2$ saturation level is 98-99%. Now nursed in air. | L.Sheldon | |
| | | | |

## CITY AND HACKNEY PROVIDER UNIT NURSING CARE PLAN

| STICK ADDRESSOGRAPH HERE | PROBLEM/NEED |
| --- | --- |
| | LINK WORD *Bronchitis* |
| | WARD: *Salter* |

| DATE | PATIENT PROBLEM/NEED | RGN SIGNATURE | REVIEW DATE |
| --- | --- | --- | --- |
| 6/1/95 | Mr and Mrs Patel appear extremely anxious since Ranjit is their first child and has not been in hospital before. | L.Sheldon | |
| | | | |
| | **GOAL** | | |
| 6/1/95 | Mr and Mrs Patel will have all their questions answered and feel more reassured. | L.Sheldon | 7/1/95 |
| | **NURSING ACTION/INSTRUCTION** | | |
| 1. | Explain Ranjit's health problem and rationale for nursing/medical interventions. | L.Sheldon | |
| 2. | Listen actively to Mr and Mrs Patel and pick up on any cues. | L.Sheldon | |
| 3. | Support Mr and Mrs Patel to continue parenting activities for Ranjit and teach them to undertake nursing activities if they wish to do so. | L.Sheldon | |
| 4. | Provide Mrs Patel with a bed next to Ranjit and show her around the parents facilities. | L.Sheldon | |
| 5. | Ensure both parents understand what is being said to them. | L.Sheldon | |
| 6. | Ascertain religious/cultural needs. | L.Sheldon | |
| | **EVALUATION** | | |
| | Mr and Mrs Patel appear more relaxed and Mrs Patel feels comfortable feeding Ranjit and recording intake on fluid chart. | L.Sheldon | |
| | | | |

**Fig. 3-6** A sample of a nursing care plan for a child admitted to hospital.

## CITY AND HACKNEY PROVIDER UNIT NURSING CARE PLAN

| STICK ADDRESSOGRAPH HERE | LINK WORD   *Felt need 7 (Peplau, 1953)*<br>*(Felt need 7 = a need to feel belonging,*<br>*participation as member of a group)*<br>CLINIC:                    *Heathway* |
|---|---|

| PATIENT'S/CLIENT'S NEED | NURSING INTERVENTION |
|---|---|
| *Tracy is unable to meet Felt Need 7. She remains entrenched in deep resentment towards what she perceives to be "betrayal" by her husband and "the other woman". The imminent breakdown of their marriage will impact on Tracy's ability to meet Felt Need 9.*<br><br>*(Felt need 9 = a need to maintain status, position, prestige and to avoid discomfort or anxiety; to identify self and to make changes in view of self in ways and at speed that facilitates favourable improvement.)* | *1. The primary nurse will spend 1 hour twice a week on one-to-one work with Tracy. The primary nurse will utilize catalytic, cathartic and supportive interventions (Heron, 1975) to enable Tracy to use these sessions to verbalize her feelings associated with the imminent breakdown of her marriage and to enable the nurse to provide a supportive relationship during this transitory phase. (Evaluate at the end of each session.)*<br>*2. The primary nurse will refer Tracy to these following activity groups which have been mutually agreed to be of therapeutic value to Tracy:*<br>*a) women's group (Monday)*<br>*b) projective art group (Tuesday)*<br>*c) movement/dance therapy group (Wednesday)*<br>*(Evaluate at the end of each week.)* |

| DATE | *25-7-94* | DATE | *25-7-94* |
|---|---|---|---|
| RMN SIGNATURE | *L.Sheldon* | RMN SIGNATURE | *L.Sheldon* |
| REVIEW DATE | *1-9-94* | REVIEW DATE | *1-8-94* |

| DATE | NURSING EVALUATION | RMN SIGNATURE | REVIEW DATE |
|---|---|---|---|
| *ACTION 1*<br><br>*Session 1* | *Tracy met with her primary nurse as agreed. The primary nurse used mostly catalyst interventions with positive results where Tracy was facilitated towards self-disclosure. Two cathartic interventions were possibly somewhat premature and brought about very angry responses from Tracy. Projection and displacement remain very evident in the way Tracy is attempting to deal with her feelings about her husband's new partner and the breakdown of her marriage. Tensions in nurse-client relations centre around the need for Tracy to draw the nurse into 'taking side' with her and the nurse's attempts to retain a more objective counsellor role. Overall, Tracy was helped towards verbalization of her feelings and she reports that she feels supported by her primary nurse. It is anticipated that Tracy will commit herself to working through her feelings with the primary nurse, although the next session will need to follow a similar structure and approach to allow trust to develop before confronting specific issues.* | *L.Sheldon* | *1-8-94* |
| *ACTION 2* | *Referrals have been made and Tracy commenced her attendance straight away. Tracy found the women's group "a little threatening" and people "too aggressive" for her to be able to use the session. Negotiated to delay attendance for two weeks and this is to be supported. The movement group seems to provide Tracy with a much needed arena to physically externalize her feelings. Art group was found by Tracy to be "calming" and "reflective". She will continue to attend these two activities.* | *L.Sheldon* | *1-8-94* |

**Fig. 3-7** A portion of a nursing care plan for an adult with mental health needs in a clinic or community setting.

| Behavioural Subsystems Involved | Observed Client Behaviour | Desired Outcome Behaviours (Goals) | | | Nursing Interventions Relating to Goals |
|---|---|---|---|---|---|
| | | Short-term | Medium-term | Long-term | Short-term |
| **Aggressive:** John's shouting and self-injurious behaviour are his main means of self-assertion, as he has no verbal communication skills. John's self-injury strategy has been successful for him, because staff find his behaviour so distressing, they try to prevent it. | As staff and clients prepare for meal time, John begins to shout and to bite his wrists. This behaviour escalates rapidly, to the point where John will bite his wrists so hard that they bleed. | The self-injurious behaviour demonstrated at meal times will be eliminated. | John will develop alternative methods of communicating his needs. | John will be able to assert himself in ways that encourage positive responses from other people, without causing himself harm. | **Self-injurious behaviour:** *Prior to each meal (while the meal is being prepared) one member of staff will spend 5-10 minutes with John using hand cream or massage oil to massage his hands and wrists. John enjoys this activity and it has been observed that he becomes more relaxed following it. During this activity, John should be gently prevented from biting his wrists.* |
| **Dependency:** John is currently dependent on his care staff to meet most of his self-care needs, including feeding and drinking. | John waits passively to be fed. He does not attempt to feed himself. | | John will be able to feed himself. | John will become less dependent on staff to meet his self-care needs. | Staff will use a graduated skills teaching programme, beginning with full physical prompts to encourage self-feeding skills. |

**Fig 3-8** A sample from a care plan for a person with a learning disability.

# CITY AND HACKNEY PROVIDER UNIT NURSING CARE PLAN

| STICK ADDRESSOGRAPH HERE | PROBLEM/NEED |
|---|---|
| | LINK WORD    *Breathlessness* |
| | WARD:    *Rudolf* |

| DATE | PATIENT PROBLEM/NEED | RGN SIGNATURE | REVIEW DATE |
|---|---|---|---|
| 12.12.94 | Mrs Browne is breathless due to a chest infection | AF Hiley | 4 hourly |
| 09.30 | | | |
| | **GOAL** | | |
| | For Mrs Browne's respirations to fall between 20-26 breaths per minute | AF Hiley | |
| | For her peak flow to record between 60-100 ml/s | | |
| | For Mrs Browne to appear less breathless, with reduced use of accessary muscles | | |
| | For her not to be cyanosed - pink lips and nail beds | AF Hiley | |
| | **NURSING ACTION/INSTRUCTION** | | |
| 1. | Administer antibiotics as prescribed | | |
| 2. | Minimise exertion by nursing Mrs Browne in bed or chair as preferred | | |
| 3. | Offer bedside commode or wheel to toilet to avoid walking | | |
| 4. | Support with pillows and table to facilitate full chest expansion | | |
| 5. | Administer prescribed oxygen 24% continuous | | |
| 6. | Perform/offer hourly mouth care | | |
| 7. | Pay attention to communication needs – anticipate needs – ask closed questions | AF Hiley | |
| 8. | Encourage expectoration – Steam inhalation – refer to physiotherapist – provide sputum pot and tissues | | |
| 9. | Spend time with Mrs Browne, answer any questions she may have, particularly concerning her illness, treatment and hospitilization | AF Hiley | |

**Fig 3-9** A sample from a nursing care plan for an adult in hospital.

**Children's Nursing
Including the family in the care plan**

It is important to include family members and/or carers in a child's care plan whenever possible. For example, the care plan of a child who is about to undergo surgery might include:
- escort the child and parents around the ward and introduce them to the child's primary nurse
- explain the procedure to the child and parents
- encourage parents to stay with the child during stressful procedures, if possible
- explain visiting hours to the parents (if they are not staying with the child)
- assess how the child's normal routine will be affected by the surgery and explain this to the parents
- provide a preadmission booklet or other informative material to the parents
- ensure parents and child understand the operation and that their consent is obtained
- after the surgery, encourage parents to alert nurses if child is in pain.

**Adult Nursing
Care plans in community nursing**

The care plan in the community setting is similar to that used in a hospital setting and nursing models are applicable to either setting. Community care plans must include the following cycle:
- assessment of client need – short, medium and long term
- assessment of carer need – short, medium and long term
- design of care plan – in negotiation with carer
- implementation of care – in negotiation with carer
- evaluation of care – client and carer outcomes
- reassessment and adaptation of care to meet changing need
- remodification of adapted plan.

**Always:**
- include the client
- include the carer
- work with other agencies from which clients may receive nursing/social care.

determine whether a specific format should be used for that particular patient/client. Even if the care plan is generally appropriate for a patient/client, the nurse must add or delete information on the preprinted form to individualize it for the patient's/client's needs. Failure to do so can result in incomplete and inaccurate care.

Core care plans are a method to streamline and augment care planning. They are not intended to replace the nursing care plan process (although some nurses believe this is a danger), but to avoid a situation in which the nurse must write the same generalized plan again and again.

Controversy exists over the use of core care plans, as they have several advantages and disadvantages. The advantages are:
- they establish clinically sound standards of care for similar groups of patients/clients, which can be useful when quality-assurance audits are conducted.
- they are easy to locate in a patient's/client's record, and thus all staff can quickly refer to them
- they teach nurses to recognize the accepted requirements of care for patients/clients
- they can improve continuity of care among professional nurses
- they save time in documentation, even though the plans must be modified for each patient/client.

The disadvantages are:
- there is a risk that the core plans inhibit nurses' identification of unique, individualized care for patients/clients
- the plans must be formally updated on a routine basis to ensure that content is current and appropriate
- staff members may develop many core plans for patients/clients seen in their institutions; thus, large

numbers of plans take up space for storage and are more costly to print than one common care plan form.

There is currently a trend among some hospitals to computerize care plans (see Chapter 5). With such a system, daily computer-generated care plans are printed and incorporate several nursing problems in a single care plan. Such a streamlined system improves the daily revision and updating of plans.

**Student Care Plans**

Nursing students learn to write and use a nursing care plan as part of their education. The **student care plan** is essential for learning the problem-solving technique, the nursing process, skills of written and verbal communication, and organizational skills needed for nursing care (Fig. 3.10). Most important, by using the nursing care plan, students can apply the knowledge gained from nursing and health care literature, and the classroom, to a practice situation.

The student care plan is more elaborate than a care plan in a hospital or community health care agency, because its purpose is to teach the process of planning care. To learn the care-planning process, the student must progress in a step-by-step manner, beginning with assessment and ending with evaluation. Student care plans vary from one educational programme to another and between beginners and more advanced students. Some educational institutions model the student care plan on the care plan used in the affiliated health care agency. The only modification may be that the teacher requires a student to include the scientific rationale for the nursing actions selected. A **scientific rationale** is the reason that, based on supporting literature, a specific nursing action was chosen.

## CITY AND HACKNEY PROVIDER UNIT NURSING CARE PLAN

| STICK ADDRESSOGRAPH HERE | PROBLEM/NEED |
| --- | --- |
| | LINK WORD   *Dry Mouth* |
| | WARD:   *Aynsley* |

| DATE | PATIENT PROBLEM/NEED | RGN SIGNATURE | REVIEW DATE |
| --- | --- | --- | --- |
| 02.12.94 | Mrs Jones has a dry, sore mouth with a furred tongue and cracked lips. This is due to recent reduced fluid intake (dehydration). | EFielding (student) | Hourly |
| | **GOAL** | | |
| | For Mrs Jones to state that her mouth is comfortable and no longer sore. For her mouth and tongue to be moist, pink and free from debris. For her lips to be moist. | EFielding (student) | |

| | NURSING ACTION/INSTRUCTION | RATIONALE |
| --- | --- | --- |
| 1. | Restore fluid balance by offering and encouraging Mrs Jones to drink 100 mls of preferred fluid hourly | Watson (1989) restoring fluid balance key factor in improving quality of oral health in dehydrated patient |
| 2. | Encourage/assist Mrs Jones to clean her teeth with toothbrush and toothpaste 8 hourly | Most effective way of removing plaque from teeth |
| 3. | Place half of 1 gram vitamin 'C' effervescent tablet on the tongue and allow to dissolve. 6 hourly during the day | Daeffler 1981 identifies risks associated with alternatives i.e. Sodium Bicarbonate and Hydrogen Peroxide. |
| 4. | Offer/encourage hourly mouth wash with water or thymol | Trentworth and Creason 1986 identify water as efficient a mouthwash as thymol—mechanical action is an important factor |
| 5. | Avoid use of lemon glycerin swabs | Crosby 1989 – lemon glycerin can increase dryness in mouth due to reactive salivation |
| 6. | Apply petroleum jelly to lips hourly | Daeffler 1981 water soluble applications preferable for cracked lips |
| 7. | Monitor and observe urine output. Record specific gravity. Maintain fluid balance chart | Amount and concentration of urine reflects level of hydration |

**Fig 3-10** A sample of a student care plan for an adult in hospital.

## PLANNING

Planning is a category of nursing behaviour in which patient/client-centred goals are established and strategies are designed to achieve the goals. During planning, priorities are set, goals are determined, and a nursing care plan is formulated. In addition to collaborating with the patient/client and family, the nurse consults with other members of the health care team, reviews pertinent literature, modifies care, and records relevant information about the individual's health care needs and clinical management.

### Establishing Priorities

After identifying the patient's/client's problems, the nurse establishes the priorities of the problems by ranking them in order of importance. **Priorities of care** are established to identify the order in which nursing interventions will be provided when an individual has multiple problems.

Establishing priorities is not merely a matter of numbering the person's problems on the basis of severity or physiological importance. Rather, it is a method by which the nurse and the patient/client mutually rank the problems in order of their importance to the individual person.

Maslow's hierarchy of needs can be useful in designating priorities (see Chapter 7). Basic physiological needs are given priority over self-esteem needs. The needs for love, esteem, and self-actualization may have a lower priority. The nurse may encounter situations in which there are no emergency physical needs but in which high priority must be given to the psychological, sociocultural, developmental, or spiritual needs of the patient/client.

Because individuals may have many problems, the nurse may not be able to work with all of them when they are identified. The nurse and patient/client mutually agree upon priorities based on the urgency of the problem, the nature of the treatment indicated, and the interaction among the problems.

Priorities can be classified as *high*, *intermediate*, or *low*. Problems that, if untreated, could result in harm to the person, and/or others, have the highest priorities. High priorities occur in the psychological and physiological dimensions, and the nurse should avoid classifying only physiological nursing problems as high priority. Intermediate-priority problems involve the non-emergency, non-life-threatening needs of the patient/client. Low-priority problems are needs that may not be directly related to a specific illness or prognosis.

Whenever possible, the patient/client should be involved in priority setting. In some situations the patient/client and nurse assign different priority rankings to the problems identified. If both place a different value on health care needs and treatments, these differences can be resolved through open communication. However, when the patient's/client's physiological and emotional needs are at stake, the nurse needs to assume primary responsibility for setting priorities.

When the nurse assigns priorities to the patient's/client's problems, the resources of the health care system, and limitations of time are considered.

Development of patient/client goals may occur with the establishment of priorities. However, for clarity and explanation, determining goals is presented in the next section.

### Establishing Goals of Care

Goals (sometimes called *expected outcomes*) are specific statements of patient/client behaviours or responses that the nurse anticipates from nursing care. After assessing and identifying the patient's/client's problem, and establishing priorities about the person's health care needs, the nurse formulates goals with the individual for each problem. The purposes for writing goals are twofold:

- to provide direction for the individualized nursing interventions
- to determine the effectiveness of the interventions.

A variety of terms are used interchangeably in the nursing literature when discussing goals and outcomes. These terms include *objectives*, *goals*, *outcome criteria*, and *outcomes*. Regardless of the terms, the purpose of this step is to identify a specific means to evaluate the patient's/client's response to nursing care (Hickey, 1990). In this text, the term *goals* is used to indicate anticipated patient/client responses.

Each goal statement must have a time frame for evaluation. The time element depends on the nature of the problem, its cause, overall condition of the patient/client, and treatment setting.

Nursing care is planned according to the patient's/client's problems, and priority setting reflects the goals of care established by the patient/client and nurse. Because each person responds uniquely to a situation, the patient's/client's goals are also unique.

Individually identified patient/client problems and priority setting help determine the goals of care.

### Role of the Patient/Client in Goal Setting

A patient/client-centred goal is a specific, measurable, and achievable objective designed to state the patient's/client's desired behaviour. Whenever possible, the patient/client must be actively involved in setting these goals and in developing the care plan.

In order for patients/clients to participate in goal setting, they should be alert and be able to participate in problem solving and decision making. When developing goals, the nurse can act as an advocate for the patient/client to prevent further deterioration in the level of health or cognitive and physical functioning.

Goals should not only meet the immediate needs of the patient/client, but should also include prevention and rehabilitation. Two types of goals are developed for the patient/client: short-term goals and long-term goals.

### Short-Term Goals

A **short-term goal** is an objective that is expected to be achieved in a short period of time, which may be less than a few hours or days. With the present health care system and shorter hospital stays, short-term goals are the direction for the immediate care plan. Long-term goals may be more appropriate for problem resolution in the community.

## Long-Term Goals

A long-term goal is an objective that is expected to be achieved over a longer period of time, usually over weeks or months. Long-term goals may be carried over in the transfer to a rehabilitation setting, a nursing home, or to the home. These goals often focus on prevention, rehabilitation, discharge, and health education. Failure to set long-term goals may prevent the client from receiving continuity of care for discharge planning.

Goal setting establishes the framework for the nursing care plan. Through goals, the nurse is able to provide continuity of care and promote optimal use of time and resources.

## Goal Steps

Goal steps are the specific, step-by-step objective that leads to attainment of the goal and the resolution of the cause of the patient/client problem. A goal statement is the measurable behavioural change of the patient/client in response to nursing care. Goals are the desired response of a patient's/client's condition in the physiological, social, emotional, developmental, or spiritual dimensions. This change in condition is documented through observable or measurable patient/client responses. Objectives within the goals help determine when a goal has been met, and later assist in evaluating the response to nursing care and resolution of the patient's/client's problems.

Goal steps have several functions:

- they provide a direction for nursing activities, because they are projected before nursing actions are formulated
- they include observable patient/client behaviours and measurable criteria for each goal
- they provide a projected time span for attaining the goal and an opportunity to state additional resources that may be required to achieve the goal (including equipment, personnel, or knowledge)
- they can be used as criteria to evaluate the effectiveness of nursing activities.

When writing goals:

- ensure that the outcome statement is written in **measurable** behaviour terms to allow the nurse to note specifically the behaviour and the type of behavioural response expected for resolution of the problem
- write the goals **sequentially**, with given time frames to provide an order for the interventions, as well as a time reference for resolution of the problem.

 **Learning Disabilities Nursing
Goal setting for people with learning disabilities**

Achieving goals can be a very slow process for people with learning disabilities. It is, therefore, necessary to consider care and the care plan in terms of years rather than weeks or months. The care plan must reflect this and must be sufficiently flexible to take account of the inevitable changes in personal circumstances that will occur. The long-term goals that are set must be supported by medium- and short-term goals that can be reviewed, revised and amended as often as necessary. Target dates should be set and individuals must be appointed to ensure that actions are carried out. The care plan must also account in advance for life changes and events, such as the transition from Education Authority support to Adult Services support.

The care that is given will probably be multidisciplinary; therefore, it is important that the care plan is also multidisciplinary. The care plan should also include some form of continual, structured risk assessment, to ensure that the plan is neither too cautious nor too adventurous.

The goals should reflect the patient's/client's needs and desires – not the carer's expectations and priorities. For example, the patient/client may want increased autonomy and to live independently. The short- and medium-term goals implied in this long-term aim include acquisition of skills such as budgeting, cooking and self-protection. The carer, on the other hand, may see the individual's long-term future as being eventual admission into some form of sheltered, residential care. The short- and medium-term goals implicit in this aim are significantly different and can be a source of conflict and misdirection.

Above all, the care plan should be realistic and pragmatic. It is better to err on the side of caution and to set achievable targets, than to be unduly optimistic and risk catastrophic failure.

 **Mental Health Nursing
Goal setting for people with mental impairment**

When a patient's/client's cognitive and physical impairments are so severe that they are unable to actively participate in goal setting, the nursing team acts on their behalf to develop patient/client-centred goals. These patients/clients may include people who are comatose, confused, or unable to make decisions, and where a place of safety needs to be found so that care can be provided.

With the move towards community mental health care, proposals for a Community Treatment Order (CTO) will become a reality. The aim of CTO is to recreate hospital support in the community setting. Nursing individual clients in community settings will demand care planning that involves both social and health care agencies. The term *careworking* will become increasingly familiar as care workers are appointed either from social or health care to coordinate packages of care for those with mental health needs.

## Guidelines for Writing Goals

The important components of a correctly written goal can be remembered by using the acronym 'STAMPS':

- specific
- time
- achievable
- measurable
- patient-partnership
- states 'who' and 'how'.

The behaviour to be achieved, or other desired outcome, is stated in **specific** terms. For example, the patient/client 'will be able to …' (perform a particular activity), physiological measurement 'will reflect that …' or the patient/client 'will state that …' (he or she feels/no longer feels).

**Time** constraints for achieving the goal are stated. For example, 'By the end of the shift Mrs White will put on her dress unaided', or 'Mr Brown will lose 1 kg before his clinic appointment in three month's time'.

The chosen goal should be **achievable** and realistic, with a reasonable chance of success. Otherwise there is a real danger of discouraging the patient/client who may become demotivated. This is where small goals steps, or several short-term goals, are particularly useful. For example, the ultimate goal for Mr Brown is to lose 38kg – taken 1-2 kg at a time, this goal becomes less daunting. The same is true of a patient/client recovering from a stroke: ultimately, the goal is to begin walking, but the first step must be to achieve sitting balance unsupported. Nothing succeeds like success – it's good for both patients/clients and nurses.

State how you will **measure** achievement of the goal; for example, how much fluid is to be drunk over the next 24 hrs, the distance you mean your patient/client to walk twice each shift, or the size of the wound. It is much more difficult to measure subjective feelings. However, the use of pain charts, for example, can help give a type of measurement, which could be adapted to other feelings. Another possibility is to ask the patient/client to state whether or not he or she is still anxious about a particular problem. Careful observation is also useful; for example, 'Mr. Smith is grimacing rarely and he no longer holds his stitches when walking', or 'Mrs Brown is no longer tearful, and is able concentrate on her knitting now'.

Any behaviour change or activity that is imposed in the goal has, at best, a limited chance of success, therefore **patient-partnership**, or patient/client consultation, is essential. Negotiation and/or teaching skills may be needed if a patient/client is reluctant to comply with care which the nurse regards as important. The best plan is useless if the patient/client will not cooperate.

Finally, the goal should state **'who'** will perform the goal and **'how'**. The patient is usually 'who' and is at the centre of the goal. The 'how' includes special considerations, such as walking with one stick, or dressing unaided.

Short, realistic goals and expected outcomes can quickly provide the patient/client and nurse with a sense of accomplishment. In turn, this sense of accomplishment can increase the patient's/client's motivation and cooperation. When establishing realistic goals, the nurse, through assessment, must know the resources of the health care unit; the family; the patient's/client's physiological, emotional, cognitive, and sociocultural potential; and the cost and resources available to reach expected goals in a timely manner. Establishing goals without assessment of patient/client, environment, or resources may produce an unrealistic plan which is frustrating for the patient/client and the nurse.

## Designing Nursing Interventions

Nursing interventions, strategies, or actions are selected after goals are established. However, implementation of these strategies occurs during the implementation phase of the nursing process (see p. 58).

Choosing suitable nursing strategies is a decision-making process. The nurse uses assessment data, priority setting, knowledge, and experience to select actions that will successfully meet the established goals.

Each expected outcome has interventions, or nursing actions. The method of intervention selection is always the same, but the types of interventions are individualized to the patient's/client's needs.

## Selecting Interventions

Selecting interventions includes the following steps:

- **deliberating** about all possible interventions to achieve the goal – during deliberation, the nurse reviews the patient/client problem, priorities, and previous experiences to select nursing interventions that have the best potential for achieving the goals. As the nurse gains experience, this deliberation process becomes more efficient and experience-based (Benner, 1984).
- **researching** textbooks and related literature – these address usual problems and nursing actions for given conditions. Although they are written in general terms, the nurse can use these resources to acquire new patient/client care knowledge. This knowledge then helps the nurse individualize the intervention.
- **collaborating** with other health care professionals helps the nurse tap the best resources and individualize the nursing actions to meet the goal. During collaboration, the nurse collaborates with the patient/client to select suitable interventions that are congruent with the patient's/client's hopes, beliefs, values, resources, and expectations.

Usually, the nurse will have more interventions than are necessary to meet the desired goal. Some are discarded as inappropriate, and some are adapted to the patient's/client's needs and abilities. As a result, the list of possible interventions is narrowed down to those suitable to the patient/client. Techniques for avoiding common mistakes in goal setting are described in Table 3-3.

## Examples of Goal Setting

The techniques defined above are illustrated in the following examples. For clarity, where the techniques occur is shown in square brackets.

**TABLE 3-3 Techniques for Avoiding Common Mistakes in Goal Setting**

**S**pecific – describes behaviour/action planned.

**T**ime – states time frame and time constraits.

**A**chievable – is realistic, not overly optimistic.

**M**easurable – states measurement form (this may be what the patient/client says he or she feels or thinks).

**P**atient partnership – goal written in consultation with patient and mutually agreed.

**S**tates "who" and "how"– who will undertake the action or behaviour (usually the patient)
– how and under what conditions the behaviour will be carried out.

1. On 1/7/94 after discussion with the patient and occupational therapist [patient-partnership], it was decided that Mr Clarke [states 'who'] would put on [specific behaviour] and correctly fasten [measurement] his shirt with only verbal assistance [states 'how'] by 21/8/94 [realistic time frame].
2. Miss Clancy [states 'who'] will correctly draw up and administer her own insulin [specific behaviour] by subcutaneous injection [states 'how'] by 21/8/94 [realistic time frame] after discussion between the patient and diabetic nurse specialist [patient-partnership].
3. Mrs Browne [states 'who'} will state [states 'how'/behaviour] that she no longer feels pain at level 3 or above [measurement] by 6PM 1/3/94 [time frame].

## Consulting Other Health Care Professionals

**Consultation** is a process in which the nurse seeks the help of a specialist to identify ways to handle problems in patient/client management or the planning and implementing of programmes. Consultation is based on the problem-solving approach. Consultation may occur at any step in the nursing process, but is needed most often in the planning and intervention steps when the nurse is more likely to identify a problem requiring additional knowledge or skills, or may need to obtain community or agency resources.

In clinical nursing, consultation is used to solve problems in the delivery of nursing care or the use of resources. Senior nurses, ward sisters and clinical nurse specialists are most frequently approached for advice about difficult clinical problems. Nurses are consulted for their clinical expertise, patient/client education skills, or staff education skills. Nurses also consult with other members of the health care team, such as physiotherapists, dietitians, and social workers.

## When to Consult

Consultation should occur when the nurse identifies a problem that cannot be solved using personal knowledge, skills, and resources. Consultation increases the nurse's knowledge about the problem, helps the nurse learn new skills, helps obtain the resources needed to solve the problem, and ensures appropriate care for the patient. After the consultation, the nurse may be able to resolve similar problems in the future. For example, a nurse encountering a patient/client with a recent colostomy should, if possible, request a consultation from a stoma therapist to determine the materials needed to clean the colostomy site and the specific techniques to use.

## How to Consult

The use of consultation is a valuable adjunct to nursing care. In clinical nursing practice, competent and experienced nurses encounter problems beyond their knowledge or experience. Professional and competent nurses recognize their limitations, seek appropriate consultation, and learn from the findings and recommendations, as they are required to do so by the United Kingdom Central Council Code of Conduct (UKCC, 1992).

## IMPLEMENTATION

In theory, implementation of the nursing care plan follows the planning component of the nursing process. However, in practice settings, implementation should begin during or directly after assessment if possible. Immediate implementation is necessary when the nurse identifies urgent needs of the patient/client, such as a threat to physiological status (for example, a cardiac arrest), psychological status (for example, a sudden death of a loved one), socioeconomic status (for example, the sudden loss of a home in a fire), or spiritual status (for example, an illness viewed as God's punishment).

**Implementation** is the delivery of nursing care, including the initiation and completion of the actions necessary for achieving the set goals: performing, assisting, or directing the performance of activities of living, counselling and teaching the person or family, giving direct care to achieve patient/client-centred goals, supervising and evaluating the work of staff members, and recording and exchanging information relevant to the person's continued health care

Implementation begins after the care plan has been developed, and focuses on the initiation of nursing interventions to achieve the goals of care. A **nursing intervention** is any act by a nurse that implements the nursing care plan or any specific objective of the plan. The patient/client may require intervention in the form of support, medication, treatment for the current condition, patient/client-family education, or treatment to prevent future health problems.

Care delivery is continuous and interacts with the other components of the nursing process. During care delivery, the nurse reassesses the patient/client, modifies the care plan, and rewrites the goals as necessary. To complete implementation effectively, the nurse has to be knowledgeable about types of interventions, and possible patient/client reactions.

Implementation puts the care plan into action; indeed, it is sometimes called *nursing action*. After the plan has been developed according to patient/client needs and priorities, the nurse performs specific nursing interventions.

A *standing order* is a written document containing rules, policies, protocols, procedures, regulations, and orders for the conduct of patient/client care in various stipulated clinical settings. Standing orders are approved and signed by the doctor in charge of care before their implementation. They are commonly found in critical care settings, where patients'/clients' needs can change rapidly and require immediate attention. An example of such a standing order is one that specifies a certain drug for an irregular heart rhythm. After assessing the patient/client and identifying the irregular rhythm, the critical care nurse (who is a registered nurse) gives the appropriate medication without needing to notify the doctor first. Standing orders are also common in the community health setting, in which the nurse encounters situations that do not permit immediate contact with a doctor. Thus, standing orders give the nurse the legal protection to intervene appropriately in the patient's/client's best interest.

Before implementing any treatment, including those included in standing orders, the nurse must use sound judgement in determining whether the intervention is correct and appropriate. Secondly, the nurse implementing any intervention is responsible to obtain correct theoretical knowledge and for having the clinical competency necessary to perform the intervention. This is also a requirement of the UKCC Code of Conduct (UKCC, 1992). Nursing responsibility is equally great for all types of interventions.

The nurse must carefully select the interventions to achieve the goals and know the way each may affect the patient/client. Several factors make decision making more difficult when choosing among nursing interventions; one is the absence of objective data concerning the probable consequences of the interventions; another factor is that nursing interventions are often not mutually exclusive from medical therapies. For example, the nurse may need to augment relaxation, massage, and guided imagery techniques with prescribed analgesics for pain management. Consultation to ensure the safety of combining these interventions would be required.

Synder (1985) proposes an **information-processing model of decision making.** The objective of this model is to characterize the sequence of the thought process used by problem solvers. The information-processing model identifies how decisions are made. A nurse can use the following components of decision making when determining nursing interventions (Synder, 1985):
- The list of all possible nursing actions
- A list of all possible consequences associated with each possible nursing action
- The determination of the probability that each of the consequences will occur

- A judgement based on the value of that consequence to the patient/client.

This model is effective in teaching students how to make clinical decisions. However, junior students or newly-qualified practitioners still need supervision from a tutor or experienced nurse, as their knowledge base may still be inadequate.

## Reassessing the Patient/Client

Assessment is a continuous process. Each time a nurse interacts with a patient/client, additional data are gathered to reflect physical, developmental, intellectual, emotional, social, and spiritual needs. When new data are assessed and a new problem is identified, the nurse modifies the nursing care plan.

The purpose of the **reassessment** is to gather new data that can affect the care to be given. If the problem has changed, then the care to be given may have to be adapted.

The reassessment phase of the implementation process provides a mechanism for the nurse to determine whether the proposed nursing action is still appropriate for the patient's/client's current condition.

## Reviewing and Modifying the Care Plan

Although the nursing care plan is developed according to the problems identified during assessment, changes in the patient's/client's condition can necessitate modification of planned nursing care. Before beginning care, review the care plan and compare it with assessment data to validate the stated problem and to determine whether the nursing interventions are the most appropriate for the clinical situation. If the patient's/client's condition has changed, and the problems and related nursing interventions are no longer appropriate, the nursing care plan needs to be modified.

Modification of the existing care plan includes several steps:
1. Reassess the patient's/client's problems in the relevant area. Date any new data entered in the care plan to inform other members of the care team of the time that the change occurred.
2. Revise the patient's/client's problems. Delete, in order, problems that are no longer relevant; add and date new problems. Because the patient's/client's condition and health care needs have changed, the priorities and goals must also be revised. Date the revisions on the care plan (Fig. 3-11).
3. Revise specific implementation methods to correspond to the new patient/client problems and goals. This revision reflects the patient's/client's present condition. The new implementation methods indicate the patient's/client's greater independence from or dependence on nursing. In addition, revised implementation will include the patient's/client's specific health care needs.
4. Evaluate the patient's/client's response to the nursing actions. If an individual's response is not consistent with the established goals, further revisions for the plan of care are required.
5. Possible alteration of the goal statement as required.

The astute nurse is sensitive to changes in the patient's/client's condition and readily incorporates these changes into the care plan. The patient's/client's state of health is dynamic and changes continuously. Therefore, the care plan needs to be flexible to incorporate all necessary changes. **An out-of-date or incorrect care plan compromises the quality of nursing care, whereas review and modification enable the nurse to provide nursing care that meets the patient's/client's needs.**

### Identifying Areas of Assistance

Some nursing situations require the nurse to seek assistance. Assistance can fall into the following categories: additional personnel, knowledge, or nursing skills. Before implementing care, the nurse evaluates the plan to determine the need for assistance and the type required.

### Additional Personnel

These situations vary. For example, a nurse assigned to care for an immobilized patient/client may need additional personnel to help turn, transfer, and position the person because of the physical work involved. The nurse also needs to determine when the personnel are needed. If the patient/client needs to be turned and repositioned every 2 hrs, additional personnel will be needed every 2 hrs. The nurse then must determine the number of people needed and the skills and knowledge they require and must discuss the need for assistance with the nurse in charge of the ward or team. Finally, the nurse needs to take time to plan care so that the additional personnel do not become overburdened.

Additional personnel may also be required when a patient's/client's condition deteriorates or when the number of patients/clients increases. In both situations the required level of nursing care may be too much for one nurse to deliver safely.

### Additional Knowledge or Skills

Some nursing situations require additional knowledge and skills. For example, a nurse needs additional knowledge when administering a new medication or implementing a new procedure. Drug information can be obtained from *The British National Formulary*, a hospital's formulary, or a hospital's own clinical procedure book. If the nurse is still uncertain about the new medication or procedure, other members of the health care team must be consulted. In addition, another nurse who has completed the procedure correctly and safely may provide assistance. The assistance can come from a staff nurse, a sister, tutor, or a nurse specialist. Although tempting, it is advisable not to ask a fellow student.

Requesting assistance occurs frequently in all types of nursing practice and is a learning process that continues throughout educational experiences and into professional development.

### Implementing Nursing Actions

The nurse uses nursing interventions to achieve the goals of nursing care and may use any of the following methods to achieve these:

* assisting in the performance of activities of living
* counselling and educating the patient/client and family
* providing care to achieve therapeutic goals
* giving care to facilitate attainment of therapeutic goals by the patient/client.

Nursing practice is composed of cognitive, interpersonal, and psychomotor skills. Each type of skill is required to implement interventions. The nurse is responsible for knowing when one of these methods is preferred over another and for having the necessary theoretical knowledge and psychomotor skills to implement each.

### Cognitive Skills

Cognitive skills involve nursing knowledge. The nurse must know the rationale for each therapeutic intervention, understand normal and abnormal physiological and psychological responses, be able to identify patient/client learning and discharge needs, and recognize the need for preventive and compensatory nursing actions.

### Interpersonal Skills

Interpersonal skills are essential to effective nursing action. The nurse must communicate clearly with the patient/client, family, and other members of the health care team. Patient/client teaching and counselling must be done to the level of the patient's/client's understanding. The nurse must also be sensitive to the patient's/client's emotional response to the illness and treatment. Use of interpersonal skills enable the nurse to be perceptive to the patient's/client's verbal and nonverbal communication (see Chapter 15).

### Learning Disabilities Nursing
### Implementing care

One of the major difficulties repeatedly encountered in caring for people with learning disabilities is that care plans are often ignored after they have been created. It is necessary, therefore, to ensure that a key worker is responsible for ensuring all planned care is given as outlined in the care plan. Much of the day-to-day work of implementing care falls upon the patient's/client's informal carer and/or unqualified staff. These people may require advice, support and instruction to enable them to contribute to the implementation of the care plan.

An important, but often overlooked, element of implementation is enabling the person with a learning disability to make choices about his or her life and supporting those decisions, often with opposition from family and care givers. This is the work of advocacy. In these situations, nurses have a role in negotiating with the patient's/client's family and care givers, and in helping them come to terms with the patient's/client's decision. Although the nurse may consider the care plan to be a carefully designed strategy, it may appear unrealistic and unnecessarily risky to the patient's/client's family. The nurse must reassure and educate the family, so they can see the benefits of the care plan and support the patient's/client's decisions.

## CITY AND HACKNEY PROVIDER UNIT NURSING CARE PLAN

| STICK ADDRESSOGRAPH HERE | PROBLEM/NEED |
|---|---|
| | LINK WORD     *Anxiety re Smokey* |
| | WARD:              *Rudolf* |

| DATE | PATIENT PROBLEM/NEED | RGN SIGNATURE | REVIEW DATE |
|---|---|---|---|
| 12.12.94 | Mrs Browne is extremely anxious about the care of her cat 'Smokey' during hospital stay | AF Hiley | 14.00 hrs |
| | Resolved 13.30 12.12.94    AF Hiley | | |
| **GOAL** | | | |
| | For Mrs Browne to say she is happy with the care arrangements for Smokey | | |
| | For Mrs Browne to demonstrate a change in behaviour that suggests she is no longer anxious – stop crying, talk to other patients, appear more relaxed | | |
| | For observations to reflect reduced anxiety BP↓130/90  P↓100 | | |
| **NURSING ACTION/INSTRUCTION** | | | |
| | | | |
| 1. | Nurse Hacket will telephone neighbour currently caring for Smokey for advice and suggestions | | |
| 2. | Nurse Hacket will telephone social worker for help and advice | AF Hiley | |
| 3. | Nurse Hacket will keep Mrs Browne informed at shift end at latest | | |
| 4. | Spend time with Mrs Browne discussing her anxieties | | |
| | | | |
| | | | |

**Fig 3-11** Updated care plan.

### Psychomotor Skills

Psychomotor skills involve the direct care needs of patients/clients such as changing a dressing, giving an injection, or suctioning a tracheostomy. The nurse has a professional responsibility to correctly complete these skills. Some of these skills may be new. If that is the case, the nurse must assess his or her present level of competency to ensure that the patient/client receives the treatment safely, by seeking assistance and supervision when necessary.

### Communicating Nursing Actions

Nursing interventions are written or communicated verbally. When written, nursing interventions are incorporated into the nursing care plan and patient's/client's medical record. The care plan usually reflects proposed nursing interventions. After the interventions are implemented, pertinent information is written in the patient's/client's record (evaluation documentation). This information usually includes a brief description of the nursing assessment, and the patient's/client's response to nursing care.

Writing the time and details of the care given documents that the procedure was completed. A summary of the patient's/client's response to the procedure evaluates its effectiveness.

Nursing interventions are also communicated verbally from one nurse to another or to other health professionals. Nurses commonly communicate verbally when changing shifts, transferring a patient/client to another unit, or discharging an individual to another health agency. Whether the nursing intervention is written or communicated verbally, the language should be clear, concise, and to the point. Chapter 15 discusses the communication skills necessary in nursing practice, and Chapter 5 describes the skills needed to record pertinent information in the patient/client's nursing record.

## Methods of Care

The nurse carries out the nursing care plan by using several methods. For example, the patient/client with bilateral arm fractures (in plaster casts), will require assistance in performing activities of living. The patient/client coping inadequately because of fear of a diagnosis requires counselling as a method of nursing intervention. An individual with a knowledge deficit needs interventions through health education. The totally immobilized or disorientated patient/client requires nursing interventions providing total patient/client care.

## Assisting with Activities of Living

**Activities of living (ALs)** are activities usually performed in the course of a normal day; such as eating, dressing, bathing, brushing the teeth, and grooming. Conditions resulting in the need for assistance with ALs can be acute, chronic, temporary, permanent, or rehabilitative. An **acute disease** is characterized by symptoms that are usually severe and that are present for a relatively short period of time, usually less than 6 months. An episode of acute disease results in recovery to a state of health and activity comparable to the state before the disease, passage into a chronic phase of the disease, or death. For example, the postoperative patient/client is unable to complete some ALs independently because of the acute health problem related to surgery. While progressing through the postoperative period, the patient/client gradually becomes less and less dependent on nurses for completing ALs.

A **chronic disease** is ongoing, and the effects may be continuous or intermittent. Although the symptoms are usually less severe than those of the acute phase of the same disease, chronic disease may result in complete or partial disability. A patient/client with partial paralysis after a cerebrovascular accident has a chronic impairment requiring long-term assistance with some ALs.

The patient's/client's need for assistance with ALs may be temporary, permanent, or rehabilitative. In the case of temporary assistance with ALs, the patient/client requires assistance during a specific time period. A patient/client with impaired mobility because of bilateral arm plaster casts has a temporary need for assistance. After the casts are removed, the patient/client will gradually assume responsibility for ALs. A patient/client with a total self-care deficit related to an injury high in the cervical spinal cord has a permanent need for assistance. It is unrealistic for the nurse to plan a rehabilitation programme with the goal that the patient/client will be able to independently complete all ALs. This patient/client may have a rehabilitative need for assistance with ALs. Through rehabilitation, the patient/client will learn new ways to perform ALs, thus becoming more independent and better able to perform self-care.

Through assessment, the nurse collects data that verify the need for assistance with ALs. As the nurse analyses this data, patient/client problems are identified that will require resolution.

## Counselling

Counselling is a process that helps the patient/client use a problem-solving process to recognize and manage stress; it also facilitates interpersonal relationships among the patient/client, family and health care team. Nurses provide counselling to help the patient/client accept actual or impending changes. Counselling may involve emotional, intellectual, spiritual, and psychological support. A patient/client and family who need nursing counselling have 'normal' adjustment difficulties and are upset or frustrated but are not psychologically disturbed. Psychologically disabled patient/clients frequently require counselling by nurses specializing in mental health nursing.

Many counselling techniques are used to foster cognitive, behavioural, developmental, experiential, and emotional growth in patient/clients. Counselling encourages individuals to examine available alternatives and to decide which choices are useful and appropriate. When individuals are able to examine alternatives, they can develop a sense of control and are better able to manage stress. To assist patient/clients in need of counselling, the nurse must be able to identify the need for counselling and possess communication skills to develop a therapeutic relationship (Sundeen *et al*, 1989).

Patients/clients or families who may require counselling include people who must adjust their lifestyle patterns, such as stopping smoking, reducing weight, or decreasing activity levels. Patients/clients coping with chronic or disabling diseases may require counselling to help them accept changes in lifestyle or body image as the disease progresses. During life-threatening illnesses, patient/clients and families may need counselling to cope with the possibility of death.

## Teaching

Both counselling and teaching involve using communication skills to effect a change in the patient/client. However, with counselling the change results in the development of new attitudes and feelings, whereas in teaching the focus of change is intellectual growth or the acquisition of knowledge or psychomotor skills (Redman, 1988).

Teaching is used to present correct principles, procedures, and techniques of health care to individuals and to inform patients/clients about their state of health (see Chapter 16). As a nursing responsibility, teaching is implemented in all health care settings. The nurse is responsible for assessing the learning needs of patient/clients and is accountable for the quality of education delivered.

The **teaching-learning process** is an interaction between the teacher and learner in which specific learning objectives are presented (Redman, 1988). Benner calls this function 'coaching' (Benner, 1984). This process provides the organizational structure and framework for patient/client education.

During assessment, the nurse determines the patient's/client's learning needs and readiness to learn. When planning, the nurse and patient/client establish goals for learning. The teaching strategies are designed to achieve the learning goal. Finally, evaluation measures the learning that has occurred. The purpose of the teaching-learning process is to develop and implement a teaching plan individualized for the patient's/client's needs, level of knowledge, and learning resources.

## Maintaining Patient/Client Safety

To achieve the therapeutic goals, the nurse initiates interventions to compensate for adverse reactions; employs precautionary and preventive measures when providing care; uses correct techniques in administering care and preparing the patient/client for special procedures; and initiates lifesaving measures in emergency situations. The following sections briefly discuss the nursing interventions in these areas. The specific knowledge and skills required to carry out these nursing procedures are detailed in subsequent chapters.

## ADVERSE REACTIONS

An **adverse reaction** is a harmful or unintended effect of a medication, diagnostic test, or therapeutic intervention. To

---

### Mental Health Nursing
### The 'normalization' process

As part of the process of 'normalization', it is important to enable people with mental disorders to become self-advocates. One aspect of the nurse's role in the normalization process is to teach clients how to establish self-help groups, committees, or networking systems so that the clients can make choices and desicions for themselves with varying levels of support. Clients should also be encouraged to discuss their treatment and care. Nurses should listen to and learn from these discussions so they may plan effective care and develop a partnership in care with the client.

---

intervene, the nurse must be aware of the potential undesired effects. For example, when administering a medication, the nurse understands the known and potential side effects of the drug. After administration of the medication the nurse assesses the patient/client for any side effects. The nurse should be aware of drugs that can counteract the side effects. For example, a patient/client may have an unknown hypersensitivity to penicillin, and develop a rash after three doses. The nurse records the reaction and stops administration of the drug. The nurse also consults the doctor about the prescription and administers an antipruritic medication to relieve the itching and an antihistamine to reduce the allergic response.

Therapeutic interventions may also have potential adverse effects. For example, bed rest will help reduce oxygen demand following a myocardial infarction, but at the same time the immobility can contribute to pressure sores unless preventive measures are taken.

Although adverse effects are uncommon, they do occur. The nurse should be aware of any potential side effects, able to recognize the presence of one, and intervene accordingly.

## PREVENTIVE MEASURES

**Preventive nursing actions** are directed at preventing illness and promoting health to avoid the need for secondary or tertiary health care. Prevention includes assessment and promotion of the patient's/client's health, application of prescribed measures such as immunizations, early postoperative mobilization, health teaching, early diagnosis and treatment, and early rehabilitation.

In the case of a patient/client who has a hypersensitivity to penicillin, for example, the nurse can implement several preventive measures. The nurse clearly indicates the penicillin allergy in relevant sections of the patient's/client's medical record (medications chart and medical records). The nurse also informs the patient/client and family about the use and availability of a Medic-Alert® bracelet, and teaches them actions to avoid the person being given penicillin again. The nurse also teaches the patient/client and family about the allergy and specific drugs to avoid.

Preventive nursing actions are used to meet the therapeutic goals of the patient/client. Through preventive actions the nurse is able to help the patient/client attain the highest possible degree of health.

## TECHNIQUES AND PROCEDURES

The administration of nursing care requires the nurse to be experienced in many **techniques**, such as administering medications, changing patients'/clients' dressings, or inserting urinary catheters. These techniques should be based on principles of safe practice. Patient/client care, both in the hospital and community, involves many techniques. Each intervention the nurse undertakes for the patient/client is carried out with a regard principles of safety.

To carry out a nursing intervention, the nurse must be knowledgeable about it, know when it is needed, its steps, and the expected outcome. In a hospital the nurse is required to complete many nursing interventions each day. Some of these nursing interventions might be new, so before entering into a new nursing intervention the nurse assesses personal competencies and determines the need for assistance, new knowledge, or new skills.

## LIFESAVING MEASURES

A **lifesaving measure** is implemented when a patient's/client's physiological or psychological state is threatened. The purpose of the lifesaving measure is to prevent death by restoring physiological or psychological equilibrium. Such measures include: administering emergency medications, instituting cardiopulmonary resuscitation, retrieving a wandering person, calming a violent patient/client, and obtaining immediate counselling for someone who is severely anxious.

The initiation of lifesaving measures is an essential component of nursing practice. As with any procedure, the nurse must be knowledgeable about the lifesaving procedure itself, when it is necessary, its steps, and its expected outcome. If an inexperienced nurse finds him or herself in a situation requiring emergency measures, the proper nursing action is to find an experienced professional.

## Providing Nursing Care to Achieve Goals

The nurse achieves the care goals by providing an environment conducive to meeting such goals; adjusting care in accordance with patients'/clients' expressed or implied needs; stimulating and motivating patients/clients, enabling them to achieve self-care and independence, and encouraging them to accept care or adhere to the treatment regimen. For each nursing intervention, the nurse and patients/clients work together to meet the goals they developed. With some interventions, the nurse assumes a more active role, and with others a more passive one.

## Creating an Appropriate Environment

Nurses can create an environment conducive to achieving the patient's/client's goals. Ideally, the nurse develops an environment that provides the individual with adequate privacy for meeting basic needs and that allows him or her to feel safe and free to interact with the health care team. An early step in creating an appropriate environment is to show patients/clients and families around the ward/department. If it is a hospital, patients/clients need to be shown to their rooms, shown how the call bell works, and introduced to other patients/clients and the care team. Patients/clients in clinics should be shown the location of restrooms and cafeterias. When a patient/client receives care in the home, the nurse should take time to acquaint the individual and his or her family with the purposes and expectations of the home visits.

## Providing Privacy

Whether patients/clients are in the hospital, outpatient clinic, or a community setting, the nurse takes measures to provide privacy. Obviously, patients/clients need privacy to carry out activities of hygiene, grooming, and elimination. In addition, they need privacy to talk with families, friends, or members of the health care team. In an environment of privacy, patients/clients feel free to share concerns, ask questions about illness and treatment, and resolve personal problems.

## Providing Flexibility in the Care Plan

Although nursing care and other therapeutic measures are designed to meet the patient's/client's needs, the nursing care plan should include some flexibility so that the individual is not placed into a fixed routine. Obviously, the degree of flexibility depends on the nature of the need, the severity of the patient's/client's disability or illness and dependence on nursing care, and the needs of other patients/clients. However, even the smallest degree of flexibility, giving the patient/client an opportunity to have some choice about the type or timing of nursing care, is valuable.

## Encouraging Independence

Patients'/clients' with chronic diseases should be encouraged to increase their levels of self-care and independence, a difficult task often disheartening for them and the nurse. To avoid discouraging patients/clients, it is best to attempt to achieve this nursing goal gradually. The care plan is implemented so that patients/clients successfully achieve one level of independence before attempting the next. This step-by-step approach is the most effective.

## Encouraging Compliance to the Care Plan

People with chronic diseases are frequently on regimens that require adherence to methods of treatment. **Patient compliance** means that patients/clients and families must invest time in carrying out the required home treatments. For example, a diabetic person must take medication regularly, eat the recommended diet, and test blood and urine as requested (Lay, 1989). Some treatment plans include the need for the patient/client and family to adjust to functional changes as a result of medications. For example, a patient/client with high blood pressure treated with atenolol occasionally feels increasingly fatigued during the early stages of treatment, or a patient/client with cancer who is undergoing chemotherapy has changes in energy level and body image as a result of the medication.

Adherence to treatment plans can also require an increased financial investment by the patient/client and family. For example, for a patient/client who has cardiac disease, a two-story house may no longer be suitable because the person is unable to climb stairs without feeling short of breath. The individual and family must decide whether or not to move to a new house.

Investments of time, money, and personal resources for a long period of time can be discouraging. The discouraged patient/client may neglect the treatment regimen. After the person begins to default, his or her health may decline.

Patient/client compliance is a thorny issue. The reality of the situation is that in some cases individuals choose to reject advice and/or nursing intervention. It is the right of any individual to do so, and this right must be respected despite personal beliefs. This does not mean that support should be withdrawn.

## HELPING PATIENTS/CLIENTS ADHERE TO THE CARE PLAN

Nurses advise the following actions to intervene and assist the person in adhering to a treatment plan:

- provide adequate discharge planning and education of the patient/client and family to help promote a smooth transition from one health care setting to another or to the home. This also helps increase the patient's/client's level of knowledge about the treatment plan.
- provide counselling to help the patient/client and family adapt to change resulting from the disease process or treatment.
- provide continuity of care as much as possible to provide a supportive professional who is familiar with the patient's/client's pattern of living, pattern of health and illness, and treatment.
- reinforce successes with the treatment plan to encourage the patient/client to keep to the regimen.

The nurse who develops the care plan may not perform all of the nursing care. Some may be delegated to another member of the health care team. The nurse delegating tasks is responsible for ensuring that each task is assigned to an individual skilled in it. The nurse is also responsible for ensuring that the delegated task is completed according to the standard of care.

## EVALUATION

The evaluation component of the nursing process attempts to measure the patient's/client's response to nursing actions and the patient's/client's progress towards achieving goals (Fig. 3-12). Evaluation is ongoing and occurs when the nurse has contact with a patient/client. The emphasis is on patient/client goals. The nurse evaluates whether the patient's/client's behaviours or responses reflect a change in his or her condition which signifies the resolution of a problem. During evaluation, the nurse may judge the success of the previous steps of the nursing process by examining the patient's/client's responses and comparing them with the behaviours stated in the goals.

### Dynamics of Evaluating the Nursing Process

While caring for patients/clients, the nurse compares observed results (for example, reduction in pain symptoms, improved knowledge of illness, alteration in physiological indications, and proper use of equipment by the patient/client) with expected goals. **Critical thinking** is required to analyse the findings of evaluative measures; for example, when evaluating a patient/client for a change in blood pressure and pulse, the nurse must apply knowledge of disease processes and physiological responses to interpret whether a change has indeed occurred. **Positive evaluations** occur when desired results are met, leading the nurse to conclude that the care plan effectively met patient/client goals. **Negative evaluations** or undesired results indicate that the

problem was not resolved, that initial goals were inappropriate, or that potential problems were not avoided. As a result, the nurse must change the care plan, and the entire nursing process sequence is repeated.

This sequence continues until problems are resolved. The nurse must realize that evaluation is dynamic and ever-changing, depending on the patient's/client's problems and condition. A patient/client whose condition continuously changes requires more frequent evaluation. In addition, priority problems are often evaluated first. For example, a nurse evaluates a patient's/client's acute pain before evaluating a knowledge deficit.

### Evaluating Goal Achievement

One purpose of nursing care is to assist the patient/client in resolving actual health problems, preventing the occurrence of potential problems, and maintaining a healthy state. Evaluating goals may aid in determining whether this purpose was accomplished. The nurse matches the patient's/client's behaviour (for example, self-administration of insulin, or relief of anxiety) or physiological response (for example, decrease in size of pressure ulcer, or fall in body temperature) with the behaviour or response specified in the goal. The initial assessment of a patient/client provides the baseline data to be used for comparison. For example, during assessment of a patient/client who has just had a broken leg set, the person may report acute pain, rate the pain 8 on a scale of 10 (see Chapter 27), and grimace during attempts to move in bed. This baseline is used by the nurse to identify the problem of pain and establish the goal, 'this patient/client will be able to move in bed without pain in 24 hrs'. One outcome may include the patient/client being able to verbalize pain as 3 on a scale of 10. After nursing actions are performed, the nurse reassesses the patient/client by measuring the subjective report of pain and observing facial expressions. The new data are compared

| DATE | CONTINUOUS EVALUATION | NURSE'S SIGNATURE |
|---|---|---|
| 02.12.94 | Mrs Jones is drinking well. She is able to drink 100 mls per hour prefering cold water and cups of tea. Mrs Jones has drunk 600 mls this morning. Mrs Jones says her mouth is less sore and much more comfortable. Her tongue is cleaner and mouth generally moist and pink, but still feels dry without mouthwash. Lips remain cracked. Urine output 350mls this morning, remains dark and concentrated. Specific gravity 1040. | E. Fielding |
| | | |
| | | |
| | | |
| | | |
| | | |

**Fig 3-12** A sample of the evaluation section from a care plan

with set goals to determine whether predicted changes have occurred. To evaluate objectively the degree of success in achieving a goal, use the following steps:

1. **Examine** the goal statement to identify the desired patient/client behaviour or response.
2. **Assess** the patient/client for the presence of that behaviour or response.
3. **Compare** the established outcome criteria with the behaviour or response.
4. **Judge** the degree of agreement between set goals and the behaviour or response.

There are different degrees of **goal attainment**. If the patient's/client's response matches or exceeds the outcome criteria, the goal is met. If the patient's/client's behaviour begins to show changes but does not yet meet specified criteria, the goal is partially met. If there is no progress, the goal is not met. A clearly defined goal with specific outcomes is easily measured.

## Evaluative Measures and Sources

Evaluative measures include the assessment skills and instruments used to collect data for evaluation. For example, observing a patient/client changing his or her stoma appliance, inspecting the skin, and inquiring about the severity of pain are all evaluative measures. The new data collected from evaluation measures are critically analysed and compared with expected goals to ascertain whether changes have occurred. After caring for a patient/client over a period of time, the nurse is able to make subtle comparisons of responses and behaviours. The accuracy of any evaluation improves when the nurse is familiar with the patient's/client's behaviour and physiological status.

The primary source of data for evaluation is the patient/client. However, the nurse also uses the family and other care givers. The importance of documentation and reporting in the evaluation process is critical. The written nursing progress notes and information shared between nurses during change-of-shift reports (see Chapter 5) should communicate a patient's/client's progress towards meeting planned goals. Each member of the health care team should have an idea of how the patient/client is progressing. Each nurse summarizes data on an ongoing basis to ensure that the person is progressing towards an improved state of health.

## Goals

A goal specifies the behaviour or response that indicates resolution of a patient/client problem or achievement of a healthy state. It is a summary statement of what is to be accomplished when all care has been delivered. Each patient/client problem in the care plan has a goal, and every goal has a time frame for evaluation. The nurse evaluates goals after comparing evaluative findings with the expected behaviour or response stated in the goal. When a goal has been accomplished, the nurse knows that interventions have been successful and that the patient/client is progressing.

As a result of hospital stays becoming shorter, many patients are now being discharged prior to the fulfilment of all goals and the resolution of all problems. When preparing a patient for discharge, appropriate revisions to the care plan are made for home or follow-up care. The nurse must clearly distinguish between goals that have been met and goals that require continued intervention. The liaison or community nurse will probably adapt the interventions to the patient's/client's home.

## Revising a Care Plan

After goals have been evaluated, adjustments to the care plan are made as indicated. If a goal was successfully met, that portion of the care plan is discontinued. Unmet and partially met goals require the nurse to repeat the nursing process sequence. After reassessment, modification or addition of patient/client problems, goals and interventions are made as needed. The nurse also redefines priorities.

## Discontinuing a Care Plan

After determining that goals have been achieved, wherever possible, the nurse confirms this evaluation with the patient/client. If both agree that the goals have been met, the nurse discontinues that portion of the care plan.

Goal achievement must be promptly documented and reported. This ensures that other nurses will not unnecessarily continue a care plan. Significant time is wasted when achieved goals are not communicated.

## Modifying a Care Plan

When goals are unmet, evaluation involves identifying the variables or factors that interfered with goal achievement. A care plan might be altered if the initial assessment was inappropriate or incomplete, or if there is a change in the patient's/client's condition, needs, or abilities. For example, when teaching self-administration of insulin, the nurse may discover that the patient/client has a literacy problem or a visual impairment that prevents the reading of insulin dosages on the syringe. As a result, original outcomes cannot be met. Thus, the nurse uses new interventions and revises outcomes to meet the goal of care.

Lack of goal achievement may also result from an error in nursing judgement or failure to follow each step of the nursing process. Patients/clients frequently have very complex problems. The nurse should always remember the possibility of overlooking or misjudging something. When a goal is not achieved, irrespective of the reason why, the entire nursing sequence is repeated to discover changes that need to be made to promote, maintain, or restore the patient's/client's health.

During evaluation, the nurse may determine that some planned interventions are designed for an inappropriate level of nursing care. If the level of care needs to be changed, a different action verb, such as *assist* rather than *provide*, may be substituted. Sometimes the level of care is appropriate, but the interventions are unsuitable because of a change in the expected outcome. In this case, the interventions should be discontinued, and new ones planned.

During care delivery, the nurse evaluates the patient's/client's response during and immediately after intervention. This is the beginning of the evaluation process. Evaluation must be integrated with ongoing nursing care activity. If the response is favourable, care continues. Re-evaluation occurs when the intervention proves unsuccessful. The nurse then examines the other components of nursing care, such as preparation of the patient/client and the environment, anticipated complications, or the use of personal or technical skills during care delivery (Hickey, 1991).

Changes in care should be guided by the nature of the patient's/client's unfavourable response. Consulting with other nurses may yield suggestions for improving the approach to care delivery. Senior nurses are often excellent resources because of their experience. Simply changing the care plan is not enough. The nurse must implement the new plan and re-evaluate the patient's/client's response to the nursing actions. Evaluation is continuous.

Occasionally, an error during care planning and delivery is discovered during evaluation. This should be anticipated. The nursing process is designed to be a systematic, problem-solving approach to individualized patient/client care, but there is a wide array of variables for each patient/client with a health care problem. Patients/clients with the same health care problem are not treated the same. Consequently, the nurse sometimes makes errors in judgement. The systematic use of evaluation provides a way for nurses to catch these errors in judgement. The nurse consistently incorporates evaluation into practice to minimize error and ensure that the most appropriate interventions are used.

Evaluation is the final step of the nursing process, a systematic method for organizing and delivering nursing care. The exclusion of evaluation from the nursing process prevents the nurse from evaluating nursing practice and determining whether the outcomes of patient/client care are beneficial. The regular application of evaluation ensures that a patient's/client's care plan is current and appropriate.

### Re-evaluating Care

Using assessment data, nurses evaluate their nursing care. If results exceed or meet the threshold, no problem has been identified. When thresholds for satisfactory care have not been met, nurses must attempt to determine the cause of problems. For example, you may set a threshold of 100% of patients having intact skin after hip surgery. When only 90% of patients meet that goal, you must determine the reasons for this. This step requires you to honestly review practice activities and look for opportunities to reinforce nursing care standards or improve practice.

### Resolving Problems

After evaluating the success in meeting established quality indicators, develop an action plan to resolve any problems. It is important to establish actions that will result in success. For example, the action of merely notifying staff that a problem exists is unlikely to change practice or improve outcomes. An action plan should be more direct. In-service seminars, revision of assessment tools, or creation of standard nursing protocols are examples of specific action steps that nurses can recommend.

### Quality Assurance

Another aspect of evaluation involves measurement of the quality of nursing care provided in a health care setting and the quality of nursing care for a patient/client. **Quality assurance** (QA) is an ongoing, systematic, comprehensive evaluation of health care services and the impact of those services on health care consumers (see Chapter 2). The emphasis is on patient/client goals and the care givers and the systems in which they practice. Legal criteria and professional standards (see panel overleaf) are often used to evaluate the quality of care. Evaluation of nursing activities can help determine the types of nursing actions performed and the level of success in achieving patient/client goals. It also helps ensure quality professional nursing practice.

### Evaluating Improvement

After implementing an action plan to improve quality of care, re-evaluate the success of the plan. Remonitoring of quality indicators will reveal whether change has occurred. The change may be positive or negative. For example, if the incidence of skin breakdown for patients/clients who have had total hip replacements decreases from previous measures, nurses have successfully improved outcomes. Similarly, if the incidence worsens during the next monitoring period, a new plan of action is needed. When desired outcomes (QA criteria) are not met, nurses reinstitute the QA process.

The results of QA activities must be communicated to other nurses and appropriate organizational departments. If findings and results are not communicated, it is unlikely that practice changes will be incorporated by all staff members. Revision of policies and procedures, modification of standards of care, or implementation of system changes are examples of the ways that an organization may respond to quality issues.

Incorporating a QA programme within a health care setting benefits:
- the patient/client – with a focus on patient/client outcomes, QA activities will lead to a selection of interventions that result in improved patient/client care.
- the professional staff – staff members learn from their own practice, identify opportunities to change practice, and gain greater satisfaction from improved patient/client outcomes.
- the organization – organizations benefit from an improved level of care delivery that reduces excessive use of resources and improves patient/client satisfaction with services.

## SUMMARY

The nurse must consult with senior colleagues to ensure that the care he or she delivers is appropriate. If the care procedure is unfamiliar to the nurse, or he or she is otherwise inexperienced, then help and guidance should be sought, in order that the patient's/client's safety is maintained.patient's/client's nursing care plan, which is based on the assessment data and the patient's/client's identified problems or needs.

The planning component results in the development of patient/client-centred goals, which detail the selected nursing interventions and the appropriate evaluation criteria for each

### Standards of Care

The Royal College of Nursing has been actively involved in establishing practice standards for a variety of patient/client groups. Standards of Care documents (available from the RCN) have been developed in conjunction with other professional and specialist groups for each area. The purpose of these documents is to provide general guidelines to help practitioners develop local care standards, and identify specific values and beliefs that are essential to providing and delivering good nursing care to these patient/client groups.

patient/client. The student nurse learns the process of planning care in the educational and the clinical settings. Although the format of the care plan varies from one educational institution to another, and from one health care setting to another, the student nurse will encounter student care plans and the institutional care plan throughout the educational process.

Planning nursing care involves a cognitive and written process. The student learns to solve a patient's/client's health care problems by selecting appropriate nursing interventions. In addition, the student learns to communicate the patient's/client's health care needs through the written care plan. Individual care plans are the result of the nurse's knowledge and expertise, as well as the knowledge and expertise gained through consulting colleagues.

During implementation, the nurse initiates and carries out the objectives of the nursing care plan. These strategies are designed to accomplish the goals set out in the nursing care plan. Where appropriate, the patient's/client's condition is reassessed. The care plan is then adapted in response to any change in the patient/client.

The evaluation process determines the effectiveness of the nursing care plan and offers nurses the information needed to ensure optimum patient/client outcomes. A systematic process of evaluation requires the nurse to use critical thinking when comparing expected outcomes with actual results. When the individual's goals have been achieved, he or she will have reached an improved level of health. If goals are unmet, the nurse analyses the cause and re-establishes a more appropriate care plan.

However, Marks-Maran (1992) emphasizes the importance of moving away from viewing nursing as a series of tasks, or as stages of the nursing process, towards a vision of nursing as a way of thinking, doing and being. She emphasizes the shift from doing (reacting) to thinking, being and doing (proacting), and from taking care (control) of patients/clients towards partnership.

## CHAPTER 3 REVIEW
### Key Concepts

- The nursing process is a method for organizing and delivering nursing care.
- Organization of the nursing process is based on four components: assessment, planning, implementation, and evaluation.
- During assessment, the nurse gathers, verifies, and communicates data about a patient/client.
- Objective data can be measured by the data collector, but subjective data are the patient's/client's or family's perceptions.
- The interviewer identifies the patient's/client's needs, risk factors, and specific changes in level of wellness and pattern of living.
- During the planning component, patient/client goals are determined, priorities are established, nursing interventions are selected, and a nursing care plan is written.
- In general, care plans include the patient's/client's problems and goals and specific actions by the nurse.
- The care plan is a written guideline for patient/client care so that the care given can be quickly understood by all members of the health care team.
- The care plan increases communication among nurses and facilitates the continuity of care from one health care setting to another.
- Care plans become part of a patient's/client's medical record.
- Correctly written nursing interventions include actions, frequency, quantity, method, and the person to perform them.
- Implementation requires the nurse to **reassess** the patient/client, **review** and possibly **modify** the existing care plan, identify areas in which assistance is needed, **implement** nursing interventions, and **communicate** nursing actions.
- After implementation, the nurse writes in the patient's/client's record a brief description of the nursing assessment, specific procedures, and the patient's/client's response to nursing care.
- Nursing actions to achieve therapeutic goals include compensation for adverse reactions, preventive measures, correct techniques for administering care, preparing the patient/client for procedures, and lifesaving measures.
- Nursing actions that contribute to the attainment of health care goals include providing a conducive environment, adjusting care to fit the patient's/client's needs, and stimulating and motivating the patient/client.
- Delegating care to other personnel involves ensuring that the individuals are skilled in the tasks and evaluating that each task was completed according to the standard of care.
- Evaluation determines a patient's/client's response to nursing actions and the extent to which goals of care have been met.
- The nurse compares the patient's/client's response to nursing actions with expected outcomes established during planning.
- Assessment data gathered during evaluation determine the need to revise and modify the care plan.
- Evaluation enables the nurse to ascertain the reason why the care plan was successful or unsuccessful.
- Evaluation involves critical thinking because the nurse determines the optimal way to deliver nursing care.

## CRITICAL THINKING EXERCISES

1. During the initial phase of assessment, you observe that your patient/client seems reluctant to answer your questions. What information do you need to understand this reluctance? What can you do to increase the patient's/client's comfort? What

changes might you make in your interview style?

2. You are assigned to provide health care to a three-generation family in your community. How do you modify your assessment tool to obtain all data for each developmental level and to assess for environmental factors that influence health promotion?

3. What skills/abilities does a junior nurse need in order to successfully write a care plan?

4. A nurse's responsibility is to plan for a patient's/client's discharge from a health care setting. Other carers, such as social workers and physiotherapists, participate in a discharge plan. Describe how goals facilitate discharge planning.

## Key Terms

Assessment, p. 38
Associate nurse, p. 36
Confidentiality, p. 42
Core Care Plan, p. 47
Evaluative measures, p. 65
Holistic care, p. 39
Implementation, p. 58
Named nurse, p.36
Nursing diagnosis, p. 46
Nursing documentation, p. 47
Nursing intervention, p. 38
Paient/client allocation, p. 36
Patient-partnership, p. 57
Planning, p. 55
Primary nursing, p. 36
Quality assurance, p. 67
Short-/long-term goals, p. 55
Student care plan, p. 54
Task allocation, p. 36
Team nursing, p. 36

## REFERENCES

Argyle EM: *The psychology of interpersonal behaviour ed 3*, Harmondsworth, 1978, Penguin.

Benner P: *From novice to expert: excellence and power in clinical nursing practice*, Menlo Park, Calif, 1984, Addiston-Wesley.

Crosby C: Method in mouth care, *Nurs Times* 85(35):38, 1989.

Daeffler R: Oral hygiene measures for patients with cancer, *Cancer Nurs* 4:29, 1981.

De La Cuesta C: The nursing process: from development to implementation, *J Adv Nurs* 8(8):365, 1983.

DOH (Department of Health): *The patient's charter*, London, 1992, HMSO.

GNC (General Nursing Council): *A statement for educational policy, circular 77/19/A*, London, 1977, GNC.

Gordon MG: *Nursing diagnosis: process and application*, ed 5, St Louis, 1994, Mosby.

Henderson V: *The nature of nursing*, New York, 1966, Macmillan.

Heron J: *Six category intervention analysis*, University of Surrey, Human Potential Resource Group, 1975.

Hickey PW: *Nursing process handbook*, St Louis, 1990, Mosby.

Kratz CR: *The nursing process*, London, 1979, Balliere Tindall.

Ley P: Improving patients' understanding, recall, satisfaction and compliance. In Broome A, editor: *Health psychology*, London, 1989, Chapman & Hall.

Manthey M *et al*: Primary nursing: a return to the concept of 'my nurse' and 'my patient', *Nurs Forum* 9(1):65, 1970.

Manthey M: *The practice of primary nursing*, Boston, 1980, Blackwell Scientific.

Marks-Maran D: Rethinking the nursing process. In Jolley M, Brykcyznska G: *Nursing care: the challenge to change*, London, 1992, Edward Arnold.

Mason G, Webb C: Nursing diagnosis: a review of the literature, *J Clin Nurs* 2:67, 1993.

Menzies EP: *The functioning of social systems as a defence against anxiety*, London, 1960, Tavistock.

Mortensen M, McMullin C: Discharge score for surgical outpatients, *Am J Nurs* 88:1347, 1986.

Pearson A: *The clinical nursing unit*, London, 1983, Heinemann.

Pearson A: Trends in clinical nursing. In Pearson A, editor: *Primary nursing*, London, 1988, Croom Helm.

Peplau HE: *Interpersonal relations in nursing*, New York, 1952, Putnam.

Redman BK: *The process of patient education*, ed 6, St Louis,1988, Mosby.

Roper N, Logan WW, Tierney AJ: *The elements of nursing*, ed 2, London, 1988, Churchill Livingstone.

Snyder M: *Independent nursing interventions*, New York, 1985, John Wiley & Sons.

Steele SM, Harmon VM: *Values clarification in nursing*, Norwalk, Conn, 1983, Appleton-Century-Crofts.

Stockwell F: *The unpopular patient*, London, 1972, Royal College of Nursing.

Sundeen SJ *et al*: *Nurse/client interaction: implementing the nursing process*, St Louis, ed 5, 1994, Mosby.

Tranterrorth P, Creason N: Nurse administered oral hygiene: is there a scientific basis? *J Adv Nurs* 11:323, 1986.

UKCC (United Kingdom Central Council): *Code of Professional Conduct*, 1992, UKCC.

Walsh M: Model example, *Nurs Standard* 22(3):22, 1989.

Walton I: *The nursing process in perspective: a literature review*, York, 1986, University of York.

Waters K: Organizing nursing care: team nursing, *Nurs Practice* 1(1):7, 1985.

Watson R: Care of the mouth, *Nursing* 3(44):22, 1989.

Webb C: Nursing diagnosis - or two steps back, *Nurs Times* 88(7):33, 1992.

Yura H, Walsh MB: *The nursing process*, ed 5, Conn, 1988, Appleton and Lange.

## FURTHER READING
### Adult Nursing

Beckman JS: What is a standard of practice: *J Nurs Qual Assur* 1(2):1, 1987.

Bower FL: *The process of planning nursing care*, St Louis, 1983, Mosby.

Brown JJ, Fanner CA, Padrick KP: Nursing's search for scientific knowledge, *Nurs Res* 33:26, 1984.

Given B *et al*: Relationships of processes of care to patient outcomes, *Nurs Res* 28(2):85, 1979.

Hegyvary ST: Issues in outcomes research, *J Nurs Qual Assur* 5(2):1, 1991.

Hunt J, Marks-Maran D: *Nursing Care plans: the nursing process at work*, Chichester 1986, Wiley.

Iyer PW, Taptich BJ, Bernocchi-Losey D: *Nursing process and nursing diagnosis*, Philadelphia, 1986, Saunders.

Lillesand KM, Korff S: Nursing process evaluation: a quality assurance tool, *Nurs Adm Q* 7(3):9, 1983.

Marek KD: Outcome measurement in nursing, *J Nurs Qual Assur* 4(1):1, 1989.

Marriner A: *The nursing process: a scientific approach to nursing care*, ed 4, St Louis, 1987, Mosby.

Peters DA, Pearlson J: Clinical evaluation: research for quality assurance, *J Nurs Qual Assur* 3(3)1, 1989.

Potter PA: An assessment tool for developing quality indicators, *J Nurs Care Qual* 6(1):30, 1991.

Sanborn CW, Blount M: Standard plans for care and discharge, *Am J Nurs* 84:1394, 1984.

Schroeder P: Directions and dilemmas in nursing quality assurance, *Nurs Clin North Am* 23(3):657, 1988.

United Kingdom Central Council: *A guide for students of nursing and midwifery,* London, 1992, UKCC.

Williams AD: Development and application of clinical indicators for nursing, *J Nurs Care Qual* 6(1):1, 1991.

## Children's Nursing

Bishop J: Sharing the caring, *Nurs Times* 84(33):60, 1988.

Casey A: A partnership with child and family, *Sen Nurs* 8(4):8, 1988.

Jay P: Paediatric intensive care – involving parents in the care of their child, *Matern Child Nurs J* 2:195, 1977.

Lewer J, Robinson H: *Care of the child,* London, 1983, Macmillan.

Muller D *et al: Nursing children – psychology, research and practice,* ed 2, London, 1992, Chapman & Hall.

Nelson L, Beckel J, editors: *Nursing care plans for the pediatric patient,* St Louis, 1987, Mosby.

Sainsbury C *et al:* Care by parents of their children in hospital, *Arch Dis Child* 61:612, 1986.

Speer E: *Pediatric care plans,* Pennsylvania, 1990, Springhouse.

White A, editor: *Caring for children,* London, 1991, Edward Arnold.

## Learning Disabilities Nursing

Blunden R *et al: Planning with individuals: an outline guide,* 1987, Cardiff Mental Handicap in Wales - Applied Research Unit.

Brown H, Smith H eds: *Normalisation: the reader for the nineties,* London, 1992, Tavistock/Routledge.

Flemming I, Tosh M: Going for goals (Nursing process and goal planning in the care of the mentally handicapped), *Nursing Mirror* 160, 15 (5): 42-45, 1985.

Shanley E, Starrs TA: *Learning disabilities: a handbook of care ed 2,* Edinburgh, 1993, Churchill Livingstone.

## Mental Health Nursing

Dalley G: *Ideologies of caring,* London, 1988, Macmillan.

Dickers A: Care management in Britain and America: a comparison, *Comm Psychiatr Nurs J*:12, 1993.

Loomis ME: Levels of contracting, *J Psychosoc Nurs* 23(3):9, 1985.

Robertson K: Unconditional discharge? *Nurs Times* 88(43):30, 1992.

Stockwell F: *The nursing process in psychiatric nursing,* London, 1985, Croom Helm.

Sundeen SJ *et al: Nurse-client interaction: implementing the nursing process,* ed 5, St Louis, 1994, Mosby.

Thomas A: No room for change, *Nurs Times* 89(16):34, 1993.

Ward M: *The nursing process in psychiatry ed 2,* Edinburgh, 1992, Churchill Livingstone.

# Health and Physical Assessment

## CHAPTER OUTLINE

Purposes of Physical Assessment

Integration of Physical Assessment with Nursing Care

Skills of Physical Assessment

Preparation for Examination

Organization of the Examination

Performing a General Survey

Guidelines for Taking Vital Signs

Body Temperature

Pulse

Respiration

Blood Pressure

Reporting and Recording Vital Signs

## LEARNING OUTCOMES

After studying this chapter, you should be able to:
- *Define the key terms listed.*
- *Discuss the purposes of the health assessment.*
- *Describe the techniques used with each health assessment skill.*
- *Make environmental preparations before an examination.*
- *List techniques used to promote the patient's/client's physical and psychological comfort during an examination.*
- *Identify information to collect from the nursing history before an examination.*
- *Discuss possible areas of patient/client assessment and suggest factors that may influence assessment findings.*
- *Discuss ways to incorporate health teaching into the examination.*
- *Conduct physical assessments correctly and in an organized fashion.*
- *Identify when vital signs should be taken.*
- *Discuss the rationale for a care plan for a patient/client with a fever.*
- *Identify steps used to assess oral, rectal, axillary, and tympanic membrane temperature.*
- *Explain the physiology for the normal regulation of temperature, blood pressure, pulse, and respirations.*
- *Identify steps used to assess pulse, respirations, and blood pressure.*
- *Identify normal vital sign values for an adult and an infant.*
- *Accurately record and report vital sign measurements.*

**H**ealth screenings involve measurement of specific physical functions or diagnostic tests to detect those individuals with a high probability of having a specific health care need (Larson, 1986). For example, blood pressure screenings detect the risk for high blood pressure. Information from health screening determines the need for more comprehensive examinations.

A complete **health assessment** involves a more detailed review of a patient's/client's condition. Using the accepted nursing model for the clinical area, the nurse collects a nursing history (see Chapter 3) and performs a behavioural and physical assessment. The health history involves an interview with the patient/client to gather subjective data about the individual's status. During the interview, the nurse can also make important observations about a patient's/client's status. The nurse uses the skills of physical assessment to make clinical judgements. The accuracy of a physical assessment influences the choice of therapies a patient/client receives and the determination of the response to those therapies. Continuity in health care improves when the nurse makes ongoing, objective, and comprehensive assessments.

During the physical assessment, the patient's/client's **vital signs** are recorded (temperature, pulse, respirations, and blood pressure). These are indicators of health. Many factors such as the temperature of the environment, physical activity, and the effects of illness cause vital signs to change, sometimes beyond a normal range. Measurement of vital signs provides data that can be used to determine a patient's/client's usual state of health (*baseline* *observations*), as well as the response to physical and psychological stress, and medical and nursing therapy. An alteration from normal may signal the need for medical or nursing intervention.

Measurement of vital signs is a routine part of the complete physical assessment. Vital signs may also be measured separately as a part of a review of the patient's/client's condition. Vital signs are a quick and efficient way of monitoring a condition or identifying the presence of problems. The basic skills required to measure vital signs are simple but should not be taken for granted. Vital signs and other physiological measurements can be the basis for clinical problem solving. Careful technique ensures accurate findings.

## PURPOSES OF PHYSICAL ASSESSMENT

The nurse uses physical assessment to:
- gather baseline data about the patient's/client's health
- supplement, confirm, or refute data obtained in the nursing history
- confirm and identify nursing analyses of patient's/client's health needs
- make clinical judgements about a patient's/client's changing health status and management
- evaluate the physiological outcomes of care.

Through the nursing history, the nurse initially gathers complete and detailed information about the patient's/client's health status. However, a person may be unaware of a physical problem, so a thorough assessment of physical status is necessary. Even if a history is complete, a physical assessment reveals information that refutes, confirms, or supplements information provided by the patients/clients or their relatives.

One assessment finding cannot conclusively reveal the nature of a health problem. In addition, each abnormal finding directs the nurse to gather additional information. Information gathered during an initial physical assessment provides a baseline of functional abilities. The baseline is not the normal range of physical findings, but rather the *pattern* of findings identified when the patient/client was first assessed. This baseline provides a comparison for future assessment findings. During a subsequent assessment, the nurse can determine whether changes in the patient's/client's condition have occurred.

### Developing Nursing Analyses and a Care Plan

Physical assessment is ongoing, and thus the care plan changes with the patient's/client's condition. The nurse monitors the individual's progress and responses to therapies, to review existing problems and to identify new problems.

Physical assessment skills allow you to judge the status of the patient's/client's health and direct the management of care. For example, you may inspect a person's skin during a bath and find it excessively dry; therefore, you do not use soap and you apply body lotion to the skin. You also revise the written care plan so that other nurses know the type of skin care to provide. Performing the mechanics of physical assessment is relatively simple. The more difficult challenge lies in using findings to make decisions.

### Evaluating Nursing Care

Physical assessment skills enhance the evaluation of nursing measures through monitoring physiological and behavioural outcomes of care. The same physical assessment skill used to assess a condition (for example, palpation of the patient's/client's pulse) can be used as an evaluation measure after care is administered (for example, an evaluation of a patient's/client's tolerance to an exercise plan). Physical assessment skills allow you to make accurate, detailed, objective measurements. The measurements determine whether the expected outcomes of care are met.

## INTEGRATION OF PHYSICAL ASSESSMENT WITH NURSING CARE

Whether a complete or partial physical assessment is performed, a physical examination should be integrated into routine care. For example, the nurse can assess the condition of the skin and other body parts during a bed bath. This practice allows more efficient use of time. Physical assessment should become automatic when nurse and patient/client interact. Physical assessment skills enable you to gather more comprehensive and relevant assessment findings.

## SKILLS OF PHYSICAL ASSESSMENT

This section provides a more detailed description of assessment skills and their application in the physical examination. In many situations, the nurse will be present when the doctor carries out a physical examination. Part of the nurse's role is to prepare the environment; however, more importantly, the nurse is present in order to support and provide information for the patient/client. Information gained by the doctor may be used by the nurse in identifying patient/client problems.

### Inspection

The nurse inspects or looks at body parts in order to detect normal characteristics or significant physical signs. An understanding of normal physical characteristics helps the nurse to distinguish abnormal findings. It is especially important to know normal characteristics of patients/clients of different ages. For example, dry, wrinkled, inelastic skin is normal in an older person, but not in a young adult. Experience is needed to recognize normal variations among patients/clients, as well as ranges of normal in an individual. **Inspection** is a simple technique, but it is often underused. For example, when hurrying to complete a bath, a nurse may fail to inspect all skin surfaces and thus overlook a rash under the patient's/client's arm. The quality of an inspection depends on the nurse's willingness to spend time doing a thorough job. To inspect body parts accurately, practice the following principles:

1. Make sure good lighting is available.
2. Position and expose body parts so that all surfaces can be viewed.
3. Inspect each area for size, shape, colour, symmetry, position, and abnormalities.
4. If possible, compare each area inspected with the same area on the opposite side of the body.
5. Use additional light (for example, a penlight) to inspect body cavities.

## Palpation

Once an inspection of a body part has been completed, findings may indicate further examination. **Palpation** is often used with or after visual inspection.

Further assessment of body parts is made through the sense of touch. The hands can make delicate and sensitive measurements of specific physical signs. Using different parts of the hand enables you to detect characteristics such as texture, temperature, and the perception of movement.

The most sensitive parts of the hand, the pads of the fingertips, are used to assess texture, shape, size, consistency, and pulsation. The patient's/client's temperature can be measured most effectively by using the dorsum or back of the hand and fingers, where the skin is thinnest. The palm of the hand is more sensitive to vibration. Position, consistency, and turgor are measured by lightly grasping the body part with the fingertips.

## Percussion

**Percussion** is a technique of tapping the body with the fingertips. The sound heard may be dull or resonant, according to the condition of the underlying organ. Percussion requires considerable skill. It is perhaps the least-used assessment skill; however, it can be very helpful in confirming other assessment findings. The nurse will often support the patient/client while the doctor uses this technique; for example, by helping the patient/client to sit forward. Through percussion, the location, size, and density of an underlying structure are determined. Percussion helps verify abnormalities reported from x-ray studies or assessed through palpation and auscultation.

## Auscultation

**Auscultation** entails listening to sounds created in body organs to detect variations from normal. Some sounds can be heard with the unassisted ear, although most sounds can be heard only through a stethoscope. You must first become familiar with the normal sounds created by the cardiovascular, respiratory, and gastrointestinal systems, such as the passage of blood through an artery. Abnormal sounds can be recognized only after normal variations are learned.

To auscultate correctly requires good hearing acuity, a good stethoscope, and knowledge of how to use the stethoscope properly. Nurses with hearing disorders should purchase stethoscopes with greater sound amplification or ask colleagues to check findings through auscultation.

Page 90 describes the parts of the acoustic stethoscope and the general use of the bell and diaphragm. The bell is best for low-pitched sounds, such as vascular and certain heart sounds, and the diaphragm is suitable for high-pitched sounds, such as bowel and lung sounds.

It is important to become familiar with the stethoscope before attempting to use it with a patient/client. It helps to practise using it with a friend. A number of extraneous sounds created by movement of the tubing or chestpiece interferes with auscultation. By deliberately producing these sounds, you can learn to recognize and disregard them during the actual examination.

## Smell

While assessing a patient/client, it is important to be familiar with the nature and source of body odours (Table 4-1). Sense of smell helps you detect abnormalities that cannot be recognized by any other means. For example, a patient/client with a plaster cast is expected to experience discomfort after an injury. However, if you note a strong odour, you will suspect that the discomfort may also be related to wound infection. The discomfort alone does not reveal the presence of infection. Findings from smell and other assessment skills allow you to detect serious abnormalities. If you notice an unfamiliar odour, a colleague may be able to identify the problem.

## PREPARATION FOR EXAMINATION

### Environment

A physical examination requires privacy. An examination room that is well equipped for all necessary procedures is preferable. However, often the examination occurs on the ward, where it may be necessary to use curtains or screens around the bed. In the home, the nurse may perform an examination in the patient's/client's bedroom.

Adequate lighting is needed for proper illumination of body parts. Ideally, an examination room should be soundproof so the patient/client feels comfortable discussing his or her condition. Eliminate sources of noise, such as televisions or radios, and take steps to prevent interruptions. The room should also be warm enough to maintain a comfortable environment.

Sometimes, it is difficult to perform a complete examination when the patient/client is in bed or on a stretcher. Special examination tables make patients/clients easily accessible and help them assume special positions. Because these tables are high and narrow, you must carefully assist the patient/client so that he or she does not fall while getting on and off. A confused, agitated, or uncooperative patient/client should not be left on an examination table without supervision.

Examination tables are often hard and uncomfortable. When the patient/client lies supine, the head of the table can be raised by about 30 degrees; a small pillow may also be provided. When examining an individual in bed, raise the bed to reach body parts more easily.

### TABLE 4-1 Assessment of Characteristic Odours

| Odour | Site or Source | Potential Causes |
|---|---|---|
| Alcohol | Oral cavity | Ingestion of alcohol |
| Ammonia | Urine | Urinary tract infection |
| Body odour | Skin, particularly in areas where body parts rub together (e.g., under arms, beneath breasts) | Poor hygiene, excess perspiration, foul-smelling perspiration |
| Faeces | Wound site<br>Vomitus<br>Rectal area | Wound abscess<br>Bowel obstruction<br>Faecal incontinence |
| Foul-smelling stools in infant | Stool | Malabsorption syndrome |
| Halitosis | Oral cavity | Poor dental and oral hygiene, gum disease |
| Sweet, fruity ketones | Oral cavity | Diabetes acidosis |
| Stale urine | Skin | Uraemic acidosis |
| Sweet, heavy, thick odour | Draining wound | Pseudomonas (bacterial) infection |
| Musty odour | Limb under plaster cast | Infection inside plaster cast |
| Fetid, sweet odour | Tracheostomy or mucous secretions | Infection of bronchial tree (Pseudomonas bacteria) |

## Equipment

Always wash your hands before preparing the equipment and before the examination. Handwashing reduces the transmission of microorganisms. The equipment needed will vary according to the parts of the body being examined and the purpose of the examination. Equipment should be readily available and arranged in order for easy use. Check all equipment to ensure it functions properly.

## Physical Preparation of the Patient/Client

The patient's/client's physical comfort is vital to the success of the examination. Before starting, ask if the patient/client needs to use the toilet. An empty bladder and bowel facilitate examination of the abdomen, genitalia and rectum, and provides the opportunity to collect urine or faecal specimens. Explain the proper method for collecting specimens, and ensure that each specimen is properly labelled.

**Physical preparation** also includes ensuring the patient/client is dressed and covered properly. If the examination is limited to certain body systems, it may be unnecessary for the patient/client to undress completely. It is essential to explain exactly how much clothing to remove and which way a gown should be worn. The patient/client should have privacy during undressing and plenty of time to finish. Walking into the room as the person is undressing causes embarrassment. Ensure that the patient/client stays warm by eliminating draughts, controlling room temperature, and providing warm blankets. Ask if the patient/client is comfortable.

## Positioning

During the examination, ask the patient/client to assume proper positions so that body parts are accessible and the patient/client remains comfortable. Table 4-2 (see p. 77) lists the preferred positions for each part of the examination. Patients'/clients' abilities to assume positions will depend on their physical strength and degree of wellness. Many of the positions, such as the lithotomy and knee-chest, are embarrassing and uncomfortable. Therefore, patients/clients should be kept in these positions for no longer than necessary. Explain the positions and assist the patient/client in attaining them. Adjust to ensure the area to be examined is accessible and no body part is unnecessarily exposed.

## Psychological Preparation of the Patient/Client

Patients/clients are easily embarrassed when asked to answer sensitive questions about bodily functions or when body parts are exposed and examined. The possibility that the examiner will find something abnormal also creates anxiety, so reduction of this anxiety may be the nurse's highest priority before the examination:

- provide a thorough explanation so the patient/client knows what to expect and what to do so that he or she can cooperate
- use simple terms when describing steps of the examination; complicated terminology confuses patients/clients and adds to their fears
- use a professional manner, but also use relaxed intonation and facial expressions to put the patient/client at ease
- during the examination, watch the patient's/client's emotional responses; for example whether his or her facial expression conveys fear or concern and whether body movements reveal anxiety (such as frequently pulling the covers around the body or tensing up as the examiner touches the body)
- remain calm and clearly explain each step of the assessment.

## ORGANIZATION OF THE EXAMINATION

A physical examination, using the skills of physical assessment, is composed of individual assessments for each body system. The extent of an examination depends on its purpose and on the patient's/client's condition. A person who comes to a clinic with symptoms of a severe chest cold will not routinely require a neurological assessment. An acutely ill person requires assessment of body systems most at risk for being abnormal. When a patient/client is admitted to the hospital, a complete examination is usually performed. People with specific symptoms or needs often require only portions of an examination.

## PERFORMING A GENERAL SURVEY

As soon as a nurse meets a patient/client, assessment begins. During the patient's/client's health history, make mental notes of the person's behaviour and appearance.

Begin the examination with a **general survey** that includes observation of general appearance and behaviour, taking vital signs, height, and weight measurements. If abnormalities are found, the affected body system is closely assessed later during the examination.

### General Appearance and Behaviour

Assessment of appearance and behaviour begins while the nurse prepares the patient/client for the examination. Information gained about general features may reveal characteristics of illness (for example, the facial appearance of a depressed patient/client). A review of general appearance and behaviour includes the following:

- **Gender and race**. A person's gender and cultural background affects the type of examination performed and the manner in which assessments are made.
- **Signs of distress**. There may be obvious signs or symptoms indicating a problem such as pain, difficulty in breathing or anxiety. These findings help to establish priorities regarding what to examine first.
- **Body type**. Observe whether a patient/client appears trim and muscular, obese or excessively thin. Body type can reflect level of health, age, and lifestyle.
- **Posture**. Normal standing posture is an upright stance with parallel alignment of hips and shoulders. Normal sitting posture involves some degree of rounding of the shoulders. Observe whether the patient/client has a slumped, erect, or bent posture. Posture may reflect mood or presence of pain.
- **Gait**. A person normally walks with arms swinging freely at the sides, with the head and face leading the body. Altered gait or uncoordinated movements can be a helpful indicator of health problems.
- **Body movements**. Observe whether movements are purposeful and note whether there are any tremors, weaknesses or lack of coordination. Also determine whether any body parts are immobile.

**Learning Disabilities Nursing**
**Physical examinations — special**
**considerations**

Undergoing a physical examination can be traumatic for anyone; irrespective of his or her mental ability. Nurses play a central role in ensuring that the necessary procedures are conducted in a manner that is as free of stress as is possible, and which maintains the privacy and dignity of the patient/client. Prior to a planned examination, the nurse must ensure that the patient/client with a learning disability is thoroughly prepared.

Verbal explanations of the procedure may not suffice for many individuals. Therefore, it may be necessary to familiarize the patient/client with the venue of the examination and the equipment to be used. Using pictures, photographs and role play may be useful components in this educative process.

Some doctors may not be familiar with the requirements of a person with learning disabilities; therefore, it is important for the nurse to be on hand before, during and after the physical examination in order to ensure:
- the patient/client fully understands the reasons for the examination
- that, if the individual refuses the examination, his or her withdrawal of real consent is recognized and respected (except in emergency, life threatening, situations)
- the patient/client is informed of the examination results in a manner that he or she can understand.

Similarly, patient's/client's parents or guardians may have difficulty understanding the purposes for, or results of, a specific examination. The nurse must be ready to offer sensible, jargon-free explanations of what is required in the patient's/client's interest.

A good example is that of a patient/client for whom a CAT scan is planned. The nurse should:
- show the patient/client the room where the scan will be conducted
- enable the patient/client to meet the specialist staff
- explain the procedure to him or her
- possibly allow the person to lie briefly in the machine and ask questions prior to the actual scan.

In the past, people with learning disabilities have often been subjected unnecessarily to invasive physical examinations which had no therapeutic value. As the patient's/client's advocate, the nurse can help reduce such incidents.

- **Age.** Age influences the normal features or physical characteristics. The ability to participate in some parts of the examination are also influenced by age.
- **Hygiene and grooming**. The patient's/client's level of cleanliness is noted by observing the appearance of the hair, skin, and fingernails. Note whether the person's clothes are clean. Grooming may depend on the activities being performed just before the examination.

- **Dress**. Culture, lifestyle, socioeconomic level, and personal preference affect the type of clothes worn. Note whether the type of clothing worn is appropriate for the temperature and weather conditions. A depressed or mentally ill person may be unable to choose proper clothing.
- **Body odour**. An unpleasant body odour may be the result of physical exercise. Poor hygiene may result in body odour, and poor oral hygiene may result in bad breath. A breath with the odour of alcohol does not always mean alcohol misuse.
- **Affect and mood**. Affect is a person's feelings as they appear to others. Mood or emotional state is expressed verbally and nonverbally. Note whether verbal expressions match nonverbal behaviour and whether the patient's/client's mood is appropriate for the situation. Observe facial expressions as questions are asked.
- **Speech**. Normal speech is understandable and moderately paced and shows an association with the person's thoughts. Note whether the patient/client talks rapidly or slowly. An abnormal pace may be caused by emotions or neurological impairment. Also observe whether the patient/client speaks in a normal tone with clear inflection of words.
- **Patient/client abuse**. The abuse or neglect of a child or older adult is becoming a serious problem. The nurse may suspect abuse while conducting a general survey. Additional assessment findings that may indicate abuse include the patient's/client's fear of the carer, parent, or child; the carer's history of violence, alcohol misuse, or drug abuse; evidence that the patient/client has suffered obvious physical injury or signs of neglect (for example, evidence of malnutrition); the carer's unemployment, illness, or frustration in caring for the person (Bennett, 1990; Royal College of Nursing, 1991).

Most nurses prefer to measure vital signs before the physical examination, because positioning or moving the patient/client during the examination can interfere with obtaining accurate values.

### Children's Nursing
### Assessing infants and children

- When obtaining histories on infants and children, gather all or part of the information from parents or guardians.
- Because parents may think they are being tested by the examiner, offer support during the examination and do not pass judgement.
- Ask the parents what they call their child, this may not necessarily be the first name on the notes, and ask the parents how they would like to be addressed.
- Use open-ended questions to allow parents to share more information and describe more of the child's problems.
- Interview older children, who can often provide details about their health history and severity of symptoms, and observe parent-child interactions.
- Treat adolescents as adults and individuals because they tend to respond best when treated as such.
- Remember that adolescents have the right to confidentiality. After talking with parents about historical information, speak alone with adolescents.

## Height and Weight

The general level of health can be reflected in the ratio of height to weight. Weight is a routine measure for patients/clients visiting doctors surgeries or clinics, and many health screenings routinely include height and weight. A nurse measures infants' and children's height and weight to assess growth and development. Before this measurement, the nurse asks patients/clients their height and weight. It may help to know their satisfaction or perceptions of body image. The nurse also determines whether they have had recent weight gains or losses. If a change exists, the nurse determines the amount, the period of time over which weight change occurred, and the cause, including

### Adult Nursing
### Assessing older adults

It is important to:
- assess what older people CAN do (not just what they cannot do)
- identify how they have coped in the past
- recognize that illness may manifest differently in older people (for example, infection will not necessarily produce pyrexia)
- understand that assessing how an older person functions may be more important than the impact of a particular disease process
- understand that normal ranges for vital signs change with age (eg, blood pressure, pulse, and temperature)
- understand that laboratory reference values change with age
- adjust the manner and pace of assessment interviews to acknowledge sight, hearing, and communication abilities of the older person.

### Mental Health Nursing
### Physical assessment of patients/clients in a mental health setting

During physical assessment, it is important to check for bruising and/or cuts. Evidence of bruising and/or cuts needs to be documented accurately on admission and further investigations may be needed to eliminate any possible internal injuries. Such evidence should also prompt the nurse to inquire whether injuries may be self-inflicted or whether the individual may have been subjected to physical abuse by someone else. Care must be exercised when questioning the patient/client on issues of abuse, as such matters are deeply personal and sensitive areas and the early stages of the nurse-patient/client encounter may not provide a safe enough environment for the individual to trust the nurse with such information.

## TABLE 4-2 Positions for Physical Examination

| Position | Areas Assessed | Rationale | Limitations |
|---|---|---|---|
| Sitting 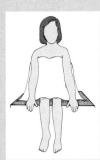 | Head and neck, back, posterior thorax and lungs, breasts, axillae, heart, vital signs, and upper extremities | Sitting upright provides full expansion of lungs and provides better visualization of symmetry of upper body parts. | Physically weakened patient/client may be unable to sit. Examiner should use supine position with head of bed elevated instead. |
| Supine 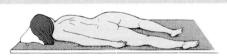 | Head and neck, anterior thorax and lungs, breasts, axillae, heart, abdomen, extremities, pulses | This is the most normally relaxed position. It prevents contracture of abdominal muscles and provides easy access to pulse sites. | If patient/client becomes short of breath easily, examiner may need to raise head of bed. |
| Dorsal recumbent 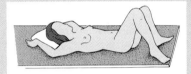 | Head and neck, anterior thorax and lungs, breasts, axillae, heart | Patients/clients with painful disorders are more comfortable with knees flexed. | Position is not used for abdominal assessment because it promotes contracture of abdominal muscles. |
| Lithotomy 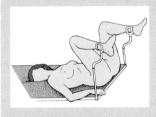 | Female genitalia and genital tract | This position provides maximal exposure of genitalia and facilitates insertion of vaginal speculum. | Lithotomy position is embarrassing and uncomfortable, so examiner minimizes time that patient/client spends in it. Patient/client is kept well draped. Patient/client with severe arthritis or other joint deformity may be unable to assume this position. |
| Sims' 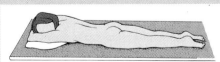 | Rectum and vagina | Flexion of hip and knee improves exposure of rectal area. | Joint deformities may hinder patient's/client's ability to bend hip and knee. |
| Prone 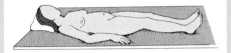 | Musculoskeletal system | This position is used only to assess extension of hip joint. | This position is intolerable for patient/client with respiratory difficulties. |
| Knee-chest 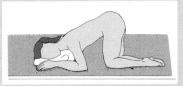 | Rectum | This position provides maximal exposure of rectal area. | This position is embarrassing and uncomfortable. Patients/clients with arthritis or other joint deformities may be unable to assume this position. |

change in diet habits, appetite, or physical symptoms (for example, nausea). A sudden loss in weight may indicate serious disease or a major change in dietary habits. It is normal for a person's weight to vary each day because of fluid loss or retention.

Patients/clients should be weighed at the same time of day, on the same scale, and in the same clothes to allow an objective comparison of subsequent weights. Individuals capable of bearing their own weight use a standing scale.

Infants can be weighed in baskets or on platform scales. Remove clothing and nappies to ensure accurate readings. The room should be warm to prevent chills. A light cloth or paper placed on the scale's surface helps prevent cross-infection.

Different techniques exist for measuring the height of weight-bearing and non weight-bearing patients/clients. Individuals who are able to stand remove their shoes. A measuring stick or tape is attached vertically to the weight scales or wall. Ask the person to stand erect, exercising good posture. On a standing scale, a metal rod, which is attached to the back of the scale, swings out and over the top of the head.

A non weight-bearing patient/client is positioned supine on a firm surface. The legs are extended straight with the soles of the feet supported upright. Place a tape measure from the soles of the feet to the vertex of the head to measure the recumbent length. Patients/clients who are unable to stand can be weighed in a sitting position.

## Integument

The skin or *integumentary system* provides the body's external protection, regulates body temperature, and acts as a sensory organ for pain, temperature, and touch. Assessment of the integument includes the skin, hair, scalp, and nails. The nurse may initially inspect all skin surfaces or may assess the skin gradually while other body systems are examined.

A large proportion of hospitalized patients are debilitated or elderly. Consequently, there are significant risks for skin lesions resulting from trauma to the skin while administering care, for exposure to pressure during immobilization, or for reaction to the various medications used in treatment. Nurses must routinely assess the skin to look for primary or initial lesions that may develop. Without proper care, primary lesions can quickly deteriorate to become secondary lesions that require more extensive nursing care. The development of a pressure ulcer, for example, can lengthen a hospital stay unless it is prevented or discovered early and treated properly (see Chapter 30). Use assessment findings to determine the type of hygiene measures required to maintain integrity of the integument (see Chapter 25). Adequate nutrition and hydration become goals of therapy if the nurse identifies alterations in the integument's status (see Chapter 21). To assess the integument, use inspection, palpation and sense of smell.

## Skin

Adequate illumination of the skin is required during assessment. If moist or draining skin lesions are present, use disposable gloves for palpation. Because the nurse inspects all skin surfaces, the patient/client must assume several positions. The examination includes inspection of the skin's colour, moisture, temperature, texture and thickness, and turgor. Vascular changes, oedema, and any lesions are noted. Skin odours are usually noted in the skin folds, such as the axilla or under the female patient's/client's breasts.

## Colour

Skin colour varies from body part to body part and from person to person. Despite individual variations, skin colour is usually uniform over the body. However, in older adults, *pigmentation* can increase unevenly, causing discoloured skin. Table 4-3 lists common variations. The assessment of colour first involves areas of the skin not exposed to the sun, such as the palms of the hands. Exposed areas such as the face and arms will be darker. Race affects skin colour, and it is more difficult to note changes such as pallor or cyanosis in patients/clients with dark skin. Usually they have lighter areas of pigmentation on the palms, soles of the feet, lips, and nail beds. Areas of increased colour (hyperpigmentation) and decreased colour (hypopigmentation) are common.

Focus on sites where abnormalities are more easily identified. For example, pallor is most easily perceived in the buccal (mouth) mucosa, particularly in individuals with dark skin. Anaemia can be detected by checking the patient's/client's inner eyelid. *Cyanosis* (bluish discolouration) is more readily seen in areas of least pigmentation such as the lips and nail beds. The best site to inspect for *jaundice* (yellow-orange discolourations) is the patient's/client's sclera. Localized skin changes, such as pallor or *erythema* (red discolouration), may indicate circulatory changes. For example, an area of erythema may be due to localized vasodilation resulting from sunburn or fever. An area of an extremity that appears unusually pale may result from arterial occlusion or oedema. It is important to ask if the patient/client has noticed any changes in skin colouring. He or she usually knows whether a change has occurred.

## Moisture

Moisture in the skin is directly related to the degree of hydration and the condition of the outer lipid layer of the skin surface (DeWitt, 1990). The hydration of skin and mucous membranes helps reveal body fluid imbalances, changes in the integument's environment, and regulation of body temperature. *Moisture* refers

**Children's Nursing**
**Skin assessment in children**

When taking the nursing history and assessing the child's physical, psychological and social well-being, the child's skin must be inspected for deviations from the norm. Skin colour may indicate a problem; rashes are common for children but scratches, bruises and sore areas must be recorded.

The distribution and sites of lesions may be relevant; for example, burrows of scabies are seen in specific sites such as between the fingers and soles of feet. Bruises are often caused by accident, but bilateral black eyes, or fingertip-like bruises on the upper arms and face are not normal and may indicate abuse.

## TABLE 4-3 Skin Colour Variations

| Colour | Condition | Causes | Assessment Locations |
|---|---|---|---|
| Bluish (cyanosis) | Increased amount of deoxygenated haemoglobin (associated with hypoxia) | Heart or lung disease, cold environment | Nail beds, lips, mouth, skin (severe cases) |
| Pallor (decrease in colour) | Reduced amount of oxyhaemoglobin | Anaemia | Face, conjunctivae, nail beds, palms of hands |
| | Reduced visibility of oxyhaemoglobin resulting from decreased blood flow | Shock | Skin, nail beds, conjunctivae, lips |
| | Vitiligo | | |
| Yellow-orange (jaundice) | Increased deposit of bilirubin in tissues | Liver disease, destruction of red blood cells | Sclera, mucous membranes, skin |
| Red (erythema) | Increased visibility of oxyhaemoglobin caused by dilation or increased blood flow | Fever, direct trauma, blushing, alcohol intake | Face, area of trauma, sacrum, shoulders, other common sites for pressure ulcers |
| Tan-brown | Increased amount of melanin | Suntan, pregnancy | Areas exposed to sun: face, arms; areola, nipples |

to wetness and oiliness. The skin is normally smooth and dry. Skin folds such as the axillae are normally moist. After excessive exercise or exposure to warm temperatures, the skin may be moist from perspiration. Dry skin is common in older adults and people who use excessive amounts of soap during bathing. Palpate the skin surface and observe mucous membranes for dullness, dryness, crusting, and flaking. Ask the patient/client about itching; excessive dryness can worsen existing skin conditions such as *eczema* and *dermatitis*. During palpation, you may locate skin lesions. If lesions ooze fluid, note the colour, odour, amount, and consistency. Always wear gloves to prevent exposure to infectious drainage.

### Temperature

The temperature of the skin depends on the amount of blood circulating through the dermis. Increased or decreased skin temperature indicates an increase or decrease in blood flow. Temperature is more accurately assessed by palpating the skin with the dorsum or back of the hand. Skin temperature may be the same throughout the body or may vary in one area, such as the localized warmth at an infected wound site or the coldness of fingers resulting from reduced blood flow. Assessment of skin temperature is a basic assessment when the patient/client is at risk for having impaired circulation (for example, after application of a plaster cast or tight bandage or after vascular surgery). In addition, a nurse can identify a Stage 1 pressure ulcer early when noting warmth and erythema of an area of the skin.

### Texture

The character of the skin's surface and the feel of deeper portions are its texture. The nurse determines whether the patient's/client's skin is smooth or rough, thin or thick, tight or supple, and *indurated* (hardened) or soft by stroking it and palpating it lightly with the fingertips. The texture of the skin is normally smooth, soft, and flexible in children and adults. However, the texture is usually not uniform throughout. The palms of the hand and soles of the feet tend to be thicker. In older adults, the skin becomes wrinkled and leathery because of a decrease in collagen, subcutaneous fat, and sweat glands.

Localized changes may result from trauma or lesions. When irregularities in texture are found, the nurse asks if the patient/client has experienced any recent injury to the skin.

### Turgor

*Turgor* is the skin's elasticity, which can be diminished by oedema or dehydration. Normally the skin loses its elasticity with age. To assess the skin turgor, a fold of skin on the back of the patient's/client's hand is pinched between the thumb and forefinger and released (Fig. 4-1). Note the ease with which the

**Mental Health Nursing**
**Munchausen's syndrome**

If a patient/client has multiple operation scars on his or her body, and has history of operations at several different hospitals, there is a possibility that the person may be suffering from a psychological condition called Munchausen's syndrome. Individuals with Munchausen's syndrome have a tendency to attempt to satisfy some psychological need through seeking surgical operations and medical treatments for non-existent physical conditions. While the nurse should be alerted to the potential of Munchausen's syndrome, this does not mean that the patient/client may not actually be physically ill and in genuine need of medical or surgical intervention.

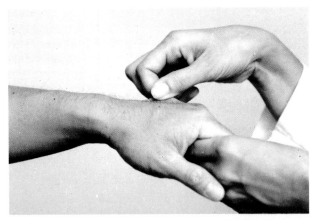

**Fig. 4-1** Assessment for skin turgor. From Canobbio MM: *Cardiovascular disorders*, St Louis, 1990, Mosby-Year Book.

skin moves and the speed at which it returns to place. Normally the skin lifts easily and snaps back immediately to its resting position. Failure of the skin to reassume its normal contour or shape indicates dehydration. Individuals with poor skin turgor do not have a resilience to the normal wear and tear on the skin. The skin tends to stay pinched or tented when turgor is poor. A decrease in turgor predisposes the person to skin breakdown.

## Vascularity

The circulation of the skin affects colour in localized areas and the appearance of superficial blood vessels. With ageing, capillaries become fragile. Localized pressure areas, found after a patient/client has lain or sat in one position, appear reddened, pink, or pale. *Petechiae* are tiny, pinpoint-sized, red or purple spots on the skin caused by small haemorrhages in the skin layers. Petechiae may indicate serious blood-clotting disorders, drug reactions, or liver disease.

## Oedema

Areas of the skin become oedematous because of a build up of fluid in the tissues. Direct trauma and impairment of venous return are two common causes of *oedema*. Direct trauma causes localized oedema. Impaired venous return causes dependent oedema, which typically collects in the feet, ankles and sacrum. Oedematous areas should be inspected for location, colour, and shape. The formation of oedema separates the skin's surface from the pigmented and vascular layers, masking skin colour. The skin often becomes stretched and takes on a shiny appearance. When pressure from the examiner's finger leaves an indentation in the oedematous area, it is called *pitting oedema*.

## Lesions

The skin is normally free of lesions, except common freckles or age-related changes such as skin tags, *keratosis* (thickening of skin), and atrophic warts. When a lesion is detected, it is inspected for colour, location, size, grouping (clustered or linear), and distribution (localized or generalized).

It helps to ask patients/clients if they have noticed any lesions, their causes, and any recent changes in their character. Many people react with fear and anxiety to rashes or other

lesions. Malignant lesions frequently undergo changes in colour and size. Abnormal lesions are reported to the doctor, because further examination will be required.

## Hair and Scalp

Good lighting allows the nurse to inspect the condition and distribution of hair and integrity of the scalp. Because many patients/clients are sensitive about personal appearance, it helps to explain the need to separate parts of the hair to detect problems. If lesions or lice are probable, wear disposable gloves to avoid infection.

Changes may occur in the thickness, texture, and lubrication of scalp hair. A number of disturbances in body function, such as a febrile illness, can result in hair loss. Scalp disease can also cause loss of hair. Baldness **(alopecia)**, or thinning of the hair, is usually related to genetic tendencies and endocrine disorders such as diabetes, thyroiditis, and even menopause (DeWitt, 1990). The hair is lubricated from the oil of sebaceous glands. Excessively oily hair is associated with androgen hormone stimulation. Dry, brittle hair occurs with ageing and with excessive use of shampoo or other chemical agents. Poor nutrition often causes development of dry, coarse, discoloured hair.

### Children's Nursing
### Assessing scalp and hair

Assessment of the scalp and hair is very important in infants or children. Cradle cap (infantile seborrhoea dermatitis) is very common in infants aged 2-3 months. It is often caused by the mother's reluctance to wash the 'soft spot'. It is readily treatable and causes minimal problems.

In older children, head lice is fairly common among all social classes and outbreaks are prevalent in schools and children's wards. Hair must be inspected and, if infected, must be treated with a preparation containing benzene hexachloride. It is important to advise that the entire family need similar treatment.

Inspect hair follicles for lice or other parasites. The three types of lice are *Pediculus humanus capitis* (head lice), *Pediculus humanus corporis* (body lice), and *Pediculus pubis* (crab lice). Head and crab lice attach their eggs to hair. The tiny eggs look like oval particles of dandruff. The lice themselves are difficult to see. Head and body lice are very small with greyish white bodies. Crab lice have red legs. The nurse looks for bites or pustular eruptions in the hair follicles and in areas where skin surfaces meet, such as behind the ears and in the groin. The discovery of lice requires immediate treatment.

## Nails

The nails can reflect an individual's general state of health, state of nutrition and occupation. Even a person's psychological state may be revealed by evidence of nails which have been bitten, possibly indicating a nervous predisposition.

The colour of nails is an indicator of blood oxygenation. A blue or purple colour to the nail beds occurs with cyanosis. A white cast or pallor can be the result of anaemia. Thin nails can be a sign of poor circulation and nutritional deficiency.

## GUIDELINES FOR TAKING VITAL SIGNS

Vital signs are a part of the information a nurse collects during assessment (see box for normal values in an adult). The nurse must be able to measure vital signs correctly, understand and interpret the values, communicate findings appropriately, and begin interventions as needed. The nurse's judgement helps determine the need for and frequency of vital sign measurement.

Vital signs are physiological data that assist the nurse in performing day-to-day care measures and critical interventions. For example, to determine whether a patient/client tolerates exercise, the nurse may assess pulse rate before and during exercise. When a patient/client experiences excessive blood loss after injury or surgery, blood pressure measurement can reveal the seriousness of the haemorrhage. Continued blood pressure checks help determine when to administer fluids or medications to restore blood pressure to normal. (See box to right for when to take vital signs.)

### Vital Signs: Normal Ranges for Adults

**TEMPERATURE**
**Oral:** 37°C
**Rectal:** 37.6°C
**Axilla:** 36.4°C

**PULSE**
60 – 100 beats/min

**RESPIRATIONS**
12 – 20 breaths/min

**BLOOD PRESSURE**
**Average:** 120/80 mmHg
**Hypertension:** Systolic above 140 mmHg
Diastolic above 90 mmHg
**Hypotension:** Systolic below 90 mmHg with signs of dizziness and increased pulse
**Orthostatic hypotension:** Fall in systolic blood pressure of 25 mmHg systolic and 10 mmHg diastolic accompanied by signs and symptoms of inadequate cerebral perfusion when arising from lying position to sitting or standing position.

## BODY TEMPERATURE

### Physiology

The body's **temperature** remains within a relatively narrow range for optimal function, despite internal extremes (for example, metabolic changes) or external conditions (for example, climatic temperature). Temperature-control mechanisms keep the body's core temperature (that is, organs within the skull, and the thoracic and abdominal cavities) in a relatively constant range, 36.1°C to 37.8°C.

A clinical thermometer registers the body's temperature. No single temperature is normal for all people. When the body's core temperature rises above normal, **hyperthermia** occurs. When the body's core temperature falls below normal, **hypothermia** occurs.

### When to Take Vital Signs

- on the patient's admission to hospital
- in a hospital according to hospital policy
- before and after a surgical procedure
- before and after an invasive diagnostic procedure
- before and after the administration of certain medications that affect cardiovascular, respiratory, and temperature-control functions
- when the patient's/client's general physical condition changes (as with loss of consciousness or increased intensity of pain)
- before and after nursing interventions influencing a vital sign (such as when a patient/client previously on bed rest ambulates or when a patient requires tracheal suctioning)
- when the patient/client reports nonspecific symptoms of physical distress (such as feeling 'funny' or 'different')

### Regulation

The balance of body temperature is precisely regulated by physiological and behavioural mechanisms. For the body temperature to remain constant, heat produced in the body must equal heat lost to the environment.

### Neural Control

The hypothalamus in the brain controls body temperature in the same way that a thermostat works in the home. A comfortable temperature is the set point at which a heating system operates. In the home a fall in environmental temperature activates the heating system, whereas a rise in temperature shuts the system down. The hypothalamus senses minor changes in body temperature. When body temperature deviates from the set point, the temperature centre of the hypothalamus activates heat loss (cooling) or heat production so that the core temperature stays in a safe physiological range.

When nerve cells in the hypothalamus become heated, impulses are sent out to reduce body temperature. The body cools itself by sweating, *vasodilation* (widening of blood vessels), and inhibition of heat production. If the hypothalamus senses that the body's temperature is too low, signals are sent out to increase heat production and conservation through *vasoconstriction* (narrowing of blood vessels), muscle shivering, and *piloerection* (erection of hairs) giving the characteristic 'goose pimples'. Lesions or trauma to the hypothalamus or spinal cord, which carries hypothalamic messages, can cause serious alterations in temperature control.

### HEAT PRODUCTION

Heat is produced in the body by metabolism, which is the chemical reaction in all body cells. Food is the primary fuel source for metabolism. Heat production is a constant process and increases when a person is active. During quiet times and rest, most heat comes from the body's core. During work, the main site of heat production is the muscles.

### Skin and Temperature Regulation

The skin helps regulate body temperature in the following ways:
- **Insulation of the body** (which affects the amount of blood

flow and heat loss to the skin) — the skin, subcutaneous tissue, and fat keep heat inside the body. When blood flow between skin layers is reduced, the skin alone is an excellent insulator. People with more body fat have more natural insulation than slim and muscular people.

- **Vasoconstriction** — in humans internal organs produce heat, and during exercise or increased sympathetic stimulation, the amount of heat produced is greater than the normal core temperature. Blood flows from the internal organs, carrying heat to the body surface. The skin is well supplied with blood vessels. In the most exposed areas of the body (the hands, feet, and ears) blood can flow directly from arteries to veins. Blood flow through the more vascular areas of the skin may vary from minimal flow to as much as 30% of the blood ejected from the heart (Guyton, 1991). Heat transfers from the blood, through vessel walls, and to the skin's surface and is lost to the environment through heat-loss mechanisms. The body's core temperature remains within safe limits.

  The degree of vasoconstriction determines the amount of blood flow and heat loss to the skin. If the core temperature is too high, the hypothalamus inhibits vasoconstriction. As a result, blood vessels dilate, and more blood reaches the skin's surface. On a hot, humid day the blood vessels in the hands are dilated and easily visible. In contrast, if the core temperature becomes too low, the hypothalamus initiates vasoconstriction and blood flow to the skin lessens. Thus, body heat is conserved.

- **Temperature sensation** — the skin is well supplied with heat and cold receptors. Because cold receptors are more plentiful, however, the skin functions primarily to detect cold surface temperatures. When the skin becomes chilled, its sensors send information to the hypothalamus, which initiates shivering to increase body heat production, inhibition of sweating, and vasoconstriction.

## Heat Loss Mechanisms

As the body produces heat, it also loses heat (Fig. 4-2). The skin's structure and exposure to the environment result in constant, normal heat loss through radiation, conduction, convection, and evaporation.

### RADIATION

*Radiation* is the transfer of heat from the surface of one object to the surface of another without actual contact between the two (Thibodeau and Patton, 1993). Heat radiates from the skin to cooler nearby objects and radiates to the skin from warmer objects. The amount of heat lost by radiation from the skin varies according to dilation of surface blood vessels when the body is overheated, and by vasoconstriction when the body is chilled.

Heat loss through radiation can be reduced by covering the body with clothing, especially dark, closely woven clothes. Radiant heat loss can be enhanced by removing clothing or by wearing light clothing that facilitates heat loss. Body positioning also affects heat loss through radiation. Because of the amount of exposed surface area, a person standing with arms and legs

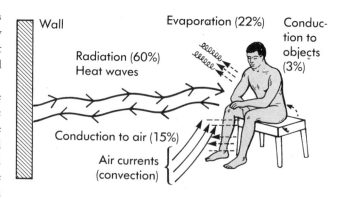

**Fig. 4-2** Mechanisms of heat loss from the body.
From Guyton AC: *Textbook of medical physiology*, ed 8, Philadelphia, 1991, Saunders.

extended radiates more heat than a person lying down in a fetal position.

### CONDUCTION

*Conduction* is the transfer of heat to any object or surface in contact with the body. Conduction accounts for a small amount of heat loss. Heat conducts through solids, gases, and liquids.

When a person sits on a chair, heat is conducted from the person's body to the chair until the surface temperature of the chair begins to rise. When the temperature of the skin and chair temperature are the same, conductive heat loss stops. If the air next to the skin is cooler than the skin's surface, the body's heat warms the air. Wearing several layers of clothing creates layers of warmed air surrounding the body, which keeps a person warm and reduces conductive heat loss. This is the rationale for advising patients/clients to wear several layers of clothing to prevent hypothermia.

Water conducts heat more efficiently than air. Thus, water used to bathe patient/clients should be above body temperature to prevent conductive heat loss. However, if the patient's/client's temperature is abnormally high (fever), the nurse can lower it by sponging the person in tepid water that is *below* body temperature. Conductive heat loss from the body will then occur.

### CONVECTION

*Convection* is the transfer of heat away from a surface, such as the skin, by movement of heated air or fluid particles (Thibodeau and Patton, 1993). Normally, a warm layer of air exists close to the skin's surface. Heated air rises from the skin and passes to cooler air by convection currents, causing a minimal amount of heat loss from the skin.

As the speed of movement of air surrounding the skin increases, the convection of heat loss from the skin increases. Normally, convective heat loss is minimal, but it can be artificially enhanced by the use of fans to promote heat loss.

### EVAPORATION

Heat energy is needed to change water from a liquid to a gas. For each gram of water that evaporates from the body surface, approximately 0.6 kilocalorie (kcal) of heat is lost (Mountcastle, 1980). The body always loses some heat and water by *evaporation*.

This occurs from the continuous, insensible loss of water from the skin and lungs. About 500-600 ml of moisture that evaporates daily from breathing and skin functions is considered *insensible water loss*. However, insensible loss occurs regardless of body temperature and thus does not play a major role in temperature regulation.

*Diaphoresis* (sweating), however, controls body temperature through evaporative heat loss. Millions of sweat glands lie deep below the dermal layer of the skin. The glands secrete sweat, a watery solution containing sodium and chloride, which passes through tiny ducts on the skin's surface. The glands are controlled by the sympathetic nervous system. When the body's temperature rises, sweat glands release sweat, which evaporates from the skin's surface to promote heat loss. Exercise causes a significant rise in body temperature to stimulate diaphoresis. Emotional or mental stress causes diaphoresis through sympathetic stimulation. When temperatures are cold, sweat gland secretion is inhibited, and body temperature is conserved. Diaphoresis is less efficient when air movement is minimal or when the humidity of the air is high.

## Behavioural Control

Behavioural regulation involves the voluntary acts that people take to maintain comfortable body temperatures. Humans alter their behaviour when exposed to temperature extremes. When the temperature in the environment falls, for example, people can add clothing, move to warmer places, raise the temperature settings on heating thermostats, increase muscular activity by running in place, or sit with arms and legs tightly wrapped together. In contrast, when the temperature becomes hot, individuals can remove clothing, stop activity, lower temperature settings on air conditioners, turn on fans, seek cooler places, or take cool showers or baths.

People with altered temperature-control mechanisms, such as infants or older adults, have difficulty with maintaining body temperature. These individuals may need assistance in changing their environments so that their exposure to temperature extremes is limited. Individuals who are ill or who have injuries that lower consciousness or cause impairment in thought processes may also be unable to recognize the need to change behaviour for temperature control.

## Factors Affecting Body Temperature

To assess temperature variations and evaluate the significance of changes from normal, the nurse must be aware of several factors that affect body temperature.

## Age

At birth, the newborn leaves a warm, relatively constant environment and enters one in which temperatures fluctuate widely. Temperature-control mechanisms are not fully developed; thus, an infant's temperature may change drastically with changes in the environment. Extra care is therefore needed to protect the newborn. Clothing must be adequate, and exposure to temperature extremes must be avoided. A newborn loses up to 30% of body heat through the head and therefore needs to wear a bonnet to prevent heat loss. When protected from environmental extremes, the newborn's body temperature is maintained within 35.5 to 39.5°C. Heat production steadily declines as the infant grows into childhood (Wong, 1995).

Temperature regulation is unstable until children reach puberty. The normal temperature range gradually drops as individuals approach older adulthood. Oral temperatures of 35°C are not unusual for older adults in cold weather. However, the average body temperature of older adults is approximately 36°C. Older adults are particularly sensitive to temperature extremes because of deterioration in thermoregulation, including poor vasomotor control (control of vasoconstriction and vasodilation), reduced amounts of subcutaneous tissue, reduced sweat gland activity, and reduced mobility and metabolism. Some of these people are especially at risk for hypothermia, in which body temperature falls below 35°C. This drop may occur when environmental temperatures fall and older adults are not physically active or are unable to heat their homes adequately.

## Exercise

Muscle activity requires an increased blood supply and an increase in carbohydrate and fat breakdown for more energy. This increased metabolism causes an increase in heat production. Any form of exercise can increase heat production and thus body temperature. After prolonged exercise, such as long-distance running, body temperatures may temporarily reach levels as high as 39 to 41°C (Petersdorf, 1980).

## Hormone Level

Women generally experience greater fluctuations in body temperature than men. Hormonal variations during the menstrual cycle cause body temperature fluctuations. Progesterone levels rise and fall cyclically during the menstrual cycle. Before this cycle, progesterone levels are low, and the body temperature falls a few tenths of a degree below the baseline level. The lower temperature persists until ovulation occurs. During ovulation, greater amounts of progesterone enter the circulatory system and raise the body temperature to previous baseline levels or higher. Plotting temperature variations during the menstrual cycle to determine when ovulation occurs can be used to predict a woman's most fertile time to achieve pregnancy.

Body temperature changes also occur in women during menopause (cessation of menstruation). Women who have stopped menstruating may experience periods of intense body heat and sweating lasting from 30 seconds to 5 minutes. This is due to the instability of the vasomotor controls for vasodilation and vasoconstriction (Bobak *et al*, 1989).

The amounts of thyroxine, triiodothyronine, adrenaline, and noradrenaline circulating in the body also affect heat production and the basal metabolic rate.

## Circadian Rhythms

Body temperatures normally change 0.5 to 1°C during a 24-hour period. However, temperature is one of the most stable rhythms in humans. Body temperature is usually lowest between 1 and 4AM (Fig. 4-3). During the day, body temperature rises steadily, until

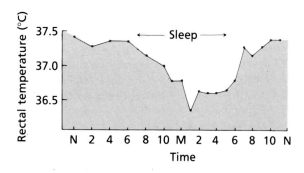

**Fig. 4-3** The 24-hour temperature cycle. From Mountcastle VB: *Medical physiology*, vol 2, ed 14, St Louis, 1980, Mosby.

about 6PM, and then declines to early morning levels. At one time, daily temperature variations were believed to be a result of greater daytime activity. However, temperature patterns are not automatically reversed in people who work during the night and sleep during the day. It takes 1 to 3 weeks for the cycle to reverse. Every patient/client has a different temperature pattern, which the nurse must assess in order to identify a change in health.

## Stress

Physical and emotional stress increase body temperature through hormonal and neural stimulation. The patient/client may experience an increased heart or respiratory rate or increased diaphoresis. These physiological changes increase metabolism, which increases heat production. Individuals who are anxious about entering a hospital or a doctor's surgery may register a higher-than-normal temperature.

## Environment

Environment influences body temperature. If the temperature is assessed in a very warm room, a patient/client may be unable to conduct heat away, and the body temperature will be elevated. If the patient/client has just been outside in the cold without warm clothing, body temperature may be low because of extensive radiant and conductive heat loss. The person may be shivering to raise body temperature. Infants and older adults are most likely to be affected by environmental temperatures because their temperature-regulating mechanisms are less efficient.

## Thermal Disorders

Thermal disorders are heat-related disorders and are not symptoms of another disease. In other words, fever and excess heat production are the *primary* problems rather than indications of infection. Thermal disorders include heat exhaustion, heat stroke, and hypothermia, in which the body is unable to maintain optimum temperature.

## Fever

The simplest definition of a **fever** or **pyrexia** is a core temperature above 38°C that is measured under resting conditions. However, because each person's temperature range varies, a fever may exist in a person whose temperature is within the normal accepted range. A true fever results from an alteration in the hypothalamic set point. Bacteria, viruses, fungi, and certain antigens are *pyrogens* (substances that cause a rise in body temperature). After pyrogens enter the body, more white blood cells are produced to help promote the body's defense against infection (Fig. 4-4). The body's immune system responds by producing endogenous pyrogens (interleukin 1) which act on cells in the hypothalamus to raise the set point in the body. After the set point is increased, physiological and behavioural mechanisms work to produce fever. During the chill phase of a fever, the body acts to produce and conserve heat. It may take several hours before the body temperature reaches the new set point. During this time, neural responses cause vasoconstriction. A person experiences chills and shivers and feels cold, even though body temperature is rising. After the body temperature reaches the new set point, the chills subside, and the person then feels warm.

During a fever, the body's metabolism increases 7% for every degree of temperature elevation. Heart and respiratory rates also increase to meet this metabolic demand. If the patient/client has a cardiac or respiratory problem, the stress of fever can be great. A prolonged fever can seriously weaken a patient/client because of exhaustion of energy stores and the increased work of breathing. Older adults are especially at risk for rapid deterioration resulting from fever because they have a diminished response to pyrogens and may already have chronic diseases causing debilitation. Confusion can result from high fevers because of reduced oxygen levels in the brain (although this condition is completely reversible in some cases). The increased metabolism places a patient/client at risk for dehydration from evaporative heat loss and possible reduced oral intake of fluids. Dehydration is a problem, especially for children because they can quickly lose large amounts of fluids in proportion to their body weight.

After the cause of the fever is removed (for example, destruction of bacteria by antibiotic medication), the

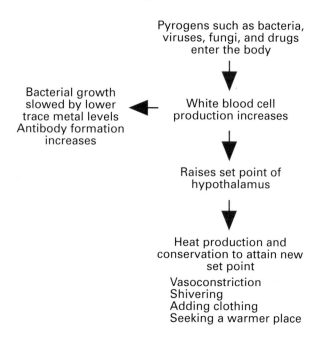

**Fig. 4-4** Mechanism of a fever.

hypothalamic set point drops and the body initiates the heat-loss mechanisms described earlier.

Fever may also result from administration of a drug. A 'drug fever' can be a hypersensitivity reaction accompanied by allergy symptoms, such as rash and itching (Hanson, 1991).

## TREATMENT ISSUES

Doctors often disagree about when to treat a fever. A fever is usually not harmful if it stays below 39°C. Research (Dinarello, 1984) suggests that fever is an important defense mechanism. Moderate fevers, those between 37 and 38°C, may help activate the body's immune system to produce antibodies. These disease-fighting agents work best at higher temperatures. Fever also fights viral infections by stimulating interferon, the body's natural virus-fighting substance. Fevers may also serve a diagnostic purpose, because the natural pattern of a fever may reveal its cause.

Most fevers in children are of a viral origin, are of brief duration, and have limited effects (Lovejoy, 1978). However, children still have unstable temperature-control mechanisms. Temperature can rise rapidly, causing dehydration or febrile seizures in children under 5 years. Some researchers believe that the *rate* of rise is more important in generating a seizure than is the absolute temperature (Leung and Robson, 1991).

Generally, the nurse needs to report elevated body temperatures to the doctor for all patients/clients. Treatment is usually indicated if the temperature is greater than 38°C (101°F), especially if the patient/client is restless or listless, has profuse diaphoresis, or exhibits other symptoms (see following section).

### Heat Exhaustion

*Heat exhaustion* occurs when a person loses excessive amounts of water and sodium from profuse diaphoresis. This condition occurs commonly in marathon runners who do not drink enough fluid. The reduction in fluid volume and electrolytes causes extreme thirst, nausea, vomiting, weakness, headache, mild disorientation, normal or slightly elevated body temperature, tachycardia, and **postural hypotension** (drop in blood pressure when a person stands or sits). Exposure to high environmental temperature causes this common heat-related illness. Placing a person immediately in a cool environment to rest, and stopping diaphoresis is the first treatment. Fluid and electrolyte replacement (see Chapter 18) will restore imbalances.

### Heat Stroke

*Heat stroke* is a dangerous condition because it has a high fatality rate. People most at risk include infants and older adults; obese people; patients/clients with cardiovascular disease, hyperthyroidism, diabetes, and alcohol dependency; patients/clients taking medications that decrease the body's ability to lose heat; and people who exercise or work strenuously in the heat (for example, athletes, construction workers, and farmers).

Heat stroke with temperatures greater than 40°C produces tissue damage to the cells of all body organs. The brain may be the first organ affected because of its sensitivity to electrolyte imbalances. Permanent central nervous system damage can occur if cooling measures are not initiated rapidly.

### Hypothermia

When a person is found ill or injured in cold weather or immersed in cold water, **hypothermia** should be suspected. This condition usually develops gradually and may not be noticed for several hours. Skin temperature drops to around 35°C and uncontrolled shivering begins. A loss of memory, depression, and signs of poor judgement may be early indications. If body temperature falls to below 34.4°C heart and respiratory rates and blood pressure begin to fall, and the skin becomes cyanotic. If hypothermia progresses, the patient/client may experience cardiac dysrhythmias, lose consciousness, and may become unresponsive to painful stimuli. In cases of severe hypothermia, a person may demonstrate clinical signs similar to death (for example, lack of response to stimuli and extremely slow respirations and pulse).

Surface areas of the skin can actually freeze when a patient/client is exposed to extremely cold temperatures without protection. This is called *frostbite*. Areas especially susceptible to frostbite include the earlobes, fingers, and toes. Permanent circulatory and tissue damage may result if ice crystals form inside the cells (Guyton, 1991).

The priority treatment for hypothermia is the conscious prevention of further decrease in body temperature and to promote natural warming. The nurse should remove wet clothes, replace them with dry ones, and wrap the person in blankets, preferably thermal, or foil 'space' blankets. In emergencies, it helps to have the patient/client lie next to a warm person. A conscious person will benefit from drinking hot liquids such as soup.

Prevention is the key for patients/clients at risk for hypothermia. Prevention involves educating the person or family and friends. Patients/clients most at risk include infants, older adults, and people debilitated by trauma, stroke, diabetes, drug or alcohol intoxication, sepsis, and Raynaud's disease (LaVoy, 1985). A mentally ill person or someone with learning difficulties may suffer hypothermia because they are unaware of the potential dangers of cold conditions. People who have inadequate home heating, poor diet, or lack of warm clothing are also at risk.

### Assessment of Body Temperature

### Sites

The mouth, rectum, and axilla are common sites for measuring body temperature. Special chemically prepared thermometer strips or patches can also be applied to the forehead. Tympanic membrane probes for temperature measurement at the ear are currently being studied. Each site has advantages and disadvantages (Table 4-4). *Oral* temperatures can be affected by a number of variables. Wait 20 to 30 minutes, for example, to measure oral temperature after a patient/client ingests hot or cold liquids or food, has been smoking, or has been involved in strenuous exercise. An oral thermometer can be used reliably as long as the person is able to close his or her mouth and breathe through his or her nose. This includes patients/clients using oxygen via nasal cannula or face mask, nasogastric tubes, and nasal endotracheal tubes (Heinz, 1985; Lukasiewicz, 1986). Oral temperature is approximately 1°C lower than core temperature. It is important that the thermometer sensor be placed as close to

**Fig. 4-5** Oral thermometer with centigrade calibration.

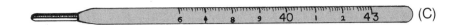

The mercury-in-glass thermometer is the most familiar. It consists of a glass tube sealed at one end and a mercury-filled bulb at the other. Exposure of the bulb to heat causes the mercury to expand and rise in the enclosed tube. The length of the thermometer is marked with centigrade calibrations (Fig. 4-5). The mercury will not fluctuate or fall unless the thermometer is shaken vigorously.

A glass thermometer is read by holding it with the fingertips horizontally at eye level, with the bulb pointed to the left. The bulb should not be touched. Touching it might bring the fingers into contact with the person's body secretions and may also cause a change in the thermometer reading. The thermometer is rotated slowly until the column of silver mercury appears. The calibrated line at the end of the mercury column is the temperature reading.

The oral thermometer is slender, allowing greater exposure of the bulb against the blood vessels in the mouth. The pear-shaped rectal thermometer has a blunt end designed to prevent trauma during rectal insertion. It usually has a blue tip. Time delay for recordings and easy breakability are disadvantages of mercury-in-glass thermometers. The length of time required to achieve an accurate recording has been the subject of several pieces of research with variations of 2 minutes up to 30 minutes recommended (McCleod-Clarke, 1989). Advantages are low price and wide availability.

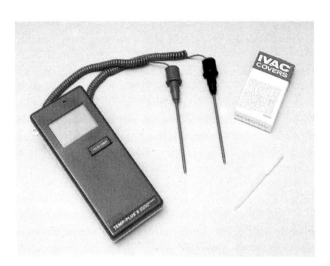

**Fig. 4-6** Electronic thermometer.

sublingual arteries as possible. Thermometer sensors should be placed in the sublingual heat pockets either side of the frenulum on the floor of the mouth. Oral temperature measurements can vary by as much as 1.7°C depending on where the thermometer is placed (Closs, 1987).

The rectal site is believed to provide the most reliable measurement because few factors can alter the results; however, the use of rectal thermometers is currently being questioned, as some practitioners believe that rectal trauma may result, and as yet research results remain inconclusive (Rogers, 1992; Morley, 1992, 1993). *Rectal* temperature is usually a few tenths of a degree higher than the oral temperature. Even within the rectum, variations of 0.1 to 0.9°C exist, depending on the position of the thermometer (Mountcastle, 1980).

The *axilla* is a commonly used site for temperature measurement. However, the time required for measurement with a thermometer and the difficulty with thermometer placement makes the axillary area less convenient and accurate. When chemical thermometer strips are used, an axillary temperature can be obtained within one minute. Axillary temperature is cooler than oral temperature.

The *tympanic membrane* is an excellent site for temperature measurement because of its highly vascular nature and easy accessibility. The problem lies in the availability of reliable, accurate, cost-efficient equipment (Davis, 1993). Several tympanic membrane thermometers are available and appear to be accurate, instantaneous, and easy to use. Tympanic membrane temperatures directly reflect core temperature.

### Thermometers

The four types of thermometer available for determining body temperature include mercury in glass, electronic, disposable, and tympanic membrane.

The electronic thermometer consists of a battery-powered display unit, a thin wire cord, and a temperature-sensitive probe covered by a disposable plastic sheath to prevent the transmission of infection (Fig. 4-6). Separate probes are available for oral and rectal use. Within seconds of insertion a reading appears on the display unit. Electronic thermometers have many advantages. They can be inserted immediately. Their readings appear within seconds, and they are easy to read. The duration of the patient's/client's discomfort is also minimized.

Disposable, single-use thermometers are thin strips of plastic with chemically impregnated paper. They are used for oral or axillary temperatures, particularly with children. They can be inserted in the same way as an oral thermometer or can be applied to the skin. The chemical dots on the thermometer change colour to reflect the temperature reading. Only 45 seconds are needed to record a temperature. Chemically treated paper thermometers are generally less accurate, but they are useful in providing a general temperature range.

Tympanic membrane thermometers are small hand-held devices similar to otoscopes, with disposable speculums, infrared sensing electronics, and liquid crystal displays (Fig. 4-7). Most are battery operated and rechargeable. Results are displayed 1 to 2 seconds after placing the speculum in the outer third of the ear canal.. Accuracy appears to be good (Shinozaki *et al*, 1988), but studies have been conflicting.

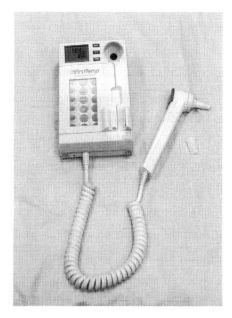

**Fig. 4-7** Tympanic membrane thermometer.

## Guidelines for Taking Temperature

When measuring body temperature at any site, follow these basic principles carefully, to maintain the patient's/client's safety and ensure accuracy in measurement:

1. Consider the best method for obtaining a temperature reading.
2. Ensure that the patient/client is comfortable and has not recently exercised or had a drink.

3. Following local policy, ensure that thermometers are cleaned with the recommended solution, or that a disposable sheath is applied.
4. Ensure that the thermometer is correctly positioned (for example, on the sublingual heat pockets either side of the frenulum under the tongue).
5. Keep the thermometer in place for the time set out in local policy, based on current research, remembering that this will vary widely according to the selected method.
6. Read and chart the result, noting and reporting any changes from baseline, or the effects of any medication.

## During Febrile Episode

The nurse caring for patients/clients with febrile conditions performs the following assessments through all stages of the febrile episode:

1. **Measure vital signs** when a fever is suspected, and as ordered (for example, every 2 to 4 hours), until body temperature returns to normal. An increase in temperature usually occurs with tachycardia (increased heart rate) and tachypnoea (increased respiratory rate). Hypertension (increased blood pressure) may be seen initially with fever, and hypotension (decreased blood pressure) may follow with prolonged, high fevers.
2. **Inspect and palpate** the patient's/client's skin and check for turgor. As a fever develops, the skin may feel cool and dry, and may look pale. At the height of the fever the skin becomes warm. After a fever begins to break, the skin is flushed, warm, and moist from sweating. Reduced skin turgor

## TABLE 4-4 Advantages and Disadvantages of Sites for Temperature Measurement

| Advantages | Disadvantages |
|---|---|
| **MOUTH** | |
| Most accessible site; more comfortable for patient/client | Should not be used for patients/clients who: <br>• could be injured by thermometer, <br>• are unable to hold thermometer properly, or who might bite thermometer, including infants or small children, confused or unconscious patients/clients, <br>• have had oral surgery, <br>• have had trauma to face or mouth, <br>• are experiencing oral pain, <br>• breathe only with mouth open, <br>• have a history of convulsions, <br>• experience shaking chills |
| **RECTUM** | |
| Thought to provide most reliable measurement | Should not be used for patients/clients who have had rectal surgery, patients/clients who have a rectal disorder such as tumour or severe haemorrhoids, patients/clients who cannot be positioned for proper thermometer placement such as those in traction, or those who are constipated |
| **AXILLA** | |
| Safest method because noninvasive | Requires nurse to hold thermometer in position; is less accurate |
| **TYMPANIC MEMBRANE** | |
| Easy access to vascular tympanic membrane, which reflects core temperature | Is costly and device is less accessible. Can be unreliable if not sealed against room air |

is a sign of dehydration. Children and older adults are especially prone to dehydration and should be observed closely.

3. **Ask** how the patient/client feels. Common symptoms of fever include headache, *myalgia* (muscle aches), chills, nausea, *photophobia* (sensitivity of the eyes to light), weakness, fatigue, and loss of appetite. A patient/client often complains of thirst.

4. **Note** vomiting or diarrhoea, which can increase fluid and electrolyte loss.

5. **Observe** the patient/client for behavioural changes, such as confusion or disorientation and restlessness or listlessness.

6. **Monitor** test results for electrolyte levels. An excessive loss of fluids will cause electrolyte imbalance (see Chapter 18). (Sodium, potassium, and chloride levels are most likely to be altered.)

7. **Inspect** the condition of the oral mucosa for dryness resulting from dehydration.

Fever involves complex physiological responses from many organ systems. Goals of care for patients/clients with fever include the following:

* attaining a sense of comfort and rest
* returning to normal body temperature
* maintaining adequate nutrition
* maintaining fluid and electrolye balance.

## PULSE

The alternating expansion and recoil of elastic arteries during each cardiac cycle creates a pressure wave (a **pulse**) that is transmitted through the arterial tree with each heart beat. You can feel a pulse in any artery lying close to the body surface by compressing the artery against firm tissue, this provides an easy way of counting the heart rate (Marieb, 1989). For cells to function normally, there must be a continuous blood flow and an appropriate volume and distribution of blood to cells that need nutrients.

### Physiology and Regulation

Blood flows through the body in a continuous circuit. The heart is a muscular pump, ejecting blood intermittently into the arterial system. Cardiac centres located in the medulla of the brainstem receive impulses from sensory receptors. These sensory impulses then cause the cardiac centres in the medulla to speed up or slow down the heart rate through sympathetic or parasympathetic innervation. For example, if there is excessive stretch of the aortic arch by an increase in blood volume, sensory impulses travel to the cardiac centre. This then triggers a reflex slowing of the heart rate through the action of the vagus nerve. This decrease in heart rate compensates for the increased blood volume. When volume returns to normal, the heart rate returns to baseline.

A person's heart rate varies throughout the day. Nevertheless, the heart functions to maintain a relatively constant circulatory blood flow. Approximately 70 to 72 ml of blood enters the aorta with each ventricular contraction *(stroke volume)*. With each stroke volume ejection, the walls of the aorta distend, creating a pulse wave that travels rapidly towards the distal ends of the arteries (Guyton, 1991). When a pulse wave reaches a peripheral artery, it can be palpated by pressing the artery lightly against underlying bone or muscle. The pulse rate is an indirect measurement of heart rate. The volume of blood pumped by the heart during 1 minute is the *cardiac output (CO)*; the product of heart rate (HR) and the ventricle's stroke volume (SV) (HR x SV = CO). In an adult, the heart normally pumps 5000 to 6000 ml of blood per minute throughout the circulation.

An abnormally slow, rapid, or irregular pulse may indicate a problem in circulatory regulation. The pathological process causing a change from the normal heartbeat may ultimately alter cardiac output.

### Assessment of Pulse

The radial and carotid arteries are the most accessible peripheral pulse sites for assessment (Fig. 4-8). When a person's condition suddenly deteriorates, the carotid artery in the neck is the best site for finding a pulse quickly. This is because the heart will continue delivering blood through the carotid artery to the brain as long as possible, whereas peripheral pulses may weaken. In non-emergency circumstances the radial artery is the most common site for assessment of pulse rate.

Assessment of other peripheral pulse sites, such as the brachial or femoral artery, is unnecessary when routinely taking vital signs. If the *radial pulse* at the wrist is abnormal or intermittent, resulting from dysrhythmias, or if it is inaccessible because of a dressing or plaster cast, the **apex contraction rate** is assessed. This is achieved by listening to the apex of the heart with a stethoscope. When a patient/client takes medication that affects the heart rate (for example digoxin), the apex pulse may provide a more accurate assessment of heart function; this is particularly useful when taken in conjunction with the radial pulse. Two nurses take these pulses simultaneously. This is termed an *apex and radial pulse*. The apex pulse is the best site for assessing an infant's or young child's pulse because the peripheral pulses are deep and difficult to palpate accurately.

In order to palpate a peripheral pulse, the first two fingers of the hand are used. The tips are the most sensitive parts of the fingers for detecting the pulsation of the arterial wall. Inexperienced students sometimes apply excessive pressure over the artery and totally obliterate the pulse. It helps to imagine the anatomical position of the artery when attempting to locate it. If the pulse is not easily located on one side, the other can be tried. The patient's/client's extremity should be kept in a relaxed position to permit full exposure of an artery. For assessment of the radial artery (Fig. 4-9), the person's wrist should be extended and relaxed. This position ensures that the artery lies superficially above the radius.

### Arterial Pulses

The nurse may be required to find pulses other than those discussed in relation to recording a heart rate. The assessment of peripheral pulses is required in patients/clients with vascular problems in their limbs; for example, following trauma to a limb, surgery or peripheral vascular disease.

To palpate the *brachial pulse*, find the groove between the biceps and triceps muscles above the elbow at the antecubital fossa.

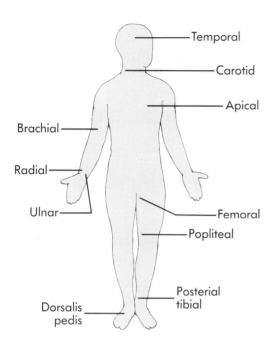

Fig. 4-8 Location of pulse points in the body.

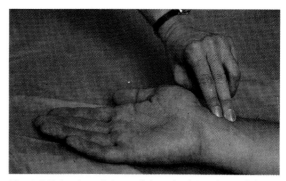

Fig. 4-9 Palpation of the radial pusle along the radial side of the forearm.

The artery runs along the medial side of the extended arm. Palpate the artery with the fingertips of the first three fingers in the muscle groove.

The femoral artery is the primary artery in the leg, delivering blood to the popliteal, posterior tibial, and dorsalis pedis arteries. It is one of the strongest arteries in an infant or small child. An interconnection between the posterior tibial and dorsalis pedis arteries guards against local arterial occlusion.

The *femoral pulse* is found most easily with the patient/client lying down with the inguinal area exposed. The femoral artery runs below the inguinal ligament, midway between the symphysis pubis and the anterosuperior iliac spine. Deep palpation may be required to feel the pulse. Bimanual palpation is effective in obese patients/clients. This technique differs from the previous description of bimanual palpation. Place the fingertips of both hands on opposite sides of the pulse site. A pulsatile sensation can be felt as the fingertips are pushed apart by arterial pulsation.

The *popliteal pulse* is found behind the knee. The patient/client should slightly flex the knee, with the foot resting on the examination table. The person may also assume a prone position with the knee slightly flexed. Instruct the patient/client to keep leg muscles relaxed. Palpate with the fingers of both hands deeply into the popliteal fossa, just lateral to the midline. The popliteal pulse is difficult to locate.

With the person's foot relaxed, locate the dorsalis pedis pulse. The artery runs along the top of the foot in a line with the groove between the extensor tendons of the great toe and first toe. Often an examiner finds the pulse by placing the fingertips between the great and first toe and slowly inching up the foot. This pulse may be congenitally absent.

The *posterior tibial pulse* is found on the inner side of each ankle. Place your fingers behind and below the medial malleolus (ankle bone). The artery is easily located with the foot relaxed and slightly extended.

### Doppler Stethoscope

Occasionally a nurse has difficulty palpating a pulse. A pulse wave may not be palpable if the person is obese, if cardiac output is reduced or if there is an obstruction of the artery. A Doppler stethoscope, a type of ultrasound stethescope, will amplify sounds, allowing the nurse to hear low-velocity blood flow (Fig. 4-10).

### Stethoscope

A stethoscope is used to assess the apex pulse. Sound waves originating from an internal organ usually reach the body's surface and are dissipated into the air. Unless the sounds are of a high amplitude, the unassisted ear cannot hear them clearly. The **stethoscope** is a closed cylinder that prevents the dissipation of sound waves as they reach the body's surface and amplifies them for the examiner. The four major parts of the stethoscope are the earpieces, binaurals, plastic or rubber tubing, and chestpiece (Fig. 4-11).

### Character of the Pulse

Assessing the radial pulse includes measuring the pulse rate, rhythm and strength. When auscultating an apex pulse, assess the heart *rate* and *rhythm* only.

### Rate

Before measuring a pulse, know the baseline heart rate for comparison (Table 4-5). Pulse rates vary, depending on age, level of activity, and a variety of other factors. The sinoatrial (SA) node in the heart is the primary pacemaker of the heart, setting the heart rate faster or slower, depending on the metabolic demands of the body (see Chapter 17). To obtain a baseline pulse, the person should be at rest during measurement of the pulse, because physical activity increases the heart rate.

Some practitioners prefer to make baseline measurements of the pulse rate as the person assumes sitting, standing, and lying positions. Postural changes cause changes in the pulse rate, resulting from alterations in blood volume and distribution and sympathetic activity. The heart rate typically increases when a person moves from a lying position to a sitting or standing position. To assess the peripheral pulse rate, count the number of

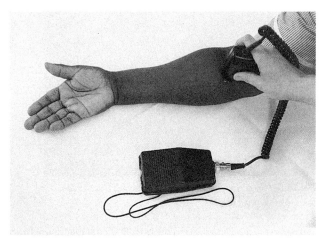

**Fig.4-10** Ultrasound stethoscope in position on brachial artery.

Photograph © 1994, Bruce Bailey/Select Photos, London.

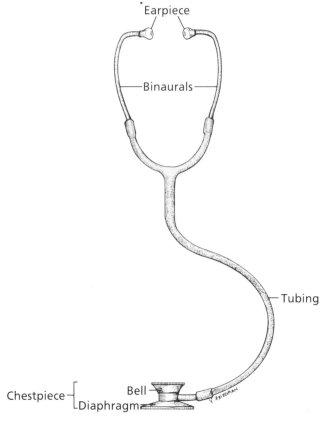

**Fig.4-11** Acoustic stethoscope.

arterial pulsations that occur in 60 seconds. The practice of taking a pulse for less than this and then calculating the number of pulsations that would have occurred in 60 seconds, should be discouraged because it is inaccurate in patients who may have an irregular or slow pulse.

Assess the apex pulse by listening for heart sounds. Try to identify the first and second heart sounds ($S_1$ and $S_2$). These arise from the closing of heart valves. At normal slow rates, $S_1$ is low pitched and dull in quality, sounding like a 'lub', $S_2$ is a higher pitched and shorter sound and creates the sound 'dub'. Using the diaphragm or bell of the stethoscope, count the number of *lub-dubs* occurring in a minute. One *lub-dub* equals one heart beat.

The apex pulse can be heard by placing the stethoscope over the 5th intercostal space in the mid clavicular line on the left side of the chest (Fig. 4-12).

The nurse may assess common variations in heart rate. **Tachycardia** is an abnormally elevated heart rate, above 100 beats per minute in adults. **Bradycardia** is a rate below 60 beats per minute in adults. The nurse should assess an apex pulse when tachycardia or bradycardia are detected at peripheral pulse sites.

### Rhythm

Successive heart beats normally occur at regular intervals. If an interval is interrupted by an early beat or if a beat is late or missed, the individual has an abnormal rhythm (*dysrhythmia*). A dysrhythmia alters the heart's ability to pump properly, particularly if it occurs repetitively. Assess dysrhythmia by palpating an interruption in the successive pulse waves or auscultating an interruption between sounds. If dysrhythmia is present, the regularity of its occurrence is assessed. It may be

### TABLE 4-5 Normal Heart Rates

| Age | Resting (Awake) | Heart Rate*<br>Resting (Sleeping) | Exercise or Fever |
|-----|-----------------|-----------------------------------|-------------------|
| Newborn | 100 - 180 | 80 - 160 | Up to 220 |
| 1 wk to 3 mo | 100 - 220 | 80 - 200 | Up to 220 |
| 3 mo to 2 yr | 80 - 150 | 70 - 120 | Up to 200 |
| 2 yr to 10 yr | 70 - 110 | 60 - 90 | Up to 200 |
| 10 yr to adult | 55 - 90 | 50 - 90 | Up to 200 |

Older adults: The heart rate slows with age, ranging from 44-108 beats per minute. Systole prolongs, as a heart rate of 120 or greater is not well tolerated. Stroke volume and cardiac output decrease (Eliopoulos, 1990).

*In beats/min.

From Gillette PC: Dysrhythmias. In Adams FH, Emmanouilides GC, editors: *Moss' heart disease in infants, children, and adolescents,* ed 3, Baltimore, 1983, Williams & Wilkins.

intermittent (occasional missed beats) or irregularly irregular (variation in frequency). Children often have a sinus dysrythmia, which is an irregular heart beat that speeds up with inspiration and slows down with expiration; this is a normal finding.

## Strength

The strength or amplitude of a pulse reflects the volume of blood ejected against the arterial wall with each heart contraction. Assessing the pulse strength is a subjective process and requires considerable practice. Normally, the pulse strength remains the same with each heart beat. A weak pulse is difficult to palpate and easy to lose during palpation. The weak pulse is thready and often rapid. A normal pulse is full, easily palpable, and not easily obliterated by the assessor's fingers. A bounding pulse is easily palpated and difficult to obliterate.

## RESPIRATION

Human survival depends on the ability of oxygen ($O_2$) to reach body cells and for carbon dioxide ($CO_2$) to be removed from the cells (Chapter 17). **Respiration** involves two distinctly different processes: external respiration, or the movement of air between the environment and lungs, and internal respiration, or the movement of $O_2$ between haemoglobin and single cells. External respiration further involves the following complex but interrelated processes: ventilation, the mechanical movement of air to and from the lungs and the exchange of respiratory gases; conduction, the movement of air through the airways of the lungs; diffusion, movement of $O_2$ and $CO_2$ between alveoli and red blood cells; and perfusion, distribution of blood through the pulmonary capillaries.

The nurse can directly assess only the process of external respiration, specifically by assessing ventilation. The rate, depth, and rhythm of ventilatory movements indicate the quality and efficiency of the respiratory process.

## Physiological Control

Breathing is generally a passive process. Normally, a person thinks little about it. The respiratory centres in the brainstem regulate the involuntary control of respiration. Adults normally breathe smoothly and uninterrupted, 12 to 18 times a minute.

Ventilation is regulated by levels of $CO_2$, $O_2$, and hydrogen ion concentration (*pH*) in the arterial blood. The most important factor in the control of ventilation is the carbon dioxide pressure ($PCO_2$) of arterial blood. An elevation in the $PCO_2$ causes the respiratory centre to increase the rate and depth of breathing. The increased ventilatory effort removes excess $PCO_2$ during exhalation. *Hypercarbia*, a chronic excess of $CO_2$ in arterial blood, can eventually depress ventilation.

Chemoreceptors located in the aorta and carotid arteries are receptors sensitive to $CO_2$, pH, and *hypoxia* (low levels of arterial $O_2$). If arterial $O_2$ levels fall, the chemoreceptors signal the respiratory centre to increase the rate and depth of ventilation. Normally, rising $PCO_2$ levels stimulate the initiation of inspiration, and falling $PCO_2$ levels have a limited impact on the control of ventilation. However, in patients/clients with chronic lung disease such as emphysema or bronchitis, the hypoxic drive to increase ventilation can become very important. These people may have chronic hypercarbia, which can suppress the normal stimulus for ventilation. A low level of arterial $O_2$ then becomes the primary stimulus to breathing for some patients/clients who have chronic lung diseases (see Chapter 17).

## Mechanics of Breathing

Although breathing is normally passive, muscular work moves the lungs and chest wall. Inspiration is more active than expiration. During inspiration the respiratory centre sends impulses along the phrenic nerve, causing the diaphragm, a thin, dome-shaped muscle connected to the lower ribs, to contract. As the diaphragm contracts it flattens and the abdominal organs move downward and forward, increasing the length of the chest cavity. At the same time, the ribs lift upward and outward, causing transverse expansion of the lungs. Fig. 4-13 shows how diaphragmatic movement affects the size of the chest cavity. During expiration, the diaphragm relaxes in the elevated position, and the abdominal organs return to their original positions. The elastic lung and chest wall also return to a relaxed state. Little energy is required to move air out of the lungs. Expiration becomes an active process only during exercise, voluntary *hyperventilation* (increased ventilation), and certain disease states (see Chapter 17).

Assess respirations by observing for normal thoracic and abdominal movements and symmetry in chest wall movement. During quiet breathing, the chest wall gently rises and falls. Contraction of the intercostal muscles between the ribs or of the accessory muscles in the neck and shoulders is not visible. Passive breathing is more diaphragmatic, as the abdominal cavity slowly rises and falls. Breathing during sleep is a good example of passive breathing using the diaphragm. Infants also use abdominal breathing.

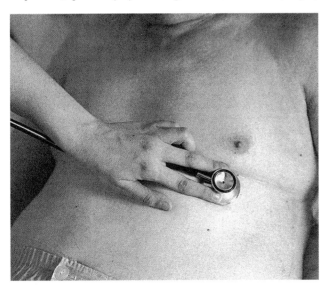

**Fig. 4-12** To hear the apex pulse, place the stethoscope over the 5th intercostal space in the mid clavicular line on the left side of the chest. Photograph © 1994, Bruce Bailey/Select Photos, London.

When breathing requires more effort, rib (costal) movement increases. The intercostal and accessory muscles work actively to move air in and out. The shoulders may rise and fall, and the accessory muscles in the neck visibly contract. Diaphragmatic movement is less noticeable when rib movement increases.

## Assessing Respirations

Respirations are the easiest of all vital signs to assess, but are often the most haphazardly measured. Sometimes a nurse merely estimates the respiratory rate. However, **recognition of a subtle change in the character of respirations is important**.

Assess respirations when the patient/client is at rest. If the patient/client is anxious, in pain, or fearful, the respirations will probably be increased in rate and depth. A skillful nurse does not let a patient/client know that respirations are being assessed. A patient/client who is aware of the nurse's intentions may consciously alter the rate and depth of breathing. Assessment is best done immediately after measuring pulse rate, with the nurse's hand still on the patient/client's wrist. The nurse should always assess respirations carefully to avoid overlooking signs that may be relevant to a patient's/client's physiological needs.

## Rate

Observe a full inspiration and expiration when counting a respiration. The respiratory rate varies with age (Table 4-6). An infant normally breathes 30 to 35 times per minute. Throughout childhood, the respiratory rate declines. Among adults, normal rates vary from 12 to 20 respirations per minute. Respiratory rates greater than 20 in adults are called **tachypnoea**. Respiratory rates less than 10 are called **bradypnoea** and may be seen normally when people sleep. *Apnoea* is the absence of breathing, which may be for a few seconds, or life threatening if prolonged. The box (next page) lists factors affecting character of respirations.

## Depth

The depth of respirations is assessed by observing the degree of movement in the chest wall. Ventilatory movements are objectively described as *shallow*, *normal*, or *deep*.

During a normal, relaxed breath, a person inhales or exhales approximately 500 ml of air (*tidal volume*). A deep respiration involves a full expansion of the lungs with full exhalation. Respirations are shallow when only a small quantity of air passes through the lungs and ventilatory movement is difficult to see.

The capacity of the lungs to take in air depends on gender and age. Lung capacity is determined by taking as deep a breath as possible and then blowing it entirely out into a *spirometer*, a device that measures air volume. The amount of air exhaled after a minimal full inspiration is the lung's *vital capacity* and is about 4800 ml of air. Men tend to have a larger vital capacity than women of the same age. Infants and young children have smaller vital capacities than adolescents and adults. With advancing age the lung loses its elasticity, and the capacity for forcible exhalation declines. Nursing care may focus on increasing the patient's/client's efforts to breathe deeply. Knowledge of the patient's/client's normal capacity to move air is helpful in planning realistic therapy.

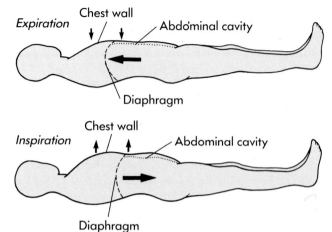

**Fig.4-13** Illustration of diaphragmatic movement during inspiration and expiration.

## Rhythm

Normal breathing is regular and uninterrupted. A regular interval occurs after each respiratory cycle. An occasional extra deep breath, a sigh, is commonly seen during quiet breathing. Infants tend to breathe less regularly. The young child may breathe slowly for a few seconds and then suddenly breathe more rapidly.

Noninvasive assessment of oxygenation is simple. An *oximeter* equipped with a probe to clip to the finger or ear can provide continuous or intermittent determinations of *oxygen saturation* (percent of haemoglobin saturated with oxygen). This provides a reliable method of assessing adequacy of oxygenation and indirectly assessing adequacy of ventilation (see Chapter 17).

Another respiratory monitoring device that aids assessment is the apnoea monitor. Apnoea monitoring is used frequently with infants in the hospital and at home to observe for prolonged apnoeic events.

## General Respiratory Characteristics

While assessing the three objective qualities of rate, depth, and rhythm, it is also important to observe factors related to the

| TABLE 4-6 Normal Respiratory Rates by Age | |
|---|---|
| **Age Group** | **Rate \*** |
| Newborn | 35 |
| 1 - 11 mo | 30 |
| 2 yr | 25 |
| 4 yr | 23 |
| 6 yr | 21 |
| 8 yr | 20 |
| 10 yr | 19 |
| 12 yr | 19 |
| 14 yr | 18 |
| 16 yr | 17 |
| 18 yr | 16–18 |
| Adult | 12–20 |

*per minute

## Factors Influencing the Character of Respirations

- Exercise. Exercise increases rate and depth to meet the body's greater $O_2$ needs.
- Acute pain. Pain increases rate and depth as a result of sympathetic stimulation (not if chest pain or trauma).
- Anxiety. Anxiety increases rate and depth as a result of sympathetic stimulation (not if chest pain or trauma).
- Smoking. Long-term smoking changes the lung's airways, resulting in an increased rate.
- Body position. Straight, erect posture promotes full chest expansion. Stooped or slumped position impairs ventilatory movement.
- Medications. Narcotic analgesics and sedatives depress rate and depth.
- Brainstem injury. Injury to the brainstem impairs the respiratory centre and inhibits respiratory rate and rhythm.

general character of respirations. Depending on the level of oxygenation, respiratory alterations may cause changes in skin colour and level of consciousness. The nail beds, lips, and skin may take on a bluish or cyanotic appearance when arterial $O_2$ levels are reduced. As oxygenation decreases, a person typically becomes more restless and anxious and tries harder to breathe.

Difficulty in breathing is *dyspnoea*. As breathing becomes laboured a person uses accessory muscles in the chest and neck to breathe. A patient/client with dyspnoea usually feels short of breath.

Sounds of breathing may indicate a respiratory disorder. Inflammation or stricture of the trachea or larynx causes obstruction to airflow. As a patient/client inhales, air passing the obstruction creates a harsh, crowing sound, or respiratory stridor, which can easily be heard without a stethoscope. Secretions in the large airways of the trachea and the bronchus can often be heard without a stethoscope. These sounds can occur during inspiration or expiration. They have a gurgling sound and are called *rhonchi* or *gurgles*. The rhythm and regularity of breaths should be noted, and also whether both sides of the chest (i.e. both lungs) are expanding symmetrically during breathing.

## BLOOD PRESSURE

**Blood pressure** is the force exerted by the blood against a vessel wall. The standard unit for measuring blood pressure is millimetres of mercury (mmHg). The measurement indicates the height to which the blood pressure can raise a column of mercury. In a cardiac cycle blood pressure reaches a peak that is followed by a trough (see Chapter 17). The peak or maximum pressure occurs during **systole** as the left ventricle pumps blood into the aorta. The trough occurs during **diastole** as the ventricles relax. Diastolic pressure is the minimal pressure exerted against the arterial walls at all times. Blood pressure is recorded with the systolic reading before the diastolic (for example, 120/80 mmHg).

## Physiology of Arterial Blood Pressure

Blood pressure reflects the balance between various factors, including cardiac output, blood volume, *peripheral vascular resistance* (resistance within the blood vessels in the periphery of the body) and blood viscosity (thickness). Each factor can affect another. For example, an increase in blood volume increases cardiac output. These factors have an impact on blood movement and blood pressure in the body and are known as *haemodynamic factors*.

The complex control of the cardiovascular system normally prevents any single factor from permanently changing blood pressure. For example, if blood volume falls, the body compensates with increased peripheral resistance due to vasoconstriction. This shunts blood to vital organs and maintains the blood pressure at a normal level. When vascular resistance increases, the blood pressure rises. The size of arteries and arterioles changes to adjust blood flow to the needs of local tissues. The smaller the lumen (internal diameter) of a vessel, the greater its peripheral vascular resistance to blood flow. When blood flow to a major organ falls sharply, peripheral arteries vasoconstrict to shunt blood back to the major vessels supplying the organ. Arterial pressure rises to push blood through narrowed vessels. In contrast, as vessels dilate and vascular resistance falls, blood pressure drops.

The blood pressure (BP) is a product of the cardiac output (CO) and peripheral vascular resistance (PR); therefore:

$$BP = CO \times PR$$

When volume increases in an enclosed space, the pressure in that space rises. Thus, as the cardiac output increases, more blood is pumped against the arterial walls, causing an elevation in blood pressure. Exercise temporarily elevates blood pressure as the demand for cardiac output increases.

The volume of blood circulating within the vascular system affects blood pressure. Most adults have a circulating blood volume of 5000 ml. Normally the blood volume remains constant. However, if volume increases, more pressure is exerted against arterial walls. The rapid, uncontrolled infusion of intravenous fluids is a typical cause of elevated blood pressure. When circulating blood volume falls to a critical level, as in the case of haemorrhage or dehydration, blood pressure falls.

## Factors Influencing Blood Pressure

Blood pressure does not stay constant. Many factors influence it throughout the day. An understanding of these factors ensures a more accurate interpretation of blood pressure readings.

## Age

Normal blood pressure levels vary throughout life. They increase during childhood. The level of a child's or adolescent's blood pressure is assessed with respect to body size and age (Task Force on Blood Pressure Control in Children, 1987). An infant's blood pressure ranges from 65-115/42-80 mmHg. The normal blood pressure for a 7 year old is 87-117/48-64 mmHg. Larger children (heavier and/or taller) have higher blood pressures than smaller children of the same age.

During adolescence, blood pressure continues to vary according to body size. However, the normal range for 10 to 19 year olds at the 90th percentile is 124-136/77-84 mmHg for boys and 124-127/63-74 mmHg for girls.

An adult's blood pressure tends to increase with advancing age. The standard norm for a healthy, middle-age adult is 120/80 mmHg. A systolic pressure below 140 mmHg and a diastolic pressure below 90 mmHg are still considered normal. The older adult's blood pressure range is 140-160/80-90 mmHg.

## Stress

Anxiety, fear, pain, and emotional stress initiate sympathetic stimulation, causing the blood pressure to rise. Sympathetic stimulation increases the heart rate, which increases the cardiac output and vasoconstriction, which results in increased peripheral vascular resistance.

## Race

US statistics indicate the rate of hypertension is higher in urban African Americans than in European Americans (National Academy of Science, 1989). The predisposition for hypertension is believed to be genetically and environmentally related.

## Medications

Some medications can directly or indirectly affect blood pressure. During blood pressure assessment, the nurse should consider whether the patient/client is receiving medication which could lower blood pressure.

## Diurnal Variation

Blood pressure levels vary over the course of a day. The blood pressure is typically lowest in the early morning. It gradually rises during the morning and afternoon, peaking in late afternoon or evening. No two people have the same pattern or degree of variation. A student may find it interesting to have a friend check blood pressure at intervals during a 24-hour period.

## Hypertension

**Hypertension** is a major factor underlying death from strokes, and it also contributes to myocardial infarctions (heart attacks). One blood pressure recording does not qualify as a diagnosis of hypertension. However, if the nurse assesses a high reading (for example, 150/90 mmHg), this should be reported and repeated.

Hypertension is often the result of thickening and loss of elasticity in the arterial walls. Peripheral vascular resistance increases within the affected vessels. As a result, blood flow to vital organs such as the heart, brain, and kidney decreases. The heart must continually pump against greater resistance.

The nurse can educate patients/clients about their risks for hypertension. People with family members who have had hypertension are at significant risk. Other risk factors for hypertension are listed in the box.

## Hypotension

**Hypotension** is generally considered present when the systolic blood pressure falls to 90 mmHg or below. Although some adults

### Risk Factors for Hypertension

- Family history of hypertension
- Obesity
- Cigarette smoking
- Heavy alcohol consumption
- Elevated blood cholesterol level
- Continued exposure to stress

have a low blood pressure normally, for the majority of people, low blood pressure is an abnormal finding associated with illness.

Hypotension occurs in disease because of the dilation of the arteries in the vascular bed, the loss of a substantial amount of blood volume, or the failure of the heart muscle to pump adequately. Hypotension associated with pallor, skin mottling, clamminess, confusion, increased heart rate, or decreased urine output may be life threatening and should be reported to a doctor immediately.

## Assessment of Blood Pressure

Blood pressure may be measured directly or indirectly. The direct method requires the insertion of a thin intravenous catheter into an artery. Tubing connects the catheter with an electronic sensor. Pressure within the artery transmits pressure along the fluid-filled tubing to the sensor, which then displays a blood pressure reading on an electronic display. Direct monitoring is used only in an operating theatre or critical care areas.

The indirect method requires use of the sphygmomanometer. The nurse may use auscultation, palpation, or both. Assessing the blood pressure indirectly by auscultation is the most common technique (see Procedure 4-1).

## Sphygmomanometer

To assess blood pressure, it is important to have equipment that functions properly, to be competent and to feel comfortable when using a stethoscope and sphygmomanometer. Procedure 4-1 describes how to measure blood pressure using a sphygmomanometer.

A **sphygmomanometer** consists of a pressure manometer, an occlusive cloth cuff enclosing an inflatable rubber bladder, and a pressure bulb with a release valve to inflate the cuff (Fig. 4-14). There are two types of manometers, mercury and aneroid. The mercury manometer is the most accurate. It is an upright tube containing mercury. Pressure created by inflation of the compression cuff moves the column of mercury upward against the force of gravity. Millimetre calibrations mark the height of the mercury column. To ensure accurate readings, the mercury column should always be at *zero* when the cuff is deflated, and it should fall freely as pressure is released. Mercury manometers are mounted on the wall or are portable. Accurate readings are made by looking at the mercury meniscus at eye level. This is the point where the crescent-shaped top of the mercury column aligns with the manometer scale. Looking up or down at the mercury results in measurement distortions.

The aneroid manometer has a glass-enclosed circular gauge containing a needle that registers millimeter calibrations. A metal

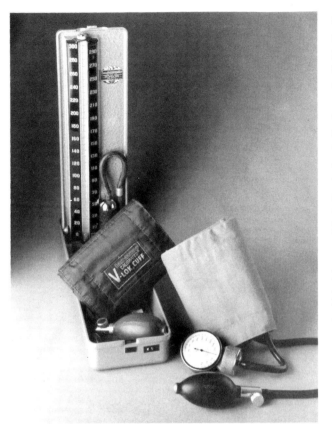

Fig.4-14 Mercury *(left)* and aneroid sphygmomanometers.

bellows within the gauge expands and collapses in response to pressure variations in the inflated cuff. Before using the aneroid model, ensure that the needle points to *zero* and that the manometer is correctly calibrated. It should be recalibrated against a perfectly working mercury manometer at least once a year. Aneroid manometers have the advantages of being lightweight, portable, and compact.

Cloth cuffs used with the sphygmomanometer come in several sizes. Ideally the width of the cuff should be 40% of the circumference (or 20% wider than the diameter) of the midpoint of the limb on which the cuff is to be used (Eliopoulos, 1984). The length of the enclosed bladder should be approximately twice the recommended width. A bladder of this length nearly encircles the arm and minimizes the risk of misapplication. In an adult the average bladder width is 19 to 20 cm, and the length is 22 to 23 cm. In children the lower edge of the cuff should be above the antecubital fossa, allowing room for placement of the stethoscope. An improperly fitting cuff causes inaccurate readings (Table 4-7).

## Auscultation

The best environment for blood pressure measurement by auscultation is a quiet room at a comfortable temperature. Try to control the patient's/client's pain, anxiety, or exertion and ask the patient/client to refrain from eating or smoking before the assessment, because these factors can cause false high readings.

Although the patient/client may lie or stand, sitting is the preferred position. Some patient/clients, especially older adults,

may experience postural or **orthostatic hypotension** (a drop of 25 mmHg in systolic pressure and a drop of 10 mmHg in diastolic pressure when moving from a lying to sitting or a sitting to standing position). Orthostatic hypotension is a common side effect of antihypertensive medications.

The procedure of taking a blood pressure requires practice using the equipment and familiarity with the sounds from the stethoscope. Many students initially experience difficulty with this, but should not be alarmed as practice does help. Under NO circumstances should a nurse pretend to hear a blood pressure, as this could have dangerous consequences for the patient. Always ask a senior nurse to check. (A teaching stethoscope, which has two sets of ear pieces, may also be used so that two people can listen simultaneously.)

## PRESSURE DYNAMICS

Indirect measurement of arterial blood pressure works on a basic principle of pressure. The external application of pressure beyond that which keeps a vessel open causes the vessel to close. For example, in a patient/client with a normal blood pressure of 120/80 mmHg, blood flows freely through the brachial artery at a systolic pressure of 120 mmHg. Inflation of the cuff gradually applies pressure to tissues surrounding the brachial artery. When the cuff pressure exceeds 120 mmHg, the artery collapses, blood flow ceases, and auscultation reveals absence of sounds. When the cuff pressure is released, the point on the manometer at which sounds reappear through auscultation is the systolic pressure.

## KOROTKOFF SOUNDS

With the stethoscope placed over the artery, listen for sounds created by blood flowing through it. In 1905, Nikolai S. Korotkoff, a Russian surgeon, first described arterial sounds. The *Korotkoff sounds* are used to assess arterial blood pressure values.

The first Korotkoff sound (Phase I) is a clear, rhythmical, tapping sound. *Onset of the sound corresponds to the systolic pressure.* With the second Korotkoff sound (Phase II), a murmur or swishing sound appears as the cuff is further deflated. As the artery distends, there is a turbulence of blood flow. With the third Korotkoff sound (Phase III), sounds become temporarily crisper and more intense. The fourth Korotkoff sound (Phase IV) becomes muffled and low pitched as the cuff is further deflated. Cuff pressure falls below the pressure within the vessel walls. *This sound is the diastolic pressure in infants and children.* The fifth Korotkoff sound (Phase V) is a disappearance of all sounds. *In adolescents and adults, this sound corresponds with the diastolic pressure.*

It should be noted that there is divided opinion as to whether the muffling or the disappearance is a more precise indicator of blood pressure (Perry, 1991).

## POTENTIAL ERRORS IN AUSCULTATION

Several causes may result in an error in blood pressure readings if the auscultation method is not performed correctly. Table 4-7 summarizes common mistakes in measurement.

## PROCEDURE 4-1 Indirect Measurement of Blood Pressure Using a Sphygmomanometer

**Sequence of Actions**

1. Ensure the patient/client is resting quietly, ideally with his or her arm resting on a table or pillow so that it is about level with the heart (see illustration). Ensure that sleeves can be pushed up above the level of the blood pressure cuff; if this cannot be done without the clothing causing a restriction in blood flow, the arm should be taken out of the sleeve.

2. Wrap the cuff of the sphygmomanometer snugly around the arm, about 2.5 cm above the anticubital space. Depending on cuff design, secure the Velcro or tuck in the cuff end.

3. To determine the maximum pressure to which the cuff should be inflated, palpate the brachial artery and inflate the cuff simultaneously. The pressure at which the brachial pulse is no longer palpable is the systolic pressure. The maximum pressure the cuff should be inflated to its systolic pressure plus 30 mmHg. The cuff should not be inflated any more than this as this will cause the patient/client extreme discomfort and avoidable pain.

4. Place the earpiece of the stethoscope in your ears and hold the bell of the stethoscope firmly over the brachial artery (see illustration).

5. Hold the rubber bulb of the sphygmomanometer in the palm of the hand with the screw between the thumb and index finger. Close the valve by tightening the screw.

**Rationale**

Maintains comfort during measurement. Placement of arm above heart level causes false low reading. Ensures proper cuff application.

Inflating cuff directly over brachial artery ensures that proper pressure is applied during inflation. Loose-fitting cuff causes false high readings.

Identifies approximate systolic pressure and determines maximum inflation point for accurate reading. Prevents auscultatory gap.

Proper stethoscope placement ensures optimal sound reception. Stethoscope improperly positioned causes muffled sounds that often result in false low systolic and false high diastolic readings.

Tightening of valve prevents air leak during inflation.

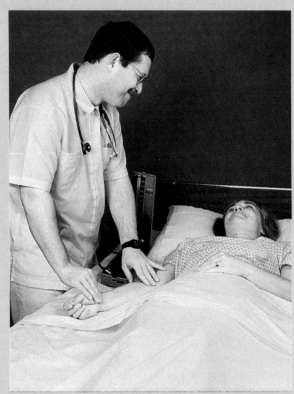

Step 1.

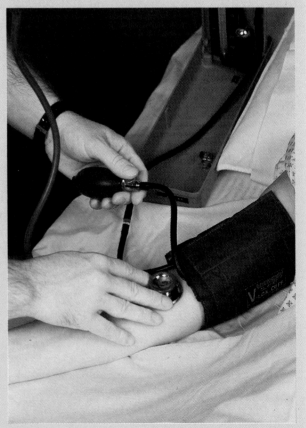

Step 4.

**PROCEDURE 4-1 (Cont'd)**  **Indirect Measurement of Blood Pressure Using a Sphygmomanometer**

| Sequence of Actions | Rationale |
|---|---|
| 6. Inflate the cuff by pumping the rubber bulb (see illustration). Continue until the manometer reads systolic pressure plus 30 mmHg. This will ensure the brachial artery is compressed. At this time, no sounds will be heard through the stethoscope. | Ensures accurate measurement of systolic pressure. |
| 7. Slowly release the pressure in the cuff by opening the screw valve. As the pressure in the cuff decreases, the artery allows some blood through. This turbulent flow can be heard by a tapping sound. Note the reading on the manometer when these sounds are heard. This is the systolic pressure. | First Korotkoff sound indicates systolic pressure. |
| 8. The sound will become more muffled as the cuff is further deflated. When the sound becomes inaudible, this is the diastolic pressure and should be read from the manometer. | Ensures accurate measurement of diastolic pressure. |
| 9. Record blood pressure in nursing notes or TPR chart. Report abnormal findings immediately. | Vital signs should be recorded immediately to ensure accuracy. |

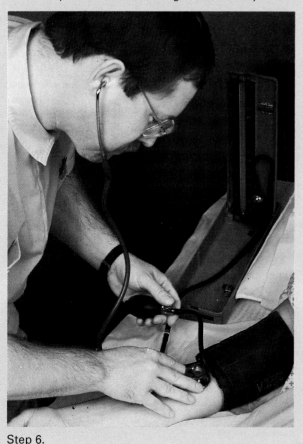

Step 6.

## Assessment of Blood Pressure in Children

Measurement and interpretation of blood pressure in infants and children is difficult for the following reasons:

- various arm sizes require careful and appropriate cuff size selection
- readings are difficult to obtain in restless or anxious infants and children
- placing the stethoscope too firmly on the antecubital fossa can cause errors in auscultation of Korotkoff sounds
- Korotkoff sounds are difficult to hear in children because of low frequency and amplitude
- blood pressure in children changes with growth and development.

## TABLE 4-7 Common Mistakes in Blood Pressure Assessment

| Error | Effect |
| --- | --- |
| Bladder or cuff too wide | False low reading |
| Bladder or cuff too narrow | False high reading |
| Cuff wrapped too loosely | False high reading |
| Deflating cuff too slowly | False high diastolic reading |
| Deflating cuff too quickly | False low systolic and false high diastolic reading |
| Stethoscope that fits poorly or impairment of the examiner's hearing, causing sounds to be muffled | False low systolic and false high diastolic reading |
| Inaccurate inflation level | False low systolic reading |
| Multiple examiners using different Korotkoff sounds for diastolic readings | Inaccurate interpretation of systolic and diastolic readings |

Use the same auscultation method for children as is used with adults. A Doppler ultrasonic stethoscope may be helpful with small children and infants. Infants or children under 5 years of age should lie supine with the arms supported at heart level. Older children may sit. Children should be relaxed and calm. A delay of at least 15 minutes before taking a reading is recommended to allow children to recover from recent activity or apprehension. Those 15 minutes can be used for other quiet nursing activities. It may help to have parents or guardians nearby.

## REPORTING AND RECORDING VITAL SIGNS

The nurse is responsible for recording all vital signs accurately and in a timely manner. When a change or abnormality is assessed, report the problem to the nurse in charge, who will then inform the doctor.

Observation, or temperature, pulse and respiration (TPR) charts are used to record vital signs. These flow charts highlight trends and deviations from the norm (Fig. 4-15). In addition to the actual vital sign values, record in the nurses' notes any accompanying or precipitating symptoms such as chest pain and dizziness with abnormal blood pressure, shortness of breath with abnormal respirations, or flushing and diaphoresis (sweating) with elevated temperature. Document any interventions initiated as a result of vital sign measurement, such as administration of tepid sponging or an antipyretic medication.

## SUMMARY

Vital signs measurements are a basic series of physiological assessments reflecting a patient's/client's health. The nurse uses these observations to make clinical decisions. Physical and psychological factors can create changes in vital signs. The nurse often decides the need for and frequency of vital sign assessment, which is not simply a routine task but rather an important part of a nurse's practice.

Before measuring any vital sign, you should understand the physiological controls governing it. Each physiological control is influenced by certain variables such as age, physical exercise, or hormonal changes. The nurse who understands the effects of these variables is better prepared to anticipate normal variations. You cannot recognize abnormalities without first knowing the norms.

Basic principles apply in the procedures for assessing vital signs accurately. The patient/client should be placed in the most comfortable position for measurements. Procedures should be explained to the patient/client to reduce anxiety. Results are recorded promptly and accurately.

Through physical assessment, the nurse makes clinical decisions that contribute to the patient's/client's health management. Information gathered during physical assessment supplements data obtained during the nursing history and from ongoing nurse-patient/client interactions. As a result of more thorough data gathering, the nurse is able to make nursing decisions with greater precision. Therefore the care plan becomes more individualized and comprehensive. Physical assessment findings also reveal whether specific nursing interventions were successful.

Before an examination begins, take the necessary steps to prepare the patient/client and setting. Take measures to ensure privacy, provide psychological and physical comfort and reduce the transmission of microorganisms. Patients/clients become active participants as you carefully explain each step of the examination. Use time during an assessment to provide important information about how patients/clients can maintain or improve their health.

## CHAPTER 4 REVIEW

### Key concepts

- Vital signs include the physiological measurements of temperature, pulse, respirations, and blood pressure.
- Use clinical judgement to determine the frequency of vital sign measurement.

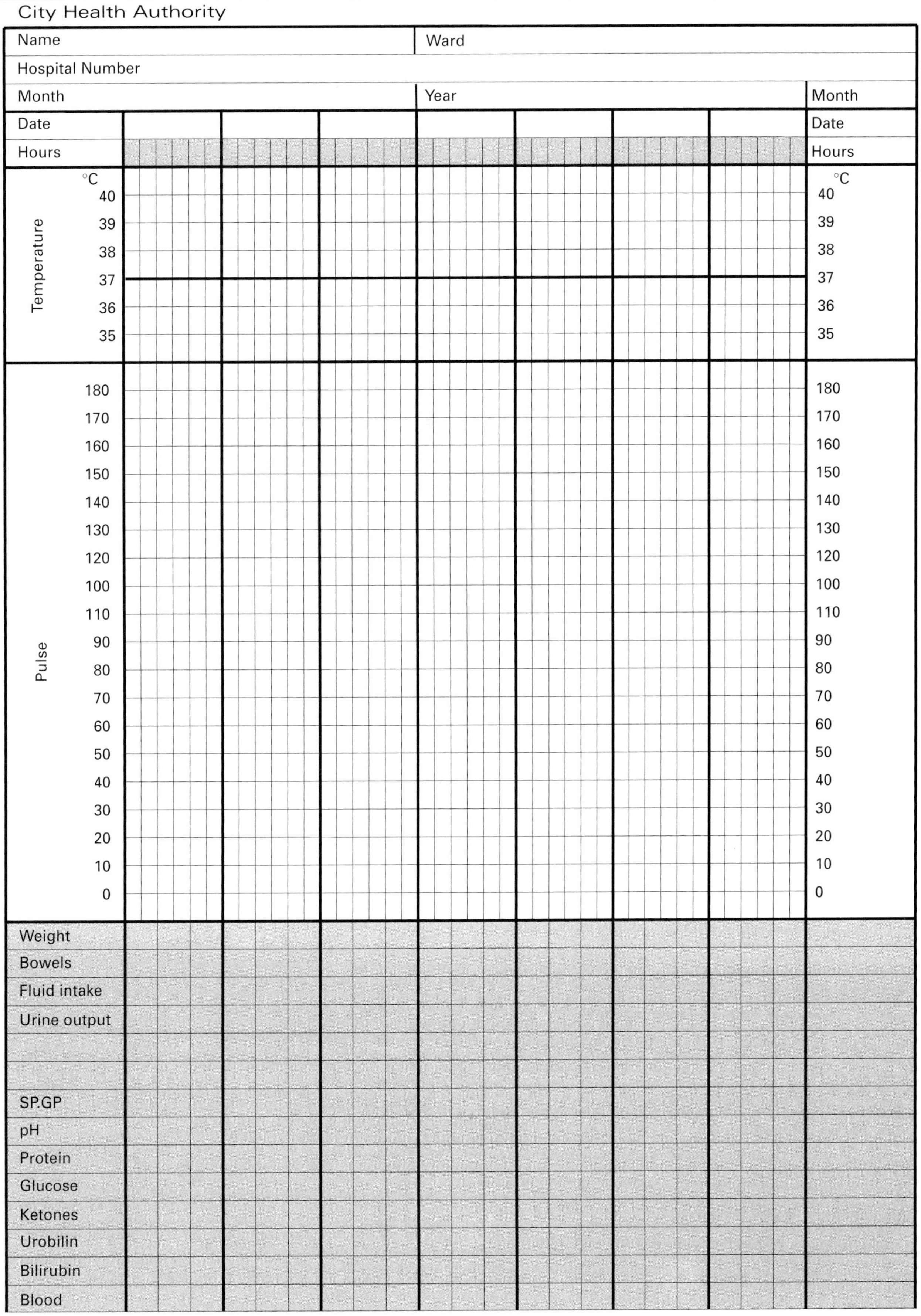

## City Health Authority

| Name | | Ward | |
|---|---|---|---|
| Hospital Number | | | |
| Month | | Year | Month |
| Date | | | Date |
| Hours | | | Hours |

Temperature

| °C | | °C |
|---|---|---|
| 40 | | 40 |
| 39 | | 39 |
| 38 | | 38 |
| 37 | | 37 |
| 36 | | 36 |
| 35 | | 35 |

Pulse

| | | |
|---|---|---|
| 180 | | 180 |
| 170 | | 170 |
| 160 | | 160 |
| 150 | | 150 |
| 140 | | 140 |
| 130 | | 130 |
| 120 | | 120 |
| 100 | | 100 |
| 110 | | 110 |
| 90 | | 90 |
| 80 | | 80 |
| 70 | | 70 |
| 60 | | 60 |
| 50 | | 50 |
| 40 | | 40 |
| 30 | | 30 |
| 20 | | 20 |
| 10 | | 10 |
| 0 | | 0 |

| Weight | |
|---|---|
| Bowels | |
| Fluid intake | |
| Urine output | |
| | |
| | |
| SP.GP | |
| pH | |
| Protein | |
| Glucose | |
| Ketones | |
| Urobilin | |
| Bilirubin | |
| Blood | |

**Fig.4-15** Temperature, pulse, and respiration chart. *Courtesy, St. Bartholomew's Hospital, London.*

- Knowledge of the factors influencing vital signs assists in interpreting abnormal values.
- Vital sign measurements provide a basis for evaluating response to nursing interventions.
- Assessment of vital signs yields the most accurate values when the patient/client is inactive and the environment is controlled for comfort.
- Normally, heat production balances heat loss to maintain body temperature.
- Assist the patient/client in attaining a normal body temperature by initiating interventions promoting heat loss or production.
- A fever is a normal defence mechanism and often does not require treatment.
- To assess cardiac function, pulse rate and rhythm are most easily and accurately measured using the radial or apex pulse.
- Assessment of respirations involves observation of ventilatory movements through the whole respiratory cycle.
- Blood pressure levels reflect the relationship among several haemodynamic variables and can be measured by auscultation.
- Changes in any vital sign can influence characteristics of the other vital signs.
- Baseline assessment findings reflect functional abilities when the nurse first assesses the patient/client and serve as the basis for comparison with subsequent assessment findings.
- Physical assessment of a child or infant requires the nurse to apply principles of physical growth and development.
- The nurse recognizes that the normal process of ageing affects physical findings collected from an older adult.
- Patient/client teaching should be integrated throughout the examination to help each person understand the implications of all findings.
- The nurse can use time more efficiently by integrating physical assessment with nursing care.
- Inspection requires good lighting, full exposure of the body part, and a careful comparison of the part with its counterpart on the opposite side of the body.
- A physical examination should be performed only after proper preparation of the environment and equipment. The patient's/client's comfort should be checked at each step of the procedure.
- The nurse assesses mental and emotional status by interacting with the patient/client throughout the examination.

## CRITICAL THINKING EXERCISES

1. During admission assessment, you need to obtain a temperature measurement on a restless 18-year-old patient who had been in a motor vehicle accident. Oral, rectal or tympanic electronic thermometers are available. What criteria do you use to select the most efficient and effective method for obtaining this patient's body temperature?

2. It is raining and your patient/client just ran into the clinic from the car park. What effect would you expect this activity to have on vital signs? When would you expect to get vital signs that are the person's 'true' values for pulse, blood pressure and respirations?

3. The previous blood pressure for your 120 kg male patient/client was taken with a regular cuff, and the reading was 170/100 mmHg. What conclusions can you make about the previous reading? What would you do to verify this reading?

4. While obtaining your patient's/client's vital signs, you palpate a rapid, irregular heart beat. Your confirm this irregularity with a one-minute apex pulse measurement. The result is a rate of 124 beats per minute with irregular rhythm. What are your anticipated follow-up activities for this patient/client?

## Key Terms

Blood pressure, p. 93
Bradycardia, p. 90
Bradypnoea, p. 92
Diastole, p. 93
Health assessment, p. 71
Health screening, p. 71
Hypertension, p. 94
Hyperthermia, p. 81
Hypotension, p. 94
Hypothermia, p. 85
Physical preparation, p. 74
Pulse, p. 88
Pyrexia, p. 84
Respirations, p. 91
Sphygmonanometer, p. 94
Stethoscope, p. 89
Systole, p. 93
Tachycardia, p. 90
Tachypnoea, p. 92
Temperature, p. 81
Vital signs, p. 71

## REFERENCES

Baker NC et al: The effect of type of thermometer and length of time inserted on oral temperature measurements of afebrile subjects, *Nurs Res* 33:109, 1984.

Bennett G: Assessing abuse in the elderly, *Geriatr Med* 20(7):49, 1990.

Bobak IM: *Maternity and gynecologic care: the nurse and the family* ed 5, St Louis, 1993, Mosby.

Closs J: Oral temperature measurement, *Nurs Times* 83:36, 1987.

Davis K: Ear temperature measurement questioned, *Nurs Times* 89(33):10, 1993.

DeWitt S: Nursing assessment of the skin and dermatologic lesions, *Nurs Clin North Am* 25(1):235, 1990.

Dinarello C: Interleukin-1, *Rev Infect Dis* 6:51, 1984.

Eliopoulos C: *Health assessment of the older adult*, California, 1984, Addison-Wesley.

Guyton AC: *Textbook of medical physiology*, ed 8, Philadelphia, 1991, Saunders.

Hanson M: Drug fever: remember to consider it in diagnosis, *Postgrad Med* 89(5):167, 1991.

Heinz J: Validation of sublingual temperature in patients with nasogastric tubes, *Heart and lung*, 14: 198, 1985.

Hollerbach AD, Sneed NV: Accuracy of radial pulse assessment by length of counting interval, *Heart Lung* 19(3):258, 1990.

Kim MJ, McFarland GK, McLane AM: *Pocket guide to nursing diagnoses*, ed 4, St Louis, 1991, Mosby–Year Book.

Larson E: Evaluating validity of screening tests, *Nurs. Res.* 35:186, 1986.

LaVoy K: Dealing with hypothermia and frostbite, *RN* 48:53, 1985.

Leung AKC, Robson WLM: Febrile convulsions: how dangerous are they? *Postgrad Med* 89(5):217, 1991.

Lovejoy F H: Aspirin and acetaminophen : a comparative view of their antipyretic and analgesic activity, *Pediatrics* 62 (suppl) : 904, 1978

Lukasiewicz P: Rectal temperatures are as accurate as oral temperatures in patients receiving oxygen therapy, *Crit Care Nurse* 6:72, 1986.

Marieb EN: *Human anatomy and physiology*, Redwood City, Calif, 1989, Benjamin/Cummings.

McCleod-Clarke J, Hockey L: *Further research for nursing*, London, 1989, Scutari.

Morley CJ *et al*: Axillary and rectal temperature measurements in infants, *Arch Dis Child* 67:122, 1992.

Morley CJ *et al*: Axillary versus rectal temperature taking, *Nurs Times* 89(4):48, 1993.

Mountcastle VB: *Medical physiology*, vol 2, ed 14, St Louis, 1980, Mosby.

National Academy of Science: *Recommended dietary allowances*, Washington DC, 1989, The Academy.

Perry IJ, Recording diastolic blood pressure in pregnancy, *Nurs Times* 87(16), 1991.

Petersdorf RC: *Disturbances of heat regulation.* In Isselbacker KJ (eds): Harrison's principles of internal medicine ed 9, New York, 1980, McGraw-Hill.

Rogers M: Temperature recording in infants and children, *Paed Nurs* 4, 1992

Royal College of Nursing: *Guidelines for nurses: abuse and older people*, London, RCN, 1991.

Shinozaki T, Deane R, Perkins FM: Infrared tympanic thermometer: evaluation of a new clinical thermometer, *Crit Care Med* 16(2):148, 1988.

Task Force on Blood Pressure Control in Children: Report of second task force on blood pressure control in children: 1987, *Pediatrics* 79:1, 1987.

Thibodeau GA, Patton K: *Anatomy and physiology*, ed 2, St Louis, 1993, Mosby.

Wong DL: *Nursing care of infants and children*, ed 5, St Louis, 1995, Mosby.

## FURTHER READING

### Adult Nursing

Boylan A, Brown P: Student Observations. Respirations. *Nurs Times* 81:38, 1985.

Boylan A, Brown P: Student Observations. Temperature. *Nurs Times* 81:36, 1985.

Boylan A, Brown P: Student Observations. The pulse and blood pressure, *Nurs Times* 81:26, 1985.

Croft PR, Cruikshank JK: Blood pressure management in adults: large cuffs for all? *J Epidemiol Community Health* 4:170, 1990.

Davis C, Lentz M: Circadian rhythms: charting oral temperatures to spot abnormalities, *J Gerontol Nurs* 15(4):34, 1989.

Dennison R: Cardiopulmonary assessment, *Nurs 86* 16:34, 1986.

Draper P: Not a job for juniors, *Nurs Times* 83(10): 58, 1987.

Dressler DK *et al*: A comparison of oral and rectal temperature measurement on patients receiving oxygen by mask, *Nurs Res* 32:393, 1983.

Durham ML, Swanson B, Paulford N: Effect of tachypnea on oral temperature estimation: a replication, *Nurs Res* 35(4):211, 1986.

Fulbrook P: Temperature measurement in adults: a literature review, *J Adv Nurs* 18:1451, 1993.

Giuffre M *et al*: The relationship between axillary and core body temperatures, *Appl Nurs Res* 3(2):52, 1990.

Griffin JP: Fever: when to leave it alone, *Nurs 86* 16:58, 1986.

McCarron K: Fever: the cardinal vital sign, *CCQ* 9 (1):15, 1986.

Nolan J, Nolan M: Can nurses take an accurate blood pressure? *Br J Nurs* 2(14):724, 1993.

Rebenson-Piano M *et al*: An evaluation of two indirect methods of blood pressure measurements in ill patients, *Nurs Res* 39:42, 1989.

Stevens S, Becker KL: How to perform picture-perfect respiratory assessment, *Nurs 88* 19:57, 1988.

### Children's Nursing

Reeves-Swift R: Rational management of a child's acute fever, *MCN* 15(2):82, 1990.

Thomas DO: Fever in children, *RN* 48:19, 1985.

Thomas SP, Groer MW: Relationship of demographic lifestyle and stress variables to blood pressure in adolescents, *Nurs Res* 35:169, 1986.

### Learning Disabilities Nursing

Bealil N, Crook S: Assessing knowledge (assessment methods for mentally handicapped people), *Nursing Times and Nursing Mirror* 1983, 1 (4): 50-1, 1987.

Dickens P et al: *Assessing mentally handicapped people: a guide for care staff*, Windsor, 1987, NFER/Nelson.

Hogg J, Kaynes NV: *Assessment in mental handicap: a guide to assessment practices, tests and checklists*, London, 1987, Croom Helm.

Jakes M: Nursing model of psychological assessment? (an assessment of the mentally handicapped), *Senior Nurse*, 8 (11): 8-10, 1988.

Steele SM, Cuto KL: The role of the clinical nurse specialist in the assessment and development of social-sexual skills of adults who are developmentally disabled, *Clinical Nurse Specialist*, 3 (3): 48-153, 1989.

Van Der Gaag AD, Lawler CA: The validation of a language and communication assessment for use with adults with learning difficulties, *Health Bulletin*, 48 (5) Sept, (R54-259), 1990.

### Mental Health

Barker P J: *Patient assessment in psychiatric nursing*, London, 1985, Croom Helm.

Ritter SAH: *Bethlem Royal and Maudsley Hospital manual of clinical psychiatric nursing principles and procedures*, London, 1989, Harper and Row, Chapter 1, Nursing Assessment, (3-12)

Thomas BL, Brooking JI: *Psychiatric nursing assessment.* In Brooking, Ritter & Thomas, A textbook of psychiatric and mental health nursing, Edinburgh, 1992, Churchill Livingstone, 225-35

Lusis SA *et al*: Nursing assessment of mental status in the elderly: *GeriatricNursing* 14 (5): 255-9, 1993.

# CHAPTER 5

# Documentation and Reporting

## CHAPTER OUTLINE

**Communication Within the Multidisciplinary Team**

**Guidelines for Good Documentation and Reporting**
*Factual*
*Accurate*
*Complete*
*Current*
*Organized*
*Confidential*

**Reporting**
*Nurse-to-nurse handover reports*
*Telephone reports*
*Transfer reports*
*Incident reports*

**Documentation**
*Purpose of records*
*Legal documentation*
*Methods of recording*
*Common record-keeping forms*
*Home-care documentation*
*Computerized documentation*

## LEARNING OUTCOMES

*After studying this chapter, you should be able to:*
- *Define the key terms listed.*
- *Explain the purposes of documentation and reporting and its importance for all members of the multidisciplinary team.*
- *Describe the purpose of a change of shift handover report.*
- *Prepare and present a change of shift report on an actual patient/client, under supervision.*
- *Identify ways to maintain confidentiality of reports and documentations.*
- *Explain how documentation data can be used to review practice.*
- *Discuss the legal implications for correct documentation and reporting.*
- *Discuss the advantages and disadvantages of standardized documentation forms.*
- *Identify factors to include when planning a patient's/client's discharge from hospital.*
- *Discuss the role of computerized documentation in the health care setting.*

As members of the multidisciplinary team (MDT), nurses must communicate information about patients/clients accurately and completely and in the most timely and effective way possible. A patient/client depends on care givers communicating effectively with one another to ensure the best quality of care. All health care providers require the same information about patients/clients so that they can plan an organized, comprehensive care plan. For example, when a patient/client experiences pain, all care givers should be informed about the nature of the pain and the most effective therapies that benefit the patient/client. Unless the person's care plan is communicated to all members of the health care team, care becomes fragmented, repetition of tasks occurs, and therapies are often delayed or even overlooked. The result of poor communication is often poor patient/client outcomes such as delayed recovery and complications that could have been avoided.

The health care environment creates many challenges for accurately documenting and reporting the care delivered to patients/clients. Regulations require health care organizations to monitor and evaluate the quality and appropriateness of patient/client care. Such monitoring requires a thorough review of the documentation in a patient's/client's record. Everything that is done for a patient/client should be documented on the appropriate record. Finally, the individual's record is a legal document and can be used in a court of law. Nurses are accountable for their actions, and as a result, information in the record must be clear and logical, describing exactly all care delivered.

The quality of care deserved by patients/clients, the standards of statutory bodies, and the legal guidelines for nursing practice make documentation and reporting two of the most important functions of a nurse. Any information about a patient's/client's care should be communicated with careful thought, maintaining **confidentiality** (see box). All members of the MDT depend on recorded and reported information. Accurate information, using effective and appropriate communication strategies, ensures continuity and quality of care.

Nurses should be aware of the United Kingdom Central Council for Nursing, Midwifery and Health Visiting's Code of Professional Conduct (UKCC), particularly point 10 which states that a nurse, midwife, or health visitor must 'protect all confidential information concerning patients and clients obtained in the course of professional practice and make disclosures only with consent, where required by the order of a court or where [they] can justify disclosure in the wider public interest'.

## COMMUNICATION WITHIN THE MULTIDISCIPLINARY TEAM

It is difficult for staff members caring for a specific patient/client to communicate with one another. The more that care givers know about the person, the better prepared they are to provide high-quality care. Care givers use a variety of ways to communicate information about patients/clients. Reports are oral or written exchanges of information shared between care givers. After completing a work shift, nurses give a verbal report to nurses on the next shift. A doctor may telephone a ward or unit to receive a verbal report on a patient's/client's progress for the day. The laboratory submits a written report describing the results of diagnostic tests for inclusion in the patient's/client's medical record, or results may be reported through the computer system and received on the unit terminal.

A **record** is a permanent, written communication that documents information relevant to a patient's/client's health care management. An example is a clinic record or chart. After each clinic visit, information about the patient's/client's health care is recorded. With each successive visit the record is available to the doctor and other members of the team. It is a continuing account of the patient's/client's health care status and needs.

### The Access to Health Records Act

The Access to Health Records Act came into effect in November, 1991. The Act enables all people over the age of 16 to see their health records, unless the health professional believes access should be denied. Access may be denied if the health professionals involved believe the information would harm the physical or mental well-being of the patient/client or another individual; if access would disclose information provided by or relating to a third party who has not yet given their permission; or if the record was compiled before November, 1991, unless this earlier information is required to make sense of a current entry. If access is denied, the patient/client can take the case to court.

From Royal College of Nursing: Access to health records: the nurse's responsibilities, *Issues in Nursing and Health*, London, 1992, Royal College of Nursing.

Information is also communicated through **discussions** among team members. Discussions may be informal or formal. They allow a review of information so that problems are identified and solutions recommended. An example is a discharge planning meeting, in which members of all disciplines (for example, nursing, social work, medicine, and physiotherapy) meet to discuss the patient's/client's progress toward established discharge goals, in conjunction with the discharge planning policy or guidelines. Good **discharge planning** is essential to community care and is a directive of the NHS Community Care Act, 1990, and the Patients' Charter (Standard 9).

**Consultations** are a form of discussion whereby one professional care giver gives formal advice about the care of a patient/client to another. For example, a clinical nurse specialist may confer with a general nurse about the best choice of therapies for controlling the side effects of chemotherapy, or a doctor may consult with a dietitian to select the best diet for a patient/client. Both consultations and meetings should be documented in a patient's/client's permanent record so that all care givers can benefit from the information and plan care accordingly.

### Children's Nursing Documentation

It is always important to include the child in the documentation process. During an initial assessment, address most of your questions to the child; then request further clarification from the parents or guardians. Children's ability and desire to be involved in this process varies. Nurses should respect the child's wishes, and avoid over-involving the child or excluding the child from the process (Alderson, 1993). Many young children choose to accept their parents' decisions; others wish to share in desisions; a few want to be the 'main decision maker' (Alderson, 1993). In most situations, both the parents and children have similar viewpoints; however, it is important to value the child as an *individual* who has the right to dictate health care needs with his or her parents' help and support.

## GUIDELINES FOR GOOD DOCUMENTATION AND REPORTING

Failure to take documentation and reporting seriously can cause many problems, such as those in the following situations:

*Mrs Blake has recently been diagnosed with diabetes mellitus. She must learn to give herself insulin injections before going home. A nurse on the day shift fails to document the teaching session about insulin administration. During the evening shift, another nurse spends time assessing Mrs Blake's learning needs because the teaching plan was not communicated. Valuable time is wasted, and Mrs Blake becomes frustrated with the nurses' failure to know her needs. Effective communication of any teaching plan or health promotion strategy should be readily available in the patient's/client's file. This will enable more effective discharge planning and liaison with the community services.*

*Mr Ryan returned from major abdominal surgery just before change of shift. The day nurse, Staff Nurse Wells, measures and records the patient's/client's observations and administers a medication for pain. The evening nurse, Staff Nurse Tally, learns during the report that Mr Ryan received an analgesic medication but is not told his response to the drug. When Staff Nurse Tally enters Mr Ryan's room, she measures his blood pressure at 90/60 mmHg. She leaves the room to check the chart because she is concerned that the analgesic has lowered Mr Ryan's blood pressure. If Staff Nurse Wells had given a thorough report, Staff Nurse Tally would have known the patient's/client's blood pressure was normally low.*

Both examples demonstrate that quality documentation and reporting are necessary to enhance efficient, individualized patient/client care, in hospital as well as in community settings. Six important guidelines must be followed for quality documentation and reporting. Documentation and reports must be:

- factual
- accurate
- complete
- current
- organized
- confidential.

## Factual

Information about patients/clients and their care must be factual. A record should contain descriptive, **objective information** about what a nurse sees, hears, feels, and smells. An objective description (for example, 'Respirations 14 per minute, regular, with normal breath sounds bilaterally') is the result of direct observation and measurement. **Factual information is less likely to be misleading or to cause misinterpretation**. The use of words such as appears, seems, or apparently is not ideal because they can lead to conclusions that cannot be supported by objective information. If a nurse documents inferences or conclusions without factual information, errors in care can occur.

**Subjective information** should be documented only when it is supported by facts. For example, the description, 'the patient/client seems depressed' does not communicate helpful information. The description does not tell another care giver whether the patient/client is withdrawing from conversation or is threatening to injure himself or herself. The phrase 'seems depressed', is a conclusion without supported facts. **Documentation should clearly explain the nurse's observations of the patient's/client's behaviours, but should not interpret those observations**. If a patient/client reports information to the nurse, it should be charted as a subjective entry, in the patient's/client's own words. For example, 'Patient/client states, "I feel so helpless being unable to do anything for myself. Sometimes I wish I could stop all of this"'. The nurse can then add any objective findings that more clearly describe the patient's/client's depression, such as crying or difficulty with sleeping.

## Accurate

A patient's/client's record must be reliable. In other words, information must be accurate so that health team members have confidence in it. The use of precise measurements ensures that a record is accurate. Descriptions such as 'Intake, 360 ml of water' are more accurate than 'Patient/client drank an adequate amount of fluid' or 'fluids encouraged'. Measurements are later used as a means to determine whether a patient's/client's condition has improved or worsened. Charting that an abdominal wound is '5 cm in length' is more accurate than 'large and gaping'. Use of an organization's accepted symbols, and system of measures (for example, metric) ensures that all staff members will use the same language in their reports and records.

It is also important that the records are accurate in the event that they are requested by a court of law or coroners court. Remembering facts several months or years later is extremely difficult and nurses may be liable to prosecution for failing to maintain accurate records. Abbreviations should not normally be used as these can be misleading, particularly for the student nurse still in the process of learning.

Correct spelling and legible handwriting are also important for accurate documentation and reporting. Terms can easily be confused or misinterpreted (for example, *dysphagia or dysphasia*). Simple spelling mistakes can also cause serious treatment errors. Medications such as digitoxin or digoxin must be spelled carefully and legibly. If a mistake is made on a medication record, a patient/client may receive the wrong medication. As a nurse, you will be responsible for administering a prescribed drug; therefore, you must be clear as to what the drug actually is, its side effects, correct dosage parameters, contraindications and its effects upon the patient/client (see Chapter 31).

An accurate entry in a record must reflect what nurses do during the time frame of the entry. *Never* chart for anyone else or let anyone chart for you. In a court of law, it would be easy for a lawyer to create doubt about care when a recorded note did not truly reflect what was done by the nurses.

Another way to ensure accuracy of records is to correctly countersign entries. An example would include registered nurses being required to countersign a note entered into the record by a student nurse. When a nurse countersigns another nurse's entry, it means that the entry was reviewed and the care given was approved. When a nurse countersigns an entry, it is important that the person administering care is clearly identified. If the record is inaccurate, both nurses can share liability for any patient/client injury that might result.

Any descriptive entry in a patient's/client's record ends with the care giver's full name and status, such as 'Sharon Day, RN' printed and signed in full. Do not use nicknames. A student nurse enters the full name and current programme status, such as 'Tom Needy, pre-registration student'. The signature holds the nurse **accountable** for information recorded.

## Complete

The information within a recorded entry or a report should be complete, containing concise and thorough information about a patient's/client's care. Concise data are easy to understand, whereas lengthy notes can be difficult to read. Sketchy or abbreviated notes may leave an impression that nursing care was hurried or incomplete and attention to detail lacking. A long report wastes time and is often boring. Clear, succinct recording and reporting gives only essential information and avoids the use of unnecessary words or irrelevant detail. A comparison of concise and lengthy record entries follows:

**Concise entry**: Left toes are warm, colour pink; nail beds show capillary return within 2 sec; dorsalis pedis pulse strong bilaterally; no inflammation; patient/client denies pain.

**Lengthy entry**: The patient's/client's left toes appear to be warm with colour pink. There is no inflammation. There is good capillary return present. Dorsalis pedis pulse in left foot is strong. The patient/client denies pain.

A good report or record is thorough, with complete information about the patient/client. Criteria for thorough communication exist for certain health problems or nursing activities (Table 5-1). The nurse makes written entries in the patient's/client's nursing record, describing nursing care administered and the person's response. An example of a thorough nurse's note follows:

> *7.15.PM Patient/client verbalizes sharp, throbbing pain localized along radial side of right wrist, beginning approximately 15 minutes ago. Pain increased with movement of wrist, slightly relieved with elevation of hand on pillow. Radial pulses equal bilaterally. Right wrist circumference 1 cm larger than left wrist. Dr Kent notified at 7.20PM, Sarah Robinson, RN.*

### Current

Delays in recording or reporting can result in serious omissions and untimely delays for needed care. For example, failure to report a drop in blood pressure can delay the administration of a critically needed medication. Legally, a late entry in a chart may be interpreted as **negligence**. Ongoing decisions about care must be based on currently reported information. Activities or findings to communicate at the time of occurrence include the following:

- observations
- administration of medications and treatments
- preparation for diagnostic tests or surgery
- change in the patient's/client's condition
- admission, transfer, discharge, or death of a patient/client
- treatment for a sudden change in condition.

Routine activities such as bathing or giving oral hygiene do not need to be charted immediately. This information is often included on continuation sheets. When describing an aspect of care, it is important to refer to the patient's/client's problem, nursing intervention, and patient's/client's response. A revision or update of a care plan should occur when the patient's/client's condition changes (see Chapter 3). It is impossible and unnecessary for a nurse to document every aspect of care in the record when it happens. Consequently, it may help to keep a worksheet or notepad close at hand when caring for several patients/clients. Writing notes while they are fresh in your mind ensures that an entry recorded later in the record will be accurate. If this is the chosen method it is important to take great care

about the location of the notepad, because patient/client information is absolutely confidential.

### Organized

Communicate information in a logical sequence. Health team members understand information better when it is given in the order in which it occurred. An organized note describes the patient's/client's condition accurately and succinctly; describes the nurse's assessment and interventions; and describes the doctor's treatment instructions in a logical order of occurrence. A disorganized note is fragmented and does not clearly explain what happened first. Poorly organized notes can lead to confusion about whether proper care was given.

### Confidential

A **confidential communication** is information given by one person to another with trust and confidence that such information will not be disclosed. The law protects information about patients/clients that is gathered by examination, observation, conversation or treatment. Nurses should not discuss patients'/clients' status with other patients/clients or staff uninvolved in their care. Nurses are legally and ethically obliged to keep information about patients'/clients' illnesses and treatments confidential. Legal action can be brought against nurses who disclose information about individuals without their consent. Only staff members directly involved in care have legitimate access to the records. Nurses and other health care professionals may have reason to use records for data gathering, research, or continuing education. These are not breaks in confidentiality as long as the records are used as specified and written permission is granted from appropriate hospital/clinic/college personnel.

A patient's/client's record is accessible to many personnel. Nurses are responsible for protecting records from unauthorized readers such as visitors. Care plans are now

**Mental Health Nursing**
**Patient/client participation**

Patients/clients in mental health care settings should be provided with the appropriate information which will enable them to make decisions about their health care. There is debate as to whether any patient/client will ever have 'equal' power in his or her relationship with health care professionals, but this must not detract mental health nurses from the important task of building a genuine and trusting relationship with the person. This relationship is important if the nurse is to address the patient's/client's needs rather than the nurse's needs.

The nursing process is a tool that works best when the person can be actively involved in his or her nursing care. Not every patient/client will wish to be involved, and not everyone will feel able to collaborate. Nevertheless, the skilful mental health nurse will strive towards a working relationship with the patient/client, whenever it is appropriate.

## TABLE 5-1 Examples of Criteria for Documentation and Reporting

| Topic | Items to Report or Record |
|---|---|
| Symptom (e.g. pain, nausea, headache, dizziness) | Description of episode<br>Length of time<br>Location of symptom<br>Severity<br>Onset<br>Precipitating factors<br>Frequency and duration<br>Aggravating and relieving factors<br>Associated symptoms |
| Sign (e.g. rash, tenderness on palpation of body part) | Location of sign<br>Description or quality of findings<br>Aggravating or relieving factors<br>Onset |
| Nursing care measures (e.g. bath, dressing change) | Time administered<br>Equipment used if appropriate<br>Patient's/client's response (positive* or negative†)<br>Nurse's observations |
| Patient/client behaviour (e.g. anxiety, confusion, hostility) | Onset<br>Behaviours exhibited<br>Precipitating factors<br>Nursing response or action<br>Patient's/client's response |
| Medication administration | Time administered<br>Any required preliminary observations (e.g. pulse and blood pressure measurements)<br>Patient's/client's response or effect of medication (positive‡ or negative§) |
| Teaching | Nursing measures taken for negative response<br>Information or topic presented<br>Method of teaching (e.g. discussion, role playing, demonstration)<br>Resources used (e.g. videotape, booklet)<br>Evidence that patient/client understands teaching (e.g. return demonstration, change in behaviour) |
| Discharge planning | Patient/client goals or expected outcomes<br>Progress towards goals<br>Need for referrals or resources<br>Patient/client and family involvement in care plan |

\* For example, patient/client denied pain during dressing change.
† For example, patient/client experienced severe abdominal cramping during enema.
‡ For example, the patient/client reports that pain is reduced after analgesic.
§ For example, rash over lower abdomen is noted.

usually kept at the patient's/client's bedside or in the individual's home. The information written concerns the day-to-day care and decisions taken about this. Many patients/clients are encouraged to write on their own care plans. However, the individual's assessment records, containing personal, family and health details, are usually kept securely by the nurses in order that confidentiality can be maintained. You should know the secure location of the record at all times. If it is misplaced, every effort should be made to find it. The record is returned to the medical records department after discharge or death of the person.

## REPORTING

Information about patients/clients is exchanged between health care team members, patients/clients, and family members. Nurses communicate information about patients/clients so that all team members can make the optimum decisions about them and their care. Reports offer a summary of activities or observations seen, performed, or heard. There are various types of reports made by nurses; the nurse-to-nurse handover report; telephone reports; transfer reports; and incident reports. With the introduction of the Access to Health Records Act 1991, individuals may view their medical records by arrangement, though patients are increasingly holding their own nursing records.

## Nurse-to-Nurse Handover Reports

The **nurse-to-nurse handover report** is carried out in various ways in different care settings. The content of reports depends to an extent on whether care is organized in a system of Primary Nursing, Team Nursing, or patient/client allocation (see Chapter 3). The report transfers essential information necessary for safe and holistic patient/client care (Riegel, 1985). The purpose of the report is to provide better continuity of care among nurses caring for a patient/client. If a dressing is changed a certain way during the day shift, it should be changed the same way on the evening shift unless the patient's/client's condition changes or the prescribed treatment changes. If one nurse finds a certain pain-relief measure more effective for a patient/client, it is important that the information be relayed to the next nurse caring for him or her so that pain control can be maintained. This information is also incorporated into the written care plan to further enhance communication between shifts. A complete report establishes the nurses' accountability and ensures that patient/client care is uninterrupted, and where possible, effective. A person who sees different nurses performing care in the same manner will trust the care givers more.

A handover report is usually given orally in person, or during rounds at the patient's/client's bedside in hospital (Fig. 5-1) or at home. Reports can also be given in ward or unit offices or other suitable venues, with staff members from both shifts participating. Reports given in person or during rounds in hospital permit nurses to obtain immediate feedback when questions are raised about a patient's/client's care. **Rounds** may involve two or more nurses going to a patient's/client's bedside to discuss the care plan or assisting with a MDT round involving doctors, dietitians, social workers and others. When nurses make rounds, the patient/client and family members should be encouraged to participate in discussions and decisions. Patients/clients and their families should feel that staff are talking with them, not about them. Discussion of sensitive issues should be held away from the bedside. In the home setting, discussions among the community nurse, GP, patient/client and family should proceed in a similar manner.

Nurses on rounds can also see the patient/client together, in order to perform assessments, evaluate progress, and determine the interventions best suited to the patient's/client's needs. These methods can also be utilized as a teaching/learning activity.

Because of the many responsibilities nurses have to assume, it is important that a handover report be conducted quickly and efficiently (Table 5-2). A good report describes the patients'/clients' health status and exactly what kind of care the patient/client will require. Significant facts about patients/clients are reviewed (for example, the condition of wounds or episodes of chest pain) to provide a baseline for comparison. Any data about patients/clients should be objective and concise. Interpretation, the result of selecting, comparing, and summarizing, is important because the nurse can report the clinical significance of the events.

An organized report follows a logical sequence. To prepare the report, gather information from the patient's/client's care plans and other appropriate documentation. The following is an example of a handover report:

*Background information:* Robert Johnson, a 32-year-old patient of Mr Lang in bed 4, is listed for a colon resection this morning. He has had ulcerative colitis for 2 years. This is his first experience with surgery. He knows he may require a colostomy.

*Assessment:* Mr Johnson expressed difficulty in sleeping last night. He had several questions about surgery. Early in the night he called for assistance several times.

*Nursing problems:* His main nursing care problems are knowledge deficit related to inexperience with surgery and anxiety related to change in body image.

*Teaching plan:* He asks appropriate questions about surgery. Mr Lang has fully explained to him that a colostomy may be necessary. Staff on the late shift explained postoperative care. I reinforced information with him early in the night. He stated that he felt less anxious.

*Treatments:* An evacuant enema was administered until 9PM. No blood was noted in the return. He complained of some abdominal cramping immediately afterwards, but that disappeared. He received temazepam 20 mg orally at 11PM. He fell asleep shortly after midnight.

*Family information:* His wife remained with him last evening until the end of visiting hours. She has returned and is with him this morning.

*Discharge plan:* Mr Johnson is a very active person at home. He plays tennis and basketball and swims. Mrs Johnson is concerned about how he might react to a colostomy. I suggested making an appointment for him to see a stomatherapist if the colostomy is performed.

*Priority needs:* Currently, Mr Johnson is relaxing in bed. The consent form has been signed. All preoperative preparation and the preoperative checklist have been completed, except for his preop medications, due on call from the operating theatre.

In the above example, the nurse gave a clear picture of Mr Johnson's anxiety about surgery and need for information. The nurse taking over Mr Johnson's care has a clear picture of the patient's/client's immediate needs. If Mr Johnson presents new information during the next shift the nurse will know that a change in Mr Johnson's condition has occurred or new problems have developed. An organized and comprehensive approach to reporting helps you anticipate the patient's/client's needs early and lessens the chance of important information being forgotten or overlooked.

When giving a report, discuss patients/clients or family members in a professional manner. It is often necessary to describe the interactions between the person, nurse, and family members in behavioural terms. Avoid using labels such as *uncooperative, difficult,* or *bad* when describing such behaviours. A good report is objective and nonjudgemental. Value-laden terms do not establish working relationships between staff members and patients/clients. Staff members may unintentionally form a prejudicial opinion about patients/clients before even meeting them. The content of reports should be pertinent to patients'/clients' health care, regardless of age, race, sexual orientation or gender. Individualized patient/client care should be performed and accurately documented at all times.

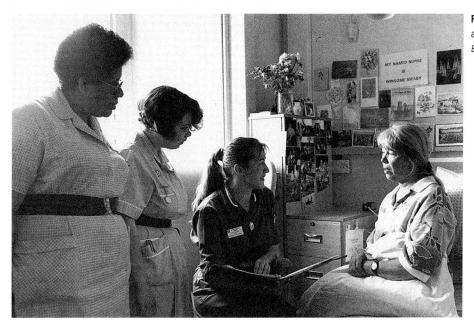

**Fig 5-1** Nurses handing over report at patient's bedside. *Photograph © Bruce Bailey, Select Photos London.*

## Telephone Reports

Members of the MDT frequently talk to one another by telephone. For example, a nurse informs a doctor of changes in a patient's/client's condition, a nurse from one ward communicates information to a nurse on another ward about a patient/client transfer, or the laboratory staff or a radiologist reports results of diagnostic tests. Information in a **telephone report** should be permanently documented in written form if significant events or changes in a patient's/client's condition have occurred. Thus, the people involved with a telephone report should be sure that the information is clear, accurate, and concise. If any doubt exists about the information conveyed over the telephone, the receiver repeats the message back to the sender.

To document a phone call, include when the call was made, who made it (if other than the writer of the information), who was called, to whom information was given, what information

| TABLE 5-2 Dos and Don'ts of Giving Handover Information in Hospital and Community Settings | |
|---|---|
| **Dos** | **Don'ts** |
| Provide only essential background information about patient/client (i.e., patient name, sex, age, doctor's diagnosis, and medical history) | Don't review all routine care procedures or tasks (e.g., bathing, scheduled medications). |
| Identify patient's/client's nursing problems and their related causes, if known. | Don't review all biographical information already available. |
| Describe objective measurements or observations about patient's/client's condition and response to health problem. Stress recent changes. | Don't use critical comments about patient's/client's behaviour, such as "Mrs Wills is so demanding". |
| Share significant information about family members as it relates to patient's/client's problems. | Don't make assumptions about relationships between family members. |
| Continuously review ongoing discharge plan (e.g. need for resources, patient's/client's level of preparation to go home). | Don't engage in idle gossip. |
| Relay to staff significant changes in the way care is given (e.g. different position for pain relief, new medication). | Don't describe basic steps of a procedure. |
| Describe instructions given in teaching plan and patient's/client's response. | Don't explain detailed content unless staff members ask for clarification. |
| Evaluate results of nursing or medical care measures (e.g. effect of massage or analgesic administration). | Don't simply describe results as 'good' or 'poor'. Be specific. |
| Be clear on priorities to which oncoming staff must attend. | Don't force oncoming staff to guess what to do first. |

was given, and what information was received. An example would be, "At 10.22 AM called laboratory; S Thomas, technician, reported Mr Rush's potassium at 3.2 mmol/l , Carol Smith, RN."

It is important to be as courteous as possible when making or receiving phone calls. Anyone calling a ward/unit/clinic should be treated as a consumer needing a service. Courtesy conveys a sense of caring and professionalism and promotes cooperation of all the team members.

### Transfer Reports

Patients/clients may transfer from one ward or unit to another. For example, individuals are transferred from intensive care units to general wards when intensive monitoring is no longer required. A **transfer report** involves communication of information about the patient/client from the nurse on the sending ward/unit to the nurse on the receiving ward/unit. The receiving ward must know the most current information about the patient/client and his or her progress. For example, if a person has undergone a surgical procedure, the receiving ward will want to know the type of procedure, information about any complications, and the patient's/client's current health status. A complete and accurate transfer report is essential for continuity of care from one ward to the next.

Transfer reports should be given in person. A transfer form is completed for nurses to document the patient's/client's status at the time of transfer. It is also important for the patient's/client's record to be up to date. A transfer report should include the following information:

- patient's/client's name, age, consultant, and medical diagnosis
- summary of progress up to the time of transfer
- current health status (physical and psychosocial)
- current nursing problems and care plan
- any treatments required immediately following transfer
- need for any special equipment.

After the sending nurse completes the transfer report, the receiving nurse should have time to ask any questions about the patient's/client's condition.

### Incident Reports

An incident is any event not consistent with the routine operation of a health care unit or routine care of a patient/client (Blake, 1984). The patient/client, visitor, or employee may be at risk when anything unusual occurs in a health care setting. Examples of incidents include patient/client falls, accidental needlestick injuries, a visitor experiencing symptoms of illness or drug errors. Changes in policies and protocols, in-service education about nursing care practice, and changes in the operation of a nursing environment are ways in which repeated incidents can be corrected. Incident reports are an important part of a hospital or clinic's quality-assurance programme.

When an incident occurs, the nurse involved in the incident or the nurse who witnesses an injury completes an **incident form**. The form is completed even though an injury does not occur or is not apparent. Most institutions have specific incident report forms (Fig. 5-2). The completed report goes to the manager or senior nurse of the ward or unit. Further action may occur, depending on the nature of the incident. For example, the occupational health department might review all incidents involving employee needlestick injuries. The hospital's legal department may review incidents when possible legal action against the hospital is expected.

When a patient/client or visitor is involved in an incident, take steps to remove the individual from risk and then begin a report describing details of the incident. A doctor examines the individual to determine whether any injury has been sustained. If a patient/client is affected, the doctor documents the examination and findings in the person's medical record. The nurse documents only an objective description of what happened and any follow-up care that occurred. The nurse reports what was actually observed.

An incident report should be concise and accurate, reporting exactly what the nurse observes and administers in the way of care, and who else was involved.

Nurses usually become involved in patient/client-related incidents at some point in their career. They must understand the purpose of incident reports and the correct way to report information. The following list provides some guidelines for correctly completing an incident report:

1. The nurse who witnessed the incident or who found the patient/client at the time of the incident should file the report immediately.
2. Describe specifically what happened in concise, objective and measureable terms.
3. Do not interpret or attempt to explain the cause of the incident.
4. Describe objectively the patient's/client's condition when the incident was discovered.
5. Report any measures taken by the nurse, other nurses, or doctors at the time of the incident.
6. Do not blame any nurse/person/doctor in an incident report.
7. Submit the report as soon as possible to the appropriate manager or senior nurse.
8. You should always be aware of what has been documented. Concealing untoward incidents, failing to keep essential records, falsifying records and breach of confidentiality are among some of the reasons for removal from the professional register (UKCC, 1993).

## DOCUMENTATION

Documentation is very important in health care today. Edelstein (1990) defines **documentation** as anything written or printed that is relied on as a record of proof for authorized persons. A written record should be a comprehensive description of the patient's/client's health status and needs, as well as the services provided for the individual's care. Good documentation reflects not only quality of care but also evidence of each health care member's accountability in giving care.

Several types of records are used to communicate information about patients/clients. Although each health care setting uses different record formats, all records contain basically the following information:

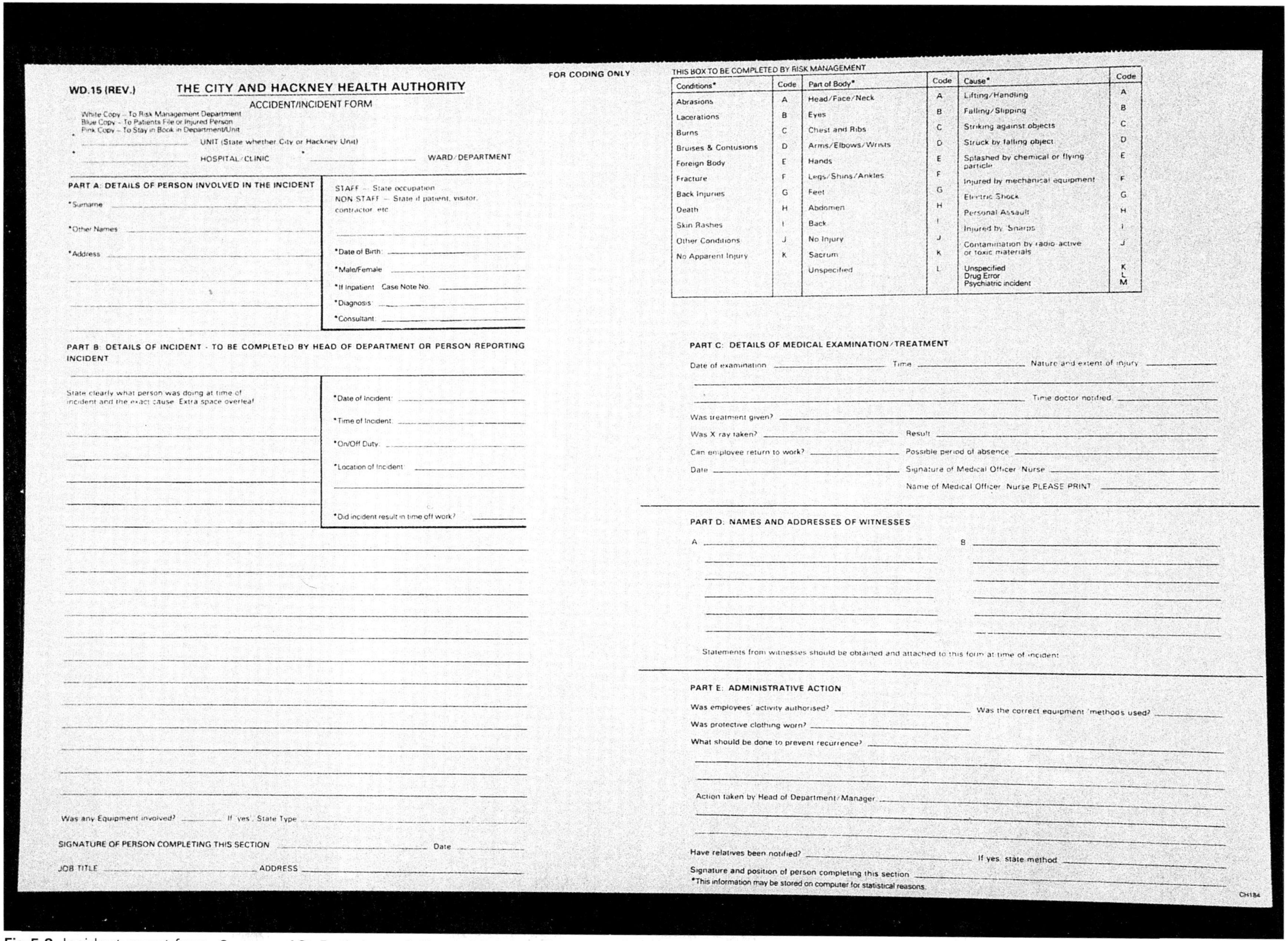

WD.15 (REV.)

THE CITY AND HACKNEY HEALTH AUTHORITY

ACCIDENT/INCIDENT FORM

White Copy – To Risk Management Department
Blue Copy – To Patients File or Injured Person
Pink Copy – To Stay in Book in Department/Unit

UNIT (State whether City or Hackney Unit)

HOSPITAL/CLINIC

WARD/DEPARTMENT

FOR CODING ONLY

THIS BOX TO BE COMPLETED BY RISK MANAGEMENT

| Conditions* | Code | Part of Body* | Code | Cause* | Code |
|---|---|---|---|---|---|
| Abrasions | A | Head/Face/Neck | A | Lifting/Handling | A |
| Lacerations | B | Eyes | B | Falling/Slipping | B |
| Burns | C | Chest and Ribs | C | Striking against objects | C |
| Bruises & Contusions | D | Arms/Elbows/Wrists | D | Struck by falling object | D |
| Foreign Body | E | Hands | E | Splashed by chemical or flying particle | E |
| Fracture | F | Legs/Shins/Ankles | F | Injured by mechanical equipment | F |
| Back Injuries | G | Feet | G | Electric Shock | G |
| Death | H | Abdomen | H | Personal Assault | H |
| Skin Rashes | I | Back | I | Injured by Sharps | I |
| Other Conditions | J | No Injury | J | Contamination by radio active or toxic materials | J |
| No Apparent Injury | K | Sacrum | K | Unspecified | K |
| | | Unspecified | L | Drug Error | L |
| | | | | Psychiatric incident | M |

PART A: DETAILS OF PERSON INVOLVED IN THE INCIDENT

*Surname

*Other Names

*Address

STAFF – State occupation
NON STAFF – State if patient, visitor, contractor etc

*Date of Birth:

*Male/Female

*If Inpatient Case Note No.

*Diagnosis:

*Consultant:

PART B: DETAILS OF INCIDENT - TO BE COMPLETED BY HEAD OF DEPARTMENT OR PERSON REPORTING INCIDENT

State clearly what person was doing at time of incident and the exact cause. Extra space overleaf

*Date of Incident:

*Time of Incident:

*On/Off Duty:

*Location of Incident:

*Did incident result in time off work?

Was any Equipment involved? If 'yes', State Type

SIGNATURE OF PERSON COMPLETING THIS SECTION Date

JOB TITLE ADDRESS

PART C: DETAILS OF MEDICAL EXAMINATION/TREATMENT

Date of examination Time Nature and extent of injury

Time doctor notified

Was treatment given?

Was X ray taken? Result

Can employee return to work? Possible period of absence

Date Signature of Medical Officer/Nurse

Name of Medical Officer/Nurse PLEASE PRINT

PART D: NAMES AND ADDRESSES OF WITNESSES

A B

Statements from witnesses should be obtained and attached to this form at time of incident

PART E: ADMINISTRATIVE ACTION

Was employees' activity authorised? Was the correct equipment/methods used?

Was protective clothing worn?

What should be done to prevent recurrence?

Action taken by Head of Department/Manager

Have relatives been notified? If yes, state method

Signature and position of person completing this section

*This information may be stored on computer for statistical reasons.

CH184

**Fig 5-2** Incident report form. Courtesy of St. Bartholomew's Hospital, London. *Photograph © Bruce Bailey, Select Photos London.*

- patient/client identification and demographic data
- informed consent for treatment and procedures
- admission nursing history
- nursing problems
- nursing care plan
- record of nursing care treatment and evaluation
- medical history
- medical diagnosis
- therapeutic orders
- medical and health discipline's progress notes
- reports of physical examinations
- reports of diagnostic studies
- summary of operative procedures
- discharge plan and summary.

## Purpose of Records

A record is a valuable source of data used by all members of the MDT. Its purposes include communication, education, assessment, research, auditing, and legal documentation.

## Communication

The record is a means by which the MDT members communicate contributions to the patient's/client's care, including individual therapies, patient/client education, and use of referrals for discharge planning. A care plan should be clear to anyone reading the chart. When a staff member is caring for a patient/client, the record should explain the measures needed to maintain continuity and consistency of care.

## Education

A patient's/client's record contains a variety of information. Students of nursing, medicine, and other health-related disciplines use these records as educational resources. An effective way of finding input about the nature of an illness and the response to it is to read the medical record. Although no two patients/clients have identical records, patterns of information can be identified in records of patients/clients who have similar problems. From this information, students can discover possible patterns to look for in various health problems or diseases and become better able to anticipate the type of care required for a patient/client.

## Assessment

The record provides data used to identify and support nursing assessment and to plan proper interventions for care. Information from the record adds to the nurse's own observations and assessment. Before caring for any patient/client, refer to the nursing records for new and relevant assessment findings.

The record provides a total picture of the patient's/client's health status. Assessment data entered by each member of the MDT do not simply describe isolated happenings. Each observation is part of a larger puzzle, which when solved reveals the patient's/client's health status. The record contains data to explain and confirm observations or refute interpretations. After inspection of a wound, for example, the nurse may conclude that it is healing poorly; the nurse checks the record, which may give

### Learning Disabilities Nursing
### Life books and diaries

Life books and diaries can help enhance the memory of people with learning disabilities. These records provide patients/clients, their carers, and health professionals with the patient's/client's personalized account of events. When these are augmented with photographs, sketches or other memorabilia, they can also serve as a valuable learning tool for patients/clients with sensory impairments.

Life books have proven useful in helping individuals make the transition from hospital to community life. They also provide care givers in the community with insight into the person's life while in hospital.

Much of the information documented and reported about people with learning disabilities refers to their behaviour; often, the antisocial, unwelcome behaviour. The need for objectivity in these cases is extremely important. Nurses should state the facts in simple terms and should not record their own conclusions. It is good practice to involve the patient/client in compiling the records; however, there may be some instances in which this is not practicable.

additional information, including the patient's/client's appetite, other descriptions of the wound's appearance, laboratory results indicating the onset of infection, and the observation of the wound on previous assessment. Any observations or interpretations made by the nurse are compared with data from the record. The record helps to explain the reasons for and implications of any findings the nurse gathers.

## Research

**Statistical data** relating to the frequency of clinical disorders, complications, use of specific medical and nursing therapies, deaths, and recovery from illness can be gathered from patient/client records (see Chapter 14). Records are a valuable resource for describing characteristics of the patient/client population.

A nurse may use patients'/clients' records during a research study to collect information on certain factors (see box). For example, if a nurse uses a different nursing therapy for pain control on a group of patients/clients, the records could provide data on the success of therapy. Recording entries that describe the number of analgesic medications used or patients'/clients' subjective reports of pain relief could be used to evaluate new pain-control measures. Nurses may also retrospectively research records of previously discharged patients/clients to identify nursing care problems. For example, a study to determine the incidence of infection in patients/clients with specific types of intravenous catheters might be performed with a review of the documentation.

## Auditing and Monitoring

A regular review of information in patient/client records provides a basis for evaluation of the quality and appropriateness of care provided in a particular health care setting. Quality-assurance and quality-improvement programmes keep you informed of standards of nursing practice required to maintain excellence in nursing care (see Chapter 2).

## Legal Documentation

A nursing record must be accurate because it is a legal document. In the case of **legal action**, the record, not the nursing care, is submitted as evidence. The record serves as a description of exactly what happened to a person. Nursing care may have been excellent; however, in a court of law, care not documented is regarded as care not done. Patients/clients are beginning to request copies of their medical records, and they have the right to read those records. Trusts and Health Authorities have policies for controlling the manner in which records are shared.

Recording should not become merely routine or superficial, nor should nurses wait until the end of a tiring day to record the patient's/client's care. Effective documentation should be performed in a timely manner with careful thought. Table 5-3 provides guidelines to ensure that a patient's/client's record is legally sound.

## Methods of Recording

The quality of documentation is constantly under review by nursing managers as they attempt to find ways to help nurses improve their documentation.

Nurses involved in the direct care of patients/clients often experience difficulties in fully documenting their patient's/client's care. These difficulties have led to more **bedside charting**. Bedside charts and care plans offer the convenience of entering information immediately after it is collected from a patient/client. They also enhance the patient's/client's participation in these processes.

The method of documenting should reflect the philosophy of the nursing service and the model of care used. It may also incorporate the standards of care and practice for the unit.

Many record-keeping methods are found within health care institutions. The difference between them is the manner in which information is organized.

It is important to avoid listing problems that are vague. Ideally, the problem should be listed in the patient's/client's own

### Patient Records and Research:

### A Position Statement

Information contained in patient records should be held in confidence and viewed only by those who are directly involved in the care of the patient. When patient information is required for clinical audit, it must be presented in an anonymous form to protect patient confidentiality. Ensuring anonymity can be undertaken by the clinician or by records staff who are employed to handle such records and have a contractual duty to respect and safeguard confidentiality.

If patient records are to be used for other research purposes, the prior consent of the patient must be obtained. The relationship of confidence exists between the clinician and the patient. It cannot be overturned by the third party, even in the form of a properly constituted ethical committee.

From Royal College of Nursing: Patient records and research — a position statement, *Issues in nursing and health*, no. 2, London, 1992, Royal College of Nursing.

terms. For example, "I have severe left-sided chest pain when I take minimal exercise".

The list of problems is identified on the appropriate nursing documentation to serve as an organizer or a basis on which to plan effective, safe care. New problems are added as they are identified. After a problem has been resolved, record the date, draw a line through the problem and its number, and sign the entry. The number for a resolved problem is not used again. This system keeps the problem list simple and meaningful. After a problem list is developed, succeeding record entries such as progress notes are identified by the problem number.

## Care Plan

A care plan is developed for each problem (see Chapter 3). The plan will be used as a central focus for the delivery of care and can be utilized by other members of the MDT. The care plan can also be used to educate the patient/client. Members of the MDT can identify the types of information or skills required by a patient/client to assume self-care or adapt to any health-related problems.

## Progress Evaluation Notes

Members of the MDT monitor and record the progress of a patient's/client's problems. Evaluation notes, continuation sheets and discharge summaries are forms used to document the patient's/client's progress. These are often useful in settings, such as ante natal clinics, or in a district nursing or health visitor setting.

## Common Record-Keeping Forms

A patient's/client's medical record may use a variety of forms to make documentation easy, quick, and comprehensive. Many forms eliminate the need to duplicate repeated data in the nursing notes. The forms present special types of information in a format more accessible than long, detailed progress notes.

## Nursing Assessment Forms

A **nursing assessment form** is a special form completed at the time a patient/client is admitted to a ward or unit. The form usually contains basic biographical data (for example, age, method of admission, and doctor), the admitting medical diagnosis or chief complaint, a brief medical-surgical history (for example, previous surgeries or illnesses, allergies, and medication history), and the patient's/client's own perceptions about illness or hospitalization. The form allows the admitting nurse to make a thorough assessment to identify relevant nursing problems for the patient's/client's care plan. Data on assessment forms provide baseline information that can be compared with changes in the patient's/client's condition. Each institution designs a nursing assessment form differently, depending on the standards of practice and philosophy of nursing care.

## Progress/Evaluation Notes

**Progress/evaluation notes** provide concise, measurable and accurate notes on the patient's/client's progress. Each of the notes made should be clearly linked with an associated nursing problem

## TABLE 5-3 Legal Guidelines for Recording

| Guidelines | Rationale | Correct Action |
|---|---|---|
| Do not erase, apply correction fluid, or scratch out errors made while recording. | Charting becomes illegible. It may appear as though you were attempting to hide information or deface record. | Draw single line through error, write word *error* above it, and sign your name or initials. Then record note correctly. |
| Do not write retaliatory or critical comments about patient/client or care by other health care professionals. | Statements can be used as evidence for poor quality of care. | Enter only objective descriptions of patient's/client's behaviour. Patient/client comments should be quoted exactly. |
| Correct all errors promptly. | Errors in recording can lead to errors in treatment. | Avoid rushing to complete charting. Ensure information is accurate. |
| Record only facts. | Record must be accurate and reliable. | Be certain entry is factual. Do not speculate or guess. |
| Do not leave blank spaces in nurse's notes. | Another person can add incorrect information in the space. | Chart consecutively, line by line. If space is left, draw line horizontally through it and sign your name at end. |
| Record all entries legibly and in ink. | Illegible entries can be misinterpreted, causing errors and legal action. Ink cannot be erased. | Never erase entries or use correction fluid, and never use a pencil. |
| If an order is questioned, record that clarification was sought sought. | If you perform an order known to be incorrect, you are just as liable for prosecution as the doctor or other professional. | Do not record "doctor made error". Instead chart that "Dr Smith was called to clarify order for — ". |
| Chart only for yourself. | You are accountable for information you enter into chart. | Never chart for someone else. |
| Avoid using generalized, empty phrases such as 'condition unchanged' or 'had good day'. | Specific information about patient's/client's condition or case can be accidentally deleted if information is too generalized. | Use complete, concise descriptions of care. |
| Begin each entry with time and end with your signature and title. | This ensures that correct sequence of events is recorded. Sign documents if accountable for care delivered. | Do not wait until end of shift to record important changes that occurred several hours earlier. Be sure to sign each entry. |

identified on the care plan. Rambling and incoherent notes cause confusion and do not monitor or evaluate nursing care. Each entry should be dated, timed, legibly written, signed, and countersigned if appropriate.

### Nursing Kardex

This system is very rarely used as a total documentation system. However, in some health care settings a modified Kardex system may still be in operation. The Kardex is a flip-over card usually kept in a portable index file at the nurses' station. Nurses may utilize the Kardex to obtain basic biographical data. An updated Kardex eliminates the need for continual referral to the chart for routine information. Information which may be found in a Kardex system includes:

* basic demographic data (for example, age and religion)
* primary medical diagnosis
* safety precautions to be used in the patient's/client's care, for example, highlighting any allergies the person may have.

However, it should be emphasized that in most cases the care plan pertaining to a particular patient/client will be housed with the person, usually at the bedside. However, personal, family and health details are kept in a more confidential manner. If a Kardex system is used, it is not normally a permanent record, rather it is used as an aide memoire. Information within the Kardex should not be a reflection of routine nursing responsibilities or standardized care.

### Standardized Care Plans

Although every professional nurse is responsible for developing an individualized care plan for a patient/client, the process of writing the plan is time consuming. Nurses caring for several patients/clients may need to write extensive care plans. Many institutions have attempted to make documentation easier for nurses with **core care plans** (see Chapter 3 for details about writing nursing care plans). The plans, based on the institution's standards of nursing practice, are pre-printed and establish guidelines that are used to care for patients/clients who have similar health problems (see example plan in Chapter 29).

When core care plans are used in a health care setting, the nurse remains responsible for an individualized approach to care. Therefore, if a core plan has an intervention that is not specifically tailored to the patient's/client's need, there should be a method to revise or alter the intervention to make it individualized. Core care plans are not meant to replace the nurse's professional judgement and decision making.

## Discharge Summary Forms

Much emphasis is placed on preparing a patient/client for an efficient and timely discharge from a health care institution. It is important to ensure that a patient's/client's discharge results in desirable outcomes, and guidelines for discharge practice are given in the Department of Health's Hospital Discharge Workbook (1994).

Ideally, discharge planning begins at admission. Nurses revise the plan as the patient's/client's condition changes. There should be evidence of involvement by both the patient/client and family members during the discharge-planning process. There should be no surprises by the time the patient/client is discharged. The person should have the necessary information and resources to return home. With the introduction of the Community Care Act, it is essential that enough notice is given to the Social Services Department and other relevant agencies, to enable effective discharge planning to take place.

At discharge, the nurse and other members of the MDT summarize the patient's/client's condition and review the care plan for the home. The patient's/client's condition should be described in relation to planned outcomes of discharge. **Discharge summary forms** make the summary concise and instructive. Many forms include a copy that is given to a patient/client, family member, or community nurse. This transfer of information ensures better continuity of self-care in the home. A summary form emphasizes previous learning by the patient/client and family. This can be an ideal time for instituting health promotion and education strategies. An individualized approach is necessary to achieve maximum health potential (see box).

### Home-care documentation

Patients/clients may need community care in a number of instances. For example, an elderly person requiring assistance with the activities of living (Roper *et al*, 1985), or a person requiring dressings to a surgical wound. The nurse documents the extent to which patients/clients require community care throughout the period that visits are made. The same principles which are applied to records and documentation in hospital are applied in the community. It is important for nurses to be open with the patient/client and family, and to share information with them. There is a growing trend toward **client-held records** in primary health care, and some records are kept at the client's home as well as in clinic. An example of one type of community record is shown in Chapter 3.

### Computerized Documentation

Computers have been widely used in hospitals and other health care settings for several years (see Chapter 2). Automated technology improves the integration of resources and the accessibility of the information to all health care personnel. The results of laboratory and diagnostic tests can be stored within the computer and displayed on the computer terminal screen with a mere push of a key.

In the past, most hospital information systems have included ordering programmes and communication systems. Nurses have been among the primary users of these systems. Supplies, equipment, stock medications, and diagnostic testing are examples of services nurses may order through a computer. **Computerized communication** systems relay information about patients/clients quickly and accurately; for example, patient/client classification, dependency levels, and test results can be organized within the computer for all individuals and made accessible when the nurse enters a name or identification number.

Currently, computers are changing the way nurses practice. The new information systems that are available can relieve nurses of repetitive clerical and monitoring tasks and increase the time available for direct patient/client care. Some programmes allow nurses to quickly enter specific assessment data, with the information automatically transferred to different reports. For example, after a nurse enters intake and output measurements for a specific time, the information is automatically transferred to shift total and daily summary records. Computers can also help reduce errors, standardize nursing practice (for example, care plans and test preparation protocols), and document patient/client care (Ford, 1990; Schroeder, 1987). Instead of

---

### Writing Discharge Summary Forms

#### Information for Community Nurses

- Familiarize and utilize the discharge planning policy.
- Describe nursing interventions (e.g. dressing changes, step-by-step wound care).
- Describe information presented to patient/client.
- Describe patient's/client's ability to perform health care skills (e.g. administering medications, use of crutches).
- Explain family members' involvement in care.
- Describe resources needed in home (e.g. Meals on Wheels, self-help devices).

#### Information for Patients/Clients:

- Use clear, concise descriptions in patient's/client's own language.
- Provide step-by-step description of how to perform a procedure (e.g. home drug administration). Reinforce explanation with printed instructions.
- Identify precautions to follow when performing self-care or administering medications.
- Review signs and symptoms of complications that should be reported to doctor.
- List names and phone numbers of health care providers that patients/clients can contact.
- List outpatient appointments.
- Provide any required/prescribed equipment and/or medications.

writing lengthy nurses' notes, nurses can select choices on a screen to automatically build a comprehensive record of an event.

It is important to know the benefits and risks of computerized documentation. All members of the MDT can access and enter data and thus generate a comprehensive database. McNeil (1979) describes the computer as a source of information superior to face-to-face reporting because the input of all individuals caring for a patient/client is available in an integrated and more complete manner than what previous shift members choose to report. Computers can reduce many tasks that take up nurses valuable time.

There are legal risks associated with computerized documentation. The main piece of legislation which covers this area is the **Data Protection Act**, 1984. Computers open the way for access to information by almost everyone. The password used to enter and sign off computer files should not be shared with another care giver under any circumstances. A good system requires frequent changes in personal passwords to prevent unauthorized persons from tampering with records. Nurses must know how to correct charting errors on a computer. Any data that has been permanently saved as part of the record should not be deleted. However, any incorrect entries or misspelt words that have not been stored can be deleted or corrected (Collins, 1990). If information is accidentally deleted, a brief explanation can be entered into the computer. Some institutions may request an incident report. Finally, printouts of computerized records should be protected. Shredding of printouts or the logging of the number of copies generated by each care giver are ways to minimize duplicate records and protect the confidentiality of patients/clients.

Since most hospitals now have automated systems nurses should be familiar with basic computer skills. Hospitals have large mainframe computer systems or individualized personal computers. A mainframe system consists of one centrally located computer with a huge memory capacity to power a variety of programs throughout the hospital.

## SUMMARY

Documentation and reporting are methods of communicating information related to health care management. In any setting the success of a care plan depends on accurate and complete reporting and precise record documentation. Effective reporting and documentation create a high level of communication, thus helping members of the MDT to have a common view of the patient's/client's problems. Nurses are the primary care providers because they have the most contact with patients/clients. The use of basic principles for accurate and comprehensive documentation and reporting will ensure the delivery of safe and effective nursing care.

## CHAPTER 5 REVIEW
### Key Concepts

- A patient's/client's health care record is written documentation of the care received.
- Accurate record keeping requires legibility, an objective interpretation of data, precise measurements, correct spelling, and proper use of abbreviations.

- The patient's/client's record is a legal document and requires accurate information. Facts should be reported, not inferences.
- A nurse's signature on an entry in a record designates accountability for the contents of that entry.
- Any change in a patient's/client's condition warrants immediate reporting to the nurse in charge, and an accurate record should be made.
- An organized record presents information logically, in order of the occurrence of events.
- All information pertaining to a patient's/client's health care management that is gathered by examination, observation, conversation, or treatment is confidential.
- The major purpose of the change-of-shift report is to maintain continuity of care.
- Rounds allow nurses to perform needed assessments, evaluate patients'/clients' progress, and determine the best interventions for a patients'/clients' needs.
- Any oral report is delivered in a professional manner emphasizing objectivity and a nonjudgemental viewpoint.
- When information pertinent to care is communicated by telephone, the information must be verified.
- Incident reports objectively describe any event not consistent with the routine care of a patient/client.
- Errors made while recording should never be erased or made illegible.
- Computerized information systems provide information about patients/clients in an organized and easily accessible fashion. However, care must be taken to protect absolute confidentiality.

## CRITICAL THINKING EXERCISES

1. Review the following brief report and identify what is missing:
   'Mr Robinson was given frusemide 80mg at 8AM as

### Key Terms

prescribed', B Sims, RN.

2. Practise completing an incident form accurately and completely. In a small tutorial group, analyse the strengths and limitations of your completed forms.

3. Gather together a collection of nursing documentation and recording charts in your own particular area of work and familiarize yourself with them.

4. Discuss who you would and would not provide patient/client information to. Give a detailed rationale for your response(s).

5. Write the following report in a more accurate and meaningful way:

'Mr Jackson has had a good morning. He has had a wash and shave and his sacral pressure sore is about the same. His right ankle is swollen. He complained of slight abdominal pain at about 10AM'.

## REFERENCES

Alderson P: *Children's consent to surgery,* Buckingham, 1993, Open University Press.

Blake P: Incident investigation: a complete guide, *Nurs Manage* 15:37, 1984.

Collins HL: Legal risks of computer charting, *RN* 53:81, 1990.

Department of health: *Hospital discharge workbook: a manual on hospital discharge practice,* BAPS, Health Publications Unit, Lancashire.

Edelstein J: A study of nursing documentation, *Nurs Manage* 21:40, 1990.

Ford J: Computers and nursing, possibilities for transforming nursing, *Comput Nurs* 8(4):160, 1990.

McNeil DG: Developing the complete computer-based information system, *JONA* 9:34, 1979.

Riegel B: A method of giving intershift report based on a conceptual model, *Focus Crit Care* 12:12, 1985.

Roper N, Logan WW, Tierney A: T*he elements of nursing, ed 3,* Edinburgh, 1990, Churchill Livingstone.

Royal College of Nursing: Access to health records — the nurse's responsibilities, *Issues in Nursing and Health* (flyer) 16, London, 1992, RCN.

Schroeder MA: Computers in nursing: applications for ambulatory care, *Nurs Econ* 5(1):27, 1987.

United Kingdom Central Council: *Code of professional conduct,* London, 1993, UKCC.

## FURTHER READING

### Adult Nursing

Albrecht CA, Lieske AM: Automating patient care planning, *Nurs Manage* 16:, 1985.

Costello S, Summers BY: Documenting patient care: getting it all together, *Nurs Manage* 16:31, 1985.

Dimond B: *Legal aspects of nursing,* London, 1990, Prentice Hall.

Dobberstein K: Attacking fuzzy documentation, *Am J Nurs* 6:559, 1986.

Gamberg D et al: Outcome charting, *Nurs Manage* 12:36, 1981.

Harkins B: Keep your eye on the patient's problems, *RN* 49(12):30, 1986.

Her Majesty's Stationary Office: *Access to Health Records Act,* London, 1991, HMSO.

Her Majesty's Stationary Office: *Data Protection Act,* London, 1984, HMSO.

Kitto J, Dale B: Designing a brief discharge planning screen, *Nurs Manage* 16:28, 1985.

Miller P, Pastorino C: Daily nursing documentation can be quick and thorough, *Nurs Manage* 20(11):47, 1990.

Nadzam DM: Documentation evaluation system: streamlining quality of care and personnel evaluations, *Nurs Manage* 18(11):38, 1987.

Napiewocki JK: Documentation: a nurse's best defence, *Prof Nurs* 1:321, 1985.

National Health Service Executive: *Keeping the records straight,* London, 1993, NHS.

Reiley PJ, Stengrevics SS: Change-of-shift report: put it in writing! *Nurs Manage* 20(9):54, 1989.

Sanborn CW, Blount M: Standard plans for care and discharge, *Am J Nurs* 84:1294, 1984.

The King's Fund Centre: *A handbook for nurse to nurse reporting,* ed 2, London, 1983.

The Medical Defence Union Ltd: *Confidentiality,* London, 1992.

The Medical Defence Union Ltd: *Medical records,* London, 1993.

Thielman DE: Report: how to say it all in a few words, *RN* 50:15, 1987.

United Kingdom Central Council for Nursing, Midwifery and Health Visiting: *Complaints about professional conduct,* 1993, UKCC.

United Kingdom Central Council for Nursing, Midwifery and Health Visiting: *Standards for records and record keeping,* 1993, UKCC.

### Learning Disabilities Nursing

Jeffree D & Cheseldine S: *Pathways to independence: checklists of selfhelp, personal and social skills,* London, 1982, Hodder and Stoughton.

Jones L: *The Kidderminster curriculum for children and adults with profound multiple learning difficulties,* Birmingham, 1989, Birmingham University.

Mulhall D: *Functional performance record,* Windsor, 1989, NFER/Nelson.

Nihira K: *AAMD adaptive behaviour scale ed 3,* Washington, 1975, American Association on Mental Retardation.

RCN : *Standards of care for nursing people with a learning disability,* London, 1992, RCN.

Whitehouse J: *Mossford assessment chart for the physically handicapped,* Windsor, 1983, NFER/Nelson.

Williams C: *The STAR profile: social training achievement record,* Kidderminster, 1986, BIMH.

### Children's Nursing

Beinadol et al: ABC method of emotional assessment and intervention, *J Emerg Nurs,* 16(2):70, 1990.

Cox P: Documentation for the life model, *Paed Nurs:*10, 1990.

Hully M, Hyne J: Using parent held records in an oncology unit, *Paed Nurs* 5(8):14, 1993.

Kleiber C, Chase L: Solving documentation problems with a pediatric flow sheet, *Pediatr Nurs* 15(3):253, 1989.

Nelson N, Beckel J, editors: *Nursing care plans for the pediatric patient,* St Louis, 1987, Mosby.

### Mental Health Nursing

Heron J: *Six category intervention analysis,* Surrey, 1975, Surrey University Human Potential Resource Group.

Reynolds et al: *Writing and reading mental health records,* London, 1992, Sage.

Ritter S: *Manual of clinical psychiatric nursing principles and procedures,* London, 1989, Harper & Row. Chap 23, Documenting nursing care.

Ritter SAH: *Bethlem Royal Maudsley Hospital manual of clinical psychiatric nursing principles and procedures,* London, 1989, Harper and Row. Chapter 23, Documenting Nursing Care, (153-157).

Sundeen SJ *et al Nurse–client interaction — implementing the nursing process,* ed 5, St Louis, 1994, Mosby.

Tunmore RGD: *Nursing care planning,* In Brooking, Ritter & Thomas, A textbook of psychiatric and mental health nursing, (235 chp 19) Edinburgh, 1992, Churchill Livingstone.

# unit 2

# The Nurse and the Patient/Client

# Growth and Development of the Individual and Family

## CHAPTER OUTLINE

## LEARNING OUTCOMES

After studying this chapter, you should be able to:
- *Define the key terms listed.*
- *Define growth and development and list the seven basic principles involved.*
- *Discuss physiological and psychosocial health concerns during the transition from intrauterine to extrauterine life.*
- *Discuss the psychosocial and cognitive development of children, from birth to adolescence.*
- *Identify factors that can disturb or promote optimal development of the child, from birth to adolescence.*
- *Discuss developmental theories of young and middle adults.*

*(Cont'd.)*

■ *Discuss the major life events and developmental tasks of young and middle-aged adults, and the childbearing family.*

■ *Discuss the physiological, cognitive and psychosocial changes occurring during the adult years.*

■ *Describe common myths and stereotypes about older adults.*

■ *Discuss biological and psychosocial theories of ageing.*

■ *State and discuss the developmental tasks of the older adult.*

■ *Describe psychosocial changes related to retirement, sexuality, housing, and death of spouse and peers, to which older adults must adjust.*

■ *Identify the differing main health concerns for every age group and suggest relevent health promotion activities.*

■ *Outline the way families change and evolve.*

■ *Discuss the relationship which the nurse may have as a health professional with individuals and their families.*

**N**ursing practice based on the principles of growth and development is organized and directed at helping children, adults and families adapt to changing internal and external conditions. For proper assessment, nurses must know the appropriate developmental expectations for each age group.

Children and adolescents, for example, must cope with changes involving all areas of development which frequently occur at the same time. The stress of these changes may cause the child to develop physical and psychosocial health problems. By helping children and adolescents achieve a necessary developmental balance, nurses can help them promote health.

During young adulthood, individuals increasingly separate from their families of origin, establish career goals, and decide whether to marry and begin families or remain single. Young adults, therefore, must adapt to new experiences. During their transition to middle age, individuals may reassess their goals in life and may add new goals.

Nursing care of older adults poses special challenges, because of the diversity in physiological, cognitive, and psychosocial health. Before assessing an older adult, nurses should be aware of the expected physical and psychosocial findings, and normal changes of ageing. However, nurses should not assume that all older adults have signs, symptoms, or behaviours representing the lower end of the health continuum.

A comprehensive knowledge of the principles of growth and development, their application to health promotion, and the effects of the family unit on the health of individual members will enable nurses to provide individualized care for every patient/client.

## DEFINING GROWTH AND DEVELOPMENT

Human growth and development are orderly, predictable processes beginning with conception and continuing until death. All individuals progress through definite phases of growth and development, but the pace and characteristics of this progression are highly individual. The ability to progress through each **developmental phase** influences a person's health. The success or failure experienced within a phase affects the ability to complete subsequent phases.

A developmental perspective helps the nurse understand *why* commonalities and variations exist and *how* they influence health. With this knowledge the nurse can provide care in a manner that addresses the patient's/client's unique needs and developmental level.

Growth and development are synchronous processes that are interdependent within the healthy individual. A person experiences both *quantitative* and *qualitative* changes in growth and development:

- **Physical growth** is the quantitative, or measurable, aspect of an individual's increase in physical measurements. Measurable growth indicators include height, weight, and dental, skeletal, and sexual age.
- **Development** describes the qualitative, or behavioural, aspects of progressive adaptation to the environment.
- **Maturation** is the process of becoming fully developed. It involves an individual's biological ability, physiological condition, and desire to learn more mature behaviours. To mature, the individual may have to relinquish previous behaviours and learning, integrate new patterns into existing behaviours, or both.
- **Sensitive periods of development** are specific spans of time during which the environment has its greatest impact on the individual (Papalia and Olds, 1989). During these periods, some form of sensory stimulation is necessary for developmental progression.

## PRINCIPLES OF GROWTH AND DEVELOPMENT

The following principles of growth and development are true for everyone:

- Individuals have adaptive potential for qualitative and quantitative changes by receiving stimuli from and giving stimuli to the environment.
- Individuals derive uniqueness from the interaction of heredity and environment.
- The primary goal of development is achievement of potential.

The basic principles of growth and development are that it is:

- Orderly – follows a set sequence.
- Directional – proceeds along the following body axes:
  (a) **cephalocaudal**, in which growth proceeds from the head to the lower parts of the body
  (b) **proximodistal**, in which development proceeds from the central (proximal) areas of the body to the outer (peripheral)
  (c) **differentiation**, in which development proceeds from simple to complex.
- **Complex**, yet predictable – occurs with a consistent pattern and chronology.
- **Unique** to individuals and their genetic potential – each individual tends to seek a maximal potential for development.
- **Ongoing process** – occurs through conflict and adaptation, and different aspects develop at different rates, creating periods of equilibrium and disequilibrium.

- **Challenging** – involves challenges for individuals in the form of certain tasks specific to age and ability.
- **Demanding** – requires practice and energy, the focus of which varies with each developmental stage and task accomplished.

## THEORIES OF HUMAN DEVELOPMENT

Theories of cognitive and psychosocial development vary in the way humans are viewed and in the aspect of development emphasized. Some theories view development as a continuous process, moving from the simple to the more complex. Others consider it as discontinuous, with alternating periods of relative equilibrium and disequilibrium. Health care professionals often use different theoretical frameworks, which may complicate communication between them. Nurses must be familiar with the common theories in order to coordinate care and communicate effectively (Table 6-1).

According to **Freud** (1905, 1920), pleasure shifts from one bodily erogenous zone to another. A child's maturation level determines when this shift occurs. If gratified either too much or too little, the child may become emotionally fixated at that stage. Freud did not specifically define 'too much' or 'too little'.

According to **Erikson** (1963), each stage has a personality crisis involving a major conflict that is critical at that time. The developing ego is greatly affected by societal and cultural influences, and the successful mastery of each conflict is built on satisfactory completion of the previous conflict. This theory recognizes the importance of heredity and environment.

**Piaget** (1952) views the development of the mind as occurring through adaptation to the environment via **assimilation** (fitting new information into existing cognitive structure or schema) and **accommodation** (changing schema to deal with new information). Cognitive development within and between stages is a function of maturation, experience, social interaction, and equilibration. Piaget emphasizes both genetics and interaction and places humans in an active learning role.

**Kohlberg** (1969) contends that cognitive development underlies the progression of a person's morality from level to level. These stages occur in the same order, regardless of culture. Individuals differ in how quickly and how far they progress through these stages.

## SELECTING A DEVELOPMENTAL FRAMEWORK FOR NURSING

Nursing patients/clients of all developmental stages is easier when planning is based on a theoretical framework which encourages organized care directed at the patient's/client's current level of functioning.

The sections which follow concentrate on physical development, cognitive development and psychosocial development from conception, through infancy, childhood, and adulthood to old age. Health issues and concerns are raised for each life stage. **Cognitive development** considers the process by which a person becomes intelligent, acquiring with growth the knowledge and ability to communicate, think, learn, do, reason and abstract. **Psychosocial development** considers the normal serial side of trust, autonomy, identity and intimacy.

Within the developmental approach patients'/clients' capabilities are emphasized, and they are actively involved in their own care. The nurse and patient/client focus on activities that foster the completion of developmental tasks and promote health.

## CONCEPTION

From the moment of conception, human development proceeds at a rapid rate. Most intrauterine health problems are caused by genetic and environmental factors. During the prenatal period, the embryo grows from a single cell to a complex, physiological being. All major organ systems develop *in utero*, with some functioning before birth. The psychosocial being also begins to emerge during gestation.

The primary carer for the healthy pregnant woman in the UK is the **midwife**. The midwife assesses, plans, and implements care on an individual basis for the pregnant woman and for the safe delivery of her child.

### Intrauterine Life

Intrauterine life generally lasts 9 calendar or 10 lunar months (see box). The organism's life begins after sexual intercourse has occurred, when the ovum is penetrated by one sperm. Fertilization takes place in the fallopian tube within 12 to 24 hours after the ovum is released from the ovary. The ovum and sperm fuse, and the material from both cell nuclei unites. The organism then has its full genetic complement in one pair of sex chromosomes and 22 pairs of autosomal chromosomes. These contain the blueprint for inherited characteristics, such as eye colour.

In some cultures, for example, in China and Korea, age is calculated from the age of conception. Individuals will thus consider themselves to be nine months older than is stated on a birth certificate. Other cultures may use a lunar calendar and this will add 10 days per year, or 1 year every 36 years to someone's age (Squires, 1991).

The fertilized ovum, or **zygote**, passes through the fallopian tube to the uterus within 4 days. By the third day a solid ball of cells, the **morula**, has formed. This solid ball soon develops a central cavity, or **blastocyst**, and cells begin to differentiate in structure and function.

Formation of a placenta enables the transfer of material between the embryo and mother, including oxygen, carbon dioxide, nutrients, and waste products.

The period of gestation is frequently divided into three time periods called *trimesters*.

### Physical Development
### First Trimester

During this trimester, processes of cellular change (differentiation) and staged organ change (development) occur at

## TABLE 6-1 Summary of Development According to Stage Theorists

### FREUD'S PSYCHOSEXUAL THEORY

| Stages and Ages | Characteristics of Stages | Theory Addendum |
|---|---|---|
| Oral-sensory (birth to 12-18 mo) (infancy) | Activities involving mouth such as sucking, biting, and chewing are chief source of pleasure. | Child deprived of sufficient sucking might attempt to satisfy this need later in life through activities such as gum chewing, smoking, and overeating. |
| Anal-muscular (12-18 mo to 3 yr) (toddlerhood) | Sensual gratification is derived from retention and expulsion of faeces. Smearing is common activity. | External conflicts may be encountered when toilet training is attempted and later result in behaviours such as constipation, tardiness, or stinginess. |
| Phallic-locomotion (3-6 yr) (preschool) | Manipulation of genitalia results in pleasurable sensations. Masturbation begins and sexual curiosity becomes evident. | Emergence of Oedipus and Electra complexes for males and females respectively, occurs. Brashness, bashfulness, and timidity may be expressions of fixation at this stage. |
| Latency (6 yr to puberty) (school-aged) | A tranquil period when Freud believed sexual drives were dormant; however, child may engage in erogenous activities with same-sex peers. | Child's use of coping and defence mechanisms emerge at this time; any sexual interest may be sublimated through vigorous play and skill acquisition. |
| Genital (puberty to adulthood) (adolescence and adulthood) | Genitalia become centre of sexual tension and pleasure. Sexual hormone production stimulates development of sexual relationships. | This is a time of biological upheaval, when immature emotional interactions often occur in early phase. In time, ability to give and receive mature love develops. |

### ERIKSON'S PSYCHOSOCIAL THEORY

| | | |
|---|---|---|
| *Trust versus mistrust* (birth to 1 yr) (infancy) Mode: taking in and getting Virtue: hope | Care giver's satisfaction of infant's basic needs for food and sucking, warmth and comfort, and love and security in consistent and sensitive manner results in trust. | When basic needs of infant are not met or are met inadequately, infant becomes suspicious, fearful, and mistrusting. This is evidenced by poor eating, sleeping, and elimination behaviours. |
| *Autonomy versus doubt and shame* (1-3 yr) (toddlerhood) Mode: holding on and letting go Virtue: will | Child begins to develop independence while gaining control over bodily functions of undressing and dressing, walking, talking, feeding self, and toileting. Self-control begins. | If toddler's developing independence is discouraged by parents, child may doubt personal abilities; if child is made to feel bad when attempts to be autonomous fail, child develops shame. |
| *Initiative versus guilt* (3-6 yr) (preschool) Mode: intrusive attack and conquest Virtue: purpose | Child develops initiative when planning and trying out new things. Behaviour of child is characterized as vigorous, imaginative, and intrusive. Conscience and identification with same-sex parent develop. | Parental restrictiveness may prevent child from developing initiative. Guilt may arise when child undertakes activities in conflict with those of parents. Child must learn to initiate activities without infringing on rights of others. |
| *Industry versus inferiority* (6-12 yr to puberty) (school-aged) Mode: doing and producing Virtue: competence | Child wins recognition by demonstrating skills and producing things, and develops self-esteem through achievements. Child is greatly influenced by teachers and school. | Feelings of inferiority may occur when adults perceive child's attempt to learn how things work to be silly or troublesome. Lack of success in school, or difficulty developing physical skills, or making friends also contribute to feelings of inferiority. |

## TABLE 6-1 Summary of Development According to Stage Theorists (Cont'd)

**ERIKSON'S PSYCHOSOCIAL THEORY**

| Stages and Ages | Characteristics of Stages | Theory Addendum |
|---|---|---|
| *Identity versus role confusion or diffusion* (puberty to 18-21 yr) (adolescence) Virtue: fidelity | Individual develops integrated sense of 'self'. Peers have major influence over behaviour. Major decision is to determine vocational goal. | Failure to develop sense of personal identity may lead to role confusion, which often results in feelings of inadequacy, isolation, and indecisiveness. Psychosocial moratorium provides extra time for making vocational decision. |
| *Intimacy versus isolation* (18-21 to 40 yr) Mode: loving Virtue: love | Task is to develop close and sharing relationships with others, which may include sexual partner. | Individual unsure of self-identity will have difficulty developing intimacy. Person unwilling or unable to share self will be lonely. |
| *Generativity versus self-absorption or stagnation* (40-65 yr) (middle adulthood) Mode: nurturing Virtue: care | Mature adult is concerned with establishing and guiding next generation. Adult looks beyond self and expresses concern for future of world in general. | Self-absorbed adult will be preoccupied with personal well-being and material gains. Preoccupation with self leads to stagnation of life. |
| *Ego integrity versus despair* (65 yr to death) (older adulthood) | Older adult can look back with sense of satisfaction and acceptance of life and death. | Unsuccessful resolution of this crisis may result in sense of despair in which individual views life as series of misfortunes, disappointments, and failures. |

**PIAGET'S THEORY OF COGNITIVE DEVELOPMENT**

| | | |
|---|---|---|
| Sensorimotor (birth to 2 yr) | Child learns about world through sensory and motor activities. | Child slowly develops concept that people and objects have permanence, even though they are no longer visible. |
| Reflex activities (birth to 1 mo) | Child exercises inborn reflexes and gains some control over them. | Modified reflexes become more efficient. Sucking is more effective and selective. |
| Primary circular reactions (1-4 mo) | Infant repeats pleasurable actions that first occur by chance. Activities focus on body of infant; coordination begins. | Eye, eye-ear, and hand-to-mouth coordination develop, and activities such as thumb sucking and bottle sucking become more intentional and proficient. |
| Secondary circular reactions (4-8 mo) | Child attempts to reproduce interesting, pleasant events in environment. Interest goes beyond body. | Infant searches for object dropped and recognizes partially hidden object. Child begins to associate two behaviours such as cradle position and feeding. |
| Coordination of secondary schemes (8-12 mo) | Child puts together skills used earlier to reach goal in new situation. | Child will crawl across room to get desired toy and search for hidden objects where they were previously hidden. |

(Cont'd)

different rates and times. Interference with growth can cause the congenital absence of an organ system or extensive structural or functional alterations. Figure 6-1 shows the approximate times of critical differentiation for some of the major organ systems and their overlapping of development.

## HEALTH CONCERNS

Agents capable of producing adverse effects in the fetus are called **teratogens**. Some teratogens produce defects only if the fetus is exposed to the agent when the vulnerable organ is developing. One such teratogen is the rubella or German measles virus, which can cause abortion, stillbirth, or defects of the eyes, ears, and heart, primarily when exposure is in the first trimester.

Some drugs are teratogenic during rapid organ growth (organogenesis) in the first trimester. Barbiturates, alcohol, hydantoins, anticonvulsants, and anticoagulants are only a few of the chemical agents associated with fetal abnormalities, and many other agents are under investigation. Benefits of any drug needed to maintain the mother's health must be weighed against potential harm to the fetus.

## Second Trimester

During the second trimester, months 3 to 6, some organ systems continue basic development, and the functional capabilities of

## TABLE 6-1 Summary of Development According to Stage Theorists (Cont'd)

### PIAGET'S THEORY OF COGNITIVE DEVELOPMENT

| Stages and Ages | Characteristics of Stages | Theory Addendum |
|---|---|---|
| Tertiary circular reactions (12-18 mo) ('trial and error') | Child actively explores world and varies actions to see novelty of object, event, or situation. Trial and error are used to problem solve. | Child might try to get toy out of small opening of container with hand first and then turn it upside down and hit it so that toy falls out. Child comprehends series of object displacements if visible. |
| Invention of new means through mental combinations (18-24 mo) ('representation') | Toddler begins creating mental images and thus can devise new ways to deal with environment. Child begins to think about events without resorting to action. | Child attains true object permanence and will search for objects they have not seen hidden; for example, toddler will look in many places for a bottle. Insight is demonstrated by looking for the bottle in refrigerator. |
| Preoperational (2-7 yr) | Child develops representational system and uses symbols such as words to represent people, places, and objects. | Preoperational concepts are limited by ability to focus on only one aspect at time (centration), and thought often seems illogical because child reasons from one specific to another (e.g. car hit dog because boy was angry with it). |
| Preconceptual (2-4 yr) | Child is primarily egocentric. Perceptual-bound and transductive thinking begin; child is animistic. | Deferred imitation (imitation of observed action after time has passed) demonstrates use of symbolism. |
| Intuitive (4-7 yr) | Child begins to work things out but cannot explain them rationally. | Intuitive concepts allow classification of items by one attribute, usually colour or shape (e.g. inability to focus on more than one characteristic at a time). |
| Concrete operations (7-11 yr) | Ability to understand law of conservation results in logical thought patterns and mental operations such as reversibility, decentering, seriation, transformation, classification of two or more attributes, and inductive and deductive reasoning. | Limitations are inability of child to understand abstractions. Child's thinking is restricted to immediate and physical. School-aged child can reason about what is but cannot hypothesize about what may be and thus cannot think about future problems (e.g. ability to play game of chess). |
| Formal operations (develops 11-15 yr, used throughout life) | Ability to think in abstract manner develops, and scientific reasoning emerges. Initially, thought is rigid, but it becomes adaptable and flexible. | Adolescent may confuse ideal with practical but, when confronted with problem (real or hypothetical), can suggest number of solutions. Ability to consider moral and political issues from variety of perspectives is present. |

### KOHLBERG'S THEORY OF MORAL REASONING

| | | |
|---|---|---|
| Premoral level (birth to 9 yr) | There is little awareness, which is socially acceptable moral behaviour. Control is external. | Infant defers to power and authority. Life is valued for number and power of possessions. |
| Punishment and obedience orientation (birth to 6 yr) | Rules of others are followed to avoid punishment. | Child integrates labels of *good* and *bad* and *right* and *wrong* into behaviour in terms of the consequences of actions. Elements of bargaining, equal sharing, and fairness are evident. Life is valued for how child can satisfy needs of others. |
| Naively egoistic orientation (6-9 yr) | Child conforms to rules out of self-interest; child reasons that reward or favour will be earned. | |

**TABLE 6-1 Summary of Development According to Stage Theorists (Cont'd)**

**KOHLBERG'S THEORY OF MORAL REASONING**

| | | |
|---|---|---|
| Conventional morality (9-13 yr) | Efforts are made to please other persons. Control is becoming internal. | Child is loyal and concerned with maintaining family expectations regardless of consequences. |
| 'Good boy, nice girl' (9-10 yr) | Desire to please and help others is foremost. Child conforms to avoid rejection. | Life is valued for how good interpersonal relationships are (identify with emotionally important persons). |
| Authority maintaining morality | Child does duty to avoid criticism by authorities. | Identification shifts to religious or social institutions such as school. |
| Postconventional level of morality (13 yr to death) | Individual attains true morality. Conduct control is internal. | Attainment of true morality occurs after formal operations have been reached. Not everyone reaches this level. |
| Contractual and legalistic orientation | Individual selects moral principles by which to live and obeys laws. | Individual is careful not to violate rights and wills of others. Moral and legal views conflict. Person will work to change laws. |
| Universal ethical-principle orientation | Individual behaves in way that respects dignity of all. | This stage is rarely attained. If internal set of ideas are violated, guilt results. |

others are refined. By the end of this trimester, most organ systems are complete and can function.

The fetus is covered with **vernix caseosa**, a cheese-like substance coating the skin. **Lanugo**, or fine hair, covers most of the body. These substances protect the thin, fragile skin and decrease in amount as gestation lengthens; thus prematurely born infants have more of these protective coverings than full-term infants.

## HEALTH CONCERNS

In the second trimester the fetal heart beat becomes audible to stethoscope auscultation, and the mother becomes aware of fetal movement. Both events are highly significant to the parents because they provide tangible evidence of the pregnancy and reassure them that the fetus is alive.

Pregnancy is often a good time for midwives to provide education about gestational events and appropriate maternal rest and nutrition.

### Third Trimester

During the last 3 months of intrauterine life, defined as the third trimester, the fetus grows to approximately 50 cm in length. Subcutaneous fat is stored, and weight increases to between 3.2 and 3.4 kg. The skin thickens, lanugo begins to disappear, and the fetal body becomes rounder and fuller.

A tremendous spurt in brain growth begins during this trimester and lasts well into the first few years of life. The central nervous system has established its total number of neurones and connections between neurones, and myelination of nerve fibres progresses at a rapid rate. Exposure to noxious agents and the absence of essential nutrients are the most common causes of damage to the central nervous system during this trimester. The

midwife can teach the woman about these factors, particularly through nutritional counselling (see Chapter 21).

At the end of the third trimester the normal fetus is physically able to make the transition from intrauterine to extrauterine life. The lungs are capable of maintaining the inflated state for gas exchange. The primitive temperature maintenance systems, reflexes, and sensory organs are ready for use.

### HEALTH CONCERNS

Thoughts of delivering a healthy infant are foremost in the mother's mind as she focuses on preparing her mind and body for the delivery. Parents often seek information and midwives provide organized parentcraft discussion groups to ensure their questions are answered.

## TRANSITION FROM INTRAUTERINE TO EXTRAUTERINE LIFE

The transition from intrauterine to extrauterine life requires rapid changes in the neonate. The midwife assesses the neonate's ability to make these changes and intervenes if necessary to ensure success. Gestational age, exposure to depressant drugs before or during labour, and the neonate's own behavioural style influence adjustment to the external environment. Consequently, initial assessment encompasses a variety of physical and psychosocial elements. The midwife also provides opportunities for the parents and child to develop close emotional ties.

### Physical Health Concerns

An immediate assessment of the neonate's condition is performed; the main concern is the physiological functioning of the major organ systems. Care is then directed at clearing the airway if necessary, stabilizing body temperature by wrapping the neonate in a warm dry towel and giving it to the mother to hold, and protecting the neonate from infection.

Preventing infection is a major concern in the care of the neonate, whose immune system is immature. Gloves are worn to handle the neonate in the delivery room and later when handling other body fluids. Good handwashing technique is the most important factor in protecting the neonate and midwife from infection. Midwives should also wear gloves when changing nappies and when handling body fluids.

The stump of the umbilical cord is an excellent medium for bacterial growth. However, cleanliness and dryness may be sufficient preventive measures. Research tends to show there is little value in cord treatment and that tap water is equally effective.

## Psychosocial Concerns

After immediate physical evaluation and application of identification bracelets, the midwife assesses the parents' and newborn's needs for close physical contact.

Merely placing the family together does not promote closeness. The parents and neonate must be capable and desirous of exploring and responding to each other. Most healthy neonates are awake and alert for the first half hour after birth, and if the parents are receptive, this is an opportune time for parent-child interaction to begin. Close body contact, often including breast-feeding, is a satisfying way for most families to start. If immediate contact is not possible, the midwife incorporates it into the care plan as early as possible, which may mean bringing the newborn to an ill parent or bringing the parents to an ill or premature child if parents and neonate have been separated.

## NEONATE

The neonatal period is the first month of life. During this stage the newborn's physical functioning is often reflexive, and stabilization of major organ systems is the body's primary task.

## Physical Development

A comprehensive assessment is performed as soon as the neonate's physiological functioning is stable, generally within a few hours after birth. At this time the midwife or health visitor measures height, weight, head circumference, temperature, pulse, and respirations and observes general appearance, body functions, sensory capabilities, and responsiveness. In addition, the midwife or health visitor coordinates screening tests and other laboratory tests as indicated by the neonate's state of health. Blood tests such as those for hypothyroidism and phenylketonuria allow early detection and treatment, thereby preventing permanent central nervous system damage.

During the first month the baby's weight increases by 100 to 200 grams per week, length by 0.6 to 2.5 cm, and head circumference by 2 cm. The neonate's heart rate gradually decreases from the fetal rate of 130 to 160 beats per minute to 120 to 140 beats per minute. The average blood pressure is 70/55 mmHg. The newborn's respiratory movements are primarily abdominal and vary in rate and rhythm, but the average rate is 30 to 50 breaths per minute. Since a neonate breathes through the nose, it is important to keep the nasal passages clear. Their axillary temperature ranges from 36.5° to 37.5°C and generally stabilizes within 24 hours after birth.

Normal physical characteristics include the continued presence of lanugo on the skin of the back; cyanosis of the hands and feet, especially during activity; and a soft, protuberant

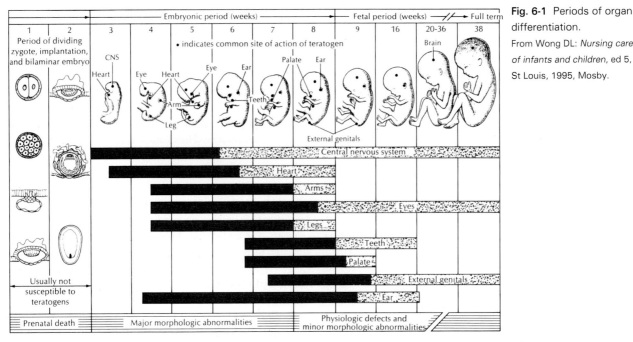

**Fig. 6-1** Periods of organ differentiation.

From Wong DL: *Nursing care of infants and children*, ed 5, St Louis, 1995, Mosby.

abdomen. Skin colour varies according to racial and genetic heritage and gradually changes during infancy. **Moulding**, or overlapping of the soft skull bones, is common during birth. The bones readjust rapidly, producing a more rounded appearance. The linear breaks, sutures, and fontanelles are usually palpable at birth.

Normal behavioural characteristics of the newborn include periods of sucking, crying, sleeping, and activity. Movements are generally sporadic, but they are symmetrical and involve all four extremities. The relatively flexed position of intrauterine life continues as the neonate attempts to maintain an enclosed, secure feeling.

Neurological function is assessed by observing the neonate's level of activity, alertness, irritability, and responsiveness to stimuli and the presence and strength of reflexes. Normal reflexes include blinking in response to bright lights and startling in response to sudden, loud noises. Their absence indicates possible trauma or central nervous system complications.

### Cognitive Development

Early cognitive development begins with innate behaviours, reflexes, and sensory functions. During this time, newborns initiate reflex activities, assimilate new objects into behaviour, and accommodate these behaviours to achieve their desires. For example, within 72 hours neonates learn to turn to the nipple. Although the infants behave of their own volition, activities learned are limited to reflex and sensory function (Nelms and Mullins, 1982).

Sensory functions contribute to cognitive development in the newborn. At birth, children can focus on objects about 20 to 25 cm from their faces and can perceive forms. A preference for the human face is apparent. Auditory and vestibular systems function from birth. These sensory capabilities allow neonates to elicit stimuli rather than simply receive it. Parents should be taught the importance of providing reciprocate sensory stimulation, such as talking to their babies and holding them to see their faces. This allows infants to seek or take in stimuli, thereby enhancing learning and promoting cognitive development.

Crying elicits a response, and care givers discriminate crying patterns. Crying therefore has significance to newborns and parents. For neonates, crying is a means of communication. Some babies cry because their nappies are wet or they are hungry or want to be held. Others cry just to make noise. Crying may frustrate the parents if they cannot see an apparent cause. With the nurse's help, parents can learn to differentiate between different crying patterns and take appropriate action when necessary.

### Psychosocial Development

During the first month of life, parents and newborns normally develop a strong bond that grows into a deep **attachment**. Interactions during routine care enhance or detract from the attachment process. Feeding, hygiene, and comfort measures consume much of the infants' waking time. These interactive experiences provide a foundation from which deep attachments form. Neonates are active participants in this process.

If parents or children experience health complications after birth, attachment may be compromised. Infants' behavioural cues may be weak or absent. Care and care giving are less mutually satisfying. Tired, ill parents have difficulty interpreting and responding to their infants. Children who have congenital anomalies are too weak to be responsive to parental cues, and those who require special care need supportive nursing care.

## INFANT

Infancy is the period from 1 month to 1 year of age. Rapid physical growth and change characterize this stage. Psychosocial development advances, aided by the progression from reflexive to more purposeful behaviour. Interaction between infants and the environment is greater and more meaningful.

### Physical Development

Steady and proportional growth of the infant is more important than absolute growth values. Charts of normal age- and sex-related growth measurements enable growth comparison with norms for a child's age. These are called centile charts. Using growth charts, you can also evaluate growth patterns by recording measurements of weight, length, and head circumference at intervals. Measurements recorded over time are the best way to monitor growth and identify problems. Single measurements are unhelpful.

Size (weight and length) increases rapidly during the first year of life; birth weight doubles by 6 months on average and triples by 12 months. Length increases rapidly, by 15 cm in the first year, decreasing to 3-8 cm per annum until adolescence. Head circumference increases proportionally.

Physiological functioning stabilizes; by the end of the first year, the heart rate is 80 to 130 beats per minute, the blood pressure is 72-110/38-72 mmHg, and respiratory rate is 30 to 35 breaths per minute. Patterns of body function also stabilize, usually there are predictable sleep, elimination, and feeding routines. Motor development proceeds steadily in a head-to-foot direction. Table 6-2 identifies developmental **milestones** in gross motor and fine motor development.

### Cognitive Development

Infants learn by experiencing and manipulating the environment. Developing motor skills and increasing mobility expand an infant's environment and, developing visual and auditory skills, enhance cognitive development. For these reasons, Piaget (1952) has named his first stage of cognitive development, which extends until around the second birthday, the *sensorimotor period*. Before the acquisition of language, the extraordinary development of the mind occurs through the child's developing senses and motor abilities. For example, a 1-month-old can follow the path of a moving object. Improved visual acuity and eye-hand coordination allow grasping and exploration of objects. In addition, rudimentary colour vision begins by 2 months and improves throughout the first year, making the environment more interesting to see and explore. The infant's hearing also progresses, allowing localization and discrimination of sounds.

## TABLE 6-2 Milestones in Infant Motor Development

|  | Gross motor | Fine motor |
|---|---|---|
| Month 3 | Lifts head and chest while prone | Grasps and briefly holds objects and takes them to mouth |
| Month 6 | Rolls over<br>Sits without support<br><br>Crawls on abdomen with arms | Uses palm grasp with finger encircling object<br><br>Transfers object from hand to mouth |
| Month 9 | Attains sitting position independently<br>Creeps on all four extremities<br>Pulls self to standing position | Picks up small objects with thumb-and-finger pincer motion. |
| Month 12 | Walks holding onto walls and furniture (cruising)<br><br>Stands alone<br><br>Takes 1-3 steps | Places tiny object, such as raisin, into container<br><br>Makes marks with crayon |
| Month 15 | Walks alone | Scribbles with crayon<br>Builds tower of two cubes |

Speech is an important aspect of cognition that develops during the first year. Infants proceed from crying, cooing, and laughing to imitating sounds, comprehending the meaning of simple commands, and repeating words with knowledge of their meaning. By 1 year, infants may not only recognize their own names but also have two- or three-word vocabularies including *Da-Da*, *Ma-Ma*, and *no*. Language development can be promoted by encouraging mothers to name objects on which their infants' attention is focused.

### Psychosocial Development

During their first year, infants begin to differentiate themselves from others as separate beings capable of acting on their own. Initially, infants are unaware of the boundaries of self, but through repeated experiences with the environment, they learn where the self ends and the external world begins. This process is slow, and infants occasionally experience brief frustrations with more frequent and consistent satisfactions. As infants determine their physical boundaries, they begin to respond to others. Two- and three-month-old infants begin to smile responsively rather than reflexively. Similarly, they can recognize differences in people when their sensory and cognitive capabilities improve. By 8 months, most infants can differentiate a stranger from a familiar person and respond differently to the two. Close attachment to the primary care givers, most often parents, is usually established by this age. Infants seek out these persons for support and comfort during times of stress. The ability to distinguish self from others allow infants to interact and socialize more within their environments. By 9 months, for example, infants play simple social games such as pat-a-cake and peek-a-boo. More complex interactive games such as hide-and-seek involving objects are possible by the age of 1.

Erikson (1963) describes the psychosocial developmental crisis for the infant as *trust* versus *mistrust*. He explains that the quality of parent-infant interactions determines development of trust or mistrust. Parents who meet needs for warmth and comfort, love and security, and food when infants express these needs promote a sense of trust, whereas those that meet the needs of infants at their own convenience or not at all allow a sense of mistrust to develop (Erikson, 1963).

### Perception of Health

The foundation for children's perceptions of their health status is established early in life. Internal body sensations and experiences with the outside world affect **self-perceptions**. The nature of this influence and the value of nursing interventions to alter later perceptions are unknown. It is known, however, that parents tend to label children who are ill in early life as more *vulnerable* than their siblings and that this labelling may affect the child's perception of his or her own health.

### TODDLER

Toddlerhood ranges from the time when children begin to walk independently until they walk and run with ease, which is approximately from 12 to 36 months. Toddlerhood is characterized by increasing independence bolstered by greater physical mobility and cognitive abilities. Toddlers are increasingly aware of their abilities to control and are pleased with successful efforts with this new skill. This success leads them to repeated attempts to control their environments. Unsuccessful attempts at control may result in negative behaviours and temper tantrums.

### Physical Development

The rate of increase in weight and length slows. By 2 years the child weighs approximately four times the birth weight. Height

**Learning Disabilities Nursing**
**Identifying developmental**
**disabilities**

The way in which parents become aware that their child is developmentally delayed, or has a learning disability, is one of the crucial factors that determines how the family comes to terms with the disability and how they meet the needs of the child.

If there is no obvious sign of a disability at birth, the realization that a problem exists can occur very gradually. For example, a mother who has a quiet, sleepy baby (and little experience of other children the same age), may be please that the baby is 'good'. She may not realize the baby has a disability until obvious milestones — such as sitting, crawling, or walking — are not achieved. In this case, the health visitor can alert the parents to potential problems early in the child's developmental process.

In another situation, a previously 'normal' child may gradually fall behind his or her peer group, developmentally. While the parents may recognize that something is wrong, it may take some time for the GP or health visitor to define the problem, unless there is a family history of a progressive degenerative condition. When a long awaited diagnosis is made, it can sometimes be a relief to the family.

Nurses and other health care professionals play a key role in helping the family cope in its own way. For some families, the diagnosis of a child's disability may lead to a sense of loss and bereavement. For others, however, it can bring unity and a sense of purpose.

during toddlerhood increases 8 to 13 cm a year, mainly as a result of increases in leg length.

The rapid development of **motor skills** allows the child to participate in self-care activities such as feeding, dressing, and toileting. In the beginning the toddler walks in an upright position with a broad-stanced gait, protuberant abdomen, and arms out to the sides for balance. Soon the child begins to navigate stairs, using a rail or the wall to maintain balance while progressing upward, placing both feet on the same step before continuing. Locomotion skills soon include running, jumping, standing on one foot for several seconds, and kicking a ball. Most toddlers can ride tricycles, climb ladders, and run well by their third birthday. Fine motor capabilities move from scribbling spontaneously to drawing circles and crosses accurately. By 3 years the child draws simple stick people and can usually stack a tower of small blocks. Improved mobility, the ability to undress, and development of sphincter control allow toilet training if the toddler has developed the necessary cognitive abilities. Health visitors can advise parents on the development of the child.

The cardiopulmonary system becomes stable in the toddler years. The heart and respiratory rates slow to 110 beats and 24 to 26 breaths per minute, and the blood pressure rises slightly to an average of 92/56 mmHg.

Most toddlers change from breast milk or formula to milk, consuming three to four glasses per day. Nutritional requirements are increasingly met by solid foods in the remaining three basic food groups (see Chapter 21).

## Cognitive Development

Toddlers' completion of the development of *object permanence* (Piaget, 1952), their ability to remember events, and to start to put thoughts into words at about 2 years of age signals their transition from Piaget's sensorimotor stage of cognitive development to the **preoperational thought** stage (Piaget, 1952). Table 6-1 outlines the basic characteristics of the three substages of cognitive development through which toddlers move between 12 and 36 months. Toddlers recognize that they are separate beings from their mothers, but they are unable to assume the view of another. They use symbols to represent objects, places, and persons.

The 18-month-old child uses approximately 10 words. The 24-month-old child has a vocabulary of up to 300 words and is generally able to speak in short sentences. "Who's that?" and "What's that?" typify questions asked during this period. Verbal expressions such as "me do it" and "that's mine" demonstrate the 2-year-old child's use of pronouns and desire for independence and control.

Because children's **moral development** is closely associated with their cognitive abilities, the moral development of toddlers is only beginning and is also egocentric. Toddlers do not understand concepts of right and wrong. However, they do grasp the fact that some behaviours bring pleasant results (positive reinforcement) and others elicit unpleasant results (negative reinforcement).

## Psychosocial Development

According to Erikson (1963), a sense of **autonomy** emerges during toddlerhood. Children strive for independence by using their developing muscles to do everything for themselves and become the master of their bodily functions. Their strong wills are frequently exhibited in negative behaviour when care givers attempt to direct their actions. Temper tantrums may result when toddlers are frustrated by parental restrictions. Socially, toddlers remain strongly attached to their parents and fear separation from them.

The child engages in solitary play during toddlerhood but also begins to participate in **parallel play**, which is playing beside rather than with another child (Piaget, 1952).

The newly developed locomotion abilities and insatiable curiosity of toddlers make them a danger to their own well-being, due to accidents, poisonings and drownings (see Chapter 19). Toddlers require close supervision at all times and parents should be extremely vigilant of the child's safety during this period.

## Perception of Health

Toddlers' perceptions of their own health are limited by their cognitive capabilities. Children increasingly recognize internal body sensations but have difficulty pinpointing their location.

During this stage, children begin to internalize the labels that parents or health care professionals give to the somatic states. That is, if the parents label particular sensations, such as abdominal discomfort, an 'illness', children begin to label related sensations similarly. At the same time, children observe and mimic parents' health care practices. *Health beliefs and practices* are therefore being significantly shaped.

## PRESCHOOL CHILD

The preschool years are a transition between toddlerhood and the school-age years. The period spans between the ages of 3 and 6 years. Physical development continues to slow, whereas cognitive and psychosocial development are rapid.

### Physical Development

Several aspects of physical development continue to stabilize in the preschool years. Heart and respiratory rates decrease only slightly to approximately 90 beats and 22 to 24 breaths per minute. Blood pressure rises slightly to an average of 95/58 mmHg. Children gain about 2 kg per year until they are 4 years old, then approximately 3 kg per year until the age of 10.

Large and fine muscle coordination improves. Preschoolers run well, walk up and down steps with ease, and learn to hop. By the age of 6, they can usually skip and throw and catch balls. Improving *fine motor skills* allow intricate manipulations. Children can copy circles, crosses, squares, and triangles. These skills make printing of letters and numbers possible.

### Cognitive Development

Preschoolers continue to master the preoperational stage of cognition. The first phase of this period, known as *preconceptual thought* (2 to 4 years), is characterized by perceptual-bound thinking, in which children judge persons, objects, and events by their outward appearance (Piaget, 1952).

Around the age of 4 years, the *intuitive phase* of *preoperational thought* develops and the child is able to think in complex terms. Egocentricity persists, but during these 3 years it begins to be replaced with social interaction. Children become aware of cause-and-effect relationships as illustrated by the statement 'The sun sets because people want to go to bed.'

Preschoolers' knowledge of the world remains closely linked to concrete experiences. Their rich fantasy life is grounded in the perception of reality. The mixing of the two aspects can lead to many childhood fears and may be misinterpreted by adults as lying when children are actually presenting reality from their perspective.

The preschooler's moral development expands to include an initial understanding of behaviours considered socially right or wrong. The child continues to be motivated, however, by the wish to avoid punishment or the desire to obtain a reward. The primary difference between this stage of moral development and that of a toddler is that a preschool child is more able to identify behaviours that elicit rewards or punishment and begins to label these behaviours as *right* or *wrong*.

Preschoolers' vocabularies continue to increase rapidly. By the age of 5, preschoolers will have a vocabulary of more than 2000 words that they can use to define familiar objects, identify colours, and express their desires and frustrations. Language is more social, and questions expand to "Why?" and "How come?" in the quest for information. Phonetically similar words such as *die* and *dye* may confuse preschool children.

### Psychosocial Development

The world of preschoolers expands beyond the family into the neighbourhood where children meet other children and adults. Their unquenchable curiosity and developing initiative lead to the active exploration of the environment, the development of new skills, and the making of new friends.

The play of preschool children becomes more socially interactive after the third birthday as it shifts from parallel to *associative play*, which involves a borrowing and lending of play material. All participants engage in similar if not identical activity; however, there is no division of labour, and all children do as they wish. Most 3-year-old children are able to play with one other child in a cooperative manner in which they make something or play designated roles such as mother and baby. By the age of 4, children play in groups of two or three, and by 5 years the group has a temporary leader for each activity.

In many play activities, preschoolers display awareness of social context. Sex-role identification is strengthening, and children most often assume roles of persons of their own sex. Children frequently mimic or repeat social experiences.

Pretend play involving imaginary situations depends on the child's ability to retain images of things that he or she has seen or heard. This sociodramatic play involving other children occupies about a third of 5-year-old childrens' playtime. Pretending allows children to learn to understand other's points of view, develop skills in solving social problems, and become more creative. Children who watch a great deal of television engage less frequently in imaginative play, possibly because they develop the habit of passively absorbing images rather than generating their own.

### Perception of Health

Little research has explored preschoolers, perceptions of their own health. Parental beliefs about health, childrens' bodily sensations, and their ability to perform daily activities help children develop attitudes about their health. Preschoolers are usually quite independent in washing, dressing, and feeding. Alterations in this independence can influence their feelings about their own health.

## SCHOOL-AGED CHILD

During these 'middle years' of childhood, the foundation for adult roles in work, recreation, and social interaction is laid. In industrialized countries, this period begins when the child starts primary school around the age of 5 years; puberty, around 12 years of age, signals the end of middle childhood. Great developmental strides are made during these early school years when children develop competencies in physical, cognitive, and psychosocial skills.

The school or educational experience expands the child's world and is a transition from a life of relatively free play to a life of structured play, learning, and work. The school and home influence growth and development, requiring adjustment by the parents and child.

### Physical Development

For the majority of children, the rate of growth during these early school years is slower than at any time since birth, but continues in a steady manner. Growth accelerates at different times for different children. The average increase in height is 30 cm per year, while the weight, which is more variable, increases by 1.8 to 3.2 kg per year. Many children double their weight during these middle years.

School provides children with the opportunity to compare themselves with large numbers of children of the same age. Regular measurement of height and weight may reveal alterations in growth that are symptoms of the onset of a variety of childhood diseases.

Boys are slightly taller and heavier than girls during these early school years. Approximately 2 years before puberty, these school-aged children experience a rapid acceleration in skeletal growth, and girls, who generally reach puberty first, begin to surpass boys in height and weight, which causes embarrassment to both sexes. These changes may begin as early as 9 years in girls but do not usually occur in boys before 12 years.

Cardiovascular functioning is refined and stabilized during the school years. The heart rate averages 70 to 90 beats per minute, the blood pressure normalizes to approximately 110/70 mmHg, and the respiratory rate stabilizes to 19 to 21 breaths per minute. Lung growth is minimal. However, by the end of this period the heart is six times the size it was at birth and has generally reached its adult size.

## Gross Motor Coordination

School-aged children become more graceful during the school years because their large muscle coordination improves and strength doubles. Most children practise the basic gross motor skills of running, jumping, balancing, throwing, and catching during play, resulting in refinement of *neuromuscular function and skills*. Physical education is important in encouraging this development. Individual differences in the rate of mastering skills and ultimate skill achievement become apparent. Individual differences in motor skills are established by participation in activities and games requiring coordinated muscle movements and innate ability.

## Fine Motor Coordination

Fine motor skills lag behind gross motor skills but progress at approximately the same rate. As control is gained over fingers and wrists, children become proficient in a wide range of activities.

Most 6-year-old children can hold a pencil adeptly and print letters and words, but by the age of 12 the child can make detailed drawings and write sentences in script.

The improved fine motor capabilities of children in middle childhood allow them to become very independent in bathing, dressing, and taking care of other personal needs, and they develop strong personal preferences in the way these needs are met. Illness and hospitalization may threaten children's control in these areas. Therefore, it is important to allow them to participate in care and maintain as much independence as possible. Children whose care demands restriction of fluids, for example, cannot be allowed to decide the amount of fluids they will drink in 24 hours, but they can help decide the type of fluids and keep an accurate record of intake.

Assessment of neurological development is often based on fine motor coordination. This assessment may include penmanship, stacking ability, and performance of sequential, rapid, alternating movements such as touching the finger to the nose and then to the examiner's finger.

## Other Changes

Other physical changes take place during the school years. A steady skeletal growth in the trunk and extremities occurs, and small- and long-bone ossification is present but not complete by the age of 12. Facial bones grow and remodel, as indicated by the presence of frontal sinuses by the age of 8 or 9. Dental growth is prominent during the school years. By the age of 12, all primary teeth have been shed, and the most of the permanent teeth have erupted.

As skeletal growth progresses, body appearance and posture change. Earlier posture, which was characterized by a stoop-shouldered, slightly lordotic stance and prominent abdomen, changes to a more erect posture.

Eye shape alters because of skeletal growth. This improves visual acuity, and normal adult 20/20 vision is achievable. Screening for vision and hearing problems is easier, and results are more reliable because school-aged children can more fully understand and cooperate with the test directions. The school nurse typically assesses the dental, visual, and auditory status of school-aged children biannually and refers those with possible deviations to a paediatrician.

## Cognitive Development

Cognitive changes provide the school-aged child with the ability to think in a logical manner about the present, but not about abstraction. The thoughts of school-aged children are no longer dominated by their perceptions, and thus their ability to understand the world greatly expands. Around 7 years of age, children enter Piaget's third stage of cognitive development (see Table 6-1), known as *concrete operations*, in which they are able to use symbols to carry out operations (mental activities) in thought rather than in action. They begin to use logical thought processes with concrete materials (objects, people, and events they can touch and see).

The mental process of *classification* becomes more complex during the school years. Young children can separate objects into groups according to shape or colour, but school-aged children understand that the same element can exist in two classes at the same time. For example, the school-aged child could be shown a group of 16 wooden green beads and four wooden red beads and asked if there were more green beads or more wooden beads. The school-aged child would recognize there were three classes of beads (red, green, and wooden) and would answer there were more wooden beads, whereas the preschool child would identify only two classes of beads and answer "green".

Middle childhood youngsters can use their newly developed cognitive skills to solve problems. Some people are better than others at problem solving because of native intelligence, education, and experience. However, all children can improve these skills. Middle school-aged children who are good problem solvers demonstrate the following characteristics: a positive attitude that the problem can be solved with persistence, a concern for accuracy, the ability to divide the problem into parts for study, and the ability to avoid guessing while searching for facts.

## Language Development

Language growth is so rapid during middle childhood that it is no longer possible to match age with language achievements. The average 6-year-old child has a vocabulary of about 3000 words that quickly expands with exposure to peers and adults and reading ability. Children improve their use of language and expand their structural knowledge. They become more aware of the rules of **syntax**, the rules for linking words into phrases and sentences. They can also identify generalizations and exceptions to rules. They accept language as a means for representing the world in a subjective manner and realize that words have arbitrary, rather than absolute, meanings. They can use different words for the same object or concept, and they understand that a single word may have many meanings. Many school-aged children use 'bad language' to gain peer status and to shock adults. By the end of this period, their use of language is similar to that of adults.

### Children's Nursing
### Effects of hospitalization on children

For children, hospitalization and illness are stressful experiences, primarily because of separation from the normal environment and significant others, a limited selection of coping behaviours, and altered states of health. However, the nurse should try to make the experience a positive one.

Nurses should assess the availability and appropriateness of experiences contributing to psychosocial development. Hospitalized infants may have difficulty establishing physical boundaries because of repeated bodily intrusions and painful sensations. Limiting these negative experiences and providing pleasurable sensations are interventions that support early psychosocial development. Extended separations from parents complicate the attachment process and increase the number of care givers with whom the infant must interact. Ideally, the parents should provide the majority of care during hospitalization. When parents are not present, an attempt should be made to limit the number of care givers who have contact with the infant and to follow the parents' directions for care. These interventions will foster the infant's continuing development of trust.

Children also need opportunities to learn and practice physical skills while in hospital. Nursing care of healthy and ill children includes an assessment of the availability of these opportunities. Although children with acute illnesses benefit from rest and exclusion from the usual daily activities, children who have chronic conditions or who have been hospitalized for long periods need ongoing exposure to developmental opportunities. The parents and nurse must weave these opportunities into the children's daily experiences, depending on their abilities, needs, and energy level.

## Psychosocial Development
## Moral Development

The need for a moral code and social rules becomes more evident as school-aged children's cognitive abilities and social experiences increase. For example, a 12-year-old child is able to consider what society would be like without rules because of his or her ability to reason logically and experience group play.

## Peer Relationships

Group and personal achievements become important to the school-aged child. Success is important in physical and cognitive activities. Play involves peers and the pursuit of group goals. Although solitary activities are not eliminated, they are overshadowed by group play. Learning to contribute, collaborate, and work cooperatively toward a common goal becomes a measure of success.

The school-aged child prefers same-sex peers to opposite-sex peers. This strong *gender identity* is evidenced by the close network of same-sex companions that a child maintains. In general, girls and boys view the opposite sex negatively. **Peer influence** becomes quite diverse during this stage of development. Conformity is evidenced in mannerisms, clothing styles, and speech patterns that are reinforced and influenced by contact with peers. Group identity increases as the school-aged child approaches adolescence.

## Sexual Identity

Freud described middle childhood as the *latency period*. He believed that children of this period had little interest in their sexuality. Today, many contemporary researchers believe that school-aged children have a great deal of interest in their sexuality and engage in hidden sex play and masturbation.

## Self-Concept and Health

During the school-aged years, identity and self-concept become stronger and more individualized. Perception of wellness is based on readily observable facts such as presence or absence of illness and adequacy of eating or sleeping. Functional ability is the standard by which personal health and the health of others are judged.

Promotion of good health practices is a nursing responsibility. Programmes directed at health education are frequently organized and conducted in the school. During these programmes, the nurse focuses on the development of behaviours that positively affect children's health status.

## Specific Health Concerns

Accidents and injuries are a major health problem affecting school-aged children (see Chapter 19). Motor vehicle accidents and accidents related to recreational activities or equipment are the leading causes of death or injury.

School-aged children are also affected by cancer, birth defects, and heart disease. In this age group, these problems have a relatively low mortality rate but a high morbidity rate compared to accidents. Infections account for nearly 80% of all childhood illnesses; respiratory infections are the most prevalent. The common cold remains the chief illness of childhood. Certain groups of children are more prone to disease, for example, homeless children, children living in poverty, children with chronic illness, children who were low-birth-weight infants, foreign-born adopted children, and children in day-care centres (Bell *et al*, 1989).

## ADOLESCENT

Adolescence is the period of development during which the individual makes the transition from childhood to adulthood, usually between 13 and 21 years. The term *adolescent* usually refers to psychological maturation of the individual, whereas *puberty* refers to the point at which reproduction becomes possible. The hormonal changes of puberty result in changes in the appearance of the young person, and mental development results in the ability to hypothesize and deal with abstractions. Adjustments and adaptations are required to cope with these simultaneous changes and the attempt to establish an adult sense of identity.

### Physical Changes and Sexual Maturation
Physical changes occur rapidly in adolescence. Sexual maturation occurs with the development of primary and secondary sexual characteristics. Primary characteristics are physical and hormonal changes necessary for reproduction, and secondary characteristics externally differentiate males from females. Four main focuses of the physical changes are summarized by Tanner (1974):
- increased growth rate of skeleton, muscle, and viscera
- sex-specific changes, such as changes in shoulder and hip width
- alteration in distribution of muscle and fat
- development of the reproductive system and secondary sex characteristics.

A wide variation exists in the timing of physical changes associated with puberty, and girls tend to begin their physical changes earlier than boys.

### Weight and Skeletal Changes
Height and weight increases usually occur during the *prepubertal growth spurt*. The growth spurt for girls generally begins between the ages of 8 and 14. Height increases 5 to 20 cm, and weight increases by 7 to 25 kg. The male growth spurt usually takes place between 10 and 16 years of age. Height increases approximately 10 to 30 cm, and weight increases by 7 to 29 kg.

Girls attain 90 to 95% of their adult height by *menarche* (the onset of menstruation) and reach their full height by 16 to 17 years of age, whereas boys continue to grow taller until 18 to 20 years of age. Fat is redistributed into adult proportions as height and weight increase, and gradually the adolescent torso takes on an adult appearance.

### Effects of Physical Changes on Peer Interaction
Adolescents are sensitive about physical changes that make them different from peers. For this reason, they are generally interested

in the normal pattern of growth and their personal growth curves. Consequently, the nurse should share this information to reassure adolescents that their own patterns are normal.

The number of eating disorders is on the rise in adolescent girls, and knowledge of growth progression may be a way to discourage radical weight-reduction activities. If an adolescent deviates radically from the usual pattern, further assessment is necessary to identify the cause. Weight extremes resulting from excessive or inadequate calorific intake are common during the adolescent years. Allowing the adolescent to see when and how the weight curve changed can be a first step in identifying the problem and implementing dietary changes.

### TIMING AND SEQUENCE OF PUBERTY
A wide variation exists between the sexes and within the same sex as to when the physical changes of puberty begin. The sequence of pubertal growth changes is the same in most individuals. The ranges of *normal* are stressed. As with increases in height and weight, the pattern of sexual changes is more significant than their time of onset. Large deviations from normal frames require investigation. For example, a 17-year-old girl who has not menstruated requires assessment and referral.

Being like peers is extremely important for adolescents. Any deviation in the timing of the physical changes can be extremely difficult for them to accept. The nurse should therefore provide emotional support for adolescents undergoing assessment of early or delayed puberty. Even adolescents whose physical changes are occurring at the normal times may seek confirmation of and reassurance about their normality.

### HORMONAL CHANGES
Visible and invisible changes take place during puberty. All of these changes are created by hormonal changes within the body when the hypothalamus begins to produce gonadotropin-releasing hormones, which signal the pituitary to secrete gonadotropic hormones. Gonadotropic hormones stimulate ovarian cells to produce oestrogen and testicular cells to produce testosterone. These hormones contribute to the development of secondary sex characteristics such as hair growth and voice changes, and play an essential role in reproduction. The changing

**Mental Health Nursing**
**Group identity and ethnic minorities**

Many adolescents born in the UK to ethnic parents face considerable problems when it comes to developing an individual and group identity. Loyalties to their peer group and family values often conflict. The values of individualism in contemporary Western first world countries often stand diametrically opposed to family values of the collective good. While many adolescents may be experiencing a Western notion of adolescence, many adolescents from ethnic backgrounds may not have that choice; finding themselves, as they frequently do, as child brides/grooms in arranged marriages, which are part of their cultural practice.
Adapted from d'Ardenne P, Mahtani A: *Transcultural counselling in action*, London, 1990, Sage.

concentrations of these hormones are also linked to acne and to body odour.

## Cognitive Development

According to Piaget (1972), changes that occur within the mind and the widening social environment of the adolescent result in *formal operations*, the highest level of intellectual development. Young people who possess sufficient neurological development to reach this stage may not attain it if they do not receive sufficient support from their cultural and educational environment, and those who are guided toward rational thinking may reach this stage early.

During this period of cognitive development, the teenager develops the ability to solve problems through formal operations (see Table 6-1). The teenager can think abstractly and deal effectively with hypothetical problems. When confronted with a problem, the teenager can consider an infinite variety of causes and solutions, and can move beyond the physical or concrete properties of a situation and use reasoning powers to understand the abstract. Development of this ability is important in the pursuit of an identity. For example, newly acquired cognitive skills allow the teenager to define appropriate, effective, and comfortable sex-role behaviours and to consider their impact on peers, family, and society. The ability to think logically about these behaviours and their outcomes encourages the adolescent to develop personal thoughts and means of expressing sexual identity. In addition, a higher level of cognitive functioning makes the adolescent receptive to more detailed and diverse information about sexuality and sexual behaviours. The complex development of thought during this period leads adolescents to question society and its values. Although teenagers have the capability to think as well as an adult, they do not have the life experiences on which to build.

## Language Skills

Language development is fairly complete by adolescence, although vocabulary continues to expand. The primary focus becomes *communication skills* that can be used effectively in various situations. Adolescents need to communicate thoughts, feelings, and facts to peers, parents, teachers, and other persons of authority.

## Psychosocial Development

The search for *personal identity* is the major task of adolescent psychosocial development. Teenagers must establish close peer relationships or remain socially isolated. Erikson sees identity (or role) confusion as the prime danger of this stage and suggests that the cliquishness and intolerance of differences seen in adolescent behaviour are defences against identity confusion (Erikson, 1968). Teenagers must become emotionally independent from their parents and yet retain family ties. In addition, they need to develop their own ethical systems based on personal values. It is important to remember that the degree to which adolescents conform to social norms and expectations is greatly influenced by the culture in which they are raised.

## Sexual Identity

Achievement of **sexual identity** is enhanced by the physical changes of puberty. In Freud's view, these physiological changes of puberty reactivate the libido, the energy source that fuels the sex drive. This is manifested by the teenager's interest in heterosexual and homosexual relationships with partners outside of the family and the practice of masturbation. The physical evidence of maturity encourages the development of masculine and feminine behaviours. If these physical changes involve deviations from the norm, the person has more difficulty developing a comfortable sexual identity. Adolescents depend on these physical clues because they want assurance of 'maleness' or 'femaleness' and because they do not wish to be different from peers. Without these physical characteristics, achieving sexual identity is difficult. Other influences are cultural attitudes and expectations of sex-role behaviour and available role models. The masculine and feminine behaviours that teenagers see affect the way that they express sexuality. Adolescents master age appropriate sexuality after feeling comfortable with sexual behaviours, choices, and relationships.

## Group Identity

Adolescents seek a **group identity** because they need esteem and acceptance. Similarity in dress or speech is common in teenage groups. Popularity is a major concern. Popularity with opposite-sex and same-sex peers is important. The strong need for group identity seems to conflict at times with the search for personal identity. It is as though adolescents require close bonds with peers so that they can later redefine themselves against this group identity.

## Family Identity

The movement towards stronger peer relationships is contrasted with adolescents' movements away from parents. Although financial independence for adolescents is not the norm in contemporary Western society, many adolescents work part-time, using their income to bolster independence.

## Moral Identity

The development of moral judgement depends heavily on cognitive and communication skills and peer interaction. Although moral development begins in early childhood, it is consolidated in adolescence because of the presence of certain skills.

Kohlberg (1964) explains moral developments in terms of stages (see Table 6-1). Adolescents can achieve the highest level of moral judgement. At this level, morality is derived from individual principles of conscience. Adolescents judge themselves by internalized ideals, which often leads to conflict between personal and group values. Group values become less significant in later adolescence.

## Specific Health Concerns

Accidents remain the leading cause of death in adolescents (about 70%) (see Chapter 19). Motor vehicle accidents, which are the most common cause of death, result in almost half the fatalities of

16 to 19 year olds (Rivara, 1988). Such accidents are often associated with alcohol intoxication or drug abuse. Other frequent causes of accidental death in teenagers are drowning, violence, and poisoning. Feelings of being indestructible lead to risk-taking behaviours.

Substance abuse is in fact a major concern to those who work with teenagers. Teenagers may believe that mood-altering substances create a sense of well-being or improve their level of performance. All adolescents are at risk for experimental or recreational substance use, but those who have unconventional values or come from unstable homes may be more at risk for chronic use and physical dependency.

Suicide is the third leading cause of death in adolescents (rates are especially high in some Asian communities) between 15 and 24 years of age; accidents and homicides are the leading causes. Depression and social isolation commonly precede a suicide attempt, but suicide probably results from a combination of several factors. Immediate referrals to mental health professionals need to be made when assessment suggests that an adolescent may be considering suicide.

Sexual experimentation is common among adolescents. Peer pressure, physiological and emotional changes, and societal expectations contribute to early heterosexual and homosexual relations. Nurses can provide sex education and counselling. The degree of sexual activity among teenagers may not change significantly, but the degree of informed, consenting participation can. Two prominent consequences of adolescent sexual activity are sexually transmitted disease and pregnancy.

## THEORIES OF ADULTHOOD

Many theorists have attempted to describe the phases of adulthood and related developmental tasks. Selected examples are presented in this section.

### Young Adulthood

Levinson *et al* (1978) identified five phases of young and middle adult development:
1. Early adult transition (ages 18 to 20), when the person separates from the family and desires independence.
2. Entrance into the adult world (ages 21 to 27), when the person tries out careers and lifestyles.
3. Transition (ages 28 to 32), when the person may modify life activities greatly.
4. Settling down (ages 33 to 39), when the person experiences greater stability.
5. The pay-off years (ages 45 to 65), a time for maximal influence, self-direction, and self-appraisal.

Theorists propose that intellectual and moral development differs between men and women. According to Gilligan (1982), women struggle with the issues of care and responsibility, and in turn their relationships progress towards a maturity of interdependence. As women progress towards adulthood the moral dilemma changes from how to exercise their rights without interfering in the rights of others to 'how to lead a moral life' that includes obligations to themselves, their families and people in general (Gilligan, 1982).

As women entered the professional arenas, they hoped to develop the caring and nurturing roles in their male colleagues (Gordon, 1991). Women have long recognized that, without caring, the perceived quality of life is changed. As a result women maintained caring in the home and educational and work environments. However, women became frustrated in their development because the responsibility of caring was not shared, and frequently nurturing became a gender-specific responsibility (Benner and Wrubel, 1989).

Another theory for young adult development has been developed by Diekelmann (1976), who proposes that young adults experience the following developmental tasks:
1. They achieve independence from parental controls.
2. They begin to develop strong friendships and intimate relationships outside the family.
3. They establish a personal set of values.
4. They develop a sense of personal identity.
5. They prepare for life work and develop the capacity for intimacy.

These theories, along with the work of Erikson (1963, 1982), provide nurses with a basis for understanding the life events and developmental tasks of the young adult. Each young adult, however, brings unique characteristics and needs to this developmental stage. A patient/client in this developmental stage presents challenges to nurses who themselves may be young adults coping with the demands of this period. Young adult nurses must be careful to recognize the needs of a young adult patient/client even if they are not experiencing the same challenges and events.

### Middle Adulthood
### Erikson's Theory
According to Erikson's developmental theory, the primary developmental task of the middle years is to achieve 'generativity' (Erikson, 1968, 1982). Generativity is the willingness to care for and guide others. Middle adults can achieve generativity with their own children or the children of close friends or through guidance in social interactions with the next generation. If middle adults fail to achieve generativity, stagnation occurs. This is manifested by excessive concern with themselves or destructive behaviour toward their children and the community.

### Havighurst's Theory
Havighurst's developmental theory has been summarized in terms of the following seven developmental tasks for the middle-aged adult (Havighurst, 1972; Rawlins *et al*, 1993):
1. Achieving adult civic social responsibility.
2. Establishing and maintaining a standard of living.
3. Helping teenage children become responsible and happy adults.
4. Developing leisure activities.
5. Relating to one's spouse as a person.
6. Accepting and adjusting to the physiological changes of middle age.
7. Adjusting to ageing parents.

## Mother and Child Nursing
### The pregnant woman and childbearing family

An important decision for most young couples is when to begin a family. Although the physiological changes associated with childbearing affect only the woman, cognitive and psychosocial changes affect the entire family, including siblings and grandparents.

### Psychological changes

Women and men who are anticipating conceiving a baby benefit from preconception health education. Advice could include information about a balanced diet, exercise, alcohol intake and the effects of smoking.

### Antenatal care

In the UK, antenatal care is available to all who need it. Midwives, obstetricians and general practitioners may give this care individually or as a team. Midwives are setting up team practices to provide continuity of care and of carer wherever possible. The aim is to maximize pregnancy outcome and minimize the stress and risk related to childbearing.

Women are encouraged to come for care eight weeks after conception and are seen at regular intervals throughout pregnancy; more frequently from 28 weeks. The health and well-being of the woman and fetus is monitored carefully and advice is given about anxieties or health problems, such as pregnancy induced hypertension, as they arise. While mortality from childbearing is low, it is still the most significant cause of death in young women.

At 36 weeks, the woman's ability to cope physically with the process of labour is assessed and decisions may be taken concerning the mode of delivery; for example, a caesarean section may be safer for mother and baby.

### Need for education

The couple are offered a series of formal parentcraft classes about pregnancy, labour, delivery, infant feeding, neonatal behaviour and other topics. These help reduce their anxiety about their ability to cope with future demands. Classes may be offered to people with special needs, such as single parents and grandparents, and may be available in different languages as needed.

### Psychosocial changes — body image

Although the physical changes are not obvious to others until the second trimester, the woman generally perceives changes in her body, such as enlargement of her breasts, during the first three months. Minor discomforts, such as morning sickness, may make her feel ambivalent about her pregnancy at first.

However, women, particularly primigravidae (pregnant for the first time), generally enjoy the second trimester. Their pregnancy is beginning to 'show' and they start to plan their maternity wardrobe. At this time, they feel the baby move and begin to fantasize about the baby's appearance. Towards the end of the pregnancy the woman may feel big, awkward and unattractive. Family and friends can reassure her and help her overcome these feelings.

### Role changes

As pregnancy advances it is normal for expectant parents to feel ambivalent about the forthcoming event. In particular, they may worry about their ability to be good parents. Parenting skills can be outlined in formal discussions, but these anxieties are best coped with by discussion and help as needed by individuals.

Another role change for the woman is the decision to be taken about her employment. For some women there may be no choice, due to lack of support at home or at work. She may have to stay at home with the baby. Selecting appropriate carers can also be a major source of anxiety for the mother who returns to work.

In the post natal period the parents might be unsure about their ability to identify and attend to the needs of the baby. The midwife may visit up to 28 days, should the parents need support. The health visitor also visits and plays a key part in supporting and establishing the family.

### Sexuality

Pregnancy does not alter a woman's sexual response and sexual activity is not harmful to the fetus. However, the couple may need to consider alternative, more comfortable positions and behaviours for their sexual needs.

Following delivery there is often a minor problem with sexuality for the couple. The mother may be tired because of her additional responsibilities and sore because of the delivery of the baby. Men have sometimes been afraid to resume sexual relationships because of the above factors. If more serious problems arise, psychosexual counselling may be needed. All couples should be advised about fertility control so that the babies they have are wanted and welcome.

## Activity Theory (Havighurst, 1963)

Successful ageing can be achieved by maintaining the values and activity patterns of middle age. Happiness in later life is achieved by denying the onset of old age and where the relationships, activities or roles of middle age are lost, it is important to replace them with new ones in order to maintain life satisfaction. This theory ignores the fact that age-related pathologies may impose limitations on activity and the option for people to take up replacement activities will, for example, depend on them having sufficient income.

## Continuity Theory (Neugarten et al, 1968)

This theory suggests that there is no marked change in the way people live their lives as they grow older but rather an increasing consistency in the way they behave. People who have been busy and active in earlier life will remain so, while those who always enjoyed a more relaxed approach are likely to continue in that fashion. On balance, this theory allows for more individuality and acknowledges the complexity of the ageing process.

## Physical Development

The young adult has achieved physical growth by the age of 20. An exception to this is the pregnant or lactating woman. Young adults are usually quite active, experience severe illnesses less commonly than older age groups, tend to ignore physical symptoms, and often postpone seeking health care. Physical characteristics of young adults begin to change as middle age approaches. Unless patients/clients have illnesses, assessment findings are generally within normal limits.

## Cognitive Development

Rational thinking habits increase steadily through the young and middle adult years. Formal and informal educational experiences, general life experiences, and occupational opportunities dramatically increase the individual's conceptual, problem-solving, and motor skills.

Identifying preferred occupational areas is a major task of young adults. When people know their educational preparation, skills, talents, and personality characteristics, occupational choices are easier, and they are generally more satisfied with their choices.

An understanding of how adults learn assists nurses in developing teaching plans for them. Adults enter the teaching-learning situation with a background of unique life experiences. Therefore, it is important to always view adults as individuals. Their compliance with regimens, such as medications, treatments, or lifestyle changes, involves decision-making processes. You should present as much information as they need to make decisions about the prescribed course of therapy.

As young adults are continually evolving and adjusting to changes in the home, workplace, and personal lives, their decision-making processes should be flexible. The more secure that young adults feel in their roles, the more flexible and open they are to change. Insecure persons tend to be more rigid in making decisions.

## Psychosocial Development

The emotional health of the young adult is related to the individual's ability to address and resolve personal and social tasks. Certain patterns or trends are relatively predictable. Between the ages of 23 to 28, the person refines self-perception and ability for intimacy. From 29 to 34 the person directs enormous energy toward achievement and mastery of the surrounding world. The years from 35 to 43 are a time of vigorous examination of life goals and relationships. Alterations are made in personal, social, and occupational lives. Often the stresses of this re-examination result in a 'midlife crisis' in which marital partner, lifestyle, and occupation may change.

During the young adult years, people generally give more attention to occupational and social pursuits. During this period, individuals attempt to improve their socioeconomic status. Upward mobility is possible through career choices. Career and personal counselling can help individuals identify career choices and set realistic goals.

Ethnic and gender factors have a sociological and psychological influence on an adult's life. An understanding of ethnicity, race, and gender differences enables the nurse to provide individualized care.

Support from the nurse, access to information, anticipatory guidance, and appropriate referrals provide opportunities for achievement of a patient's/client's potential. Since health is not

## Mental Health Nursing
### Psychosocial concerns in middle adulthood

Two common psychosocial health concerns of the middle adult are anxiety and depression.

*Anxiety:* adults often experience anxiety in response to the physiological and psychosocial changes of middle age. Such anxiety can motivate the adult to rethink life goals and can stimulate productivity. For some adults, however, this anxiety precipitates psychosomatic illness and preoccupation with death. In this case the middle adult views life as being half or more over and thinks in terms of the time left to live (Rawlins *et al*, 1993).

Clearly a life-threatening illness, marital transition, or job stress increases the anxiety of the client and family. The nurse may need to use crisis-intervention or stress-management techniques to help the patient/client adapt to the changes of the middle adult years.

*Depression:* depression is common among adults in the middle years and may have many causes. The risk factors for depression are listed in Table 6-3. Menopause is no longer believed to be the only cause of depression. Depression that occurs during the middle years, often referred to as agitated depression, is characterized by moderate-to-high anxiety, bizarre physical complaints, and paranoid ideation (formation of a mental concept or image). Depression may be worsened by the abuse of alcohol or other substances. The nurse may need to refer a severely depressed patient/client for specialized psychotherapy.

merely the absence of disease but involves wellness in all human dimensions, the holistic, humanistic nurse acknowledges the importance of the young adult's psychosocial needs as well as needs in other dimensions.

The young adult must make decisions concerning career, marriage, and parenthood. Although each person makes these decisions based on individual factors, the nurse should understand the general principles involved in these aspects of psychosocial development to assess the young adult's psychosocial status.

## Career

Many adults devote a major portion of their energy and interest to their chosen career. Therefore, a successful **vocational adjustment** is important in the lives of most men and women. Successful employment not only ensures economic security but also leads to friendships, social activities, support, and respect from co-workers.

Two-career marriages are increasing. The two-career marriage has benefits and liabilities. In addition to increasing the family's financial base, the person who works outside the home is able to expand friendships, activities, and interests. However, stresses may occur in a two-career family. These stressors result from a job transfer to a new location; increased expenditures of physical, mental, or emotional energy; child care demands; or household needs.

## TABLE 6-3 Risk Factors for Depression in the Middle Years

| Risk Factor | Characteristics |
| --- | --- |
| Sex | Female |
| Age | Women: declines after early 50s |
| | Men: increases after late 50s |
| Social isolation | Absence of intimate, confiding relationships after change in the nature of relationship with parents, children, and spouse |
| Losses | Parental deprivation or loss of mother before age 14 |
| | Other losses during midlife such as job loss, career difficulties, marital problems, and physical changes |
| | Departure of last child from home |
| Family history | History of depression in family or origin |

From, Rawlins RP, Williams SR, Beck CM: *Mental health – psychiatric nursing: a holistic life-cycle approach*, ed 3, St Louis, 1993, Mosby.

## Marriage

Young adults go through a period of being single before getting married, or forming long-term relationship. Social pressure to get married is not as great as it once was. Today, it is socially acceptable for a young adult to leave home and live in an apartment or to own a home without first marrying.

Another cause for the increased single population is the expanding career opportunities for women. Women enter the job market with greater career potential and have greater opportunities for financial independence. It is also becoming more socially acceptable for single individuals to live together outside of marriage. Similarly, it has become more socially acceptable for married couples to separate or divorce if they find their marital situation unsatisfactory.

Every couple's relationship is unique and no rules guarantee a successful marriage. When establishing a household and family, the married couple must begin to work as a team. They have the following tasks:

- establishing an intimate relationship
- deciding on and working toward mutual goals
- establishing guidelines for power and decision-making issues
- setting standards for extrafamily interactions
- finding companionship with other people for a social life
- choosing morals, values, and ideologies acceptable to both.

These major tasks require considerable maturity and self-esteem. When accomplished, however, they provide the foundation for a stable relationship. Growth in marriage extends over many years. Success in solving the formidable problems that occur in any marriage offers marital partners insight into each other.

A marital relationship generally passes through three developmental stages. The establishment stage begins at cohabitation and continues as the couple attempts to function as a dyad (pair). They learn patterns of sexual expression and ways to live intimately with each other. They must learn styles of conflict resolution, decision making, and role patterns. In addition, each partner may experience a sense of loss of individuality and self in the transition from *me* to *we*.

## Sexuality

The psychodynamic aspect of sexual activity is as important as the type or frequency of sexual intercourse to young adults. Young adults usually have emotional maturity to complement the physical ability and are therefore able to develop *mature sexual relationships*. Masters and Johnson (1970) have contributed important information about the physiological characteristics of the adult sexual response.

Sex is considered by Maslow (1970) to be a basic physiological need that generally takes priority over higher-level needs. Sexual needs, and the manner in which they are met, are influenced by age, sociocultural background, ethics, values, self-esteem, and level of wellness. The concept of sexuality encompasses more than sex as a need, and includes consideration of aspects of the individual, such as appearance, relationships and gender-based roles (Roper, 1983). Psychological beliefs and expectations give feelings of pleasure and satisfaction to adults. To maintain total wellness, adults should be encouraged to explore various aspects of their sexuality and be aware that their sexual needs and concerns evolve. Today, young adults are at risk for sexually transmitted diseases; as a result, they need education regarding the mode of transmission, prevention, and symptom recognition and management.

## Specific Health Concerns

Young adults are generally active and have no major health problems. However, their lifestyles may put them at risk for illnesses or disabilities during their middle or older adult years. In addition, infertility is a problem for many young adults.

## Risk Factors

Risk factors for the young adult's health originate in the community, lifestyle, and family history. These risk factors fall into the following categories:

- **Violent death and injury** — violence is the greatest cause of mortality and morbidity in the young adult population. Death and injury can occur from physical assaults, motor vehicle or other accidents, and suicide attempts.

- **Substance abuse** — substance abuse directly or indirectly contributes to mortality and morbidity in young adults. Intoxicated young adults may be severely injured in motor-vehicle accidents that may result in death or permanent disability to other young adults, as well.

Dependence on stimulant or depressant drugs can result in death. Overdose of a stimulant drug ('upper') can stress the cardiovascular and nervous systems to the extent that death occurs. The use of depressants ('downers') can lead to an accidental or intentional overdose and death.

It is a misconception that drug abuse occurs only among adolescents. Cocaine is increasingly used by young adults who have families and responsible jobs.

- **Unwanted pregnancies** — unplanned pregnancies, although more common among adolescents, can also have long-term physical and emotional effects if they occur in the young adult years. Unplanned pregnancies are a continual source of stress. Often young adults have educational and career goals that take precedence over family development. Interference with these goals can affect future relationships and later parent-child relationships.

- **Sexually transmitted diseases** — sexually transmitted diseases include syphilis, gonorrhoea, genital herpes, and acquired immunodeficiency syndrome (AIDS). These diseases may occur in sexually active persons. Recently, sexual activity with multiple partners has decreased. Many young adults are seeking to establish meaningful relationships before engaging in sexual activity.

Sexually transmitted diseases have immediate effects such as discharge, discomfort, and infection. They may also lead to chronic disorders, which can result from genital herpes; infertility, which can result from gonorrhoea; or even death, which results from AIDS.

- **Environmental or occupational factors** — a common environmental or occupational risk factor is exposure to airborne particles, which may cause lung diseases and cancer. Such lung diseases include silicosis from inhalation of talcum and silicon dust, pneumoconiosis from inhalation of coal dust, and emphysema from inhalation of smoke. Cancers resulting from occupational exposures may involve the lung, liver, brain, blood, or skin.

## Infertility

**Infertility** is the man's, woman's, or couple's inability to conceive. To most health care professionals, it is the inability to conceive after a year or more of regular sexual intercourse. An estimated 10 to 15% of all couples are infertile (Bobak and Jensen, 1991). However, about half of the couples evaluated and treated in infertility clinics become pregnant. In about 10 to 20% of couples the cause of infertility is unknown, and they remain infertile. In the remaining 30% the cause of the infertility is diagnosed, but they remain infertile because of endometriosis, blocked fallopian tubes, or decreased sperm motility.

## MIDDLE-AGED ADULT

### Physical Development

Major physiological changes occur between 40 and 65 years of age. The most visible changes are greying of the hair, wrinkling of the skin, and thickening of the waist. Balding commonly begins during the middle years, but it may also occur in young adults. Often these physiological changes have an impact on **self-concept** and **body image**. The most significant physiological changes during middle age are menopause in women and the climacteric in men.

### Menopause

Menstruation and ovulation occur in a cyclical rhythm from adolescence into middle adulthood. *Menopause* is the disruption of this cycle, primarily because of the inability of the neurohumoural system to maintain its periodic stimulation of the endocrine system. The ovaries no longer produce oestrogen and progesterone, and the blood levels of these hormones drop markedly. Menopause typically occurs between 45 and 60 years of age.

### Climacteric

The *climacteric*, or andropause, occurs in men in their late 40s or early 50s. It is caused by decreased levels of androgens. Throughout this period and thereafter, a man is still capable of producing fertile sperm and fathering a child. However, penile erection is less firm, ejaculation is less frequent, and the refractory period is longer.

### Cognitive Development

Changes in the cognitive function of middle-aged adults are rare except with illness or trauma. The middle-aged adult can learn new skills and information and some adults enter educational or vocational programmes to prepare themselves for entering the job market or changing jobs.

### Psychosocial Development

The psychosocial changes in the middle-aged adult may involve expected events, such as children moving away from home, or unexpected events, such as a marital separation or the death of a spouse. These changes may result in stress that can affect the adult's overall level of health.

### Career Transition

Career changes may occur by choice or as a result of changes in the workplace or society. In recent decades, middle-aged adults more often change occupations because they are bored with their present employment. In some cases, technological advances or other changes force middle-aged adults to seek new jobs. Such changes, particularly when unanticipated, may result in stress that can affect health, family relationships, self-concept, and other dimensions.

### Sexuality

The onset of menopause and the climacteric can affect the sexual health of the middle-aged adult. Menopause results in cessation of ovulation and the ability to conceive. A woman may desire more sexual activity because pregnancy is no longer possible. A man may notice changes in the strength of his erection and a decrease in his ability to experience repeated orgasm. Both may experience stresses related to sexual changes or a conflict between their sexual needs and self-perceptions and social attitudes or expectations.

### Family

Psychosocial factors involving the family may include marital changes, transition of the family as children leave home, and the care of ageing parents.

### MARITAL CHANGES

Marital changes that may occur during middle age include death of a spouse, separation, divorce, and the choice of remarrying or remaining single. A widowed, separated, or divorced patient/client goes through a period of grief and loss in which it is necessary to adapt to the change in marital status.

If a single middle-aged adult decides to marry, the stressors of marriage are similar to those for the young adult. In addition, the couple may have to cope with the social expectations and pressures related to marriage.

### FAMILY TRANSITIONS

The departure of the last child from the home may be a stressor. Many parents welcome freedom from child-rearing responsibilities, whereas others feel lonely or without direction because of this change. Eventually, parents must reassess their marriage and are able to resolve conflicts and plan for the future. Occasionally, this *readjustment phase* may lead to marital conflicts, separation, and divorce. Increasing numbers of women will find themselves having to look after elderly relatives (Leonard and Speakman, 1986).

### CARE OF AGEING PARENTS

Housing, employment, health, and economic realities have altered the traditional **social expectations** between generations in families. The middle-aged adult and the older adult parent may have conflicting priorities related to their relationship. Negotiations and compromises are useful in defining and resolving such problems. Nurses care for middle-aged and older adults in the community, long-term care facilities, and hospitals. The nurse can help identify the health needs of both groups and can assist the multigenerational family in determining the health and community resources available to them as they make decisions and plans.

### Specific Health Concerns

Physiological concerns include stress, level of wellness, and the formation of positive health habits.

Because middle-aged adults experience physiological changes and face certain health realities, their perceptions of health and health behaviours are often important factors in maintaining health. Today's complex world makes individuals more prone to stress-related illnesses such as heart attacks, hypertension, migraine headaches, ulcers, colitis, autoimmune disease,

backache, arthritis, and cancer.

When adults seek health care, the nurse's focus on the goal of wellness can guide patients/clients to evaluate health behaviours, lifestyle, and environment. Attention to risk factors that can be altered to improve the patient's/client's health can increase the quality of life and add years to it.

### Changing Health Habits

Health teaching and health counselling are often directed at improving **health habits**. The more fully the nurse understands the dynamics of behaviour and habits, the more likely interventions will help the patient/client to achieve or reinforce health-promoting behaviours.

To help patients/clients form positive health habits the nurse becomes a teacher and facilitator. By providing information about how the body functions and how habits are formed and changed, you raise the person's level of knowledge regarding the potential impact of behaviour on health, but you cannot change patients'/clients' habits. Patients/clients have control of and are responsible for their own behaviours. You can explain psychological principles of changing habits and offer information about health risks, and you can also offer positive reinforcement (such as praise and rewards) for health-directed behaviours and decisions. Such reinforcement increases the likelihood that the behaviour will be repeated. Ultimately, however, the patient/client decides which behaviours will become habits of daily living.

### Health Promotion

Community health programmes for young and middle-aged adults are designed to prevent illness, promote health, and detect disease in the early stages. Nurses can make valuable contributions to the community's health by taking an active part in the planning of screening and teaching programmes.

Family planning, birthing, and parenting skills are programme topics in which adults might be interested. Health screening for diabetes, hypertension, eye disease, and cancer is a good opportunity for the nurse to perform assessment and provide health teaching and health counselling.

Health education programmes can promote changes in behaviour and lifestyle. As a health teacher, you offer information that will enable the person to make decisions about health practices. During health counselling the nurse and patient/client design a plan of action that addresses the person's health and well-being. Through objective problem solving, you help the person grow and change.

Regardless of the age of its members and its structure, the family faces certain health tasks. The nurse as health teacher and counsellor understands the autonomy of the family and supports it while promoting family health.

## OLDER ADULT

In the UK, older adulthood is considered, chronologically, to occur after the age of retirement (previously 60 years for women, now 65 years, and 65 years for men). As life expectancy increases,

## THE SOCIAL LIFE CYCLE

FIRST AGE – the age of childhood and socialization.
SECOND AGE – the age of paid work and family raising.
THIRD AGE – the age of active, independent life beyond work and parenting.
FOURTH AGE – the age of eventual dependence.

Adapted from: The British Gas Report on Attitudes to Ageing (1991)

the part of the lifespan after retirement can potentially be 15 to 20 years or more. For many people, the concept of being 'old' is linked to ill health and disability. However, these tend to be relatively low in the retired population until the age of 75, after which the incidence of both acute and chronic illness increases (OPCS, 1988). Bernard (1990) suggests that the period of life following retirement is potentially one of the most stable periods of a person's life.

It is useful to view the lifespan in terms of social status constructs, rather than in chronological terms (see above). This acknowledges the diversity of individuals in later life and the different rates at which people age.

Increasingly, older adulthood is being recognized as a phase of life that brings new experiences and opportunities for development. This challenges the commonly held view of later life solely as a period of decline.

The increase in life expectancy and decrease in the birth rate have resulted in an increase in the number and proportion of older people in the total population. In 1990, the population of the UK was 57,411,000, which included 10,490,000 (18.27%) over pensionable age (OPCS, 1992).

Older adults, normally those older than 75, are the main users of health and social care services. Nurses are required to promote health, facilitate self-care and give care to dependent people in a variety of settings. It is important to be properly prepared for this role by knowing the biological, and psychosocial changes that occur in older adulthood, in order to meet individual needs prior to planning and giving care.

### Cognitive Development

Cognitive ability encompasses intelligence, learning, and memory, and enables individuals to cope with environmental change. A large study by Schaie (1989) that spanned several years and involved different cohorts of older people, demonstrated that cognitive function is subject to fluctuations throughout the lifespan, and is influenced by motivation, opportunities for development and confidence in one's abilities. Decrements in intellectual ability, as measured by intelligence tests, are due to changes in the central nervous system and these are more noticeable after age 75. Tasks relying on speed are affected most. As with many other areas of ageing, however, there is significant individual variation.

Memory is also subject to change. Although memory loss is not inevitable, it does affect an increasing number of people as they grow older. Recall in older people slows, because the speed of information processing decreases with age. A study by Holland and Rabbit (1991) suggests that the *quality* of daily social

## Myths, Stereotypes and Ageism

We live in an age-segregated society which often excludes extensive personal contact between people in different age groups. Many of us have grandparents and even great grandparents who may influence our view of what ageing is about. On the other hand, we may believe that their experience is atypical because it does not comply with some of the more common views of later life. These views are often acquired as a result of adopting stereotypical images of older people and their lives. These stereotypes are frequently used as a means of attempting to relate to our fellow beings (Featherstone and Hepworth, 1990). A stereotype is not necessarily a negative image (though it is more commonly so) when it is used to describe an older person. Stereotypical images of older people often focus on the unwelcome aspects of ageing, such as physical and mental decline, and negative personality traits, which are assumed to be characteristic of older people. Generally, these negative stereotypes are based on myths about ageing. It is therefore essential that all nurses involved in the care of older adults examine their own preconceptions about ageing and clarify their values surrounding their own ageing. **Nursing care based on false perceptions is unlikely to be effective and may even be detrimental to the older person.** Therefore, nurses need to distinguish between myth and reality, in order to identify accurately the older person's strengths and weaknesses.
Common beliefs about ageing are:

* ageing brings an end to productivity
* older people normally wish to disengage from society
* older people are rigid or inflexible in their thinking and are set in their ways
* 'senility' or mental impairment is an inevitable part of ageing
* ill-health is a normal part of ageing
* older people are unhappy because they are old
* older people are neglected by their family
* older people are asexual
* older people are unable to learn new things
* older people are isolated and lonely.

These notions, most of which are quite false, have led to the concept of **ageism** — discrimination against older people, simply because they are old. Butler (1969) suggests that ageism also reflects a fear of ageing by those who are still young, and serves as a means of distancing themselves from what is seen as inevitable decline.

Ageism is endemic in today's society and resides in everyone — including those who are themselves old (Scrutton, 1989). The result is that both the old and their professional carers often accept, without question, the socially constructed view of old age, not because it is a reality, but because our social beliefs are powerful enough to become self-fulfilling.

Nurses are part of this same society and will carry their values, attitudes and beliefs about older people into the workplace. As a profession, nurses must to be ever mindful of the way in which they contribute to the myths and stereotypes of older people.

### Disengagement Theory (Cumming and Henry, 1961)

This was the first major psychosocial theory that challenged the view of ageing as inevitable physical and psychological decline. The authors regarded *disengagement* as a universal and inevitable process: society withdraws from the older person because of the need to fit younger people into the positions once occupied by older people, who are no longer as useful and dependable as they were. Older people themselves choose to retreat because of an awareness of their diminishing capacities and short time left before death. The whole process results in the maintenance of equilibrium within society.

This theory caused much controversy and its critics suggested that it embodies the notion that older people have little to offer. However, Townsend (1981) has suggested that the structured dependency created by government policy makers gives the theory some currency; for example, as a result of fixed retirement ages.

experience significantly affects the older person's memory; those who are cognitively unimpaired and living in their own homes are more likely to use memory in decision making for everyday living, and this helps keep the process in good order. Cohen and Faulkner (1984) suggest that most areas of memory hold up well in old age and that deficits are minimal. Decrements are more marked for telephone numbers, postcodes, names of acquaintances and information that is learned by rote.

Social gerontologists have attempted to explain the general processes of psychosocial adjustment related to ageing (see box).

## Cognitive Impairment

Mental health problems affect a comparatively small number of older adults, despite the fact that some people believe that mental impairment is inevitable. It is important to distinguish between permanent and temporary impairment and to be clear about the correct use of the term confusion. Sometimes, for example, confusion and dementia are used interchangeably; this is incorrect. Confusion is not a diagnosis, but a symptom. Older people presenting with cognitive impairment should receive a full assessment, so that an accurate diagnosis and appropriate treatment and care are given. It is essential to differentiate between an episode of delirium (an acute confusional state), dementia (reversible and irreversible) and depression.

## Dementia

Brooking (1986) defines dementia as 'a steadily progressive and usually irreversible decline in previously normal mental function which is associated with detectable brain pathology'. It impairs memory, skills, control of emotions and social behaviour, and the ability to solve day-to-day problems. It is estimated to affect 7% of the population over 65 and 20% over 80 (Copeland, 1990). Alzheimer's disease is the most common form of dementia and accounts for 50% of cases. Multi-infarct dementia accounts for 20% and a combination of both conditions affects another 20%. With careful and supportive nursing management, patients/clients with chronic brain disorders can be helped to maintain function.

## Delirium

Brooking (1986) describes delirium as 'an acute or subacute alteration in previously normal mental function which is often temporary and reversible, associated with impaired brain function, usually secondary to a pathological process outside the nervous system'. The person becomes disconnected from his or her immediate surroundings and misinterprets reality. The condition is made worse by increased anxiety. Older people are particularly susceptible to the development of delirium, due to age-related changes in organ function. The main causes are stroke, infection and metabolic disorders. Lipowski (1983) suggests that between one-third and one-half of hospitalized older adults are likely to be delirious at some point during their admission. Delirium is likely to become more common, due to the rising numbers of very old people. Timely recognition falls within the remit of nursing assessment and subsequent skilful nursing interventions can reduce emotional stress for both the patient/client and relatives. Manipulation of the environment, attention to communication and ensuring continuity are the key areas for focusing nursing care. After reversible confusion is resolved, nurses should provide an opportunity to discuss the experience and its meaning to the patient/client and family.

## Depression

The prevalence of depression in people aged over 65 is 10-15% (Gurland *et al*, 1980). It can often be missed, particularly if it is believed to be inevitable. Depression may also be less obvious because of altered presentation. For example, mental slowing, lack of interest and memory problems may be attributed to ageing, both by the older person and by health professionals. Nurses can provide support by facilitating therapeutic communication, mobilizing family and social support, and encouraging medical staff to prescribe antidepressants. Given the chance, older people are thought to respond to treatment as well as any other age group (Allen and Baldwin, 1994).

## Therapeutic Approaches to Cognitive Impairment
### REALITY ORIENTATION

This involves sensitive and simple repetition of essential information to reinforce time, place and person and manipulation of the environment to provide supportive orientation cues. Access to calendars, clocks, television and newspapers, was found to minimize confusion in post-operative orthopaedic patients (Williams *et al*, 1985).

### VALIDATION THERAPY

**Validation therapy** is a technique used with severely confused and disoriented older adults. The goal is to provide a sense of dignity and self-worth and validate patients'/clients' feelings. Clients are not confronted with their inappropriate behaviours. Rather, the nurse attempts to meet older adults in their reality and find the meaning behind the behaviours. Confused older adults gain a positive sense of self because the nurse validates feelings.

## TASKS FOR LATER MATURITY

- to adjust to decreasing physical strength
- to adjust to retirement and decreased income
- to adjust to the death of one's spouse
- to establish links and friendships with one's age group
- to adopt and adapt to social roles in a flexible way
- to establish satisfactory living arrangements.

Adapted from Havighurst RJ: Successful ageing. In William RH *et al*, editors: *Process of ageing*, vol 1, New York, 1963, Atherton.

## Psychosocial Development

A developmental approach to the human lifecourse assumes that psychological growth can occur at any point on the life continuum. Prior to Erikson's (1963) theory of **lifespan development**, later life was viewed in terms of decline rather than growth. Erikson's final task for older adulthood was 'integrity' versus 'despair'; that is, to accept life as it has been lived and to be able to look back on it with satisfaction. The alternative to this is to hold feelings of disgust and bitterness at one's failures, but yet to realize that it is too late to make amends. This theory is useful in helping nurses to understand the behaviour, priorities and aspirations of older adults.

Havighurst (1963) describes developmental tasks that are specific to life transitions (see above).

The majority of older people are retired from full-time paid work. It is important to acknowledge, however, that retirement is a twentieth century phenomenon and as such can be viewed as a social construction of industrialized societies. Prior to the mid-nineteenth century, it was usual for people to work until they were physically incapable to do so. Retired people who are in good health are still able to contribute to society in a variety of ways, such as by caring for children and dependent relatives, supporting friends and neighbours, and volunteering for public service and charitable organizations. Those who are financially secure are able to contribute to the economy by purchasing goods and services.

Pre-retirement planning is critical, because retirement can last for up to 30 years. This should include sources of retirement income, place of residence, use of time, and activities for health maintenance. Although the financial position of retired people is slowly improving due to occupational pensions and increased home ownership, in 1991 54% of retired people still relied upon state benefits for 75% of their income (Tinker, 1992).

Most older adults are faced with the deaths of spouses, friends, siblings, and sometimes children, as well as their own mortality. Nurses play a valuable role in supporting them throughout the grieving process (see Chapter 11).

The many role changes and events characteristic of later life are frequently viewed in terms of loss. For example, loss of role and income as a result of retirement; the loss of a spouse and siblings; or the loss of one's home and a move to institutional care. However, this picture is unduly negative. Older people have had lifelong experience in adapting to change, and are likely to have a repertoire of successful coping methods. Nevertheless, the effects of such changes should not be underestimated, and older people may need help and support from nurses to adjust to their changed circumstances, even if they view the transition as a gain rather than a loss.

Some older people may experience multiple losses, which may undermine their confidence and self-esteem. Nurses working with these people must recognize these circumstances, and help rebuild the person's self-confidence by identifying and building on the person's strengths and abilities. Finally, it is important that nurses do not impose their own judgements on what might appear to be unwelcome life changes. For example, the death of a spouse might be a relief and release from an unsatisfying marriage; the move to a nursing home may bring a welcome sense of security and opportunities for companionship. Each event should be judged in accordance with its meaning for the individual involved.

## Housing and Environment

Housing and environment have a major impact on the health of older adults. It is widely acknowledged that the majority of older adults wish to remain in their own homes (Wenger, 1987). However, increasing disability or frailty, which is sometimes combined with pressure from relatives, may result in a move to a relative's home, a smaller dwelling, sheltered housing or to a residential or nursing home. Choice of relocation is largely governed by the person's level of disability. A change in living arrangements may require an extended period of adjustment, during which support from nurses can be invaluable. The environment can support or hinder physical and social functioning, enhance or drain energy, and complement or tax existing physical changes such as hearing or vision. Whenever possible the environment should be modified to increase independence and functional ability, and thus the quality of life. Simple measures such as colour coding, increased illumination and appropriate furniture can facilitate independence (see Chapter 19).

## Body-Image Interventions

The way older adults present themselves has a significant impact on body image and self-confidence. Some physical characteristics of older adulthood are socially desirable, such as distinguished-looking grey hair. Other features are also impressive, such as a lined face that displays character, or wrinkled hands that convey a lifetime of hard work. Too often, however, society sees older people as incapacitated, deaf, obese, or shrunken in stature. When older adults have acute or chronic illnesses, the related physical dependence makes it difficult for them to maintain body image. A nurse with stereotypes about the appearance of older adults may give little attention to grooming or hygiene. Consequences of illness and ageing that threaten the older adult's body image include invasive diagnostic procedures, pain, surgery, prosthesis, loss of sensation in a body part, skin changes, dependence on life-sustaining medication, denture odour, loss of scalp hair, and incontinence.

The older adult does not choose to have an objectionable appearance. Nurses have a direct influence on the patient's/client's appearance. The importance to the older adult of presenting a socially acceptable image must be considered. It

## TABLE 6-4 Normal Physical Changes of Ageing

| System | Normal Findings |
| --- | --- |
| **Integument** | |
| Skin colour | Spotty pigmentation in areas exposed to the sun; pallor even in absence of anaemia |
| Moisture | Dry, scaly condition |
| Temperature | Cooler extremities; decreased perspiration |
| Texture | Decreased elasticity; wrinkles; folding, sagging condition |
| **Fat distribution** | Decreased amount on extremities; increased amount on abdomen |
| **Hair** | Thinning and greying on scalp; often decreased facial hair in men; possible chin and upper lip hair in women |
| **Nails** | Decreased growth rate |
| **Head and neck** | |
| Head | Sharp and angular nasal and facial bones; loss of eyebrow hair in women; bushier eyebrows in men |
| Eyes | Decreased visual acuity; decreased accommodation; reduced adaptation to darkness; sensitivity to glare |
| Ears | Decreased pitch discrimination; diminished light reflex; diminished hearing acuity |
| Nose and sinuses | Increased nasal hair; decreased sense of smell |
| Mouth and pharynx | Use of bridges or dentures; decreased sense of taste; atrophy of papillae of lateral edges of tongue |
| Neck | Nodular thyroid gland; slight tracheal deviation resulting from muscle atrophy |
| **Thorax and lungs** | Increased anteroposterior diameter; increased chest rigidity; increased respiratory rate with decreased lung expansion; increased airway resistance |
| **Heart and vascular system** | Significant increase in systolic pressure with slight increase in diastolic pressure; usually insignificant changes in heart rate at rest; common diastolic murmurs; easily palpated peripheral pulses; weaker pedal pulses and colder lower extremities, especially at night |
| **Breasts** | Diminished breast tissue; pendulous, flabby condition |
| **Gastrointestinal system** | Decreased salivary secretions, which may make swallowing more difficult; decreased peristalsis; decreased production of digestive enzymes, including hydrochloric acid, pepsin, and pancreatic enzymes; constipation; reduced motility |
| **Reproductive system** | |
| Female | Decreased oestrogen; decreased uterine size; decreased secretions; atrophy of epithelial lining of vagina |
| Male | Decreased levels of testosterone; decreased sperm count; decreased testicular size |
| **Urinary system** | Decreased renal filtration and renal efficiency; subsequent loss of protein from kidney; nocturia; decreased bladder capacity; increased incontinence |
| Female | Urgency and stress incontinence resulting from decrease in perineal muscle tone |
| Male | Urinary frequency and retention resulting from prostatic enlargement |
| **Musculoskeletal system** | Decreased muscle mass and strength; bone demineralization (more pronounced in women); shortening of trunk as result of intervertebral space narrowing; decreased joint mobility; decreased range of motion; enhanced bony prominences |
| **Neurological system** | Decreased rate of voluntary or automatic reflexes; decreased ability to respond to multiple stimuli; insomnia; shorter sleeping periods |

Modified from Ebersole P and Hess P: *Toward healthy aging: human needs and nursing response*, ed 4, St Louis, 1994, Mosby.

takes little effort to assist the patient/client with combing hair, cleaning dentures, shaving, or changing clothing. Nurses should also be sensitive to odours in the environment. Odours created by urine and some illnesses may be present. By controlling odours, the nurse may prevent visitors from shortening their stay or not coming at all.

### Sexuality

Sexuality is increasingly recognized as important in the care of older adults. All older adults, whether healthy or frail, need to express sexual feelings. Sexuality involves love, warmth, sharing, and touching, not just the act of intercourse. Sexuality is linked with identity and validates the belief that people can give to others and be appreciated by them.

Ensure that care is directed at helping the patient/client maintain sexual health. This requires integration of physical, emotional, intellectual, and social aspects of the sexual being. Success will enhance personality, communication, and love (Woods, 1983). To help the older adult achieve or maintain sexual health, it is important to understand the physical changes in sexual response.

As discussed earlier, the libido does not decrease, although frequency of sexual activity may decline. An older woman who does not understand physical changes affecting sexual activity may be concerned that her sex life is nearly over with the onset of menopause. The older man may feel the same when he discovers a change in the firmness of his erection, has a decreased need for ejaculation with each orgasm, or has a longer recovery period between episodes of intercourse.

In addition to physical changes affecting sexual functioning, many older adults take drugs that depress sexual activity, such as antihypertensives, antidepressants, sedatives, or hypnotics. In addition, some drugs, such as tranquillizers and antidepressants, increase libido in older adults.

## Maintaining Psychosocial Health

The following interventions and considerations can be useful in facilitating the psychosocial health of older adults.

### Therapeutic Communication

With therapeutic communication the nurse perceives and respects the patient's/client's uniqueness. The nurse who communicates effectively will be accepted as one who shares a genuine concern for the patient's/client's welfare.

The nurse cannot simply enter a patient's/client's environment and immediately establish a therapeutic relationship. The nurse must first be knowledgeable and skilled in communication techniques. The nursing student can practise these techniques with other students (see Chapter 15).

### Touch

Touch is the first sense to become functional. It provides knowledge about others throughout life. In all cultures, gentle touch conveys affection and friendliness. Often, older adults who are victims of social isolation are deprived of the touching that was an important part of earlier life.

Touch is a therapeutic tool nurses can use to help comfort older adults. It can provide sensory stimulation, reduce anxiety, orient the person to reality, relieve physiological and emotional pain, and give comfort during the dying process (Barnett, 1972).

An older adult who is isolated, dependent, or ill; who fears death; or who lacks self-esteem has a greater need for touch. The patient/client may invite touch by reaching for a nurse's hand. Often, older men are wrongly accused of sexual advances when they demonstrate this need. It is important to recognize that the patient/client may be suffering from touch deprivation. However, it is important not to use touch in a condescending way, such as a pat on the head or a gentle squeeze. Touch should convey respect

and sensitivity and the nurse should not be surprised if the patient/client reciprocates because of an unmet need for intimacy.

## A Biographical Approach to Nursing Assessment

A biographical approach to nursing assessment involves taking a patient's/client's life history as part of the assessment process and using the salient aspects of the story to interpret his or her current needs. Nursing assessment is usually concerned with determining aspects of the patient's/client's present lifestyle and circumstances. This is often solely confined to the activities of living. Consequently, assessments are usually concerned with the identification of problems rather than strengths. This may lead care givers to focus on that which is pathological and decremental, often to the exclusion of the individual's remaining strengths and abilities. Johnson (1976) points out that older people themselves may view their present situation in a different light to that of the professional; if placed in the context of a life history, the reasons for this may become apparent.

A life history, however, is not told quickly and time constraints in acute care settings prevent the collection of biographical details from every person. A complete depth of understanding is not always required but when a serious situation arises which may lead to a radical change in lifestyle, biographical knowledge can be utilized. It is important to recognize when biographical details might help clarify present concerns and help identify the true focus for care.

### Life Review

Butler (1963) described life review as the 'universal occurrence of an inner experience of reviewing one's life'. It happens as an important part of trying to make sense of one's life as it has been lived. Older people are sometimes accused of living in the past, particularly when they talk about significant life events from long ago. Before Butler's reassessment of reminiscence, it was thought to be an unwelcome sign of cognitive deterioration. However, it is now viewed in a more positive light and nurses can facilitate this discussion of past events. Butler believes that approaching death prompts the need to review a life. It is a backward-looking process which is set in motion by looking forward to death. It may lead to a deeper understanding of past events or provide an opportunity to come to terms with events which have previously not been well accepted. Butler also warns that, for a minority, the process of life review may result in a sense of failure to make reparation with the past and in turn this may lead to depression. If this is identified, medical referrals should be made so that the older person receives appropriate treatment.

### Reminiscence

Reminiscence, as a therapeutic approach to ageing, also has its roots in Butler's (1963) early writing. Older people are encouraged to reminisce about their past life either in one-to-one or group situations. Items of clothing, everyday objects, pictures, readings and even sounds and smells can be used to trigger past memories. The prime purpose of using reminiscence as a therapy is to maintain a person's identity with the premise that past roles and achievements combine to confirm an individual's identity. At a time when there might be few opportunities to take on new roles, particularly for older people in institutional care, reminiscing cannot only confer a sense of self esteem, but can also be an entertaining and pleasurable occupation. A study by Coleman (1986) however, indicates that not everyone wishes to participate in reminiscence. Some people find it too painful and others have other sources of self-esteem. Nurses should be mindful of this when attempting to get a group together.

## Physical Development

Physiological changes vary with each person. Table 6-4 describes general physiological changes anticipated in older adults. These physiological changes are not pathological processes; they occur in all people but at different rates and depend on life circumstances Any changes can alter the presentation of illness (for example the first sign of a chest infection may be delirium rather than a raised temperature). It is important to learn these age-related changes, in order to accurately assess health health and to provide appropriate information support and care.

## Chronic Health Concerns in Older Age

It is estimated that 66% of adults over 75 have a long-standing illness and that in 50% of adults the illness limits their lifestyle (DOH, 1992b). Common causes of chronic health problems in older age are arthritis, cardiovascular disease (hypertension, coronary heart disease and cerebrovascular accident – stroke), respiratory disease, cancer and sensory impairment (see Chapter 26). Nurses should be familiar with chronic health problems common in older adults and should acknowledge that the majority of older adults are interested in their health and wish to take charge of their lives.

## Sensory Impairments

Older adults usually experience changes in vision, hearing, taste and smell which are often the result of age related changes (see Chapter 26).

## Oral Health

Oral health in older adults is gradually improving, although 86% of people over 80 are edentulous. It is also likely to take more than 50 years before the total population retain some of their natural teeth for life (Todd and Lader, 1991). The presence of natural teeth or a well-fitting set of dentures can improve nutritional intake, help maintain clear speech and enhance physical appearance. Nurses can help prevent dental and gum disease through education about routine oral care.

## Nutrition

Older active adults require a daily energy requirement of 2000 kilocalories, though this decreases in response to illness, reduction in the basal metabolic rate and decreased exercise (see Chapter 21). It is important to ensure that the diet of older people is nutritionally adequate particularly if they are eating less food.

## Exercise

Older adults should be encouraged to maintain physical exercise and activity, as a means of delaying or even reversing physical decline. This can be achieved by carrying out some physical activity for 20-30 minutes at least two or three times each week. Examples of suitable exercise would be brisk walking, golf, gardening, bowls, ballroom dancing and swimming. Also, people who smoke should be encouraged to give up (Carnegie Trust, 1992). It is important, however, that people who have not exercised for some time have a medical check before they begin, in order to be able to match the exercise programme to their level of fitness.

## Drug Effects

Older adults are the major consumers of prescribed and over-the-counter medications. See Chapter 31 for details on altered drug handling and how nursing interventions can reduce drug interactions, unwanted side effects and increase compliance.

## THE FAMILY
## Current Trends

The **family** is an important **institution** in society. Hareven (1982) suggests that there is no such thing as the family, only families and that any family will go through a series of different 'types' over time.

Families are made up of individuals and all individuals go through life cycles. Infants become boys and girls who become adolescents and, subsequently, men and women. The end of that life cycle is death.

Today, couples tend to have one or two children soon after marriage. Less time is spent bearing children but more time is spent in rearing them. In addition, women are more likely to have long periods of caring for elderly relatives. The increased separation of home from work creates many problems for men and women with young children. The number of single parent families has also risen, resulting from either a conscious choice not to marry or the breakdown of a marriage.

The health status of family members influences family functioning and family functioning in turn influences its own and society's perception of health both physical and psychological. The health of the family is influenced by its relative position in society (i.e. its social class, economic resources, and ethnic and racial background). Inequalities in society affect the family and its members (Townsend and Davidson, 1980).

Families have been compared to a homeostatic system (Bowen, 1972) where a change in the functioning of one family member results in compensatory changes in the functioning of other members. Even though the family is but one of many emotional systems in which the individual is involved, it is probably the most intense and influential. Our notions of relationships with people arise in our early relationships with our families. To a greater or lesser extent our individual physical, cognitive, and emotional development is inextricably tied up in our early family experiences.

Families are sometimes described as 'functional' or

'dysfunctional'. A well-functioning family is a flexible organization which can shift roles, levels of responsibility, and patterns of interaction as it goes through life cycles. Dysfunctional families lack these characteristics.

The nurse will have his or her own experiences of family life and these will shape his or her attitude towards patients/clients and the many types of family life he or she will encounter. Social policies governing health and social services will have an impact on families and individuals (DOH, 1989). If the nurse is to practise holistic care, he or she must be aware of individual and family development within the context of an ever evolving society.

## SUMMARY

It is helpful for the nurse to understand each of the developmental phases in the lifespan and how the physiological, cognitive and psychosocial dimensions of these interact to influence health. An awareness of the relationship between these dimensions and the health of patients/clients will facilitate an holistic approach to their care pertinent to their age or developmental stage. This knowledge can also be applied in the advocation of suitable health-promotion activities, enabling nurses to provide more personalised care and to work with patients/clients in helping them to anticipate and adjust to the changes which they experience. An understanding of each developmental phase enables nurses to identify areas of particular concern for patients/clients, and to be aware of interpersonal/familial factors in planning nursing care. Nurses, midwives and health visitors have key roles within the health team, caring for individuals through all transitions, from birth to old age.

## CHAPTER 6 REVIEW
### Key Concepts
- People progress through similar chronological stages of growth and development but at an individual pace and with individual behaviours.
- A developmental perspective helps the nurse understand commonalities and variations in each stage and the impact that they have on the patient's/client's health.
- Growth and development are influenced by the inner forces of heredity and temperament and the outer forces of family, peers, life experiences, and environmental elements.
- Physiological, cognitive, and psychosocial development continues throughout the neonate, infant, toddler, and preschool periods, and the nurse must be familiar with normal parameters to determine potential problems and promote normal development.
- The nurse recognizes that the child's perception of health and health behaviours begins early and assists the parent and child in establishing healthy patterns that will continue for the entire life span.
- The developmental theories of Freud, Erikson, Piaget, and Kohlberg help explain the individual aspects of development for each patient/client.

- The major psychosocial developmental task of the school-aged child is the development of a sense of industry, which is gained through personal achievements and results in positive self-esteem.
- Physical growth during the school years is slow and steady until the skeletal growth spurt just before puberty.
- Changes in growth pattern may indicate the onset of disease.
- The adolescent is able to solve complex mental problems, use deductive reasoning, and hypothesize about the future.
- Adolescents begin the long process of emancipation from their parents and need parental support to accomplish this.
- Adult development involves orderly and sequential changes in characteristics and attitudes that adults experience over time.
- Many changes experienced by the young adult are related to the natural process of maturation and socialization. Maturity is reached when the young adult attains a balance of growth in the physiological, psychosocial, and cognitive areas.
- Young adults are in a stable period of physical development, except for changes related to pregnancy.
- Emotional health of young adults is correlated with the ability to address and resolve personal and social problems.
- Midlife transition begins when a person becomes aware that physiological and psychosocial changes signify passage to another stage in life.
- Two significant physiological changes of the middle years are menopause in women and the climacteric in men.
- Cognitive changes are rare in middle age except in cases of illness or physical trauma.
- Psychosocial changes for middle aged adults may be related to career transition, sexuality, marital changes, family transition, and care of the ageing parent.
- Health concerns of middle aged adults commonly involve stress-related illnesses, health assessment, and adoption of positive health habits.
- Myths and stereotypes portray older adults as ill, rigid in thinking, institutionalized, poor, unable to learn, and without sexual needs.
- A nurse's attitudes toward older adults affects the quality and level of care.
- The psychosocial theories of ageing, which include the disengagement, activity, and continuity theories, attempt to describe the effects of lifestyle, personality, and environmental factors on longevity.
- Psychosocial changes affecting the older adult include retirement, sexuality, the deaths of one's spouse and peers, and changes in living arrangements.
- The older adult and family require nursing interventions to help them cope with the dying process.

## CRITICAL THINKING EXERCISES
1. Between the ages of 7 and 11, children develop concrete operations, according to Piaget. How might the nurse assess the progress that a particular child is making towards this development?
2. In what ways might decisions about transferring care back to informal carers in the community place families under stress?

3. Outline some of the challenges facing an elderly Asian couple growing old in the UK where they witness differences in their ideas of growing old and those of their children and grandchildren who have grown up in the UK.

4. What kinds of health advice might benefit two young adults with learning difficulties who wish to get married, settle in their own home and eventually start their own family?

5. What sorts of mental health concerns are likely to arise for a middle-aged business executive and his family when he is made redundant and continues to remain unemployed for the foreseeable future?

6. Mrs Jones, an 80-year-old woman, visits her GP practice and is seen by the practice nurse. She is taking eight different medications, prescibed by two consultant doctors. She tells the nurse that she is not feeling well. What advice should the nurse give and what action should the nurse take?

## Key Terms

Ageism, p. 141
Attachment, p. 127
Autonomy, p. 129
Cognitive development, p. 121
Developmental phase, p. 120
Family institution, p. 146
Group identity, p. 134
Health habits, p. 140
Lifespan development, p. 143
Maturation, p. 120
Milestones (developmental), p. 127
Moral development, p. 129
Motor skills, p. 129
Peer influence, p. 132
Physical growth, p. 120
Psychosocial development, p. 121
Self concept/body image, p. 139
Self-perceptions, p. 128
Sexual identity, p. 134
Social expectations, p. 140
Vocational adjustment, p. 137

## REFERENCES

Allen H, Baldwin R: What do you do when she's depressed? *Care of the Elderly* 6(3):98, 1994.

Barnett K: A survey of the current utilization of touch by health team personnel with hospitalized patients, *Int J Nurs Stud* 9:195, 1972.

Bell D *et al*: Illness associated with child day care: a study of incidence and cost, *Am J Public Health* 79(4):479, 1989.

Benner P, Wrubel J: *The privacy of caring: stress and coping in health and illness*, Menlo Park, Calif, 1989, Addison-Wesley.

Bernard M: Changing the image of retirement, *Nursing the Elderly* Nov/Dec , 1990.

Bobak IM, Jensen MD: *Essentials of maternity nursing*, St Louis, 1991, Mosby.

Bowen M: Towards differentiation of oneself in one's own family. In Framo JL, editor: *Family interactions*, New York, 1972, Springer.

Brooking JI: Dementia and confusion in the elderly. In: Redfern SJ, editor: *Nursing elderly people*, Edinburgh, 1986, Churchill Livingstone.

Butler RN: The life review: an interpretation of reminiscence in the aged, *Psychiatry* 26:65, 1963.

Butler RN: Ageism: another form of bigotry, *Gerontol* 9:234, 1969.

Carnegie Trust: *Health: abilities and wellbeing in the third age*, Folkestone, Kent, 1992, Bailey Management Services.

Cohen G, Faulkner F: Memory in old age: good in parts, *New Scientist* Oct. 11, 1984.

Coleman PG: Adjustment in later life. In Bond J, Coleman P, editors: *Ageing in society*, London, 1990, Sage Publications.

Copeland JRM: Epidemiological aspects of the mental disorders of old age. In Bergener *et al*, editors: *Challenges in ageing*, London, 1990, Academic Press.

Cumming E, Henry WE: *Growing old: the process of disengagement*, New York, 1961, Basic Books.

d'Ardenne P, Mahthani A: *Transcultural counselling in action*. London, 1990, Sage Publications.

Department of Health: *The health of elderly people*, London, 1992a, HMSO.

Department of Health: *The health of the nation*, London, 1992b, HMSO.

Diekelmann JL: The young adult: the choice is health or illness, *Am J Nurs* 76:1276, 1976.

Ebersole P, Hess P: T*oward healthy aging: human needs and nursing response*, ed 4, St Louis, 1994, Mosby.

Erikson EH: *Childhood and society*, ed 2, New York, 1963, Norton.

Erikson EH: *Identity: youth and crises*, New York, 1968, Norton.

Erikson EH: *The life cycle completed: a review*, New York, 1982, Norton.

Featherstone M, Hepworth M: Images of ageing. In Bond J, Coleman P, editors: *Ageing in society,* London, 1990, Sage Publications.

Freud S : *A general introduction into psychoanalysis*, New York, 1969, Pocket Books.

Gilligan C: *In a different voice*, Cambridge, Mass, 1982, Harvard University Press.

Gordon S: *Prisoners of men's dreams: striking out for a new feminine future*, Boston, 1991, Little, Brown & Co.

Gurland B et al: The epidemiology of depression and dementia in the elderly: the use of multiple indicators of these conditions. In Cole, JO, Barrett J, editors: *Psychopathology in the aged*, New York, 1980, Raven Press.

Hareven T: *Family time and industrial time*, New York, 1982, Cambridge University.

Havighurst RJ: Successful aging. In William RH et al, editors: *Process of aging*, vol 1, New York,1963, Atherton.

Holland CA, Rabbitt Patrick MA: Ageing memory: use versus impairment, *Br J Psychol* 82:29, 1991.

Johnson ML: That was your life: a biographical approach to later life. In Carver V, Liddiard P, editors: *An ageing population*, Buckingham, 1976, Open University Press.

Kohlberg L: Development of moral character and moral ideology. In Hoffman, ML and Hoffman LNW, editors: *Review of child development research*, vol 1, New York, 1964, Russell Sage Foundation.

Kohlberg L: Stages and sequence: the cognitive-development approach to socialization. In Goslin A, editor: *Handbook of socialization theory and research*, Chicago, 1969, Rond McNally.

Leonard D, Speakman MA: Women in the family: companion or caretakers. In Beechey V, Whitelegg E, editors: *Women in Britain today*, Milton Keynes, 1986, Oxford University Press.

Levinson D et al: *The seasons of a man's life*, New York, 1978, Knopf.

Lipowski ZJ: Transient cognitive disorders (delirium, acute confusional states) in the elderly, *Am J Psychiatr* 140(11), 1983.

Maslow AH: *Motivation and personality*, New York, 1970, Harper & Row.

Masters WH, Johnson VE: *Human sexual responses*, Boston, 1970, Little, Brown & Co.

Nelms BC, Mullins R: *Growth and development: a primary health care approach*, New Jersey, 1982, Prentice Hall.

Neugarten BL, Havighurst RJ, Tobin SE: Personality and patterns of ageing. In Neugarten BL, editor: *Middle age and aging,* Chicago, 1968, University of Chicago Press.

Office of Population Census and Surveys: *Population trends,* London, 1992, HMSO.

Papalia DE, Olds SW: *Human development,* ed 4, New York, 1989, McGraw-Hill.

Piaget J: Intellectual evolution from adolescence to adulthood, *Hum Devel* 15:1, 1972.

Piaget J: *The origins of intelligence in children,* New York, 1952, International Universities Press.

Rawlins RP, Williams SR, Beck CM: *Mental health and psychiatric nursing: a holistic life-cycle approach,* St Louis, 1988, Mosby.

Rivara FP: Motor vehicle injuries during adolescence, *Pediatr Ann* 17:107, 1988.

Schaie KW: The hazards of cognitive ageing, *Gerontol* 29(4), 1989.

Scrutton S: *Counselling older people,* London, 1989, Edward Arnold.

Squires A: Multicultural healthcare and rehabilitation of older people, London, 1991, Edward Arnold.

Tanner JM: Sequence of events in the somatic changes of puberty. In Grunbach MM et al, editors: *Control of the onset of puberty,* New York, 1974, John Wiley & Sons Ltd.

Tinker A: *Elderly people in modern society.* London, 1992, Longman Group Ltd.

Todd JE, Lader D: *Adult dental health,* London, 1991, HMSO.

Townsend P: The structured dependency of the elderly: a creation of social policy in the twentieth century, *Ageing & Society* 1:5, 1981.

Townsend P, Davidson N: *The Black Report,* Harmondsworth, 1980, 1982, 1992, Penguin Books.

Roper N, Tierney A, Logan W: *Using a model for nursing,* Edinburgh, 1983, Churchill Livingstone.

Wenger C: Support networks: change and stability, Bangor, 1987, The Centre for Social Policy Research and Development, University College of North Wales.

Williams MA *et al*: Reducing acute confusional states in elderly patients with hip fractures, *Res in Nurs and Health* 8:329, 1985.

Wong DL: *Nursing care of infants and children,* ed 5, St Louis, 1995, Mosby.

Woods NF: *Human sexuality in health and illness,* ed 3, St Louis, 1983, Mosby.

## FURTHER READING

### Adult Nursing

Bond J, Coleman P: *Ageing in society,* London, 1994, Sage.

British Medical Association: *All our tomorrows: growing old in Britain — report of the BMA's Board of Science & Education,* London, 1986, British Medical Association.

Cheal D: *Family and the state of theory,* London, 1991, Harvester Wheatsheaf.

Falkner E, Tanner M, editors: *Human growth: a comprehensive treatise,* ed 2, New York, 1986, Plenum.

Halsey AH: *Change in British society,* Oxford, 1986, Oxford University Press.

Hardey M, Crow G: *Lone parenthood: coping with constraints and making opportunities,* London, 1991, Harvester Wheatsheaf.

Meade K: *Challenging the myths: a review of pensioners' health,* London, 1986, Pensioner Link.

Pascall G: *Social policy: a feminist analysis,* London, 1986, Tavistock.

Redfern S, editor: *Nursing elderly people,* Edinburgh, 1991, Churchill Livingstone.

### Children's Nursing

Axline V: *Dibs, in search of self,* Harmondsworth, 1964, Pelican.

Ball JA: Mothers need nurturing too, *Nurs Times* 84(17):29, 1988.

Bowlby J: *Attachment and loss II: separation, anxiety and anger,* London, 1969, Hogarth Press.

Bowlby J: *The making and breaking of affectional bonds,* London, 1979, Tavistock.

Bowlby J: *Attachment and loss: loss, sadness and depression,* London, 1980, Hogarth Press.

Haley J : *Leaving home,* New York, 1980, McGraw Hill.

Hayes CD, editor: *Risking the future: adolescent sexuality, pregnancy, and childbearing,* vol 1, Washington, DC, 1987, National Academy Press.

Kitzinger S: *The crying baby,* London, 1990, Penguin.

Lee E et al: Stressful life events and accidents at school, *Pediatr Nurs* 15(2):140, 1989.

Rew L: The relationship between self-care behaviors and selected psychosocial variables in children with asthma, *J Pediatr Nurs* 2(5):333, 1987.

Riesch, SK, Forsyth, DM: Preparing to parent the adolescent: a theoretical overview, *J Child Adolescent Psychiatr Mental Health Nurs* 5(1):32, 1992.

Winnicott DW: *Babies and their mothers,* London, 1988, Free Association Books.

### Learning Disabilities Nursing

Beresford B: *Positively parents: caring for a severely disabled child,* London, 1994, HMSO.

Hogg J: *Profound retardation and multiple impairment vol 3: Development and learning,* Beckenham, 1986, Croom Helm.

Levitt S: *Basic abilities: a whole approach. A developmental guide for children with disabilities,* London, 1994, Souvenir Press.

Tizard B ed: *Vulnerabilitiy and resilience in human development: a festschrift for Ann and Alan Clarke,* London, 1992, Jessica Kingsley.

### Mental Health Nursing

De'Ath E: Families and their differing needs. In Street E, Dryden W: *Family therapy in Great Britain,* Milton Keynes, 1988, Oxford University Press.

Gearing B, Johnson M, Heller T, editors: *Mental health problems in old age,* Milton Keynes, 1989, Oxford University Press.

Gilbert LA: Female development and achievement, *Issues Mental Health Nurs* 5(1/4):5, 1983.

Golan N: *Passing through transitions,* London, 1981, Collier MacMillan.

Herzog D, Newman KL, Yeh C et al: Body image satisfaction in homosexual and heterosexual women, *Int J Eating Dis* 2(4):391, 1992.

Holder D: Boys will be boys, *Independent on Sunday,* 16 May, 1992.

Stafford-Clarke D: *What Freud really said,* Harmondsworth, 1983, Penguin.

Thomas VG: Body-image satisfaction among black women, *J Soc Psychol* 129 (1):107, 1988.

# Health and Human Needs

## CHAPTER OUTLINE

## LEARNING OUTCOMES

After studying this chapter you should be able to:
- *Define the key terms listed.*
- *Discuss each component of Maslow's hierarchy of needs.*
- *List the eight basic physiological needs of all human beings.*
- *Describe assessment techniques for identifying unmet needs.*
- *Identify actual or potential conditions that threaten fulfilment of a patient's/client's needs.*
- *Describe relationships among the different levels of needs.*
- *State factors that influence individual need priorities.*
- *Describe the fundamental nursing implications concerning unmet needs.*

**B**asic human needs are matters such as food, water, safety, and love that are necessary for survival and health. Although each person has additional, unique needs, everyone has the same basic human needs. The extent to which basic needs are met determines a person's level of health and position on the health-illness continuum (Roper *et al*, 1983). Nurses are therefore concerned with ensuring that basic human needs are met.

Maslow's **hierarchy of basic human needs** is a theory that nurses can use to understand the relationships among basic human needs when providing care. Maslow has assigned priorities to basic needs. According to his theory, certain human needs are more basic than others; that is, some needs must be met before others. For example, a starving person is more likely to seek food than to engage in activities that increase self-esteem.

The hierarchy of human needs arranges the basic needs in five levels of priority (Fig. 7-1). The most basic, or first, level includes **physiological needs** such as air, water, and food. The second level includes safety and security needs, which involve physical and psychological security. The third level contains love and belonging needs, including friendship, social relationships, and sexual love. The fourth level encompasses esteem and self-esteem needs, which involve self-confidence, usefulness, achievement, and self-worth. The final level is the need for self-actualization, the state of fully achieving potential and having the ability to solve problems and cope realistically with life's situations.

Through life experiences an individual's basic human needs may be unmet, partially met, or wholly fulfilled. According to this theory, a person whose needs are all met is healthy, and a person with one or more **unmet needs** is at risk for illness or may be unhealthy in one or more of the human dimensions.

The hierarchy of needs is a theoretical model; that is, the priorities given to human needs are generally true of people but not necessarily true of all individuals. Thus, the hierarchy of needs can still be applied to individuals who seem to have different priorities. When providing care to individuals with unmet needs, the nurse should always take into account their personal priorities, as well as other factors, such as environment and social interactions, that influence how well needs can be met.

Patients/clients entering the health care system generally have known and unrecognized unmet needs, or they may be unable to continue meeting their own needs. A person brought to an accident and emergency department experiencing cardiac arrest has an unmet need for air, the most basic physiological need. An older woman in a high-crime area may be concerned about physical safety and, while hospitalized, may have a need for psychological security from fear that her home will be burgled. A widowed housewife whose children have moved away may feel that she does not belong or is not loved. Nurses in all practice settings encounter patients/clients whose needs might be unmet. Nursing care includes helping patients/clients, and often the family, meet these needs.

The hierarchy of needs is a useful way for nurses to evaluate and understand the needs and behaviours of a patient. Although one need may take priority over another (such as restoration of an adequate airway before education that will help the patient/client adjust to an emotional conflict), the nurse simultaneously assesses needs on different levels. An example is helping a patient meet the need for social belonging while also helping achieve adequate nutrition. The nurse assesses the patient's/client's needs, within the framework of any nursing model being used, and then considers how to use the nursing process and mutual goal setting to help the patient.

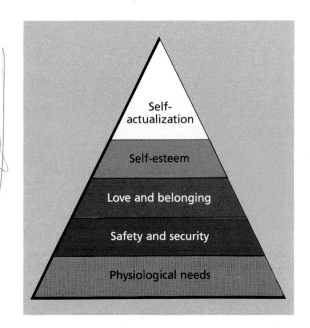

**Fig.7-1** Maslow's hierarchy of needs.

## PHYSIOLOGICAL NEEDS

Physiological needs have the highest priority in Maslow's hierarchy. An individual who has several unmet needs generally seeks first to fulfil physiological needs (Maslow, 1970). For example, a person who lacks food, safety, and love usually searches for food before seeking love.

Physiological needs are necessary or important for survival. Detailed explanations of these physiological needs can be found in subsequent chapters. Humans have eight such needs: oxygen, fluid, nutrition, temperature, elimination, shelter, rest, and sex. The very young, very old, poor, ill, and handicapped frequently depend on others for meeting basic physiological needs. The nurse often has a role in helping these patients/clients meet those needs. In some instances, individuals may not recognize that they are not meeting their basic needs; for example, those with mental illnesses or a learning disability.

### Oxygen

**Oxygen** is an essential physiological need. The body depends on oxygen for moment-to-moment survival. Some tissues, such as skeletal muscle, can survive for a time without oxygen through **anaerobic metabolism**, a process by which these tissues provide their own energy in the absence of oxygen. In long-distance running, for example, the runner's skeletal muscles undergo anaerobic metabolism so that the available oxygen can be used by more vital organs such as the heart, brain, and lungs.

Tissues that carry out only **aerobic metabolism**, the process of providing energy in the presence of oxygen, depend totally on oxygen for survival. The brain, for example, cannot function without oxygen for longer than 4 to 5 minutes.

Oxygen must be adequately delivered from the environment to the lungs, the bloodstream, and finally the tissues. At any point in their lives, patients/clients are at risk for not meeting their oxygen needs. The need can be acute, as with a cardiac arrest, or chronic, as with the disease emphysema.

### Nursing Assessment

Nurses continually evaluate patients'/clients' oxygenation to determine whether this need is being met. This assessment is basically the same in chronic and acute situations. Patients/clients may be confused or lethargic because the level of oxygen in their blood and tissues is decreased. When oxygen needs are unmet, people are often unable to lie flat because of air hunger and are forced to remain upright so that gravity can assist in lung expansion. Patients/clients breathe quickly to deliver more oxygen to their lungs, and respirations are usually shallow. Frequently, this effort fatigues the person rather than meeting the need for oxygenation. Other signs of inadequate oxygenation include nasal flaring and sternal, substernal, and suprasternal retractions. Patients/clients appear to be struggling for air.

Patients/clients with progressive, long-term decreases in tissue oxygen levels show **cyanosis**, a bluish discolouration of skin and mucous membranes caused by decreased oxygen in the blood. Cyanosis is a late sign of poor oxygenation, so the nurse should be aware of the earlier, more subtle indicators.

## Nursing Implications

Oxygen has the highest priority of all physiological needs because many organs such as the brain and heart cannot survive without it. The nurse must be able to assess the need for oxygen and meet it. For example, a nursing assessment of *anxiety* is supported by the defining characteristic of *hyperventilation*. During hyperventilation, there is a decrease in the intake of oxygen and an increase in the expiration of carbon dioxide. The person becomes more anxious and confused and may feel a tingling of the hands and feet, numbness around the lips, and dizziness. The nursing intervention is directed at controlling the imbalance of respiratory gases by having a patient/client breathe into a paper bag, which will cause the person to re-breathe carbon dioxide and slow the respiratory rate. After the patient/client has adequate oxygen, the nurse may use reassurance, teaching, and counselling to help control anxiety.

In other instances the nurse uses specific techniques to help the patient/client meet oxygen needs. For example, a 50-year-old man has a long smoking history and a medical diagnosis of chronic obstructive airways disease. Nursing assessment documents chronic breathlessness and a requirement of 1 L/min of oxygen every night administered through a nasal cannula. Identifying a problem of chronic breathlessness, the nurse develops a care plan so that the patient/client has adequate opportunity to meet needs for hygiene, nutrition, and rest. The nurse also teaches the patient/client to rest in a position that increases respiratory volume and thus the level of oxygen.

Nursing measures to meet oxygen needs range from emergency cardiopulmonary resuscitation for cardiac arrest, to supportive measures such as administration of oxygen to patients/clients with pulmonary disease during exercise (see Chapter 17).

---

### Mental Health Nursing
### Basic needs and mental illness

When working with people who have a mental illness, it is important to appreciate that many of them are unable to recognize their basic needs and are unable to meet these needs or to articulate them to carers. For example:

**Safety**: this need is paramount in people with a mental illness or who are in severe mental distress. Individuals may self-inflict injuries or may take their own life.

**Food and fluids**: people with mental illness or severe mental distress may not be able to meet their intake of food or fluids. This can negatively affect their health. Some adolescents use food and fluid as a symbol of protest about their intrapsychic pain and their disillusionment with their life.

**Belonging**: mental distress and mental illness still attract negative labels in our society, and affected individuals are frequently ostracized. Many people with mental health needs feel alienated from their family, friends and peers, and this repeated rejection leads them to distrust the world around them.

## Fluids

The human body requires a *balance* between intake and output of fluids. Fluids are taken in by mouth, or parenterally, and fluids leave the body from the intestines, lungs, skin, and kidneys. Patients/clients of any age can have unmet fluid needs, but the very young and very old have the greatest risk. Severely ill, traumatized, or handicapped people are also more likely to have unmet fluid needs.

Dehydration and oedema indicate unmet fluid needs. **Dehydration** is the excessive loss of water from body tissues; it is accompanied by a disturbance of body electrolytes. Dehydration may result from excessive and prolonged fever, vomiting, diarrhoea, trauma, or any condition that causes a rapid fluid loss. **Oedema** is the abnormal accumulation of fluid in the interstitial spaces of tissues, pericardial sac, intrapleural space, peritoneal cavity, or joint capsules. Oedema is also accompanied by a disturbance of electrolytes and may occur in a nutritional, cardiovascular, renal, malignant, traumatic, or other disorder that results in a rapid accumulation of fluids.

### Nursing Assessment

The nurse examines patients/clients for actual or potential **fluid and electrolyte imbalance**. Poor skin turgor, flushed dry skin, decreased tears or salivation, a coated tongue, decreased urine output, confusion, and irritability indicate dehydration. Skin turgor is the normal elasticity of the skin, which becomes lax with dehydration; when grasped and raised between two fingers, the skin slowly returns to its former position.

The dehydrated patient's/client's skin is dry because the body transfers fluid to the circulation and vital organs. The skin may be flushed because of an elevated body temperature that can accompany dehydration. The tongue is coated and dry. A dehydrated person may cry but not have tears. **Oliguria**, a diminished ability of the kidneys to form and excrete urine, is frequently caused by dehydration. Because of the fluid and associated electrolyte imbalances, mental status is altered, and the patient/client may be irritable and confused. In cases of severe dehydration the patient/client may even be comatose.

Excessive body fluids most commonly manifest as oedema. Oedema may be caused by decreased serum protein levels; severe burns; altered functioning of the cardiovascular, renal, or hepatic system; or drugs. Oedema is usually observed in lower body regions; when the person is standing, oedema is seen in feet and legs. The patient/client with oedema may also have a daily weight gain, breathlessness, or an increased heart rate.

### Nursing Implications

The overall nursing goal for patients/clients with unmet fluid needs is to restore body fluid and electrolyte balances. The nurse uses simple or complex measures to meet this goal. For example, during assessment the nurse documents diarrhoea without vomiting and arrives at the nursing opinion of *increased risk of fluid volume deficit*. An appropriate nursing intervention is to increase the person's oral intake of fluids. If fluid loss is greater, as with a severe burn, the nursing opinion is *fluid volume deficit*, and nursing interventions are more complex and may include carrying out the doctor's prescription for administration of intravenous fluids.

## Children's Nursing
## Basic human needs for children

An infant requires someone to meet the needs for food, shelter, fluids, adequate temperature, and elimination. As the individual grows and progresses developmentally, the ability to satisfy physiological needs is increased. A 2-year-old who wants a drink of water usually knows where water is and how to get it. Although the child's efforts may not be very efficient, if the motivation is great enough the child will meet the need alone, or by enlisting help.

When the nursing assessment reveals findings consistent with *fluid volume excess,* nursing actions restrict the patient's/client's fluid intake and facilitate elimination of fluids from the body (see Chapter 18).

## Nutrition

The human body has an essential need for nutrients (see Chapter 21), although it can survive without food longer than without fluids. As with other physiological needs, **nutritional needs** may be unmet in a person of any age.

The body's metabolic processes control digestion, storage of nutrients, and elimination of waste products. Digestion and storage of nutrients are essential in meeting the body's nutritional demands.

After food is eaten, digestive processes break down nutrients into usable compounds such as glucose, amino acids, and fatty acids, which meet immediate nutritional needs. Glucose is a body sugar that satisfies immediate energy requirements. Nutrients not needed immediately are stored as glycogen, protein, and fat.

When a person skips a meal, eats insufficiently or sporadically, or fasts, the body uses its stored reserves to meet nutritional needs. Glycogen, stored in the liver and muscles, is used first because it is readily available and can be quickly converted to glucose. If the person still has not eaten when glycogen is depleted, the body begins to use stored protein and fat.

The body also needs vitamins and minerals to function with full efficiency. For example, deficiencies in vitamin C impair wound healing. Deficiencies in calcium and vitamin D retard bone growth and bone metabolism.

## Nursing Assessment

To determine whether patients/clients are meeting nutritional needs, the nurse considers body weight and many other factors. Patients/clients with appropriate body weight may still have nutritional deficits. Nutritional assessment should include measurement of body muscle mass, laboratory data, and food intake patterns. Signs and symptoms indicating that individuals are not meeting nutritional needs include failure to grow or gain weight, unplanned weight loss, fatigue, pallor, and recurring mouth and gum sores.

## Nursing Implications

Patients/clients require adequate nutrition to carry out activities of living, promote wound healing, and maintain wellness. In some cases the nurse takes a direct role in meeting patients'/clients' nutritional needs. For example, when caring for infants with the syndrome known as *failure to thrive* the nurse and health care team assume total responsibility for nutrition.

Sometimes a nurse assists in meeting nutritional needs through teaching. An adult who eats more than normal body requirements and has recently diagnosed insulin-dependent diabetes mellitus, for example, needs to be taught to balance nutritional needs, insulin intake, and exercise habits.

To help individuals meet their nutritional needs, the nurse must understand the digestive and metabolic processes of the body. The nurse may use various nutritional supplements and techniques to correct nutritional deficits (see Chapter 21).

## Temperature

The body can function normally within only a narrow **temperature** range, 37°C ± 1°C (Mountcastle, 1980). Body temperatures outside this range can result in injuries, permanent effects such as brain damage, or death.

The body can temporarily regulate temperature by certain mechanisms. For example, a person shivers when moving from a warm environment to one of 10°C. This adaptive response can temporarily increase body temperature.

## Nursing Assessment

The body has a physiological response to extreme temperatures. Prolonged exposure to cold decreases the rate of metabolism and use of oxygen. If body temperature is lowered beyond the point at which the body can adapt, heart rate and respirations decrease, consciousness decreases, the person is more difficult to arouse, the skin is pale and cold, and urinary output decreases. A localized exposure to cold in a severe winter may lead to frostbite. **Frostbite** is a traumatic effect of extreme cold on the skin and subcutaneous tissues and is first displayed as distinct pallor. Blood circulation in the area is impaired, leading to decreased oxygen in tissues. This may cause tissue death.

Prolonged exposure to heat increases the body's metabolic activity and increases tissue oxygen demand. Extreme or prolonged heat exposure can also have specific physiological effects. Local exposure to heat can result in first-, second-, or third-degree burns. Overexposure to the sun can lead to **sunstroke** (also called heatstroke), which is characterized by a high temperature, convulsions, and coma. Heatstroke may be a risk during prolonged hot weather, particularly for children and older people. Symptoms are elevated body temperature, dehydration, and fluid and electrolyte imbalances. If this condition is untreated the person becomes disoriented and confused, enters a coma, and dies.

## Nursing Implications

Nursing care for patients/clients exposed to extreme heat or cold is directed at restoring normal body temperature. In addition, the nurse helps patients/clients avoid exposure to heat or cold. Elderly people in the community are at risk of **hypothermia** and nurses have a role in identifying those at risk and advising on preventative measures.

To treat frostbite, the nurse gently warms the affected area. The nurse does not rub the area in an attempt to increase circulation because this action can further damage skin and underlying tissues. An individual with sunstroke needs emergency treatment to reduce body temperature. Nursing measures include a tepid sponge bath, fluid replacements, and medications (see Chapter 4 for temperature assessment).

## Elimination

The **elimination of waste** materials is one of the body's metabolic processes. Waste products are eliminated by the lungs, skin, kidneys, and intestines.

The lungs primarily eliminate carbon dioxide, a gas formed during tissue metabolism. Most carbon dioxide is carried to the lungs by the venous system and excreted through breathing. If a patient/client has difficulty eliminating this gas (for example, with acid-base imbalances that originate in the pulmonary system), nursing measures are needed to prevent severe impairment or death.

The skin eliminates water and sodium, most noticeably as sweat. This also assists in temperature regulation because evaporation of sweat lowers body temperature. Sweat cannot always be seen, but the skin excretes water continuously, about 200 ml a day. A patient/client with an elevated temperature or prolonged exposure to hot, humid weather has an increased water loss from the skin. The nurse considers water loss from the skin when caring for a patient/clients with actual or potential dehydration.

The kidneys are the body's primary means of excreting excess body fluids, electrolytes, hydrogen ions, and acids. Urinary elimination normally depends on fluid intake and circulatory blood volume; if either is decreased, urinary output decreases. Urinary output is also changed in people with kidney disease, which affects the quantity of urine and the content of waste products within the urine. Kidney disease can be life threatening.

The intestines eliminate solid waste products and some fluid from the body. The elimination of solid waste by bowel evacuation usually becomes a pattern at 30 to 36 months of age.

## Nursing Assessment

A patient/client whose urinary elimination needs are unmet may become incontinent or develop urinary tract infection. *Incontinence* can occur because the person is unable to perceive the urge to urinate, as when waking from general anaesthesia or after severe head injury or spinal cord injury. Incontinence may also occur if an immobilized person is unable to reach a bedpan or obtain assistance.

Unmet urinary elimination needs also result in fluid and electrolyte imbalances. A *fluid volume deficit* such as that occurring with dehydration or shock may lead to an imbalance in waste products eliminated by the kidneys. An electrolyte imbalance may result from an acute or chronic kidney disorder.

A patient's/client's unmet needs for bowel elimination may lead to changes in the pattern of elimination or diet intake. Changes in bowel elimination patterns can result in *bowel incontinence*, *constipation*, and *diarrhoea*. Altering the diet intake of fluids and foods can also change elimination patterns and needs.

## Nursing Implications

Nursing care assists the patient/client in meeting elimination needs. Nursing intervention may be simple, such as providing privacy or changing the diet, or complex, such as inserting a catheter or administering an enema. When helping patients/clients meet urinary and bowel elimination needs, a nurse uses his or her knowledge of anatomy and physiology, as well as specific skills and techniques (see Chapters 22 and 23).

## Shelter

All humans need **shelter**. Although most people have some kind of shelter, sometimes it is substandard and does not offer full protection. Disasters such as floods and fire can render an entire community homeless. Agencies such as the Red Cross, Salvation Army and homeless centres are resources in helping individuals obtain shelter.

## Nursing Assessment

Often the nurse can identify **environmental risk factors** in a patient's/client's home that may indicate that shelter needs are not being met. These include exposure to temperature extremes, as in a poorly insulated, draughty home or a poorly ventilated home. Others may involve physical safety of the home and its environment. A home with a leaky roof and an unprotected home in a high-crime neighbourhood are inadequate shelters. The most extreme example of unmet shelter needs is homelessness. Homeless people are often those most at risk of ill health.

Patients/clients with limited financial, social, and family resources are also at risk of unmet shelter needs. Frequently, such individuals are older or handicapped or have limited job skills. They may feel trapped in their environment because they are unaware of resources that can help them relocate.

When assessing whether a patient/client is meeting shelter needs, the nurse identifies risk factors for illness or injury. Environments that are dirty may attract insects or rodents that can increase the risk of illness. If a home is poorly lit or cluttered, there is an increased risk of accidental injury. In addition, overcrowding and lack of cleanliness are predisposing factors to communicable diseases, such as tuberculosis.

## Nursing Implications

In many situations, it is unrealistic for a nurse to seek new shelter for a patient/client and family. However, the nurse makes referrals to community agencies that can help. Community agencies can enforce standards for rented housing and help a patient/client pay bills or make home repairs. Such agencies can also help the person identify alternatives for shelter.

The nurse can help the patient/client make changes within the home to make it healthier. For example, rails can be installed in a bathroom for an individual who has mobility problems. Health promotion often involves teaching patients/clients about the relationship between home environment and health.

## Rest

Every individual has a basic physiological need for regular **rest**. The amount of sleep needed varies, depending on the person's quality of sleep, health status, activity patterns, lifestyle, and age.

An individual with chronic disease requires more rest than a healthy person of the same age. Pregnancy, lactation, and health status changes such as surgery also increase the need for rest. Physical and emotional stress may also increase a person's need for rest. Rest and sleep often provide temporary relief from stress. However, rest can also be a non-productive method for resolving stress, because a patient/client may depend on it as an escape.

## Nursing Assessment

With insufficient sleep, a person's appearance and behaviour change. Circles under the patient's/client's eyes and a dishevelled appearance are signs of such change. The person may also have less energy, seem less motivated, be more irritable or withdrawn, stare into space, have difficulty concentrating, and be restless.

## Nursing Implications

When possible, the nurse should plan care to fit the patient's/client's usual **sleep-wake cycle**. Any bedtime habits, such as walking, bathing, reading, or drinking milk, should be incorporated into the care plan.

Frequently, rest patterns are changed by illness or pain. The nurse uses specific methods to promote comfort and relieve pain so that the patient's/client's need for rest can be anticipated and met. If the individual is unable to sleep and rest because of other factors, such as lifestyle or chronic stress, the nurse directs care at resolving the cause while helping meet these needs (see Chapter 20).

## Sex

Sex is considered by Maslow (1970) to be a basic physiological need that generally takes priority over higher-level needs. **Sexual needs**, and the manner in which they are met, are influenced by age, sociocultural background, ethics, values, self-esteem, and level of wellness.

The concept of sexuality encompasses more than sex as a need, and includes consideration of aspects of the individual, such as appearance, relationships and gender-based roles (such as breadwinner or homemaker) (Roper *et al*, 1983). Health professionals are giving increasing attention to sexuality as a component of health and nurses take sexuality needs into consideration as they become more knowledgeable about them (Webb and Askham, 1987). Sexuality can be affected by illness, chronic conditions, and hospitalization (Webb, 1985).

## Nursing Assessment

Paralysis, mastectomy, or any change in physical appearance can affect how people feel about themselves as sexual beings. This change in physical appearance can result in an altered body image (Price, 1990) and can impair the expression of sexuality or sexual needs.

Patients/clients unable to meet sexual needs may indicate in their behaviour that these needs are unmet. Alternative expressions might include sexual language, masturbation, or exposure of sexual organs. Other patients/clients might flirt or redirect sexual need to physical exercise, overeating, or overwork.

Individuals who experience depression, grief, or lifestyle changes are at risk for having unmet sexual and sexuality needs. For some patients/clients, the meeting of sexual needs is only temporarily interrupted. For others, especially those with severe physical disability, sexual needs may be unmet for longer and may resolve only with specific help or counselling.

## Nursing Implications

Nursing care designed to resolve *changes in sexuality patterns* or *sexual dysfunction* must consider the patient's/client's developmental level, values, habits, level of health, sexual partner, and preferred sexual practices. There are situations where standardized advice or literature can help, for example following myocardial infarction or prostatectomy (Murray *et al*, 1989; Ewles and Simnet, 1992). Not all nurses feel competent to discuss sexual needs with patients/clients, but it is important to recognize a person's sexual needs so that appropriate support can be made available. This may be in the form of a trained and experienced nurse, a counsellor, or a sexual therapist.

## SAFETY AND SECURITY NEEDS

Next in priority after the patient's/client's physiological needs are needs for physical and psychological safety and security.

### Physical Safety

An infant enters the world totally dependent on others for needs and physical safety. As the infant grows and develops, greater independence is gradually achieved. Adults are generally able to provide for their physical safety, but the ill and handicapped may need help.

Maintaining physical safety involves reducing or eliminating threats to body or life. The threat may be illness, accident, danger, or environmental exposure. When ill, a patient/client may be vulnerable to complications such as infection and therefore depends on professionals in the health care system for protection.

Meeting physical safety needs sometimes takes precedence over meeting a physiological need. For example, a nurse may need to protect a disoriented patient from falling out of bed before providing care to meet nutritional needs.

## Nursing Assessment

When assessing the physical safety needs of a patient/client, the nurse considers actual and potential threats. Patients/clients with limited movement or total immobilization of an extremity are at risk for developing joint contractures, skin breakdown, and muscle atrophy. Patients/clients taking medication are at risk for side effects. Patients/clients with indwelling intravenous lines or urinary catheters are at risk for secondary infections.

Patients/clients with acute or chronic illnesses, disability, or handicaps may need help meeting safety needs. The nurse assesses the total environment, whether it is the individual's home or a hospital, to identify potential or actual threats.

Health problems in other dimensions may also present a safety risk to an individual. Patients/clients under emotional stress, for example, may behave in a manner that might threaten their safety. A socially isolated patient/client may be unaware of environmental factors that threaten physical safety.

## Nursing Implications

The best way to select strategies that maintain the patient's/client's safety is the early identification of defining characteristics to support the actual or potential problem of risk for injury. For example, nurses teach parents about common risks to their children throughout the developmental stages and the nurse teaches patients/clients receiving medication or therapy about side effects, interaction effects, and potential hazards of treatments, as well as the desired effects. The nurse individualizes education for patients/clients and families to assist in meeting their safety needs.

In addition, the nurse increases the individual's physical safety in a health care setting by maintaining beds in the low position with the call bell or light within easy reach. The hospital or home bedroom is uncluttered so that the individual can easily move about without risk of injury. Lastly, frequent observation of the patient/client maintains continual assessment of physiological and psychosocial status and complications or threats that can be reduced (see Chapter 19).

## Psychological Safety

To be safe and secure psychologically, a person must understand what to expect from others, including family members and health care professionals. The person must also know what to expect from procedures, new experiences, and encounters within the environment. Everyone feels some threat to psychological safety with new and unfamiliar experiences. A student entering university may feel insecure, a person starting a new job may feel threatened by having to interact with unfamiliar people, and a patient/client about to undergo a diagnostic test may be threatened by the technology involved. In such cases, people generally do not directly state that their psychological safety is threatened, but their conversation may indirectly reveal their feelings.

## Nursing Assessment

Assessment of psychological safety is often difficult because the nurse may have to interpret the patient's/client's language and behaviours. Because a perceived threat causes stress, the individual may act in various ways to adapt to the stress. The patient's/client's behaviour may change radically. For example, an outgoing, active person may become withdrawn, or a previously cooperative patient/client may suddenly refuse to participate in care. Most patients/clients want to be active and cooperative, and a drastic change in behaviour is a clue that some threat to phychological safety may be felt.

## Nursing Implications

The nurse can use teaching methods to reduce a threat to psychological safety, particularly when the potential threat includes a change in role, a change in body image, or an invasive diagnostic or surgical procedure. Because people often fear the unknown or have unrealistic expectations about it, telling patients/clients and their families what to expect greatly reduces anxiety and increases their participation in health care.

Healthy adults are generally able to meet physical and psychological safety needs without help from health care professionals. However, ill or handicapped people are more susceptible to threats to physical and emotional well-being, so the nurse intervenes to help protect them from harm.

**Learning Disabilities Nursing**
**Expressing sexuality**

When working with people who have a learning disability, it is important to recognize that many of them are unable to identify or meet their own basic needs or to articulate them to carers. It must also be recognized that in certain situations carers will also fail to recognize, or may deny the existence of, some basic needs such as sexuality.

There are two contradictory myths concerning the sexuality of people with learning disabilities. The first is that their sexual appetites are uncontrollable if roused; the second is that they are generally childlike and asexual. Neither of these statements is accurate, but both have created a situation in which many people have grown up in ignorance of their own physical sexuality and without an opportunity to learn socially acceptable ways of expressing themselves sexually, without exposing themselves to exploitation and abuse.

The full extent of how little regard and respect is shown for people with learning disabilities as sexual beings is demonstated by the issues surrounding sterilization of women with learning disabilities, and their perceived inability to parent. There is also evidence that indicates a high vulnerability to sexual abuse within this patient/client group.

## LOVE AND BELONGING NEEDS

The next priority after physiological and safety needs is the need for **love and belonging**. People generally need to feel that they are loved by their family and that they are accepted by peers and the community. This need generally arises after physiological and safety needs are met, because only when individuals feel safe and secure do they have the time and energy to seek love and belonging, and to share that love with others (Rogers, 1961).

Even a person who is generally able to meet needs for love and belonging is often unable to fulfil them when illness or injury occurs. It becomes even more difficult in the hospital. The person is forced to adapt to aspects of the health care system such as organization, routines, environmental limitations, and visiting hours. As a result, there is little time or energy left to meet the needs for love and belonging with family or significant others.

## Nursing Assessment

A patient/client of any age in any health care setting may have difficulty meeting love and belonging needs. The ways in which these unmet needs are manifested depend on the individual. The patient's/client's behaviour may be similar to the reactions of a person responding to stress.

Discussion with the family is important as the nurse compares the individual's needs for love and belonging with fulfilment of these needs. The nurse may identify changes in the family or in a relationship with a family member that can provide insight into the patient's/client's needs for love and belonging.

Physical and behavioural changes may indicate that a person is unable to meet love and belonging needs. The patient's/client's appearance and hygiene habits may change. A normally well-groomed person may seem uncaring about appearance. The person may complain of physical ailments such as headaches or gastrointestinal problems when separated from family. Sleep and eating habits may also change.

Conversation often demonstrates that needs for love and belonging are not being met. A hospitalized patient/client may speak often of family or friends expected to visit. In addition, a patient/client who becomes anxious because family or friends have not yet visited may attempt to cope with unmet needs by insisting that it does not matter. A child separated from parents because of illness or injury may seem to adopt the nurse as a surrogate parent. A patient/client may attempt to interact with the nurse as a close friend or may even become possessive about the amount of time spent with the nurse. All of these behaviours are manifestations of the normal need for love and affection.

If a person's need persists for a long period without being met, behaviour may change in more noticeable ways. A usually mild-tempered person may become easily irritated. An outgoing person may withdraw from interaction with co-workers and friends. The person's work habits may change, leading to increased absenteeism or over commitment to the job.

## Nursing Implications

The nursing care plan for patients/clients should include means by which needs for love and belonging can be met. For example, if the patient/client is a young child who will be hospitalized for a long time, the care plan should include specific opportunities for the child and family to interact. The mother or father may wish to remain overnight, and parents should always be given this option. Where possible, children should be cared for at home.

A patient/client *experiencing social isolation* caused by illness or injury cannot meet needs for love and belonging in the usual ways. If opportunities for social interaction are limited, the patient/client may have a sense of not belonging and begin to withdraw. The nurse can take specific actions to help the person maintain social contacts and thus meet love and belonging needs. A hospitalized patient/client may benefit from short social visits by members of the health care team. Resources in the community may help. For example, an older person can be helped to meet the need for contact through a senior citizens' group.

Finally, the nurse works with patients/clients and families to adapt care plans to help individuals meet their needs for love and belonging. The more actively involved patients/clients are in developing care plans and the more control they have over the environment while receiving care, the easier it is for them to meet these needs.

## ESTEEM AND SELF-ESTEEM NEEDS

People need a stable sense of self-esteem, as well as the feeling that they are held in regard by others. The need for self-esteem is linked to the desire for strength, achievement, adequacy, competence, confidence, and independence. People also need recognition or appreciation from others. When both of these needs are met, a person feels self-confident and useful. If needs for self-esteem and

esteem of others are unfulfilled, a person may feel helpless and inferior (Maslow, 1970).

## Nursing Assessment

A change in roles may threaten self-esteem. The change may be anticipated, such as retirement, or sudden, such as an injury. A change in independence and relationship with others occurs with role changes. A person who was formerly independent may become more dependent, and relationships with others may become strained. A person may become more dependent on family members, social agencies, or health care professionals and may begin to question usefulness and importance. The person may lose self-esteem. If no longer functioning in a former role, such as that of a coal miner, a person may feel that the esteem of others is lost as well.

Changes in body image, such as those caused by illness or injury, may also influence self-esteem. Body image changes include obvious changes such as the amputation of a leg and nonobservable changes such as a hysterectomy. Normal developmental changes such as puberty or menopause can change a person's image.

It is not the magnitude of a change in body image or role that affects self-esteem, but rather how the person perceives the self after the change. A person's sense of self-esteem and the esteem of others therefore depend on values and beliefs, support from others, and self-concept.

There are many indications of unmet needs for self-esteem or the esteem of others. A person who feels helpless or inferior may defer all decisions rather than express wishes. The patient/client may become self-critical or seem unusually lethargic or apathetic about anything involving the self, including appearance. The person's general attitude may be summed up as a feeling of hopelessness. In some cases a patient/client with low self-esteem may avoid or ignore opportunities for actions that could increase self-esteem because of the possibility of failure. The loss of self-esteem can thus become a self-fulfilling prophecy.

### Mental Health Nursing
### Psychological safety

Most individuals have the capacity to evaluate their encounters with life events. In general, the more a person desires the unattainable, the greater their feelings of negativity when they do not get what they want.

In addition, there is the issue of tolerance, where the individual acknowledges that an undesirable event has happened, believes that the event should occur empirically and, if it cannot be modified, will pursue other goals.

Finally, there is the question of acceptance, where the individual accepts him/herself and others as fallible beings and that the world is highly complex and exists according to laws which are frequently outside their personal control.

Dryden W: *Counselling individuals: the rationale-emotive approach* London, 1987, Taylor & Francis.

A person feeling the lack of esteem of other people may test others by making statements that call for their approval or praise. Conversely, the patient/client may act in a way that prevents such approval if little self-esteem is present and the person is certain of failure.

### Nursing Implications

Helping to resolve *low self-esteem* can begin with the first contact between patient/client and nurse. From the beginning the nurse must convey respect for the patient/client as an individual. Even though the patient/client may have different beliefs and values, the nurse needs to accept, not judge, the person's values.

If patients'/clients' self-concepts are changed by illness or injury, nursing care involves improving self-concept and body image. Specific nursing actions depend on individuals' support systems and personalities, the cause of altered self-concept, and available resources. If patients' levels of self-esteem are so low that they fail to care for themselves, the nurse may have to help meet other needs, such as those for nutrition and safety, while taking steps to increase self-esteem.

## NEED FOR SELF-ACTUALIZATION

Self-actualization is the highest level of needs in Maslow's hierarchy of human needs. It is by self-actualization that people achieve their fullest potential (Maslow, 1970).

Self-actualized people have multiple characteristics (see box). They have a mature multidimensional personality, frequently they are able to assume and complete multiple tasks, and they achieve fulfilment from the pleasure of a job well done. They do not totally depend on the opinions of others about appearance, quality of work, or problem-solving methods. Although they may have failings and doubts, they generally deal with them realistically.

Present needs, environment, and stressors influence how well people meet their need for self-actualization. Self-actualization is possible when there is a balance among the patients'/clients' needs, stressors, and ability to adapt to changes of the body and environment.

### Assessment

Illness, injury, loss of a loved one, change in role, and change in status can threaten or disturb self-actualization. A loss of self-actualization occurs when a person can no longer achieve the fullest potential because of the limitations imposed by the illness or injury. This loss may result in behavioural changes. The patient/client may feel frustrated because the illness prevents decision making, creativity, and independent problem solving. Instead, because of the illness, the person is forced to be more self-centred, more dependent on others, and motivated more by external factors.

### Nursing Implications

The major focus for nursing care is to restore the patient/client as much as possible to a self-actualized state. Nursing care is planned to encourage the individual to make decisions when possible, particularly in regard to health care. Thus, the nurse seeks the

**Mental Health Nursing**
**Eight ways to 'self-actualize'**

1. Experiencing fully, vividly, selflessly, with full concentration and total absorption.
2. Viewing life as a process of choices.
3. Acknowledging that the self does exist and is allowed to emerge.
4. When in doubt, be honest.
5. Daring to listen to oneself and choosing what is constitutionally right for oneself.
6. Commitment to going through an arduous and demanding period of self-preparation to realize one's possibilities.
7. An awareness that peak experiences are transient moments of ecstasy which cannot be bought, sought or guaranteed.
8. Finding out who one is; opening oneself to explore psychopathology.

*Maslow AH: the farther reaches of human nature, Harmondsworth, 1971, Penguin.*

involvement of the patient/client when planning and delivering nursing care.

Because the self-actualized person tends to be creative and highly individual in many ways, nursing care should include the opportunity to fulfil creative needs. The individual should be encouraged to continue with specific projects, and if the patient/client is hospitalized, time should be set aside for them.

The patient's/client's need for privacy must be respected and met. When in good health the self-actualized person generally has a strong need for privacy. An illness, especially in a hospital setting, can greatly reduce privacy. Nurses can help meet this need by planning health care so that privacy will not be interrupted during specific times.

## APPLICATION OF BASIC NEEDS THEORY

Maslow's theory of human needs can provide a basis for nursing care of patients/clients of all ages and in a variety of health settings. When the nurse applies this theory in practice, however, the focus is on the needs of the individual rather than rigid adherence to Maslow's hierarchy. Maslow's hierarchy is a generalization about the need priorities of most but not all people. In all cases, an emergency physiological need takes precedence over a higher-level need. With one patient/client the need for self-esteem may be a higher priority than a long-term nutritional need, whereas for another person, this may be reversed. To provide the most effective care, the nurse needs to understand relationships among different needs for the individual. Furthermore, although the hierarchy of needs suggests that one need should be met before another, nursing care often addresses two or more at the same time.

### Relationships Among Needs

In some nursing situations, it is unrealistic to expect a patient's/client's basic needs to be fulfilled in the fixed hierarchical order. For example, a person enters the health care system with a chronic respiratory infection. While providing care, the nurse learns that the patient has not eaten adequately, slept well, or maintained social relationships since his wife died 2 years before. In this case the person has several unmet needs, including the physiological needs for nutrition and rest and needs for love and a sense of belonging. For the patient/client, these separate needs are closely related. Nursing care in this situation would not simply be directed to helping the person meet the higher-priority needs for nutrition and rest because these needs in part occurred because the patient/client was not meeting lower-priority needs. Nursing care focuses also on assisting this person through the grieving process so that, after grief and loneliness have been resolved, former eating and sleeping habits will be regained and thus these physiological needs will be met.

An opposite relationship among similar needs may be true of a different patient/client. For example, a woman is receiving treatment for severe arthritis and often feels pain or discomfort during certain activities. Because of this, she has changed her habits and no longer visits family members and friends. The nurse realizes that the woman also has unmet needs for love and belonging. These two sets of needs are clearly related and the nurse provides care directed at meeting both. In this situation, however, the priority is to provide relief from pain, which will then allow the woman to return to former activities that meet the love and belonging needs.

For different individuals, needs on different levels may be related in different ways. Some people may give sexual need a higher priority than the need for love, whereas for others, sexual need is deferred until the need for love is met. Similarly, people with unmet needs for self-esteem may be unable to seek fulfilment of the need for love if their self-esteem is so low that they feel inferior and fear rejection. In these and many other ways, needs on different levels may be closely related for individuals. When assessing needs and planning care, the nurse must not assume that a lower-level need always takes priority. As with all other aspects of providing care, the nurse individualizes the nursing care plan to provide for the unique needs and desires of the patient/client.

## Simultaneous Meeting of Needs

The nurse provides care for patients/clients with many needs because illness often disrupts the ability to meet needs on different levels. After identifying patients'/clients' specific needs, the nurse generally has to set **priorities** to help them meet these needs. However, setting priorities does not mean that the nurse provides care for only one need at a time. The nurse does not, for example, simply begin with the first need in the hierarchy and move up only after the first has been met. In emergency situations, of course, physiological needs take precedence, but even then the nurse is aware of other needs. Even in an emergency the nurse considers patients'/clients' higher-level needs.

A young man who is hospitalized with paraplegia resulting from a severed spinal cord, for example, needs assistance in meeting physiological needs. However, he may also have low self-esteem related to his condition. The nurse is faced with the challenge of simultaneously meeting his physiological needs and need for self-esteem because he may not eat properly or participate in physical care if he does not feel good about himself. The nurse should not offer the person false hope about future recovery. However, while planning care to meet physiological needs the nurse can include measures that will help restore self-esteem.

## Factors Influencing Need Priorities

Ideally, nursing care can be directed at meeting several needs simultaneously. In practice, though, one need often takes precedence over another, and priorities must be determined so that care can be more focused and effective. Life-threatening situations always take priority, and unmet physiological needs that pose a threat to life certainly have a high priority. In other situations the nurse considers factors that influence the priority of needs for an individual.

A person's personality and mood affect the perception of and ability to meet a particular need. A depressed person may react negatively to a suggestion for an activity that could increase self-esteem, although in another mood the person might respond with enthusiasm. Thus, when providing care to help meet several needs, the nurse can adjust the care plan to correspond most effectively to the patient's/client's personality and mood.

Some needs must be deferred until the person is in better health. A patient/client recovering from an acute gastrointestinal infection should not be encouraged to resume physical activities related to needs for self-esteem until needs for physical safety and security have been met by achieving full health. Similarly, a diabetic patient/client whose condition is unstable may have to defer other needs until nutritional needs related to insulin therapy are satisfied.

The patient's/client's perception of needs varies among socio-economic and cultural groups. In addition, the individual's perception of some needs, such as sexual needs, varies between the sexes and within different developmental levels. The nurse considers the patient's/client's perception of needs when planning care and does not impose personal perceptions about priorities.

The patient's/client's family structure can influence the way needs are satisfied. A mother may, for example, place the needs of an infant before her own, such as when she interrupts a meal or sleep to feed the child.

When setting need priorities, the nurse considers that basic needs are interrelated. Physiological functioning is closely related to body systems, environment, values, ethics, and culture. One need does not occur independently of others. For example, if nutritional needs are unmet for a long time, a person begins to show signs of malnutrition, the body deteriorates, weakness occurs, and the person is unable to recognize or meet the lower-priority needs of safety, love, and self-esteem. Needs are interrelated in unique ways for each person, and the nurse considers such relationships in planning care. Rather than rigidly following the hierarchy of the human needs theory, the nurse involves the individual and family in planning so that need priorities are not neglected.

## SUMMARY

Healthy adults are usually able to meet most of their basic needs. As an adult ages or becomes ill or handicapped, the risk of not being able to meet basic needs increases.

Maslow's theory proposes that a hierarchical relationship exists among different levels of human needs. A person entering the health care system may have one or more unmet needs at different levels. Nursing care addresses all patient/client needs. Essential, life-sustaining needs generally take priority over others. The patient's/client's different needs may be interrelated in unique ways, and the nurse considers the patient's/client's priorities. Nursing care may be directed at meeting several needs simultaneously. The care plan is based on the nurse's assessment of the extent to which the individual is meeting, and is able to meet, all needs.

Nursing involves providing care for the whole person. The nurse applies knowledge about the body systems and about the individual's family, social system, emotions, values, ethics, and goals of health care. In this way the theory of human needs corresponds to nursing's holistic perspective by addressing the patient's/client's needs in the physiological, psychological, sociocultural, developmental, and spiritual dimensions. The basic needs theory is appropriate and applicable in primary health care (community health), psychiatric, outpatient, and institutional settings, including critical-care wards and rehabilitation centres. This theory can provide a basis for nursing care for individuals of all ages and developmental stages, from the neonate to the older adult patient/client. The human needs theory is therefore a set of concepts important for the nurse's understanding of health and illness and the patient's/client's position on the health-illness continuum.

## CHAPTER 7 REVIEW
### Key Concepts
- Basic human needs are the needs for things such as oxygen, food, water, safety, and love required to survive and be healthy.
- Some human needs are more necessary to survival than others and must be met first.
- Maslow's hierarchy is a theoretical representation of the levels of basic needs.
- Very young, very old, chronically ill, and handicapped people are generally less able than others to meet needs without assistance.
- The highest priority is given to physiological needs, including

### Key Terms

Basic human needs, p. 151
Elimination of waste, p. 155
Environmental risk factors, p. 155
Esteem and self-esteem needs, p. 158
Hierarchy of basic human needs, p. 151
Love and belonging needs, p. 157
Oxygen, p. 152
Physiological needs, p. 152
Priorities of need, p. 152
Safety and security needs, p. 156
Self-actualization, p. 159
Sexual needs, p. 156
Shelter needs, p. 155
Sleep wake cycle, p. 156
Temperature, p. 154
Unmet needs, p. 152

oxygen, fluid, nutrition, temperature, elimination, shelter, rest, and sex.
- Oxygen is the most essential physiological need. A chronic or acute oxygen need can be identified by confusion, lethargy, rapid and shallow respirations, an inability to lie flat, nasal flaring, sternal retractions, a decreased level of consciousness, and cyanosis.
- Fluid needs require a balance between the intake and output of fluids. Dehydration or oedema indicates unmet fluid needs.
- Dehydration may result in flushed and dry skin, poor skin turgor, a coated tongue, dry mucous membranes, decreased saliva, decreased tears, and oliguria.
- Oedema may result in the swelling of a dependent body part, weight gain, shortness of breath, increased heart rate, and smooth, shiny skin.
- Nutritional needs require an adequate intake of foods to allow the body to carry on metabolic processes. Unmet nutritional needs may be indicated by weight loss or failure to grow or gain weight, fatigue, pallor, and recurring sores in the mouth and gums.
- The body is able to function within only a small temperature range. Unmet temperature needs may result from exposure to cold or heat.
- Elimination needs involve the body's removal of excess fluids and wastes. The body meets these needs by elimination through the skin, lungs, kidneys, and intestines.
- The need for shelter is a physiological need. Unmet needs can be identified through assessment of the environment.
- Sleep and rest needs vary, depending on the individual's quality of sleep, age, health status, activity patterns, and lifestyle. Unmet needs may result in a decreased level of energy, dishevelled appearance, irritability, decreased concentration, and restlessness.
- People have different needs related to sexuality at different times in life, and the manifestation of unmet sexual needs can take many forms.
- Safety and security needs include physical and psychological safety and the need to prevent complications.
- Patients/clients in the health care system may be unable to meet their needs for love and belonging because of changes in relationships with others and the separation often imposed by illness.
- Self-esteem and the self-actualization needs can be threatened by changes that occur with changes in role, body image, illness or injury.
- To apply basic needs theory in practice, the nurse considers the relationships between the patient's/client's specific needs, sets priorities for meeting needs by considering the individual's priorities, and when possible and necessary assists the person in simultaneously meeting needs on different levels.

### CRITICAL THINKING EXERCISES
1. When meeting patients'/clients' basic needs how do you establish priorities of care?
2. How do you determine when to meet psychosocial needs before physiological needs?

3. What information do you require to design a care plan to meet several basic needs simultaneously?

## REFERENCES

Dryden W: *Counselling individuals: the rationale-emotive approach,* London, 1987, Taylor and Francis.

Ewles L, Simnet I: *Promoting health: a practical guide,* Middlesex, 1992, Scutari Press.

Maslow AH: *Motivation and personality,* ed 2, New York, 1970, Harper & Row.

Murray R, Zeutner J, Howells C: *Nursing concepts for health promotion,* Hertfordshire, 1989, Prentice Hall.

Mountcastle VR: *Medical physiology,* ed 14, St Louis, 1980, Mosby–Year Book.

Price B: *Body image, nursing concepts and care,* Hemel Hempstead, 1990, Prentice Hall.

Rogers C: *On becoming a person,* Boston, 1961, Houghton Mifflin.

Roper N, Logan W, Tierney A: *Using a model for nursing,* London, 1983, Churchill Livingstone.

Webb C: *Sexuality, nursing and health,* Chichester, 1985, John Wiley & Sons.

Webb C, Askham J: Nurses' knowledge and attitudes about sexuality in health care — a review of the literature, *Nurs Education Today* 7:75, 1987.

## FURTHER READING

### Adult Nursing

Maslow AH: *Toward a psychology of being,* ed 2, New York, 1968, Van Reinhold.

Maslow AH: Toward a humanistic biology, *Am Psychol* 24:724, 1969.

Roper N, Logan W, Tierney A: *The elements of nursing,* ed 3, London, 1990, Churchill Livingstone.

### Children's Nursing

Bowlby J: *Attachment and loss,* Volume II, Gretna, LA, 1975, Pelican.

Muller DJ, Harris PJ, Wattley LA *et al: Nursing children research and practice,* 3e, London, 1992, Chapman and Hall.

Wong D: *Nursing care of infants and children,* 5e, St Louis, 1995, Mosby.

### Learning Disabilities Nursing

Brown H, Craft A, editors: *Thinking the unthinkable: papers on sexual abuse and people with learning difficulties,* London, 1989, FPA Education Unit.

Craft A, editor: *Mental handicap and sexuality: issues and perspectives,* Tunbridge Wells, 1987, Costello.

### Mental Health Nursing

Asher R, Malingering. In Black N, Boswell D, Gray A *et al: Health and disease,* Milton Keynes, 1984, Oxford University Press.

Garland A: In a panic, *Nurs Times* 88(52):25, 1992.

Kinchin D: Telephobia, *Nurs Times* 88(52):27, 1992.

Priestley P, McGuire J, Flegg D *et al: Social skills and personal problem solving: a handbook of methods,* London, 1982, Tavistock.

Satre JP: *Existentialism and humanism,* London, 1973, Eyre Metheun.

Tschudin V: Support yourself, *Nurs Times* 86(12):40, 1990.

# Culture, Ethnicity, and Religion

## CHAPTER OUTLINE

## LEARNING OUTCOMES

After studying this chapter, you should be able to:
- *Define the key terms listed.*
- *Discuss the importance of cultural awareness in the provision of quality care.*
- *Define transcultural communication.*
- *Discuss ways in which culture may influence the nurse-patient/client relationship.*
- *Understand migration and its implications for health care planning and provision.*
- *Explain how demography and ethnicity influence health and access to health care.*
- *List the diverse health needs of different ethnic and cultural groups.*
- *Discuss different religious beliefs and how these may influence the health beliefs and care of the patient/client.*

Never before have ethnic and cultural understanding been more necessary for nursing. Nurses have a diverse heritage as a result of different ethnic, cultural and religious backgrounds. Similarly, patients/clients are from diverse ethnic, cultural and religious backgrounds. Quality care and clinical effectiveness demand an understanding of the patient's/client's ethnic background, sociocultural history, and an understanding of the individual's religious and health beliefs.

Sensitivity to the patient's/client's unique health practices and health beliefs enables nurses to maximize their therapeutic and health promotion roles. Effective rapport and communication with patients/clients enhance nurses' ability to assess health needs, provide skilled nursing intervention, and solve problems in culturally sensitive ways. Understanding culture, ethnicity and religion is crucial for planning and providing effective health care.

### THE IMPORTANCE OF TRANSCULTURAL COMMUNICATION

**Transcultural communication** occurs when people attempt to understand another person's point of view from that person's cultural frame of reference. Effective transcultural communication is facilitated by understanding the differing values and core principles, as well as by identifying commonalities. After reaching a cultural understanding, the nurse must consider how the patient's/client's cultural perspectives might affect negotiated care plans and implementation of the nursing process. In the past decade, international nursing research has emphasized the importance of considering cultural factors when delivering nursing care.

The developments in **transcultural nursing** represent an effort by nurses from varying cultural backgrounds and clinical specialties to develop the knowledge and skills needed to provide care that is clinically effective, appropriate and sensitive to the patient's/client's needs.

## HOW CULTURE INFLUENCES HEALTH BELIEFS

A broad range of health and illness beliefs exist in a **multicultural society** such as in the UK. Many of these beliefs have roots in the cultural, ethnic, religious and social background of the person, family, and community. When experiencing an illness or crisis, a person may use a modern or a **traditional approach** to prevention and healing, or may use a combination of approaches. The nurse who demonstrates reflective and clinically effective practice will enhance patient/client satisfaction, as well as advance the art and science of nursing.

When reflecting on your own culture and on the patient's/client's, ask yourself these questions:

- Who am I from a cultural perspective? Who is the patient/client from a cultural perspective?
- What is my heritage? What is the patient's/client's heritage?
- What are the health traditions of my heritage? What are the health traditions of the patient's/client's heritage?
- What cultural phenomena interact with my health care perspectives? What cultural phenomena interact with the patient's/client's health care perspectives?
- Where are the gaps between the patient's/client's health care needs and my perspectives of the patient's/client's health care needs?
- What particular conflicts exist between the patient's/client's health care beliefs and my health care beliefs?

It is essential that nurses explore these questions and form patient/client relationships which are free from cultural stereotypes. The cultural values and beliefs of the patient/client must be determined so that health care can be delivered within that person's cultural context. Consider this example:

*Mrs B, a patient/client of Caribbean origin was diagnosed as having high blood pressure. During consultation, Mrs B was advised to eat plenty of fish and less red meat, and to make other dietary adjustments. The patient/client complied with the advice but, instead of eating fresh fish, ate dried cod fish which is considered a delicacy in her country of origin. Because dried cod has a large amount of salt, Mrs B's blood pressure increased rather than decreased. During further consultation she was criticized for non-compliance with therapeutic advice. However, when Mrs B was counselled by a nurse from a similar cultural background, the nurse asked her how much dried cod she was eating. Mrs B reported that she ate dried cod*

**Adult Nursing**
**Cultural influences on health practices**

Cultural background influences individual beliefs, values, and customs. It influences entry into the health care system and personal health practices. For example, health visitors and others within primary health care are becoming increasingly concerned about the health of Asian and black women. A study undertaken by Mori (1993) for City and East London FHSA found that Asian, black and other ethnic minority groups are disadvantaged in relation to some aspects of health and health care. A previous study by Ibrahim and Hersi (1988) found that between the ages of two weeks and 15 years some black females are circumcised, which can adversely affect sexual function in later years.

*every day. The nurse then explained that Mrs B should eat fresh fish and taught her about the effects of a high salt diet on high blood pressure.*

This example clearly demonstrates the need to understand the patient's/client's normal cultural behaviour and to recognize behavioural responses to illness.

## CULTURE, ETHNICITY AND DEMOGRAPHY

**Culture** represents *nonphysical* traits, such as values, beliefs, attitudes, customs, and shared beliefs about the causes of illness, remedies and illness prevention. Many cultures exist in the UK. Although nurses must be aware of diverse *cultural groups* and be familiar with their basic characteristics, it is essential that patients/clients are assessed as *individuals*, because the characteristic beliefs of a cultural group are not necessarily shared by each individual in that group. However, the patient's/client's background may be used as a framework for providing culturally sensitive nursing care.

It is generally accepted that **ethnicity** may be associated with a long shared history or a common cultural tradition. Characteristics of ethnicity might include common:

- geographic origin, or a small number of common ancestors with shared values, customs, traditions and beliefs
- language and dialect
- literature, folklore and music
- religion
- food preferences.

In some cases, ethnicity may refer to a minority group within a larger host community. People from the same ethnic group often have a sense of uniqueness. These characteristics extend from family, to neighbourhood and community. However, ethnicity is not just related to people who are not of the indigenous population, or to simple factors such as skin colour. Ethnicity is a sense of *identification* associated with a cultural group's common social and cultural heritage in terms of race, language, religion and geographic origin (Horton and Karmi, 1992).

### Mental Health Nursing
### Defining mental health across cultures

The characteristics of mental health vary with individuals and social values, and may be defined differently by different societies (Kaplan, 1971). Kaplan defines 'mental health' as the 'quality of the interacting process' through which individuals relate themselves to the world. Yet, there are problems in defining mental health, because the parameters of mental health are not constant; mental health is an individual and personal matter and the standards of normal behaviour vary with time, place, culture and the expectations of society. Hence, there is wide variation in adaptive patterns and behavioural repertoires, depending on culture, subculture, ethnic group and family group (Jackson, 1967).

Mental health is also influenced by external factors, such as socioeconomic circumstances and physical health. For example, black people in the UK experience a disproportionate amount of long-term stress (unemployment, racism, poor housing, unrewarding roles in society) that increases their incidence of mental distress.

Consideration of a person's ethnic background may reveal alternative explanations for disturbed behaviour, because some genetic disorders are common in some ethnic groups. For example, Tay-Sachs' disease (common in the Jewish community) and Batten's disease (common among some Bengali people) may affect behaviour in some patients/clients.

Northern Ireland accounting for fewer numbers in every group. For Northern Ireland, censusdata concentrated on religious rather than ethnic group, and therefore detailed information is not currently available. For this reason, the following statistics refer to Great Britain (which excludes Northern Ireland). Between 1988-1990, the total ethnic minority population in Great Britain was about 2.58 million, an increase of 18% from 1981 (Jones, 1993). Figure 8-1 shows the estimated size of different ethnic minority populations in Great Britain in 1991.

The 1991 census was the first to collect information on the ethnic composition of the British population. The census found the population of Great Britain to be nearly 54.9 million, of which the ethnic minority population was just over 3 million or 5.5%. People of South Asian origin account for nearly one-half of this figure (2.6%), with Indians being the largest individual ethnic minority group. Black Caribbeans form the second largest group (slightly larger than the total Pakistani group), while Bangladeshis and Chinese each account for about 5% of all people from ethnic minorities (Centre for Research in Ethnic Relations, 1991).

As people from ethnic minorities have assimilated into British society, differences in the patterns of illness and disease, compared with those seen in the white population, have been identified by health and social services providers. Recent epidemiological data indicate that, when compared with the white population, people with different genetic and cultural backgrounds show a different pattern of disease and therefore require health services which are appropriate and sensitive to their needs.

The development of ethnic monitoring data within the UK has led to some debate on ethnicity. Some people believe ethnicity is related to minority ethnic groups within a larger host community; however, from a sociocultural perspective, we all belong to an ethnic group (Senior, 1965). A person is born into an ethnic group, but may also adopt characteristics of another ethnic group. For example, a child whose parents were born in a different country from where the family now resides may adopt the ethnicity of the host community; thus the child may consider himself or herself to be of different ethnicity from his or her parents.

Health and illness can be interpreted in terms of beliefs, expectations and personal experiences. Every ethnic group has its own beliefs and practices about health and illness. There are many approaches to health and illness, and people base their responses on beliefs and on cultural, religious, and ethnic backgrounds. The responses are culture-specific, based on patient's/clients' experiences and perceptions.

### Ethnic Minority Populations of the United Kingdom

Following the second World War, the main flow of migration to the UK was from Southern Ireland, Europe, and the New Commonwealth — primarily the Caribbean and the Indian subcontinent. People from black and **ethnic minority communities** now account for approximately 5.5% of the total population in the UK. Of this figure, the majority (over 6%) are located in England, with Wales (1.5%), Scotland (1.3%) and

### Learning Disabilities Nursing
### Culture, ethnicity and learning disabilities

Services for people with learning disabilities are currently structured essentially for white Anglo-Saxon English people. Consequently, people from large ethnic minority populations in the UK whose culture is not Anglo-Saxon may have difficulty accessing services.

In cultures where there is a fatalistic acceptance of an individual's learning disability, people may have little motivation to locate or use available services and facilities. In some of these cultures, women with learning disabilities are likely to be particularly disadvantaged.

In meeting the needs of a person with learning disabilities, it is important to understand and respect his or her cultural and ethnic background. It is easy to cause offence without realizing it — for example, by offering a pork pie to a Muslim or Hindu patient/client; or by a male nurse addressing himself directly to the female members of a family, a practice which is not acceptable in some cultures. Nurses should seek advice on the cultural and religious prescriptions of their patients/clients and should maintain contact with relevant community associations and religious leaders.

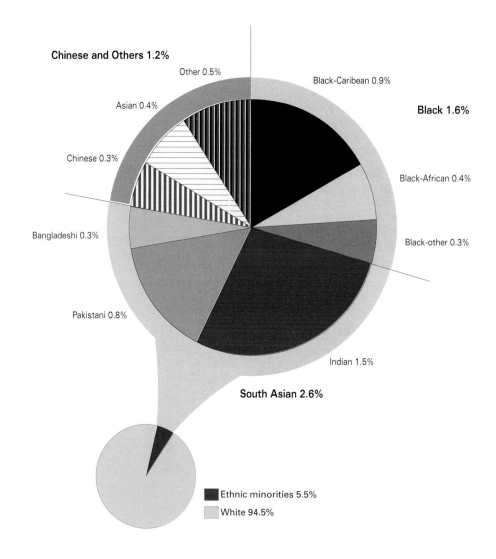

**Fig. 8-1** Ethnic group composition of Great Britain, 1991 as a percent of total population.
Source of data, Centre for Research in Ethnic Relations: *Ethnic Minorities in Great Britain: Settlement Patterns*, NEMDA 1991
Census Statistical Paper No. 1, Coventry, University of Warwick.

## Place of Birth

Forty-six percent of the ethnic minority group population were born in Great Britain, compared with 97% of the white population. Of the various minority ethnic groups, people of Afro-Caribbean (57%), other/mixed (53%), and Pakistani (50%) origin are most likely to have been born in Great Britain (Jones, 1993). Thirty-two percent of Bangladeshi people and 34% of African-Asian people were born in the British Isles. In contrast, approximately 74% of the Chinese population were born abroad. Of these, most were born in the New Commonwealth and Pakistani countries, and approximately 26% were born in the 'rest of the world', which includes China.

For all minority ethnic groups, the younger the age group, the higher the proportion of people born in the British Isles. Of all children under 16 from ethnic minority communities, 87% are born in the British Isles (Jones, 1993). Fig. 8-2 shows the general age distribution of the ethnic minority population compared to the white population in Great Britain.

## Regional patterns

There is considerable variation in the geographic distribution of ethnic minority populations in Great Britain. With the largest percentage of ethnic minorities living in England, more than one-half live in the southeast of England (compared to about 30% of white people); and four-fifths of this group live in Greater London. The other major concentration is in the West Midlands, mainly within the former metropolitan county (Fig. 8-3). This region contains over 14% of the total British ethnic minority population, but only 9% of the white population. Elsewhere, only West Yorkshire and Greater Manchester have a larger ethnic minority population than white population. The proportion in each of the three broad ethnic categories is highest in Greater

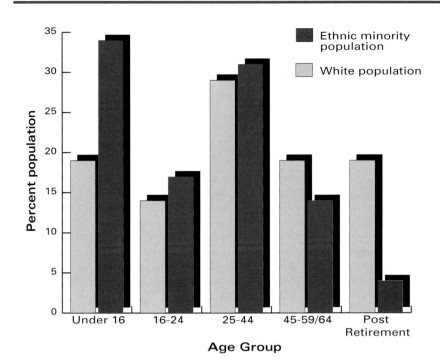

**Figure 8-2** Age distribution by ethnic group.
Source of data, Jones T: *Britain's Ethnic Minorities*, London, PSI Publishing, 1993.

London and the West Midlands metropolitan county. The black groups are most strongly represented in these two counties together with the metropolitan counties of the North West, Yorkshire and Humberside. In contrast, South Asians are much more widely distributed throughout Britain, with major concentrations in the East Midlands, Yorkshire and Humberside, and the North West. They form the largest ethnic minority group in most counties in Britain, except in Merseyside and Wales. Most people of mixed ethnic origin live in the South East, West Midlands, and North West (Centre for Research in Ethnic Relations, 1991).

## County-scale variations in ethnic minority composition

A regional analysis of ethnic minority populations demonstrated that most live in major conurbations and that most of these conurbations have a diverse ethnic mix.

Among local districts in Great Britain, Birmingham contains the largest number of people from minority ethnic groups, but there is a larger concentration of minority ethnic groups in Greater London. In Brent, nearly half the population is from minority ethnic groups, with Indians comprising the largest group (one sixth of the total borough population). Also notable is the very high concentration of Bangladeshis in Tower Hamlets, where they represent nearly 25% of the population. Black Caribbeans are the largest single ethnic group in south and central London, and Indians are more strongly represented in the northern and outer boroughs (Centre for Research in Ethnic Relations, 1991).

## Demographic differences between ethnic minority groups

According to the 1991 report, *The State of the Public Health*, from the Chief Medical Officer for Health (Calman, 1991), the following have been documented among ethnic groups in the UK:

- a higher rate of coronary heart disease mortality in people born in the Indian subcontinent.
- a higher rate of stroke mortality in people born in the Caribbean, the African Commonwealth and the Indian-subcontinent.
- rates of tuberculosis decrease more slowly in Indian, Pakistani and Bangladeshi people when compared to the indigenous white population.
- higher rate of schizophrenia in Caribbean people living in England (up to six times higher than the general population, and when compared with people living in Jamaica; the rate of mental illness in Asian people is reported to be lower, but there is recognition that health needs might not be fully identified).
- higher rates of perinatal mortality in Pakistani-born women and higher rates of congenital malformations in all Asian groups, but a lower sudden post-neonatal death of unknown cause in Asian people.

The Office of Population and Census Surveys (OPCS) is currently conducting a further study of morbidity statistics collated from general practice that will provide patient morbidity data by economic, family and housing status by ethnicity.

## FACTORS THAT INFLUENCE THE HEALTH OF ETHNIC MINORITY POPULATIONS
### Housing

It is widely accepted that adequate housing is one of the parameters of healthy living, but currently neither sufficient qualitative nor quantitative data exist for in-depth analysis of the relationship between housing and health in the UK. There is clear evidence, however, of a correlation between poor housing conditions and ill-health (Heginbotham, 1985). Housing can be a

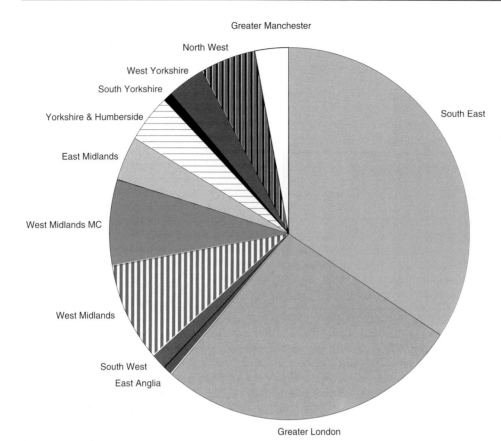

**Figure 8-3** Ethnic minorities in England by region, 1991. Source of data, Centre for Research in Ethnic Relations: *Ethnic Minorities in Great Britain: Settlement Patterns*, NEMDA 1991 Census Statistical Paper No. 1, Coventry, University of Warwick.

source of short-term stress and significant long-term problems. Poor housing is often associated with poor environmental amenities, such as play space for children. Research has shown that housing problems are a significant source of stress, depression and schizophrenia and that the role and place of housing in contributing to psychiatric and physical morbidity has been undervalued in past decisions of health care (Heginbotham, 1985).

## Education

Education is also distributed inequitably in some areas of the UK and it could be argued that inequalities in income and education are linked to the continuing inequality in health across social classes. Lefcowitz (1983) suggests that the level of education is more important than income in explaining health, and that the more education an individual has, the more frequently that person will see the doctor and the more medical services will be consumed when the person is in need. Furthermore, educated people are more likely to adopt lifestyles consistent with good health (Lefcowitz, 1983).

## Inherited diseases
### Hypertension

It is well established that people of Afro-Caribbean ethnic origin are much more likely to suffer from hypertension. Analysis of hospital admission data and screening surveys in the US and at several centres in the UK have identified the prevalence of hypertension among Afro-Caribbean people (Langford, 1981; Sever, 1981). These studies have found that, allowing for the standardization of age, black people are six times more likely than white people to have hypertension, and that these results are reflected in mortality rates for hypertension-related diseases.

Review of both Langford's and Sever's studies suggests that the causes of hypertension are not well understood. In an attempt to explain the difference between black and white populations, arguments have supported both environmental and genetic causes. But in the absence of a causal relationship, no preventive programmes have been devised, and in the absence of known symptoms to the general public, people with high blood pressure do not report themselves to be ill. Although it is generally assumed that hypertension will be identified in the course of consultations with the GP, many people may not consult their GP frequently.

## Diabetes

Diabetes mellitus (type II) is known to be one of the five leading causes of death by disease in the West Indies. This form of the disease tends to occur in families. There is some evidence that West Indians are more likely than others to develop diabetes, but this is only becoming apparent as more people reach the peak age for onset of the disease (Nikolardes *et al*, 1981). The prevalence of diabetes in people of Asian and Caribbean origin living in the

**Table 8-1 Diseases: Ethnic connection**

| Ethnic group | Disease |
| --- | --- |
| English | Cystic fibrosis, pernicious anaemia |
| Irish | Lung cancer, tuberculosis |
| Jewish | Tay–Sachs' disease, Niemann–Pick disease |
| Italians | Congenital hip dislocation |
| Asians | Lactose intolerance, rickets, tuberculosis |
| Afro-Caribbeans | Catarrhal child syndrome, hernias (eg. umbilical) |

Adapted from: Qureshi B: *Transcultural medicine: dealing with patients from different cultures*, London, 1994, Kluwer Academic Publishers.

UK is twice that of the general population (Cruickshank, 1989). There is a fivefold increase of type II diabetes in Asians (Simmons *et al*, 1989).

## Sickle Cell Disease

Sickle cell is an inherited disease which is most common in Afro-Caribbean people, although it is also found in people from the Mediterranean, Middle East and India. If a child inherits a sickle cell gene from one parent only, he or she is said to have sickle cell trait. If sickle cell genes are inherited from both parents, the child has sickle cell disease. The haemoglobin of people with sickle cell disease is abnormal and, when the red blood cells release their oxygen into the tissues, they become sickle or crescent-shaped. They may block small blood vessels, causing severe pain. Also, because the cells are fragile, they may disintegrate. If this situation becomes severe, the patient/client becomes anaemic.

People with sickle cell are particularly at risk when undergoing general anaesthetic. Those from high-risk races, particularly children, may be automatically screened on admission to hospital. Genetic counselling may be offered to parents.

## Thalassaemia

Thalassaemia is also an inherited disorder of haemoglobin synthesis, and is most common in peoples of Mediterranean origins and those from South East Asia.

## Tay–Sachs' Disease

Tay-Sachs' disease and Niemann-Pick disease are enzyme abnormalities, which cause eye and brain disorders. These are found most commonly in children of Jewish origin, who usually die within the first few years of life. Genetic counselling and bereavement support are required in such circumstances (Qureshi, 1994).

## THE INTERACTION OF ETHNIC MINORITIES WITH HEALTH SERVICES

The diverse needs of our changing population are the result of a variety of **sociocultural changes**. One of these changes was the 'post-war boom'. After the war, the UK was short of skilled labour and large numbers of migrant workers came to work as labourers on the railways, farms, and in foundries and other industries. Although the UK was keen to facilitate the migration of skilled and semi-skilled workers, it made no long-term plans for the health and welfare of the immigrants or their children and families. Consequently, various factors contributed to the poor mental and physical health of the immigrants. In addition to poor housing and living conditions, their self-esteem was diminished by working in jobs which were not commensurate with their skills, and through educational discrimination against their children, who invariably spoke other languages and were rated 'educationally inferior' on the culturally-biased educational psychological tests used in the UK (Fryer, 1985).

Patients/clients and their advocates have argued that health care in the UK is both eurocentric and discriminatory to people from black and minority populations. The health care has been described as inadequate, inappropriate, and inaccessible to many people from black and minority ethnic communities.

The initial response of the National Health Service (NHS) to new immigrants is prompted by Immigration Officers who refer the new immigrants to the Medical Officer of Health of the area to which they are relocating (McNaught, 1983). Early interaction of immigrants with the NHS involves both an educational and screening service. The Health Department's procedure is to visit the immigrants as soon as possible after arrival in order to:

- give information about local medical services, including the need for and the procedure for registering with a GP.
- test for immunity to TB, including chest x-ray, with immunization to follow, if necessary.
- encourage registration of children with the Local Education Authority.
- arrange medical examinations for children entering school in order to discover defects requiring remedial treatment, establish the presence of any disease requiring treatment, and commence required immunizations (Dodge, 1969).

Care of people from ethnic minority communities was implemented in varying standards until the reorganization of the NHS in 1974. Since 1974, the Local Authority Health Service has been integrated with the District Health Service; the role of the Medical Officer of Health has been redefined, and reports relating to the health of ethnic minority people have been discontinued (Yellowes, 1980). Recently, NHS purchasers have begun to consider the service delivery implications from cultural perspectives.

### Access to Health Care

Health services are being delivered to an increasingly **multiracial** and **multicultural** society. However, it is only recently that formal strategies have been published to meet the needs of this diverse population. In 1993, the Secretary of State, Virginia Bottomley, reported:

> I am determined to ensure . . . equal access to services for all sections of the community. The services may not always reach people from ethnic minorities as comprehensively as they should . . . Health Authorities need to recognize and respond to people's different needs and expectations. This will depend on a whole range of factors, such as, geographical location, age, health status and socioeconomic background. Race is also a very important consideration in commissioning for health care.

A higher proportion of women than men from ethnic minorities come into contact with the health services in their communities, largely because they have undertaken caring roles (GLC Ethnic Minorities Committee Report, 1985). Although black women interact with the health services in the same way as non-black women (Whitleg, 1982), it is clear that they do not have equal access to the health services. Dungate (1984) suggests that black and ethnic minority people do not have equal access to the statutory and voluntary services, are not referred from hospitals and other agencies, and that health services are often organized around the needs of white people and are of little practical help to black and ethnic minority communities.

Fenton's (1985) survey demonstrated the inequality of access in relation to further referrals within the health services. The survey found that Asian and Afro-Caribbean people had more difficulty than white people in gaining access to services beyond primary care. Where they were referred to hospital, black people often reported facing more difficulties in their relations with hospital staff than with their GPs.

## Use of Health Services

West Indians tend to prefer private medical practitioners to National Health Service doctors. To the West Indian, a full medical examination, whatever the complaint, is considered an important part of the treatment process.

Fenton's (1985) survey of the welfare of Afro-Caribbean and South Asians in Bristol found that a significant majority of Afro-Caribbean people are likely to seek a second, private opinion after consulting their GP, either because of dissatisfaction with their own GP, or because of a feeling that buying the time of the practitioner is the only way to ensure proper attention. Fenton noted that some Afro-Caribbean people reported feeling that they were treated as second-class citizens in medical situations; some reported the tendency among doctors and receptionists to patronize black people (Fenton, 1985).

These perceptions were partly corroborated by a survey reported by Tucket, whose analysis of more than 1000 general practice consultations demonstrated that Afro-Caribbean people were, on average, given shorter consultations and were less likely than other patients/clients to be given clear information and explanations by their GPs (Tucket *et al*, 1985).

Currently, data about ethnicity of patients/clients are not readily collected in the NHS; information is therefore scarce and mainly confined to *ad hoc* studies (Calman, 1991). It is not yet

### Adult Nursing
### Cultural considerations: naming systems

Naming systems vary in different parts of the world. Names may be personal and individual, or they may indicate family or clan, a class or caste, a gender or a religion.

Personal names may have particular significance within a nation, tradition or religion.

Family or clan names may appear after the first name (as in Britain) or before (as in China). In very small villages in some countries, there may be only two or three clans, and family names are not necessary. In some societies the family name is passed through the male, in others through the female. In some cases married women retain their family name in addition to their married name.

Class or caste may be indicated by names. For example, Patel is a middle-class Hindu name. Double-barrelled names in Britain traditionally had upper class associations.

Religion can also also be significant in the awarding of names. Sikh boys are called 'singh' meaning 'lion', while girls are called 'kaur' meaning 'princess'. Sometimes these names are used as a surname, for example Mr Singh or Mrs Kaur. In Islam the names Mohammed, Allah and Ullah may be placed before a personal name.

Gender can also be indicated in names. In Islam, female personal names may be followed by Begum or Bibi, which are courtesy titles. For Hindus, Shrimati (Mrs) or Kumari (Miss) are courtesy titles. In Sikhism, it is the religious name which indicates gender rather than the personal name. For example Rajinda-Singh.

Squires A (ed); *Multicultural Health Care and Rehabilitation of Older People*, 1991, London, Edward Arnold.

possible to give a full explanation of the differences, and until ethnic monitoring of service users is fully implemented, analysis will be incomplete.

## HEALTH CARE PLANNING FOR ETHNIC MINORITY POPULATIONS
### Access to Care

Interacting and coping with the health care system in the UK is a continuous struggle for many people from black and ethnic minority groups. Invariably, their struggle is made worse by a lack of service provision, inadequate access to health care, and discrimination. Even second and third generation black offspring from settlers who came to the UK in the 1950s are not given clear information of where to go for support or help, and are not told of the benefits to which they are entitled. Most access to health information is through informal networks such as family, friends and colleagues; however, this communication breaks down when there is displacement of families, poor interaction between communities, and discrimination. Consequently, there is a need to develop other methods of communicating health information to people who may otherwise have difficulty obtaining and assessing the information. It is important for nurses to be appropriately informed about health information for people from ethnic minorities, such as *Services on Health and Race Exchange* (SHARE), published regularly by the King's Fund Centre. This type of information helps improve services for black and ethnic minority communities and helps decrease discrimination in health care delivery.

## Providing Appropriate Care

There is increasing recognition of the need for health services to address particular needs of black and ethnic minorities living in the UK, and to take positive steps to eliminate discrimination within the Health Service (NAHAT, 1988). Discrimination is defined as 'less favourable treatment of individuals or groups on the grounds of culture, colour, race, ethnicity, religious or national origin' (NAHAT, 1988). Discrimination might occur unintentionally in service provision; for example, when health care intervention is inappropriate and insensitive. Nurses must eliminate discrimination in nursing care by ensuring patients/clients have:

- respect for the patient's/client's standards of dignity and privacy.
- information in languages of ethnic minority communities.
- available link workers, interpreters and advocates.
- available women doctors for women patients.
- respect for and facilities for religious observance and access to spiritual advisers.
- appropriate diet, such as halal meat or vegetarian meals.

*The State of the Public Health: Chief Medical Officer of Health Report* (Calman, 1991) promoted full commitment to equal access to health services for members of black and ethnic minority communities:

- ensuring that members of black and ethnic minority communities understand the health service, what it offers, and when and how they can use it, and
- ensuring that all health services, including preventative services, are appropriate to the health care needs of the local population (including the black and ethnic minority population) and that they are delivered in a manner that is culturally sensitive.

## Health Care Expectations

Diverse cultural and ethnic groups have varying expectations of health care, which is often demonstrated in their use of alternative health care. A significant number of multi-ethnic people in the United Kingdom use a combination of holistic health care therapies (see Chapter 32). Some of the commonly used alternative therapies include acupuncture, aromatherapy, Bach flower remedies, healing, herbal medicine, homoeopathy, reflexology and massage, and osteopathy.

## THE EFFECTS OF RELIGION ON HEALTH BELIEFS

**Religion** is a belief in a divine or superhuman power (or powers) to be obeyed and worshipped as the creator and ruler of the universe. Ethical values and **religious beliefs and practices**

### Children's Nursing
### Cultural considerations

It is important for nurses to be aware of differing attitudes towards children and to the cultural and religious beliefs and practices, and political ideologies which inform and influence attitudes about children (Crompton, 1992).

For example, current practice in infant feeding and child nutrition should focus on multicultural perspectives, rather than eurocentric perspectives. Since carers are motivated to influence their child's nutrition by doing what is good for the child, it is imperative that nurses understand the nutritional value of foods that are eaten by various ethnic groups. Such an understanding will enable nurses to give ethnic-sensitive nutritional information from which the client can make an informed choice.

further clarify ethnicity by providing a frame of reference and a perspective within which to organize information (Abramson, 1980). Religious teachings help formulate a meaningful philosophy and system of practices through a system of beliefs, practices, and social controls having specific values, norms, and ethics that vary between religious groups. Some religious practices are health related. For example, some religions teach that adherence to a code or mandate is conducive to harmony and health, and that breaking it may cause disharmony or illness (Thernstrom, 1980).

Health belief models are firmly rooted in religious philosophies, cultural patterns and value systems. The nurse's understanding of a range of common religious philosophies can be of much comfort for patients/clients in health and illness. Some of the most common religions among ethnic minorities in the UK are described below.

### Judaism

**Judaism** is not only a religion, but a religion of a race of people. Jewish people live all over the world and their skins are of varying colours. Despite this diversity, Neuberger (1994) claims that there is a strong sense of loyalty and peoplehood among Jews.

Jewish people regard Abraham as the first of three patriarchs who, together, were the founding fathers of the people of Israel. The Old Testament describes events through generations which led to the Exodus of Moses from Egypt. Moses and his people wandered the wilderness for 40 years before reaching the promised land. These events, however historically accurate, have made an enormous impact on Jewish religious practices. Examples of these are the observance of the Sabbath as the day of rest (as the slaves and animals rested in Egypt), the festival of the Passover (when the hand of God passed over Jewish households during one of the plagues affecting Egyptian people), or the offering of the bitter herbs (to represent the bitterness of slavery in Egypt).

Neuberger (1994, states that Jewish people, however orthodox, liberal or unpractising they seem, would find comfort in some tangible links with their roots. Examples of this might be the lighting of candles on a Friday evening at the start of the

Sabbath, a gift of unleavened bread at Passover, or a visit from a rabbi. Neuberger also emphasizes that Jewish people may feel offended by crucifixes hung on walls, or to be asked to kneel for prayer, as this is not a Jewish custom.

There are day-to-day customs which, if nurses sensitively observe, can make immense difference to the experience of the Jewish person's encounter with health care. For example, to Jewish people food can represent a connection with here-and-now reality, and life as it is. There may also be food restrictions, for example not to eat 'forbidden' foods such as pork or shellfish, not to eat meat and milk at the same meal or with the same utensils, or to eat only 'fit' or kosher food.

## Christianity

The fundamental tenet of **Christianity** is the belief in the historical existence of Jesus of Nazareth, who was born in Bethlehem about 2000 years ago. Christians believe that Jesus was born of a Jewish family and gave the last years of his life to teaching and miracle-working. His followers believed him to be the 'Annointed One' or Jewish Messiah. To many of his followers, Jesus was proclaimed 'The Son of God', and many Christians believe that Jesus is the Being through whom they approach God.

The two universally recognised Christian festivals are Christmas (when the birth of Jesus is celebrated) and Easter (when his death and resurrection are celebrated). During Lent, which lasts for 40 days and nights and prepares for Easter, many Christians will intentionally deprive themselves of a particular food or pleasure in a recognition of the belief that Jesus wandered for 40 days and nights in a wilderness in order to prepare for his crucifixion. Lent is a time when Christians may reassess themselves and work towards being 'better individuals' in the sight of Jesus. Whitsun, or Pentecost, celebrates the entering of the Holy Spirit into the disciples of Christ, enabling them to speak in 'tongues', or various languages, and thus spread the word of Christianity throughout the world.

Virtually all Christians believe in an afterlife, although concepts and descriptions of this vary. Some also contrast Heaven and Hell.

Christian religions take various forms:

- The Roman Catholic Church believes that the Pope is the spiritual descendent of Saint Peter. For practising Roman Catholics, Holy Communion is a regular practice, and, if an individual is unable to attend church, services at the bedside can be offered. If the person is dying 'the sacrament of the sick' or 'the last rites' should be offered. To Roman Catholics, the Virgin Mary is of great importance. Patients may derive comfort from a statues or rosaries.
- The Protestant Churches, developed during revolution against Catholic traditions, take many names and follow various forms of worship. The Church of Scotland and the Free Church differ in practices from the Church of England. As always, it is important to sensitively check with the patient and family what nurses can do, or organise, by way of religious support, or the facilitation of religious observances or practices.

- The Quakers (or religious Society of Friends) have no clergy but may be comforted by an overseer from the local Friends Meeting House.
- Other groups such as Plymouth Brethren, Jehovah's Witnesses and Mormons, which are not formally Christian, will need similar sensitivity to their beliefs and practices.

## Buddhism

**Buddhism** is a philosophy and a system of ethics. Buddhists believe in reincarnation and therefore conduct their lives by principles to avoid being demoted in the next life. Central to Buddhist principles are right thoughts, right words, right action and right direction. The ultimate goal of the Buddhist is to escape the eternal cycle of life and death and to attain a state of higher understanding. Buddhist laymen are obliged to observe five precepts: no killing, no stealing, no sexual misconduct, no falsehood and abstention from intoxicating substances (Silas). Buddhism promotes love for all living beings and respect for all forms of life. Buddhist practices are also based around charity, hospitality and self-discipline. Although there are several Buddhist sects, the two main schools are the Mahayana, found in China and Japan, and Therevadada, mainly found in South East Asia (Karmi, 1992).

The Therevadada celebrate the most important Buddhist festivals: the birth; the enlightenment; and the entry to Nirvana (death) of the Buddha on the day of Vesak. In addition to these dates, the Mahayana celebrate Ullambana (All Souls) and New Year as important festivals.

Nurses should be aware of the physical environment of the Buddhist, whose religious observance requires meditation and chanting. Incense is often burned during meditation. There are no specific dietary regulations, but many Buddhists are vegetarians through personal choice. Cremation is the preferred death rite for the Buddhist (Karmi, 1992).

## Hinduism

**Hinduism** is both a social system as well as a set of religious beliefs and its practices vary, depending on the Hindu's caste and the place from which he or she originated. It is believed that the caste or social status of the Hindu is determined by individual karma, which relates to rewards for good deeds and punishment for wrong doings.

Hindu festivals revolve around the moon. Important festivals are: Mahashivaratri, the birth of Shiva; Ram Naumi, the birth of Rama and the incarnation of Vishnu; Janmastanmi, the birth of Krishna; and Diwali, the festival of light.

A practising Hindu requires support from nurses and health care professionals to enable fasting. Some Hindus fast every week; some less often. In some cases, fasting may include eating only 'pure' foods, such as fruits, rather than complete abstinence.

Most Hindus do not eat meat or fish. Some castes which are considered to be lower may eat meat, but neither pork (because the pig is considered to be a scavenger) nor beef (because the cow is considered a sacred animal). Strict vegetarians may not eat eggs, as they are considered to be a potential source of life, or cheese which is made from animal rennet. They may also avoid onions and garlic, which are considered to be harmful stimulants.

A significant proportion of Hindus avoid tea, coffee and alcohol. It is always best to ask the patient/client about dietary regulations rather than to make assumptions (Karmi, 1992).

Nurses should be aware of the patient's/client's need for spiritual purity and physical cleanliness. Most Hindus prefer showers rather than baths, and gold is often worn next to the skin to ward off disease. It is important to ask the person's permission before removing any jewellery, because the item may have important personal, religious or cultural significance.

Wherever possible, the nurse should enable women patients/clients to be examined by women doctors. Cremation is the preferred death rite and, while post mortem examination is not prohibited, many Hindus consider the act to be highly disrespectful (Karmi, 1992).

## Islam

The literal meaning of **Islam** is a *submission to the wills of Allah.* Mekka (Mecca) in Saudi Arabia is the place of pilgrimage and the birthplace of the prophet Mohammed, and it is towards Mekka that Muslims face when praying. The Qur'an (Koran), the Holy Book of Islam, is believed to be the divine revelation from Almighty Allah.

Islam's foundation is grounded in five duties or pillars which guide the practising Muslim:

- Shahadah, a declaration of faith.
- five daily prayers which are preceded by ritual ablutions.
- fasting during Ramadam, one month of abstaining from food and drink from dawn to sunset (except women who are menstruating, pregnant or breast feeding, pre-adolescent children and people who are ill).
- Zakat, the giving of alms.
- Hajj, the pilgrimage to Mekka.

**Muslims** need the nurse's support to maintain general cleanliness. Where possible, bidets in bathrooms are ideal for the provision of water to necessitate ablutions prior to praying.

Muslims are required to eat halal meat, which means that the animal must be slaughtered according to strict Islamic laws. Pork is forbidden, as well as alcohol (Karmi, 1992).

Nurses need to be sensitive to the needs and practices of Muslims, such as:

- maintaining general cleanliness by providing bathrooms or water for ablutions and providing halal meat.
- supporting patients/clients during Ramadam who have special dietary needs such as diabetics or those with a gastric ulcer.
- supporting modesty of patients/clients – Muslim women may prefer to be examined in the presence of their husbands, and the dignity of the unmarried woman needs appropriate sensitivity.
- respecting religious observances, for example, dying Muslims may wish to face Mekka.
- enabling family and friends to sit in a quiet environment with the dying person, as they may wish to read the holy Qur'an or other appropriate supplications.
- supporting dying patients/clients and their families by placing

the dying individual onto his or her right side with the foot of the bed facing Mekka; in the event of death, mortuary staff should be asked to remove the Christian cross and candlesticks from the chapel altar and replace them with appropriate religious artifacts (Karmi, 1992).

## Sikhism

Sikh means disciple or follower. Sikhs are monotheistic and there is no priesthood. They believe in transmigration of the soul and in reincarnation. There is a strict code of discipline within which each individual strives to know God, to be kind, truthful and generous. There is also a strong sense of community in the gurdwara (Sikh temple). Local sikhs gather not only to worship, but also to share information and celebrate special occasions such as births and marriages. When a sikh person is ill at home or admitted to hospital, sikh leaders from the local gurdwara may visit the patient/client.

**Sikhism** embraces specific symbols of faith which should be respected by nurses. These are kes (uncut hair), kangha (a small comb worn in the hair under the turban), kara (a steel bangle), kirpan (a symbolic dagger) and kacha (special shorts or underpants).

## Chinese Religions and Customs

In China, religions are not as clearly differentiated as in the Western World. Religions may be based on Islam, Buddhism or Christianity. Broadly, it is suggested that the 'philosophical' expression within **Chinese religions** derives from a fusion of Confucianism, Taoism and Buddhism. The three chinese religions have four main aspects in common. These are:

- a belief in the goodness of human nature
- a belief in spiritual enlightenment and self-improvement through learning and training
- the view of the gods as personifications of the forces of nature
- the lack of appealing to devine revelation in order to support their teachings (Neuberger, 1994).

## New Age Spirituality

In recent decades, some people in the UK have looked beyond religious boundaries towards an idea of spirituality. They believe that people can be spiritual without believing in, or practising, a particular religion. Atheists, for example, do not believe in the presence of a creator, agnostics believe that the presence of a creator is difficult to prove.

Spirituality can be described as a state of awareness of one's eternal being which is formless, timeless and not confined to space at any particular time. Spirituality is a feeling of infinite worth in which 'the higher self' transcends human perceptions of religion and human limitations, and taps into the collective consciousness of humankind. Through spirituality, people find the inner strength to cope with adversity in life. Spirituality is about unconditional love for one's self and others; a commitment to working in harmony with life's purpose; recognising that every event and circumstance is an opportunity for growth and learning. Spiritual experiences enable one to find meaning and insight to life.

People often use visualisation, channelling or meditation to access their inner wisdom and inner knowing, and to sort out the questions and doubts of the rational mind. Inner knowing is fulfilled with inner contentment and transcends the thoughts of the rational mind. Faith, belief, unconditional love, non-judgement and trusting in the power of the universe are examples of this view spirituality.

## Nursing Care and Religion

Individual beliefs and practices are aspects of care which require a great deal of sensitivity.

Neuberger (1994) emphasizes this individuality and suggests that in many religions there is an orthodox, or traditional, movement, and one which is more liberal, or progressive. Divisions in religion may derive from a country or area or origin, for example Shi'ite or Sunni Muslims, and Sephardi or Ashkenazi Jews. Similarly, there are many variations of Christianity, such as Roman Catholic and Protestant.

Attaching a religious label to an individual may actually give little indication as to the care they would wish to receive. For example, some people might describe themselves as Jewish, Church of England, or Muslim and gain comfort or security from this. However, nurses could then assume that these individuals may follow certain rituals (for example, praying, cleansing or fasting) and could ask well-intentioned questions about how the rituals could be incorporated into care. Patients who do not follow the suggested rituals could then feel that the nurses are prying when they ask questions.

Despite the multifarious and profound sensitivities attaching to this aspect of care, it is often the case, as Neuberger (1994) highlights, that individuals and their families will be pleased if nurses take an interest in their religious and cultural life; particularly if the questions are asked in a spirit of genuine enquiry. This aspect of care also offers tremendous potential for enrichment of the understanding of nurses and an exciting field for new learning.

### Key Terms

Buddhism, p. 172
Chinese religions, p. 173
Christianity, p. 172
Culture, p. 164
Ethnic minorities/populations, p. 165
Ethnicity, p. 164
Hinduism, p. 172
Individuality/individual beliefs, p. 173
Islam, p. 173
Judaism, p. 171
Multicultural society, p. 164, 169
Multiracial society, p. 169
Muslim, p. 173
Religion/religious beliefs and practices, p. 171
Sikhism, p. 173
Sociocultural change, p. 169
Traditional approach to healing, p. 164
Transcultural communication, p. 163
Transcultural nursing, p. 164

## SUMMARY

Nurses need to be aware of and sensitive to the cultural needs of patients/clients when caring for them at home or in hospital. The body of transcultural nursing is rapidly growing, and it is imperative that nurses from all cultural backgrounds be aware of nursing implications in this area. The practice of nursing today demands that the nurse identifies and meets the cultural needs of diverse groups; understands the social and cultural reality of the patient/client, family, and community; develops expertise to implement culturally acceptable strategies to provide nursing care; and identifies and uses resources available and acceptable to the patient/client (Boyle, 1987).

## CHAPTER 8 REVIEW
### Key Concepts

- Before assessing the cultural background of a patient/client, nurses should assess how they are influenced by their own cultures.
- The way that cultural background and religion may influence behaviours, attitudes, and values depends on many factors, and thus may not be the same for individual members of a cultural group.
- The patient/client-centred concept of nursing is evolving through patient/client focused care and other models of nursing.
- The way a person seeks to meet basic human needs is influenced by culture, and may also be influenced by religious beliefs; therefore, the planning and implementation of nursing interventions should be adapted as much as possible to the individual patient/client.
- Nurses who are involved in purchasing and contracting processes need to analyse demographic factors in order to inform the process.

## CRITICAL THINKING EXERCISES

1. What benefits might an understanding of health belief models of diverse cultures bring to the development of nursing knowledge and skills?
2. What role does demographic information play in purchasing and commissioning of health care?
3. How might a nurse's knowledge of religious observance support culturally sensitive nursing?
4. How might a patient's/client's spiritual connections be enhanced within health care environments?
5. Ms. Recvaditch recently arrived from Bosnia as a refugee. She has been admitted to hospital for the first time in her life. She appears apprehensive. What might nurses do to help her adjust to this strange environment?
6. Mr Jabar is a practising Muslim and on a clear liquid diet. He refuses to eat the jelly that he is served. What intervention would be helpful in respect to his diet?
7. What could be done by nurses to ensure that patients/clients are not given appointments on key religious days and festivals?

# REFERENCES

Abramson HJ: *The Harvard encyclopedia of American ethnic groups,* Cambridge, Mass, 1980, Harvard University Press.

Bottomley V: Secretary of State for Health: My new year resolution for the NHS, *Health Service Journal,* 103 (5334):43, 1993.

Boyle JS: The practice of transcultural nursing, *Transcultural Society Newsletter* 7:2, 1987.

Calman K: *The state of the public health,* Chief Medical Officer of Health Report, 1991, HMSO.

Centre for Research in Ethnic Relations: NEMDA 1991 Census Statistical Paper, Coventry, 1991, University of Warwick.

Crompton M: *Children and counselling,* London, 1992, Edward Arnold.

Cruikshank JK: Diabetics: contrast between peoples of black (West African), Indian and white European origin. In Cruikashank JK, Beevers DG, editors: *Ethnic factors in health and disease,* London, 1989, Wright.

Dodge JS: *The field worker in immigrant health,* New York 1969, Staples Press.

Dungate M: *A multi-racial society: the role of voluntary organisations,* London, 1984, Bedford Square Press.

Fenton S: *Race, health and welfare: Afro-Caribbean and South Asian people in central Bristol,* Health and Social Services Department of Sociology,1985, Bristol University.

Fryer P: *The history of black people in Britain,* London, 1985, Pluto Press.

GLC: *Ethnic minorities committee report: ethnic minorities and the Health Service in London,* London, 1985, GLC.

Heginbotham C: Health and housing. In *Hospital and Health Services Review,* 81 (5): 218, 1985.

Horton CR, Karmi G: *Guidelines for implementation of ethnic monitoring in health service provision,* London, 1992, Northeast and Northwest Thames Regional Health Authority.

Ibrahiam A, Hersi A: *London Black woman's health action project annual report 1987-1988,* London, 1988, Bethnal Green Hospital.

Jackson RD: Play, paradox and people: the myth of normality. *Medical Opinion and Rev* 3:28, 1967 London.

Jones I: *Britain's ethnic minorities,* London, 1993, PST Publishing.

Kaplan L: *Education and mental health,* New York, 1971, Harper & Row.

Karmi G: *The ethnic health file: a guide for health professionals who care for people from ethnic backgrounds,* London, 1992, Northeast and Northwest Thames Regional Health Authority.

Langford HG: Is blood pressure different in back people? *Post Graduate Medical Journal* 57:748-754, 1981.

Lefcowitz MJ: Poverty and health on re-examination, *Inquiry* No 10, 3-13, 1983.

McNaught: *Race and health care in the United Kingdom,* Occasional Papers in Health Service, London, 1983, HMSO.

Mori L: *East London health: research study conducted for City and East London FHSA,* London, 1993, Mori.

National Association of Health Authorities and Trusts: *Action not words: a strategy to improve health services for black and minority ethnic groups,* Birmingham, 1988, NAHAT.

Neuberger J: *Caring for dying people of different faiths 2e,* London, 1994, Mosby.

Nikolardes et al: West Indian diabetic population of a large inner-city diabetic clinic, *British Medical Journal* 21(11):81, 1981.

Qureshi B: *Transcultural medicine: dealing with patients from different cultures,* London, 1994, Kluwer Academic Publishers.

Senior C:*The Puerto Ricans: strangers then neighbors,* Chicago, 1965, Quadrangle Press.

Sever PS: Racial differences in blood pressure: genetic and environmental factors,

*Post Graduate Medical Journal* 57:755-759, 1981.

Simmons D, Williams DR, Powell MJ: Presence of diabetes in a predominantly Asian community: preliminary findings of the Coventry diabetic study, *BMJ*, 298:18-21, 1989.

Squires A: *Multicultural health care and rehabilitation of older people,* London, 1991, Edward Arnold.

Thernstrom S: *The Harvard encyclopedia of American ethnic groups,* Cambridge, Mass, London, 1980, Harvard University Press.

Tucket et al: *Meetings between experts,* London, 1985, Tavistock Publications.

Whitleg J: *Inequalities in health care: problems of access and provision,* London, 1982, Straw Barnes.

Yellowes P: *Medical examination of immigrants,* London, 1980, Department of Health and Social Services.

## Further Reading
### Adult Nursing

Au K, Au W: *Working with Chinese carers: a handbook for professionals working with Chinese carers,* London, 1992, Health Education Authority.

Balarajan R, Raleigh S: *Ethnicity and health: a guide for the NHS,* London, 1993, DOH.

Henley A: *Caring for Sikhs and their families: religious aspects of care ,* Cambridge, 1983, National Extension College. (Asians in Britain series)

Henley A: *Caring for Muslims and their families: religious aspects of care,* Cambridge, 1983, National Extension College. (Asians in Britain series)

Mares P: *Health care in multiracial Britain,* Cambridge, 1985, Health Education Council and National Extension College.

Waldergrave W: Government's commitment to ethnic minority issues, London, 1991, DOH Press Release H91/627.

### Childrens Nursing

Alderman C: A Colour-Blind Health Service (Action for sick children report on child health services for ethnic minorities) *Nursing Standard.* 17 (3): 18-19), 1993.

Arnold E & James M: Trading black families for black children in care: a case study. *New Community.* 417-425, 1989.

Black J: *Child health in a multicultural society,* London, 1989, British Medical Journal.

Duggan M B *et al:* Iron status, energy intake, and nutritional status of health in young Asian children. *Archives of Disease in Childhood,* 66 (12): 1386-9, 1991

Hodge S: Disorders of children of ethnic minorities, *Maternal and Child Health.* 10 (4): 114-), 1985.

Niederhauser V P: Health care of immigrant children: incorporating culture into practice, *Pediatric Nursing* 15 (6): 569-74, 1989.

Weller B F: Cultural aspects of children's health and illness, In Lindsay B Ed: *The child and the family: contemporary nursing issues in child health and care.* London, 1994, Bailliere Tindall.

### Learning Disabilities Nursing

Baxter C, et al: *Double discrimination: issues and services for people with learning difficulties from black and ethnic minority communities,* London, 1990, King's Fund Centre.

Gunaratnam Y: *Dekhbaal lai pukkar/call for care,* London, 1992, Health Education Authority.

Manchester Council for Community Relations and the King's Fund Centre: *Awaaz,* Manchester, 1990, MCCR.

McCalman J: *The forgotten people: carers in three minority ethnic communities in Southwark,* London, 1990, King's Fund Centre.

## Mental Health Nursing

Burke A (ed): Is racism a causatory factor in mental illness? *Int J Social Psych* 30(1):2, 1984.

Burke A: Racism and psychological disturbance among West Indians in Briatin, *Int J Social Psych* 30(2):50, 1984.

Fernando S: Racism as a cause of depression, *Transcultural Psych* 30:41, 1984.

Fernando S: *Race and culture in psychiatry,* Beckenham, 1988, Croom Helm.

Lipsedge M, Littlewood R: Transcultural psychiatry. In Granville-Grossman (ed): *Recent advances in psychiatry,* Edinburgh, 1979, Churchill Livingstone.

Littlewood R, Lipsedge M: Acute psychotic reactions in Caribbean-born patients, *Psychol Med* 2:303, 1981.

Littlewood R, Lipsedge M: *Aliens and alienists: ethnic minorities and psychiatry,* New York, 1982, Penguin USA.

Littlewood R, Lipsedge M: Some social and phenomenological characteristics of psychotic immigrants, *Psychol Med* 2:289, 1981.

Mama A: Mental health and black women, *GLC Women's Committee* issue 23, 1985.

Mitchell J: *What is to be done about illness and health?* Harmondsworth, 1984, Penguin.

Wilson M: *Mental health and Britain's black communities,* London, 1993, King's Fund Centre.

# Health and Illness

## LEARNING OUTCOMES

After studying this chapter, you should be able to:
- *Define the key terms listed.*
- *Discuss the definition of health and related concepts.*
- *Discuss the health-illness continuum, high-level wellness, agent-host-environment, health belief, evolutionary-based, and health-promotion models.*
- *Describe internal and external variables that influence an individual's health beliefs and practices.*
- *Describe health-promotion and illness-prevention activities.*
- *List and discuss the three levels of preventative care.*
- *List and explain four interrelated kinds of risk factors.*
- *Describe variables influencing illness behaviour.*
- *List and discuss the stages of behaviour a patient/client may manifest during adjustment to illness.*
- *Describe the impact of illness on the patient/client and family.*
- *Discuss the nurse-patient/client relationship in health and illness.*

In the past, most individuals and societies have viewed good health or wellness as the opposite of or absence of disease. This attitude towards health remains popular with many health professionals. It assumes that people are normally healthy and that people with disease are unhealthy and in an abnormal state. This simple, either-or attitude can be easily applied; a person is considered healthy or ill, with no range in between. Nevertheless, this attitude ignores states of health *between* disease and good health. Also, it emphasizes the physiological dimension of a person, considering only the body as ill or healthy. In addition, this limited view overlooks the complex interrelationships between the physiological, emotional, intellectual, sociocultural, developmental, and spiritual dimensions.

Since Nightingale's time, there has been an association between the practice of nursing and the concept of health (Tripp-Reimer, 1984). Today's health and medical care services are shaped largely by the way health professionals and consumers define health and illness (Weitzel, 1989; Balog, 1982).

Health care professionals' definitions serve as bases for determining about the types and quality of health care services that should be provided. Not all health care professionals, however, agree on the definition of these concepts. Consumers of health care frequently view their health as an absence of disease, and the better people believe their health to be, the more active they are in maintaining those levels of health (Yarcheski and Mahon, 1989; Weitzel, 1989).

However, the definition of good health or wellness, from a health care worker's perspective, may not always correspond with a patient's/client's concept. Each patient's/client's concept of health and health care practices is unique and based on lifestyle, cultural background, spiritual beliefs, and economic and psychosocial status. Therefore, to provide individualized care for the patient/client, the nurse needs to be aware of variables influencing health beliefs and practices.

People also have different attitudes about illness and react to it in different ways (Downie *et al*, 1991). Medical sociologists call the reaction to illness, **illness behaviour**. The nurse needs to understand the way that patients/clients react to illness and the way that illness affects patients/clients and families. Illness can have an enormous impact on them. The nurse who recognizes this impact and the factors involved can take steps to minimize the effects of illness and assist the patient/client and family in maintaining or returning to the highest level of functioning.

The nurse also identifies actual and potential **risk factors** that predispose a person or group of people to illness (Roper *et al*, 1983). Risk factors are genetic, behavioural, environmental, gender, and age-related items that predispose an individual to an increased risk for disease. Types of risk factors are discussed later in this chapter. Nursing actions involving health promotion and illness prevention assist the patient/client not only in maintaining and increasing the existing level of health but also in achieving an optimal level of health.

The nurse assesses all dimensions of the whole person, including the physical, intellectual, emotional, developmental, and spiritual aspects (Orem, 1991). The nurse also observes interactions with family and community. To assist the patient/client in health maintenance and promotion, illness prevention, and adaptation to the changes that illness produces in every dimension of functioning, the nurse must understand all these dimensions (Edelman and Mandle, 1990).

## DEFINITION OF HEALTH

Good health or wellness is not merely the absence of illness. Defining good health is difficult, because each person has a personal concept of health. Health is a state of being that people define in relation to their own values.

The World Health Organization (WHO) defines health as a "state of complete physical, mental and social well-being, not merely the absence of disease or infirmity" (WHO, 1947). This definition of health has not been universally accepted by health care workers. Those opposed to it believe that it is unrealistic, because people from underdeveloped countries and many persons of low economic status would not be considered healthy (Fuchs, 1974). In addition, the WHO definition is difficult to use when trying to determine scientifically who is or is not healthy, or to determine the point at which a person becomes ill rather than healthy (Breslow, 1972).

The WHO definition, however, has the following characteristics that promote a more positive **concept of health** (Edelman and Mandle, 1990):

1. A concern for the individual as a total system.

**Children's Nursing**
**Children's beliefs about health and illness**

Children's knowledge of, and attitudes towards, health and illness change with age. It is important for health professionals to be aware of development and related beliefs, and to respond accordingly. For example, young children may feel that illness is a punishment and that all illnesses are contagious. Nurses should be aware of such development-related beliefs when talking to young children and when educating parents and carers.

2. A view of health that identifies internal and external environments.

3. An acknowledgment of the importance of an individual's role in life.

Another issue related to defining health is the unique ideas, convictions and attitudes of each patient/client towards health, which involves much more than the absence of illness or disability. To help patients/clients identify and reach health goals, the nurse must discover and use information about their concepts of health. As a result, health goals may be different for each patient/client.

Nurses also differ on their definitions of health. They plan care based on a definition of health and accepted standards of health care. In the Roper *et al* (1983) model of nursing each individual experiences different levels of health along a **dependent/independent** continuum. Health is related to how an individual can perform activities of daily living in relation to dependence and independence (Fig. 9-1).

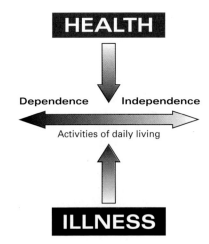

**Fig. 9-1** Health: dependence/independence continuum based on the activities of daily living (*Roper et al, 1983*).

Health in its broadest sense is a dynamic state in which the individual adapts to changes in internal and external environments to maintain a state of well-being. The *internal environment* includes many factors that influence health, including genetic and psychological variables, intellectual and spiritual dimensions, and disease processes. The *external environment* includes factors outside the person that may influence health, including the physical environment, social relationships, and economic variables. Because both environments change continuously, the person must adapt to maintain a state of well-being.

*Health* and *illness* therefore must be defined in terms of the individual. Health can include conditions that the patient/client or nurse may have previously considered to be illness. For example, a person with epilepsy who has learned to control seizures with medication and who functions at home and at work may now not consider himself or herself ill. Health is also closely related to an individual's lifestyle, and some illnesses can be considered to be the result of that lifestyle. A patient/client who experiences constant stress may have frequent gastrointestinal upsets. In such a case, treating the condition may have no effect on the pattern of behaviour, and the person may not even consider a gastrointestinal upset an illness at all if it seems a 'normal' or usual aspect of life. A health professional's rigid attitude towards health and illness, in which the whole person is not considered, may have little meaning for such a person's future health.

Therefore, because the attitudes of a patient/client and nurse towards health may not coincide exactly, the nurse can use the nursing process as a tool to work with the patient/client and family to mutually establish goals of care and plan individualized care (see Chapter 3).

## MODELS OF HEALTH AND ILLNESS

A model is a theoretical way of understanding a concept or idea. Because health and illness are complex concepts, models are used to understand the relationships between these concepts and the patient's/client's attitudes towards health and health practices.

**Health beliefs** are a person's ideas, convictions, and attitudes about health and illness. Health beliefs may be based on factual information or misinformation, common sense or myths, or reality or false expectations. Because **health behaviours** usually result from health beliefs, they can positively or negatively affect health. **Positive health behaviours** are activities related to maintaining, attaining, or regaining good health and preventing illness. Common **positive health behaviours** include immunizations, proper sleep patterns, and adequate exercise, diet, and nutrition. **Negative health behaviours** include practices actually or potentially harmful to health, such as smoking, drug or alcohol abuse, poor diet, and refusal to take necessary medication.

A patient's/client's health beliefs depend on many factors, including perception of the level of health, modifying factors such as demographics, personality, and perception of benefits resulting from positive health behaviours. Health models usually incorporate many of these components.

### High-Level Wellness Model

First developed in the late 1950s and revised by Dunn (1977), the *high-level wellness* model is orientated towards maximizing the

health potential of an individual. This model requires the individual to maintain a continuum of balance and purposeful direction within the environment. It involves progress towards a higher level of functioning, an open-ended and ever-expanding challenge to live at the fullest potential. There is continued integration of health practices by the individual at increasingly higher levels throughout life (Dunn, 1959, 1977; Pender, 1987).

Nursing models of wellness are directed at behavioural change and have been successful in nurse-managed centres for older adults (Gilpatrick, 1989; Smith and Sorrell, 1989). In the *behavioural change* approach to wellness, nurses implement nursing interventions that help patients/clients modify selected high-risk behaviours. These interventions are in broad categories and are based on principles of adult learning (Gilpatrick, 1989).

Health care directed at helping a patient/client achieve *high-level wellness* emphasizes health-promotion and illness-prevention activities rather than treatment for illness. High-level wellness is a dynamic process, not a passive, static state.

The high-level wellness model can also be applied to family and community health. Families and communities have many functions, and high-level wellness involves successful functioning in an integrated manner.

### Agent-Host-Environment Model

The *agent-host-environment* model of health and illness originated in the community health work of Leavell *et al* (1965) and has since been expanded as a model for describing the cause of illness in other health areas. According to this approach, the level of health or illness of an individual or group depends on the dynamic relationship of the agent, host, and environment.

The **agent** is any internal or external factor that by its presence or absence can lead to disease or illness. Agents can be biological, chemical, physical, mechanical, or psychosocial. The presence of these agents does not mean a person will become ill, but an agent must be present (or absent, as in a lack of adequate nutrition) for a particular illness to occur.

The **host** is the person or persons who may be susceptible to a particular illness or disease. Host factors are physical or psychosocial situations or conditions putting an individual or group at risk for becoming ill. Examples of such factors are the host's family history, age, or lifestyle.

The **environment** consists of all factors outside of the host. Physical environment includes economic level, climate, living conditions, and elements such as light and sound levels. Social environment consists of factors involving a person's or group's interaction with others, including stress, conflicts with others, economic hardships, and life crises such as the death of a spouse.

The agent-host-environment model emphasizes that health and illness depend on the dynamic interaction of all three variables. Community health nursing has further developed the interaction between agent-host-environment into a causal model for addressing the health needs for homeless families (Fig. 9-2). This model, first developed by Pesznecker (1984) and recently reported by Berne *et al* (1990), proposes that health-promoting or health-damaging responses are shaped by interaction between the individual or group and the environment and that the responses are further mediated by public policy. For example, homeless persons are faced with a variety of stressors or agents that can affect their levels of health; exposure to inadequate shelter, crime, and exposure to nature's elements increase the homeless patient's/client's risk for illness.

The agent-host-environment model has been expanded into a general theory of the multiple causes of disease. Until recent decades, it was commonly believed that single causes of a disease could be identified. Infectious diseases in particular were thought to have single causes; the agents (for example the bacteria or viruses) were considered solely responsible. It is now recognized that most diseases have multiple causes, as the agent-host-environment model demonstrates. The theory of the multiple causes of disease is important to nurses because nursing emphasizes holistic care of the patient/client, which is based on knowledge of environmental, psychosocial, and lifestyle factors.

## Health-Belief Model
Rosenstock's (1974) and Becker and Maiman's (1975) **health-belief model** (Fig. 9-3) addresses the relationship between a person's belief and behaviours. It provides a way of understanding and predicting how patients/clients will behave in relation to their health and how they will comply with health care therapies. The three components of this model are:

1. **Individual's perception of susceptibility to an illness**. For example, a patient/client needs to recognize the familial link for coronary artery disease. After this link is recognized, particularly when one parent and two siblings have died in their fourth decade from myocardial infarction, the patient/client may perceive the personal risk of heart disease.

2. **The individual's perception of the seriousness of the illness**. This perception is influenced and modified by demographic and sociopsychological variables, perceived threats of the illness, and cues to action (for example, mass media campaigns and advice from family, friends, and medical professionals).

3. **The likelihood that a person will take preventive action** is the person's perception of the benefits and barriers to taking action. Preventive action may include lifestyle changes, increased adherence to medical therapies, or a search for medical advice or treatment. However, if a complex treatment regimen is prescribed, this may be perceived as too burdensome by the person.

The health-belief model helps nurses understand factors

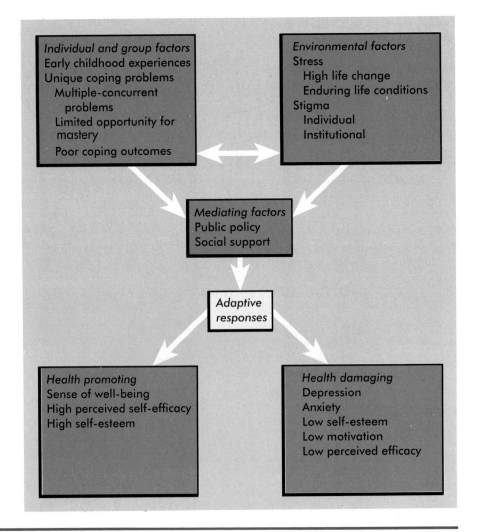

**Fig. 9-2** Adaptational model of poverty. Adapted from Pesznecker E: *Public Health Nurs* 1(4):237, 1984.

influencing patients'/clients' perceptions, beliefs, and behaviour and plan care that will most effectively assist patients/clients in maintaining or regaining health and preventing illness.

## Evolutionary-Based Model

The *evolutionary-based* model of health and viability is supported by the principle that illness and death sometimes serve an evolutionary function (Dixon, Dixon, 1984). The model (Fig. 9-4) interrelates the following elements:

- **Life events**, which reflect developmental variables and variables associated with chance, such as accidents or relocation.
- **Life-style determinants**, which are personal and learned adaptive strategies that an individual uses to make lifestyle changes.
- **Evolutionary viability** within the social context, which reflects the extent to which individuals function to promote survival and well-being (Dixon, Dixon, 1984).
- **Control perceptions**, which reflect the extent to which a person can influence the circumstances of life.
- **Viability emotions**, which are affective reactions developed from life events or lifestyle determinants.
- **Health outcomes**, which are the physiological, behavioural, and psychological states resulting from viability emotions and the other factors within the model.

With this model, nursing interventions can be developed for all six of the above patient/client dimensions. The full scope of clinical experience may require assisting patients/clients to regain a sense of viability. This is particularly important in nursing because of the opportunity for long-term contact with the patient/client and family (Dixon and Dixon, 1984).

## Health-Promotion Model

The *health-promotion* model proposed by Pender (1982, 1984) was designed to be a "complementary counterpart to models of health protection". Health promotion is directed at increasing a patient's/client's level of well-being (Pender, 1987). The model focuses on three functions (Fig. 9-5). It identifies factors (for example, demographic and social) that enhance or decrease participation in health promotion. The model also organizes cues into a pattern to explain the likelihood of a patient's/client's participation in health-promotion behaviours. The focus of this model is to explain the reasons individuals engage in health activities. It is not designed for use with families or communities. This model has been tested with a variety of populations because it is a reliable indicator of health promotion.

## VARIABLES INFLUENCING HEALTH BELIEFS AND PRACTICES

Nurses need to understand the variables that can influence patients'/clients' health beliefs and practices. Internal and external variables can influence how a person thinks and acts. Understanding the way in which these variables affect a

patient/client allows the nurse to plan and deliver individualized care for that patient/client.

## Internal Variables

Internal variables include a person's developmental stage, intellectual background, perception of personal functioning, and emotional and spiritual factors.

### Developmental Stage

A person's thought and behaviour patterns change throughout life. The nurse must consider level of growth and development when using the patient's/client's health beliefs and practices as a basis for planning care. For example, a young child is not generally able to recognize the potential seriousness of illnesses and needs to be motivated to act in ways beneficial to a treatment plan or to develop habits for illness prevention. An adolescent's emotional development may influence personal beliefs about health-related matters such as the use of contraception, and the nurse thus uses different techniques of teaching than would be used for a young adult. Knowledge of the stages of growth and development helps the nurse predict the patient's/client's response to the present illness or the threat of future illness. The planning of nursing care is then adapted to these expectations, as well as to the patient's/client's abilities to participate in self-care.

### Intellectual Background

A person's beliefs about health are shaped in part by intellectual variables, including knowledge (or misinformation) about body functions and illnesses, educational background, and past experiences. These variables influence a person's thoughts. In addition, cognitive abilities shape the way a person thinks, including the ability to understand factors involved in illness and to apply knowledge of health and illness to personal health practices. Cognitive abilities also relate to a person's developmental stage. A nurse considers intellectual background when trying to understand a patient's/client's beliefs about health and health practices so that these variables can be incorporated into nursing care.

### Perception of Functioning

The way a person perceives physical functioning affects health beliefs and practices. For example, people with chronic heart conditions perceive their levels of health differently than people who have never had major health problems. As a result, the health beliefs and practices of these people tend to be different. In addition, individuals who have successfully recovered from severe acute illnesses may change health beliefs and practices as a result of those illnesses.

When nurses assess a patient's/client's level of health, they gather subjective data about the way the patient/client perceives physical functioning, such as level of fatigue, shortness of breath, or pain. They also obtain objective data about actual functioning such as blood pressure, weight and height measurements. This information allows nurses to plan and implement individualized care effectively.

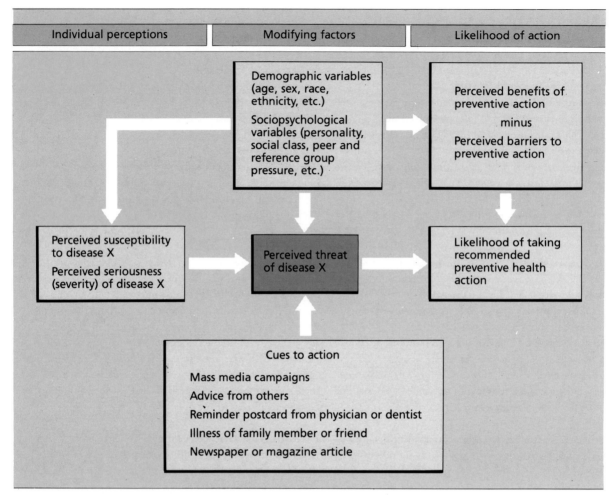

Fig. 9-3 Health belief model. From Becker MH, Maiman LA: *Med Care* 13(1):12, 1975.

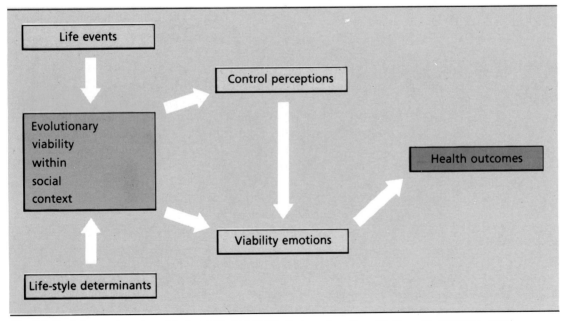

Fig. 9-4 Evolutionary-based model of viability and health. Redrawn from Dixon JK, Dixon JP: *ANS* 6(3):1, 1984.

## Emotional and Spiritual Factors

Emotional and spiritual factors also influence health beliefs and practices. A person experiencing a stress response with each change in life tends to respond to any sign of illness, such as worrying that the illness is life threatening. A person who generally is very calm may have little emotional response during illness, whereas an individual unable to cope emotionally with the threat of illness may deny the presence of symptoms and not take therapeutic actions. For example, a man who is breathless and coughs frequently may blame this condition on cold weather if he cannot emotionally accept the possibility of a respiratory illness. Many people have strong emotional reactions against even thinking about the risk of cancer and will deny symptoms and refuse to take preventive action. Other illnesses are more emotionally acceptable, however, and the person will be more

likely to acknowledge the symptoms and seek appropriate care.

If religious beliefs include the belief that physical health is necessary for spiritual health, patients'/clients' health practices will reflect that belief. On the other hand, if their religious beliefs require refusal of certain kinds of medical treatment, health care may be avoided. In some cases, patients/clients may believe that illness is a deserved punishment and thus do nothing to regain or maintain health. Thus, as with emotional variables, a nurse must understand patients'/clients' spiritual values to involve them effectively in nursing care.

## External Variables

External variables influencing a person's health beliefs and practices include family practices, socioeconomic factors, and cultural variables.

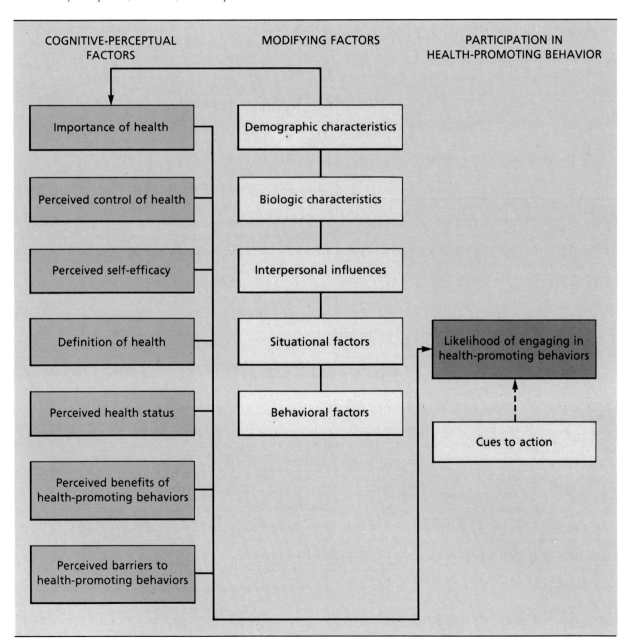

**Fig. 9-5** Health promotion model. From Pender NJ: *Health promotion in nursing practice, ed 2,* Norwalk, Conn, 1987, Appleton & Lange.

## Family Practices

The way that patients'/clients' families use health care services generally affects their health practices. Healthy families generally seek ways to help all members achieve their highest potential. Flexibility in healthy families encourages members to change role responsibilities. For example, men can assume some household and child-care responsibilities. Members are able to perform temporarily each others tasks (deChesnay and Magnuson, 1988).

If a child's parents treated every virus and illness as a potentially severe disease and immediately sought health care, the child generally does the same in adulthood. A person with this type of family background would be more likely to stay home from school or work with a cold, whereas others would attempt to carry on as usual. Likewise, adult patients/clients are also more likely to practise prevention if their families did so. For example, people whose parents took them for annual check-ups as children are more likely to take their own children for regular checkups.

## Socioeconomic Factors

Social and psychosocial factors can increase the risk for illness and influence the way that a person defines and reacts to illness. Psychosocial variables include the stability of the person's marital or intimate relationship, lifestyle habits, and occupational environment.

A person's social network is also related to health behaviour (Steele, 1982; Parsons, 1958). Neighbours, peers, and co-workers

---

### Children's Nursing
### Health promotion needs of children

Promoting health in children, in its broadest sense, means promoting health for the family unit. Children's nurses work in partnership with the family to promote self-care or to facilitate family care when the child has not developed maturity to undertake self-care. The nurse plans interventions to ensure the family unit is maintained.

---

are often aware of a person's level of health, and if the person is unexpectedly absent from work or a planned activity or is experiencing a symptom of illness, a member of the social network may encourage medical attention. A person generally seeks approval and support from social groups, and this desire for approval and support affects health beliefs and practices. For example, if it is socially acceptable in a particular peer group for teenage girls to smoke, the pressure to conform may be stronger than the concern about smoking being harmful to health.

Economic factors, like social factors, can affect a patient's/client's level of health by increasing the risk for disease, by influencing how a person lives and by limiting compliance with a prescribed treatment plan because of a lack of resources or poor living conditions.

Epidemiological studies have shown that people at low economic levels have a greater risk for pulmonary disease, cancer, and diabetes mellitus than people at higher levels (Goldsmith, 1975; Davidson, 1971). In addition, a large number of people at low economic levels live in urban areas and therefore have a greater risk for disease because of their environment.

## Cultural Background

Sociocultural differences between patients/clients and nurses can affect the nurse-patient/client relationship and the quality of nursing care delivered (Anderson, 1987). If nurses are not aware of their own and other cultural patterns of behaviour and language, they may not be able to recognize and understand a patient's/client's behaviour and beliefs and may have difficulty in interacting with the patient/client. For example, a patient/client from a culture that strongly values and expects close, warm, and supportive family relationships may experience cultural conflict with a nurse who does not value or has not experienced close kinship ties (Leininger, 1977). The nurse must identify and incorporate cultural factors into a patient's/client's care plan to avoid conflict between goals and methods of care and the patient's/client's cultural background.

## HEALTH PROMOTION AND ILLNESS PREVENTION

Nurses emphasize health promotion and illness-prevention activities as important forms of health care. Nurses assist patients/clients in maintaining good health and improving their levels of health instead of merely providing care after illness occurs. Health promotion and illness prevention are closely related concepts and, in practice, overlap to some extent. Activities involving **health promotion** help patients/clients maintain or enhance their present levels of health. Activities for **illness prevention** protect patients/clients from actual or potential threats to health. Both types of activities are future orientated. The difference between them involves motivations and goals. Health-promotion activities motivate people to act positively to reach the goals of more stable levels of health. Illness-prevention activities motivate people to avoid declines in health or functional levels.

Health-promotion activities can be passive or active. With **passive strategies of health promotion**, individuals gain from the activities of others without doing anything themselves. The fluoridation of municipal drinking water and the fortification of milk with vitamin D are two examples of passive health-promotion strategies.

With **active strategies of health promotion**, individuals are motivated to adopt specific health programmes. Weight reduction and smoking cessation programmes require patients/clients to be actively involved in measures to improve their present and future levels of wellness while decreasing the risk of disease.

Health-promotion and illness-prevention activities have become an important focus of health care. Although scientific and medical advances since the 1940s have resulted in cures for many infectious diseases, there are still no cures for many chronic diseases. Thus, there is greater motivation for preventing the occurrence of these diseases.

**Adult Nursing
Cultural influences on health
practices**

Cultural background influences individual beliefs,
values, and customs. It influences entry into the health
care system and personal health practices. Particular
sensitivities are needed in contraceptive or family
planning advice. For example, to a Muslim woman
menstruation is a curse and she will refuse to have a
vaginal examination, an intrauterine device insertion,
or the use of pessaries during this time. Some Chinese
women may not like the contraceptive pill, preferring to
use a Chinese remedy from an alternative practitioner.

**Learning Disabilities Nursing
Health promotion in people with
learning disabilities**

People with learning disabilities have the same rights
and responsibilities as anyone else. It is therefore
reasonable for a person with a learning disability to
take the same care of his or her health. In this context,
the targets identified by the four Health Departments
are equally relevant to people with learning disabilities.
The major difference lies in the input necessary to
ensure that people with learning disabilities eat
sensibly, exercise regularly, learn to recognize
hazardous situations, develop healthy interpersonal
relationships, do not smoke, and do not become
accidentally pregnant or infected with a sexually
transmitted disease.

**Access to appropriate information:** The key to
success in health promotion for people with learning
disabilities is role modelling of people who are
significant to them. When these patients/clients see a
carer eating junk food or smoking, or hear them
boasting about casual sex, then it should not be
surprising that they wish to emulate this behaviour.

**Healthy eating:** Patients/clients living independent
or semi-independent lifestyles in the community are at
risk for unhealthy eating behaviours. The difficulties of
budgeting and cooking healthy meals on a limited
budget makes these individuals more likely to eat 'junk'
food, which is high in damaging fatty acids and
deficient in vitamins and minerals.

**Social skills training and sex education:** It is sensible
and most productive to teach these issues using a
'lifestyle' approach. For example, teach the individual
about assertiveness skills (including the right to say
'no'), before teaching him or her about contraception.
Because some patients/clients have difficulty in
generalizing information, it is best not to focus on
specific issues. Instead, it is better to tackle these
issues in the context of relationships and
responsibilities (Johnson, 1987; RCN, 1991).

**Parenting skills:** Whether or not people with
learning disabilities can or should parent is a
controversial issue. Many couples (where either or
both partners have a learning disability) make a
positive choice not to have children because they
recognize their own limitations. Other couples actively
choose to have children — a decision that may cause
anxiety and concern for family members and health
professionals. It is critical that people with learning
disabilities who choose to become parents receive
parentcraft training. Such training takes account of
their own experiences and provides continual support
for the parent and his or her ability to care for the child.

Pender (1987) has developed the Lifestyle and Health Habits
Assessment (LHHA), which is divided into 10 sections (see box).
The assessment tool uses yes and no responses. The rating in each
section, as well as the total score, provides the information
necessary to design an individualized health-protection and
health-promotion programme for the patient/client. Use of the
LHHA may increase the patient's/client's awareness of living
patterns and assist in motivating behaviour changes (Pender,
1987).

The goal of a **total health programme** is to improve a
patient's/client's level of well-being in all dimensions, not just
physical health. Total programmes are based on the belief that
many factors can affect level of health. Health can be influenced
by individual practices such as poor eating habits and little or no
exercise. It can also be affected by physical stressors, a poor living
environment, exposure to air pollutants, and an unsafe
environment. Psychological stressors and hereditary factors can
also influence level of health. Total health-promotion
programmes are directed at changing lifestyle by developing
habits that can improve level of health. The following categories
are identified as important determinants of health status
(Edelman and Mandle, 1990):

- smoking
- nutrition
- alcohol use
- habitual drug use
- driving
- exercise
- sexuality and contraceptive or barrier use
- family relationships
- risk-factor modification
- coping and adaptation.

Some health-promotion and illness-prevention programmes
are operated by health care agencies. Others are independently
operated. Many businesses have developed health-promotion
activities for employees. Likewise, universities and community
centres offer health-promotion and illness-prevention
programmes. Nurses may be actively involved in these
programmes or may serve as consultants or give referrals. The
goal of these activities is to improve health through preventive
health services, environmental protection, and health education.

Health-promotion and illness-prevention activities are
important to the consumer and the health care provider. Whether
an activity uses the active or passive strategy, the goal is to
maintain or improve the level of physical, emotional, intellectual,
social, developmental, and spiritual well-being. Although
activities are often organized in specific programmes, nurses in all
areas of practice often have opportunities to assist patients/clients

**Categories of Lifestyle and Health Habits Assessment***

- General competencies of self-care
- Nutritional practices
- Physical or recreational activities
- Sleep patterns
- Stress management
- Self-actualization
- Sense of purpose
- Relationship with others
- Environmental control
- Use of health care system

*The complete LHHA and the rating scale are described in detail in Pender NJ: *Health promotion in nursing practice*, ed 2, Norwalk, Conn., 1987, Appleton & Lange.

in adopting activities to promote health and decrease risks of illness.

## Levels of Preventative Care — Primary Health Care

Nursing care orientated to health promotion and illness prevention can be understood in terms of health activities on the primary, secondary, and tertiary levels (Table 9-1).

## Primary Prevention

**Primary prevention** is true prevention; it precedes disease or dysfunction and is applied to patients/clients considered physically and emotionally healthy. It is not therapeutic, does not use therapeutic treatments, and does not involve symptom identification (Edelman and Mandle, 1990). Activities are directed at decreasing the probability of specific illnesses or dysfunctions. In addition, primary prevention includes health education programmes, immunization, or physical and nutritional fitness activities. Primary prevention can be provided to an individual or to a general population, or it can focus on individuals at risk for developing specific diseases.

## Secondary Prevention

**Secondary prevention** focuses on individuals who are experiencing health problems or illnesses and who are at risk for developing complications or worsening conditions. Activities are directed at diagnosis and prompt intervention, thereby reducing severity and enabling the patient/client to return to normal health at the earliest possible point (Pender, 1987; Edelman and Mandle, 1990). A large portion of secondary level nursing care is delivered in the home, hospital, or specialist unit in order to prevent complications. Secondary prevention includes screening techniques and treatment of early stages of disease to limit disability by averting or delaying the consequences of advanced disease.

## Tertiary Prevention

**Tertiary prevention** occurs when a defect or disability is permanent and irreversible. It involves minimizing the effects of the disease or disability by interventions directed at preventing complications and deterioration (Edelman and Mandle, 1990).

Activities are directed at rehabilitation rather than diagnosis and treatment (Pender, 1987). Care at this level aims to help patients/clients achieve as high a level of functioning as possible, despite the limitations caused by illness or impaired functioning. This level of care is called preventative care because it involves prevention of further disability or reduced functioning. A nurse who provides tertiary care to a recently blinded person, for example, not only assists the patient/client in adapting to the disability through activities such as teaching techniques to perform personal hygiene, but also directs attention to the goal of preventing future problems such as accidents in the home or potential problems with child rearing.

## RISK FACTORS

A **risk factor** is any situation, habit, environmental condition, physiological condition, or another variable that increases the vulnerability of an individual or group to an illness or accident. For example, a person whose father and paternal grandfather died of acute myocardial infarctions in their forties is at risk for coronary disease. Likewise, members of a community exposed to industrial air pollution are at risk for developing pulmonary disease. Risk factors include variables other than physical conditions. For example, a person who has experienced emotional stressors over a long period risks developing many kinds of illness.

The presence of risk factors does not mean that a disease state will develop, but risk factors increase the chances that the individual will experience a particular disease. Risk factors can occur in different aspects of a person's internal or external environment. Nurses and other health care professionals are concerned with them for several reasons. Risk factors play a major role in how a nurse identifies a patient's/client's health status. They can also influence health beliefs and practices if a person is aware of their presence. Identifying risk factors is also important for health-promotion and illness-prevention activities; such identificaton allows modification or elimination of the risk factors.

Risk factors can be placed in the following interrelated categories: genetic and physiological factors, age, physical environment, and lifestyle.

### Genetic and Physiological Factors

Physiological risk factors involve the physical functioning of the body. Certain physical conditions, such as being pregnant or overweight, place increased stress on a person's physiological systems (for example, the circulatory system), increasing susceptibility to illness in these areas. Heredity, or genetic predisposition to specific illness, is a major physical risk factor. For example, a person with a family history of diabetes mellitus is at risk of developing the disease later in life. Other documented genetic risk factors include family histories of cancer, coronary disease, and renal disease.

### Age

Age increases susceptibility to certain illnesses. For example, the risk of cardiovascular disease increases with age for both sexes.

## TABLE 9-1 The Three Levels of Prevention

| Primary Prevention | Secondary Prevention | Tertiary Prevention |
|---|---|---|
| **Health Promotion** | **Early Diagnosis and Prompt Treatment** | **Restoration and Rehabilitation** |
| Health education<br>Good standard of nutrition adjusted to developmental phases of life<br>Attention to personal development<br>Provision of adequate housing and recreation and agreeable working conditions<br>Marriage counselling and sex education<br>Genetic screening<br>Periodic selective examinations | Case-finding measures: individual and mass<br>Screening surveys<br>Selective examinations<br>Cure and prevention of disease process to prevent spread of communicable disease, prevent complications, and shorten period of disability | Provision of hospital and community facilities for retraining and education to maximize use of remaining capacities<br>Education of the public and industries to use rehabilitated people to the fullest possible extent<br>Selective placement<br>Work therapy in hospitals<br>Use of sheltered workshops and social education centres |
| **Specific Protection** | **Disability Limitations** | |
| Use of specific immunizations<br>Attention to personal hygiene<br>Use of environmental sanitation<br>Protection against environmental hazards<br>Protection from accidents<br>Use of specific nutrients<br>Protection from carcinogens<br>Avoidance of allergens | Adequate treatment to arrest disease process and prevent further complications<br>Provision of facilities to limit disability and prevent death | |

Modified from Leavell H, Clark AE: *Preventive medicine for doctors in the community*, New York, 1965, McGraw-Hill.

The risks of birth defects and complications of pregnancy increase after age 35. Many kinds of cancer pose a greater risk for people aged over 65 than for younger people. Age risk factors are often closely associated with other risk factors such as family history and personal habits. For example, a 60-year-old man who has smoked for 40 years is at a greater risk for developing lung cancer than a 30-year-old man who has smoked for 10 years.

## Environment

The physical environment in which a person works or lives can increase the likelihood that certain illnesses will occur. For example, some kinds of cancer and other diseases are more likely to develop when industrial workers are exposed to certain chemicals or when people live near toxic waste disposal sites. Screening for these environmentally based risk factors is directed at the short-term effects of the exposure and the potential for long-term effects (Edelman and Mandle, 1990).

Air, water, and noise pollution increase the risk of illness. High crime rates or overcrowding can also lead to stresses that make individuals more susceptible to disease.

In the home the physical environment may include conditions that pose risks to an individual or family. Unclean, poorly heated or cooled, or overcrowded dwellings increase the likelihood that infections and other diseases will be contracted and spread. Within the family, conflicts or other problems may create stressors that put individual members or the family as a whole at increased risk of illness.

## Lifestyle

Many activities, habits, and practices involve risk factors; the stresses of life crises and frequent lifestyle changes are also risk factors. Health practices and behaviours can have positive or negative effects on health. Practices with potential negative effects are risk factors; these include overeating or poor nutrition, insufficient rest and sleep, and poor personal hygiene. Other habits that put a person at risk for illness include smoking, alcohol or drug abuse, and activities involving a threat of injury such as skydiving or mountain climbing. Some habits are risk factors for specific diseases. For example, excessive sunbathing increases the risk of skin cancer, and eating a high cholesterol diet increases the risk of cardiovascular disease.

Emotional stress can be a risk factor if it is severe or prolonged, or if the person is unable to cope adequately with it. In such a case, emotional stress may increase the chance of illness. Emotional stressors may occur with events such as divorce, pregnancy, and arguments. Any area of life that leads to long-term emotional stress can be a risk factor. Job-related stresses, for example, may overtax a person's cognitive skills and decision-making ability, leading to 'mental overload' or 'burnout'.

Holmes and Rahe (1967) developed a classic **social readjustment rating scale** that correlates life changes with the risk of illness. Their research has shown that there is a greater risk for illness when a person has encountered a major life event change or multiple changes.

Adjustments that patients/clients must make in hospitals and other health care settings also involve a risk for further illness. Volicer (1974) developed a **hospital stress rating scale** that closely parallels the Holmes and Rahe scale. The objective of this scale is to predict the risk of a long hospital stay, complications, and pain; all of these factors may be linked to further disability or prolonged illness. The hospital stress rating scale assigns a numerical value to actual or potential stressors experienced during hospitalization. The higher the total score, the greater the risk that complications will develop, that pain medications will be necessary, and that the hospital stay will be prolonged. A high score on the scale does not mean that a patient/client will experience complications or a long hospital stay. However, it does predict general risks and therefore helps a nurse identify risks so that nursing interventions can be developed to reduce hospital stress and the incidence of complications (Volicer, 1974).

## ILLNESS AND ILLNESS BEHAVIOUR

Illness is not merely the presence of a disease process. Illness is a state in which a person's physical, emotional, intellectual, social, developmental, or spiritual functioning is diminished or impaired compared with that person's previous experience. Cancer is a disease process, but one patient/client with leukaemia who is responding to treatment may not perceive herself or himself as ill and may continue to function as usual, whereas another patient/client with breast cancer who is preparing for surgery may perceive herself as ill and be affected in dimensions other than the physical.

Illness therefore is not synonymous with disease. Although nurses must be familiar with different kinds of diseases and their treatments, they are concerned more with illness, which may include disease but also the effects on functioning and well-being in all dimensions.

People who are ill generally act in a way that medical sociologists call **illness behaviour**. Illness behaviour involves the ways people monitor their bodies, define and interpret their symptoms, take remedial actions, and use the health care system (Mechanic, 1982). If individuals perceive themselves to be ill, illness behaviours can serve as coping mechanisms. For example, illness behaviour may be a means of obtaining reassurance. A person who has been off work for a week because of illness may need to be reassured that his employer missed his or her contribution and that others care about him or her (Lambert and Lambert, 1987). The health care team can also be a source of support and reassurance for patients/clients. This support is particularly important for patients/clients with chronic diseases. People with severe cardiac impairments who are unable to care for themselves look to the health team for support. Patients/clients may need reassurance that the inability to care for themselves is due to the physical disease and not to a lack of motivation or desire. In addition, illness behaviour can result in patients/clients being released from roles, social expectations, or responsibilities. For a housewife, for example, the 'flu' may be a temporary release from child care and household responsibilities.

### Mental Health Nursing
### Illness behaviour

The history of mental illness in Europe and certainly in the UK has been one of incarceration of those diagnosed as insane in large Victorian workhouses and asylums, thereby separating the insane from the rest of the 'sane' population. The move towards the closure of many of these large mental institutions from the 1960s has meant the decarceration of many long stay patients/clients. In the case of many of these patients/clients, the long periods of institutionalization have conditioned them to entrenched 'illness behaviour' which leaves them poorly equipped to deal with life outside of institutions, and many have lost the ability to define health in their own terms.

Barham P, Hayward R: *From the Mental Patient to the Person* London, 1991, Tavistock/Routledge.

## Variables Influencing Illness Behaviour

Just as health behaviour is affected by internal and external variables, so is illness behaviour. To understand the patient's/client's behaviour and plan individualized care, the nurse needs to understand the influences of these variables. They are complex in their origins and effects.

### Internal Variables

Important internal variables influencing the way patients/clients behave when they are ill are their perceptions of symptoms and the nature of the illness itself. If patients/clients believe that the symptoms of their illnesses disrupt their normal routine, they are more likely to seek health care assistance than if they do not perceive the symptoms to be disruptive. If patients/clients believe that the symptoms are serious or perhaps life threatening, they are also more likely to seek assistance. People awakened by crushing chest pains in the middle of the night generally view this event as a symptom of a potentially serious and life-threatening illness and will probably be motivated to seek assistance. However, such a perception can also have the opposite effect. Individuals may fear serious illness, react by denying it, and not seek medical assistance.

A patient's/client's illness behaviour can also be affected by the nature of the illness. Acute illnesses involve symptoms of relatively short duration that are usually severe and that may affect functioning in any dimension. Chronic illnesses persist over a long period, usually longer than six months, and can affect functioning in any dimension. Several variables influence the illness behaviour of a person with a chronic illness. The patient/client may fluctuate between a state of maximal functioning and serious recurrences that may be life threatening. If a chronic illness cannot be cured and the symptoms are only partially relieved by therapy, the patient/client may not be highly motivated to comply with the therapy plan.

Patients/clients with acute illnesses are more likely to seek health care and comply readily with therapy. Chronically ill people may become less actively involved in their care, may experience greater frustration, and may comply less readily with care. Because nurses generally spend more time with chronically ill people than do other health care professionals, they are in the unique position of being able to assist these patients/clients in overcoming problems related to illness behaviour.

## External Variables

External variables influencing a patient's/client's illness behaviour include the visibility of symptoms, social group, cultural background, economic variables and social support.

The visibility of the symptoms of an illness can affect body image and illness behaviour. For example, a person who has a weeping sore on the lip may seek assistance sooner than a person with a sore throat because people may comment on the sore, the sore changes the person's appearance, and the weeping requires continual care.

Patients'/clients' social groups may assist them in recognizing the threat of illness or support the denial of potential illness. For example, two 35-year-old women in two different social groups have identified breast masses while performing breast self-examination; both discuss the finding with their friends. The first woman's friends might encourage her to seek medical attention to determine whether a biopsy is necessary, whereas the second woman's friends might tell her that the lump probably represents only fibrocystic disease and that she does not need to rush to a doctor. These examples show the influence that friends may have on an individual. The patient's/client's interaction with family members, peers, and others may have similar results and these are known as lay referral systems.

Illness behaviour can be interpreted and explained in terms of personal experiences and expectations. Cultural and ethnic socialization teaches an individual how to be healthy, recognize illness, and be ill. Meanings attached to health and illness are related to the basic culture-bound values by which a person defines a given experience and perception (Spector, 1991).

Western culture has emphasized a specific, systematic, causal explanation for trying to understand disease. In addition, the effects of disease and its interpretation also vary according to cultural circumstances. For example, there is a higher mortality rate from measles in underdeveloped countries than in Western cultures (Moore *et al*, 1980). Therefore, to develop individualized therapy, a nurse needs to understand a patient's/client's cultural background.

Economic variables also influence the way that a patient/client reacts to illness. Because of economic constraints, an individual may delay treatment and in many cases continue to work, rear children, or go to school.

Social support has been linked to health practices such as seat belt use, exercise, nutrition, smoking cessation, and health screening practices (Muhlenkamp and Sayles, 1986). Research notes that patients/clients react positively to social support during participation in positive health practices (Hubbard *et al* 1984). Thus, persons who view themselves as being part of a social group and having emotional and personal resources on which they can rely are more likely to practice positive health behaviours.

These internal and external factors can interact in various

ways to influence how people behave when ill and how and when they seek health care. Mechanic (1982) summarized the influences on illness behaviour in a list of 10 primary determinants (see box below). A nurse who knows the variables that affect illness behaviour can better understand such behaviour. Nursing care can then be planned and delivered in a way that involves patients'/clients' resources so they are restored to maximal levels of health.

### Ten Determinants of Illness Behaviour

- The visibility and recognizability of the illness' symptoms
- The extent to which the person perceives the symptoms as serious (the person's estimate of the present and future risks)
- The person's information, knowledge, and cultural assumptions and understanding related to the perceived symptoms
- The extent to which symptoms disrupt family, work, and social activities
- The frequency of the appearance of the symptoms and their persistence
- The extent to which others exposed to the person tolerate the symptoms
- The extent to which basic needs are denied because of the illness
- The extent to which meeting other needs competes with illness responses
- The extent to which the person gives other possible interpretations to the symptoms
- The availability and physical proximity of treatment resources and the psychological and monetary costs of taking action (including costs in time and effort, as well as costs such as stigma, social distance, and feelings of humiliation)

Modified from Mechanic D: *Symptoms, illness behaviour, and help seeking,* New York, 1982, Prodist.

## IMPACT OF ILLNESS ON PATIENT/CLIENT AND FAMILY

Illness is never an isolated life event. The patient/client and family must deal with changes resulting from illness and treatment. Each patient/client responds uniquely to illness, and therefore nursing interventions must be individualized. The patient/client and family commonly experience behavioural and emotional changes, as well as changes in roles, body image, self-concept, and family dynamics.

Environment, personal behaviours, and psychosocial factors play an interactive role in illness and health. The health care professional can no longer focus only on physical functioning. Assessment from a biopsychosocial perspective is more comprehensive and results in more specific planning and interventions (Shaver, 1985).

### Behavioural and Emotional Changes

People react differently to illness or the threat of illness. Individual behavioural and emotional reactions depend on the nature of the illness, the patient's/client's attitude towards it, the reaction of others to it, and the variables of illness behaviour.

Short-term, non-life-threatening illnesses evoke few behavioural changes in the functioning of the patient/client or family. A husband and father who has a cold, for example, may lack the energy and patience to spend time in family activities and may be irritable and prefer not to interact with his family. This is a behavioural change, but the change is subtle and does not last long. Some may even consider such a change a normal response to illness.

Severe illness, particularly one that is life threatening, can lead to more extensive emotional and behavioural changes, such as anxiety, shock, denial, anger, and withdrawal. These are common responses to the stress of illness. The nurse develops interventions to assist the patient/client and family in coping with this stress because the stressor itself cannot usually be changed.

## Impact on Family Roles

People have many roles in life such as wage earner, decision maker, professional, and parent. When an illness occurs, the roles of patient/client and family may change. Such a change may be subtle and short term or drastic and long term. An individual and family generally adjust more easily to subtle, short-term changes. In most cases they know that the role change is only temporary. For example, the mother of two preschool children has a viral infection, and her illness continues for a week; during this time, she gives up her roles of housewife and child care provider. Initially, she may welcome giving up these roles to be able to care for herself. As she gets better, however, she begins to look forward to resuming her roles.

With short-term role changes, a patient/client does not go through prolonged adjustment phases. Long-term changes, however, require an adjustment process similar to the grief process. The patient/client and family often require specific counselling and guidance to assist them in coping with the role changes.

## Impact on Body Image

Body image is the subjective concept of physical appearance. Some illnesses result in changes in physical appearance, and patients/clients and families react differently to these changes. The reactions of patients/clients and families to changes in body image depend on the following:

- the types of changes (for example, loss of a limb, a special sense, or an organ)
- their adaptive capacity
- the rate at which changes take place
- supportive services available.

When a change in body image occurs, such as that resulting from a leg amputation, the patient/client generally adjusts in the following phases: shock, withdrawal, acknowledgment, acceptance, and rehabilitation. Initially, the patient/client may be shocked by the change or impending change and may depersonalize it and talk about it as though it were happening to someone else. As the patient/client and family recognize the

reality of the change, they become anxious and may withdraw, refusing to discuss it. Withdrawal is an adaptive coping mechanism that can assist the patient/client in making the adjustment. As the patient/client and family acknowledge the change, they move through a period of grieving. At the end of the acknowledgment phase, they accept the loss. During

**Children's Nursing**
**Coping with chronic illness in children**

Families with children who have been diagnosed with a chronic /long-term health problem can experience a number of grief reactions. Once they have accepted the problem it must remain a nursing priority to ensure that the family copes with each other as well as with the sick child. Austin (1990) recommends that a model for care is utilized, such as an ABCX model — this assesses five major concepts about a family, which are: family demands, adaptive resources, coping, attitude towards the illness and adaptation. Whatever model is used it must clearly assess characteristics of family coping or not coping, and intervention must be targeted accordingly.

rehabilitation, the patient/client is ready to learn how to adapt to the change in body image through use of a prosthesis or changes in lifestyle and goals (Price, 1993).

## Impact on Self-Concept

Self-concept is an individual's mental image of themselves, including how they view their strengths and weaknesses in all aspects of their personalities. Self-concept depends in part on body image and roles but also includes other aspects of psychological and spiritual self. The impact of illness on the self-concept of patients/clients and family members may be more complex and less readily observed than role changes.

Self-concept is important in a person's relationships with other family members. A patient/client whose self-concept changes because of illness may no longer meet the expectations of the family, leading to tension or conflict. As a result, family members may change their interactions with the patient/client. For example, the patient/client may no longer be part of the family's decision-making process or may not be perceived as being able to provide emotional support to other family members or friends. Finally, the patient/client may be left out of social functions. In the course of providing care, a nurse is able to observe changes in the patient's/client's self-concept, or in the self-concepts of family members, and develop a care plan to help them adjust to the impact of illness.

## Impact on Family Dynamics

Because of the effects of illness on the patient/client and family, family dynamics often change. Nursing interventions need to be directed towards the family and patient/client (Reeder, 1991). Family dynamics is the process by which the family functions, makes decisions, gives support to individual members, and copes with everyday changes and challenges. If a parent in a family becomes ill, family activities and decision making often stop as the other family members wait for the illness to pass, or they delay action because they are reluctant to assume the ill person's roles or responsibilities. In some cases of prolonged illness, the family often has to shift to a new pattern of functioning, a change that can lead to emotional stress. Young children, for example, may experience a strong sense of loss if either parent is hospitalized or is unable to provide affection and a sense of security. Emotional difficulty may continue even when the other parent or family members are successful in assuming the roles and responsibilities of the hospitalized parent. If a parent of an adult becomes ill and cannot carry out his or her usual activities, the adult child often assumes many of the parent's responsibilities and in essence becomes a parent to the parent. Such a reversal of the usual situation can lead to stress, conflicting responsibilities for the adult child, or direct conflict over decision making.

Illness can disrupt a family's pattern of living, just as it can disrupt the functioning of the patient/client in all dimensions. A nurse must view the whole family as a patient/client and plan care to meet the same goal that must be met for the ill person to regain the maximal level of functioning and well-being.

## SUMMARY

The concepts of health and illness continuously change. Health is not merely the absence of illness or disability. It is a dynamic state in which individuals adapt to internal and external environments to maintain well-being. To provide effective nursing care and assist patients/clients in regaining and maintaining high levels of wellness, nurses must understand patients'/clients' concepts of health and their health beliefs and practices.

Health care professionals and consumers are emphasizing health-promotion and illness-prevention activities, which are designed to help patients/clients reduce the risks of illness and maintain maximal health.

When people become ill, their behaviours change. If the illnesses are serious enough for people to enter the health care system and receive nursing care, a nurse should be able to identify the factors influencing behaviour and the impact of illnesses on patients/clients and families. Nursing care is thus directed at preventing illness and promoting health, helping patients/clients adjust to illnesses and their impact, and helping regain maximal functioning.

## CHAPTER 9 REVIEW
### Key Concepts

- A healthy individual adapts to changes in the internal and external environment and thus maintains a state of well-being in all dimensions.
- An illness may be a disease, but it also includes reduced functioning in any human dimension.
- A person's state of health or illness should be considered in relation to individual values, personality, and lifestyle rather than measured by any absolute standard.

- The high-level wellness model describes health as an integrated method of functioning orientated at maximizing an individual's potential.
- The agent-host-environment model describes disease or illness as the result of the dynamic interaction of factors related to the agent, host, and environment. No one factor is the cause of disease or illness.
- The health-belief model considers factors influencing health beliefs. This model helps nurses understand and predict the behaviours of patients/clients in seeking or complying with health care.
- The evolutionary-based model of health and viability is based on the principle that illness and death sometimes serve as evolutionary functions.
- The health-promotion model is directed at increasing an individual's level of well-being and self-actualization.
- Health beliefs and practices are influenced by internal variables, including developmental stage, intellectual background, perception of functioning, and emotional and spiritual factors, and by external variables, including family practices and socioeconomic and cultural factors.
- To individualize care and ensure maximal participation in it, the nurse considers the patient's/client's health beliefs and practices when planning care.
- Health-promotion activities maintain or enhance a person's health.
- Illness-prevention activities protect against risk factors and thus maintain a person's level of health.
- Nursing incorporates health-promotion and illness-prevention activities rather than simply treating illness after it occurs.
- Primary preventative care helps healthy people maintain and increase their levels of health.
- Secondary preventative care helps ill people avoid complications or further health problems.
- Tertiary preventative care helps patients/clients adapt to or overcome disability or reduced functioning caused by illness.

### Key Terms

Active strategies of health promotion, p. 184
Concept(s) of health, p. 178
Dependent/independent continuum, p. 178
Health behaviours, p. 179
Health-belief and practices, p. 179
Health promotion, p. 184
Health-belief model, p. 180
Hospital stress rating scale, p. 188
Illness behaviour, p. 178, 188
Illness prevention, p. 184
Negative health behaviour, p. 179
Passive strategies of health promotion, p. 184
Positive health behaviours, p. 179
Primary prevention, p. 186
Risk factor, p. 178
Secondary prevention, p. 186
Social readjustment rating scale, p. 187
Tertiary prevention, p. 186
Total health programme, p. 185

- Risk factors threaten a person's health, influence health practices, are important considerations in illness-prevention activities and are commonly associated with genetic or physiological variables, age, environment, and lifestyle.
- Illness behaviour, like health practices, is influenced by many variables and must be considered by the nurse when planning care.
- Illness can have many effects on the patient/client and family, including behavioural and emotional changes and changes in roles, body image, self-concept, and family dynamics.
- To plan and implement holistic nursing care that assists in attaining states of maximal functioning and well-being, a nurse must consider all of the effects of an illness on a patient/client and family.

## CRITICAL THINKING EXERCISES

1. You are working in a junior school. You're asked to design a health promotion programme for the 10-year-old group. You initially focus on diet and exercise. How do you begin to design the programme? What resources do you need?
2. One of the students in your college/university seeks your advice for smoking cessation programmes. How do you identify appropriate resources? Which programmes would be suitable for this person? What information does the patient/client need about the potential programmes?
3. Assess your own lifestyle. Identify three areas for change. Select one area, determine what needs to change, how to identify resources to promote change, how to select and implement the resources, and how to evaluate the effectiveness of the change.
4. Describe how you would educate school children about an area of mental health, such as coping with stress.

## REFERENCES

Anderson JM: The cultural context of caring, *Can Crit Care Nurs J* 4(4):7, 1987.

Austin S: Assessment of coping mechanisms used by parents and children with chronic illness, *MCN* 15: 98,1990.

Balog JE: The concepts of health and disease: a relativistic perspective, *Health Values* 6:7, 1982.

Barham P, Hayward R: *From the Mental Patient to the Person*. London, 1991, Tavistock/Routledge.

Becker MH, Maiman LA: Sociobehavioural determinants of compliance with health and medical care recommendations, *Med Care* 133(1):121, 1975.

Berne AS et al: A nursing model for addressing the health needs of homeless families, *Image J Nurs Sch* 22:8, 1990.

Breslow L: A quantitative approach to the World Health Organization definition of health: physical, mental and social well-being, *Int J Epidemiol* 1:347, 1972.

Davidson JK: Diabetes in socio-economically deprived neighborhoods. In American Diabetes Association: *Diabetes mellitus: diagnosis and treatment*, New York, 1971, The Association.

deChesnay M, Magnuson N: How healthy families cope with stress, *AAOHN J* 36:361, 1988.

Dixon JK, Dixon JP: An evolutionary-based model of health and viability, *ANS* 6(3):1, 1984.

Downie R, Fyfe C, Tannahill A: *Health promotion models and values*, Oxford, 1991, Oxford University Press.

Dunn H: What high level wellness means, *Health Values* 1:9, 1977.

Dunn HL: High-level wellness for man and society, *Am J Public Health* 49:789, 1959.

Edelman CL, Mandle CL: *Health promotion throughout the life span*, ed 2, St Louis, 1990, Mosby.

Fuchs VR: *Who shall live? Health, economics, and social choice*,

New York, 1974, Basic Books.

Gilpatrick DM: Moving patients/clients toward wellness: behavioural change, *Clin Nurs Spec* 3(1):25, 1989.

Goldsmith JR: Health effects of air pollution, *Basics RD* 4(2):4, 1975.

Holmes TH, Rahe RH: Social readjustment rating scale, *J Psychosom Res* 11:213, 1967.

Hubbard P, Muhlenkamp AF, Brown N: The relationship between social support and self-care practices, *Nurs Res* 33:266, 1984.

Johnson P: Becoming real: a developmental approach to relationship education. In Craft A, editor: *Mental handicap and sexuality: issues and perspectives*. Tunbridge Wells, 1987, Costello.

Lambert CE, Lambert VA: Psychosocial impacts created by chronic illness, *Nurs Clin North Am* 22:527, 1987.

Leavell HR et al: *Preventive medicine for the doctor in his community*, ed 3, New York, 1965, McGraw-Hill.

Leininger M: Cultural diversities of health and nursing care, *Nurs Clin North Am* 12(1):5, 1977.

Mechanic D: The epidemiology of illness behaviour and its relationship to physical and psychological distress. In Mechanic D: *Symptoms, illness behaviour, and help seeking*, New York, 1982, Prodist.

Moore LG et al: *The biocultural basis of health: expanding views of medicine anthropology*, Prospect Heights, Ill, 1980, Waveland Press.

Muhlenkamp AF, Sayles JA: Self-esteem, social support and positive health practices, *Nurs Res* 35:334, 1986.

Orem, D: *Nursing concepts of practice*, ed 4, St. Louis, 1991, Mosby.

Parsons T: Definitions of health and illness in light of American values and social structures. In Joco EG, editor: *Patients, physicians, and illness*, New York, 1958, Free Press.

Pender NJ: *Health promotion and nursing practice*, Norwalk, Conn, 1982, Appleton-Century-Crofts.

Pender NJ: Health promotion and illness prevention. In Werley HH and Fitzpatrick JJ, editors: *Annual review of nursing research*, New York, 1984, Springer.

Pender NJ: *Health promotion in nursing practice*, ed 2, Norwalk, Conn, 1987, Appleton & Lange.

Pesznecker BL: The poor: a population at risk, *Public Health Nurs* 1:237, 1984.

Price B: Profiling the high risk altered body image patient, *Senior Nurs*, 13(4): 17, 1993.

Reeder JM: Family perception: a key to intervention. In American Association of Critical-Care Nurses: *AACN clinical issues in critical care nurse*, 1991, The Association.

Roper N, Logan W, Tierney A: *Using a model for nursing,* London, 1983, Churchill Livingstone.

Rosenstock I: Historical origin of the health belief model, *Health Educ Monogr* 2:334, 1974.

Royal College of Nursing: *AIDS — a proactive approach.* London, 1991, Scutari.

Shaver JF: A biopsychosocial view of human health, *Nurs Outlook* 33:186, 1985.

Smith JM, Sorrell V: Developing wellness programmes: a nurse- managed stay-well centre for senior citizens, *Clin Nurse Spec* 3(1): 198,1989.

Spector RE: *Cultural diversity in health and illness,* ed 3, Norwalk, Conn, 1991, Appleton & Lange.

Steele RL: Social networks as a means of health maintenance, *Health Values* 6(6):6, 1982.

Tripp-Reimer T: Reconceptualizing the construct of health: integrating emic and itic perspectives, *Res Nurs Health* 7:101, 1984.

Volicer BJ: Patient's perceptions of stressful events associated with hospitalization, *Nurs Res* 2(3):235, 1974.

Weitzel MH: A test of the health promotion model with blue-collar workers, *Nurs Res* 38:99, 1989.

World Health Organization Interim Commission: *Chronicle of WHO* Geneva, 1947, The Organization.

Yarcheski A, Mahon N: A causal model of positive health practices: the relationship between approach and replication, *Nurs Res* 38:88, 1989.

## FURTHER READING

### Adult Nursing

Alexy B: Goal setting and health risk reduction, *Nurs Res* 34(5):283, 1985.

Bowling A: *Measuring health: a review of quality of life measurement scales,* Milton Keynes, 1991, Open University Press.

Collier JAH: Developmental and systems perspectives on chronic illness, *Holistic Nurs Pract* 5(1):1, 1990.

Ferrans CE, Powers MJ: Quality of life index: development and psychometric properties, *ANS* 8(1):15, 1985.

Fries JF: The future of disease and treatment: changing health conditions, changing behaviours, and new medical technology, *J Prof Nurs* 2(1):10, 1986.

Hyman RB, Woog P: Stressful life events and illness onset: a review of crucial variables, *Res Nurs Health* 5:155, 1982.

Milsum JH: Health, risk factor reduction and life-style changes, *Fam Community Health* 3:1, 1980.

Pollock SE: Human responses to chronic illness: physiologic and psychosocial adaptation, *Nurs Res* 35:90, 1986.

Seedhouse D: *Health: the foundations for achievement,* Chichester, 1986, John Wiley & Sons Ltd.

Volicer BJ: Perceived stress levels of events associated with the experience of hospitalization: development and testing of a measurement tool, *Nurs Res* 22:491, 1973.

Volicer BJ, Bahannon MW: A hospital stress rating scale, *Nurs Res* 24:354, 1975.

Wolinsky FD: *The sociology of health: principles, professionals and issues,* Boston, Little, Brown, 1980.

### Children's Nursing

Elser C: It's OK having asthma — young children's beliefs about illness. In Glasper A, editor: *Childcare: some nursing perspectives.* London, 1991, Wolfe.

Elser C: What children think about hospitals and illness. In Glasper A, editor: *Childcare: some nursing perspectives.* London, 1991, Wolfe.

Haggerty  R J: Life stress, illness and social support, *Development Medicine and Child Neurology* 22:391, 1980.

Hall D, Editor: *Health for all children: a programme for child health surveillance.* Oxford, 1989, Oxford University Press.

Hergenrather J, Rabinowitz: Age-related differences in the organisation of children's knowledge of illness. *Developmental Psychology* 66: 952, 1991.

Hull D: Children's health. *BMJ* 303:514, 1991.

Mayall B, Foster M: *Childhealth care.* Oxford, 1989, Heinemann Nursing.

Open University Press: Experiencing and explaining disease. In *Health and disease,* Milton Keynes, 1985, Open University Press.

Rutter M: Stress, coping and developments: some issues and some questions. *J of Child Psych,* 22(4): 323, 1981.

Wald N H (ed): *Antenatal and neonatal screening.* Oxford, 1984, Oxford University Press.

World Health Organization. Child mental health and social development. *WHO Technical Report Series,* no 613. Geneva, WHO, 1977.

Wykes, Hewison J, editors: *Childhealth matters,* Milton Keynes, 1991, Open University Press.

### Learning Disabilities Nursing

Craft A, editor: *Mental handicap and sexuality: issues and perspectives.* Tunbridge Wells, 1987, Costello.

Tymchuck A, Andron L, Tymchuck M: Training mothers with mental handicaps to understand behavioural and developmental principles, *Mental Hand Res* 3(1):51, 1990.

Tymchuk A, Andron L: Clinic and home parent training of a mother with mental handicap caring for three children with developmental delay, *Mental Hand Res* 1(1):24, 1988.

### Mental Health Nursing

Barnes M, Maple NA: *Women and mental health,* Birmingham, 1992, Venture Press.

Black N, Boswell D, Gray A: *Health and disease — a reader* (parts 1, 2 & 6), Milton Keynes, 1984, Oxford University Press.

Boyle M: *Schizophrenia — a scientific decision.* London, 1990, Routledge.

Department of Health: *Key area handbook — mental illness (The Health of the Nation),* 1992, DOH.

McBean S: Health and health promotion — consensus and conflict. In Perry A, Folley M, editors: *Nursing: a knowledge for practice.* London, 1991, Edward Arnold.

Rose J, Holmes S: Changing staff attitudes to the sexuality of people with mental handicaps: an evaluative comparison of one- and three-day workshops, *Mental Hand Res* 4(1):67, 1991.

Royal College of General Practitioners. Prevention of psychiatric disorders in general practice. *Report from general practice,* no20. London, 1981 RCGP.

Szasz T: *The myth of mental illness.* London, 1981 Granada Books.

Wright H, Giddey M, editors: *Mental health nursing* (parts 1, 2, & 3), London, 1993, Chapman & Hall.

# Stress and Adaptation

## LEARNING OUTCOMES

After studying this chapter, you should be able to:

- *Define the key terms listed.*
- *Discuss the role and limitations of physiological adaptation mechanisms in maintaining homeostasis.*
- *Discuss four models of stress as they relate to nursing practice.*
- *Describe how adaptation occurs in each of the six dimensions of an individual.*
- *Describe two forms of local physiological adaptation response.*
- *Describe the three phases of the general adaptation syndrome.*
- *Identify common physiological indicators of stress.*
- *Identify developmental factors that may lead to stress for each different age group.*
- *List and discuss behaviours that are responses to stress and their relationship to ego defence mechanisms.*
- *Discuss the effects of prolonged stress on each of the dimensions of a person's functioning.*
- *Describe stress-management techniques that nurses can help patients/clients use and that can benefit nurses themselves.*

Every person experiences forms of stress throughout life. Stress can provide the stimulus for change and growth and, in this respect, some stress can be positive. However, too much stress can result in poor judgement, physical illness, and inability to cope.

Various disciplines such as nursing, physiology, psychology and sociology have attempted to define stress within the boundaries of that specific discipline. However, each group has worked in isolation from the other groups, leading to a disparity in the literature about stress. Stress is a phenomenon that affects the physical, developmental, emotional, intellectual, social and spiritual dimensions of an individual (Lindsay and Carrieri, 1986). Therefore, the nurse should consider all of these factors within each step of the nursing process (see Chapter 3).

## CONCEPTS OF STRESS

### Stress and Stressors

Everyone experiences stress from time to time. Normally a person is either able to adapt to long-term stress, or to cope with short-term stress until it passes. Stress can place heavy demands upon a person, and if the person is unable to adapt, physical and mental illness can result.

Stress is any situation in which a non-specific demand requires an individual to respond or take action (Selye, 1956; Lindsay and Carrieri, 1986). It involves physiological and psychological responses. Stress can lead to negative or counterproductive feelings, or can threaten emotional well-being. It can threaten the way a person normally perceives reality, solves problems, or thinks in general. It can alter people's relationships, their sense of belonging, general outlook on life, attitude towards loved ones, job satisfaction, ability to solve problems, and health status.

An individual's perception or experience of a major change initiates the **stress response**. The stimuli preceding or precipitating the change are called **stressors**. Stressors may be physiological, psychological, social, environmental, developmental, spiritual, or cultural, and represent an unmet need. Stressors can generally be classified as internal or external. Internal stressors originate inside a person (for example, a fever, a condition such as pregnancy or menopause, or an emotion such as guilt). External stressors originate outside a person (for example, a marked change in environmental temperature, a change in family or social role, or peer pressure) (Riehl and Roy, 1980). The relationship between the person and the environment is thus interactive.

## Physiological Adaptation

Physiological adaptation to stress is the body's ability to maintain a state of relative balance. This adaptive ability is a dynamic form of equilibrium in the body's internal environment. The internal environment constantly changes and the body's adaptive mechanisms continually function to adjust to these changes and thus to maintain equilibrium, or homeostasis.

**Homeostasis** is maintained by physiological mechanisms that control body functions and monitor body organs. For the most part, these mechanisms are controlled by the nervous and endocrine systems and do not involve conscious behaviour. The body makes adjustments in heart rate, respiratory rate, blood pressure, temperature, fluid and electrolyte balances, hormone secretions, and level of consciousness – all directed at maintaining adaptation.

## Mechanisms of Physiological Adaptation

When a person becomes aware of an unmet physiological need, such as food or warmth, deliberate actions can meet the need. For the most part, however, adaptation involves adjustments that the body makes automatically to maintain equilibrium. These homeostatic mechanisms are self-regulatory; in other words, they are automatic. In a person with an illness or injury, however, the mechanisms may not be able to maintain and sustain homeostasis.

Physiological mechanisms of adaptation function through negative feedback, a process by which the controlling mechanism senses an abnormal state, such as lowered body temperature, and makes an adaptive response, such as initiating shivering to generate body heat. Three of the major mechanisms used in adapting to a stressor are controlled by the medulla oblongata, the reticular formation, and the pituitary gland.

### Mental Health Nursing
### Post-traumatic stress

In many parts of the UK's inner cities, there are large groups of refugees from many war-torn nations. Many of these people suffer from post-traumatic stress as a result of being casualties of war and having witnessed the destruction of their family and lifestyle. Many experience stress at a level which most of us may never encounter and may not begin to comprehend. Adjusting to a new life in a new country is often extremely difficult for these refugees.

Adapted from: Kareem J, Littlewood R: *Intercultural therapy*, Oxford, 1992, Blackwell Scientific Publishers.

## MEDULLA OBLONGATA

The medulla oblongata controls vital functions necessary to survival. These include heart rate, blood pressure, and respiration. Impulses travelling to and from the medulla oblongata can increase or decrease these vital functions. For example, regulation of the heart beat is the result of sympathetic or parasympathetic nervous system impulses travelling from the medulla oblongata to the heart. The heart rate increases in response to impulses from sympathetic fibres and decreases with impulses from parasympathetic fibres.

## RETICULAR FORMATION

The reticular formation is a small cluster of neurones in the brainstem and spinal cord. It also controls vital functions and continuously monitors the physiological status of the body through connections with sensory and motor tracts. For example, certain cells within the reticular formation can cause a sleeping person to regain consciousness or increase the level of consciousness when a need arises.

## PITUITARY GLAND

The pituitary gland, a small gland attached to the hypothalamus, supplies hormones that control vital functions. The pituitary gland produces hormones necessary for adaptation to stress (see Fig. 10-1 on p. 200). In addition, the pituitary gland regulates the secretion of thyroid hormones through thyroid stimulating hormone. It also regulates gonadal hormones via follicle stimulating hormone and luteinizing hormone. Hormone secretion, like other homeostatic mechanisms, is normally regulated by negative feedback, which continuously monitors hormone levels in the blood. When hormone levels drop, the pituitary gland receives a message to increase hormone secretion. When hormone levels rise, the pituitary gland decreases hormone production.

## Limitations of Physiological Mechanisms of Adaptation

Physiological mechanisms of adaptation work together through complex relationships in the nervous and endocrine systems and other body systems to maintain a relative constancy within the body. In a healthy person, these mechanisms affect physiological balance, and the body's needs are met. However, physiological mechanisms of adaptation can provide only short-term control over the body's equilibrium. They cannot adapt to long-term changes in hormone secretion or vital functions. Thus illness, injury, or prolonged stress can decrease the adaptive capacity. Decreased functioning can result in continued but inadequate homeostatic control or breakdown of the feedback mechanism that allows control. Either form of decreased function can result in further illness or death.

In severe stress situations, for example, the pituitary gland supplies the body with the necessary hormones (see Fig. 10-1) and the autonomic nervous system is triggered into action by the hypothalamus. However, these hormones may be insufficient in quantity to provide the physiological energy necessary for coping. In this case the person's condition deteriorates, and functioning declines. The feedback mechanism of homeostatic control may break down because of organ abnormality.

## Models of Stress

Models of stress are used to identify the stressors for a particular individual and to predict that person's responses to them. Each model emphasizes a different aspect of stress and may guide the nurse when working with a patient/client with unhealthy, nonproductive responses to stressors.

## Response-Based Model of Stress

The *response-based* model is concerned with specifying the particular response or pattern of responses that may indicate a stressor. Selye's model of stress (1976) is a response-based model that defines stress as a nonspecific response of the body to any demand made on it. Stress is demonstrated by a specific physiological reaction, the GAS (general adaptation syndrome). Thus the response of a person to stress is purely physiological and is never modified to allow cognitive influences.

This model does not allow for individual differences in response patterns and this lack of flexibility may produce some difficulties for nurses because individual differences must be identified in the assessment phase.

## Adaptation Model

The *adaptation* model proposes that four factors determine whether a situation is stressful (Mechanic, 1962; Riehl and Roy, 1980). The ability to cope with stress, the first factor, usually depends on the person's experience with similar stressors, support systems, and overall perception of the stressor.

The second factor deals with the practices and norms of the person's peer group. If the peer group considers it normal to talk about a particular stressor, the patient/client may respond by complaining or worrying about it. This response may help adaptation to the stress, or the patient/client may respond in this way simply to conform to peer group behaviour.

The third factor is the impact of the social environment in assisting an individual to adapt to a stressor. For example, a junior student who may have a sexually transmitted disease may confide this fear to a senior student, who may then support this student to seek a consultation at a clinic. In this example the resources of the older student and the clinic offer the means of reducing the severity of the stressor.

The adaptation model is based on the understanding that people experience anxiety and increased stress when they are unprepared to cope with stressful situations. Using this model and appropriate informative interventions (Heron, 1989), nurses can help patients/clients and families to reduce the effects of stress in all human dimensions.

## Stimulus-Based Model

The stimulus-based model focuses on disturbing or disruptive characteristics within the environment. The classic research that identified stress as a stimulus has resulted in the development of the social readjustment scale (see Chapter 9), which measures the effects of major life events on illness (Holmes and Rahe, 1976).

The stimulus-based model focuses on the following assumptions:
1. Life change events are normal, and they require the same type and duration of adjustment.
2. People are passive recipients of stress, and their perceptions of the event are irrelevant.
3. All people have a common threshold of stimulus, and illness results at any point after the threshold.

As with the response-based model, the stimulus-based model does not allow for individual differences in perception and response to stressors.

## Transaction-Based Model

The *transaction-based* model views the person and environment in a dynamic, reciprocal, interactive, relationship (Lazarus and Folkman, 1984). This model, developed by Lazarus and Folkman, views the stressor as an individual perceptual response rooted in psychological and cognitive processes. Stress originates from the relationship between the person and the environment. This model focuses on stress-related processes such as cognitive appraisal and coping (Dryden, 1987).

## Factors Influencing Response to Stressors

The response to any stressor depends on physiological functioning, personality, and behavioural characteristics, as well as the nature of the stressor. The nature of the stressor involves the following factors:
1. Intensity
2. Scope
3. Duration
4. Number and nature of other stressors.

Each factor influences the response to a stressor. A person may perceive the intensity or magnitude of a stressor as minimal, moderate, or severe. The greater the magnitude of the stressor, the greater the stress response. Likewise, the scope of a stressor can be described as limited, medium, or extensive. The greater the scope of a stressor, the greater the response of the patient/client to it (Lazarus and Folkman, 1984).

## ADAPTATION TO STRESSORS

Stress can affect the physical, emotional, intellectual, developmental, social or spiritual dimensions of an individual. Adaptive resources exist in each of these dimensions, and assessment should consider the whole person, as well as any family or community influences on adaptation.

There are many forms of adaptation. Physiological adaptations make possible a physiological homeostasis. A similar process of adaptation may occur in the psychological or social dimensions.

Adaptation is thus an attempt to maintain optimal functioning when a stimulus from the internal or external environment causes a departure from the balanced state of the organism. Adaptation involves reflexes, automatic body mechanisms for protection, coping mechanisms, and instincts

### Learning Disabilities Nursing
### Causes of stress

There are many specific factors that can cause stress in people with learning disabilities. For example, living in a group home with people who have violent, challenging behaviour; the death of a carer; the transition from one care provision system to another; or adhering to a care plan that requires intellectual, emotional and social development at a pace which may be frightening for the client. Nurses must be aware of these and other stress factors, and must observe for signs of stress in their clients. Because some types of stress are an unavoidable fact of daily life, nurses must ensure their clients learn constructive and healthy ways to deal with it.

(Selye, 1976; Riehl and Roy, 1980). A stressor that stimulates adaptation may be short term, such as a fever, or long term, such as the death of a loved one. To function optimally, a person must be able to respond to such stressors and adapt to the required demands or changes. Adaptation requires an active response from the whole person.

Like an individual, a family or group may need to adapt to a stressor. Intra family dynamics and the family's interactions with the world at large may hinder or aid adaptation (Laing, 1964; Skynner, 1976).

## Dimensions of Adaptation
### Physical Dimension

Physiological adaptation is the process by which the body responds to a stressor to maintain functioning compatible with survival. Physiological adaptive responses are stimulated by demands in the internal environment, such as a fever or inflammation, or in the external environment, such as changes in altitude or ambient temperature. A physiological response to stress may be limited to a particular body area, or it may involve the entire body. The sections on local and general adaptation syndromes will discuss physiological adaptive responses in more detail.

### Developmental Dimension

Each developmental stage involves particular tasks and thus potential stressors (see Chapter 6). A young adult, for example, may have to adapt to stressors such as establishing a career and rearing children. At the same time, each developmental stage is characterized by potential adaptive resources by which an individual can respond to stress (Erikson, 1980). For example, an older adult, because of greater past experience with certain stressors, may be better able to adapt than a young adult.

### Emotional Dimension

Adaptation in the emotional dimension involves the use of normal psychological coping mechanisms to resolve stress. Everyone has a different personality and every patient/client copes with stress in a different way. Although certain basic forms of psychological adaptation are common there will be times when

some adaptive responses may seem bizarre to the nurse. Adaptive behaviour is most successful when it leads to a sense of discovery and creativity. A person may not always be happy and content when adapting to stress, but the goal of adaptation is growth.

## Intellectual Dimension

A person's intellectual dimension includes not only development and education but also perceptions of other people and the world, problem-solving ability, communication patterns, and past coping strategies. Intellectual adaptive responses include gathering information, solving problems, and communicating with others to adjust.

Intellectual adaptation can be strongly influenced by emotions. If people are unable to adapt emotionally to the changes necessitated by illness, for example, they may be less able to adapt intellectually by learning more about their conditions. Similarly, success in emotional adaptation can lead to more effective intellectual adaptation.

### Mental Health Nursing
### Women and stress

In their study of depressed women in South East London, Brown and Harris (1978) concluded that stressors such as social isolation, loss of mother, and coping with a young growing family, contributed to depression in the study population. Stressors are likely to be worse for women of various ethnic backgrounds, where English is not their first language and where their ethnic background makes them visible targets for abuse. The mental health needs of such women are frequently not recognized or acknowledged; partly because of the ethnocentricity of health and social care professionals, and partly because of the inability or reluctance of individuals to articulate their distress, due to language or cultural barriers.

Adapted from: d'Ardenne P, Mahtan A: *Transcultural counselling in action*, London, 1990, Sage.

## Social Dimension

Everyone has social relationships with others, for example partners, family members, co-workers, and peers. This network can be important in helping a person adapt to stressors. The social group may provide psychological support and can help direct a person to resources for coping with stress. For example, friends often can help a person adjust to the death of a loved one by encouraging the person to express feelings. In addition, organized social groups, such as Alcoholics Anonymous, can help people adapt to specific stresses in the social dimension.

A person's social dimension is often closely interrelated with other dimensions. For example, a patient/client who is unable to cope emotionally with stress may withdraw from contact with people who can assist him or her in adapting.

## Spiritual Dimension

A person's spiritual dimension can include beliefs about a supreme being, a feeling of oneness with nature and the world as a whole, and a positive sense of life's meaning and purpose. These beliefs can be a powerful resource for adapting to stress (see Chapter 8).

## RESPONSE TO STRESS

The total person is involved in responding and adapting to stresses. Most research into stress responses, however, focuses on psychological or emotional and physiological responses, even though these dimensions overlap and interact with the other dimensions.

When stress occurs, a person uses physiological and psychological energy to respond and adapt. The amount of energy required and the effectiveness of the attempt to adapt depend on the intensity, scope, and duration of the stressor and the number of other stressors. The stress response is adaptive and protective, and the characteristics of this response are the result of integrated neuroendocrine response.

### Physiological Response

The classic research by Selye (1956) has identified the two physiological responses to stress: the **local adaptation syndrome (LAS) and the general adaptation syndrome (GAS)**. The LAS is a response of a body tissue, organ, or part to the stress of trauma, illness, or other physiological change. The GAS is a defence response of the whole body to stress.

### Local Adaptation Syndrome

The body produces many localized responses to stress. These include wound healing (see Chapter 30). All forms of the LAS share the following characteristics:

1.  The response is localized; it does not involve entire body systems.
2.  The response is adaptive, meaning that a stressor is necessary to stimulate it.
3.  The response is short term. It does not persist indefinitely.
4.  The response is restorative, meaning that the LAS assists in restoring homeostasis to the body region or part.

The reflex pain response (see Chapter 27) and the inflammatory response (see Chapter 30) are examples of the LAS.

### General Adaptation Syndrome

The GAS is a physiological response of the whole body to stress. It involves several body systems, primarily the autonomic nervous system and the endocrine system. Some textbooks refer to the GAS as the neuroendocrine response. The GAS consists of the alarm reaction, the resistance stage, and the exhaustion stage (Fig. 10.1).

### ALARM REACTION

The *alarm reaction* involves the mobilization of the defence mechanisms of the body and mind to cope with the stressor. Hormone levels rise to increase blood glucose and blood volume and thereby prepare the person to act and to make energy available for adaptation. Increased levels of adrenaline and noradrenaline result in an increased heart rate, increased blood flow to muscles, increased oxygen intake, **increased blood glucose** and greater mental alertness.

This extensive hormonal activity prepares the person for the **flight-or-fight response**. Cardiac output, oxygen intake, and respiratory rate are increased; the pupils of the eyes are dilated to produce a greater visual field; and the heart rate is increased for more energy. Other changes occur to prepare the person to act. With this increased mental energy and alertness, the person is prepared to flee or fight the stressor.

During the alarm reaction the person is faced with a specific stressor. The person's physiological response is extensive, involving major systems of the body, and it may last from a minute to many hours. If the stressor is extreme or remains for a long time, there may be a threat to life. If the stressor is still present after the initial alarm reaction, the person progresses to the second phase of the GAS, resistance.

### RESISTANCE STAGE

In the *resistance stage* the body stabilizes, and hormone levels, heart rate, blood pressure, and cardiac output return to normal. The person is attempting to adapt to the stressor. During this stage, the body's ability to fight infection is reduced and wound healing is delayed. If the stress can be resolved, the body repairs damage that may have occurred. However, if the stressor remains present, as in continued blood loss, debilitating disease, or long-term severe mental illness, and adaptation is impossible, the person enters the third phase of the GAS, exhaustion.

### EXHAUSTION STAGE

The *exhaustion stage* occurs when the body can no longer resist stress and when the energy necessary to maintain adaptation is depleted. The physiological response is intensified, but the person's energy level is compromised and adaptation to the stressor diminishes. The body is unable to defend itself against the impact of the stressor, physiological regulation diminishes, and if the stress continues, death may result.

### Psychological Response

Exposure to a stressor results in psychological and physiological adaptive responses. As people are exposed to stressors, their ability to meet their basic needs is threatened. This threat, whether actual or perceived, can produce frustration, anxiety, and tension (Freud, 1984). Psychological adaptive behaviours assist the person's ability to cope with stressors. These behaviours are directed at stress management and are acquired through learning and experience as a person identifies acceptable and successful behaviours.

Ego defence mechanisms (first described by Freud) are unconsciously motivated behaviours that can be constructive or destructive. **Constructive behaviours** can help individuals to protect themselves from failings such as anxiety and to accept the challenge to resolve conflict.

**Destructive behaviours** can occur when ego defence mechanisms become distorted. These can affect reality orientation, problem-solving abilities, personality, and, in severe circumstances, the ability to function. Anxiety can be constructive (in that it gives a signal for action) or destructive (if a person is unable to act to remove the stressor).

Psychological adaptive behaviours are also referred to as **coping mechanisms**. Such mechanisms can be ego-defensive, or can be task oriented, involving the use of direct problem-solving techniques to cope with the threats.

### Task-Oriented Behaviours

**Task-oriented behaviours** involve using cognitive abilities to reduce stress, solve problems, resolve conflicts, and gratify needs (Stuart and Sundeen, 1991). Task-oriented behaviours enable a person to cope realistically with the demands of a stressor. The three general types of task-oriented behaviour are attack behaviour, withdrawal behaviour, and compromise.

## NURSING CARE AND ADAPTATION TO STRESS

Each patient/client has specific perceptions and responses to stress. A person's perception of a stressor is based on beliefs and

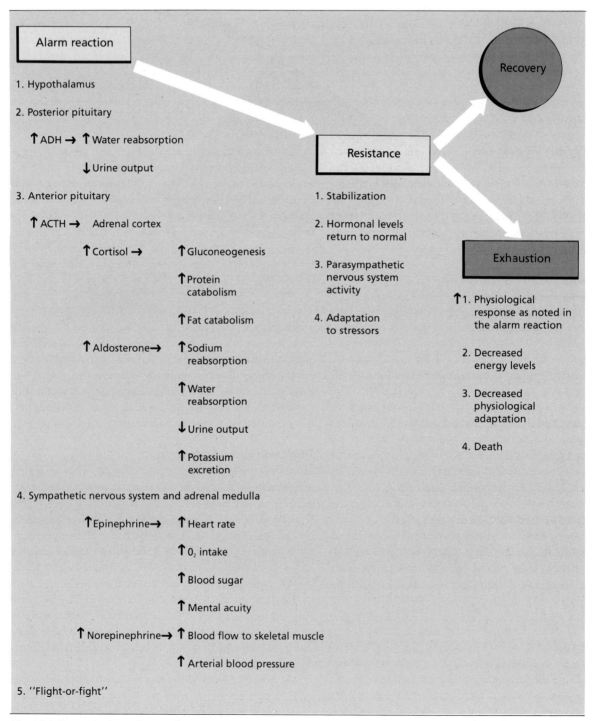

Fig. 10-1 General adaptation syndrome.

### Children's Nursing
### Stress and maternal behaviour

An infant's capacity to cope with frustration and stress was found to be highly correlated with the following characteristics of maternal behaviour:
- the amount of physical contact a mother gave her infants
- the extent to which a mother's way of holding her infant was adapted to the infant's characteristics and rhythms
- the degree to which the mother's soothing techniques were effective
- the extent to which the mother stimulated and encouraged the infant; whether to respond socially, to express his or her needs, or to make developmental progress
- the extent to which materials and experiences given an infant were suited to the infant's individual capacities
- the frequency and intensity of expression of positive feelings towards the infant from the mother, father and others

Adapted from Yarrow LJ (1963), quoted in Bowlby J: *Attachment*, Gretna, LA, 1971, Pelican.

norms, life experiences and patterns, environmental factors, family structure and function, developmental stage, past experiences with stress, and coping mechanisms. The nurse may not always be able to identify with the patient's/client's sense of distress. However, the nurse needs to regard the person's feelings as real and valid, without attempting to impose judgements. The nurse as a professional has a duty to carry out a thorough nursing assessment (see Chapter 3).

## Physiological Indicators

Physiological indicators of stress are objective and more readily identified (see box). These parameters can be commonly observed or measured. However, they are not always observed all the time in all patients/clients experiencing stress, and they vary with individuals. Vital signs are usually altered (see Chapter 4), and the patient/client may appear restless or may be unable to concentrate. These indicators can appear at any stage of stress. The duration and intensity of the symptoms are directly related to the perceived duration and intensity of the stressor. Physiological indicators arise from a variety of systems. Therefore the assessment of stress involves collecting data from all systems.

The link between psychological stress and disease is frequently called the mind-body interaction. Research has shown that stress can affect illness and disease patterns. At the turn of the century, infectious diseases were the leading causes of death but, since then, improved living conditions, increased knowledge of nutrition, better sanitation methods and antibiotics have lowered the death rate. Now the leading cause of death in Western cultures is ill health resulting from lifestyle stressors.

During any stage of stress, there may be physical complaints such as nausea, vomiting, diarrhoea, or headache. Physical appearance may be changed; posture may be slumped, hygiene

and grooming may be poor, and style of dress may change. Prolonged stress has been linked with cardiovascular and gastrointestinal diseases. Additionally, some cancers and immunological disorders, as well as fatigue, burnout, and irritability, have been associated with prolonged, unresolved stressors (Greer, 1979; Leidy, 1990).

Mild stress situations do not usually produce chronic physiological damage, but moderate and severe stress can create a risk of short-term illness, or a worsening of a chronic condition. **Mild stress situations** are stressors that everyone encounters regularly, such as a traffic jam or criticism from a superior. Such situations usually last a few minutes to a few hours. By themselves, these stressors are not significant risks for symptom development. However, multiple mild stressors over a short time can increase the risk of illness (Holmes and Rahe, 1976).

**Moderate stress situations** last longer, from several hours to days. For example, an unresolved disagreement with a co-worker, work overload, new job expectations, or the prolonged absence of a family member are moderate stress situations.

**Severe stress situations** are chronic situations that may last several weeks to several years, such as continual marital disagreements, prolonged financial difficulties, or long-term physical illness. The more intense and longer the stress situation, the higher the health risk (Wheeler, 1989). The development of stress-related disease can be examined in terms of the health-illness continuum (Fig. 10-2). As a person's stress increases, stress behaviours increase gradually, and this situation can decrease both energy and adaptive responses.

Identifying the mind-body interaction is crucial for predicting the risk of stress-related illness. A nurse can often consider the effects of a stressful lifestyle or event and assess the individual's coping mechanisms.

## Developmental Indicators

Prolonged stress can affect the ability to complete developmental tasks. In any developmental stage an individual normally encounters tasks and engages in behaviours characteristic of the stage (Erikson, 1980). Prolonged stress can interrupt or impede passage through the stage. In extreme forms, prolonged stress can lead to maturational crises, which can generate stress and, if unresolved, may lead to mental distress or illness.

Infants or young children generally encounter stressors at home. When nurtured in responsive, empathetic environments, they are able to develop healthy self-esteem and ultimately learn healthy adaptive coping responses (Wheeler, 1989). However, either the absence of parental figures or parental failure to provide the security needed to develop a sense of trust can be stressors. In later life, there may be chronic distrust, resulting in withdrawal and limited interpersonal relationships. Alternatively, when parents or the environment prevent children from developing a sense of autonomy, the children may experience stress, indicated by excessive dependence on others.

Preschool children normally develop by exploring their surroundings, exploring differences between boys and girls, and developing a conscience. Children are ashamed when caught being 'bad' and want to be told when they are 'good'. An indicator of stress at this stage may be passive, inactive behaviour towards the environment.

Children of school age normally develop a sense of adequacy. They begin to realize that the accumulation of knowledge and the mastery of skills can help them to accomplish goals. Self-esteem develops through friendships and sharing with peers. At this stage, stress can be indicated by an inability or unwillingness to develop friendships.

Adolescents normally develop a strong sense of identity but at the same time need to be accepted by their peers. Adolescents with strong social support systems report an increased ability to problem solve and adjust to stressors, but adolescents without social support systems frequently report increased physical and behavioural symptoms (Elkind, 1970; Marcia, 1968). There are many stressors in this age group, including conflicts involving sexual drive and expected standards of behaviour. Prolonged conflict may indicate indecision and confusion, rebellion, depression, or anxiety.

> ### Children's Nursing
> ### Helping children cope with stress
> Accurate assessment is fundamental in helping parents and their children deal with stressful experiences. It is essential to identify family strengths and deficiencies in order to guide intervention that will encourage the optimum development of all family members (Austin, 1990).

Young adults are in transition from youthful experiences to adult responsibilities. They must prepare for careers, for living alone, and perhaps for starting families. Conflicts may develop between work and family responsibilities. Stressors include conflicts between expectations and reality.

A child or adult with physical or intellectual special needs may not react to stress in the same way as other children.

Adults in their middle years are usually involved in family building, creating stable careers, and perhaps caring for older parents. They are generally able to control desires and in some cases substitute the needs of spouses, children, or parents for their needs. Stress can result, however, if they feel that too many responsibilities have been placed on them. A recent trend is looking at the impact of stressors of the family care giver's role. The middle years have been called the *sandwich generation* in which adults are frequently responsible for chronically ill parents while raising their own families. Because of the stressors involved, care givers have reported increases in fatigue, minor illnesses (for example, colds and influenza), depression, and dissatisfaction with family interaction (Friedemann, 1990; Gass, 1989).

Older adults are commonly faced with adapting to changes in family and perhaps to the deaths of spouses. Older adults must also adjust to changes in physical appearance and physiological functioning. In addition, the stress of decreasing social interactions, as friends die or become unable to maintain contact, and retirement often brings more change. Prolonged fear and stress can be indicated in older adults by worsening of pre-existing chronic illness, which may cause further stress on family or social relationships (Bahr, 1981; Gass, 1989).

## Physiological Indicators of Stress

- Elevated blood pressure
- Increased muscle tension in neck, shoulders, back
- Elevated pulse and increased respiration
- Sweaty palms
- Cold hands and feet
- Slumped posture
- Fatigue
- Tension headache
- Upset stomach
- Higher-pitched voice
- Nausea, vomiting, and diarrhoea
- Change in appetite
- Change in urinary frequency
- Abnormal laboratory findings: elevated adrenocorticotropic hormone, cortisol, and catecholamine levels and hyperglycaemia
- Restlessness: difficulty falling asleep or frequent awakening
- Dilated pupils

## Psychosocial Indicators

Psychosocial changes are direct and sometimes obvious results of prolonged stress. Frequently a nurse can observe the emotional impact of stress through changes in behaviour.

Stress affects emotional well-being in many ways (see box). Everyone's personality involves a complex relationship among many factors and so the reaction to prolonged stress depends on support systems, prior experience with stressors, coping mechanisms, and the overall stress response. A change in behaviour should alert a nurse, family member, or friend that the person needs help in adapting to stress. Ideally, coping problems should be anticipated and preventive measures taken, but often it is difficult to anticipate unique psychosocial reactions to stress.

## Cognitive Indicators

Prolonged stress can have cognitive indicators. A person's ability to acquire new knowledge or skills can be impaired. For example, a patient/client with a chronic illness may have difficulty learning about the illness or treatment. Prolonged stress can also affect role performance, for example, a person may even be unable to continue employment. Stress can also impede communication between a patient/client and other people or even with a family where they may be unable to resolve conflicts.

## Spiritual Indicators

People use spiritual resources to adapt to stress in many ways, but stress can also threaten a person in the spiritual dimension. Severe stress could result in anger at the person's supreme being, or the individual may view the stressor as a punishment. Stressors such as acute illness or the death of a loved one may threaten a person's meaning of life or may precipitate a spiritual crisis, during which the person may act destructively towards self and/or others. A nurse should never judge the appropriateness of religious feelings or practices, but should assist the patient/client in using spiritual resources in order to adapt.

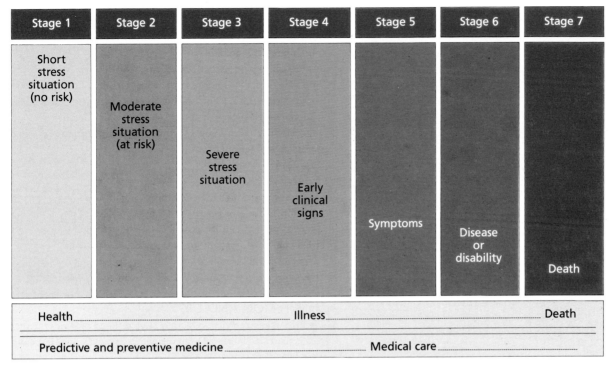

| Stage 1 | Stage 2 | Stage 3 | Stage 4 | Stage 5 | Stage 6 | Stage 7 |
|---|---|---|---|---|---|---|
| Short stress situation (no risk) | Moderate stress situation (at risk) | Severe stress situation | Early clinical signs | Symptoms | Disease or disability | Death |

Health............................................................ Illness................................................ Death

Predictive and preventive medicine.................................... Medical care...................................

Fig. 10-2 Stages of illness development in stress-related diseases.

## Reducing Stressful Situations

It is unrealistic to try to eliminate all stressors. However, the nurse can reduce some stressors and thereby provide the individual with a greater sense of control. Pender (1987) identifies five methods to assist in reducing stressful situations: habituation, change avoidance, time blocking, time management, and environment modification.

## HABITUATION

Every person has unique habits and routines that help accomplish day-to-day activities. According to Pender (1987), 'Routines reduce the need for expenditure of physical and psychological energy, resist change, and thus serve as a stabilizing force'. Illnesses, crises, or spells of hospitalization disturb a patient's/client's routine, thereby disturbing the pattern of living and resulting in greater energy expenditure.

During actual or potential stress an established routine can be effective in supporting energy conservation. An example of this might be a woman who has chosen to stay at home to raise children and is now sending her youngest child to school. Although she anticipated this change, she may now be unable to obtain a job in her field. She may express a fear about being 'unable to get anything done at home'. In this situation the person's habits have been disrupted, and a new routine has not been developed. A plan that assists her in developing a new routine consistent with her goals could reduce the stress, and is likely to enhance the quality of parenting.

## CHANGE AVOIDANCE

**Change avoidance** is merely limiting unnecessary and avoidable changes. For example, a father of two children (school age) is divorcing his wife and is experiencing stress-related symptoms.

At the same time his company is pressuring him to relocate. This man and his children are experiencing a change in family structure; therefore it may be wiser to postpone a relocation than to multiply changes and, potentially, stressors.

Tension created by multiple changes increases the response to stress. The capacity for upsetting a person's well-being increases with each distressing change. Deliberately reducing or postponing changes that result in tension can assist the patient/client in dealing more constructively with unavoidable change.

Controlled or self-initiated changes can provide a challenge for an individual. The person can then turn the challenge into personal growth such as can be seen in increased coping strategies or increased self-confidence.

## TIME BLOCKING

Time blocking is a technique in which an individual has a specific period of time to focus on, and adapt to, stressors. The major advantage of time blocking is that the person establishes a period of time in which to address specific goals or concerns and reduce the sense of time urgency. In addition, the individual can use the remaining time and resources more effectively because the level of anxiety is reduced.

## TIME MANAGEMENT

People who use time efficiently generally experience less stress related to social, family, and job activities. For some people, **time-management** techniques may include establishing an order of priorities for a list of tasks. This technique can be beneficial for people unable to get anything done because there seems to be too much to do.

Another time-management technique is learning to say 'no' to potential disruptions (Dickson, 1989). Time management may

### Behavioural and Emotional Indicators of Stress

- Anxiety
- Depression
- Burnout
- Increased use of chemical substances
- Change in eating habits, sleep, and activity patterns
- Mental exhaustion
- Feelings of inadequacy
- Loss of self-esteem
- Increased irritability
- Loss of motivation
- Emotional outbursts and crying
- Decreased productivity and quality of job performance
- Tendency to make mistakes (i.e. poor judgement)
- Forgetfulness and blocking
- Diminished attention to detail
- Preoccupation (i.e. daydreaming or 'spacing out')
- Inability to concentrate on tasks
- Increased absenteeism and illness
- Lethargy
- Loss of interest
- Proneness to accidents

also include scheduling appointments realistically to avoid rushing from task to task or meeting to meeting.

Controlling the demands of others is essential for effective time management. Few people are able to meet all of the requests made by others. It is important to learn to recognize which requests can be realistically met, which are impossible to meet, and which are negotiable.

## ENVIRONMENTAL MODIFICATION

Realistic changes in environment can reduce stressful situations. For example, job stress can be reduced by avoiding situations and people that produce stress. Changing factors in the home in order to reduce housework or to provide safety measures can reduce stress.

When people have realistic control over their environments, stress is mediated. After the minimal or moderate stressors are mediated the individual is better able to resolve severe stressors.

## Decreasing Physiological Response to Stress

In general, **stress-management** techniques involve health-enhancing habits that can reduce the impact of stress on physical and mental health. These are often commonsense approaches that provide a basis for low-stress living. General pre-requisites for stress management include regular exercise, humour, good nutrition and diet, adequate rest, and relaxation techniques.

## REGULAR EXERCISE

A regular exercise programme improves muscle tone and posture, controls weight, reduces tension, and promotes relaxation. In addition, exercise reduces the risk of cardiovascular disease and improves cardiopulmonary functioning.

A person who has a history of chronic illness, who is at risk for developing an illness, or who is over the age of 35 should begin a physical exercise programme only after discussing it with

a doctor. In general, for a fitness programme to have positive physical effects, a person should exercise at least 3 times a week for 30 to 40 minutes.

Exercise programmes are effective in decreasing the severity of stress-related conditions such as hypertension, obesity, tension headaches, fatigue, mental exhaustion, irritability, and depression. Adults particularly need routine exercise plans because they are occupied with rearing children, developing careers, and establishing homes.

## HUMOUR

Humour shared within the context of a mutually respecting relationship may alleviate some of the feelings of stress. In one study, Warner (1990) investigated the way that nursing students used humour to mediate stressors associated with clinical practice. Humour in this instance allowed the students to regulate stressful emotions and alter a stressful person-environment relationship.

## NUTRITION AND DIET

Nutrition and exercise are closely related. Food provides the fuel for activity and increased exercise, which improves circulation and the delivery of nutrients to body tissues.

Poor dietary habits can worsen a stress response and make a person irritable, hyperactive, and anxious. This impairs the ability to meet personal, family, and job responsibilities (see Chapter 21).

## REST

An established, habitual pattern of sufficient rest and sleep is also important for managing stress. A person experiencing stress should be encouraged to allow time for rest and sleep. Sleep not only refreshes the body but also helps a person become mentally relaxed. An individual may need specific help in learning to relax to fall asleep.

## RELAXATION TECHNIQUES

Progressive relaxation with and without muscle tension and imagery reduces the physiological and emotional components of stress. Relaxation techniques are learned behaviours and require training and practice sessions (MacDonald and Wallace, 1980) (see Chapter 32). After the patient/client becomes skilled at these techniques, tension is reduced and physiological parameters are changed.

## Improved Behavioural and Emotional Responses to Stress

Behavioural and emotional responses to stress can be mediated by the use of support systems, crisis intervention, and enhancement of self-esteem.

## SUPPORT SYSTEMS

The quote, "No man is an island," (from a meditation by John Donne) is of particular importance for stress management. A support system of family, friends, and colleagues who will listen and offer advice and emotional support is beneficial to a person experiencing stress. **Support systems** can reduce stress reactions and promote physical and mental well-being. Nursing research has documented the correlation of positive social supports and the reduction of symptoms in chronic diseases (Mays, 1988; Fiore *et al*, 1986).

Nurses can use various methods to help patients and clients build support networks, such as encouraging family members to visit, making support groups available, encouraging involvement in religious or social groups, and encouraging recreational activities. Nurses can use a range of therapeutic communication skills (Heron, 1975) to encourage individuals to express their feelings and identify causes of stress. Referrals may also be made for patient/client or problem-centred counselling. Alternatively, psychotherapy or cognitive therapy may be accessed by the patient/client.

## CRISIS INTERVENTION

**Crisis intervention** is a therapeutic technique for helping someone resolve a particular, immediate stress problem. Crisis intervention does not involve an in-depth analysis of a situation but addresses the immediate, urgent need for stress reduction. The goal is to restore the person as quickly as possible to the pre-crisis level of functioning in all dimensions.

Crises occur when people encounter problems or stress situations with which they are unable to cope in usual ways but which may lead to growth or stagnation.

Patients/clients and nurses are at risk for two types of crises, situational and developmental. A *situational crisis* arises suddenly in response to an external event or conflict involving a specific circumstance. Symptoms associated with situational crises are transient, and the episode is brief. Situational crises include giving birth, major role changes, acute physical illness, physical assault or rape, family changes such as remarriage or the death of a family member, and unexpected unemployment.

A *developmental crisis* occurs when a person is unable to complete the developmental tasks of a psychosocial stage and is therefore unable to continue developing. A developmental crisis can occur at any point in life if circumstances prevent a person from meeting the challenge of a particular stage. The development and maintenance of self-concept is a complex process which involves self-concept, self-esteem and body image as inter-related concepts.

Self-concept is the psychic representation or identity of an individual. It is a dynamic combination formulated over years and based on the following sources:

- Reaction of others to the infant's or child's body and behaviour
- Ongoing perceptions of others' reaction to the self
- Experiences with self and others
- Personality structure
- Perceptions of psychological and sensory stimuli that impinge on the self
- Prior and new experiences
- Present feelings about the physical, emotional and social self
- Expectations about self.

Body image is a personal mental picture of an individual's body, including the external, internal and postural images. These mental images are not necessarily consistent with the actual body structure or appearance. Body image includes attitudes, emotions and personality reactions to the body as an object in space, with a distinct boundary and separate from all others and the general environment (Schilder, 1951). Body image develops gradually over years as children learn about their bodies and their structures, functions, abilities and limitations.

**Self-esteem** is the evaluation that an individual customarily maintains of self and conveys to others by verbal or overt behavioural expressions. This judgemental feeling includes approval or disapproval and indicates the extent to which an individual believes in personal capabilities, significance, value, success and worth (Coopersmith, 1967). Self-esteem involves the acceptance of self because of basic worth and despite limitations.

## Stress and the Nurse

Rapid changes in society, health care technology, and health care knowledge, as well as changes in the nursing profession, can place demands which far exceed the nurse's ability to cope with stress. **Job stress** can result from a series of factors at work that interact with the worker to disrupt psychological or physiological balance and decision making.

Job stress frequently results in a condition called **burnout**, which is characterized by a decreased concern for the people with whom one is working. During burnout, the individual experiences physical and emotional exhaustion. The job or profession no longer has any positive rewards. The individual may also experience anger and apathy while on the job.

Nurses are at risk for job stress as a result of three factors. First, new graduates generally have high expectations that may not be met in the workplace, leading to frustration. Second, nurses usually work in close contact with others, specifically, patients/clients and other health care professionals. Such continuous interaction can lead to conflicts and other stresses. Finally, the workplace itself increases the risk for job stresses. When these stressors become insurmountable, the employee's desire to change jobs becomes greater (Parasuraman, 1989). Therefore if the stressors can be reduced by the institution or employee, the turnover rate can be reduced (Menzies, 1988; Melia, 1987). Nurses, as people, are no different from the patients/clients with whom they work. Socialization into the job often means that nurses deny their feelings of stress for fear they may be judged to be less than able in their role.

Nurses can reduce stressors by using the same stress-management techniques that they teach patients/clients. These commonsense techniques improve physical and mental well-being, enabling nurses to cope more successfully with stressors. In addition, nurses should identify specific stressors in their workplaces and if possible eliminate or minimize them, for example, with membership schemes, staff support groups, peer support, co-counselling, and adequate supervision (Melia, 1987).

## SUMMARY

Each person reacts to stress differently, according to perception of the stressor, personality, prior experience with stress, and use of coping mechanisms. Various models of stress help the nurse understand causes and responses to stress.

Prolonged stress can affect level of health, resulting in physical or mental illness. Stress-management techniques are directed at changing a person's reactions to stressors. Through the use of health-promotion and health-maintenance strategies, nurses can help patients/clients manage stress successfully.

## CHAPTER 10 REVIEW
### Key Concepts
- Physiological adaptive mechanisms are controlled by the medulla oblongata, reticular formation, and pituitary gland.
- Prolonged stress decreases the adaptive capacity of the body.
- Stress is physiological or psychological tension that can affect a person in any or all human dimensions.
- An individual may encounter stressors in the internal or external environment.
- Stressors necessitate change or adaptation so that a state of equilibrium can be maintained.
- A person's response to stress is influenced by the intensity, duration, and scope of the stressor and by the number of stressors present at one time.
- A person adapts to stress by using resources in the physical and developmental, emotional, intellectual, social, and spiritual dimensions.
- The two forms of physiological response to stress are the local adaptation syndrome and the general adaptation syndrome.
- The local adaptation syndrome involves several specific responses to stress, including the reflex pain response.
- The general adaptation syndrome involves a multisystem physiological response to stress.
- The three stages of the general adaptation syndrome are the alarm reaction, the resistance stage, and the exhaustion stage.
- Psychological responses to stress include task-orientated behaviours and ego-defence mechanisms.

- Task-orientated behaviours include attack behaviour, withdrawal, and compromise.
- Ego-defence mechanisms are unconscious behaviours that offer a person psychological protection from stressful feelings or events.
- Stress has an impact on the onset, course, and outcome of illness.
- Prolonged stress decreases the ability to adapt to the stress and affects the person in all dimensions.
- People generally learn to use short- and long-term strategies to cope with stress.
- Stress-management techniques include health-enhancing habits, crisis intervention, and methods of reducing job stress.

## CRITICAL THINKING EXERCISES
1. Craig Johnson is 26 years old and has a high-level management position in an advertising firm. He states that he enjoys his job, but it has been 'very stressful for the last month'. He has noted increased gastrointestinal problems and headaches and reports an increase in alcohol consumption. What strategies can the nurse design to assist in reducing Mr Johnson's response to stress?
2. Calvin Kleiger had a myocardial infarction yesterday. What are the important physiological responses to stress that can increase the risk for further cardiac damage? What nursing measures can reduce these stress responses?
3. While visiting a family, a district nurse notes that a young mother appears exhausted and expresses difficulty in managing her three-month-old baby who is continually crying. What strategies can the nurse suggest to reduce this young mother's level of fatigue?
4. What forms of supportive strategies may be helpful for those members of the family who have to live with children with severe learning difficulties and challenging behaviours?

### KEY TERMS
Adaptation, p. 197
Burnout, p. 205
Change avoidance, p. 203
Constructive behaviours, p. 199
Coping mechanisms, p. 200
Crisis intervention, p. 205
Destructive behaviours, p. 199
Flight-or-fight response, p. 199
General adaptation syndrome (GAS), p. 199
Homeostasis, p. 196
Job stress, p. 199
Local adaptation syndrome (LAS), p. 199
Mild stress situations, p. 201
Moderate stress situations, p. 201
Self-esteem, p. 205
Severe stress situations, p. 201
Stress response, p. 195
Stress-management, p. 204
Stressors, p. 195
Support systems, p. 204
Task-orientated behaviours, p. 200
Time-management, p. 203

### REFERENCES
Austin J: Assessment of coping mechanisms used by parents and children with chronic illness, *MCN* 15: 98, 1990.

Bahr R: Management of common stressors in the later years, Responding to stress: *Community health in the '80's* , London, 1981, NLN publications.

Coopersmith S: *The intecedents of self esteem*, San Francisco, 1967, Freeman.

Dickson A: *A woman in your own right,* London, 1989, Quartet Books

Dryden W: *Counselling individuals: the rationale-emotive approach*, London, 1987, Taylor and Francis.

Elkind D: Erik Erikson's eight ages of man, *New York Times Magazine* 16, 1970.

Erikson E: *Identity and the life cycle*, New York, 1980, Norton.

Fiore J et al: Social support as a multifaceted concept: examination of important dimensions for adjustment, *Am J Community Psychol*, 14(1), 93, 1986.

Freud S: *The ego and the id*, Harmondsworth, 1984, Penguin.

Friedemann M, Andrews M: Family support and child adjustment in single-parent families, *Issues in Comprehensive Paed Nurs* 13 (4): 289, 1990.

Gass KA, Chang AS: Appraisal of bereavement: coping resources and psychosocial health dysfunction in widows and widowers, *Nurs Res* 38(1):31, 1989.

Greer A, Morris T, Pettingale KW: Psychosocial response to breast cancer: effect on outcome, *Lancet* 13: 785, 1979.

Heron J: *Six category intervention analysis*, University of Surrey: 1975, Human Potential Resource Group.

Holmes T, Rahe R: The social readjustment scale, *J Psychosomatic Res*, 12:213, 1976.

Laing R D: *Sanity, madness and the family*, London, 1964, Penguin.

Lazarus RS, Folkman S: *Stress appraisal and coping*, New York, 1984, Springer-Verlag.

Leidy NK, Ozbolt JG, Swain MAP: Psychophysiological processes of stress in chronic physical illness: a theoretical perspective, *J Adv Nurs* 15 (4): 478, 1990.

Lindsey AM, Carrieri VK: Stress Response. In Lindsey AM, Carrieri VK (editors): *Pathological phenomenon in nursing: human response to illness*, Philadelphia, 1986, Saunders.

MacDonald Wallace J: Stress and tension control, *Nurs* 1(10):451, 1980.

Marcia JE: The case history of a conduct: ego identity status. In Vinacke E (editor): *Readings in general psychology*, New York, 1968, Van Nostrand-Reinhold.

Mays RM: Family stress and adaptation, *Nurs Practitioner* 13(8):52, 1988.

Mechanic D: *Students under stress*, Illinois, 1962, Freepress.

Melia K: *Learning and working : the occupational socialisation of nurses*, London, 1987, Tavistock Publisations Ltd.

Menzies Lyth I: *Containing anxiety in institutions*, London, 1988, Free Association Books.

Parasuraman S : Nursing turnover: an integrated model, Res *Nurs Health* 12: 267, 1989.

Pender NJ: *Health promotion in nursing practice*, Connecticut, 1987, Appleton & Lange.

Riehl JP, Roy C (editors): *Conceptual models for nursing*, New York, 1980, Appleton-Century-Crofts.

Schilder P: *Image and appearance of the human body*, New York, 1951, International Universities Press.

Selye H: *The stress of life*, New York, 1956, McGraw-Hill.

Selye H: *The stress of life*, ed 2, New York, 1976, McGraw-Hill.

Skynner R: *One flesh separate persons*, London, 1976, Constable.

Stuart GW, Sundeen SJ: *Principles and practice of psychiatric nursing*, St Louis, 1991, Mosby-Year Book.

Warner SL: Humor: a coping response for student nurses, *Arch Psych Nurs*, 5(1):10, 1990.

Wheeler K: Self psychology's contribution to understanding stress and implications for nursing, *J Adv Med Surg Nurs* 1(4):1, 1989.

## FURTHER READING

### Adult Nursing

Bond M: *Stress and self awareness: a guide for nurses*, London, 1986, Heinemann.

Byass R: *Soothing body and soul*, *Nurs Times* 84(24):9, 1988.

Cava R: *Dealing with difficult people*, London, 1990, Piatkus.

Lindop E: Individual stress among nurses in training: why some leave while others stay, *Nurs Ed Today* 11:110, 1991.

Mackenzie Stuart A: Stress and organic disease, *Nurs* 1(10):437, 1980.

Makin PE, Lindley PA: *Positive stress management*, London, 1991, Kogan Page.

Powell TJ, Enright SJ: *Anxiety and stress management*, London, 1990, Routledge.

Thomas M: Stress and mental illness, *Nurs* 1(10):438, 1980.

Wen J: *Managing anxiety: a guide to anxiety management training*, Birmingham, 1985, Prepare Publications.

Williams C: Empathy and burnout in male and female helping professionals, *Res Nurs Health*, 12:169, 1989.

### Children's Nursing

Axyline V: *Play therapy*, London, 1989, Churchill Livingstone.

Bowlby J: *Attachment and loss*, Volume 11, Gretna, LA, 1975, Pelican.

Bowlby J: *Child care and the growth of love*, London, 1965, Penguin.

Crompton M: *Children and counselling*, London, 1992, Edward Arnold.

David H: *Counselling parents of children with chronic illness or disability*, London, 1993, British Psychological Society.

Garmez Y: Stressors of childhood. In Garmez Y, Rutter N (editor): *Stress, coping and development in children*, New York, 1983, McGraw-Hill.

Gillham B, Plunkett K: *Child psychology — the child to five years*, London, 1982, Hodder & Stoughton.

Hall D: *Beyond separation*, 1979, Routledge & Kegan Paul.

Hornby G: *Counselling in child disability: skills for working with parents*, London, 1994, Chapman and Hall.

Johnson K: *Trauma in the lives of children*, 1989, Macmillan.

Muller DJ *et al*: *Nursing children, research and practice* 2e, London, 1992, Chapman and Hall.

Sandstrom C: *Psychology of childhood and adolescence*, London, 1979, Penguin.

Wolfe S: *Children under stress*, London, 1981, Penguin.

### Learning Disabilities Nursing

Halliday S *et al*: Caring for people with severe learning difficulties in ordinary houses: issues of staff stress & support, *Mental Handicap*. Dec, 1992

Hubert J: *Home-bound: crisis in the care of young people with severe learning difficulties*, London, 1991, Kings Fund Centre.

McCubbin A M: Family stress and family strengths: a comparison of single and two parent families with handicapped children, *Research in Nursing and Health*. 12: 101-110, 1989.

Pahl J *et al*: *Families with mentally handicapped children: a study of stress and of service response*, Kent, 1984, University of Kent.

Sinason V: *Mental handicap and the human condition: new approaches from the Tavistock*, London, 1992, Free Association.

Stuttard R: When mental problems overlap, (stress and the mentally handicapped) *Parents Voice*, 35 (3): 14-15, 1985.

Turk V, Francis E: An anxiety management group: strengths and pitfalls, (with a group of mentally handicapped adults) *Mental Handicap*, 18 (2): 78-81, 1990.

### Mental Health Nursing

Cava R: *Dealing with difficult people*, London, 1990, Piatkus.

Skynner R: *One flesh separate persons*, London, 1976, Constable.

Stuart GW, Sundeen SJ: *Principles and practice of psychiatric nursing*, St Louis, 1991, Mosby-Year Book.

Thomas M: Stress and mental illness, *Nurs* 1(10):438, 1980.

Vinacke E (editor): *Readings in general psychology*, New York, 1968, Van Nostrand-Reinhold.

# CHAPTER 11

# Loss, Death, and Grieving

---

## CHAPTER OUTLINE

**Loss, Death, Grief, and Nursing**
*Loss*
*Grief, mourning and bereavement*
*Concepts and theories of the grieving process*

**Nursing Care and Grief**
*Assessment*
*Planning care*
*Implementation*
*Evaluation*

---

## LEARNING OUTCOMES

After studying this chapter, you should be able to:
- ◼ *Define the key terms listed.*
- ◼ *Identify the nurse's role in assisting patients/clients with problems related to loss, death, and grief.*
- ◼ *List the five categories of loss.*
- ◼ *Compare and contrast the phases of grieving described by Engel, Kübler-Ross, and Martocchio.*
- ◼ *Define and compare anticipatory grief, grief after loss, and resolved grief.*
- ◼ *Identify personal, psychological, and social factors that influence the patient's/client's grief response.*
- ◼ *Describe the roles of care planning, therapeutic communication, and other nursing interventions in meeting the dying person's comfort needs.*
- ◼ *Explain ways for the nurse to assist and support the family in caring for a dying person.*
- ◼ *Discuss the purposes of a hospice.*
- ◼ *Discuss important factors in caring for the body after death.*
- ◼ *Discuss the role of the nurse's own loss experience as it influences care of the grieving.*

**B**irth, loss, and death are universal and individually unique events of the human experience. Life is a series of losses and gains. A child beginning to walk gains independence with mobility. An older person with visual and hearing changes may lose self-confidence. Illness and hospitalization frequently cause losses.

A nurse works with many people who experience different types of loss. Coping mechanisms determine the person's ability to face and accept loss. Grief is a natural response to loss. The nurse assists patients/clients in understanding and accepting loss so that life can continue. Death is the greatest loss any individual can sustain, whether it be the person's own, or that of someone close. When a person becomes terminally ill, others are reminded of their own mortality. The style of dying reflects a person's style of living, and attitudes about death depend upon a person's beliefs and emotional strengths.

## LOSS, DEATH, GRIEF, AND NURSING

Nurses need to understand loss and grief, since death is a frequent reality in many nursing care settings. Most nurses interact daily with patients/clients and families experiencing loss and grief. Nurses also experience personal loss as patient/client-family-nurse relationships end through transfer, discharge, recovery or death. Nurses may find that it is easy to relieve physical symptoms associated with illness and death; however, it is difficult to become involved in meaningful interpersonal relationships to support a person who is suffering or dying. Personal feelings, values, and experiences influence the extent to which nurses can support individuals and families during loss or death. Self-awareness – exploring personal attitudes, feelings, and values – is necessary before nurses can use a sensitive, therapeutic approach with others. Developing the art of being with the grieving and dying requires an inner strength that arises from knowledge of and a positive belief in self. Formulation of a philosophy of life helps nurses function during difficult times. Knowledge of the concepts of loss and the grieving process enables nurses to use creative interventions to promote health, prevent illness and to support patients/clients who are dying or facing loss.

## Loss

A person experiences loss in the absence of an object, person, body part or function, or emotion that was formerly present. Losses may be actual or perceived. **Actual losses** are easily identified, as with the child whose playmate moves away or the adult who loses a marriage partner through divorce. **Perceived losses** are less tangible and are easily misunderstood, such as the loss of confidence or prestige. The more invested in what is lost, the greater the feeling of loss. A person may experience *maturational loss* (loss resulting from normal life transitions, for example, a child going off to school for the first time), *situational loss* (loss occurring suddenly in response to a specific external event, such as the sudden death of a loved one) or both. The child learning to walk loses the infant-like body image, the woman experiencing menopause loses the ability to bear children, and an unemployed person may lose self-esteem.

**Personal loss** is any significant loss that requires adaptation through the grieving process. Loss occurs when something or someone can no longer be seen, felt, heard, known, or experienced. The type of loss influences the degree of stress. For example, the loss of an object might not generate the same stress as the loss of a significant other. However, individuals respond to loss differently. The death of a family member would be expected to cause more stress than the loss of a pet, but for an older person living alone, the death of a pet that has been a constant companion would possibly cause more emotional stress than that of a cousin who has not been seen for years. The type of loss is significant to the grieving process; yet the nurse must recognize that **each person's interpretation of a loss is highly individualized**.

There are five categories of loss: loss of an external object; loss of a known environment; loss of a significant other; loss of an aspect of self; and loss of life. Nurses may encounter a person who has experienced more than one type. For the hospitalized chronically ill adult, Lewis (1983) describes many potential permanent losses (see box). Loss threatens self-esteem, security and sense of worth. The nurse must recognize the meaning of each loss to a patient/client and its impact on physical and psychological functioning.

### Loss of an External Object

Loss of an external object involves any possession that is worn out, misplaced, stolen, or ruined by disaster. For a child the object may be a toy or a blanket; for an adult it may be a piece of jewellery or an article of clothing. The extent of grieving that a person feels for a lost object depends on its value, the sentiment the person attaches to it, and the object's usefulness.

### Loss of a Known Environment

The loss associated with separation from a known environment includes leaving a familiar setting for a period or relocating permanently; examples include moving to a new neighbourhood or city, starting a new job, or hospitalization. Loss through separation from a known environment may occur through maturational or situational circumstances and through injury or illness.

Confinement within an institution results in isolation from routine events. The rules of a hospital create an environment that is often impersonal and demoralizing. The loneliness of an unfamiliar setting may threaten self-esteem and make grieving more difficult.

### Loss of a Significant Other

Significant others include parents, spouses, children, siblings, teachers, clergy, friends, neighbours, and colleagues. Celebrities and well-known athletes may be significant others for young people. Research shows that many people regard pets as significant others (Lee, 1992). Loss occurs as a result of separation, moving, running away, promotion at work, and death.

### Loss of an Aspect of Self

The loss of an aspect of self may include a body part, physiological function, or psychological function. Loss of a body part may include an eye, breast, or limb (Parkes, 1991). Loss of physiological function includes loss of urinary or bowel control, mobility, strength, or sensory function. Loss of psychological function includes loss of memory, humour, self-esteem, self-confidence, power, respect, or love. The loss of these aspects of self may result from illness, injury, or developmental and situational changes. Such a loss lessens the individual's well-being. A person not only experiences grief over the loss but may experience permanent changes in body image and self-concept.

### Loss of Life

People who face death live, feel, think, and respond to events and people around them until the moment of death. Concern is often not about death itself but about pain and loss of control. Although most people are afraid of death, the same issues will not be equally important to each person. Each person responds differently to death. For people who have lived alone and suffered long terminal illnesses, death may be a relief. Some perceive death as an entry into an afterlife to be reunited with loved ones in paradise. Others fear separation, abandonment and loneliness.

### Grief, Mourning and Bereavement

**Bereavement** is the state of thought, feeling, and activity that follows loss. It includes grief and mourning. **Grief** is a form of sorrow that follows the perception or anticipation of a loss of one

---

### Children's Nursing
### Caring for dying children

Caring for dying children requires the nurse to be aware of the developmental stage the child has reached and be aware that dying children generally know about death. It is also important to develop an awareness of the individual perception of that particular child. The nurse can use this information to plan care to meet the needs of the child and family.

## Potential Losses in Chronic Illness

- Health
- Independence
- Sense of control over life
- Privacy
- Modesty
- Body image
- Relationships
- Established roles inside and outside the home
- Social status
- Self-confidence
- Possessions
- Financial security
- Means of productivity and self-fulfilment
- Lifestyle
- Plans or fantasies for the future
- Fantasy of immortality
- Money
- Daily routine
- Sleep
- Sexual functioning
- Leisure activities

Modified from Lewis K: Potential losses in chronic illness. *J Rehabil* 49: 8, 1983.

### Learning Disabilities Nursing
### Addressing bereavement issues

Research has shown that adults with learning disabilities have a sophisticated understanding of the concept of death (McEvoy, 1989), and that they grieve in much the same way as anyone else (Oswin, 1981). However, carers and care givers are often reluctant to discuss death and bereavement with these clients. For example, during a family crisis, the family may place the family member with a learning disability into respite care, so that they may address the crisis without having to take care of, or worry about, the disabled family member. When a death occurs, the family often decide that it is in the client's best interest not to attend the funeral or return home until everything is over, because they think these events will be too upsetting for him or her. This denies the person with learning disabilities the opportunity to work through his or her own grief and to use established rituals to come to terms with the loss.

Increasing attention is now being given to helping people with learning disabilities to work through death and bereavement. These needs are also being addressed for clients and carers who live in long-term residential settings, such as group homes, because emotional attachments and bonds are frequently strong in these environments.

### Mental Health Nursing
### The impact of relocation

As a result of policy decisions by successive governments affecting the balance between institutional and community care, many older adults and people with mental health needs have been moved from longstay institutions into alternative homes within the community. These moves can require significant adjustment or grief for the individual who is relocated.

Schulz and Brenner (1977) found that individuals who were relocated involuntarily consistently suffered from some form of setback in personal adjustment, while those who moved from choice maintained, or even improved, on some of the indicators they used in their research.

Schulz and Brenner concluded that:
- the greater the choice the less negative the effects of the relocation
- the more predictable the move, the less negative the effects of the relocation
- pre-relocation preparation programmes appear to increase the predictability of the new environment, and effectively contribute to improved health.

or more valued or significant objects. These responses often include helplessness, loneliness, hopelessness, sadness, guilt, and anger. **Mourning** is the process that follows a loss and includes working through grief. The processes of grief and mourning are intense, internal, painful, and lengthy.

Grief involves thoughts, feelings, and behaviours. Its purpose is to enable adjustment to a new way of life, which takes time.

The grieving person will try a variety of strategies in order to cope. Worden (1991) describes the following tasks of grief that facilitate healthy adjustment to loss:
- accepting the reality of the loss
- experiencing the pain of grief
- adjusting to an environment that no longer includes the lost person, object, or aspect of self
- re-investing emotional energy.

These tasks are not sequential. In fact, grieving people may work on all four tasks simultaneously, or only on one or two as priorities. Nurses can assist patients/clients and families in working through these tasks.

In the past, society discouraged openness during grief. Unhappy children were told not to cry when playmates moved away; awkward adolescents were told not to be embarrassed about sudden growth spurts, and dying people were told to remain calm and dignified. Changes in attitudes, beliefs, and values have promoted more open expressions of grief. For example, nurses learn to seek support from peers in expressing their concerns about dealing with terminally ill patients/clients. Similarly, family members seek support from carers to express anger and fear over loss. Grieving can lead to new understandings that promote growth. A person can grow from experiences of loss through openness, encouragement of others, and adequate support.

## Concepts and Theories of the Grieving Process

Grief is a normal response to any loss. Behaviours and feelings associated with the **grieving process** occur in individuals suffering from losses such as a physical deformity or the death of a close friend. They also occur when an individual faces his or her own death. Both the person undergoing the loss and the family experience grief.

There is no *right* way to grieve. The concept and theories of grief (Table 11-1) are only tools that can be used to anticipate the emotional needs of individuals and families; they can assist when planning interventions in order to help patients/clients understand and deal with their grief.

It is not helpful for a nurse to classify the patient's/client's grief; that is, the nurse should not identify a person as experiencing a certain phase of grief or working on a certain grief-related task. **The nurse's role is to assess the characteristics of grieving, recognize the influence of grief on behaviour, and provide empathetic support.**

### ENGEL'S THEORY

Engel (1964) proposed that the grieving process has three phases that can be applied to grieving and dying people.

During the first phase, the individual denies the reality of the loss and may withdraw, sit motionless, or wander aimlessly. To observers, it may seem that the person has not realized the implications of the loss. Physical reactions may include fainting, nausea, diarrhoea, rapid heart rate, restlessness, insomnia, and fatigue.

In the second phase the individual begins to feel the loss acutely and may experience desperation. Suddenly, anger, guilt, frustration, depression, and emptiness occur. Crying is typical as the individual becomes preoccupied with the loss. Crying seems to involve both an acknowledgement of the loss and the regression to a more helpless and child-like status (Engel, 1964).

During the third phase, inevitability of the loss is acknowledged. Anger or depression is no longer needed. The loss is clear to the individual, who begins to reorganize life. By experiencing these phases a person moves from a lower to a higher level of emotional and intellectual integration. New self-awareness is also developed.

### KÜBLER-ROSS' STAGES OF DYING

The framework provided by Kübler-Ross (1969) is behaviour orientated and includes five stages:

- **Denial** – the individual acts as though nothing has happened and may refuse to believe that a loss has occurred. Statements such as 'No, that can't be so', and 'It can't be happening to me!" are common.
- **Anger** – the individual resists the loss and may feel frustrated and angry, or may experience a sense of helplessness and loss of control. To be angry, we need a focus to vent our feelings towards. Sometimes this focus may be those who care for us most, including family, friends, professionals or even ourselves.
- **Bargaining** – postponement of the reality of the loss. The individual may attempt to make a deal in a subtle or overt way to prevent the loss. The person frequently seeks the opinions of others during this stage. A hospitalized patient/client may show model behaviour because of a belief that the staff will find a cure if he or she is a good patient/client.
- **Depression** – occurs when the loss is realized and the full impact of its significance is apparent. This stage may be accompanied by overwhelming loneliness and withdrawal. The depression stage provides an opportunity to work through the loss and begin problem solving.
- **Acceptance** – physiological reactions cease, and social interactions resume. Kübler-Ross defines acceptance as coming to terms with the situation rather than submitting to resignation or hopelessness.

### MARTOCCHIO'S PHASES OF GRIEVING

Although the grieving process has a predictable course and distinctive symptoms, no two people progress through it in the same way or over the same time. A person progresses and then regresses until the loss is finally resolved. Martocchio (1985) describes five phases of grief that have overlapping boundaries and no expected order. The duration of grief is variable and depends on the factors influencing the grief response. Intense reactions of grief usually subside within 6 to 12 months, and active mourning may continue for 3 to 5 years. The saying, 'Once

### TABLE 11-1 Comparison of Three Theories of the Grieving Process

| Engel (1964) | Kübler-Ross (1969) | Martocchio (1985) |
|---|---|---|
| Shock and disbelief | Denial | Shock and disbelief |
|  | Anger | Yearning and protest |
| Developing awareness | Bargaining | Anguish, disorganization, and despair |
|  | Depression | Identification in bereavement |
| Reorganization and restitution | Acceptance | Reorganization and restitution |

bereaved, always bereaved' is still true. To expect individuals to progress in a particular way over a specified time would be incorrect, inappropriate, and possibly harmful.

## ANTICIPATORY GRIEF

**Anticipatory grief** refers to accomplishing part of the grief work before the loss. For example, a hospitalized woman waiting for a mastectomy may have begun the grieving process when the lump in her breast was discovered. Before admission, she may have begun to work through the phases of disbelief and anger. When the nurse meets her, she may be developing awareness of the significance of the loss. In the same way, a family member commonly experiences anticipatory grief before the loss of a loved one. Nurses also feel anticipatory grief while caring for a person who is dying. Anticipatory grief can be beneficial if it aids progression towards a healthier emotional state after the loss.

### Complicated Grief

Some individuals find it more difficult to grieve than do others. A normal, healthy movement through their bereavement does not occur. They become 'stuck' or their emotions become greatly exaggerated. Hence their grief is prolonged.

Parkes (1991) highlighted some risk factors from his own work and others' which may predict those who are at risk of prolonged or complicated bereavement:

- multiple, sudden, unexpected, or untimely deaths
- previous mental health problems
- low self-esteem or trust in others (often developed in childhood)
- insecurity
- absent or rejecting parents (this predisposes the children to depression after bereavement in adult life)
- heavily reliant partner who loses his or her spouse
- compulsively self-reliant individuals.

Exaggerated or prolonged grief responses should be identified (Kim *et al*, 1991).

Some indicators of unresolved or **complicated grief** include the following:

- overactivity without a sense of loss
- alteration in relationships with friends and family
- hostilities against specific people
- agitated depression with tension, agitation, insomnia, feelings of worthlessness, extreme guilt, and even suicidal tendencies
- diminished participation in religious and ritual activities related to the patient's/client's culture
- inability to discuss the loss without crying (particularly more then one year after the loss)
- false euphoria.

Often, individuals with **prolonged grief** require long-term support, referral to psychiatric help or counselling. The outlook may then be positive.

## NURSING CARE AND GRIEF

### Assessment

Assessment of the individual and family begins by exploring the meaning of the loss to them. This is done by collecting objective and subjective data. The nurse interviews the patient/client and family, observes their responses and behaviours, and then communicates openly, emphasizing listening skills. The nurse should be alert for nonverbal cues. Initial impressions are validated with the individual and family so that effective interventions can be developed.

The nurse must assess how the patient/client *is* reacting rather than how the patient/client *should be* reacting. Sequences of behaviour or phases may either occur in order, be skipped, or recur. Many variables affect grief. Assessment of these variables provides the nurse with a broad database from which to individualize care.

### Factors Affecting Grief

### PERSONAL CHARACTERISTICS

Personal characteristics influence the response to loss; for example age, sex, socioeconomic status and education. The nature of the relationship with the lost object, the characteristics of the loss, cultural and spiritual beliefs, support systems, and the potential for goal achievement also affect the person's response.

### Age

Age plays a role in the recognition and reaction to loss, for example an infant is not usually able to understand loss and death until he or she is able to recognize familiar persons, form an attachment to a consistent carer (usually the mother), and demonstrate anxiety concerning strangers. After a trust bond has been formed between the parent and child, even a temporary loss can cause profound anxiety and resistance.

A toddler's cognition is still not sufficiently developed to understand death. The child's self-centredness and difficulty in separating fact from fantasy prevent comprehension of an absence of life. The toddler experiences anxiety over loss of objects, such as a favourite toy, and separation from parents or the familiar setting of the home.

The processes and responses of grieving of preschool children differ little from their elders, although they lack the capacity to put their thoughts, feelings, and memories into words. Their **grief responses** are quite variable (Raphael, 1983). The preschooler may not fully comprehend the finality of death and may view it as a reversible process. They may ask seemingly inappropriate questions and for weeks repeatedly inquire about the whereabouts of the dead person (Rando, 1984).

School-aged children are aware of their bodies and will grieve over loss of a body part or function. At this age, they are conscious of differences between themselves and others and are strongly affected by such a loss. The school-aged child associates misdeeds or bad thoughts with causing death and may feel intense guilt over the loss of a significant other. Unlike younger children, however, the school-aged child can understand logical explanations about death. The child's concept of death is one of destruction. At the age of 6 or 7 years the child associates death with ghosts or evil spirits. By the age of 9 or 10 the child recognizes the universality of death. The child may acquire an unusual fear of the unknown when a death in the family occurs or when faced with a terminal illness.

Physical attributes and strengths are important to most adolescents. Acute grief may be felt when loss of a body part or function occurs as well as concern that he or she may face rejection by peers. Adolescents have an adult comprehension of the concept of death. Yet they are the least likely of any age group to accept the loss of life, particularly their own. The rejection of death is related to the adolescent's developmental task of establishing identity, independence and purpose in life.

The young adult relates loss to its significance with regard to status, role, and lifestyle. A loss of job or economic well-being, divorce, or a physical impairment causes considerable grief and threatens success. A young adult's concept of death is largely a product of religious and cultural beliefs. The death of a young adult is perceived as especially tragic by society because it is the loss of a life at the brink of realized potential.

It is during middle age that individuals become aware that youthfulness and physical fitness cannot be taken for granted and consequently, may become sensitive to the physical changes of ageing. The individual may begin to re-examine his or her life and consider the options available in order to gain fulfilment. Adults often take time to consider life and death. Any loss in physical function can give rise to grief. A middle-aged adult often associates actively with friends, particularly if his or her children have left home. Loss of significant others creates a significant threat to lifestyle. The career-oriented adult has usually reached a professional peak. Any loss of job or ability to perform a job causes considerable grief.

Research has shown that older people think and talk about death more readily than younger people. Kalish and Reynolds (1976) suggest that older people are socialized by the deaths of their peers towards accepting their own death. It has been found that older people tend to use particular coping strategies, such as anticipatory thought. Humour is also a coping strategy used by many older people and nurses are often unprepared for this (Burnside, 1988).

Following the death of a spouse, older people may need support in order to adjust to their new circumstances. Cartwright and Bowling (1982) found that older widows and widowers needed social support (from family, friends, or groups such as CRUSE), practical support (such as transport, telephone, or finance) and health support (from the primary health care team). Studies have also demonstrated that the need for support can be as great one year after bereavement, when the reality of the loss and the new circumstances are experienced daily.

If the older person's self-esteem can be maintained this can help reduce the negative effects of the stresses following bereavement (Johnson *et al*, 1986).

### Children's Nursing
### Unfinished business

A dying child often may feel guilty at upsetting his or her family and siblings. The child may have some degree of unfinished business to deal with before his or her death. Issues such as having a row with a sibling, feeling jealous or upsetting parents all constitute unfinished business that will need to be dealt with in order for the child to feel comfortable during the last few days. A child's unfinished business is as important as that of an adult. The nurse must assist the child and family by promoting openness between all members and supporting the family at this very difficult time.

## Gender Roles

Reaction to loss is influenced by social expectations of male and female roles. In many Western cultures, it is generally more difficult for men to express grief openly. The nurse must be alert to this and verify with the patient/client feelings, reactions, and the personal meaning attached to the loss. Men and women attach different significance to body parts, functions, interpersonal relationships, and objects.

The nurse's own thoughts and feelings with regard to gender roles should also be assessed. Such a self-assessment helps a nurse be more supportive. The nurse's expectations should never influence his or her attitude toward the patient/client and family.

## Socioeconomic Status

Loss is universal, experienced by everyone, regardless of socioeconomic status. Assessment of socioeconomic status is essential because it influences the ability to build options and use support mechanisms when coping with loss. Generally, a lack of financial support, education, or occupational skills magnifies the stresses on the griever. The nurse should assess the socioeconomic status of the patient/client to determine realistic options and provide appropriate resource information.

## NATURE OF RELATIONSHIPS

The characteristics of the relationship severed and the functions that the deceased person performed in the griever's life are critical variables in the grief experience. It has been said that to lose your parents is to lose your past, to lose your spouse is to lose your present, and to lose your child is to lose your future. Empirical evidence supports the theory that the loss of a child creates the most intense grief response (Rando, 1984). A child's death is often traumatic because it is premature. Parents often feel guilty and blame themselves.

The reaction to the loss of a parent depends on the quality of the relationship. The death of a parent who was the most nurturing will probably cause the greatest grief for a child. The loss of a parent in adulthood is influenced by the psychological relationship, degree of attachment, and age of parent.

The meaning of the relationship to the griever will influence the grief response, whether the loss is due to death, separation, or divorce. Those who strongly depend on the lost person often have

**Mother and Child
Supporting the family after
stillbirth**

Some parents find release in writing about their feelings at the time of delivery — adding to it in a diary form as feelings change. At The Princess Anne Hospital in Southampton one midwifery sister has a 'Memory Book' which a few mothers have contributed to over the months and years since their babies have died. It is well worn by the many who have found comfort from reading another's account of experiences similar to their own. When a 'contributor' returns for a subsequent delivery the book may be pored over and as feelings are relived, further healing takes place.

*From Jolly J: Missed beginnings: death before life has been established, London, 1987, Mosby.*

more problems than others as they try to part with the lost relationship and establish new ones. A relationship characterized by extreme ambivalence, for example death of a spouse after a stormy marriage, is more difficult to resolve than one that is not.

One of the most stressful events in life is loss of a spouse. If marital partners usually shared household responsibilities, the loss of one leaves the other with incomplete skills and total responsibility. If children still live at home, the remaining parent may become emotionally overloaded with the extra responsibilities. The loss of a sexual partner may affect the remaining spouse's perception of sexuality and desire for sex. The loss of a spouse also makes it difficult for the survivor to establish new friendships.

Hampe (1975) studied the needs of spouses when attempting to cope with their partner's impending death. Those identified include the need:

- to be with the dying person
- to be helpful to the dying person
- to receive reassurance concerning the spouse's comfort
- to be informed of the spouse's condition
- to be informed of the impending death
- to ventilate emotions
- to receive comfort and support from the family
- to receive acceptance, support, and comfort from health care professionals.

The nurse who is able to anticipate a family's needs during loss and grief and assess the manner of adjustment to the loss is better equipped to provide emotional support. The nurse can assist by obtaining from doctors the information sought by families about their loved one's condition.

## SOCIAL SUPPORT SYSTEM

The support that individuals receive is based on their value to the members of the social system and the manner and circumstances of their loss. The visibility of a loss, such as the loss of a home resulting from disaster, often brings support from unexpected sources. The visibility of a loss, such as a facial deformity, may cause the loss of support from family or friends, thus augmenting

its severity. People experiencing less visible or invisible losses, such as early miscarriage, or losses that are often considered socially unacceptable, such as the imprisonment of a family member or the death of a gay partner, often experience a lack of or loss of support from family or friends. Those patients/clients who are unable to receive nonjudgemental compassion and support will lose the vital aid that allows them to deal with grief. Lack of support usually leads to difficulty in successful grief resolution (Rando, 1984).

The timing of social support is crucial. Support must be available and used as the griever advances through the mourning process. This requires active sharing by the bereaved individual and the supporters. However, it is common for grievers to not use the support offered (Rando, 1984).

## NATURE OF THE LOSS

The ability to resolve grief depends on the meaning of the loss and the situation surrounding the loss. The ability to accept help influences whether the bereaved will be able to cope with the loss. The visibility of the loss influences the support received. The duration of a change (that is, whether it is temporary or permanent) affects the amount of time spent in re-establishing physical, psychological, and social equilibrium.

Rando (1984) coined the term *death surround* to describe factors that influence the survivor's ability to undertake grief work, this includes the location, type, and reason for the death and the degree of preparation for it. Ideally, the survivor feels that the circumstances are appropriate; for example, the deceased had a fulfilled life and died in familiar surroundings, and the mourner

**Mental Health Nursing
Grieving and dementia**

Carers of a loved one with a dementing illness experience a grieving process. They may mourn the loss of the personality of the relative/friend whom they have known and loved for many years. The experience of grieving for this loss when the loved one is still alive and present can be frightening and bewildering.

One man wrote after the death of his wife, who had dementia, 'It was like going to her funeral every day'. Carers may experience:

- **denial and numbness** when being told that there is no cure – carers may filter what they remember and accuse professionals of not explaining fully, or they may refuse to listen and walk away
- **anger and resentment**, which may be directed at health care staff – when exhausted by the physical and emotional demands of caring, carers may express their anger by shouting or physical violence
- **guilt** – which may arise from the overwhelming demands on them, particularly those who have other family members who need time and consideration
- **depression** – arising from isolation, feeling trapped and helpless to change the situation
- **acceptance** – which is an ongoing process, but can be facilitated by emotional support and practical assistance

*Adapted from Riggans L: Living with loss, Nurs Times 88(27):34, 1992.*

## Dimensions of Hope

- **Affective:** sensations and emotions (e.g. feelings of confidence, attraction to the desirable outcome) that are part of hoping.
- **Cognitive:** the processes by which a person wishes, imagines, perceives, thinks, learns, or judges in relation to hope.
- **Behavioural:** the actions a person takes to directly achieve hope, which may be physiological, psycho-social, cultural or spiritual.
- **Affiliative:** a person's sense of involvement beyond self. (Social interaction, mutuality, attachment, and intimacy compose affiliation. There is a relationship with others.).
- **Temporal:** the person's experience of time (past, present, and future) in relation to hoping.
- **Contextual:** hope perceived within the context of life as interpreted by the person. (Life situations influence and are part of hope. An actual or potential loss may be the context in which hope arises.).

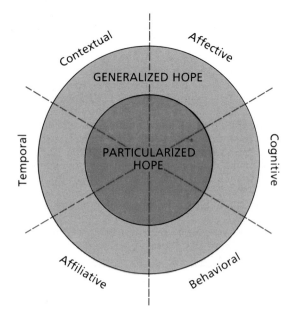

**Fig 11-1** Spheres and dimensions of hope.

From Dufault K, Martocchio BC: *Nurs Clin North Am* 20: 379, 1985.

had the opportunity and time to prepare for the loss and complete **unfinished business**. However, sudden and unexpected loss can lead to slower recovery from grief. Deaths by violence through suicide, murder, or self-neglect are even more difficult to accept. A prolonged, painful illness may leave the survivor emotionally exhausted. Studies show that survivors of patients/clients who died from short-term chronic illnesses (less than 6 months in duration) coped better than those whose loved ones died of a prolonged chronic illness (longer than 6 months in duration) (Rando, 1984).

### CULTURAL AND SPIRITUAL BELIEFS

Values, attitudes, beliefs, and customs are cultural aspects that influence reaction to loss, grief, and death. The expression of grief generally arises from the cultural background and family dynamics. Culture influences each person differently (see Chapter 8). A nurse avoids stereotyping patients/clients by culture and uses self-assessment so that judgemental or prejudicial reactions can be avoided.

Spiritual or religious beliefs include practices, rites, and rituals. An individual may find solace and meaning in losses through spiritual beliefs. Frequently, a grieving person turns to religion for strength and support (Reed, 1986). The nurse should be alert to the significance of religious practices, not only for the person but also for the family. Through the use of words and actions, the nurse can indicate sensitivity to these needs. Through openness in responses, the nurse can determine coping mechanisms used and plan appropriate interventions. For example, members of the Jewish faith remain in a dying person's presence to witness death and be assured that everything possible is done. If a Catholic person is seriously ill, a priest should be notified to provide the sacrament of Anointing of the Sick. This is offered in order to strengthen the person so that he or she can be restored to health or make the act of death a final sharing in the union with Christ.

For some individuals, loss triggers questions about the meaning of life, personal values, and beliefs. Typically this is shown by the 'why me?' response. Internal conflicts concerning religious beliefs may also occur.

### GOALS

Loss is any change in a person's situation that reduces the probability of achieving goals. It is critical to understand the patient's/client's goals in relation to the loss experienced. Important goal characteristics include the number of goals, centrality of particular goals, number of pathways to goal achievement, compatibility of goals, and change in goal characteristics (temporary or permanent). The more goals a person has, the more likely the person is able to adapt to the loss of only one. The more central the goal, the greater the grief; for example, a woman who has been training to become a ballerina could be more devastated by the amputation of her leg than by diagnosis of a potentially life-threatening illness. If a person has many pathways or options to achieving goals, then he or she has more than one coping strategy. If one is not available, the patient/client can use another. Goals shift with loss and change; for individuals to make this shift, they must have hope. Hope has been noted as of great importance to the patient/client (Herth, 1989; O'Connor, 1990).

### HOPE

**Hope** is a multidimensional, changing life force. It is characterized by a confident, yet uncertain expectation of achieving a goal (Dufault and Martocchio, 1985). Hope is not a single act but a complex series of thoughts, feelings, and actions that frequently change. Patients/clients facing terminal illness or serious loss, as well as their families, experience different dimensions of hope. According to Dufault and Martocchio, hope has six dimensions: affective, cognitive, behavioural, affiliative, temporal, and contextual (Fig. 11-1).

The process of hope involves moving through these dimensions. Dufault and Martocchio also describe two spheres of hope, generalized and particularized. *Generalized* hope is broad and directed at a future beneficial development, for example, a person with generalized hope may often say 'I always hope for the better'. *Particularized* hope is concerned with a specific outcome or state of being (for example, living until a couple's anniversary or a loved one's birthday). A person with particularized hope specifies something as important and is motivated to cope with obstacles that interfere with it.

Awareness of the **dimensions of hope** (see box) helps the nurse support a patient's/client's hope. This can help facilitate grieving associated with terminal illness.

## PHASES OF GRIEF

Observation of grieving patients/clients allows the nurse to make inferences about effects of the loss. No two people grieve in exactly the same way. However, there are distinct patterns. People in shock and disbelief act differently from those who achieve reorganization and restitution. Individuals may move back and forth through phases of grief until final resolution. It is useful to think of the final phase as one of *becoming comfortable with loss*, rather than *recovery*.

The distinguishing factors of this type of grief are its intensity and duration, and the degree to which it interferes with functioning. The grieving process can be made more difficult by factors such as sudden loss, or type of death. Patients/clients can become unable to overcome their feelings of loss. It is here that the nurse should refer the person to more appropriate support, for example counselling or psychotherapy.

## INDIVIDUAL AND FAMILY EXPERIENCES

The meaning of death varies widely for individuals, due to many variables, including the setting in which the death occurred. Nurses care for dying patients in hospitals, nursing homes, hospices, or in the patient's/client's own home. Nurses observe patient/client behaviours towards staff and families. Individuals' responses to death influence the choice of therapies.

The **intensity of coping** and the rate at which individuals pass through the experience of grief are influenced by the amount of time that elapses between their first awareness of impending death and the moment itself. In an intensive care unit, patients/clients generally recover or die quickly. Death may be sudden and unexpected, and patients/clients and families have little time for expressing grief. In contrast, the process of dying is usually gradual in wards, hospices or units for terminally ill patients/clients. Patients/clients have more time to work through grief.

An individual will experience many emotions, depending on the phase of dying or grief. Each emotion serves a purpose. However, the person's responses determine the interventions to be used by the nurse in order to relate to the patient/client. For example, as the individual and family begin to come to terms with the inevitability of death, the nurse can encourage the patient/client to discuss feelings about leaving family members behind. This will not work if the person is expressing feelings of anguish and despair.

The nurse observes for behaviours that may indicate grief.

Physical symptoms should also be noted. Gastrointestinal disturbances such as indigestion, nausea and vomiting, anorexia, or a recent change in weight may indicate grieving. People experiencing bereavement may also complain of difficulties in sleeping. Fatigue and a reduced activity level may also be present.

The patient's/client's death takes place in a social context. Even during the dying phase the family begins to reorganize itself; the person is no longer available to fulfil the same number and types of roles. The nurse assesses the family's grief process, recognizing that they may be dealing with different aspects of grief than the patient/client.

### Planning Care

Dying patients/clients require special consideration when nursing care plans are formulated. The need to grieve is one of many problems for these individuals. Patients/clients with terminal illnesses that cause deformities or physical disabilities will probably undergo alterations in body image or self-concept. Examples are patients/clients with leukaemia who receive drugs that cause loss of hair and those with bone cancer who may become disabled because of chronic pain. As the person's condition worsens, the nurse assesses areas relevant to basic needs such as alterations in comfort, alterations in elimination, ineffective breathing, or sensory alterations. Owing to the nature and severity of terminal illness, physical assessment data are collected frequently. The importance of psychological assessment must never be forgotten.

Grieving is a natural response to loss. Grieving has a therapeutic value, enabling people to think through their losses, recollect their thoughts, and resume life with new insights and direction. In addition, the physiological, emotional, developmental, and spiritual needs of the person must be considered.

Goals for a person dealing with loss are to resolve grief, accept the reality of the loss, regain a sense of self-esteem, and

### Useful Addresses

**BACUP**
**(British Association of Cancer United Patients)**
Information Service
Bath Place
Rivington Street
London EC2A 3JR

**Cancer Relief Macmillan Fund**
Anchor House
15/19 Britten Street
London SW3 3TZ

**Compassionate Friends**
6 Denmark Street
Bristol
B31 5DQ

**CRUSE**
CRUSE House
126 Sheen Street
Richmond
Surrey

renew normal activities and relationships. Physiological needs must also be met. During planning, the nurse has several resources, including family members, significant others, other team members, and community support groups.

When caring for dying individuals, the nurse's responsibilities extend to physical needs and unique psychological and social problems. The nurse must try to spend more time with the dying person, to listen to expressions of grief, and to maintain his or her quality of life. It is important that the nurse does not become distanced from dying patients/clients. Additional goals for dying patients/clients include:

- gaining and maintaining comfort
- maintaining independence in daily living activities
- maintaining hope
- achieving spiritual comfort
- gaining relief from loneliness and isolation.

The three most crucial needs of the dying person are control of pain and depressing symptoms, preservation of dignity and self-worth, and love and affection (Rando, 1984). Nurses are in a unique position to address these needs. Their presence can provide comfort and reduce anxiety. Nurses can structure routines and surroundings so that the person feels a sense of security and control over his or her life and environment. Nurses can support the person's self-esteem by asking for opinions regarding care. Nurses can enable families to make decisions with the patient/client, thereby encouraging mutual decision making. This may help prepare the family for when the person may not be able to make choices. As circumstances and the illness change, the patient/client will change as well. Each patient/client and family should be treated as unique, with recognition that their needs, fears, hopes, expectations, and concerns will change throughout the illness. Continuing re-evaluation and planning is essential.

The dying patient/client may be concerned with the circumstances and grief of those left behind. In addition to requiring help with problems related to the illness and its emotional stresses, individuals often need assistance with financial problems, changes in social and sexual relationships, and difficulties in dealing with the hospital. The formation of an interdisciplinary team is critical. The team usually involves the patient/client, family, doctors, nurses, psychologists, social workers, clergy, pharmacists, physiotherapists and occupational therapists, dietitians, and volunteers. Using an interdisciplinary perspective, the nurse can address many potential practical problems before they become overwhelming.

## Therapeutic Communication

Nursing care of the grieving patient/client begins with establishing the *significance of the loss*. This is difficult if the person is unwilling to express feelings or is experiencing shock or denial. The nurse observes the response to loss and then attempts to identify the person's strengths in dealing with it. The nurse must allow adequate private time with the patient/client and family to promote open communication and build up a therapeutic relationship. The nurse should convey acceptance of all grief reactions. For example, if a patient/client begins to cry,

the nurse quietly remains ready to offer comfort, rather than abandoning him or her at the time of need. Acknowledging grief through touch and concern promotes trust.

If patients/clients choose not to share feelings or do not wish to be touched, the nurse conveys a willingness to be available when needed. When the nurse acknowledges patients'/clients' beliefs and values, a therapeutic relationship may evolve. Occasionally, a person may need to begin to resolve grief before he or she can discuss the loss. It is also important to recognize patients'/clients' normal styles of dealing with difficult situations. If they do not normally talk about their feelings, they are unlikely to discuss feelings regarding loss.

When considering a person's potential reactions to loss, the nurse is alert to expressions of denial, anger, depression, or guilt. Initial denial is normal. If the nurse encourages the person to face the loss too soon, the nurse may precipitate a reaction that can cause depression, emotional disorganization, or further withdrawal from reality. The nurse often becomes the target of patient/client or family anger. Although it is difficult not to take anger personally, the nurse should be prepared to encounter expressions of anger or guilt. In an effective relationship the nurse must deal with personal feelings before encouraging the patient's/client's expression of anger. The nurse must let the individual and family know that such expressions are normal.

The nurse should try not to erect barriers to communication (see Chapter 15). Communication is blocked by denying the patient's/client's grief, providing false reassurance, or avoiding discussion of the problem. The nurse should attempt to support the person's expressions of anger by staying close, maintaining eye contact and remaining silent. Sometimes, it is more appropriate to do nothing and just be present. The nurse should not give advice or analyse causes for loss or behaviour.

When a patient/client demonstrates a readiness to move on to the *awareness phase*, the nurse might explain the recognized grief reactions. Anticipatory guidance provides an important normalizing function for the individual and family. Effective listening techniques, as well as communication of concern and understanding, also help the patient/client move through the grieving process.

No topic that a dying person wishes to discuss should be avoided. The person is more likely to talk about death with someone who listens. The patient/client may initially test the nurse by offering a statement that does not express true concerns.

It is important to let the patient/client discuss his or her concerns. The nurse responds to questions as honestly and as positively as possible. The nurse may use several strategies to support hope (see box). The strategies chosen will depend on the person's dimensions of hope (Dufault and Martocchio, 1985).

When all hope is lost, there may be premature psychological and then physical surrender to the environment. This depends on the individual's perception of self-worth and effectiveness. The nurse supports hope by helping the person retain control, dignity, and self-esteem. This is done by focusing on the present and immediate future, by emphasizing remaining potential and abilities, and by structuring life events to promote a sense of predictability and continuity. The nurse looks for opportunities to foster accomplishments that cause satisfaction and anticipation. The nurse encourages the patient/client and family to reminisce about previous joys and fulfilments.

As the grieving person moves towards the *resolution* or *reorganization phase*, the nurse can encourage discussion of the effects of the loss on the patient's/client's life and perceptions of the situation. The nurse may share with the patient/client and family the signs of resolution. The nurse should encourage the person to loosen ties with the past and to look ahead.

The nurse has limitations with regard to providing appropriate interventions for grieving patients/clients. The nurse may not have sufficient time to address all of the needs of terminally ill patients/clients. Consequently, it is important to utilize other resources within the health care setting and community. When other professionals are needed, the nurse explores with the patient/client and family alternatives in selecting resource people, such as Macmillan Nurses, community staff, or groups to enhance grief work. Self-help, bereavement, and parent groups are available in some areas. Signs of *unresolved grief* and complicated grief may require referral to a psychologist, psychiatrist, or counsellor.

## Maintaining Self-Esteem

Nursing interventions focus on promoting a sense of identity, dignity, and self-esteem. The nurse can help by listening, responding quickly and positively to requests, maintaining confidentiality, and providing comfort and support. The quality and quantity of the time spent with the person are important in creating a therapeutic environment for the grieving process. Davitz and Davitz (1980) have explored the characteristics of nurses who have highly refined empathy. They identified the relationship with the patient/client as the core of nursing. Measures that provide comfort and support should be implemented in a caring, pleasant manner to reinforce the person's feelings of self-worth and dignity and to decrease the fear of rejection, isolation, and sense of hopelessness.

Self-esteem and dignity complement each other. Dignity is the ability to maintain self-concept. The disabilities of dying patients/clients may threaten dignity. Care givers often take control of these individuals' lives. Taking away the right to make decisions about care fosters hopelessness and feelings of despair, and some patients/clients may lose their will to live. To maintain self-esteem, individuals must believe that their opinions are valuable, particularly with regard to decisions that affect their impending death.

The nurse can promote self-esteem by placing the patient/client in control of self-care decisions. Cleanliness, a lack of body odours, attractive clothing, and personal grooming (shaving or well-groomed hair) promote a sense of worth. The nurse who manages the person's physical care must display an attitude of respect and helpfulness rather than encourage dependence or guilt.

## Promoting Return-to-Life Activities

As individuals begin to accept their losses, it is important to encourage them to return to their normal lifestyles. If patients/clients and families are able to express grief openly and progress through the grief process with support and understanding, resolution of grief is easier. Depending on the nature of the loss, many demands may be placed on family resources.

The nurse can help by encouraging individuals to participate in decisions about relationships and resources for the future. The identification of usual lifestyle practices helps bring a sense of closure to the loss.

## Implementation

### Promoting Comfort

Nursing care of the terminally ill can be demanding and stressful. However, helping a dying person retain dignity is one of nursing's greatest rewards. A person may experience many symptoms for months before death occurs. The nurse can share the dying

### Nursing Implications for Promoting Hope

**AFFECTIVE DIMENSION**
- Convey an empathetic understanding of patients'/clients' worries, fears, and doubts.
- Reduce the degree to which patients/clients become immobilized by concerns.
- Build on patient/client and family strengths of patience and courage.

**COGNITIVE DIMENSION**
- Clarify or modify hoping persons' reality perceptions.
- Offer information about the illnesses or treatments, correct misinformation, and share the experiences of others as a basis of comparison.

**BEHAVIOURAL DIMENSION**
- Help patients/clients use personal and family resources in relation to hope.
- Balance levels of independence, interdependence, and dependence when planning care.
- Enhance patients'/clients' self-esteem and capabilities; give praise and encouragement appropriately.

**AFFILIATIVE DIMENSION**
- Strengthen or foster relationships that provide hope.
- Help patients/clients know that they are loved, cared for, and important to others.

**TEMPORAL DIMENSION**
- Attend to patients'/clients' experiences.
- Use patients'/clients' insights from past experiences and apply them to the present.

**CONTEXTUAL DIMENSION**
- Provide the opportunity to communicate about life situations that encourage hope.
- Encourage discussion about desired goals, reminiscing, reviewing values, and reflecting on the meaning of suffering, life, or death.

**SPIRITUAL DIMENSION**
- Provide care which is sensitive to cultural or religious beliefs and practices.
- Arrange whatever spiritual support is requested.

person's suffering and intervene in a way that improves his or her quality of life. A dying patient/client must be cared for with respect and concern (see box). Although the Dying Person's Bill of Rights is an American document, it gives a useful framework for care in the United Kingdom.

The nurse provides a variety of comfort measures for the terminally ill person (Table 11-2). Pain control is important since pain alters sleep, appetite, mobility, and psychological function. Fear of pain is common; early relief from pain allows the person to have more energy available for maintaining quality of life activities. Providing comfort for terminally ill individuals also involves controlling the symptoms of disease or the side-effects of the therapies administered.

Personal hygiene is a routine part of keeping the terminally ill person comfortable. The person will eventually depend on the nurse or family for basic needs and may be embarrassed by this dependence. Whenever possible, patients/clients should make their own decisions about care.

---

## The Dying Person's Bill of Rights

- I have the right to be treated as a living human being until I die.
- I have the right to maintain a sense of hopefulness, however changing its focus may be.
- I have the right to be cared for by those who can maintain a sense of hopefulness, however changing this might be.
- I have the right to express my feelings and emotions about my death in my own way.
- I have the right to participate in decisions concerning my care.
- I have the right to expect continuing medical and nursing attention even though cure goals must be changed to comfort goals.
- I have the right not to die alone.
- I have the right to be free from pain.
- I have the right to have my questions answered honestly.
- I have the right not to be deceived.
- I have the right to have help from and for my family in accepting my death.
- I have the right to die in peace and dignity.
- I have the right to retain my individuality and not be judged for my decisions, which may be contrary to the beliefs of others.
- I have the right to discuss and enlarge my religious and/or spiritual experiences, whatever these may mean to others.
- I have the right to expect that the sanctity of the human body will be respected after death.
- I have the right to be cared for by caring, sensitive, knowledgeable people who will attempt to understand my needs and will be able to gain some satisfaction in helping me face my death.

From Barbus AJ: The dying person's bill of rights, *Am J Nurs* 75(1): 99, 1975.

## Maintaining Independence

Choosing the right location for care is very important for the dying patient/client. There are alternatives to the acute hospital, for example hospice care. Many patients/clients prefer to be in their own home.

Most dying patients/clients achieve some satisfaction from being as self-sufficient as possible. Allowing the person to perform simple tasks such as washing, putting on glasses, and eating helps to maintain dignity and a sense of worth. When a person becomes physically unable to perform self-care, encourage participation in decision making to give him or her a sense of control. Look for nonverbal cues that suggest unwillingness to participate in care. Do not force participation, particularly if physical limitations make it difficult. The family must also encourage the person to make decisions because they often have a tendency to take over. When caring takes place in the home, normal routines can be re-established to help create a sense of control.

## Preventing Loneliness and Isolation

When the nurse is detached and avoids discussion of the situation, dying patients/clients may experience overwhelming loneliness. It is important to remain in the domain of caring rather than coping, if you are to provide support for the dying patient/client. In the traditional medical ethos, cure is seen as success, but if the nurse can see good care as success, then the death of the patient/client will not mean failure.

The process of dying may cause patients/clients to be seen as unpleasant. If conditions cause offensive odours, incontinence, confusion, or aggressiveness, nurses may avoid patients/clients. In some hospitals, dying people may be nursed in private rooms to avoid exposing others to suffering. The room may be dimly lit, the curtains may be drawn, and sounds are reduced. Without meaningful sensory stimulation, dying people probably feel abandoned and isolated. This may also encourage nurses to withdraw from such patients/clients.

To prevent loneliness and sensory deprivation the nurse must intervene to improve the quality of the environment. Dying individuals should not be routinely placed in side rooms in out-of-the-way locations. Patients/clients feel a sense of involvement when sharing a ward and watching the nurse's activities. The person can then share in the companionship of other patients/clients and visitors. When the person dies, however, the nurse should give attention to the remaining patients/clients, since watching a person die can be frightening. The death of a patient/client may create feelings of mortality and trigger a grief reaction in other patients/clients.

Perhaps most important in preventing loneliness is involvement with family members and friends. In the home, family and friends can interact more easily with the person. In a hospital or extended care facility, visitors should be allowed to remain with the dying person at any time. If several family members visit, a private room may be necessary. The dying person becomes particularly lonely at night and may feel more

## TABLE 11-2 Promoting Physical Comfort in the Terminally Ill Person

| Cause of Discomfort | Nursing Implications | Rationale |
|---|---|---|
| **PAIN**<br>Usually chronic and severe. Often requiring morphine. | Assess using a pain assessment tool [80% of patients/clients have more than one pain, 34% more than four (Twycross, 1972)]. | To assess cause to enable appropriate analgesia administration.<br>To monitor effect of treatment. |
| **Relieving Pain** | Ensure adequate dose of analgesia is prescribed for 'breakthrough' pain. | To prevent pain reoccurring without immediate treatment and 'pain-fear' cycle. |
| | Analgesia is prescribed using the *Analgesic Ladder* (WHO, 1990) (see Fig. 30-9)<br>— by the mouth<br>— by the clock<br>— by the ladder | Using this principle prevents patients/clients being prescribed analgesia from the same group (or strength)  Analgesia can also be given IM, SC, PR. |
| | Consider other pain control methods (i.e. position, massage, guided imagery). | Pain is a multi-faceted concept. Analgesia alone may not achieve total comfort. |
| **CONSTIPATION**<br>Many analgesics (particularly morphine) can cause constipation. | Laxatives should always be prescribed and administered regularly to patients/clients on morphine(usually co-danthrusate). | Almost all patients/clients on morphine will become constipated (Regnard and Tempest,1992). |
| Nutritional intake and disturbance of normal routine may contribute. | Provide preventive care where possible (e.g. diet and fluids). | |
| **Relieving Constipation** | Assess problem. Consider performing a rectal examination. | To determine cause and appropriate treatment. |
| | If rectum is empty, continue oral laxatives.<br>Exclude obstruction. | |
| | Hard faeces present: lubricate using glycerine suppositories or soften using oil enema. | |
| | Soft faeces present: stimulate bowel movement with bisacodyl suppositories. | Softening faeces alone may not enable patient/client to defecate. |
| **MOUTH PROBLEMS**<br>**Infected mouth** | Assess mouth (check for signs of infection, particularly white patches).<br>Give prescribed anti-fungal if necessary [ketoconazole 200 mg once daily clears 90% of problems and is more effective than nystatin [Regnard and Tempest, 1992)]. | To determine if candida is present. |
| **Dirty Mouth** | Clean teeth and mouth with soft toothbrush (Howarth, 1977).<br>Clean mucosa helped by gentle effervescent solution, e.g. 1:1 cider and soda water. | Less trauma caused by this method. |

(cont'd)

## TABLE 11-2 Promoting Physical Comfort in the Terminally Ill Person

| Cause of Discomfort | Nursing Implications | Rationale |
|---|---|---|
| **MOUTH PROBLEMS** (cont'd) | | |
| **Dry Mouth** | Reduce dryness using crushed ice, frozen tonic water, pineapple chunks (unsweetened canned), etc. | Pineapple contains proteolytic enzyme (annase) which helps clean mouth. |
| **Painful Mouth** | Relieve pain where possible. Difflam® mouthwash. | Anti-inflammatory action and analgesic 1-2 hrs. Causes minimum numbness (Kim *et al*, 1985). |
| | Topical chlorine salicylate gel. | |
| **Dry, Cracked Lips** | Promote comfort using petroleum jelly, lip salve, or high moisture lipstick. | Prevent moisture loss from lips caused by breathing through mouth, dehydration or inability to self-moisten. |
| **NAUSEA AND VOMITING** | | |
| Complex problem and distressing. Multiple causes. | Assess underlying causes. | Success relies upon when appropriate anti-emetic treatment can be commenced (Regnard and Comisky, 1992). |
| | Give prescribed anti-emetic. Provide reassurance, support and mouth care. | |
| | Consider alternatives, e.g. aromatherapy, 'sea bands'. | P6 acupressure may provide anti-emesis (Dundee and McMillan, 1991). |
| **FATIGUE** | | |
| Increased metabolic rate due to metabolic demands of cancer, causing weakness and fatigue. | Set mutual goals with patient/client after identifying valued or desired tasks, and conserve patient's/client's energy for only those desired tasks. Provide frequent rest periods in quiet environment. Time and pace nursing activities to conserve patient's/client's energy. | |
| **DIARRHOEA** | | |
| May arise from disease (e.g. colon cancer), drugs, or impacted faeces causing overflow. | Assess cause. Check for impacted faeces. | |
| | Review medication. Maintain patient/client dignity. | Treat as for constipation. Often occurs due to over-prescription of laxatives. |
| | Maintain intact skin. Terminally ill patients are vulnerable to infection. May require stool specimen. | |
| **REDUCED NUTRITIONAL/ FLUID INTAKE** | | |
| There is no evidence to suggest that reduced diet or fluids causes discomfort (Regnard and Tempest, 1992), although the social role of food and fluids must not be forgotten. | Suggest small portions of food and drink following patient's/client's likes and dislikes. Food presentation is important (Williams and Copp, 1990). Alcohol often stimulates appetite. | |
| **BREATHLESSNESS** | | |
| Can be frightening experience. | Increase air movement over patient's/client's face (e.g. using fan). | Reduces demand for ventilation without causing respiratory depression (Heyse-Moore, 1984). |
| | Reassure patient/client, use relaxation techniques. Administer oxygen via nasal cannula or mask. Consider administering systemic or nebulized opioids (Young and Daviskas, 1989). | |

secure if someone stays at the bedside. The nurse should know how to contact family members if a visit is requested or the person's condition worsens.

The person must have someone who can share the dying experience. Nurses should not feel guilty if they cannot always provide this support. However, care may require long intervals of time with the patient/client. Try to stay with dying patients/clients when needed and show concern and compassion. To provide the care needed by the dying person, it may be necessary to ask for help from other nurses.

## Promoting Spiritual Comfort

Providing **spiritual comfort** means much more than asking spiritual advisers to visit. As death approaches, the person often seeks comfort by analysing values and beliefs related to life and death. A dying person tries to find purpose and a meaning to life before surrendering to death (Conrad, 1985) and often feels guilty if life is perceived to be unfulfilled. Consequently, the person often asks for forgiveness, either from the supreme being or family members. Additional spiritual needs are hope and love (Conrad, 1985). The nurse and family can assist in understanding and expressing hope. Love can best be expressed through kind, compassionate care. The nurse or family can provide spiritual comfort by using therapeutic communication skills expressing empathy.

The nurse must feel comfortable about personal spiritual beliefs and values before offering support. The nurse should never impose his or her own personal beliefs or practices on patients/clients or families. Attentive listening encourages patients/clients to express feelings, clarify them, and accept death. When patients/clients seek spiritual advisers but do not have their own, the nurse makes referrals (see Chapter 8).

## Supporting the Grieving Family

Family members must be supported through the dying and death of their loved one and, at the same time, be encouraged to provide support. In an institutional setting, families often have greater difficulty in giving support. The nurse must recognize the value of family members as resources and assist them in working with the dying person.

At home the family becomes closely involved in the person's care. A terminal illness places heavy demands on social and financial resources. The emotional strain often disrupts normal communication. The family may become afraid to interact with the person. Benoliel (1985) describes circumstances that make it difficult for families to cope with the demands of terminal illness. These include a lengthy period of dying, difficulty in controlling symptoms, unpleasant sights and smells, limited coping resources, and poor relationships with care givers; when a child is dying it may be even more difficult for the family to cope.

Acknowledging grief is the nurse's first step in developing a supportive relationship with the family. The family senses the nurse's concern and should be more willing to share feelings.

Before using family members as resources, determine whether they want to be involved; some do not. Assess the family's role as observer, comforter, or care giver; their roles may often change.

## Dying People of Different Faiths

Each religion will have its own traditions and rituals at the time of death. It is fundamentally important to ask the dying person and/or family what arrangements they would like to be made, and how they would like the nursing care to be offered.

Some examples are given below, but further details can be found in *Caring for dying people of different faiths*, by Julia Neuberger (1994).

**Hinduism** – The dying person's family often requests that they remain near the bedside. Especially significant is the dying person's eldest son, even if he is young. The family may bring coins or clothes, or read passages from holy books.

After death the relatives, including the eldest son, may wash the body. If the dead person is female the washing will generally be carried out by women. The family may pour water into the dead person's mouth or dress the body in new clothes.

**Islam** – Special prayers, recited in Arabic, may be said for the dying person. The prayers may include the declaration of the faith that there is no god but God and Mohammed is his Messenger. The dying person and family face Mecca when praying.

After death the body is washed by members of the family according to Islamic tradition. Males are washed by males and females by females.

**Judaism** – There are no last rites in Judaism, although often a dying Jew will ask to see a Rabbi. It is important to ask whether the dying person would like to see an orthodox Rabbi or a reform/liberal Rabbi.

After the death, it is traditional to close the eyes and lay the arms straight at the sides. this should preferably be done by members of the family, or by other Jews. However, if family or other Jews are not present, it is permissible for this to be done by members of staff (Neuberger, 1994). The 1960 guidelines by the Sexton's Office of the United Synagogue Burial Society state that the corpse should be wrapped in a plain sheet, without any religious emblem, and then placed in a special room for Jewish bodies, or a mortuary.

**Roman Catholic** – When dying, a Roman Catholic person will generally ask to see a Priest in order to make a confession and to receive the Sacrament of the Sick.

The dying person or family may request that, after death, the dead person's hands be placed in an attitude of prayer, holding a crucifix, rosary or flower (Sampson 1982).

## Hospice Care

A desire to change traditional care for the dying led to the establishment of hospices. Most patients/clients in hospices have 6 months or less to live.

There are several types of hospice programmes. Acute-care hospitals and long-term care facilities often have separate units or designated beds for hospice care. A trained interdisciplinary team works with patients/clients and families. In addition, there are voluntary and charitable hospices that care only for the terminally ill.

A hospice programme emphasizes **palliative care**, which is the

**Adult Nursing
Suggestions for involving the family in the care of a dying patient/client**

- Assist in planning a visiting rota for family members to prevent patient/client and family from becoming fatigued.

- Allow young children to visit a dying parent or grandparent when the person is able to communicate.

- Be willing to listen to family complaints about the patient's/client's care and feelings about the person.

- Help family members learn to interact with the dying person (e.g. using attentive listening, avoiding false reassurances, conducting conversations about normal family activities or problems).

- Support family members if they want to help with care measures such as feeding, bathing, and straightening bed linen. Recognize that family members are often more successful than nursing staff in persuading the patient/client to eat.

- When the family becomes fatigued with care activities, relieve them from their duties so that they can acquire needed rest and support. Refer them to resources for meals and lodging.

- Support the act of grieving between patient/client and family. Provide privacy when preferred. Do not discourage open expression of grief between family and patient/client.

- Provide information daily with regard to the patient's/client's condition. Prepare the family for sudden changes in the person's appearance and behaviour.

- Communicate news of impending death when the family is together, if possible. Remember that members can provide support for one another. Convey the news in a private area and be willing to stay with the family.

- As death nears, help the family stay in communication with the dying person through short visits, caring silence, touch, and telling the patient/client of their love.

- After death, assist the family with decision making, such as selection of an undertaker, transport for family members, and collection of the patient's/client's belongings.

control of symptoms and psychological support rather than curative treatment of disease. The patient/client and family participate in care. Patient/client care can be coordinated between the home and hospice setting. Efforts are directed at keeping the person at home as much as possible. The family becomes the primary care giver, administering medication and treatment, and the palliative care team provides psychological and physical resources needed for family support. Most patients/clients wish to be at home. The support of the District or Macmillan Nurse, who is specifically trained in this area, can make this possible.

## Evaluation
## Care after death

Usually the doctor is responsible for certifying the death in the medical records. The time of death and a description of therapies or actions taken are described in the medical record. The doctor may request permission from the family for a **post-mortem**. Post-mortems are required in circumstances of unusual death (for example, violent trauma or unexpected death in the home).

If sudden death occurs, organ donation may be appropriate. Discussions of donations should be performed in a sensitive and caring manner. A trained staff member, often a nurse, discusses donation with families or guardians, making certain that they understand that donation is an option and that it is not compulsory. The regional transplant unit should then be contacted.

The nurse may lay-out the person's body after death, performing this last service with dignity and sensivity. However, it is vital to check with the family first, since some faiths and cultures have important rituals concerning how the body is treated (Neuberger, 1994). The family may wish to be involved. After death the body undergoes a number of physical changes (Table 11-3). The body should be cared for as soon as possible after death to prevent tissue damage or disfigurement. If the family requests organ donation, appropriate measures must be taken immediately.

Offer the family the opportunity to view the body. It may help to suggest that this is an opportunity to say goodbye to their loved one, especially if they were not present at the time of death. If the family decides to view the body, assure them that they will not be alone and that you will be glad to accompany them or will request whomever they would like. Spend as much time as possible assisting the grieving family and offer to contact other support services, such as social services and the spiritual adviser.

Before the family views the body, prepare it and the room to minimize the stress of the experience. Prepare the body by making it look as comfortable as possible:

- insert the person's dentures to maintain normal facial features; a rolled-up towel under the chin keeps the mouth closed. Remove this before the family visits.

- wash soiled body parts, dress the body in a clean gown, comb or brush the hair, and cover the body to the shoulders with clean linen.

It is important to respect the religious and cultural beliefs of the deceased and his or her family. Touching the body could be very offensive to the family. If in doubt, contact the family regarding religious practices before doing anything.

After the body is prepared, invite the family into the room. The nurse or family member should be there to provide emotional support. It is important not to rush the family while they spend time with the deceased.

Nurses are also responsible for disposing of the deceased's personal belongings and noting this on the property list. The nurse can check with the patient's/client's family about taking the belongings or ensure that they are transported with the deceased. No clothing, dentures, plants, gifts, hair pieces, or other personal

## TABLE 11-3 Physiological Changes after Death

| Change | Related Interventions |
|---|---|
| Stiffening of body (rigor mortis), developing 2 to 4 hr after death (involves contraction of skeletal and smooth muscle from lack of adenosine triphosphate) | Before rigor mortis develops, position body in normal anatomical alignment, close eyelids and mouth, and insert dentures in mouth. |
| Reduction in body temperature with loss of skin elasticity (algor mortis) | Remove tape and dressings gently to avoid tissue breakdown. Avoid pulling on skin or body parts. |
| Purple discolouration of skin (livor mortis) in dependent areas from breakdown of red blood cells | Elevate head to prevent discolouration. |
| Softening and liquifying of body tissues by bacterial fermentation | Move body to cool place in hospital mortuary or other designated area. |

items are discarded. No jewellery or religious icons (including bracelets) should be removed without the family's permission.

## LAST OFFICES

The procedure for preparing the body to leave the ward or unit is called **last offices**. The body is washed, and personal grooming performed. All equipment is removed. A label is attached to the body to ensure identification. The body is dressed in a shroud and wrapped in sheets covered by tape. Increasingly, bodies are being placed in specially designed waterproof bags to prevent the possibility of contamination from body fluids.

Families may like to be involved in the washing and personal grooming. Religious practices must always be observed and will vary — always consult the family. Bodies do not need to be dressed in shrouds. The person's own nightclothes could be used — ask the family's permission and preferences.

## AFTER THE DEATH

The family must collect the death certificate from the doctor, and then must register the death with the local registrar. When this has been completed, they may contact a funeral director of their choice who will guide them through the funeral preparations.

### Caring for the Nurse

Nurses working with critically or terminally ill people also experience grief. Grief is the natural response to loss, and each loss needs to be grieved. When nurses experience multiple losses and fail to adequately process them, they can experience **bereavement overload**. They experience frustration, anger, guilt, sadness, helplessness, anxiety, depression, and feelings of being overwhelmed. Self-care is critical to survival. Nurses need to do for themselves what they do for their patients/clients and families. They need to mourn their losses. This can be done on an individual basis and as part of a larger group caring for the person. Nurses need to develop personal support systems that allow time away from the care-giving setting, opportunities to share feelings in nonjudgemental, open relationships, and use stress-management techniques that restore energy (see Chapter 10). Sometimes the health care organization provides opportunities for staff to get together for mutual support and for closure and grieving over the loss of a patient/client. Nurses' roles in the care of the dying and bereaved are filled with experiences that bring grief and stress. They must attend to the need for relief from these

demands. Unrelieved grief and stress can lead to diminished well-being and inability to care for others. It is no longer considered improper for nurses to share a tear with families and patients providing it is genuine and unobtrusive. However, the nurse must not forget that his or her primary role is to support others.

### Grief Resolution

Although **resolution** of grief may require months or years, most individuals are under a nurse's care for only a short period of time. The nurse may become frustrated when, just as the person or family begins to express grief, the person leaves the health care unit or dies. Grieving is an individual process, and resolution of loss does not follow a set schedule.

## SUMMARY

Categories of loss include loss of an aspect of self, an external object, a significant other, a known environment, and life. The nurse interacts daily with patients/clients and families experiencing loss. Knowledge of the concepts and theories of loss, death, and the grieving process provides a framework for the nursing process. The nurse's responses and interactions with patients/clients and families create the climate for openness in expressing grief. The nurse explores patients'/clients' strengths and support systems by listening, being available when needed, and conveying respect for values and beliefs. A trusting relationship creates a therapeutic environment that encourages expression of grief and fosters dignity and self-esteem. Understanding promotes growth and paves the way for effective care of grieving or dying patients/clients and their families.

## CHAPTER 11 REVIEW
### Key Concepts

- The grieving process involves a set of emotional, cognitive, and behavioural responses to an actual or perceived loss.
- Individuals experience different aspects of the grieving process at different times.
- The phases of the grieving process vary among theories but progress from distress and shock to resolution and acceptance.
- Dying may lead to a grief response similar to that with other kinds of losses.
- The individual's perception of a loss is influenced by many

factors, including developmental stage, beliefs, roles, relationships, and socioeconomic status.

- Therapeutic communication helps the nurse assist the grieving and the dying person in coping with loss.
- Nursing care of the grieving and dying patient/client should promote a sense of identity, dignity, and self-esteem.
- Nursing care can assists the patient/client in resolving grief and accepting the loss.
- Nursing care of the terminally ill individual focuses on promoting comfort and improving the quality of remaining life.
- As death approaches, a person reviews and analyses values and beliefs pertinent to the meaning of life and death.
- A nurse must assess whether family members are willing to be involved in a dying patient's/client's care before using them as resources.
- Care after death involves caring for the body with dignity and sensitivity.
- Preparing the body to leave the ward or unit is called *last offices*.
- The nurse's own loss history influences responses to patient/client losses.
- Nurses who work with critically or terminally ill patients/clients experience loss and grief.
- Nurses need to be aware of and mourn their own losses on an ongoing basis to avoid bereavement overload.

## CRITICAL THINKING EXERCISES

1. You are caring for a 16-year-old male accident victim, who lost his right leg in the accident. It has been 2 weeks since the accident, and you notice that he has become progressively withdrawn. He has refused to undertake any physiotherapy or do anything for himself. You suspect that he is grieving, but are not sure. Describe how you would approach the person and what you would assess.

2. Mrs Sullivan, aged 75 years, seems to be depressed. When you enquire as to how she is, she tells you that she lost her husband of 50 years 6 months ago. Her children have been telling her that she should sell her house and get on with her life. She feels that there must be something wrong with her because she "just can't forget" her husband. What would your response be and what would you teach her about the grieving process?

3. Amir Kazi, a devout Muslim, is expected to die within two weeks. How would you prepare for his death in order to ensure that his religious and cultural wishes are respected?

4. You have been spending a lot of time with Mr Charles; your mentor informs you that you are spending far too much time with him. His condition has progressively deteriorated, and you find yourself thinking about him all the time. You do not trust anyone else to give him the care you know he needs. Your mentor comments on your attachment to the patient/client and asks you to reflect on what is influencing your response to the patient/client. What factors might influence a nurse to become overly attached to a patient/client

and how would you deal with this situation?

5. Mr Carlson's family has decided to take him home during the last days of his illness because they do not want him to die in the hospital. They realize that he requires total care. His wife is handicapped, and both children work full time. What would you need to teach the family and what will they need to consider before taking him home? What services would you contact?

6. Outline some of the concerns the community psychiatric nurse may have concerning an elderly widower who is approaching the first anniversary of his wife's death?

### Key Terms

Actual loss, p. 210
Anticipatory grief, p. 213
Bereavement overload, p. 215
Bereavement, p. 210
Complicated grief, p. 213
Grief response, p. 213
Grief, p. 210
Grieving process, p. 212
Hope, p. 216, 217
Intensity of coping, p. 217
Last offices, p. 225
Mourning, p. 211
Palliative care, p. 225
Perceived loss, p. 210
Personal loss, p. 210
Post-mortem, p. 224
Prolonged/unresolved grief, p. 213
Resolution, p. 225
Spiritual comfort, p. 223
Unfinished business, p. 213

## REFERENCES

Barbus AJ: The dying person's bill of rights, *Am J Nurs*, 75(1):99, 1975.

Benoliel JQ: Loss and terminal illness, *Nurs Clin North Am* 20:439, 1985.

Burnside I, editor: *Nursing the aged*, ed 2, New York, 1988, McGraw Hill.

Cartwright A, Bowling A: *Life after death — a study of the elderly widowed*, London, 1982, Routledge & Kegan Paul.

Conrad NL: Spiritual support for the dying, *Nurs Clin North Am* 20:415, 1985.

Davitz L, Davitz J: *Nurses' responses to patients' suffering*, New York, 1980, Springer-Verlag.

Dufault K, Martocchio BC: Hope: its spheres and dimensions, *Nurs Clin North Am* 20:379, 1985.

Dundee JW, McMillan C: Postive evidence for P6 acupuncture antiemesis, *Postgrad Med J* 67:417, 1991.

Engel GL: Grief and grieving, *Am J Nurs* 64:93, 1964.

Hampe SO: Needs of the grieving spouse in a hospital setting, *Nurs Res* 24:113, 1975.

Herth KA: The relationship between level of hope and level of coping response and other variables in patients with cancer, *Oncol Nurs Forum* 16:67, 1989.

Heyse-Moore L. Respiratory systems. In Saunders C: *The management of terminal disease*, ed 2, London, 1984, Edward Arnold.

Howarth H: Mouth care procedures for the very ill, *Nurs Times* 73(10):354, 1977.

Johnson RJ, Lund DA, Dimond MF: Stress, self-esteem and coping during bereavement among the elderly, *Soc Psychol* 49 (3): 273, 1986.

Jolly J: *Missed beginnings: death before life has been established*, London, 1987, Austen Cornish Publishers Ltd.

Kalish RA, Reynolds DK: *Death and ethnicity: a psychocultural study*, Los Angeles, 1976, Southern California Press.

Kim JH et al: A clinical study of benzydamine for the treatment of radiotherapy-induced mucositis of the oropharynx, *Int J Tissue React* 7:215, 1985.

Kim MJ, McFarland GK, McLane AM: *Pocket guide to nursing diagnoses*, St Louis, 1991, Mosby.

Kübler-Ross E: *On death and dying*, New York, 1969, Macmillan.

Lee L, Lee M: *Absent friends: coping with the loss of a treasured pet*, London, 1992, Henson Press.

Lewis K: Potential losses in chronic illness, *J Rehabil* 49(8), 1983.

Martocchio BC: Grief and bereavement: healing through hurt, *Nurs Clin North Am* 20:327, 1985.

McEvoy J: Investigating the concept of death in adults who are mentally handicapped, *Br J of Mental Subnormality* 35(69):15, 1989.

Neuberger, J: *Caring for dying people of different faiths*, London, 1994, Mosby.

O'Connor AP: Understanding the cancer patient's search for meaning, *Cancer Nurs* 13:167, 1990.

Oswin M: *Bereavement and mentally handicapped people: a discussion paper*, London, 1981, King's Fund Centre.

Parkes CM: *Bereavement: studies of grief in adult life*, Middlesex, 1991, Pelican.

Rando TA: *Grief, dying and death*, Champaign, Ill, 1984, Research Press.

Raphael B: *The anatomy of bereavement*, New York, 1983, Basic Books.

Reed PG: Religiousness among terminally ill and healthy adults, *Res Nurs Health* 9:35, 1986.

Regnard C, Comisky M: Nausea and vomiting in advanced cancer, *Palliative Med* 6:146, 1992.

Regnard C, Tempest S: *A guide to symptoms relief in advanced cancer*, Manchester, 1992, Haigh & Hochland.

Riggan L: Living with loss, *Nurs Times* 88(27):34, 1992.

Sampson C: *The neglected ethic: religious and cultural factors in the care of patients*, London, 1982, McGraw-Hill.

Schulz R, Brenner G: Relocation of the aged — a review and theoretical analysis, *J Gerontol* 32(3):323, 1977.

Twycross RG: Principles and practice of pain relief in terminal cancer, *Update* 5(2):115, 1972.

Williams J, Copp G: Food presentation and the terminally ill, *Nurs Standard* 4:29, 1990.

Worden JW: *Grief counselling and grief therapy*, New York, 1991, Springer-Verlag.

World Health Organization: *Cancer pain relief and palliative care: report of a WHO Expert Committee*, WHO Tech Rep Series No. 804, Geneva, 1990, The World Health Organization.

Young IH, Daviskas E: Effects of low-dose nebolized morphine on exercise in patients with chronic lung disease, *Thorax* 44:387, 1989.

## FURTHER READING

### Adult Nursing

Bowlby J: *Loss, sadness and depression*, Middlesex, 1981, Penguin.

Bruss CR: Nursing diagnosis of hopelessness, *J Psychosoc Nurs* 26:29, 1988.

Callanan M, Kelley P: *Final gifts: understanding and helping the dying*, Sevenoaks, 1992, Hodder & Stoughton.

Dickenson D, Johnson M et al: *Death, dying and bereavement*, London, 1993, Sage.

Fallowfield L: *The quality of life: the missing bereavement in health care*, London, 1990, Souvenir Press.

Mulhern RM: When there's no treatment left but the truth, *RN* 49:26, 1986.

Musgrave CF: The ethical and legal implications of hospice care: an international overview, *Cancer Nurs* 10:183, 1987.

Neuberger J; *Caring for dying people of different faiths*. London, 1994, Mosby.

Stickney SK, Gardner ER: Companions in suffering, *Am J Nurs* 84:1491, 1984.

Tyner R: Elements of empathetic care for dying patients and their families, *Nurs Clin North Am* 20:393, 1985.

Wegmann JA: Hospice home death, hospital death, and coping abilities of widows, *Cancer Nurs* 10:148, 1987.

### Children's Nursing

Anthony S: *The discovery of death in childhood and after*, Middlesex, 1971, Penguin.

Dominica F: Reflection on death in childhood, *BMJ* 294:108, 1987.

Langor M: Meanings of death to children. In Fifol H: *New meanings of death*, New York, 1977, McGraw-Hill.

### Learning Disabilities Nursing

Birchinall P, Jenkinson R: Death of a friend, *Nurs Times* 89(50):65, 1993.

Kennedy J: Bereavement and the person with a mental handicap, .*Nurs Stand* 4(6):36, 1989

O'Nians R: Support in grief, *Nurs Times* 89(50):62, 1993.

### Mental Health Nursing

Davis L: Facing death, *Social Work Today* 10:45, 16, 1979.

Downing AB, Smoker B: *Voluntary euthanasia*, London, 1986, Peter Owen.

Illich I: *Limits to medicine*, Harmondsworth, 1977, Pelican.

Kalish RA: *Death, grief and caring relationships*, ed 2, Monterey, 1985, Brooks/Cole.

Levine S: *Who dies: an investigation of conscious living and conscious dying*, Bath, 1986, Gateway Books.

Parkes CM, Weiss RS: *Recovery from bereavement*, New York, 1983, Basic Books.

Parkes CM: Bereavement, *B J Psych* 146:11-17, 1985.

# unit 3

# Professional Nursing Concepts and Processes

# Values and Ethics

## LEARNING OUTCOMES

After studying this chapter, you should be able to:
- *Define the key terms listed.*
- *Describe how values are formed at different stages of development.*
- *Compare and contrast modes of value transmission.*
- *Discuss how values influence behaviour.*
- *Discuss the importance of caring in professional nursing practice.*
- *Explain the relationship between the nurse's values and decision making in practice.*
- *Describe the process of values clarification and discuss the advantages of values clarification in nursing.*
- *Use a values clarification strategy to examine personal values.*
- *Discuss techniques used to help patients/clients to clarify values.*
- *Discuss the influence of ethics on nursing practice and describe the five central ethical principles*
- *Identify the purposes of a code of professional conduct.*
- *Identify and apply principles of ethics to clinical situations.*
- *Suggest benefits of using a decision-making model and list the four main questions used to gather data.*

Professional nurses constantly have to make decisions about patients'/clients' care and well-being. They also have to help patients/clients to make decisions. Most importantly, they have to collaborate with doctors, nurses and other carers in making decisions which influence the way in which interventions are carried out. Nurses also implement care prescribed by doctors and therapists and are accountable for implementing these. Nurses must judge the appropriateness of any therapy.

Decisions are based in part on a person's conscious or subconscious values. A **value** is a belief about the worth of a given idea or behaviour. Values are standards which influence behaviour. An individual's needs, the culture and society in which a person lives and the significant others to whom the individual relates, are a reflection of personal values. Values vary from person to person, developing and changing as a person grows and matures.

Nurses relate to both personal and professional sets of values. As individuals, nurses have the right to express and act on their values (Bernal, 1985). Many values that nurses hold (for example, beliefs in the importance of human dignity, independence, or positive human relationships) can influence a patient's/client's care. Each patient/client also has a value system of unique personal needs and preferences. Conflict between nurses' and patients'/clients' values may lead to **ethical dilemmas**. Nurses therefore need to understand their own values and those of their patients/clients. A systematic analysis of value systems helps nurses to act in a more professional and knowledgeable way.

The threats posed by illness cause individuals to reassess values relating not only to illness but to most aspects of living. Nurses frequently help patients/clients to clarify personal values, reorder priorities, minimize conflict, and achieve consistency among values and behaviours related to preventing illness, promoting health, and living more resourcefully and satisfyingly within their given settings.

**Ethics** is the study of personal and professional behaviour related to 'good' and 'right', and 'bad' and 'wrong'. Ethics arises in situations of challenge and change where many different factors are involved, and the outcome usually cannot be predicted.

The health care system has undergone dramatic changes in recent years. As a result, nurses work in health care settings which generate a variety of ethical situations. Many factors contribute to the complexity of today's health care environment. Advances in technology, coupled with restraints on resources, are the primary reasons for the changing scope of nursing activities. As a result, conflicts arise for nurses providing care within these environments. It is not only situations involving euthanasia, informed consent, and quality of life which present ethical dilemmas to nurses. Daily challenges of rights and responsibilities make today's nurses more aware and more accountable as well as more willing to exercise their responsibility in making decisions at many levels.

Nurses maintain a primary commitment to patients/clients. At the same time nurses are accountable to doctors (whose orders they carry out), other health team members (with whom they work), the institutions (which employ them) and their profession (which registers them). Today, patients/clients are more aware of their rights within the health care system and this demands adaptability and openness from health care workers. Nurses frequently act as the liaison between patients/clients and other health care team members to ensure that the individual's rights are honoured and that patients/clients know and understand their options. Patients/clients seek information from nurses to understand their choices; nurses are asked to assist them in decision making.

Daily and frequent personal contact with patients/clients place nurses in a unique position compared with other health care professionals. Nurses are present when the most basic human activities are performed (such as bathing and toileting) when dressings are changed, medications are given, and when physical assessment takes place. Establishing and maintaining a relationship with the patient/client therefore forms the foundation of nursing ethics. This aspect will be stressed in the text as it is basic to the more holistic approach to care which is less tied to the medical model.

## THE NATURE AND FUNCTION OF VALUES

A person is in part identified by the values he or she holds. Values represent a way of life. They are expressed as behaviours that a person tries to maintain (Omery, 1989). The total number of values a person possesses is probably relatively small and tends to be organized into systems. Values may be conscious or subconscious. An individual may express values openly or may demonstrate them through verbal and nonverbal behaviours.

Values can be divided into three levels of expression: beliefs, attitudes and values themselves.

**Beliefs** are based more on faith than facts. Beliefs go beyond the obvious but have their basis in facts. Examples of such beliefs are that patients/clients will get better with care, that nursing is worthwhile work, and that people are trustworthy (Tschudin, 1992).

An **attitude** is a feeling towards a person, object, or idea (Steele, 1986). A person's attitudes are relatively constant. A person evaluates whether the person, object, or idea is good or bad, positive or negative. A person may have an attitude about certain ideas but without valuing them. Attitudes can and do influence behaviour.

**Values** are beliefs upon which a person acts and which then become the standards for guiding actions, developing and maintaining attitudes towards relevant objects, morally judging self and others, and comparing self and others (Rokeach, 1973). Values have a strong motivational component that directs conduct. There are only a few values (for example, friendship, quality of health, religious freedom, or material gain) that a person consciously acknowledges as important and significant in influencing life. Only a few values consistently and predictably have an impact on behaviour and no two individuals give equal importance to the same values. The values that hold the greatest importance in shaping thoughts and actions are a part of a person's unique identity.

Values related to one another form a **value system**. Examples of value systems are those related to religion and health. Rokeach (1973) describes value systems as learned principles and rules to allow choice and guide decisions. Zuzich (1978) speaks of 'standards of conduct' to describe the value system that a person holds and uses for making judgements.

A person's values about health determine the use of resources and choices made about health care during a time of illness. For example, eating a balanced diet, exercising, and seeking early medical attention during illness are the result of a person's value of health. The behaviours a person assumes as a result of personal values should be realistic. For example, a young man with severe heart disease cannot set unrealistic expectations for the maintenance of physical strength and endurance. A realistic value system allows the person to be flexible and attain greater satisfaction from the beliefs, attitudes, behaviours, and feelings influenced by personal values.

Values may be classified as *intrinsic* or *extrinsic* (Steele, 1986). Intrinsic values are related to the maintenance of life such as the value of food, or friendship. Values categorized as extrinsic originate from outside a person and are not essential to the maintenance of life. For example, values associated with the choice of an occupation are extrinsic. Some values appear less important than others, depending on the type of choices a person must make or the priority of the values held.

A person's perceptions of other individuals are influenced by personal values. When meeting someone for the first time, for example, a person notes the other person's behaviour. Values direct a person's responses towards another. The nurse may perceive a sick person's value of maintaining courage during a time of suffering. If the patient/client expresses a need to stay strong in the presence of family members, the nurse respects this by making the patient/client as comfortable as possible and having basic needs met before family members visit.

Values shape reactions to others and form a basis for evaluating human interaction and relationships.

## FORMATION OF VALUES

Values are learned through observation. An individual observes not only behaviour but also the setting in which it occurs and the response it creates. For example, a student nurse closely observes a clinical teacher's actions at the patient's/client's bedside and the person's reactions. If the patient/client remains relaxed and accepting as the teacher administers care, the student learns to value being a competent and caring nurse. The teacher's competence and caring as a professional nurse are incorporated into the student's value system.

Values are also acquired through doing or creating something. After repeatedly doing something, a person looks back on such situations to determine what behaviours led to the desirable effects and how other people responded to those behaviours. The student nurse who receives praise after performing a task well will probably continue to value high standards of achievement. Repeated reinforcement results in the student becoming a skilled practitioner.

But most of all, values are acquired through suffering — both one's own suffering and that of other people (Frankl, 1962). Frankl argues that the most important goal in life for every person is to find meaning and that this is achieved through values. We do not *give* meaning to situations and experiences, but *discover* meaning in them. Thus when caring for people who are suffering we discover the meaning of caring. When suffering ourselves, we discover our own values of life, health, friends, religions, etc. People who have discovered their values of life live more purposefully. Values of health are only truly discovered through experiencing ill-health, or threats to the health of oneself or others.

Brill (1973) has summarized the way in which values are learned or acquired:

1. A particular circumstance demands a reaction from an individual.
2. The individual responds on a trial-and-error basis or on the basis of principle.
3. The individual selects an effective response.
4. The individual comes to believe that this is the 'right' response because it works for him or her.
5. The individual believes that people who respond differently in the same situation are 'wrong'.

People learn values by observing and interacting with others. Individuals have values that they believe to be important for a satisfying life. They often transmit their values to others in an effort to influence their attitudes and behaviours.

### Modes of Value Transmission

Values are learned over a lifetime. This is not a deliberate process whereby individuals consciously choose the values they wish to have. Values become a part of an individual during socialization in the family, school, work, religious, and other social groups. When children observe parents, family, and friends, they internalize behaviours which become the foundation of their value system. When appreciating people, they experience the values of others and incorporate them into their own systems.

The people who influence a child are generally unaware of the way they transmit their values. For example, if a mother consistently demonstrates honesty in dealings with others, her child will probably see the value of telling the truth. The child becomes honest without the mother's insistence or threat. However, the process of imposing values can be deliberate, as when a parent says to a child who has lied, "You should be ashamed of yourself. Good children don't lie".

There are five traditional modes of value transmission (Table 12-1); modelling, moralizing, laissez-faire, responsible choice, and reward and punishment. Each mode has profound implications for childhood behaviour and acquisition of values.

When **modelling** values, people act in such a way as to show others the preferred mode of behaviour. People acquire values from a variety of role models, but the implications of such modelling on the young may be that children imitate their parents in an initial wish to be like them, and that parents, in turn, may purposefully choose to model socially acceptable behaviour.

The approach of **moralizing** in order to acquire values is very authoritarian in that it has been identified as the mode through which parents and teachers force children to conform to their standards of right and wrong.

The **laissez-faire** mode describes the way in which people can acquire values by behaving informally without restrictions or limitations. This mode may lead to a freedom for parents and children, and inspires creativity. Parents refrain from discipline. The inadequacy of this model is that no-one assumes responsibility for the child's behaviour.

**Responsible choice** suggests a balance of freedom and restriction which allows children to select values that lead to personal satisfaction and parental support. This favours *discussion* of choices, and values are not strictly imposed by parents.

**Reward and punishment** serves to control behaviour. Offering rewards for certain valued actions strengthens this. Individuals may choose either mode of value transmission, with the clear implication that using rewards can be seen to be a positive mode of valuing, but using punishment may teach that violence is acceptable.

### Influence of Development on Values Formation

Value formation, modification, and reaffirmation occur throughout a person's life. Cognitive and emotional levels of

## TABLE 12-1 Modes of Value Transmission

| Descriptions | Implications |
| --- | --- |
| **MODELLING**<br>People act in way to show others the preferred way to behave.<br><br>People acquire values from a variety of role models. | Children initially wish to be like their parents, and thus parents can model values they perceive as significant.<br>Modelling may not lead to socially acceptable behaviour (e.g. viewing another's aggressive behaviour).<br>Unless a parent points out the most desirable values, children can follow any role model. |
| **MORALIZING**<br>Parents and teachers hold standards for right and wrong and rigidly enforce children to conform to their sets of values. | This approach can be very authoritarian.<br>Moralizing parents may be unwilling to consider alternative values for children.<br>With this approach, one way is often the only way.<br>Young people reared by moralizing adults often have difficulty with making independent choices. |
| **LAISSEZ-FAIRE**<br>At times, people acquire values by behaving informally without restrictions or limitations. | Parents want children to be free to explore a variety of life experiences.<br>Children are encouraged to be inquisitive and learn from experiences.<br>Parents may refrain from discipline.<br>Limitation is that no-one assumes responsibility for children's behaviour.<br>Conflict and confusion may arise if children have no direction. |
| **RESPONSIBLE CHOICE**<br>Balance of freedom and restriction allows children to select values that lead to personal satisfaction and parental support. Children's choices are more limited as compared with the laissez-faire approach. | Values are not imposed by parents.<br>As children choose values, parents, other family members, and teachers allow them to explore within boundaries new behaviours and their consequences.<br>Children who can freely discuss their behaviour and its effects will learn to understand their own values. |
| **REWARD AND PUNISHMENT**<br>Offering rewards for certain valued behaviour serves to control behaviour. When children fail to assume certain behaviours, parents administer punishment. | Parents may choose to use either form of value transmission more frequently.<br>Using rewards can be a positive response to strengthen preferred values.<br>Punishment may teach that violence is acceptable. |

development influence the way in which values are learned, maintained and passed on (see boxes).

## Sociocultural Influences

Values are formed in social settings where the educational, socioeconomic, spiritual, and cultural backgrounds of people vary. Leininger (1978) describes culture as 'a way of life belonging to a designated group of people'. A culture can have subcultures – small groups that assume an identity of their own – that have similarities to the larger culture (Steele, 1986). In the UK there are many subcultures (for example, Geordie, Cockney, Highlander) that share some values with the larger culture while adopting some values unique to their subculture (see Chapter 8).

It is difficult to establish norms for any subculture because no absolute agreement about acceptable values exists within a particular subculture. Nurses are expected to respect the values of the patient/client, even when their cultural backgrounds differ.

A particular culture's value orientation influences the way in which members pursue health care. Individuals as social groups face a certain number of problems, and there are a finite number of solutions to those problems. Individuals in certain cultural groups may seek health care for the slightest problem, whereas those in other groups seek care only when their condition is serious.

To give effective care, nurses must understand the influence of cultural traditions on health behaviours, response to stress, use of health care services and adjustment to illness. The professional care givers' value systems almost certainly differ from those of their patients/clients. However, nurses must also realize that no single culture agrees on what is 'right' or 'wrong'. Nurses need to respect **cultural orientation** but also look further into and try to understand patients'/clients' uniqueness.

## VALUES IN PROFESSIONAL NURSING

Nurses assist patients/clients in various life situations. Virginia Henderson (1964) defined nursing as:

*"assisting... individual(s), sick or well, in the performance of those activities that contribute to health or its recovery, that (they) would perform unaided if (they) had the necessary will, strength, or knowledge. And to do this in such a way as to help (them) gain independence as rapidly as possible".*

Since nursing care involves people, it is important for nurses to understand the human values that facilitate the giving of help (Raatikainen, 1989). Nurses have their own individual set of values which are the result of personal choice and learning. Society's values regarding how people should be cared for also influence nurses. Finally, the values of the institutions in which nurses are employed also influence practice. When nurses' personal and professional values are similar, they readily assume a professional role. When personal and professional values differ, nurses can become dissatisfied. The central values that direct nurses in clinical decision making and support of patients/clients may not always be clear. However, many authors identify one particular value involved in the nurse-patient/client relationship, namely *caring* (Table 12-2).

### The Value of Caring

There is an important link between the value of caring and nurses' views on people and their human dignity (Fry, 1989). **Caring** involves a sense of dedication to another person. When unable to care for patients/clients, nurses can no longer deliver the nurturing activities designed to assist people. Such a situation creates a dilemma for nurses and can be a serious source of dissatisfaction. Changes within the health care delivery system have created situations which threaten nurses' ability to exercise caring towards patients/clients. Specialization in health care has led to a subdivision of tasks by care givers; this often leads to depersonalization. Health care institutions and even society expect nurses to do more with fewer resources; yet nurses often lack the autonomy and authority to decide how care will be provided (Kurtz and Warry, 1991).

Advanced technology often endangers a humane approach to nursing care when the nurse gives more importance to monitoring of equipment than to sustaining the nurse-patient/client relationship. Caring benefits both the nurse and the patient/client. Kurtz and Warry (1991) argue that caring makes curing possible. However, caring is more than simply being concerned for another person. For caring to influence a nurse's practice, it must be integrated as a standard of performance in all care activities. Fry (1988) and Veatch (1987) identify four criteria which define caring as a moral value that serves as an ethical standard for nursing practice:

1. Caring must be viewed as an ultimate or overriding value to guide one's actions.
2. Caring must be considered a universal value and, hence, must be applied to all people in similar circumstances.
3. Caring must be considered prescriptive in that certain

**Children's Nursing
Forming values at different life stages**

**Infants:** Infants rely on their parents for physical and emotional care. Although infants do not possess an ability to reason, they acutely sense the emotions and behaviours of people around them. The manner in which parents react to their children is often a function of their parents' values. Infants begin to grow in emotional security through prompt and consistent responses of the parents to their needs.

**Toddler:** A toddler learns acceptable behaviour by imitating others and seeking approval. As the child strives for a sense of autonomy, an identity forms, shaped by the values of the people with whom the child associates. The parents balance the child's need for independence against the need for safety and protection. The setting of appropriate limits allows the toddler to continue identity development at this crucial age of character formation.

**Preschool Child:** The preschool child is at the stage of cognitive development when concept formation begins. Concepts are objects, events, and experiences that have acquired meaningful labels: dogs bark, trees have leaves, a mother holds and comforts. The child can understand the terms right or wrong as applied to single acts. If repeatedly told not to hit or push playmates, the child learns that this act is wrong but does not yet have an abstract understanding of all 'wrong' behaviours. Parents must provide kind, fair, and consistent limits for behaviour and help direct the child towards behaviours that they value.

**School-Aged Child:** The school-aged child is exposed to diverse groups of people with a variety of values. Parents usually encourage the child to be involved in activities at home and outside the home. Goal setting and achievement are incorporated, promoting values related to being a good person, doing right, avoiding harm, and choosing adequately between activities. Important behaviours are being involved in problem solving and living by choices.

**Adolescent:** Adolescence is a critical developmental period that provides rapid and varied learning experiences. Adolescents' primary concerns are to achieve a balance between personal identity and the identity established with peers. Owing to rapid physical and psychosocial development, adolescents frequently doubt themselves and the values they have been taught. As adolescents mature and the physical and emotional changes stabilize, they examine and incorporate values learned from parents and teachers. However, because their social contacts expand greatly, adolescents are no longer limited by parental values.

behaviours (for example, empathy, support, compassion, and protection) are preferred.

4. Caring must be other-regarding in that it must consider the human flourishing of others and not just one's own welfare.

Caring is an all encompassing part of nursing. Specific professional behaviours demonstrate a nurse's commitment to

### Adult Nursing
### Developing values

The mature adult is able to examine, maintain, and change values based on continuing life experiences and the acquisition of new knowledge. Marrying, rearing children, and choosing a career often require young adults to redefine their values.

Middle-aged adults often redefine self-concepts (the 'mid-life crisis') to adapt to the needs of later life. Middle-aged adults whose values have been reinforced have a growing sense of security. However, the onset of ageing can also pose a threat to adults who see their values of youth and vitality no longer applying to themselves.

During late adulthood, an individual faces significant changes in life, including retirement from work, the physical alterations of ageing, and the loss of close friends and family. The older adult may see many personal values threatened, as it becomes more difficult to stay active and maintain meaningful interpersonal relationships. It is therefore essential for the adult to remain open to new ideas and values so that the opportunity for growth and satisfaction exists despite advancing age.

### Mental Health Nursing
### Ethical issues

Ethical issues in mental health care settings can range from issues of availability of resources, to issues of individual forms of treatment and care. Mental health nurses have traditionally worked from a humanistic perspective which is dependent on human qualities, such as respect, empathy, and trust. Because mental health nurses attempt to work in partnership with patients/clients, they may sometimes find themselves in contradiction with the demands and wishes of other disciplines. Nurses who are more patient/client-oriented will work with the person and carers in ways which return the maximum autonomy for the patient/client. To do this, the nurse must use good communication skills to build a relationship with the patient/client and carers, and must utilize opportunities when the client is lucid to gain an understanding of the patient's/client's preferences and choices.

caring and excellence in practice. The United Kingdom Central Council, in its *Code of Professional Conduct* (1992a), sees this caring for nurses, midwives and health visitors to be encapsulated in the following:

- safeguarding and promoting the interests of individual patients and clients;
- serving the interests of society;
- justifying public trust and confidence; and
- upholding and enhancing the good standing and reputation of the professions.

The American Association of Colleges of Nursing (1986) recommends seven values essential for professional nurses (Table 12-3). These values equate largely with the ethical principles outlined below. In assigning priority to these values when making decisions, professional nurses are able to see how personal attributes (virtues) influence and direct professional care.

## VALUES AND
## CLINICAL DECISION MAKING

Nurses identify needs and make clinical judgements on the basis of both subjective and objective information which they collect about a patient/client. The decision-making process involves critical thinking and is an important nursing responsibility. Each patient's/client's needs must be analyzed individually so that correct decisions are made about care.

A nurse's personal and professional values influence clinical decision making. When a nurse values equality, the care delivered to a patient/client will be based on that person's needs and should be provided in a nondiscriminatory way. Nurses usually believe that life is intrinsically valuable and with it goes a paramount right which must be protected at all costs. Within this belief, however, some nurses may hold to a principle of the sanctity of

life and may therefore find it difficult to assist with abortion; others defend a principle of quality of life and those nurses may for instance find it easier to withhold treatment from a terminally ill patient/client. Taylor (1985) warns that decision making can become biased when quality of life becomes the sole criterion in health care. Differences in social and economic class can define quality of life in a variety of ways. For example, intelligent, socially accomplished and technically skilled health carers may become biased when considering the type of care that an uneducated, illiterate, or physically handicapped person would seek.

Nurses care for individuals who possess unique values about life and the human experience. Patients'/clients' values must therefore be respected. This is why it is important that nurses know their own values and the ways in which they interact with the values of patients/clients. To make intelligent and thoughtful decisions about care, nurses must be aware of the influence which values have in decisions.

## VALUES CLARIFICATION

Since individuals are not always consciously aware of their values, they can have difficulties when making choices or when they feel forced to change their values. In addition, individuals must realize the implications that their values have for their own behaviour. Yet people do not suddenly become aware of their values, and many people are unable to define their values clearly or meaningfully. To achieve an awareness of personal values, individuals use cognitive processes of values clarification.

**Values clarification,** or valuing, is a process of self-discovery that helps people to gain clearer insights into their values. It is not a set of rules that interferes with conscientious decision making. Values clarification does not imply that a specific set of values should be accepted by all people. It is also not a method of indoctrination of religious, moral, or cultural standards. When clarifying values in given situations, people learn what choices to

## TABLE 12-2 Caring as a Foundational Value of Nursing

| Definition | Central Concepts |
|---|---|
| **WATSON** | |
| Caring is a foundation of nursing as a human science. It requires commitment on the part of the nurse to protect human dignity and preserve humanity. | Nurse-patient/client relationship (caring as value of central importance). Caring as mode of being, natural state of human existence. Caring as required for one to care for self or others. Caring occurring in society to serve human needs. |
| **NODDINGS** | |
| To care may mean to be charged with protection, welfare, or maintenance of something or someone. Person-to-person encounter results in joy as basic human need. | Receptivity (acceptance by care giver of person cared for). Relatedness (relation of care giver to one cared for as fact of human existence). Responsiveness (commitment of care giver to one cared for). |
| **FRANKENA** | |
| Caring involves respect for people. It is basis of normative human judgements in general. | Respect (caring requiring identifiable form of response on part of care giver to person cared for). |
| **ROACH** | |
| Caring is the human mode of being. Individuals care because they are human beings. | Professional caring has five components: compassion, competence, confidence, conscience and commitment. |

Adapted from Kurtz RJ, Warry J: *Nurs Forum* 26(1):4, 1991, and Roach MS: *The human act of caring*, Ottawa, 1987, Canadian Hospital Association.

make when alternatives are presented and how to determine whether the choices are rationally made. The result of valuing is greater self-awareness and personal insight.

Raths *et al* (1979) pioneered values clarification as an approach to appraisal of values. Valuing involves three steps: choosing, prizing, and acting (see box). Using values clarification, the person ranks personal values in hierarchical order. The resultant hierarchy reveals to the individual a personal value system that provides a guide for personal conduct, lifestyle, and interpersonal interactions.

**Choosing:** first, the person must choose personal values freely. The freedom to select from among alternatives allows a person to cherish the final choice. However, the individual must understand the alternatives. Consider the following example:

An older woman who suddenly lost her husband, shares her concerns with a community nurse. It is clear that she has several choices; continue to live alone and grieve alone for her husband; move in with her daughter and share the grieving with her, even though this may mean moving away from friends who may also help her to grieve, but in a different way; or stay at home and socialize with male and female companions, thus coping with her grief in yet a different way. The nurse helps the woman to examine her choices without passing judgement or offering advice. A clear understanding of all the alternatives and their consequences will ensure that the woman's final choice is the right one for her.

**Prizing:** this is showing private and public satisfaction with the value chosen. A person holds a value in esteem by feeling good about a choice. A nurse can help a patient/client to use values clarification so that the person is able to affirm personal values in the presence of significant others. When the widow decides on the last option of socializing again after her husband's death, she prizes her decision by sharing it with her daughter and friends. By announcing personal values, a person reaffirms their importance or relevance.

**Acting:** acting on a chosen value consolidates its acceptance. Acting requires translating values into behaviour. The widow may start by attending local social events and enrolling as a volunteer at a local hospital. Raths *et al* (1979) suggest that people should act consistently and regularly on chosen values. It would be important for the widow to pursue opportunities regularly and to spend time with friends and acquaintances. It may, however, also be difficult to act consistently on a chosen value. For example, a patient/client who values independence may be too disabled by illness to function safely alone. The nurse may then be able to help the patient accept limitations and see what possibilities exist within these for self-care activities. The nurse can help clarify situations and alternatives for patients/clients so that they can act on the best possible choices.

## Values Clarification Versus Ethical Decision Making

Values clarification is inadequate as a guide for solving ethical dilemmas (Bernal, 1985). There are often conflicts in values among health care professionals and patients/clients that lead to ethical dilemmas. For example, a patient/client may decide not to have surgery for lung cancer. The doctor believes surgery is the

## TABLE 12-3 Essential Nursing Values and Behaviours*

| Essential Values | Attitudes and Personal Qualities | Professional Behaviours |
| --- | --- | --- |
| ALTRUISM<br>Concern for the welfare of others | Caring<br>Commitment<br>Compassion<br>Generosity<br>Perseverance | Gives full attention to the patient/client when giving care.<br>Assists other personnel in providing care when they are unable to do so.<br>Expresses concern about social trends and issues that have implications for health care. |
| EQUALITY<br>Having the same rights, privileges, or status | Acceptance<br>Assertiveness<br>Fairness<br>Self-esteem<br>Tolerance | Provides nursing care based on the individual's need irrespective of personal characteristics.<br>Interacts with other providers in a non-discriminatory manner.<br>Expresses ideas about the improvement of access to nursing and health care. |
| AESTHETICS<br>Qualities of objects, events, and persons that provide satisfaction | Appreciation<br>Creativity<br>Imagination<br>Sensitivity | Adapts the environment so that it is pleasing to the patient/client.<br>Creates a pleasant work environment for self and others.<br>Presents self in a manner that promotes a positive image of nursing. |
| FREEDOM<br>Capacity to exercise choice | Confidence<br>Hope<br>Independence<br>Openness<br>Self-direction<br>Self-discipline | Honours individual's right to refuse treatment.<br>Supports the rights of other providers to suggest alternatives to the plan of care.<br>Encourages open discussion of controversial issues in the profession. |
| HUMAN DIGNITY<br>Inherent worth and uniqueness of an individual | Consideration<br>Empathy<br>Humanness<br>Kindness<br>Respectfulness<br>Trust | Safeguards the individual's right to privacy.<br>Addresses individuals as they prefer to be addressed.<br>Maintains confidentiality of patients/clients and staff.<br>Treats others with respect regardless of background. |
| JUSTICE<br>Upholding moral and legal principles | Courage<br>Integrity<br>Morality<br>Objectivity | Acts as a health care advocate.<br>Allocates resources fairly.<br>Reports incompetent, unethical, and illegal practice objectively and factually. |
| TRUTH<br>Faithfulness to fact or reality | Accountability<br>Authenticity<br>Honesty<br>Inquisitiveness<br>Rationality<br>Reflectiveness | Documents nursing care accurately and honestly.<br>Obtains sufficient data to make sound judgements before reporting infractions of organizational policies.<br>Participates in professional efforts to protect the public from misinformation about nursing. |

*The values are listed in alphabetical rather than priority order.
From American Association of Colleges of Nursing: *Essentials of college and university education for professional nursing,* Washington, DC, 1986, The Association. Reprinted from American Nurses Association: *Code for nurses,* Kansas City, Mo, 1976, The Association.

patient's/client's only choice. The nurse may believe in an individual's autonomy but is unsure whether this patient/client has made a rational decision.

When many different values are expressed in a situation, values clarification will probably not resolve the dilemma. Each person may benefit from knowing the other's values; yet they may not agree on the final decision. **Ethical decisions** require a clear analysis of many factors. It must be assumed that some values are better than others. Until health care professionals and patients/clients in such a situation can jointly agree on one overriding value, such as patient/client autonomy, ethical decisions cannot be made easily.

### Strategies for Values Clarification
A system of strategies can help to make valuing more insightful, practical and meaningful for the person whose values are unclear. These **values clarification strategies** are exercises to help individuals to clarify personal values using the three steps of valuing. Nurses can use the strategies with patients/clients or for personal values clarification.

## Three Steps of Values Clarification

### Choosing one's beliefs and behaviours

- Choosing from alternatives
- Choosing freely
- Considering all consequences

### Prizing one's beliefs and behaviours

- Prizing and cherishing the choice
- Publicly affirming the choice

### Acting on one's beliefs

- Making the choice part of one's behaviour
- Acting with a pattern of consistency and repetition

Modified from Raths LE, Harmin M, Simon SB: *Values and teaching,* ed 2, Columbus, Ohio, 1979, Merrill.

## Sentence Completion

This strategy (see top, right box) helps nurses determine and explore their own attitudes, beliefs, interests, and goals, which are indicators of their personal values. The completed sentences can be shared with a group to give nurses an opportunity to affirm their choices.

## Rank Ordering

This strategy requires the selection of priorities among a list of different values, such as money, work and respect (see middle, right box). The nurse can develop a similar exercise to help patients/clients to order their values in specific situations. This strategy demonstrates that many issues require more consideration of values than is usually given in decision making.

## Health Value Scale

This is an exercise for setting value priorities (see lower, right box). It consists of 10 values that a patient/client ranks in order of importance. The patient/client ranks items in a way that accurately reflects a personal value hierarchy. If health is ranked in one of the top four positions, the person places a high value on health. The value placed on health is moderate if ranked *5, 6,* or *7* and low if ranked *8, 9,* or *10.* Information obtained from this exercise can help the nurse to plan health care teaching methods. Another way to complete this exercise is by having the patient/client freely name 10 values and then to establish a priority for them.

## Nurses' Values Clarification

When values clarification is used for personal benefit, personal growth and professional satisfaction can be gained. During contacts with patients/clients, peers, doctors, and other health care professionals, the nurse's values are constantly challenged and tested. Examples of challenges are:

- How does the nurse show a willingness to be accountable for actions as a professional?
- How does the nurse's attitudes about patients/clients influence the care provided?
- When another nurse performs some action unsafely, what should be done?

## Sentence Completion

Complete the following sentences. Use them to examine your feelings and values.

- I believe I succeed as a nurse when...
- A patient/client has a right to...
- I wish the director of nursing would...
- Doctors and nurses work together best when...
- I fail as a nurse if I cannot...
- The most difficult patient/client is one who...

Modified from Simon SB et al: *Values clarification: a handbook of practical strategies for teachers and students,* New York, 1978, Hart.

## Rank Ordering

Choose 3 things from the 14 choices below that give you the most satisfaction in your work.

1. To be excited by what you are doing
2. To help others solve problems
3. To contribute to society with worthwhile work
4. To be recognized as an authority
5. To motivate yourself
6. To figure things out
7. To work within a structured situation
8. To think through new solutions
9. To have choice about time
10. To make a lot of money
11. To work in a team
12. To work out-of-doors
13. To be respected for your work
14. Other _____

From Ross R: *Prospering woman,* San Rafael, Calif, 1982, Whatever Publishing.

## Health Value Scale

Below you will find 10 values listed in alphabetical order. Arrange the values in order of their importance as guiding principles in your life. Study the list carefully and choose the one value that is most important to you. Write the number *1* in the space to the left of that value. Write the number *2* for the value that ranks second in importance. Continue in the same manner for the remaining values until you have included all ranks from *1* to *10.* Each value will have a different rank.

- ____ A comfortable life (a prosperous life)
- ____ An exciting life (a stimulating, active life)
- ____ A sense of accomplishment (lasting contribution)
- ____ Freedom (independence, free choice)
- ____ Happiness (contentedness)
- ____ Health (physical and mental well-being)
- ____ Inner harmony (freedom from inner conflict)
- ____ Pleasure (an enjoyable, leisurely life)
- ____ Self-respect (self-esteem)
- ____ Social recognition (respect, admiration)

Modified from Uustal DB: *Am J Nurs* 78:2058, 1978.

The nurse has difficulty in assuming the role of a professional when personal values are unclear and poorly conceived. Values clarification helps a nurse to explore values and decide whether to act on beliefs. The nurse is able to establish more effective relationships with patients/clients and is more able to meet their needs after clearly defining personal values. Thus, values clarification facilitates decision making and problem solving.

Values clarification can be used by nurses and other health care workers who face similar value conflicts daily. Sharing values about patients/clients, their families, and colleagues assists nurses in recognizing their commonly held values. This sharing helps nurses understand the behaviour of colleagues. Communication also becomes more open when dealing with controversial issues.

### Patients'/Clients' Values Clarification

Valuing is a useful tool to help patients/clients and families adapt to the stress of illness and other health-related problems. The nurse helps patients/clients to look at emotional issues and to clarify their meaning and significance. Values clarification helps patients/clients gain awareness of personal priorities, identify ambiguities in values and resolve major conflicts between values and behaviour. Communication with patients/clients becomes more effective because the nurse is able to focus attention on patients'/clients' comments and the reasons for them. Patients/clients become more willing to express problems and true feelings, and in this way the nurse is able to establish an individualized care plan.

Nurses play an important role in educating patients/clients about health-promoting behaviours. Patients/clients are frequently taught facts and concepts about their conditions, but their behaviours remain unchanged. The nurse who learns about patients'/clients' values is able to devise a more successful teaching programme. Giving patients/clients meaningful and practical information increases the likelihood that they will assume behaviours which promote well-being.

### Values Clarification as a Tool in Patient/Client Care

Merely encouraging the patient/client to express feelings may provide inadequate information if the real problem is a conflict in values. For example, a middle-aged man who has just been given a diagnosis of a terminal illness sees his values of health, economic security, and family unity threatened. When encouraged to discuss his feelings, he may be unable to describe clearly how he feels. The nurse who is familiar with values clarification can help this patient/client to define values, clarify goals, and seek solutions.

### The Nurse's Role

Helping patients/clients to clarify values is not an attempt at psychoanalysis. **The nurse's role is to shape responses to the patient's/client's questions or statements to stimulate introspection.** Clarification of verbal responses comes from the awareness that the valuing process will motivate a patient/client to examine personal thoughts and actions. Such responses can help the person to choose a value freely, consider alternatives, prize the choice, affirm the choice with others, act on the choice, and incorporate into life the behaviours that reflect the particular value.

## PROVIDE A CLARIFYING RESPONSE

When the nurse responds to clarify a point, it should be brief, selective, nonjudgemental, thought provoking, and spontaneous. A good clarifying exchange between the nurse and patient/client lasts only a short time. The nurse's response makes the patient/client think about values after the exchange. Clarifying responses are used only when values-conflict is the issue; for example, when the nurse explains a medical procedure, an attempt at values clarification is not required. A nurse needs to make a clarifying response only in situations in which no right or wrong answer exists. Situations lacking answers are mainly those involving beliefs, aspirations, feelings, and attitudes.

**Be nonjudgemental.** The nurse's response does not judge the patient's/client's values. The person will be unable to find satisfaction in personal values if the nurse moralizes or advises about choices. The nurse's response must evoke the individual's own creative thinking. For example, a patient/client might be undecided about whether to seek another doctor's opinion about a medical problem. If the nurse chides that person for daring even to ask if this should be considered, more questions may be raised than resolved. Instead, the nurse could explain the hazards of proposed surgery and advise the patient/client that there may be no need to seek another opinion, but that it is the patient/client who must live with the choice of doctors. The focus must be on the individual and the possible outcomes of the decision.

**Be spontaneous, but not contrived.** A nurse's spontaneity helps a patient/client to think creatively. The nurse often has little warning when the patient/client asks for help with solutions to a values dilemma. With experience, a nurse can learn to make clarifying responses without advanced planning. For example, a patient/client has been encouraged by doctors to undergo experimental surgery but has been unable to make a decision. The patient/client may ask the nurse, "What should I do?". The nurse should respond, "This is obviously a difficult decision for you. Have you weighed the pros and cons?". Although the response is consciously and deliberately designed to stimulate thought, it should not appear contrived.

Values clarification can occur in any setting. The bedside, a clinic office, or the home are all places where patients/clients express their feelings. Valuing is often more successful when the nurse has the opportunity for repeated contact with patients/clients. It is difficult for the nurse to help patients/clients meaningfully to achieve each step of the valuing process when little time is spent giving care to them.

Ultimately, the patient/client perceives that valuing provides personal satisfaction. Values clarification promotes effective reasoning and decision making. The patient/client becomes more aware of the way that values influence actions, and this awareness is an essential component of problem solving.

## CASE STUDY

Mr James, a 73-year-old man, is in hospital after fracturing his ankle at home. Mr James' daughter is concerned about her father's welfare and wants Mr James to live with her family. The daughter has voiced concern to the nurse that Mr James is incapable of caring for himself. Mr James' rehabilitation has progressed well. One day, Mr James asks the nurse, "What should I do? I know my daughter worries about me, but I don't want to be cared for like a child".

The nurse realizes that Mr James is experiencing a conflict in his values for his independence, love for his daughter, and health. The nurse thinks that the values clarification process might help Mr James to make his choice. She suggests this to Mr James as a means of choosing from the alternatives available.

**Choosing from Alternatives**. The nurse's way of helping depends partly on Mr James' age, education, and level of maturity. Mr James is alert, knowledgeable about his needs, and capable of making decisions for himself. He has also demonstrated motivation in his rehabilitation. The nurse presents the alternatives, as she perceives them, to Mr James. He is helped by having them spelled out clearly and simply.

**Examining All Consequences**. Mr James loves his daughter and knows that the offer to join the daughter's family is genuine. Mr James says that he has many friends in his block of flats and that moving to his daughter's home would make it very difficult for him to socialize with his friends. Mr James' flat is on the second floor, which requires him to climb two flights of stairs. A downstairs flat will soon be vacant.

The nurse says, "Perhaps it would be helpful to weigh the advantages and disadvantages of joining your daughter against moving into the downstairs flat". When making this suggestion, the nurse carefully avoids letting her own values influence Mr James' thinking (because she has a close relationship with her own mother and has been very happy when they shared her house on extended visits).

**Choosing Freely**. The next day, the nurse enters Mr James' room while he is eating his breakfast. Her goal is to ascertain whether Mr James was able to make a decision on his own. Mr James says, "I've decided to move into the downstairs flat". The nurse asks, "Was this a difficult choice to make?".

**Prizing the Choice**. Mr James acknowledges that he does not want to hurt his daughter's feelings; however, he knows his decision was the best one. "I still have many friends and while I have been in hospital they have all encouraged me to stay in the flat. I still feel spry and able to take care of myself." The nurse recognizes that it is important for Mr James to be satisfied with his choice and expresses this to him.

**Affirming the Choice**. It is important that Mr James is able to speak out in support of his decision. He may need assistance from the nurse in thinking of ways to affirm the choice. An appropriate response by the nurse might be, "What will be the best way to share your decision with your daughter?" Mr James replies, "My daughter and son-in-law are coming to visit me this evening. I've decided to let them know then".

**Acting on the Choice**. Mr James has made the decision to retain his independence. He is able to share his choice and the rationale for it with his daughter. The nurse using values clarification recognizes Mr James' need to act on his decision. She asks, "What can you do to begin planning for your move?"

Mr James telephones the landlord to confirm his decision and to arrange for his new flat. He is going to stay with his daughter for two weeks after discharge from the hospital. Meanwhile, he will have the opportunity to select new paint and wallpaper for the flat. Mr James' value of independence remains alive in the measures he has taken to accomplish his move.

**Acting with a Pattern**. A month after discharge, Mr James returns to outpatients for a check-up. He calls into the ward and looks for the nurse. She is interested to learn whether Mr James has continued to retain his independence; for independence to be meaningful to Mr James, it must become integrated into his lifestyle. The nurse asks, "Was your choice to remain on your own the right one?" Mr James responds, "For now, yes. I am feeling much better and I have many friends to help me. My daughter visits every week. You know, though, I do have to be cautious in the way I walk around. I know one day I may have to live with my daughter."

As Mr James becomes physically more dependent, a conflict may arise between the independence he prizes and his ability to act on that value. The value of the genuine love and concern expressed by Mr James' daughter may become a higher priority than the value of independence. Mr James' maturity will be reflected in his eventual ability to modify his values. As he becomes more physically dependent, he needs to adapt his values accordingly. Mr James will still be alert and capable of making decisions. The daughter's ability to provide a safe environment for her father without compromising Mr James' ability to make his own decisions should prove to be mutually satisfying.

This case study shows a nurse who is well versed in values clarification. In fact, it takes time to develop values clarification as a tool for a patient's/client's care. Nurses cannot attempt to help a patient/client to explore values unless they have insight into their own. Values clarification can be a valuable means of helping a patient/client to sort out true feelings and beliefs and gain a better awareness of goals in life.

## DEFINITION OF ETHICS

**Ethics** reflects the principles or standards which govern proper conduct related to professional behaviours. The values of the patient/client, nurse, and society interact to set the environment for ethical behaviour. If the value systems of all those involved are not cohesive, ethical dilemmas can occur. A dilemma is a choice between alternatives. Ethical dilemmas require the nurse to make challenging and difficult decisions about the optimum way to care for patients/clients.

For example, nurses have an obligation to "act always in such a manner as to promote and safeguard the interests and well-being of patients and clients" (UKCC, 1992a) and to prevent harm. An ethical dilemma can arise from conflict between these two values. The nurse can help a patient/client with terminal lung cancer by providing the prescribed narcotic to reduce pain and provide comfort, but that same action may also cause harm by hastening death from respiratory depression. In this example, the situation may be further complicated by family members who may have expressed their concerns relating to the side effects of the narcotic and asked the nurse to withhold the drug or administer a less effective medication. In this example, a dilemma remains, even if the family and patient/client agree on the administration of the narcotic; the nurse still has to choose between the beneficial effects of providing the prescribed narcotic and avoiding the harmful side effects.

An understanding of ethical decision making will assist nurses in making effective and proper decisions which will benefit the patient/client and themselves. As nurses develop these decision-making skills, they can also help patients/clients manage their own decisions related to health care.

### Ethics in Nursing

The primary imperative of nursing is to improve the quality of the lives of those who seek or receive nursing services (Curtin, 1986). The rapidly changing scene in health care means that nurses have to make many ethical decisions not only in direct patient care, but also in how that care is organized and directed by the institution. As nurses become ethically more aware and active, they are more able to challenge traditions and concepts which may militate against effective and humane care.

There are three types of ethics:

- **Normative** ethics raises questions about what is right or what ought to be done in situations which call for ethical decisions. This type is concerned with the study of principles of right and wrong conduct for professionals and what codes and statements should apply.
- **Descriptive** ethics presents a factual narrative of ethical behaviour. Descriptive studies do not produce moral judgements on these behaviours. This type is considered by researchers and anthropologists.
- **Metaethics** is concerned with theoretical issues of meaning and justification. It is the portion of ethics which centres on the extent to which judgements are reasonable or otherwise justifiable.

Nursing ethics is a discipline which is gradually emerging alongside medical ethics. Nursing ethics has its basis in person-centred approaches to helping and is built largely on the work of feminist writers such as Gilligan (1982) and Noddings (1984). These authors have stressed the importance of relating and relationships in caring. Their work is closely allied to that of some men who stressed the ideas of responsibility (Niebuhr, 1963) and empathy (Rogers, 1980). This has meant that nursing ethics as a discipline is making an impact by highlighting the emotional and 'soft' aspects of feelings, and simply being human, alongside principles and standards which consider reason and rationality. **Nursing ethics is thus making a stand for a more holistic approach to ethics just as nursing itself is also focusing on holistic care.** Since these issues are evolving, rather than already being part of the culture and tradition, there are inevitable differences of views and values which arise in decision making.

## NURSES' CODES OF ETHICS

Nursing has developed codes of ethics which determine the profession's standards of conduct. These codes describe the goals and values of the nursing profession. Students must make a commitment to uphold these obligations when they become nurses (see Chapter 1).

A code is a set of ethical principles generally accepted by members of the profession. These principles guide and shape the profession and its workers, but **a code is not law and therefore cannot be cited for specific situations. It is the interpretation of the code for specific situations which is important**.

The two codes that apply to nurses in the UK are the International Council of Nurses *Code for Nurses* (1973) (see box) and the United Kingdom Central Council *Code of Professional Conduct for Nurses, Midwives and Health Visitors* (1992a) (see Chapter 1). The UKCC has also published a number of advisory documents (for example, *Confidentiality*, 1987; *Exercising Accountability*, 1989; *The Scope of Professional Practice*, 1992b) which should be read in conjunction with the *Code*. The language and emphasis between the International and UKCC codes differs, due largely to the fact that one code is for a specific country and situation, and the other is more generally applicable worldwide.

## ETHICAL PRINCIPLES

Since ethics is about 'good' and 'right', **ethical principles** try to capture what is meant by this in clear terms. Two schools of ethics have generally dominated ethical thinking in the West (see box):

- **Deontology** (*Deontos*: Greek = duty) starts from the point of view that laws and rules govern behaviour and that therefore people 'ought' to keep them out of a sense of duty to society. The actions themselves are of the greatest importance. This theory can be summed up with the questions: what is my duty? or what does the law say I ought to do?
- **Teleology** (*Telos*: Greek = goal, end) considers that the consequences of actions matter more than the actions themselves. This can be summed up in the question: what are the consequences? Utilitarianism is the best-known branch of this school. The main concern of Utilitarianism is 'the greatest good for the greatest number' and that the outcome

---

**Deontology (Nonsequentialism)**

Duty Ethics
    What does the law demand?
    What is my duty?

**Teleology**

    What is the goal?

    A branch of Teleology is Utilitarianism:
        What brings happiness?
        'The greatest good for the greatest number.'

## International Council of Nurses Code for Nurses

- The fundamental responsibility of the nurse is fourfold: to promote health, to prevent illness, to restore health, and to alleviate suffering.
- The need for nursing is universal. Inherent in nursing is respect for life, dignity, and the rights of man. It is unrestricted by considerations of nationality, race, creed, colour, age, sex, politics, or social status.
- Nurses render health services to the individual, the family, and the community, and coordinate their services with those of related groups.

NURSES AND PEOPLE
- The nurse's primary responsibility is to those people who require nursing care.
- The nurse, in providing care, promotes an environment in which the values, customs, and spiritual beliefs of the individual are respected.
- The nurse holds in confidence personal information and uses judgement in sharing this information.

NURSES AND PRACTICE
- The nurse carries personal responsibility for nursing practice and for maintaining competence by continual learning. The nurse maintains the highest standards of nursing care possible within the reality of a specific situation.
- The nurse uses judgement in relation to individual competence when accepting and delegating responsibilities.
- The nurse when acting in a professional capacity should at all times maintain standards of personal conduct which reflect credit upon the profession.

NURSES AND SOCIETY
- The nurse shares with other citizens the responsibility for initiating and supporting action to meet the health and social needs of the public.

NURSES AND CO-WORKERS
- The nurse sustains a cooperative relationship with co-workers in nursing and other fields. The nurse takes appropriate action to safeguard the individual when his/her care is endangered by a co-worker or any other person.

NURSES AND THE PROFESSION
- The nurse plays the major role in determining and implementing desirable standards of nursing practice and nursing education.
- The nurse is active in developing a core of professional knowledge.
- The nurse, acting through the professional organization, participates in establishing and maintaining equitable social and economic working conditions in nursing.

From International Council of Nurses: *ICN code for nurses: ethical concepts applied to nursing*, Geneva, 1973, ICN.

should be 'happiness'.

When these two schools are applied to nursing, it is possible to see that even small situations can be approached in two different ways. Consider this example:

Mr Carlton has multiple fractures after an accident at work.

Nurses have to spoon-feed him as he has both arms in plaster. This is a time-consuming activity. Nurse Raso approaches her task as one of duty, that is, it is her duty as a nurse to feed Mr Carlton and therefore her action is right even if it monopolizes one nurse for a long time at every meal. Nurse McPhee considers that Mr Carlton will get better quicker (and therefore will be able to feed himself) if he is spoon-fed regularly at every meal, regardless of the time it takes.

If these two theoretical schools are strictly followed, they are both consistent. They may lead to the same result although they started from almost opposite ends. More often there is a synthesis of the two schools and they are not treated as exclusive. It is important, however, to realize that because of the different cultures and values between health care professionals, severe differences of opinion regarding the care of patients/clients can occur.

Because of the different approaches of these two schools, there is also a difference of emphasis on their main component. Deontology stresses the individual person's duty to society; Teleology stresses that happiness should be the outcome of any action performed. The ethical principles generally agreed to apply to all people are not questioned by these two schools; only the approach to them is different. Nurses need to be familiar with general ethical principles in order to understand patients/clients and their own positions as professionals. They also need to be aware of principles applying more specifically to health care. Nursing ethics consistently stresses that anything which integrates and makes whole by relating to everything and everyone is desirable.

Five principles can be seen to cover ethical behaviour in all walks of life. Thiroux (1980) has put them in the following order (see box).

## Ethical Principles

The Principle of the Value of Life
The Principle of Goodness or Rightness
The Principle of Justice or Fairness
The Principle of Truth Telling or Honesty
The Principle of Individual Freedom

Adapted from: Thiroux JP: *Ethics, theory and practice,* ed 2, Encino, Calif, 1980, Glencoe Publishing.

### The Principle of the Value of Life

Thiroux (1980) sums up the **principle of the value of life** with the phrase: "Human beings should revere life and accept death". This principle is logically put at the beginning because life is what all people have in common and it is only because of this that people can and should act ethically. The quality of life of people differs, but morally all people are the same. No distinctions should therefore be made between people because of "ethnic origin, religious beliefs, personal attributes, the nature of their health problems or any other factor" (UKCC, 1992a). Where such distinctions are made people generally act unethically, and

**Adult Nursing
Euthanasia**

Most nurses will be confronted at some point with the issue of euthanasia (Downing and Smoker, 1986). Medical science can now prolong life, often beyond the point where there is any meaning or value to the individual and/or their family. An individual may wish to determine the stage at which he or she wishes to hasten what is perceived to be an inevitable, undignified and meaningless process.

Euthanasia remains illegal in the United Kingdom, but debates about its legalization will continue. The primary task of nurses is to become increasingly skilful at listening to individuals' expression of feelings. When a nursing assessment indicates mental health problems, such as clinical depression, it is important to act promptly to obtain appropriate treatment of his or her personal problems.

The nurse must, regardless of his or her personal views, respect and work within the definitions of the law. The resolution of personal and legal issues surrounding euthanasia will not be easy.

in health care nurses should endeavour to eliminate these distinctions.

Principles are not absolutes, but *near*-absolutes (although Deontologists might argue that duty is absolutely necessary to maintain the fabric of society). When considering the value of life it is clear that this principle is infringed at many levels: abortion, euthanasia, suicide, capital punishment, war and killing in self-defence are all examples. The quotation "thou shalt not kill; but need'st not strive officiously to keep alive" (Clough, 1862) applies to many nursing situations and becomes more apt as medical technology increases.

This principle is referred to as the principle of the 'value' of life in contrast to the 'sanctity' of life because sanctity can be misused to the exclusion of any other view. Speaking of the 'value' of life does not diminish its sanctity; on the contrary, it sets human life in the wider context of all life, including plants and animals, and indeed the life of the universe. Medical ethics, as well as nursing ethics, will have to concern itself much more with the notion of the 'value of life' in the future in the light of diminishing resources and increasing demands for life-saving and life-prolonging possibilities. The voice of nurses and nursing will be an important element.

One of the aspects of this principle is that people should be respected. '**Respect for persons**' means that individuals treat themselves and others in a way which is inherently human. As all people share life in common, so the destiny of this humanity depends on how people treat each other. The awareness of one's own and other people's values (as decribed previously) is basic to this debate. When people are respected fundamentally, then all the other principles are most likely also kept, that is, any actions done are done rightly, with justice and honesty and without pressure. Nurses often find this a difficult precept as their values of health and life can differ markedly from that of their patients/clients. A person with lung cancer who continues to smoke or a patient with diabetes who cannot stop eating cream

cakes are two examples. Arguing and reasoning may help; but this is where it becomes obvious that some ethical principles militate against other principles; that is, the principle of the value of life against the principle of justice or fairness (should patients who do not comply with treatments continue to be cared for?).

## The Principle of Goodness or Rightness

Generally speaking, people have to be 'good' to perform 'right' actions. The question therefore is, what is a 'good' person? Over the centuries 'virtues' have been described by various religious, ethical, philosophical and cultural systems to highlight certain aspects of importance. Many of these are listed in Table 12-3.

If life is what people have in common, then the **principle of goodness and rightness** requires that people should contribute to make this life as good and happy as possible. Everyone has to contribute to this effort, because everyone's contribution counts. This is why the learning of values is of such importance.

It is not possible to be totally 'good', that is, it is not possible to demand of people to keep this principle absolutely. But knowing what is possible should help people to attain at least some of the personal attributes. A code of conduct is for professionals the guideline which describes some of the ways in which 'goodness' can be recognized.

Sometimes even 'good' people cannot achieve the 'right' action despite every effort made. Ethics has always maintained that the *intention* behind an action should also be considered. Therefore the notion of **conscience** is important. Conscience is seen as an inner guide which people recognize and usually disregard only in acute situations. However, people who are constantly forced to act against their conscience learn to disregard this subtle counsel and may either become cynical or may burn out.

Any action is 'right' if it is either done from duty (Deontology) or leads to good outcomes (Teleology); an action is not 'right' if either of these are not evident. If a mother, who is poor and has difficulty feeding two children, finds herself in a shop where she is unobserved and helps herself to a loaf of bread, there are two ways of looking at the outcome: her duty (Deontology) as a citizen asks her to keep the law and not to steal, therefore her action is wrong. But her commitment to her children has as a goal (Teleology) to feed them better. The opportunity presented coincides with her goal and therefore her action could be justified. Her virtues or personal attributes and her conscience may be in conflict. Her action is ethical or not in so far as she also respects the other principles: the value of life, justice, honesty and freedom.

Medical ethics has used this principle to stress **beneficence** (doing good) and **nonmaleficence** (avoiding harm). Generally, nonmaleficence takes precedent over beneficence. In clinical situations, however, it is often difficult to draw the line between not inflicting harm and preventing or removing harmful situations. For example, a nurse who immunizes children for diphtheria, whooping cough, and tetanus inflicts some degree of harm or pain; however, the benefit of being protected against whooping cough is more important. Similarly, surgery can be seen to inflict harm; however, the benefit of removing a tumour or diseased part generally outweighs the harm related to the risk of surgery. Nursing is less strictly concerned with always avoiding harm and doing good because an ethic of caring takes these aspects into consideration in the relationship between nurse and patient/client.

## The Principle of Justice or Fairness

'Good' and 'right' do not only have to be done, they also have to be *seen* to be done. People and society at large have to benefit from being 'good' and acting 'rightly'.

The principle of **justice or fairness** requires treating others fairly and giving people their due. However, distributive justice is difficult to apply, because:

- Not everyone is equal in every way. Sometimes there are situations in which one person should receive a greater or lesser share than another.
- Resources are limited. There is not always enough for each person to receive an equal share.

Some of the suggestions that have been made to aid equal distribution include contracts, individual need, individual effort, ability to pay, social contribution, and merit. In daily life, different bases for distribution are used for different settings. Welfare payments are made based on individual need, but jobs and promotions are usually based on achievement and merit (Davis and Aroskar, 1983). The distribution of nursing care is determined by the individual needs of patients/clients and by nurses who establish priorities for each person's needs. Certain patients/clients require skilled nursing care more than others. To live and avoid permanent disability, these people are usually more seriously ill and require immediate intervention. For example, a person who is admitted to the neurological unit after suffering head trauma usually requires immediate assessment and surgical intervention to prevent brain damage associated with oedema or haemorrhage. Other patients/clients who are more physically stable are cared for as the nurse makes time for other necessary nursing activities such as discharge teaching and routine care. The criteria of need, added to the patient's/client's prognosis, is basic to the practice of triage, most widely utilized in this country in accident and emergency departments, or in other areas when resources are in short supply.

Unequal treatment to patients/clients always requires justification. Should a patient/client who does everything possible to improve health be cared for differently from someone who refuses to follow medical restrictions? The principle of justice supports the argument that there should be at least equal initial access to health care for assessment of the patient's/client's needs. This view has limitations, but it supports a more critical evaluation of distribution of scarce health care resources.

Much of the debate about justice is intensified because of the increasing insistence on **rights** in every sphere of life. The Patient's Charter (DOH, 1992) has made users and providers of health care more aware of standards which should be achieved. With rights always go responsibilities. Many people insist on certain rights, but the corresponding responsibility is not always available, thus only complicating the problem.

One of the virtues particularly associated with the principle of justice or fairness is courage: the courage to speak up and stand up for justice. The notion of patient advocacy is also allied to this principle. Nurses are often acutely aware that they work in situations of inequality, or consider treatments prescribed as unjust or unfair. In such situations they do not only have a right to be heard themselves; they must also consider their responsibilities and act accordingly.

## The Principle of Truth Telling or Honesty

The principle of **truth telling or honesty** is perhaps the most delicate one to keep and achieve. Truth is many-sided and one person's 'truth' is not necessarily also another person's 'truth'. A patient/client who begs, "tell me the truth", may not want to know what the nurse knows about the situation. The nurse may know that Ms Browning has cancer of the middle third of the oesophagus, Stage 3, with bilateral nodes but no evidence of distant metastases. To the nurse this presents a complex 'truth' of prognosis and treatment possibilities and probabilities which may not mean anything to Ms Browning. To her the 'truth' may not consist of physiology, but relates to her job, her independence and her social life. In time she may want to understand her treatments better by wanting to know about anatomy and physiology.

Truth is so important because all relationships — in families, business and industry — depend on it. But because relationships are delicate, truth is often vulnerable. Two aspects of this principle are therefore particularly concerned with truth: confidentiality and informed consent.

**Confidentiality** ensures a patient's/client's privacy. So that care can be beneficial, much information has to be available to nurses, but not all of this information is confidential. If a patient/client has given some information and the nurse is not sure if it is confidential, it is always best to ask the patient/client if there is any objection to this being passed on to other team members. In most cases there is no objection.

The UKCC document *Confidentiality* (UKCC, 1987) lists four categories under which information may be disclosed:

(a) with the consent of the patient/client;

(b) without the consent of the patient/client when the disclosure is required by law or order of a court;

(c) by accident;

(d) without the consent of the patient/client when the disclosure is considered necessary in the public interest.

It is the last category which will present most problems to nurses. This is another case when ethical principles can be in competition with each other. When this happens, either a values-clarification exercise (see p. 234) or applying a model of ethical decision making (see p. 235) may help. In category (d) it is generally accepted that the public interest takes precedence over the private interest.

Brown *et al* (1992) have described *discretion* as "the virtue of coping well with confidentiality, secrecy and privacy". Since confidentiality has much to do with communication, a discreet nurse is also a nurse who communicates well.

**Informed consent** (see also Chapters 13, 14) involves all the principles so far mentioned:
- value of life — the person is respected for what he or she is
- goodness or rightness — nothing should be done to or for patients/clients without consent; that is, only what is right should be done in the first instance and patients/clients should not be 'assaulted' with unwanted or unnecessary treatments
- justice or fairness — all patients/clients should be informed to the point of being able to make informed choices, not only articulate or intelligent people
- truth telling or honesty — information given must be as unbiased and complete as possible, and communication as open as possible
- individual freedom — once the information has been given and the patient/client wants to refuse a particular treatment or procedure, this should be accepted and the patient/client should not be pressurized.

Properly administered, informed consent helps patients/clients to understand all their options.

Nurses are often asked to explain or interpret what a doctor has told a patient/client, perhaps after a ward round or after a clinic visit. Patients/clients tend to be reluctant to ask many questions in formal settings. It is later, in an informal talk with a nurse, that fears and misunderstandings are voiced. Nurses are then sometimes reluctant to give more detailed information than a patient/client already has, so as not to influence the patient/client. It will depend largely on the relationship between nurse and the individual concerning how and what is said. Nursing ethics stresses caring, in which compassion and commitment play a large part and, with good communication, fears on both sides may be overcome and used to make each other more at ease.

### The Principle of Individual Freedom

Thiroux (1980) places the **principle of individual freedom** last in his list, not because it is least important, but because more than the others, this principle is bounded by all the others. Freedom is not absolute; if it were, everyone would do exactly as they please. But there has to be freedom of thought, belief and speech. Personal and social values are to some extent a matter of free choice, but they also have to be kept within the bounds of the possible.

People develop as individuals only because of freedom. They express themselves freely and choose lifestyles and careers freely. When people become ill or incapacitated, their freedom is usually drastically cut and this presents problems at many levels. It is important that nurses are aware of this.

The principle of individual freedom (or autonomy) means that individuals are able to act for themselves to the level of their capacity (Fowler, 1989). A respect for autonomy is not possible when a person is unconscious. Patients/clients must be able to participate in decision making. If they cannot speak for themselves, during emergencies, there is presumed consent because (Fowler, 1989):

- it is reasonable to assume that an injured or ill person would want treatment
- health care providers have a social contract based on social trust that requires that patients/clients be treated and not abandoned if they cannot speak for themselves.

When beneficence (the duty to do good) overrides the patient's/client's autonomy, the result is paternalism. **Paternalism** is doing what the health professional believes is in the patient's/client's best interests, regardless of the individual's own determinations. These two elements frequently conflict. An example of this situation is an elderly woman who is alert but forgetful and unsteady on her feet. In the past she has fallen, and the nurses are concerned for her safety. The woman does not remember to call for assistance; therefore the nurses have suggested that she has the sides of her bed raised for safety. The woman is unsettled by the side rails. In this situation, a care plan should include specific changes of activity and attention.

## RESPONSIBILITY AND ACCOUNTABILITY

Nurses assume responsibility and accountability for nursing care provided. **Responsibility** refers to the execution of duties associated with the nurse's particular role. These responsibilities must be commensurate with the level of education and training of a nurse or student. The *UKCC Code of Professional Conduct* (UKCC, 1992a) gives nurses the responsibility to acknowledge any limitations in knowledge and competence and to decline any duties or responsibilities unless able to perform them safely and in a skilled manner. When carrying out any nursing action, such as a dressing or a bath, the nurse is responsible for assessing the patient's/client's need for the action, doing it safely and correctly, and evaluating the response. A nurse who acts in a responsible manner gains the trust of patients/clients and other professionals.

**Accountability** means being answerable for one's own actions. A nurse is accountable to self, the patient/client, the profession, the employer, and society (see box). If a wrong dose of medication is given, the nurse is accountable to the patient/client who received it, the doctor who ordered it, the employer who sets standards of expected performance, and society, which demands professional excellence. To be accountable, the nurse acts according to the professional code of ethics. Thus, when an error is made, the nurse reports it and initiates care to prevent further injury. Accountability calls for an evaluation of a nurse's effectiveness in practice. Professional accountability serves the following purposes:
- to evaluate new professional practices and reassess existing ones
- to maintain standards of health care
- to facilitate personal reflection, ethical thought, and personal growth on the part of health care professionals
- to provide a basis for ethical decision making.

Accountability requires an evaluation of the nurse's performance in providing nursing care. Accountability is ensured when the quality of care can be measured. The profession's code

## Maintaining Professional Accountability

### SELF
- Report any personal conduct that endangers patients/clients.
- Stay informed of current nursing practice theory and issues.
- Make judgements based on facts.

### PATIENT/CLIENT
- Provide patients/clients with accurate information about care.
- Conduct nursing care in a manner that ensures patient/client safety and well-being.

### PROFESSION
- Maintain ethical standards in practice.
- Encourage peers to follow the same.
- Report a colleague's unethical behaviour.

### EMPLOYING INSTITUTION
- Follow policy and procedures defined by the institution.

### SOCIETY
- Maintain ethical conduct in the care of all patients/clients in all settings.

of conduct is one such measure; local standards and policies ensure local measures.

## PROCESS FOR RESOLVING ETHICAL PROBLEMS

Ethical reasoning is similar to all decision making processes, such as, for example, the nursing process. Ethical dilemmas occur as a result of conflict between moral principles which support different courses of action. Any choices made in an ethical dilemma have far-reaching effects on the perceptions of human beings and definition of personhood, relationships with others, and people and society as a whole.

Curtin and Flaherty (1982) have outlined the characteristics which distinguishing ethical problems from other problems in the health care setting. These characteristics are:

- the problem cannot be resolved solely through a review of scientific data
- the problem is perplexing — the person cannot easily think logically or make a decision about the problem
- the answer to the problem will have great relevance for several areas of human concern.

Consider the following example of the interrelatedness of these problems:

*Nurses are caring for a middle-aged man with AIDS. He is married and has informed the staff that his wife is his next of kin, but due to different lifestyles and jobs they live almost separate lives, meeting only occasionally at weekends. There are a number of male and female friends visiting. The patient has specifically requested that nobody is to be given any health details without his express consent. Nurses are concerned that any sexual partners should be aware of his*

*diagnosis as this could affect the partners. Should the nurses tell his wife, who has asked several times to be informed of his diagnosis and thus act out of their health promotion role; or should they respect the patient and keep confidentiality? Should they try to persuade the patient that he must inform the concerned people himself, thus using persuasion and imposing their own values? Should they ask the doctors to persuade him, too?*

The nurses are in a position between patient and visitors, trying to satisfy everybody, including themselves and their duties as carers with a public role. The nurses must decide how best to resolve this dilemma.

## METHODOLOGY FOR DECISION MAKING

Each ethical dilemma will be different. However, in any setting a model for ethical decision making can increase the probability that all factors are weighed equally (see box). The above example of the patient with AIDS will be used in applying the following decision-making model, which is outlined in the form of four questions:

1. ***What is happening?*** Identify the problem by asking further questions:
   - Who are the people concerned?
   - What are the relationships between them (in this case, the nurses' relationships with the patient and his family and visitors are vitally important)?
   - What factors influence the problem? What feelings are paramount?
   - What fears influence the people?
   - What memories of similar situations might influence the present situation?
   - Which of the ethical principles are mainly involved? In what way? Is it a question of duties or outcomes?

   Gather as much data as possible. Allow all concerned to voice their views, values, misgivings and anxieties. Involve all concerned (this might include the patient/client in this example; in other examples it normally would include the patient/client). This is the longest and most important aspect of the process and the one which will most influence the outcome.

2. ***What would happen if...?*** Look at the possibilities by asking more questions:
   - What outcome might there be if confidentiality would be broken?
   - What might happen if a nurse accidentally broke confidentiality under pressure?
   - What would happen if the patient were persuaded to conform to pressure?
   - What would happen if no action were taken?
   - What would the expected outcomes be of all the known possibilities?
   - Which basis for a decision is the best one: duty, goals — and whose duty; whose goals?
   - What interpretation is given to responsibility?

**A Framework for Ethical Decision Making**

What is happening?
- Consider all the people concerned.
- What are their roles?
- What are their feelings, memories, relationships?
- What ethical theories are evident?
- Which ethical principles are mainly involved?

What might happen, if...
- What might be the outcomes of any courses of action?

What is the fitting answer?
- Having explored 'What is happening?', what is the response to this situation, concerning these people?
- The fitting answer is the one which is most creative for the people in the present situation.

Adapted from: Niebuhr HR: *The responsible self*, New York, 1963, Harper & Row.

3. *What is the fitting answer?* An answer is fitting if the facts and the relationships between people have been interpreted in creative ways which enhance the humanity of all the people concerned. This should be the aim of the decision making process. An answer is not necessarily 'right', but it should always be fitting in the present circumstances. Such an answer is not reached lightly and is therefore not arbitrary, even if in similar circumstances the answer might be quite different.

4. *What has happened?* Ethical decisions have longlasting effects on the people and situations concerned. A decision will have to be carried out and this brings about an immediate change; in this example it might be a conference with the patient to explain the problem, more communication with the people involved, and perhaps a need to help several people with counselling. This question may, however, only be answered fully a long time later. For the nurses concerned in this example, it may be answered when they have another ethical problem to face and can see what they learned from this one in how to make more effective ethical decisions. Thus the outcome will have been 'fitting' for them and for the patient.

No two ethical dilemmas are the same. Using a systematic model for ethical decision making increases the probability that all ethical values and principles are reviewed, as well as the feelings and relationships of the people involved. Taking an action which is decisive is then easier. It is often essential that a nurse does not act alone when presented with a dilemma concerning a patient/client. Communicating with others is vital as most problems and dilemmas involve many people. A systematic approach to ethical decision making allows nurses to practise in a professional manner and to increase the ability to deal with complex, ethical situations.

## LOCAL RESEARCH ETHICS COMMITTEES (LRECS)

With an increase in the professionalization of nursing has come an increase in research carried out by nurses. Any research by health professionals which involves patients/clients is subject to review by a Local Research Ethics Committee (LREC) (see Chapter 14). The Department of Health has issued guidelines in the form of a document *Local Research Ethics Committees* [HSG(91)(5), DOH, 1991] which outlines the establishment, function and administrative framework of LRECs; the ethical principles to which they should have regard and the particular groups of subjects with which they might have to deal. LRECs are normally set up by and responsible to a district health authority, trust, or family health services authority. Nurses who want to undertake research should apply to the secretary of a LREC who will help in meeting the set criteria for submitting a proposal.

According to the DOH guidelines, members of a LREC should be drawn from both genders and from a wide range of age groups and should include hospital medical staff, nursing staff, general practitioners and two or more lay people. These committees exist for the purpose of research, but not for general ethical decision making; this remains the duty and privilege of individuals and groups of health care workers.

## SUMMARY

A person's unique set of values influences personal decisions and actions. Although values may be acquired and held unconsciously, a person's conscious awareness of values helps in reaching decisions and avoiding conflicts. A patient/client who is conscious of personal values related to health and health behaviours is able to participate fully in health care, and nurses conscious of their own values are better able to help patients/clients to clarify values and make decisions.

Individuals form values through observation and experience, noting the responses evoked by their own and others' behaviours. Values are acquired from parents and other family members in a continuous process which begins in infancy. Values are transmitted through various modes: modelling, moralizing, laissez-faire, responsible choice, and reward and punishment. While maturing and recognizing that life poses a variety of changes, a person must remain open to new ideas and their influence on personal values.

Nursing involves caring for human beings. The values of caring, respect for others, equality, and human dignity are important in enabling a nurse to assist patients/clients most effectively. An individual who enters the profession of nursing possesses a personal set of values. If these values complement those of professional nursing, the role of a nurse is more easily ensured. However, societal, institutional, and patient/client values can create conflicts for nurses, making decisions about the individual's care difficult. Having a clear understanding of personal and professional values helps nurses to become more committed to excellence in nursing practice. Values clarification is the use of various strategies to explore the meaning of values and behaviours. The valuing process involves choosing, prizing, and acting on one's beliefs. When values are clearly detailed and positively affirmed, the patient/client and nurse are more able to make objective decisions about health care.

Ethics is the study of 'good' and 'right' generally, and how these relate to professional practice in particular. Nurses work in situations which pose complex and sometimes conflicting problems related to patient/client care. Ethical behaviour develops from the values that nurses hold throughout their lives.

Nurses practise ethically by following the codes of their profession. Nurses study and integrate the ethical principles of the value of life, goodness or rightness, justice or fairness, truth telling or honesty and the elements associated with them of respect for persons, beneficence, nonmaleficence, rights and responsibilities, confidentiality and informed consent. Responsible and accountable nurses maintain competency when practising. Nurses are responsible in the first instance to the patient/client, but also to doctors, the employing authority, the profession and society.

In their daily work, nurses are placed in a variety of situations in which ethical questions arise. They use a systematic method to identify and attempt to resolve these problems. Ethical dilemmas are not easily resolved, and the decisions are difficult to make. The challenge posed to nurses by this is to develop even more ethical awareness and action.

## CHAPTER 12 REVIEW

### Key Concepts

- When nurses can clearly differentiate their personal values from their professional values, they are better able to help patients/clients to understand their values.
- Values provide a standard for acceptable behaviour.
- A person acquires values after observing behaviours which prove successful for others.
- A child acquires values from parents, other family members, school, and religious and other social institutions.
- Value formation begins in the early developmental stages and continues throughout life.
- The value of caring facilitates the giving of help to another human being.
- Values clarification is a process that promotes an understanding of personal values.
- A person must be able to choose values freely from available alternatives and understand the consequences of choosing.
- A nurse who assists a patient/client in clarifying values and making decisions does so non-judgementally.
- The nurse's role has become multifaceted, and this has increased the number and diversity of ethical dilemmas that a nurse encounters in practice.
- Patients/clients have the right to safe and effective nursing care.
- A code of professional conduct directs nurses' activities to promote and safeguard the interests and wellbeing of patients/clients assigned to their care.

- Professional nurses have a commitment to patients/clients, other health care professionals, their own profession, the employing authority, and society to provide high-quality care.
- An ethical nurse maintains skilled competency and assumes responsibility for nursing care.
- Responsibility refers to the scope of function and duties a nurse is required to perform.
- Accountability means being answerable for one's own actions.
- When nurses witness acts that may endanger patients/clients, they are obliged to report them.
- A systematic approach to ethical decisions making allows nurses to practise in a professional manner and to increase the ability to deal with complex, ethical situations.

## CRITICAL THINKING EXERCISES

1. It has been very difficult to care for Mr Adegbuyi, a 26-year-old patient who was severely injured in a motorcycle accident. He has been unconscious since reaching the hospital. Although Mr Adegbuyi is still alive on a ventilator, there is little hope of survival. The nurse from the day shift reports that the family has been complaining about the care Mr Adegbuyi is receiving. She notes, "They are just so ungrateful". Julie Wells is the nurse caring for Mr Adegbuyi during the evening shift. She spends extra time positioning her patient and making him comfortable. The above situation describes an attitude, value, and potential ethical dilemma. Identify each.

2. Mr Liles has been told he has cancer and that chemotherapy is his only choice of treatment. The client's brother died 2 years earlier after receiving extensive chemotherapy. The side effects of the medication caused Mr Liles' brother to be very uncomfortable. A nurse assists Mr Liles in values

### Key Terms

Beneficence, p. 242
Caring, p. 233
Conscience, p. 242
Deontology, p. 240
Ethical decisions, p. 240
Ethical dilemmas, p. 229
Ethical principles, p. 229
Ethics, p. 239
Goodness/rightness (principle of), p. 242
Individual freedom (principle of), p. 244
Justice/fairness (principle of), p. 243
Nonmaleficence, p. 242
Paternalism, p. 244
Respect for persons, p. 242
Rights, p. 243
Teleology, p. 240
Truth telling/honesty, p. 243
Value of life (principle of), p. 241
Value system, p. 230
Value, p. 234, 236
Values clarification, p. 234, 236

clarification. What are his choices and how might he be able to prize and act on each?

3. Compare and contrast a nurse's 'accountability' with a nurse's 'responsibility'.

4. A married woman with adult children and grandchildren works as a nurse at a local hospital. She had indicated to her husband that she does not want life-prolonging procedures administered unless it would enable her to function as a relatively 'normal' person. In discussion with colleagues she had also said the same. The woman has a stroke and is admitted to the hospital where she is employed. Routine treatment procedures do not produce the desired results. The family authorized treatment which required use of a respirator and a feeding tube for a time after the procedure. The family was aware that without the treatment she had no hope of living; with the treatment there was a fifty-fifty chance of recovery. The procedure was initiated. After several days it was clear that the procedure was not effective and that the patient/client would remain comatose. Some hospital staff feel that once a treatment is initiated it cannot be withdrawn. For this situation:

a. What is happening?

b. Consider all the people, events and circumstances in this dilemma.

c. Imagine the feelings and memories which might be important for the people concerned.

d. State which ethical principles and theories are involved, and explain them. If there is more than one, contrast the relationships among them.

e. Imagine what might happen if certain courses of action were followed.

f. What is the fitting answer? What is, in this situation, the answer which is most creative for the people concerned?

5. A 20-year-old person is training to become a registered nurse. The student plans marriage and a family. The student's training includes clinical practice allocations on each ward and department of a teaching hospital. One ward has a number of patients being treated for AIDS. The student cares about people, including self and the family to be. The student wants to provide the best nursing care possible; yet this person is hesitant to care for patients with AIDS. For this situation:

a. What is happening?

b. Consider all the people, events and circumstances in this dilemma.

c. Imagine the feelings and memories which might be important for the people concerned.

d. State which ethical principles and theories are involved, and explain. If there is more than one, contrast the relationships among them.

e. Imagine what might happen if certain courses of action were followed.

f. What is the fitting answer? What is, in this situation, the answer which is most creative for the people involved?

6. Based on your experience, describe a situation which presents an ethical dilemma to you as a nurse. Then, using the information in this chapter, critically assess the various aspects of the dilemma.

## REFERENCES

American Association of Colleges of Nursing: *Essentials of college and university education for professional nursing,* Washington, DC, 1986, The Association.

Bernal EW: Values clarification: a critique, *J Nurs Educ* 24:174, 1985.

Brill NI, *Working with people, the helping process,* Philadelphia, 1973, Lippincott.

Brown JM, Kitson AL, McKnight TJ: *Challenges in caring,* London, 1992, Chapman & Hall.

Clough AH: *The Latest decalogue,* 1865.

Curtin LL: The nurse as advocate: a philosophical foundation for nursing. In Chinn P, editor: *Ethical issues in nursing,* Rockville, Md, 1986, Brady.

Curtin LL, Flaherty MJ: *Nursing ethics: theories and pragmatics,* Norwalk, Conn, 1982, Appleton & Lange.

Davis A, Aroskar M: Perspectives on ethical-moral principles. In Davis A, Aroskar M, editors: *Ethical dilemmas in nursing practice,* ed 2, Norwalk, Conn, 1983, Appleton & Lange.

Department of Health: *Local research ethics committees* (HSG(91)5), London, 1991, Department of Health.

Department of Health: *The patient's charter,* London, 1992, HMSO.

Downing AB, Smoker B: *Voluntary euthanasia: experts debate the rights to die,* London, 1986, Peter Owen.

Fowler M: Ethical decision making in clinical practice, *Nurs Clin North Am* 24(4):956, 1989.

Frankl V: *Man's search for meaning,* New York, 1962, Pocket Books.

Fry ST: The ethic of caring: can it survive in nursing? *Nurs Outlook* 36(1):48, 1988.

Fry ST: Toward a theory of nursing ethics, *ANS* 11(4):9, 1989

Gilligan C: *In a different voice,* Cambridge, Mass, 1982, Harvard University Press.

Henderson V: The nature of nursing, *Am J Nurs* 64:62, 1964

International Council of Nurses: *Code for nurses: ethical concepts applied to nursing,* Geneva, 1973, ICN.

Kurtz RJ, Warry J: Caring ethic: more human kindness, the care of nursing science, *Nurs Forum* 26(1):4, 1991.

Leininger M: *Transcultural nursing: concepts, theories, and practices,* New York, Chichester, 1978, Wiley & Sons.

Niebuhr, HR: *The responsible self,* New York, 1963, Harper and Row.

Noddings N: *Caring - a feminine approach to ethics and moral education,* Berkeley, CA, 1984, University of California Press.

Omery A: Values, moral reasoning and ethics, *Nurs Clin North Am* 24(2):499, 1989.

Raatikainen R: Values and ethical principles in nursing, *J Adv Nurs* 14:92, 1989.

Raths LE, Harmin M, Simon SB: *Values and teaching,* ed 2, Columbus, Ohio, 1979, Merrill.

Rogers CR: *A way of being,* Boston, Mass, 1980, Houghton Mifflin Co.

Rokeach M: *The nature of human values,* New York, 1973, Free Press.

Ross R: *Prospering woman,* San Raphael, Calif, 1982, Whatever Publishing.

Simon SB *et al: Values clarification: a handbook of practical strategies for teachers and students,* New york, 1978, Hart..

Steele SM: AIDS: Clarifying values to close in on ethical questions, *Nurs Health Care* 7(5):246, 1986.

Taylor SG: The effect of quality of life and sanctity of life on clinical decision making, *AORN J* 41:924, 1985.

Thiroux JP: *Ethics, theory and practice* ed 2, Encino, CA, 1980, Glencoe Publishing.

Tschudin V: *Ethics in nursing: the caring relationship,* ed 2, Oxford, 1992, Butterworth Heinemann.

Uustal DB: Values clarification in nursing: application to practice, *Am J Nurs* 78:2058,1978.

United Kingdom Central Council: *Confidentiality,* London, 1987, UKCC.

United Kingdom Central Council: *Exercising accountability,* London, 1989, UKCC.

United Kingdom Central Council: *Code of professional conduct,* London, 1992a, UKCC.

United Kingdom Central Council: *The scope of professional practice,* London, 1992b, UKCC.

Veatch RM Fry ST: *Case studies of nursing ethics,* Philadelphia, 1987, Lippincott.

Zuzich A: Some frameworks for ethical development. In Reilly DE, editor: *Teaching and evaluating the affective domain in nursing programs,* Thorofare, NJ 1978, Slack.

## FURTHER READING

### Adult Nursing

Beauchamp TL, Childress JF: *Principles of biomedical ethics,* ed 3, Oxford, 1989, Oxford University Press.

Benjamin M, Curtis J: *Ethics in nursing* ed 2, Oxford, 1992, Oxford University Press.

Edwards BJ, Haddad AM: How we help nurses handle questions of ethics, *RN* 50(9):14, 1987.

Faulder C: *Whose body is it? The troubling issue of informed consent,* London, 1985, Virago.

French DG: Ethics: nurse, am I going to live? *Nurs Manage* 15:43, 1984.

Fry S: Toward a theory of nursing ethics, *Adv Nurs Sci* 11(4):9, 1989.

Gillon R: *Philosophical medical ethics,* Chichester, 1992, John Wiley & Sons.

Glover J: *Causing death and saving lives,* Harmondsworth, 1988, Pelican Books.

Grady C: Ethical issues in providing nursing care to human immunodeficiency virus-infected populations, *Nurs Clin North Am* 24(2):523, 1989.

International Council of Nurses: *ICN code for nurses: ethical concepts applied to nursing,* Geneva, 1973, Imprimeries Populaires.

Jones SR: *Ethics in midwifery,* London, 1993, Mosby.

Lanik G, Webb AA: Ethical decision making for community health nurses, *J Community Health Nurs* 6(2):95, 1989.

Roach MS: *The human act of caring,* Ottawa, 1987, The Canadian Hospital Association.

Scott RS: When it isn't life or death, *Am J Nurs* 85:19, 1985.

Seedhouse D: *Ethics: the heart of health care,* Chichester, 1989, Wiley & Sons.

Singleton J, McLaren S: *Ethical foundations of health care,* London, 1995, Mosby.

Thompson JE, Thompson HO: Teaching ethics to nursing students, *Nurs Outlook* 37(2):84, 1989.

Viens DC: A history of nursing's code of ethics, *Nurs Outlook* 37(1):45, 1989.

Weeks LC *et al:* How can a hospital ethics committee help? *Am J Nurs* 89:651, 1989.

### Children's Nursing

Alderson: A new approach to ethics: demystifying ethics in the care of adolescents, *Child Health* 1(5): 187-192, 1994.

Alderson P: Children's consent to surgery, *Paediatric Nursing* 3(10): 10-13, 1991.

Atherton TM: *The rights of the child in health care,* In Lindsay R Ed. The Child and family: contemporary nursing issues in child health and care. London, 1994, Bailliere Tindall.

Brykczynska G ed: *Ethics in paediatric nursing,* London, 1989, Chapman and Hall.

Brykczynska G: Informed consent, *Paediatric Nursing* 1(5): 6-8, 1989

Charles-Edwards L: Who decides? *Paediatric Nursing* 3(10): 6-8, 1991

Doyle L, Wilsher D: Towards guidelines for withholding and withdrawal of life prolonging treatment in neonatal medicine, *Archives of Disease in Childhood* 70:1 (supp) 66-70, 1994.

Dunn PM: Appropriate care of the newborn: ethical dilemmas, *Journal of Medical Ethics,* 19 (2): 82-4, 1993.

Korgaonkar G et al: Children and consent to medical treatment, *British Journal of Nursing* 2(7): 383-4, 1993.

### Learning Disabilities Nursing

Kay B: Learning disabilities, basic value, *Nursing Times,* 90: 58-59, 1994

Royal College of Psychiatrists, Royal College of Nursing, British Psychological Society: *Behaviour modification: report of a joint working party to formulate ethical guidelines for the conduct of programmes of behaviour modification in the National Health Service,* London, 1980, HMSO.

Sinclair L, Griffiths M: *Medical genetics and mental handicap.* In Clarke A ed: Genetic counselling: practice and principles, London, 1994, Routledge.

Spriggs L: Is reproduction a right?, *Community Care,* April 26, 1990.

Tarbuck P: Ethical standards and human rights , (challenging behaviour and control and restraint techniques), *Nursing Standard* 7 (6): 27-30, 1992.

### Mental Health Nursing

Barker PJ: *Ethical issues in mental health,* London, 1991, Chapman and Hall.

Carpenter MA: The process of ethical decision making in psychiatric nursing practice, *Issues in Mental Health Nursing* 12, 1994.

Raatikainen R: Values and ethical principles in nursing, *J Adv Nurs* 14:92, 1989.

Ritter S: *Ethical Issues,* In Ritter S: Bethlem Royal and Maudsley Hospital Manual of Clinical Psychiatric Nursing Principles and Procedures, London, 1989, Harper and Row, 263-8.

Shields PJ: The consumer view of psychiatry, *Hospital & Health Service Rev* 81:117, 1985.

Szasz T: Psychiatric justice, *Br J Psych* 154:864, 1989.

Tschudin V ed: *Nursing people with special needs, part 2,* section in Tschudin, London, 1994, Scutari.

# Legal Issues

## CHAPTER OUTLINE

### Legal Framework
*Sources of law*
*Systems of law*
*Lawyers*

### Legal Concepts Applied to Nursing
*Assault*
*Battery*
*Informed consent*
*Negligence*
*Confidentiality*
*Death and dying*
*Organ donation*
*Living wills and health care surrogates*

### Legal Safeguards in Nursing Practice
*Registration*
*Student nurses*
*Doctors' orders*
*Incident reports*
*Contracts of employment*

### Legal Issues in Speciality Practice Areas
*Nursing children*
*Nursing in intensive care units*
*Nursing people with a mental illness or a learning disability*
*Nursing older adults*

## LEARNING OUTCOMES

After studying this chapter, you should be able to:
- ▪ *Define the key terms listed.*
- ▪ *Describe the legal framework and how laws are adapted.*
- ▪ *Compare and contrast criminal law and civil law.*
- ▪ *Explain legal concepts that apply to nurses.*
- ▪ *Describe the legal responsibilities and obligations of nurses.*
- ▪ *Discuss the implications of informed consent, negligence, duty of care, and confidentiality in the provision of nursing care.*
- ▪ *Identify legal issues related to the care of the dying patient/client.*
- ▪ *Be aware of legal issues involved in the nurse's relationship with other health care workers, employer, and patients/clients.*
- ▪ *Describe the uses and purpose of an incident report.*
- ▪ *Give examples of legal issues that arise in general nursing practice and in speciality areas.*

**M**any nurses view the law with apprehension because they are largely unaware of its effect on their work. There is an increasing emphasis on the rights of patients/clients and it is important that nurses understand the nurse's legal obligations and responsibilities to patients/clients in order to provide effective nursing.

## LEGAL FRAMEWORK

### Sources of Law

The law is a composite framework of all the rules and regulations by which society governs itself. Society needs a legal framework to deal with disputes and problems in an orderly fashion, and to provide an outline for the behaviour of individuals. The law is flexible and is adapted according to society's demands, either through the legislative process or through judicial decision. The law in England and Wales differs from the law in Scotland and Northern Ireland although all are subject to the same jurisdiction of Parliament. There are two basic sources of law — legislation and judicial precedent.

#### Legislation

Parliament drafts legislation, which becomes law after receiving the royal assent. The legislation is codified in Acts of Parliament which are also known as *statutes*. These Acts of Parliament set out the law in a particular area and specify the penalties that can be applied by the courts if the Act is broken.

Every year, for example, an Act of Parliament is passed that lays down the amount of tax that is to be paid and the penalties that follow if the tax is not paid. This source of law is known as *statutory law.*

Some Acts of Parliament delegate responsibility to

organizations outside the government. The United Kingdom Central Council for Nursing, Midwifery and Health Visiting (UKCC) is a body that was formed following an Act of Parliament in 1979. The UKCC is obliged to keep a register of qualified nurses as part of a delegated duty from Parliament.

## Judicial Precedent

If a dispute arises over the interpretation of a statute, the matter is considered by the courts and a **judicial decision** is made by a judge. When a problem occurs which is not covered by any statute, the courts also have authority to hand down judgements which then become law. The judicial decisions formulated by judges form a body of law which is binding. Much of the law relating to nursing practice arises from judicial reasoning and decision making. A judge's decision can be appealed by taking the case to a higher court, generally the Court of Appeal or, from there, to the House of Lords which has the final say. This source of law is known as **common law**.

## Systems of Law
## Criminal Law

The **criminal law** determines how a society as a whole should behave. Criminal law is contained in statutes. A **crime** is an offence against society that violates a law. The Theft Act, for example, sets out the definition of theft and lays down the maximum penalty that can be imposed by the court if an offender is found guilty. All criminal cases must pass through the magistrates court even when it is apparent from the outset that a referral to the Crown Court will be necessary. There is a magistrates court in every town. The magistrates are people chosen from the community to make an initial assessment of every criminal case. Magistrates usually sit in a group of three. They are not lawyers. Magistrates have limited powers when assessing a criminal case and if the case falls outside these powers, it is referred to the Crown Court. Generally, magistrates can hear cases where the maximum penalty that could be imposed is 6 months' imprisonment or an unlimited fine.

In the Crown Court there is a judge and a jury of 12 members chosen at random from the community. The judge directs the hearing and ensures that the jury understands the law that needs to be considered. The jury decides if the defendant is guilty or not guilty. If a finding of guilt is made, the judge will decide what sentence will be passed within the limits laid down by the statute involved. A defendant can appeal to the Court of Appeal against what might have been a harsh sentence and the Court of Appeal has power to reduce the sentence.

A defendant cannot appeal against the jury's verdict of guilt unless there was some error in the judge's summary of the law which might have incorrectly influenced the jury. A jury can find a defendant guilty if the burden of proof is satisfied. The burden of proof is on the prosecution to prove guilt **beyond all reasonable doubt**.

## Civil Law

The **civil law** is concerned with the protection of the individual rights of members of society. A **tort** is a civil wrong committed against a person or property. Civil law covers everything that is not criminal in nature and as such is concerned with a much greater variety of issues; civil rights, divorce, disputes about wills, libel, nuisance, assault, battery and claims for injury are some of the matters dealt with by civil law. When one person has an individual complaint against another, the matter will be considered by the civil courts. For example, if a nurse is injured at work and wants to sue his or her employer, this will be dealt with in the civil courts. These are different from the criminal courts and separate rules and procedures exist. Most civil law disputes are heard in a county court. A single judge listens to both sides and makes a decision which is binding on both parties. The burden of proof in civil cases is lower than in criminal law. In a civil case a party has to prove the case on a **balance of probabilities** in order to succeed.

There is no need to involve a jury, as the matter is personal to the parties and does not require the judgement of society. The historical exception to this non-jury system is **libel**. A jury is required to hear libel cases and if a finding of libel is made the jury decides how much compensation the aggrieved party should receive.

Complex civil cases are handled by the High Court. Such cases can be commenced directly in the High Court and do not need to pass through the County Court. As in criminal cases, appeals against a possible error of law are made to the Court of Appeal or the House of Lords.

## Lawyers

The professional people who work in the law are called **lawyers** and include **barristers, solicitors, judges** and **legal executives**. Solicitors deal directly with clients and provide legal advice and assistance. If a hearing is to take place in the Crown Court or High Court, the solicitor will choose a barrister to present the case before the judge. Barristers wear traditional wigs and gowns when appearing in court. Barristers have specialist training in advocacy. Solicitors can appear as advocates in the magistrates court and the county court, but are not allowed in open court, in the Crown Court or High Court. Clients cannot approach a barrister directly for assistance and must always instruct a solicitor. A barrister is not allowed to talk to the client unless the solicitor is present.

There is a debate over whether solicitors and barristers should merge, as is the case in much of Europe and America. After 10 years, a barrister can apply to become a QC (Queens Counsel). These barristers deal with cases of great complexity or cases requiring special advocacy skills such as murder trials. Solicitors and barristers can apply to become judges although there are very few solicitors who have done so.

Legal executives work in solicitors' offices. They have less training than solicitors and work under supervision, although they often handle case loads as great as a solicitor.

## LEGAL CONCEPTS APPLIED TO NURSING

The nurse deals with many people, including the patient/client and family, doctors, other nurses and other health care professionals, as well as the employer. In any nurse-patient/client relationship several legal issues may arise. The public is better informed than in the past about health and illness, and more information is available to all users of the health services of their rights, through publications such as the *Patients' Charter*. Nurses are obliged to act in the patient's/client's interests under the UKCC code of conduct, which places a responsibility on nurses to protect the rights of patients/clients. It is necessary for nurses to be aware of the legal concepts that apply to their work.

## Assault

**Assault** is any wilful attempt or threat to harm another person, coupled with the ability to actually harm that person. The person believes harm will come as a result of the threat. Since most of the medical-legal case law concerns patients who have suffered actual harm, it would be unusual for a nurse to be charged with assault alone, although this is possible.

## Battery

**Battery** is any intentional touching of another person's body without his or her consent. Injury is not a requirement. Battery is both a crime and a tort. If a nurse attaches fetal electrodes during labour without asking the mother's consent, a claim of battery could be made. The important issue is consent. In some situations consent is implied, for example, if a nurse says "I have your injection for you, Mr Jones", and he holds out his arm, he is giving **implied consent** for the injection. It is unimportant whether the procedure that constitutes battery benefits the patient/client. In the American case in 1905 of *Mohr v Williams* the patient gave written consent for surgery on his right ear. After the patient was anaesthetised, the surgeon discovered that the left ear was more seriously affected and he operated on the left ear. The patient sued because surgery was performed on the 'wrong' ear and was successful. This was despite the fact that he actually benefited from the surgery. Underpinning the context of battery is the issue of *informed consent*.

## Informed Consent

**Informed consent** is a person's agreement to allow something to happen (for example surgery) based on a full disclosure of facts needed to make an intelligent decision. This includes knowledge of risks involved, benefits and consequences of refusal (see Chapter 29). The law has long recognized that individuals have the right to be free from bodily intrusion. In the celebrated American case of *Schlöendorff v Society of New York Hospital* decided in 1914, the court observed that "every human being of adult years and sound mind has a right to determine what shall be done with his body". The doctrine of informed consent not only requires that a person be given all relevant information required to reach a decision regarding treatment but also that the person be capable of understanding the relevant information and does in fact give consent. Anyone who performs a procedure on a patient/client without informed consent may be found liable in battery.

The important case of *Sidaway v Board of Governors of the Bethlem Royal Hospital*, heard in the Court of Appeal in 1985,

### Adult Nursing
### Informed consent for experimental treatment/procedures

If someone participates in an experimental treatment programme, an even more detailed and stringently regulated informed consent form should be used. These forms may be developed with the local ethics committee which gave approval to the research programme initially. The patient/client should always be given the option of withdrawing from the experiment at any time.

### Mental Health Nursing and Learning Disabilities Nursing
### Informed consent

Recent developments in public policy have emphasized the importance of informed consent and of assisting people with mental deficiencies to live the most autonomous and fulfilled lives possible, subject to continuing disability. An improved balance has been demanded between the paternalism inherent in compulsory interventions and respecting the autonomy of the individual.

decided that doctors should decide the extent of information required to enable a patient to come to a decision about treatment in accordance with the current standard adopted by a responsible body of medical opinion. In this case, the patient underwent an operation in her neck and suffered damage to the spinal column. The risk of such damage occurring was put between 1–2%. The patient was not informed of this risk. She sued and claimed that she was not informed sufficiently, prior to the operation, to give informed consent. In the future, some surgical procedures will be carried out in the community. Nurses should be aware that the same obligations concerning consent should be observed in community settings, as well as in hospital settings.

However, the Court of Appeal found that in 1974 no neurosurgeon would have felt obliged to inform a patient of this risk, as it was so small. It was for the doctor to determine the extent to which risks associated with the treatment were to be disclosed, in accordance with the currently accepted medical standard.

A signed consent form is recommended for any hazardous procedure such as surgery, some treatments such as chemotherapy, and any form of research. Written consent is not proof that the consent is *informed* or *valid*, but it can be useful evidence that a discussion between the doctor and the patient/client took place.

The following factors must be assessed before a consent can be a **valid consent**:

1. The person must be an adult and mentally competent.
2. The consent must be given voluntarily. No forceful measures may be used to obtain it.
3. The person giving consent must understand the procedure and any risks outlined by the doctor.

**Children's Nursing**
**Informed consent for children**

Parents are usually the legal guardians of children and are the persons who must sign consent forms. Occasionally a parent or guardian refuses treatment for a child. In these cases the court may intervene on the child's behalf. The practice of making a child a ward of court, administering necessary treatment, and then returning legal guardianship to the parents is relatively common in such cases. Where there is conflict the hospital can ask for the child to be made a ward of court. This means that the court assumes parental control and that any decision of the court will overrule that of the parents. At the end of the case the custody and guardianship of the child returns to the parents.

A nurse involved in such a case should inform the nursing manager, who will enlist the aid of the appropriate hospital administrator.

**Adult Nursing**
**Informed consent in complicated cases**

In some instances, obtaining informed consent is difficult. If the patient/client is unconscious, for example, consent must be obtained from a person legally authorized to give consent on the patient's/client's behalf. If a person has been declared legally incompetent in judicial proceedings, consent must be obtained from the person's legal guardian. In emergency situations, if it is impossible to obtain consent from the patient/client, the procedure required to benefit the patient/client (or perhaps to save a life) may be undertaken without liability for failure to obtain consent. In those instances, the law presumes the patient/client would wish to be treated.

4. The person giving consent must have the opportunity to have all questions answered satisfactorily.

If a patient/client is deaf or has some other impediment in communication (such as speaking a foreign language), an interpreter should be available to explain the terms of consent. Most hospitals have developed their own consent forms.

Because nurses do not perform surgery or direct the medical procedure, obtaining consent should not fall within the nursing duty. However, in many hospitals the nurse assumes responsibility for confirming consent. When a nurse takes a consent form for a patient/client to sign, the nurse should ask if the patient/client understands the procedure for which consent is being given. If the patient/client denies understanding, or the nurse suspects the individual does not understand or has some unanswered questions or doubts about the procedure, the nurse must notify either the doctor or the manager and inform the patient/client of this. The patient's/client's right to self determination gives them the right to receive clear information with which to make decisions for informed consent. In the future, some surgical procedures will be carried out in the community. Nurses should be aware that the same obligations concerning consent should be observed in community settings, as well as in hospital settings.

A patient/client refusing surgery or other medical treatment must be informed about any harmful consequences. If the patient/client persists in refusing, the rejection should be written and signed by the doctor and the patient/client.

## Negligence

Nurses are responsible for performing all procedures correctly and exercising professional judgement as they carry out their own tasks and those ordered by a doctor. Any nurse who does not meet accepted standards of practice or care, or who performs duties in a careless fashion, runs the risk of being negligent. **Negligence** is a civil tort. If nurses give care that does not meet appropriate standards, they may be held **liable** for negligence.

Negligence may involve carelessness, such as not checking a patient's/client's identity and consequently administering the wrong medication (read *UKCC Code of Professional Conduct* for additional details).

However, carelessness is not always the cause. If nurses perform procedures for which they have not been trained and do it carefully but still harm the patient/client, a claim of negligence could be made. In an action for negligence the following criteria must be established.
1. The nurse (defendant) owed a duty of care to the patient/client (plaintiff).
2. The nurse broke that duty by failing to act as a reasonable nurse.
3. The patient/client was injured.
4. The injury was a result of the nurse's failure to carry out the duty.

## The Duty of Care

This legal concept was established in the 1932 case of *Donoghue v Stevenson*. In this case, a woman in a tea shop purchased a bottle of ginger beer which, she later discovered, contained the remains of a decomposed snail. The court held that the manufacturers of the ginger beer owed her a **duty of care** to produce an uncontaminated drink. If a patient/client is being nursed on a specialist bed which breaks, it would be possible for the patient/client to consider bringing an action against the bed manufacturers, even though the contract to supply and maintain the bed will be between the hospital and the manufacturers. This would be in addition to the hospital's duty of care to maintain equiptment in safe working order.

## Breaking the Duty of Care

The duty of care is broken if a nurse fails to act as a reasonable nurse could have been expected to act in the same situation. If a nurse fails to record details of a patient's/client's temperature, or records it inaccurately, it would appear that the duty of care has been broken. The test for the standard of behaviour required to assess whether a duty of care has been broken was formulated in the case of *Bolam v Friern Barnet Management Committee* in 1957.

The standard of care required is that of a reasonable nurse acting in accordance with the practice accepted at that time as proper by a responsible body of nursing opinion.

## Causation

A nurse may break a duty of care and the patient may be injured but in order to establish negligence it is necessary to show a link between the two. In *Barnett v Chelsea and Kensington*, three night watchmen visited an Accident and Emergency Unit in the early hours of the morning complaining of sickness and vomiting. It later transpired that their tea flasks had been laced with arsenic. The nurse in Accident and Emergency rang the doctor to ask for advice and was told by the doctor to inform the men to see their GP later that day. One man died before seeing his GP and his wife sued the hospital for negligence. The court found that the nurse had acted in accordance with her duty of care to the men by seeking advice from the doctor and that she had not breached her duty of care and could not be held negligent.

The court found that the casualty doctor should have examined the men at the hospital, and that any reasonable doctor would have done so. By failing to act in accordance with a generally accepted standard, the doctor had broken his duty of care. However, the evidence showed the man would have died of poisoning in any event, even if the doctor had seen him. The failure to treat was not in itself a sufficient cause of injury, in this case death, for a finding of negligence against the doctor.

## Professional Standards of Care

The UKCC produces a code of conduct which all nurses are required to follow. Failure to do so may lead to a hearing before a Professional Conduct Committee. If a nurse fails to carry out his or her tasks competently, and a patient/client suffers harm, there will be no negligence if the link of causation cannot be established. This does not mean, however, that the nurse may not be called to account for his or her actions before the UKCC. The professional standards of the UKCC, therefore, require a higher standard of practice of a nurse than the civil law of negligence.

## Time Limits

An action in negligence must be commenced within three years of the date of the accident. If an adult patient/client suffers unforeseen injuries on 1 January 1995, the time limit will expire on 1 January 1998.

If a child is injured the law allows that child three years to commence an action after the age of majority is reached. If a child aged six is injured the time limit will expire three years after the child becomes 18 years old, i.e. 21 years of age. It is for this reason that the records of children are kept for a much longer period of time than those of adults.

Where a person is injured but cannot know it (as in the case of asbestos poisoning) the three year time limit runs from the first occasion the person was aware of the problem. This usually follows a visit to a GP where a diagnosis may be made.

## Vicarious Liability

It is possible for a patient/client to sue a nurse directly in an action for negligence. Generally, however, a patient/client will sue the hospital or employing institution in which the nurse works under the principle of **vicarious liability**. This principle allows the employer to be sued for actions of an employee which may be negligent. It is assumed that an employer should ensure the competency of its staff and should be able to take responsibility for negligent acts or omissions. When an aggrieved patient/client sues the employing hospital in negligence where injury has been caused by a nurse, it is always open to the patient/client to add the nurse as a second defendant. The nurse will need separate legal representation and it is advisable for all nurses to ensure adequate protection against such an occurrence.

Most trade unions now carry indemnity insurance as part of the services provided for their membership. This protects a nurse if a finding of negligence is made against the nurse and an order made that compensation be paid to the patient/client. Indemnity insurance would meet the cost of compensation and the legal fees incurred.

## Confidentiality

People are entitled to confidential health care. All aspects of care should be free from unwanted publicity or exposure to public scrutiny. Patients/clients may have a claim for breach of **confidentiality** when their private health affairs, with which the public has no concern, have been publicized.

An example of a breach of confidentiality is the release of information to an unauthorized person, such as the media or the patient's/client's employer. Gossip about a patient's/client's activities is another form of breach of confidentiality. A nurse should respect a wish not to inform a patient's/client's family of a terminal illness.

An individual's right to confidentiality may conflict with the public's right to information; for example, a threat or benefit to public health may override the individual's right to privacy. One of the fundamental obligations owed by a nurse to a patient/client is to respect the information disclosed by the patient/client. In some circumstances, however, disclosure of information to a third party may be legally justified.

When a patient/client is in the care of more than one person, it is assumed that the individual assents to all the appropriate health care team being properly informed so that they can carry out their duties in a competent manner.

Some diseases such as smallpox and cholera are required to be notified to the local authority and these are listed in an Act of Parliament. Recent cases have arisen where a health care worker has been diagnosed with an infectious illness which some parts of the media feel should be made public. If a nurse believes that information is about to be disclosed which relates to his or her own health, it is possible to ask the court to grant an injunction forbidding such publication. If the information has been published in advance, it is open to the person named to sue in civil law for breach of confidentiality and to ask for compensation.

In the case of *X v Y* in 1988, a national newspaper intended to publish information about two doctors who were being treated for AIDS. The employing hospital asked the court for an injunction. The newspaper argued that it was in the public

**Adult Nursing**
**Issues related to community**
**practice**

Important issues surround how much authority a health care professional has as a visitor in a patient's/client's home in relation to the patient's/client's treatment and other safety aspects of care. A hospital may have safety and treatment issues covered by local protocols. Nursing in the community, however, presents a much wider range of settings for nursing practice and may not be so easily defined in a local protocol.

**Patient's/Client's Authority**
A nurse in the community may wrongly believe that because care is offered in a patient's/client's home it must be carried out in the precise way that the client wishes. Care should be planned and delivered in a partnership incorporating the nurse, the patient/client, and any carers involved. The nurse endeavours to create a climate in which there is mutual trust and respect. If this is the case, it is highly unlikely that there will be unresolvable disagreement between the nurse, patient/client, or carer.

In rare instances, the nurse and patient/client may have differing opinions regarding the way a particular aspect of care is given. For example, a heavy patient/client who is paraplegic requires lifting in and out of bed. The nurse may decide that the most appropriate way to deliver this care safely is to use a hoist; however, the patient/client may feel more secure if the nurse lifts him or her manually.

If the situation regarding care cannot be resolved and the patient/client refuses to cooperate in using the hoist, the nurse must then decide whether the care option the patient/client requests is safe for both the patient/client and the nurse. If either the nurse or patient/client is at personal risk of injury, the nurse is not obliged to carry out the patient's/client's instructions.

This example is only an illustration of a potential problem that might occur in a patient's/client's home. Good communication and partnership between the nurse, the patient/client, and the carer should ensure that such cases are avoided.

**Confidentiality**
There are situations in which a patient's/client's notes are held in the home, and the health care professional enters data and refers to these notes in the presence of the client. It is very important that the nurse indicates to the client that records are kept with regard to the client's care and that these records may be shared with other professionals within the primary care team. The nurse should indicate this to the client at the onset of their relationship. The nurse should discuss the content of the records with the client as they are entered.

Sometimes, information crucial to care may be given to the nurse by a family member or carer who requests that the details are kept private, either from the client or from other team members. The nurse must decide how to deal with this information in the client's best interest. There is an ethical dilemma to be resolved, which involves the nature of the open relationship between the client, the nurse, and the carer or family member, and the right of the client to know the information. It is usually best if the nurse tries to persuade the giver of the information that the information should also be shared with the client.

If the nurse colludes with a carer or family member in keeping information from the client, the nurse risks destroying the trusting relationship between himself or herself, and the client. For this reason, the nurse should encourage openness among all parties.

In some exceptional instances, the nurse may consider that sensitive information should not be recorded in records held at home, and so may set up parallel notes at the health centre or surgery. An example of this may be information relating to care for a client who is HIV positive.

---

interest to publish and that this defence justified any breach of confidence. The court rejected this argument and found that the defence of the public interest was not so strong as to allow publication.

There are cases in which information is given about a major medical breakthrough, as with the first heart transplant cases or the first test-tube baby. In such cases it could be argued that the public interest defence outweighs the breach caused by revealing the information.

The nurse should not attempt personally to decide the legality of disclosing information requested by a third party. Any request for such information should be referred to senior management to ensure that a breach of confidentiality does not occur.

## Death and Dying
Many legal issues surround the event of **death**, including a basic definition of the actual point at which a person is considered dead. The law accepts that death occurs when there is an absence of brain stem function, even if other body organs still function.

This definition is useful when there is a question of whether to continue life support. Nurses must be aware of the legal definition of death and document all events that occur while the patient/client is in their care.

Ethical and legal questions (see Chapter 12) are raised by the issue of euthanasia. **Active euthanasia,** such as intentionally administering a lethal dose of morphine to a patient/client to cause death, is illegal and would constitute murder. Doctors have been convicted of murder for acting in this way.

The more problematic area of **passive euthanasia**, such as removing breathing support or withholding nutrition from a comatose patient with irreversible brain damage, raises legal questions about death and dying that were discussed at length in the House of Lords in *Airedale v Bland NHS Trust* in 1993.

## Organ Donation
Legally competent persons are free to donate their bodies or organs for medical use. Consent forms are available for this purpose. When someone has died, The Human Tissue Act 1961

sets out the requirements that need to be satisfied before the hospital can proceed to remove any part of the body. The Act states that authorization for removal must be given by a person in possession of the corpse. It is generally considered that this person is the hospital administrator, although the Act is not clear on this. If it can be shown that the deceased person had not expressed an objection to organ donation and that the surviving relatives do not object, then consideration can be given for organ removal.

The 1961 Act therefore provides an opting out approach to organ donation. Such donation can take place unless it can be shown that either the deceased person expressed a wish to the contrary or that a relative objects.

Many people carry a donor card expressing their willingness to provide organs and, although these are not required, it is a useful way to determine the intention of the deceased person very shortly after his or her death. **Organ and tissue donation** remains voluntary. Donor cards are easily obtainable and need not be witnessed.

## Living Wills and Health Care Surrogates

In light of the consideration being given to the rights of the terminally ill and people in a persistent vegetative (permanently comatose) state, the nurse may find that patients/clients have made provision for **advance directives** or **health care surrogates**. If they have not, they may ask the nurse to provide information about them.

**Living wills** are documents instructing doctors to withhold or withdraw life-sustaining procedures in patients/clients whose death is imminent. The procedures are considered to prolong the dying process rather than to promote life. Living wills have increasing legal force as an expression of self-determination by a patient/client, and should be given respect.

Individuals may, in advance of illness, appoint someone to make health care decisions if and when the individual is no longer able to make decisions on his or her own behalf. These people are known as health care surrogates. They do not need to be medically qualified or related to the patient/client.

## LEGAL SAFEGUARDS IN NURSING PRACTICE

## Registration

All nurses are required to be registered with the United Kingdom Central Council for Nursing (UKCC). Registration provides certainty of qualification and also allows nurses to offer special skills to the public. Registration can be suspended or revoked by the UKCC if a nurse's conduct violates provisions contained in the Code of Conduct (see Chapter 1) for example, nurses who perform illegal acts, such as taking controlled substances, are at risk of being removed from the register as well as facing criminal charges. When an allegation of misconduct is made, the nurse must be notified of the charges and permitted to attend hearings in which evidence can be presented. These hearings are not court proceedings, but are conducted by the UKCC in accordance with

strict rules on procedure under the Nurses, Midwives, and Health Visitors Act 1979, as amended in 1993. This Act allows a nurse to appeal to the High Court if an error in law occurs at the hearing.

## Student Nurses

If a patient/client suffers harm as a direct result of a student nurse's actions or lack of action, the liability for any charge of negligence may be shared between the student, the tutor, the hospital or other work place, or the teaching institution.

Student nurses should never be assigned to tasks for which they are unprepared, and should be carefully supervised by tutors or senior nurses as they learn new procedures. The teaching institution has a responsibility to monitor the acts of student nurses. Nurse tutors are usually responsible for teaching and observing students, but in most situations sisters, charge nurses and staff nurses may share these responsibilities. Every teaching institution and work place should provide clear definitions of responsibility.

In addition to encountering legal problems in the care of patients/clients, nurses may share responsibility for errors made by doctors and other health care personnel.

## Doctors' Orders

The doctor is responsible for directing medical treatment. Nurses are obliged to follow doctors' orders unless they believe the orders are in error, would be detrimental to patients/clients, or conflict with the nurse's own practice. Therefore, all orders must be assessed, and if one is determined to be erroneous or harmful, further clarification from the doctor is necessary. If the doctor confirms the order and the nurse still believes that it is inappropriate, a senior nurse should be informed. A written memorandum to the senior nurse detailing the events in chronological order should protect the nurse from any potential action in negligence.

The senior nurse should help resolve the questionable order. A nurse carrying out an inaccurate order may be legally responsible for any harm suffered by the patient/client, if the nurse was aware of the problem.

The doctor should write all orders, and the nurse must make sure that they are transcribed correctly. Verbal orders are not recommended because they leave possibilities for error. If a verbal order is necessary (during an emergency for example), it should be written and signed by the doctor as soon as possible; usually within 24 hours. This applies to both hospital and community care.

The difficult area regarding doctors' orders involves an order of 'do not resuscitate' (DNR) for a terminally ill patient/client. Many doctors are reluctant to write such orders because they fear legal repercussions. If a doctor has documented in the notes that the patient's/client's condition is deteriorating and that the decision not to administer cardiopulmonary resuscitation had been made, the doctor can justify the decision. Unless the doctor decides that such a discussion would be detrimental to the patient's/client's condition, the order should be discussed with the patient/client. In such cases the doctor should also discuss the order with the family. A DNR order should be written, not given verbally. Doctors should regularly review DNR orders in case the patient's/client's condition warrants a change. The British Medical Association and Royal College of Nursing have produced a joint statement on the issues affecting both doctors and nurses in this area (RCN/BMA, 1993).

### Incident Reports

An **incident report** is completed when something arises that could or did cause an injury to the nurse or the patient/client, or something occurred that was not consistent with good care (see Chapter 19). For example, if a nurse administers an incorrect dose of medication or if a patient/client falls out of bed, the nurse should complete an incident report. Most hospitals provide specific forms for this purpose. The nurse records all of the details of the incident. A doctor may need to examine either the patient/client or the nurse if an injury has occurred, and will indicate on the incident form any immediate diagnosis or treatment.

Many nurses are reluctant to complete incident forms because they believe these reports harm their employment records. However, incident forms are valuable for risk management and quality assurance. By reviewing incident reports, managers can assess areas of risk to patients/clients or to staff. For example, if a certain problem has occurred repeatedly across the hospital with a particular piece of equipment, the incident report will highlight any difficulties. With this system steps can be taken to identify and correct problems that could compromise care. An incident report should be completed as soon as the event or error has been discovered. In this way the incident report will record a written, contemporaneous statement of the facts of the incident.

If at some later date the nurse's actions are called into question, either by the UKCC or by a civil court hearing a case of negligence, it will be much easier to prove what actually happened by referring to the incident form than by trying to rely on the recollections of staff.

### Contracts of Employment

A **contract of employment** can be oral or written. It is better in a written form, as this gives more certainty to the extent of terms agreed between the parties. An oral contract is as legally binding as a written contract, but may be more difficult to prove. A **breach of contract** occurs if either party fails to carry out agreed obligations. By accepting a job, a nurse enters into an agreement with an employer. The nurse will perform professional duties competently and abide by the policies and procedures of the employer. In return, the employer pays for the nurse's services and also provides facilities and equipment in proper working order to enable the nurse to provide efficient and competent care.

## LEGAL ISSUES IN SPECIALITY PRACTICE AREAS

Legal liabilities exist in all areas of nursing practice. Any nurse working in a specialized field should study the legal issues relevant to that area of practice. Space does not permit a complete discussion of all legal liabilities, but a few issues involved in some practice areas are discussed in the following sections.

### Nursing Children

Paediatric nursing involves care of the newborn and young children, both in hospital (by children's nurses) and in the community (by midwives, nurses, and health visitors). There may be many legal issues involved in the care of an infant.

One important legal issue that has been discussed in recent years relates to the treatment of severely handicapped infants. Many of these cases involve infants born with Down's syndrome. In *R v Arthur* (1981) Dr Arthur was charged with the murder of a three-day-old baby born with Down's syndrome. When the baby was born, the parent discussed the condition with the doctor and decided, in view of the baby's handicap, that they did not wish him to live. Dr Arthur prescribed a sedative drug which was known to suppress appetite, and ordered nursing care only. The doctor's defence was that he had given the sedative as a 'holding operation' to test whether the child would live or die naturally. If the child was strong enough to survive, the doctor would then be able to institute invasive therapy. The doctor was acquitted.

Although the nurses and parents were aware of the treatment prescribed for this child, and of its potential outcome, they were not prosecuted for accessory to murder.

The court has held that there may be circumstances in which it is not necessary to sustain a child who is not dying where the current prospect of life is demonstrably so awful that it would in effect be worse to stay alive. In the case of *Re B* in 1981 a Down's syndrome baby was born with duodenum atresia and needed life-saving surgery. The parents did not feel the child should survive and the doctor agreed. The court considered the case and decided that the child should be given necessary treatment, as there was not sufficient evidence that the baby would have such an appalling existence as to justify non-treatment.

In the later case of *Re J* (1990) a very low birth weight child had severe and gross handicaps, was in great pain, and required a great deal of medical treatment. The court decided that treatment to prolong the child's life need not be given. The child should be given antibiotics if he developed a chest infection but need not be

**Children's Nursing**
**Protection of children**

The Children's Act (1989) sets out a number of principles relating to the protection of children.

**Children's nurses should:**
- work with parents to enable them to care for their children to the best of their ability,
- ensure that when working with children they listen to each child, provide appropriate information and take account of the child's wishes and feelings, and
- identify children in need and, where appropriate, refer to social services, and cooperate with the social services department and educational department to meet the health needs of the children.

reventilated if his breathing stopped. It is important to distinguish between **life-saving treatment** and **life-sustaining treatment**.

In each case, the court had to decide what would be in the child's best interests, and as such, had power to overrule the wishes of the parents or the views of the doctors. There is a presumption on the part of the court in favour of maintaining life, unless there are extreme reasons not to do so. It would seem that an assessment of the quality of life of such babies should include criteria such as anticipated life expectancy, capacity to interact with others, and degree of pain suffered.

This is a difficult area, and nurses should ensure that they receive adequate support from their managers in dealing with these particular instances. Nurses should be aware that the courts have power to intervene in all cases where a dilemma arises between the parents and the health care team over any proposed course of treatment.

## Nursing in Intensive Care Units

Nurses working in intensive care settings are also legally accountable for performing their duties. Intensive care nurses require additional training and ongoing education to provide them with information about advances in care methods.

Possible legal problems for intensive care nurses are associated with the use of electronic monitoring devices. No monitor can be considered totally reliable, and the nurse must not completely depend on it.

The staffing ratio in an intensive care setting is usually set by the hospital and may be one nurse for each patient, depending on the severity of the patient's conditions. These recommendations are made because of the intensity of care required by such patients. These patients require careful observation and assessment of their conditions, the many treatment procedures, and medication. If a nurse is assigned to three or four intensive care patients and feels unable to give appropriate care, the nurse should make his or her concerns known immediately by telephoning the appropriate manager and by recording the telephone call on each of the patient's notes. If a nurse does not do this and a patient suffers harm, the nurse may be liable for failing to inform of a shortage of staff.

## Nursing People with a Mental Illness or a Learning Disability

Mental disorder covers a wide range of conditions, including mental illness and learning disabilities. Many people who have a form of mental disorder are subject to compulsory interventions in their own interest and in the interests of other people.

### Learning Disabilities Nursing
### Mental Health Act 1983

A minority of people with learning disabilities are admitted for assessment and/or treatment under the 1983 Mental Health Act. When this occurs, it is usually because the person has displayed behaviour that brought him or her into contact with the police and judicial system, and admission to hospital is considered more appropriate than a custodial sentence.

Compulsory admission to mental health facilities and the separate concept of compulsory treatment are considered on the basis of a 'best interests' test and a 'dangerousness' test.

The general principles of law in relation to consent depend upon someone having the mental capacity, or state of mind, to agree or disagree with the proposed treatment. The law requires that a choice is given to patients/clients to agree to or to refuse treatment. A choice cannot be genuine if it is induced by fraud, or deceit, or if insufficient information is given about the possible consequences of a choice. Equally, a choice cannot be made genuinely if there is not the mental capacity to make it. This does not mean that anyone with a mental disorder is deemed by law as automatically incapable of making a choice. But there are many mental conditions which, depending on fluctuations in capacity, prevent proper judgement. At such stages the law intervenes and states that in certain circumstances treatment can be given without consent. The Mental Health Act 1983 gives the power (subject to certain procedures) for doctors and nurses to impose treatment, even if the patient/client can understand the alternative and the consequences, but simply refuses. It should be noted that the powers to impose treatment cover only treatment for mental disorder. This excludes physical disorder. A patient/client detained under the Mental Health Act 1983 who develops a physical disorder cannot have that physical disorder treated under the Mental Health Act. The exception to this is where treatment can be given under the common law doctrine of necessity where the intention is to save a life or prevent serious danger to health.

Certain treatments can never be imposed without consent. For example, section 57 of the Mental Health Act 1983 states that psychosurgery and the surgical implantation of hormones for reduction of the male sex drive cannot be imposed upon a patient without his consent, and if an approved doctor and two approved people, who are not medical practitioners, have certified that the individual is capable of understanding the nature and the effects of the treatment.

## Nursing Older Adults

Many of the legal issues surrounding the care of nursing older people relate to requests to nurses to assist in the dying process. Under the Suicide Act 1961, it is an offence to assist someone to commit suicide. Doctors have been prosecuted for attempted murder by administering large doses of medication which they knew had the effect of relieving intense pain but at the risk of causing death.

All mentally competent patients/clients have the **right to refuse treatment**, and this right was upheld by the Court of Appeal in *Re T* in a case heard in 1992. It is accepted that a competent adult can refuse medical treatment even if the potential effect of non-treatment is that he or she will die. When an individual refuses to receive treatment and subsequently does die, the court has confirmed that such a person is not committing suicide. While a valid refusal would be accepted in terms of medical treatment, it is less clear whether a patient/client may validly refuse basic nursing care. For example, could a terminally ill patient/client who had refused any further medication also

**Learning Disabilities Nursing Guardianship**

The concept of *guardianship*, addressed in the Mental Health Act 1983 (sections 7–10), is of particular importance to people with learning disabilities. Although it is rarely used, the purpose of guardianship is to provide a guardian for a person who is unable to ensure his or her own welfare, or presents a danger to others. The guardian has the power to determine where the individual lives; to ensure the individual attends medical treatment, occupation or training; and to ensure access is given at the individual's residence to doctors and social workers. For example, guardianship might be applied for when a person with a learning disability is living with his or her family of origin, but is clearly not being well cared for, is unable to protect himself or herself from neglect, and the family resists interventions from health and social services professionals, leading to grave concern for the health and well-being of the person with the learning disability.

Failure to institute the powers of guardianship may result in tragic situations that could otherwise have been prevented (Fennell, 1989).

refuse nursing treatment for pressure sores?

It is the responsibility of the nurse to ensure that the greatest amount of respect for the autonomy of the older patient/client is granted. Older people who suffer from dementia may have fluctuating periods in which they can make decisions concerning their treatment and well-being, and other periods when they are unable to do so. Nurses should be sympathetic to these fluctuations in lucidity and should be prepared to respect the fullest wishes of the patient/client when they are capable of determining how they wish to conduct their affairs.

Some older patients/clients ask nurses to witness wills that they have made while in hospital or a nursing home. Nurses should first assess whether a policy has been produced by the employing institution to determine how they should respond to such requests. If a nurse wishes to witness the will of a patient/client it is necessary to follow specific legal requirements. A will must be signed by the person making it, who is capable of understanding the content and intention. The requirements for witnessing are that the person making the will (the testator) signs and dates it in the physical presence of two witnesses who then each take it in turn to sign the will themselves in the presence of the other witness and the testator. Failure to follow this procedure renders the will invalid. A person witnessing a will cannot receive any gift in the will. If a testator wishes to leave a gift to a nurse, that nurse must consider, on professional grounds, whether it is appropriate to accept the gift.

## SUMMARY

There are many legal issues confronting nurses today. Nurses should not view the law with apprehension, but rather as a helpful structure to defining nursing practice. Nurses who are aware of

their legal rights and obligations are better prepared to care for patients/clients and to be more confident when approaching new situations.

Nursing standards of care may define appropriate nursing. Some standards are stated in general terms such as those provided by professional nursing organizations or the UKCC. If nurses act within the accepted standards of care at all times, their chances of being adversely involved in litigation are reduced.

Some legal issues, such as the necessity for informed consent and awareness of the possibility of negligence, are involved in almost every branch of nursing. Other legal issues are confined to specific areas; however, regardless of the situation, nurses are responsible for knowing the fundamental principles of law that apply to their own area of nursing practice.

## CHAPTER 13 REVIEW

### Key Concepts

- With increased emphasis on patients'/clients' rights, nurses in practice today must understand their legal obligations and responsibilities.
- Nurses should act and speak in an appropriate manner to avoid frightening, coercing or physically intimidating patients/clients, so as to avoid a charge of assault.
- A nurse must obtain a patient's/client's consent before touching that person otherwise the nurse commits battery, which is both a crime and a tort.
- Informed consent allows physical procedures to be carried out in a lawful manner, without risk that a claim of battery may be made.
- Nurses are not responsible for obtaining informed consent for any surgery or other medical procedure before the procedure is performed. They may be responsible for confirming that informed consent has been given.
- In emergency situations, informed consent is not necessary if it is impossible to obtain consent from the patient/client.
- A nurse can be found liable for negligence if the following criteria are established: the nurse (defendant) owed a duty to the patient/client (plaintiff), the nurse did not carry out that duty, the patient was injured, and the nurse's failure to carry out the duty caused the patient's/client's injury.
- The legal standard of care required by the civil law may be lower than the standard of care required by the UKCC.
- The employer generally assumes responsibility for the negligence of the employees, under the principle of vicarious liability.
- All patients/clients are entitled to confidential health care and freedom from unauthorized release of information. Otherwise, nurses may be liable for breach of confidentiality. A defence would be that the release was in the public interest.
- Legal issues involving death include the definition of death and the awareness of issues arising for comatosed patients.
- A mentally competent adult can legally give consent to donate specific organs.
- Student nurses do not have the same responsibilities as qualified nurses. They should be assigned only the tasks for

which they are prepared, and should be carefully supervised.

- Nurses are responsible for performing all procedures correctly and for exercising professional judgement as they carry out doctors' orders. Otherwise, the nurse may be liable for negligence.
- Nurses are obliged to follow doctors' orders unless they believe the orders are in error, could be detrimental to patients/clients or conflict with the nurse's own professional obligations.
- Nurses are encouraged to file incident reports in all situations when someone could or was likely to be hurt. These reports are used for risk management as well as for providing evidence of the situation that took place.
- Nurses practising in specialized areas are legally accountable for performing specialized duties and therefore require additional training and ongoing education.
- All nurses should know the law that applies to their particular area of practice.

## CRITICAL THINKING EXERCISES

1. Mrs Lee has leukaemia and has been hospitalized for acute anaemia. She is married and has two young daughters. The doctor has ordered blood transfusions to assist Mrs Lee over her crisis. However, Mrs Lee's religion prohibits her from receiving blood transfusions. She has told you that she does not wish to have any blood transfusions. You have noted this on her records. Her husband has stated that, although he does not share her religion, he will concur with her wishes. Without the transfusion, Mrs Lee will die. The doctor had told you that he will declare a medical emergency and order you to initiate the transfusions as soon as Mrs Lee slips into a coma from lack of oxygen.

a) What risks do you face if you administer the transfusion?

b) What should you do?

c) Would your answer change if Mrs Lee was admitted in a coma and there was no information regarding her wishes concerning blood transfusion?

2. Mr Andrews is an 80-year-old man, who was admitted for gall bladder surgery. He is recuperating. On the day that the doctor allows him to walk down the corridor with assistance,

### Key Terms

Active/passive euthanasia, p. 256
Advance directives, p. 257
Assault, p. 253
Battery, p. 253
Breach of contract, p. 258
Confidentiality, p. 255
Death, p. 256
DNR ('do not resuscitate') order, p. 257
Duty of care, p. 254
Implied consent, p. 253
Informed consent, p. 253
Judicial decision, p. 252
Legislation, p. 251
Liable, p. 254
Libel, p. 252
Life-saving or sustaining treatment, p. 259
Living will, p. 257
Negligence, p. 254
Organ/tissue donation, p. 257
Right to refuse treatment, p. 259
Valid consent, p. 253
Vicarious liability, p. 255

he asks you to help him do so. Mr Andrews has an anti-embolism hose and he has slippers in his locker. You get Mr Andrews out of bed and assist him to walk down the corridor, which has a newly buffed linoleum floor. You forget to put on his slippers, although you knew about them. While walking down the hall, you turn to look out of the window at a commotion in the car park. As you are looking, Mr Andrews' foot slips out from under him, and he falls to the floor, breaking his hip. Identify the elements of negligence and use this case to apply those elements.

3. Mrs Cooper has recently been diagnosed as HIV positive. She has three children aged 7, 6, and 4. Her partner left when he learned of her diagnosis. The health visitor is in constant contact with Mrs Cooper. When completing the requisite forms to transfer care of the youngest child (soon to attend school) to a school nurse, the health visitor indicated that Mrs Cooper is HIV positive. The school nurse informed the head of the school.

## REFERENCES

(Law Reports can be accessed through libraries in Law Departments of University Colleges, or through the Law Society, Chancery Lane, London. Law Reports from other countries may not be available in the UK.)

*Airedale NHS Trust v. Bland* [1993] 1AU ER 821.

*Barnett v. Chelsea & Kensington HMC* [1969] IQB 428.

*Bolam v. Friern Barnet Management Committee* [1957] 2 ALL ER 118.

*Donoghue v. Stevenson* [1932] AC 562.

Fennell P: The Beverley Lewis case: was the law to blame? *New Law J* 139:1557, 1989.

*Mohr v. Williams, 95 Minn 261, 1905.*

In *Re B* (a minor) [1981] 1WLR I421.

In *Re J* (a minor) (wardship: medical treatment ) [I990] 3 ALL ER 930.

In *Re T* (adult: refusal of treatment) [1992] 3 WLR 782.

*Schloendorff v. Society of New York Hospital, 211 MY 125, 1914.*

*Sidaway v. Board of Governors of the Bethlem Royal Hospital* [I985] 1 ALL ER 643.

Royal College of Nursing/British Medical Association: *Cardiopulmonary resuscitation*, London, 1993, RCN/BMA.

R - V - Arthur, 1981, 12 BMLR.

## FURTHER READING

### Adult Nursing

Brazier M: *Medicine, patients and the law*, ed 3, London 1992, Penguin.

Burnard P, Chapman CM: *Professional and ethical issues in nursing: the code of professional conduct*, ed 2, London, 1993, Scutari Press.

Dimond B: *Legal aspects of nursing,* New York, 1990, Prentice Hall.

Dimond B: Who cares for the future?, *Elderly Care* 5(3):14, 1993.

Dimond B: Extracting consent, *Elderly Care* 5(2):14, 1993.

Kennedy I: *Treat me right — essays in medical law and ethics,* Oxford, 1991, Clarendon Press.

Mason, McCall Smith: *Law and medical ethics,* ed 3, London, 1991, Butterworths.

Dimond B: A case of false imprisonment, *Elderly Care* 5(1):18, 1993.

Greengross S: *The law and vulnerable elderly people,* London, 1986, Age Concern.

Royal College of Nursing: Living wills — guidance for nurses, *Issues Nurs Health* 4: 1992.

Tingle J: Making the law, *Nursing Times,* 87 (31): 52, 1991.

## Children's Nursing

Atherton TM: *The rights of the child in health care,* In Lindsay R Ed. The Child and family: contemporary nursing issues in child health and care. London, 1994, Bailliere Tindall.

Korgaonkar G et al: Children and consent to medical treatment, *British Journal of Nursing* 2(7): 383-4, 1993.

Stainton Rogers W, Rocef J: *Children's rights and children's welfare: a guide to the law,* London, 1994, Hodder & Stoughton.

Dimond B: Legal aspects of paediatric nursing, *Nursing Times* 85(30): 70-71, 1989.

## Learning Disabilities Nursing

Ashton GR, Ward AD: *Mental handicap and the law,* London, 1992, Sweet & Maxwell.

Gunn MJ: *Sex and the law: a brief guide for staff working with people with learning difficulties 2nd ed,* London, 1991, FPA.

Letts P: Consent to treatment: should the courts intervene, *Comm Nurs* 6 (2): 20, 1992.

Roberts G, Griffiths G: *What can we do?, The legal framework of community care services for people with learning disabilities,* London, 1993, National Development Team.

## Mental Health Nursing

Bluglass RA: *Guide to the Mental Health Act 1983,* Edinburgh, 1983, Churchill Livingstone.

Bourne J: *Looking after the financial affairs of people with mental incapacity,* a report by the Comptroller Auditor, London, 1994, National Audit Office.

Carpenter MA: *Accountability in professional practice,* Killen S, The Mental Health Acts-the United Kingdom and Eire. In Wright H and Giddey M eds. Mental Health nursing: from first principles to professional practice. London, 1993, Chapman and Hall, 353-63; 413-32.

Carson D: Negligence: defining responsibilities, *Professional Nurse,* 141, 1987.

Derrick S: What are the legal implications of extended nursing roles, *Professional Nurse,* 350, 1989.

Gostin L, Rassaby E: *Representing the mentally ill and handicapped: a guide to mental health review trbunals,* Sunbury, 1980, MIND.

# Research

## CHAPTER OUTLINE

**Scientific Research in Nursing**
*Acquiring knowledge*
*Nursing and the scientific method*
*Definitions of scientific and nursing research*
*Nursing research and the nursing process*
*Nurse researchers*

**Ethical Issues in Research**
*Rights of human subjects*
*Rights of other research participants*

**Nursing Research in Nursing Practice**
*Identifying research studies*
*Locating research studies*
*Critiquing research studies*
*Identifying clinical nursing problems*
*Using findings in nursing practice*

## LEARNING OUTCOMES

After studying this chapter, you should be able to:
- ■ *Define the key terms listed.*
- ■ *Compare the various ways to acquire knowledge.*
- ■ *List the characteristics of methods of investigation.*
- ■ *Compare methods for developing new nursing knowledge.*
- ■ *Define nursing research.*
- ■ *Compare the research process with the nursing process and discuss the core objectives of each.*
- ■ *Explain the rights of human research subjects.*
- ■ *Explain the rights of individuals who participate in human research studies.*
- ■ *Describe the components of a research report.*
- ■ *Discuss methods of locating research reports in nursing and related areas.*
- ■ *Explain how to critique a research article or report.*
- ■ *Describe the characteristics of an area of clinical nursing in which research may lead to improved patient/client care.*
- ■ *List the criteria for using research findings in nursing practice.*

Over the last 30 years, many nursing leaders and organizations have made considerable efforts to increase nurses' awareness of the importance of conducting nursing studies and using research as a foundation for practice.

In 1972 the Committee on Nursing stated that "... a sense of the need for research should become part of the mental equipment of every practising nurse or midwife". In 1986 the United Kingdom Central Council for Nursing, Midwifery and Health Visiting (UKCC) implemented Project 2000, an educational framework that supports the development of **research awareness**, **research-based practice** and development of the **'knowledgeable doer'** in all nurses. Until the 1970s, nursing studies focussed on the roles and characteristics of nurses rather than on problems in delivering professional care to patients/clients (Gortner, 1980). This has changed considerably over the last three decades, and a vast amount of research into crucial nursing problems is being pursued.

The impetus for increased interest in clinical nursing problems may have arisen in part from the *Code of Professional Conduct* (UKCC, 1992a). The Code states that each registered nurse, midwife and health visitor must ensure that no action or omission within their practice "... is detrimental to the interests, conditions or safety of patients and clients", that they should acknowledge any limitations in their knowledge and competence, and that they should " ... decline any duties or responsibilities unless able to perform them in a safe and skilled manner" (UKCC, 1992a).

The term *research* is not used explicitly, but it is implicit within these statements through the emphasis upon registered practitioners to ensure that they are **knowledgeable, competent,** and **skilled** in their actions, and that no omissions in the care of their patients/clients occurs.

A second document, *The Scope of Professional Practice* (UKCC, 1992b), was also published to support the UKCC *Code of*

*Professional Conduct*. This document made the use of research explicit by stating:

> The practice of nursing, midwifery and health visiting requires the application of knowledge and the simultaneous exercise of judgement and skill. Practice takes place in a context of continuing change and development. Such change and development may result from advances in research leading to improvements in treatment and care. . .

## SCIENTIFIC RESEARCH IN NURSING

### Acquiring Knowledge

Human beings acquire knowledge in many ways. A person continuously takes in and processes numerous pieces of information to understand experiences. The scientific researcher also seeks to explain or understand reality, but the scientist's process of acquiring knowledge is systematic and logical. This process, or scientific method, is the foundation of research. Scientific research is the most reliable and objective of all methods of gaining knowledge.

### Methods of Learning

**Tradition:** This type of learning occurs when one generation passes knowledge to the next. For example, children often learn about traditional holidays such as Christmas, Ramadan or Passover through traditional or customary family practices. In nursing, certain traditional methods of practice such as the change-of-shift report and other daily hospital work practices are passed from one practitioner to the next. Tradition is an efficient way of learning, although it can also limit the ability to seek new ways of doing things. If tradition becomes so ingrained that a person does not question the custom, then other, more appropriate or efficient ways may be overlooked.

**Actively seeking information:** Knowledge is also acquired by seeking information from experts in a particular field. Experts are often asked to solve problems or answer questions. For example, people often seek an accountant's help to fill out tax forms. Similarly, student nurses often seek the advice of nurse teachers and practising nurses when assessing and caring for patients/clients. Authority, like tradition, is not infallible, although it is commonly treated as absolute truth.

**Experience:** Without experience, a person would have to relearn a procedure every time it was performed. Practice leads to the development of routines that help build skills. For example, a student nurse taking a blood pressure measurement for the first time may feel awkward and unsure of hearing the sounds, but with practice the student's technique and confidence improve. Although experience is an important way of learning, it has limitations. A person may continue to do something simply because it was learned that way and may overlook improved or other ways of doing the same thing. If experience causes a person to learn something incorrectly, the person uses knowledge inappropriately.

**Trial and error**: This is yet another way of gaining knowledge. Making mistakes or repeatedly trying various ways of accomplishing something will eventually result in problem solving. This method of learning is practical, but it is unsystematic and often a haphazard way of learning. **In nursing, because patients'/clients' health status depends on nursing actions, trial and error is not an appropriate way of acquiring new knowledge.**

**Scientific method:** This is the most advanced, objective means of acquiring knowledge. It is characterized by systematic, orderly procedures that, although not without fault, seek to limit the possibility for error and minimize the likelihood that any bias or opinion by the researcher might influence the results of research and thus the knowledge gained. Polit and Hungler (1991) describe the characteristics of scientific investigation as follows:

1. The steps of planning and conducting an investigation are undertaken in a systematic, orderly fashion.

2. Scientists attempt to control external factors that are not under direct investigation but that can influence a relationship between phenomena they are studying. For example, if a scientist was studying the relationship between diet and heart disease, other characteristics such as stress would have to be eliminated as contributing factors to this disease.

3. Evidence that is part of reality **(empirical data)** is gathered directly or indirectly through use of the human senses and is the basis for discovering new knowledge.

4. The goal is to understand phenomena in such a way that the knowledge gained can be applied generally, not just to isolated cases or circumstances.

5. Scientists strive to conduct investigations that contribute to testing or developing theories, thereby advancing the knowledge that can be applied towards increasing understanding of people, places, or life events.

### Nursing and the Scientific Method

Compared with other ways of acquiring knowledge, the scientific method is more orderly and objective in its approach. Nurses use this approach to develop knowledge. In the past, much of the information used in nursing practice was borrowed from biology, physiology, psychology, and sociology. Often, this information was applied to nursing without testing or comparing ways for caring for patients/clients. For example, nurses use several methods to help a patient/client sleep. Interventions such as giving a person a warm drink, making sure that the bed is clean and comfortable, preparing the environment by dimming the lights, and talking to a worried or anxious patient/client are frequently used nursing measures and, in general, are logical, common-sense approaches. However, when these measures are considered in greater depth, questions may arise about their applications for different patients/clients in different situations.

Research provides a way for nursing questions and problems to be studied in greater depth. Frequently, nurses rely on personal experience or the statements of nursing experts. If an intervention works for most patients/clients, the nurse may be satisfied with this success without questioning whether there might be a better way. If the intervention is not successful, the nurse might use an approach practised by a colleague or try a different sequence of accepted measures. Even if an intervention discovered with this approach is effective for one or more patients/clients, it may not be appropriate for other patients/clients in other settings. Approaches need to be tested to determine the measures that work best with specific patients/clients.

## Definitions of Scientific and Nursing Research

According to Kerlinger (1986), **scientific research** is a systematic, controlled, empirical, and critical investigation of natural phenomena guided by theory and hypotheses about the presumed relations among such phenomena. Several factors affect scientific research. When scientists use systematic, controlled methods for studying events or problems, they have more confidence that the results are accurate and are not influenced by opinion or belief. These studies are well organized and follow a specific procedure. For a study to be empirical, the evidence collected must come from objective findings. In addition, other researchers should be able to examine the evidence and see the same **phenomena** (results). To guide the design of a research study, scientists create a hypothetical proposition **(hypothesis)** about what they expect to see before conducting the study. Finally, scientists generally study the way that characteristics or events are different or the way that one event causes another.

When reading research studies, nurses should avoid interpreting results in terms of cause and effect, because there is a difference between cause and effect and other kinds of relationships. For example, as people get older, they tend to lose their hair, and their skin becomes wrinkled. These factors are related to each other as part of the ageing process, but neither causes the other. Researchers often study such relationships without being able to determine why or how these changes take place.

**Biomedical research** is concerned mainly with discovering the causes and treatments of disease. In contrast, **nursing research** is directed towards helping well people improve their health status and stay healthy, as well as assisting patients/clients who are sick or disabled by an illness to maintain or improve their health. Nursing also focuses on the full range of human responses (which sometimes do not lend themselves to scientific methodology), rather than solely biological or physical responses.

Gortner identified the need to distinguish between 'nursing research' and 'research in nursing'. *Nursing research* is concerned with the process of caring and the problems encountered while practising nursing, while *research in nursing* is concerned with studying the nursing profession (Gortner, 1975). Reflecting upon Gortner's discussion and the definition of research offered by Kerlinger (1986), nursing research may be defined as: *the systematic and critical investigation of the process of caring and/or the problems met whilst practising nursing that may be explained by theory.*

The International Council of Nurses (1986) supports the need for nursing research as a means for improving the health and welfare of people. Nursing research is a way to identify new knowledge, improve professional education and practice, and use resources effectively. The effects of preoperative teaching on

> ### Children's Nursing
> ### Examples of research
> The effects of hospitalization on children have been studied extensively; Quinton and Rutter (1976), for example, found that multiple hospital admissions increased the risk of psychiatric problems later in life, and that this risk increased if the first admission occurred in the pre-school year.
> Experiments by Visitainer and Wolfer (1975), demonstrated that children who were prepared effectively for hospitalization through hospital tours, play activities and films, reacted more positively to the experience and were less anxious.
> Research has also shown that positive adaptive behaviour is facilitated when the child is well supported by parents (Sylva and Stein, 1990; Hawthorne, 1974; Hayes and Knox, 1984).

postoperative recovery, for example, is an area that has been studied extensively. Some of the earliest studies undertaken in the UK (Hayward, 1975; Boore, 1978) examined the responses of patients/clients to a surgical experience. Teaching patients/clients what they can expect on the day of surgery and in the immediate postoperative period is now a widely accepted and implemented nursing measure.

Because nurses are interested in acquiring knowledge about a wide range of human needs and responses to health problems, nursing research uses many methods to study clinical problems (see box on p.266).

The hallmark of scientific research is the experiment. In a true experimental study, the conditions under which a measure is investigated are tightly controlled. The study usually includes a control or **comparison group**, which does not receive the nursing measure being investigated. The results for this group are compared with those of a study or **experimental group**, the group that receives some form of treatment or intervention. The **subjects**, people selected for the comparison and experimental groups, are chosen at random from among those eligible for the study. Designing an experiment to study physical causes of disease is less difficult than designing an experiment that also includes psychological or social aspects of health. For example, to study the relationship between postoperative anxiety and preoperative teaching, the researcher can control one psychological factor by using only subjects having surgery for the first time. However, the researcher cannot control other experiences that the patients/clients may have had, such as hearing a friend's 'horror' stories about surgery or reading about surgical experiences in the newspapers. These psychological factors that cannot be controlled may influence the subject's level of anxiety.

Nursing studies use many methods for investigating clinical problems; some may be similar to the experimental approach. Other methods may be similar to those used in the social sciences, such as anthropology and sociology. The amount of knowledge known about the problem and the type of problem being investigated are some factors that determine the methods used. Nursing is a practice discipline that deals with unique physical, emotional, and social problems that people experience in regaining, maintaining, and promoting health. Carper (1978) describes the following patterns of knowing in nursing:

1. Empirics: the science of nursing.
2. Aesthetics: knowledge about the art of nursing.
3. Personal knowledge: concrete, experiential knowing.
4. Ethics: moral nursing knowledge.

Each pattern represents a necessary but incomplete approach to the problems that nurses face in clinical practice.

Experimental approaches to studying a problem require that the information about human subjects be collected and quantified in a prescribed manner. **Quantitative research** is concerned with *qualifying* or *measuring*, as the term suggests. Quantitative research attempts to demonstrate and present findings as numbers, frequencies and statistics (Cormack, 1991). **Qualitative research** is concerned with the nature of something and explores individual situations, incidents and phenomena (Cormack, 1991). Knowledge collected through qualitative research methods does not involve the statistical organization and interpretation of information; rather it involves the discovery of important *characteristics* and the way that these might be related. For example, a qualitative research study might involve interviews assessing patients'/clients' perceptions of a teaching programme. Findings would not prove that one method of teaching is better than another. Yet data would reveal perceived characteristics of the programme. When qualitative methods are used, the investigator uses first-hand strategies such as open-ended interviews, observation, and case histories to study people under natural conditions as they are dealing with the reality of their health situation.

There are many terms used within research reports, journals and books that become more familiar as an individual's knowledge of research increases. It is beyond the scope of this chapter to define them all; however, there are three terms that should be considered at this point.

**Generalization** refers to the researcher's ability to make general statements concerning the application of their findings to the general population. The extent to which this can be claimed is dependent upon the size of the sample, how representative this sample is in relation to the general population, and how clearly all aspects of the research are reported.

**Reliability** refers to the extent to which the findings of particular tools and techniques would have been produced by a different researcher or a different sample of subjects.

**Validity**, a term which is as important as reliability, refers to the extent that a particular research technique is able to measure or describe what it is supposed to measure or describe (Bell, 1987).

## Nursing Research and the Nursing Process

The **research process** (Seaman, 1987; Abdellah and Levine, 1986) consists of phases or steps that can be compared and contrasted with those of the nursing process. Both are problem-solving processes used by nurses in practice (Table 14.1), but they are very different. The nursing process is used to determine health needs and plan nursing care for patients/clients. It is used as a basis for gaining and using information about patients/clients

---

## Types of Research

**HISTORICAL RESEARCH**
Systematic collection and critical evaluation of data relating to past events

**EXPLORATORY RESEARCH**
Initial study designed to develop or refine research questions or to test and refine data-collection methods

**EVALUATION RESEARCH**
Study that tests how well a programme, practice, or policy is working

**DESCRIPTIVE RESEARCH**
Study in which the objective is to accurately identify characteristics of persons, situations, or groups and the frequency with which certain events or characteristics occur

**EXPERIMENTAL RESEARCH**
Study in which the investigator controls the independent variable and randomly assigns subjects to different conditions

**QUASI EXPERIMENTAL RESEARCH**
Study in which subjects cannot be randomly assigned to treatment conditions, although the researcher controls the independent variables

**CORRELATIONAL RESEARCH**
Study that explores the inter-relationships among variables of interest without any active intervention by the researcher

---

to help them restore, maintain, or promote health (see Chapter 3). Depending on the nursing assessment, knowledge from a number of disciplines may be used in the nursing process to help patients/clients solve particular health problems.

In contrast, the research process is used to gain knowledge that can be used in other, similar situations. Nurses may want to learn why a particular event happens, or the best way to provide care for patients/clients with a certain health problem. The research process is used to gain knowledge that can be applied to a whole group or class of patients/clients.

During assessment, the nurse caring for a patient/client with sleeping difficulties determines factors that might interfere with the ability to sleep. These may include the patient's/client's concern about health status, pain, a noisy environment, or a messy or uncomfortable bed. After assessing these aspects, the nurse formulates patient/client goals, plans interventions, implements these interventions, and evaluates the subjective and objective evidence that indicates whether the patient/client is able to sleep.

In contrast, a researcher studying sleeping difficulties seeks new information that can be applied to more than one patient/client. For example, a nurse notices that many patients/clients seem to have a difficult time sleeping the night before a particular diagnostic procedure. Based on work with these patients/clients, the nurse determines that most of them express concerns about the results of the test. In this situation the

## TABLE 14-1 Comparison of Phases of the Nursing Process and the Research Process

| Nursing Process | Research Process |
|---|---|
| Assessment | Select the topic and identify the research problem. |
| | Formulate a summary of the proposed research. |
| | Review the literature for theory and other related studies. |
| | Define concepts and variables to be studied. |
| | Determine ethical implications of the proposed study. |
| | Identify assumptions and limitations. |
| Planning | State hypotheses about expected observation or questions to be studied. |
| | Describe the research design and methods for data collection. |
| | Define the study population and sample. |
| | Determine how to process, analyse, and summarize data. |
| | Plan for communicating findings. |
| Implementation | Collect data from subjects. |
| Evaluation | Analyse and interpret data. |
| | Communicate findings in written and other forms. |

Data from Seaman CH: *Research methods: principles, practice and theory for nursing,* Norwalk, 1987, Appleton-Century-Crofts; Abdellah FG, Levine E: *Better patient care through nursing research* , ed 3, New York, 1986, Macmillan.

nurse might design a research study in which some of the patients/clients receive the usual nursing care and others receive care based on relieving anxiety. After collecting information about the effects of the usual care for one group and the new approach for the other, the nurse researcher compares the results to determine whether patients/clients who received the new care had less difficulty sleeping than those who received the normal care. If the patients/clients receiving the new care slept better, the nurse has acquired new knowledge about how generally to help patients/clients.

### Nurse Researchers

In 1993 the Department of Health published the *Report of the Taskforce on the Strategy for Research in Nursing, Midwifery and Health Visiting*. This document was to provide a basis for discussion and action. Four key issues were identified:

1. Research and development priorities
2. Research education and training
3. Dissemination and implementation of research findings
4. Careers in research.

Although this report does not specify particular research priorities, it states that two objectives must be pursued simultaneously. These objectives are "to facilitate more and better research into nursing" and "to enhance the research skills and experience of nurses, health visitors and midwives so as to increase their involvement in research in nursing... " (Department of Health, 1993).

Nurses conduct research in a variety of settings, including institutions, such as hospitals, and within the community in

clients' homes. Student nurses and practitioners may be asked to participate in studies that investigate patient/client outcomes and the effectiveness of nursing care. Data are collected to determine the impact that nurses have on achievement of patient/client care objectives in a particular clinical setting. Since the results of such research are usually applicable only in one institution, this is not scientific research as discussed earlier. However, such research is important to the institution because the nursing department can use it to demonstrate the contributions made by nurses to patient/client care.

Clinical nursing research should be undertaken by nurses trained to conduct scientific investigations. Generally, nurse researchers hold master's and doctoral degrees. A student nurse asked to participate in a nursing study as a subject or by collecting data is entitled to receive information about the qualifications of the person conducting the study. The researcher's educational background and biographical details give some information about the person's qualifications. An experienced researcher is usually more qualified to undertake a complex, long-term project than an inexperienced researcher. Nurses new to research may, however, make important contributions by assisting with data collection, conducting replicated studies (studies previously performed elsewhere), or by conducting less complex studies.

## ETHICAL ISSUES IN RESEARCH

### Rights of Human Subjects

There may be occasions when research may conflict with the purpose of nursing practice, which is to meet specific patients'/clients' needs. In such cases the researcher is responsible

## Research in Nursing: Support for education and training

There are currently three main sources of support for training and education in nursing research:

**Department of Health**: offers **nursing research studentships** for graduate nurses to pursue full-time postgraduate study, and **postdoctoral nursing fellowships** for research in health services. Both types of awards are offered annually and are advertised in the professional press.

**Economic Social Research Council (ESRC)**: provides research and training opportunities aimed at social scientists. However, it offers two types of studentships that are relevant to the nursing professions: 1) **advanced coursework** studentships, in which students pursue a master's course and 2) **research studentships**, in which students pursue a doctorate.

**Medical Research Council**: offers postgraduate training for medical sciences, including **advanced course studentships, research studentships** and **appointments to MRC research units**. It also offers **senior clinical fellowship schemes**, designed for clinicians planning careers in academic medicine, and the **senior research leave fellowship**, which enables academic staff who are permanently employed in universities to concentrate on a research project for two or three years.

Funding for research and training is also available through higher education institutions, as well as through commercial, public sector, and charitable sponsorships.

Adapted from: Royal College of Nursing, *Strategy for Research in nursing, midwifery and health visiting*, London, 1993, Royal College of Nursing.

## Summary of Guidelines for Undertaking Research from the Royal College of Nursing

- The research must be necessary to contribute to knowledge or extend knowledge that is already available
- informed consent must be obtained from the subject, their relative, or their legal guardian
- the subjects must be assured protection against physical, mental, emotional or social injury
- confidentiality or restriction on the use of information must be assured and adhered to
- the researcher should seek advice on the ethical aspects of the research and where necessary must seek the approval of the appropriate ethics committee
- the researcher must possess the knowledge and skills compatible with the demands of the investigation, must make the results available and where possible prevent their misuse
- the researcher has the responsibility for the advancement of the theory and methods of the science in which he or she is working
- those learning to do research must work only under the guidance of an experienced researcher.

for structuring the investigation to avoid or minimize harm to the subjects. Although it is not always possible to anticipate all potential undesirable effects, researchers are obligated to inform everyone involved about the known potential risks.

The Royal College of Nursing (RCN) produced guidelines for nurses undertaking research, those in positions of authority and those practising in places where research is carried out (RCN, 1977) (see box).

**Informed consent** means that research subjects are (1) given full and complete information about the purpose of the study, procedures, data collection, potential harm and benefits, and alternative methods of treatment; (2) capable of fully understanding the research and the implications of participation; and (3) assured of free choice in giving consent, including the right to withdraw from the study at any time.

**Confidentiality** means that the privacy of subjects will be respected. Anonymity (refusal to disclose one's name) is often used to ensure privacy and, if promised, must be respected.

Not all research undertaken in clinical areas involves experimentation with human subjects. Research that does not use a new treatment with subjects may involve minimal or no risk to patients/clients. For example, a survey designed to measure patients'/clients' perceptions of stress in intensive care units holds little risk for participants. Nonetheless, a major responsibility of the **ethics committee** is to determine the risk status of all research projects. The nurse's responsibility is to protect the

patients'/clients' rights at all times.

Ethics committees work in different ways and usually include various health professionals within their membership. Some include a lay member to represent the views of the public. These committees review proposals for research with the primary purpose of protecting the potential subjects.

## Rights of Other Research Participants

Student and practising nurses may be asked to participate in research as data collectors or may be involved in the care of patients/clients participating in a study. All participants, including health care professionals caring for patients/clients, have the right to be fully informed about the study, its procedures (including informed consent and risk factors), and any physical or emotional injury that patients/clients could experience as a result of participation. Often the physical risks are more obvious than the emotional risks. Depending on the problem being studied, patients/clients may be asked to give highly personal and intrusive information. Because this type of research can lead to anxiety or stress for some individuals, the researcher should prepare all participants, including nurses delivering care, for this possibility and assist them in coping with the effects. Any student, nurse, or other participant has the right to refuse to carry out any research procedures if concerned about their ethical aspects.

Besides dealing with the harmful effects of a research project, nurses may be faced with other ethical dilemmas (Brink and Wood, 1988). For example, some people may feel they have to participate in an investigation to please the health care professionals on whom they depend for care. They may feel that they will receive inferior care if they refuse to participate. **Research ethics** require that patients/clients should not be made to feel that they are obliged to participate in a study. The ultimate decision rests with the person. Withholding proper care or in any way implying that care will be withheld from those who refuse to participate is unethical.

Another ethical dilemma in research involves withholding a new intervention from individuals who might benefit from its use. In an experiment investigating a new intervention, for example, the experimental group may receive the new intervention while the comparison group receives the usual care. In such cases, patients/clients in the comparison group are deprived of a new treatment that could be beneficial to them. One way of managing this dilemma is to offer the new nursing care to the comparison group after data necessary to the experimental study have been collected.

## NURSING RESEARCH IN NURSING PRACTICE

### Identifying Research Studies

When reading nursing literature, the practising or student nurse must be able to differentiate a research report or article from other types of writing. This may not be as simple as it seems. Even if the title has the word *research* in it, the article does not necessarily report the results of a research study. The nurse can determine whether an article reports a research study only by examining its contents.

Sometimes, however, an article's title can give a clue to its contents. Phrases such as *a study of* or *comparison of* suggest a research report. The abstract and the introductory paragraphs of an article can also indicate whether the article is based on research. An **abstract** is a short summary of the purpose of a study, the subjects included in the research, the way the study was conducted, and the results obtained in the investigation. An abstract is often very brief and does not contain all essential information from the article. The first few paragraphs of the article should provide further clues about whether it describes a research study. Phrases such as *the purpose of this study was* and *this research was carried out to determine* are indications that the article is a research report. If the article describes only the author's experience with a particular aspect of nursing care, it probably is not a research article. In addition to the abstract, a typical research report has the following parts:

1. **Introduction:** an introductory section presenting the purpose, a summary of literature used to formulate the study, and the hypotheses tested.

---

### Finding Research Articles: What Resources Are Available?

#### Journal Indexes
**Cumulative Index to Nursing and Allied Health Literature (CINAHL):** published bimonthly, contains listings from over 300 English-language nursing and allied health journals. Also available as a computerized database, e.g. CD ROM.

**International Nursing Index:** published four times a year, contains listings from over 200 nursing journals from around the world.

**Index Medicus:** an international index published monthly, includes listings from approximately 2900 biomedical journals, including about 60 nursing journals.

**Nursing Research Abstracts:** a quarterly journal of abstracts included in the DHSS Index of Nursing Research (see below).

#### Computerized Indexes and Literature Search Services
**Index of Nursing Research:** an on-line database (DHSS-Data) provided by the Department of Health/Department of Social Security library. Includes abstracts of research about nurses/nursing or conducted by nurses.

**ENB Health Care Database:** a database of support materials for nursing education

**MEDLINE:** a database available through the Medical Literature Analysis and Retrieval System (MEDLARS). Information in this system is retrieved from Index Medicus and the International Nursing Index.

**Nursing Practice Database:** contains data from nurses and midwives in the NHS on best practice. Available from the DHS.

#### Journals
*Advances in Nursing Science*
*Applied Nursing Research*
*International Journal of Nursing Studies*

*Journal of Advanced Nursing*
*Nursing Research*
*Research in Nursing and Health*
*Western Journal of Nursing Research*

#### Libraries and Other Facilities
The British Library Medical Information Service
Document Supply Centre
Boston Spa
Wetherby
West Yorkshire LS23 7BQ

ENB Resource and Careers Service
Woodseats House
764 Chesterfield Road
Sheffield S8 0SE

Health Visitors Association Library
50 Southwark Street
London SE1 1UN

Kings Fund Institute
126 Albert Street
London NW1 7NF

MIDIRS Midwives Information and Resources Service
9 Elmdale Road
Clifton
Bristol BS8 1SL

Royal College of Midwives Library
15 Mansfield Street
London W1M 0BE

Royal College of Nursing Library
20 Cavendish Square
London W1M 0AB

---

2. **Methods:** description of the methods used to conduct the study, including the sample (what or who was studied), and to collect data, including the device or instrument used to measure empirical information.
3. **Results:** description of the results obtained in the study, including any statistical tests used to analyse data.
4. **Discussion:** presentation of the author's interpretation of the results, including conclusions and implications that can be drawn from the study.
5. **Reference list:** articles used to support the study's methodology.

If the report is written by one of the researchers in the study, it is a **primary source**. Any other article about the study is considered a **secondary source** (for example, an article in which the author was not directly involved in conducting the study but collected the information from a primary or another secondary source). Most nursing textbooks are secondary sources of information. Authors of these texts incorporate knowledge and information gathered from nursing and related literature, including research written by original investigators.

The fact that a report is a primary source does not guarantee its accuracy, which depends on the ability of researchers to be scientific, impersonal, and impartial in conducting studies. However, a primary source does report firsthand knowledge, whereas a secondary source may include another person's interpretation of the original work.

## Locating Research Studies

Students and practising nurses often need to find research articles on subjects that interest them. In the health care field, a number of resources are useful when searching the literature for research articles (see box).

To locate primary research sources related to a particular subject, the first source is the journals where original research reports are usually published. The most efficient way to locate research articles is to consult an **index of journal articles**. These indexes are generally found in reference sections of medical and nursing libraries. Each index uses a list of key words that form subject headings and subheadings: article listings are grouped or organized under these headings. For example, a person might find subject headings such as *pain* or *primary nursing*, whereas subheadings might include *physiology* or *history* respectively. An author listing is also available, making it possible to find articles published during a certain time period by a particular person. Articles on a particular subject are found by first checking the subject headings to see whether the key term listed in the index matches the subject. The key term listing may also lead to other subject groupings that contain articles similar in content. Using an index may at first seem time consuming, but it is generally faster than looking through many journals trying to find articles pertinent to the subject.

Many nursing and medical libraries provide computerized searches for articles. A list of articles and abstracts is transmitted over telephone lines within hours of being requested. Computer searches generally involve a user's fee. Reference librarians have

information about this type of resource.

Some nursing journals publish research studies. Although not all articles published in these journals are research reports, most issues are devoted to primary reports of nursing studies. Other nursing journals also publish original reports of research studies. For example, *Heart and Lung,* a specialty journal, often includes research reports. Recently, more specialty practice journals appear to be publishing research articles.

Secondary literature sources such as books can be helpful in finding primary research sources. Student nurses seeking research articles should use reference lists or bibliographies at the end of textbook chapters. To document the scientific basis for their writing, authors frequently cite primary sources as references, and these references are a valuable resource for student nurses who want more information.

## Critiquing Research Studies

**Critiquing** research means reviewing it and making judgements about its strengths, weaknesses and value. This process helps nurses identify whether the research study has implications for nursing practice. Many books and journals discuss reading and reviewing using a variety of approaches (Cormack, 1991; Hawthorn, 1983; Morrison, 1991; Polit and Hungler, 1991; Treece and Treece, 1986). The particular format or plan for the critique may vary, but there are certain areas that should always be covered. Here, we will use Cormack's (1991) suggested format with the addition of one area (data analysis):

**Title:** This should clearly indicate the content, but should be concise and informative.

**Author(s):** The author's professional and academic background should be explored, identifying whether they have the appropriate experience and qualifications to undertake such a study. For example, have they clinical experience within the field they are exploring? The place of employment is also useful when exploring whether the research was undertaken through practice related interest, as part of the researchers' role, or whether the research was sponsored.

**Abstract:** This provides a brief overview of the research and enables you to decide whether the research is useful prior to reviewing the entire piece of research study.

**Introduction:** This should provide a clear synopsis of the problem, the rationale for undertaking the study, and any limitations to the study.

**Literature Review:** This should present strengths and weaknesses of previous research studies, and should support the rationale for this study. Literature reviews should progress from general issues to the specific issue of the study. The date of the previous studies published should be considered and, if the references are dated, the author should provide some discussion of this. A complete literature review should not omit any topic of the research.

**The Hypothesis:** If the use of a hypothesis is appropriate it should be clearly stated in terminology that enables the hypothesis to be tested.

**Operational Definitions:** The author(s) should clearly define any terms used within the research that may be ambiguous. This prevents misinterpretation and confusion.

**Methodology:** This should provide a clear discussion of the research approach chosen and its appropriateness to the research study. This should be supported by relevant literature.

**Subjects:** It is important that enough detail about the research subjects is provided in order for the findings to be judged as applicable to a particular problem or patient/client group. This should include information such as age, sex, race and culture.

**Sample Selection:** Information about the size of the sample and how it was chosen are also important in judging the value of the research findings. Any criteria for selection or omission should also be indicated.

**Data Collection:** The methods of data collection should be clearly stated, and should be compatible with the methodology chosen and the information being sought. A discussion of validity and reliability should be provided and whether instruments used have been pilot tested.

**Ethical Considerations:** All research reports should have a discussion of the ethical issues. This should include consent of participants, approval from the ethics committee, confidentiality, and anonymity.

**Data Analysis:** The methods of data analysis should be presented, should indicate how the data are to be used, and should indicate whether the data were analysed by hand or using equipment such as computers.

**Results:** Results from the study should be clearly and logically presented. The results presented should also provide answers to all the research questions identified. If statistical tests have been used, these should be appropriate to the study.

**Discussion:** All the results are discussed, drawing upon the relevant literature and identifying their implications to the study. The discussion should be objective, should identify limitations or weaknesses in the study, and should provide suggestions for improvements in the study.

**Conclusions:** The conclusions arise from the discussion and should be supported by the results. Conclusions that have not arisen from the data should be omitted.

**Recommendations:** This section usually has two purposes: 1) to indicate the implications of the findings to practice and 2) to recommend further study that is needed in relation to the whole topic or to an aspect that has been highlighted within the study.

Learning to find and read nursing research studies is not a simple task, but nursing research is based on principles of logic, and with a thoughtful approach, the nursing student can learn to understand and evaluate nursing research studies.

## Identifying Clinical Nursing Problems

Diers (1979) defined a **clinical nursing problem** as "a difference between two states of affairs: a discrepancy between the way things are and the way they ought to be, or between what one knows and what one needs to know to eliminate the problem". The following questions are raised by this definition:

1. Given the nursing interventions recommended for patients/clients with a particular health care problem, how might the suggested care be improved so that the results or outcomes of care are better?

2. Given the knowledge about how to provide nursing care, what additional information would be needed to plan new interventions for individuals with a particular health care problem?

Unanswered questions and the desire to improve nursing practice can provide the stimulus for conducting a research study.

Experience can make it possible to identify a researchable clinical nursing problem, but a nurse does not need to have years of clinical practice to identify a nursing problem. Sometimes a person who is relatively new in a situation can more easily see how things could be improved than those who have more experience and who take present conditions for granted. The nurse also considers whether the problem frequently occurs in a particular patient/client group, whether it can be consistently and accurately measured, and whether a possible nursing solution might change the way care is delivered (Fuller, 1982).

Sometimes student nurses or practising nurses think their ideas about nursing problems for study are not worthwhile unless they are certain that the proposed clinical study would make a radical change in patient/client care. However, research efforts also may have to refine ideas about a clinical problem before the investigator can test alternative nursing interventions. In fact, some nurse researchers think that more investigative work needs to be done to describe the patient/client response before research is designed to test an alternative intervention. In addition, the researcher may have to devise correct ways for measuring results before the study can proceed. All these factors may discourage a nurse from undertaking a nursing research project. On the other hand, such projects can be viewed as stimulating challenges because much information has yet to be scientifically tested for its relevance to nursing practice.

## Using Findings in Nursing Practice

To use findings in clinical practice, the nurse must be aware of the problems already studied. Therefore nurses should read journals that contain research reports, as well as textbooks and other sources, in nursing and related fields.

Not all research related to clinical nursing problems can or should be applied in practice. The nurse must judge the *scientific worth* of a study before considering its use in practice. This chapter can provide only a foundation for judging the worth of a research study. Other aspects that should be considered follow (Stetler and Marram, 1976; Stetler, 1985):

1. The amount of substantiating evidence provided by other scientific studies that have obtained similar results.

2. Determination of whether the subjects and environment in the study are similar to the clients for whom the nurse provides care in the particular practice setting.

3. The theoretical basis for present nursing care and the effectiveness of current theory in solving clinical nursing problems.

4. The feasibility of applying findings, including ethical and legal limitations, institutional policy, changes in the organization of nursing services that might be required, and potential costs in time, money, and equipment.

The nurse must make judgements that involve validating the scientific soundness of a study, comparatively evaluating whether any use can be made of the findings, and deciding on the type of application that would be appropriate (Stetler, 1985).

In order for nursing research to have a positive impact upon practice there needs to be identification of a clinical nursing problem (Morse and Conrad, 1983). The problem area chosen must have an established research base, be relevant to practice, and be reliably evaluated by nurses in clinical settings. When selecting the problem area, the nurse is concerned with whether a solid research base exists for changing practice, the scientific merit of the studies that constitute the research base, and the potential risk to the patient/client in implementing the practice change. The final phases include developing a clinical protocol that can be used to implement the change and clinically evaluating the outcomes of the new nursing care to determine its effectiveness.

Nurses often participate in quality assurance (QA) or quality improvement (QI) studies that evaluate the processes and outcomes (results) of nursing care (see Chapter 3). These studies measure how well nursing interventions are being implemented with specific patients/clients by examining expected outcomes related to the nursing process protocols and procedures of a specific setting.

The knowledge base developed by investigators provides a means for examining nursing measures and outcomes. By examining the quality of care provided for patients/clients in their own setting and changing care as needed, based on knowledge developed in studies, nurses can use research to improve the quality of care.

Nurses should not change from accepted to unproven ways of providing patient/client care without careful deliberation and consultation with colleagues. Experimenting with new nursing measures is inappropriate, especially if an increased risk to the patients'/clients' health is possible.

Some people estimate that the half-life of knowledge in the health care field is about five years. This means that half of what nurses learn today may be out of date in five years. By developing skills necessary to read and understand nursing research studies, nurses can remain up to date throughout their careers.

## SUMMARY

Research is an essential part of the nursing process because it is an advanced, objective method of gaining new knowledge about human needs and people's responses to illness, treatments, therapies, and other health-related factors. The research process, a problem-solving method, involves a number of phases from the identification of a problem through the development and testing of hypotheses to the analysis, interpretation, and communication of findings. To gain new knowledge in a variety of nursing areas, nurses conduct clinical research in many settings, involving many kinds of research subjects whose rights must carefully be protected.

Nurses indirectly involved in conducting research also gain from nursing research findings. Nurses therefore must develop skills for locating and identifying research studies and for organizing research information for clinical application. The successful use of research findings in practice depends on the skills of the nurse to judge the scientific worth of a study, determine whether findings can be applied to a particular clinical setting and group of patients/clients, and consider other practical issues such as ethical implications, institutional policies, and implementation costs. These skills are important for all nurses because of the continuously evolving nursing knowledge base needed to practise professional nursing in all settings.

## CHAPTER 14 REVIEW
### Key Concepts

- People acquire knowledge through tradition, from authorities in a field, through experience, by trial and error, and through application of the scientific method.
- The scientific method is the most objective method of gaining new knowledge.
- A scientific investigation is an orderly, planned, and controlled way of studying reality that can be applied to general situations and contributes to the testing of theories about people, places, or life events.
- Nursing research is conducted to study the physical or psychosocial responses of people of all ages in health and illness.
- An experimental research study controls factors that could influence the results, includes comparison and experimental treatment groups of subjects, and uses random means for selecting study subjects.
- A qualitative research study organizes information in narrative format so that phenomena can be described and patterns of relationships can be discovered.
- Participation of human subjects in research studies requires the researcher to obtain informed consent of study subjects, maintain the confidentiality of subjects, and protect subjects from undue risk or injury.
- The researcher conducting a study is required to inform all people assisting in the study about the purposes of the research and to prepare them for any adverse effects the subjects could experience.
- Research reports are most commonly found in specialized journals.
- A number of indexes for the health care field are available for finding research articles.
- A critique of a piece of research should enable the nurse to identify when, how, where and by whom the study was undertaken, and who and what was studied. It should also enable the nurse to judge the strengths, weaknesses and value to practice of the study.
- A researchable clinical nursing problem is one that is not satisfactorily resolved by present nursing interventions, occurs frequently in a particular group, can be consistently and accurately measured, and has a possible solution within the realm of nursing practice.
- To determine whether research findings can be used as a basis for nursing practice, the nurse should consider the scientific

worth of the study, the substantiating evidence provided in other studies, the similarity of the research setting to the nurse's own clinical practice setting, the status of current nursing theory, and factors affecting the feasibility of application.

## CRITICAL THINKING EXERCISES

1. A nurse is concerned about learning to properly clean a pressure ulcer. Explain the benefits to the patient/client if the nurse learns how to clean the ulcer by the scientific method versus trial and error.

2. Consider research into the 'nurse-patient/client' relationship from the perspective of using the following methods:
   (i) an experimental approach
   (ii) an observation/participation approach
   (iii) a survey approach.

3. If you were participating in a study that tested a new medication, what information do you believe should be included in order to obtain a patient's/client's consent?

4. If you thought a piece of research could be valuable to your practice discuss how you would be able to justify its use to your colleagues. What specific points would you need to document?

## Key Terms

Abstract, p. 269
Comparison group, p. 265
Confidentiality, p. 268
Critiquing, p. 270
Empirical data, p. 264
Ethics committee, p. 268
Experimental group, p. 265

Generalization, p. 266
Hypothesis, p. 265
Index of journal articles, p. 270
Informed consent, p. 268
Knowledgeable doer, p. 263
Phenomena, p. 265
Primary source, p. 270
Qualitative research, p. 266
Quantitative research, p. 266

Reliability, p. 266
Research awareness, p. 263
Research ethics, p. 268
Research process, p. 266
Research-based practice, p. 263
Secondary source, p. 270
Subjects, p. 265
Validity, p. 266

## REFERENCES

Abdellah FG, Levine E: *Better patient care though nursing research*, ed 3, New York, 1986, Macmillan.

Bell J: *Doing your research project: a guide for first-term researchers in education and social science*, Milton Keynes, 1987, Open University Press.

Boore J: *Prescription for recovery*, London, 1978, Royal College of Nursing.

Brink PJ, Wood MJ: *Basic steps in planning nursing research: from question to proposal*, ed 3, North Scituate, 1988, Duxbury Press.

Carper BA: Fundamental patterns of knowing in nursing, *ANS* 1:13, 1978.

Cormack DFS: *The research process in nursing*, ed 2, Oxford, 1991, Blackwell Scientific.

Department of Health: *Report of the taskforce on the strategy for research in nursing, midwifery and health visiting*, London, 1993, DOH.

Diers D: *Research in nursing practice*, Philadelphia, 1979, Lippincott.

Fuller ED: Selecting a clinical nursing problem, *Image* 14: 60, 1982.

Gortner SR: Research for a practice profession, *Nurs Res* 24(3): 193, 1975.

Gortner SR: Nursing research: out of the past and into the future, *Nurs Res* 29:204, 1980.

Hawthorn PJ: Principles of research: a checklist, *Nurs Times* 79(23):40, 1983.

Hawthorn PJ: *Nurse – I want my mummy*, London, 1974, Royal College of Nursing.

Hayes V, Knox J: The experience of stress in parents of children hospitalised with long-term disabilities, *J Adv Nurs* 9(4):333, 1984.

Hayward J: *Information – a prescription against pain*, London, 1975, Royal College of Nursing.

International Council of Nurses: *Nursing research: ICN position statement*, Geneva, 1986, The Council.

Kerlinger FN: *Foundations of behavioural research*, ed 3, New York 1986, Holt, Rinehart & Winston.

Morrison P: Critiquing research, *Surg Nurs* 4(3):20, 1991.

Morse JM, Conrad A: Putting research into practice, *Canadian Nurs* 79(8):40, 1983.

Polit DV, Hungler BP: *Nursing research: principals and practice*, ed 4, Philadelphia, 1991, Lippincott.

Royal College of Nursing: *Ethics related to research in nursing*, London, 1977, RCN.

Royal College of Nursing: *Strategy for research in nursing, midwifery and health visiting*, London, 1993, RCN.

Quinton D, Rutter M: Early hospital admissions of later disturbance of behaviour; an attempted replication of Douglas' findings, *Dev Med Child Neurol*, 18:447, 1976.

Seaman CH: *Research methods: principles, practice and theory for nursing*, Norwalk, 1987, Appleton-Century-Crofts.

Stetler C: Research utilization: defining the concept, *Image* 17:40, 1985.

Stetler CB, Marram G: Evaluating research findings for applicability in practice, *Nurs Outlook* 25:559, 1976.

Sylva K, Stein A: Effects of hospitalisation on young children, *Child Psychol Psychiatr Newsletter* 12(1):3, 1990.

Treece EW, Treece JW: *Elements of research in nursing*, ed 4, St Louis, 1986, Mosby.

United Kingdom Central Council for Nursing, Midwifery and Health Visiting: *Code of professional conduct*, ed 3, London, 1992a, UKCC.

United Kingdom Central Council for Nursing, Midwifery and Health Visiting: *The scope of professional practice*, London, 1992b, UKCC.

Visitainer H, Wolfer J: Psychological preparation for surgical paediatric patients: the effects on children's and parent's stress responses and adjustments, *Paediatrics* 52(2):107, 1975.

## FURTHER READING
### Adult Nursing

Armitage S: Research utilisation in practice, *Nurs Education Today* 10:10, 1990.

Bergman R (editor): *Nursing research for nursing practice: an international perspective*, London, 1990, Chapman & Hall.

Bostram AC et al: Staff nurses' attitudes towards nursing research: a descriptive survey, *J Adv Nurs* 14:915, 1989.

Brett JL: Use of nursing practice research findings, *Nurs Res* 36(6): 344, 1987.

Clark E: *Research awareness: module 2 sources of nursing knowledge*, London, 1987, Distance Learning Centre.

Clark JM, Hockey L (editors): *Further research for nursing: a new guide for the enquiring nurse*, London, 1989, Scutari.

Clifford C, Gough S: *Nursing research – a skills based introduction*, London, 1990, Prentice Hall.

Ford JS, Reutter LI: Ethical dilemmas associated with small samples, *J Adv Nurs* 15:187, 1990.

Glaser BG, Strauss AL: *The discovery of grounded theory: strategies for qualitative research*, Chicago, 1967, Aldine Press.

Hagell EI: Nursing knowledge: a woman's knowledge, a sociological perspective, *J Adv Nurs* 14:226, 1989.

Hunt M: The process of translating research findings into nursing practice, *J Adv Nurs* 12:101, 1987.

Meyer JE: New paradigm research in practice: the trials and tribulations of action research, *J Adv Nurs* 18(7):1066, 1993.

Moser CA, Kalton G: *Survey methods in social investigation*, London, 1971, Heinemann Educational.

Norton PG et al (editors): *Primary care research: traditional and innovative approaches*, London, 1991, Sage Publications Ltd.

Pollack L, Tilley S: Submitting for approval, *Senior Nurs* 8(5):24, 1988.

Seaman CCH, Verhonick PJ: *Research methods for undergraduate students in nursing*, New York, 1982, Appleton-Century-Croft.

Sims J: Nursing research: is there an obligation on subjects to participate? *J Adv Nurs* 16(11):1284, 1991.

Walsh M, Ford P: *Nursing rituals: research and rational practice*, London, 1989, Heinemann.

Webb C: Action research: philosophy, methods and personal experiences, *J Adv Nurs* 14: 403, 1989.

## Children's Nursing

Department of Health: *Overview of research in the provision and utilisation of the child health services*, London, 1984, HMSO.

Hawthorn PJ: *Nurse – I want my mummy*, London, 1974, Royal College of Nursing.

Hayes V, Knox J: The experience of stress in parents of children hospitalised with long-term disabilities, *J Adv Nurs* 9(4): 333, 1984.

Nicholson H: Medical research with children, in *Ethics, law and practice*. Oxford, 1986, Oxford University Press.

Roche S, Stacy M: *Overview of research on the care of children in hospital*, Warwick, 1992, University of Warwick.

Sylva K, Stein A: Effects of hospitalisation on young children, *Child Psychol Psychiatr Newsletter* 12(1):3, 1990.

Weithorn L, Campbell S: The competence of children and adolescents to make informed treatment decision, *Child Dev* 53:1589, 1982.

## Learning Disabilities Nursing

Atkinson D: Research interviews with people with mental handicaps, *Ment Handicap Res* 1(1):75, 1988.

Atkinson D, Williams F, editors: *Know me as I am – an anthology of prose, poetry and art by people with learning difficulties*, London, 1990, Hodder & Stoughton.

Brechin A, Walmsley J: *Making connections: reflecting on the lives and experiences of people with learning difficulties*, London, 1989, Hodder & Stoughton.

Flynn M: Adults who are mentally handicapped as consumers: issues and guidelines for interviewing, *J Ment Deficiency Res* 30:369, 1986.

Law Commission: *Mentally incapacitated adults and decision making: a new jurisdiction*. Consultation paper no. 128, London, 1993, HMSO.

Siegelman CK et al: When in doubt, say yes: acquiescence in interviews with mentally retarded persons, *Ment Retard* 19:53, 1981.

Wilkinson J. 'Being there': a way to evaluate life quality, starting with a person's feelings and daily experience. In Brechin A, Walmsley J, editors: *Making connections*, London, 1990, Hodder & Stoughton.

## Mental Health Nursing

Brooking J (editor): *Psychiatric nursing research*, Chichester, 1986, John Wiley & Sons.

Littlewood, R: Psychiatric diagnosis and racial bias, *Soc Sci Med* 34:2,141, 1992.

Pollack L: *Community psychiatric nursing, myth or reality*, Harrow, 1989, Scutari.

Reason P, Rowan J (editors): *Human inquiry: a source book of new paradigm research*, Chichester, 1981, John Wiley & Sons.

# Communication

## CHAPTER OUTLINE

## LEARNING OUTCOMES

After studying this chapter, you should be able to:
- Define the key terms listed.
- Describe differences between the three levels of communication.
- Discuss the six elements involved in the communication process.
- Identify characteristics of verbal and nonverbal communication.
- Discuss the functions and benefits of communication in the nurse-patient/client relationship as part of the nursing process.
- Identify factors that promote or inhibit communication.
- Give examples of techniques that promote therapeutic communication.
- Be aware of potential barriers to effective communication.
- Explain the dimensions of a helping relationship.
- List and discuss the phases of a therapeutic helping relationship.
- Discuss nursing care measures for patients/clients who need special consideration with communication.

Communication is the basic element of human interactions that allows people to establish, maintain, and improve contacts with others. Since communicating is something people do every day, they often mistakenly think it is simple. However, communication is a complex and multifaceted process that involves behaviours and relationships and allows individuals to associate with others and the world around them. It is an ongoing, dynamic series of events in which meaning is generated and transmitted.

**Communication** refers to nonverbal and verbal behaviour within a social context and includes all symbols and clues used by people in giving and receiving meaning (Satir, 1983). A teacher's descriptions, a student's question, or a nurse's gestures create responses in those who observe, listen, and interact. Communication refers not only to content but also to feelings and emotions that people may convey in a relationship. A nurse *listening* to an anguished husband whose wife has died is an example of communication. Consequently, not only does communication convey information but it also influences a relationship; it is an act of sharing.

Nursing is based on establishing a caring and helping relationship. Many theoretical systems for nursing are based on this interpersonal process. Nursing theorists emphasize communication as an integral part of the unique function of nursing (Peplau, 1952; Roper *et al*, 1990). Sarvimaki (1988) describes nursing as communicative interaction and believes that the foundation of nursing lies in the 'communicative attitude'. This attitude is manifested in the striving for mutual understanding, coordination, and cooperation. Instead of striving for control over patients/clients by manipulating them to behave in specific ways or by defining success as setting and meeting predetermined, definite goals, communicative interaction emphasizes patients/clients as partners and is aimed at reaching a shared understanding.

A critical component of nursing practice is the ability to communicate effectively. A nurse uses a wide range of communication techniques with patients and clients. Fritz *et al* (1984) point out the advantages to nurses of using effective communication skills. They help generate trust between the nurse and patients/clients, prevent legal problems in practice, and provide the nurse with professional satisfaction. Communication is also a means for bringing about change. The nurse listens, speaks, and acts to negotiate change that promotes patients'/clients' well-being. Communication is also the foundation of the relationship between the nurse and other members of the health team. For example, the quality of the communication between the nurse and doctor influences the outcome of patient/client care. Knaus *et al* (1986) discovered that the lowest death rates in hospitals were related to interaction between the nurse and doctor and the resulting coordinated response to the patients'/clients' needs rather than to administrative structure, specialization, or teaching status. Consequently, poor working relationships and failure to communicate can lead to serious problems for the nurse and patients/clients and can threaten the nurse's professional credibility. The process of communication cannot be simply memorized and put into practice. It is complex and requires a persistent and conscious application of principles.

## LEVELS OF COMMUNICATION

Communication occurs at intrapersonal, interpersonal, and public levels. **Intrapersonal communication** occurs within an individual. It is self-talk or an internal dialogue that occurs constantly and consciously. The goal of intrapersonal communication is self-awareness, which is influenced by self-concept and feelings of self-worth. Positive self-concept and self-awareness that come through internal dialogue can help nurses express themselves appropriately to others. For example, when a nurse encounters a patient/client in hospital and thinks, "I'll try changing his position", or, "She looks distressed, I'll spend some time with her", the communication is intrapersonal.

**Interpersonal communication** is the interaction that occurs between two people or in a small group. It is often face-to-face and is the type most frequently used in nursing situations. Individuals communicating are continuously aware of one another. Healthy interpersonal communication allows problem solving, sharing of ideas, decision making, and personal growth. In nursing, there are many situations that challenge interpersonal communication skills. Meetings with staff members, doctors, social workers, and therapists test the nurse's communication skills with people who may have different opinions and experiences. Being a member of a nursing committee challenges the nurse's ability to express ideas clearly and decisively. Interpersonal communication is the heart of nursing practice. A

**Adult Nursing**
**Communicating with older adults**

Communication is more than talking and listening or reading and writing; it is a tool for social interaction that can aid understanding. This is particularly evident in older adults who often suffer a 'silence barrier' on three levels: social, emotional, and physical (Dreher, 1987). Social barriers include the loss of spouse or friends through death or separation and a restrictive living location when they change residence or children move away. For some older adults, the cost of transportation or a telephone may further restrict social interaction (Cartwright and Bowling, 1982).

Lowered self-esteem can result in emotional barriers. Using good communication skills, particularly active listening and friendly therapeutic touch, can help relieve or diminish feelings of isolation and vulnerability. For older adults not inhibited by cost, telephoning can be a good method for maintaining contact with family and friends if travel and distance are barriers to communication.

Physical barriers can also occur; gradual changes in the body's muscles and nerves that affect voice, articulation, and hearing may result in slower and less precise speech. Sensory alterations such as a decreasing hearing acuity and an increasing threshold for intensity or loudness may prevent the older adult from receiving messages clearly. This can be complicated by ill-fitting hearing aids and poorly fitting dentures. Particular illnesses that are more common in older adults than in other age groups, such as cancer, stroke, and degenerative neurological diseases, can also distort speech and language. Motor disturbances such as dysarthria interfere with clarity of pronunciation. Many elderly people adapt to the sensory losses (see Chapter 26) and can learn to communicate effectively. When obvious deficits exist, the nurse maximizes existing motor and sensory function so that the person can communicate more effectively.

nurse can help a patient/client by communicating at an interpersonal level.

**Public communication** is interaction within large groups of people. Giving a lecture to a roomful of students and speaking to a consumer group on health education are examples of public communication. Being a competent communicator with an audience requires the ability to envisage oneself speaking to a group. Special platform skills such as use of posture, body movements, and tone of voice help a person express a point.

## ELEMENTS OF THE COMMUNICATION PROCESS

Examination of the components of the communication process helps a person understand communication. A model can simply and graphically demonstrate complex processes, but it can also oversimplify. A model provides the student nurse with a framework for observing, understanding, and predicting what occurs as two people communicate.

A communication model must incorporate several principles.

Communication is *complex*, involving many verbal and nonverbal symbols and messages exchanged between people. Communication is a *process*. After a patient/client and nurse begin to communicate, each subsequent message or thought has its base in what was said before (Fritz *et al*, 1984). Messages may be sent intentionally or unintentionally. Often, a person conveys messages about personality or attitude without being aware of it. Communication is a *response* between two or more people as they send and receive stimuli or messages.

Communication occurs on a social level, with participants engaged in intrapersonal and interpersonal contact. The process is dynamic, with the meaning of messages negotiated by participants. During communication, the person may or may not be aware of each element of communication (Fig. 15-1). During casual conversation participants do not bother to analyse the meaning of every gesture or word. For example, a person may become quite animated, using hands to express an idea without consciously thinking, "I'll wave my hand to stress this point". The nurse, however, learns to be conscious of each element of the communication process. In this way, the nurse can interact effectively with patients/clients and remain aware of the communication's effect on them. Because of the interaction between sender and receiver involved in communication, the model tends to oversimplify a complex process. However, each element is crucial. Information and meaning can be gained or lost if any element is altered.

## Referent

The **referent** or stimulus motivates a person to communicate with another. It may be an object, experience, emotion, idea, or act. Individuals who consciously consider the referent during intrapersonal interaction can carefully develop and organize messages.

## Sender

The **sender**, also called the *encoder*, is the person who initiates the interpersonal communication or message. The sender puts the referent such as an idea into a form that can be transmitted and assumes responsibility for the accuracy of the content and the emotional tone of the message. The role of sender may switch back and forth between participants at any time during the course of the communication.

## Message

The **message** is the information that is sent or expressed by the sender. The most effective message is clear and organized and is expressed in a manner familiar to the person receiving it. An appropriate amount of information must be given, and the receiver must be ready to hear the message. For example, professional jargon (technical terminology used by health care providers) needs to be reserved for interactions between professionals and not between nurses and patients/clients. Similarly, teaching would be inappropriate if nurses tried to teach the patient/client everything in one session or teach the person to manage, for example, a colostomy when he or she is unwilling to look at the stoma. The message may comprise verbal and nonverbal language symbols (for example, spoken words, facial expressions, or gestures). Unfortunately, not all symbols have universal meaning; therefore difficulties in communication may occur with the message if the sender is not aware of this factor and does not seek clarification.

## Channels

The message is sent along a channel of communication. **Channels** are means of conveying messages, such as through visual, auditory, and tactile senses. The sender's facial expression visually conveys a message. The spoken word travels via auditory channels. Placing a hand on an individual while communicating uses the channel of touch. Generally, the more channels the nurse uses to send a message, the better the individual will understand it. For example, when attempting to relieve pain, the nurse verbalizes concern, expresses a sense of compassion, and perhaps repositions the patient/client gently to lessen the pain, or offers an analgesic.

## Receiver

The **receiver**, also called the *decoder*, is the person to whom the message is sent. For communication to be effective, the receiver must perceive or become aware of the message. The message from the sender then acts as one of the receiver's referents. It prompts the receiver to decode and respond to the sender's message. The nurse learns to engage in intrapersonal communication to analyse and interpret the person's comments. Ideally, the sender's intention is perceived by the receiver. There is no guarantee that this will occur, because words and symbols have multiple meanings. However, the more that the sender and receiver have in common, the more likely that the sender's meaning will be communicated.

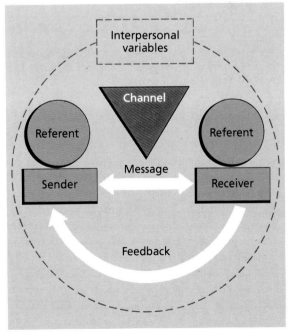

**Fig. 15-1** Communication as an active process between sender and receiver.

## Feedback

Communication is an ongoing process. The receiver returns a message to the sender. This **feedback** helps to reveal whether the meaning of the message is received. Mere intent to communicate is insufficient to ensure that a message is accurately received. The receiver's verbal and nonverbal response sends feedback to the sender to reveal the receiver's understanding of the message. To be effective, the two must be sensitive and open to each other's message, clarify the message, and modify behaviour accordingly. In a social relationship, both persons involved assume equal responsibility for seeking openness and clarification, whereas in the nurse-patient/client relationship the nurse assumes major responsibility.

## MODES OF COMMUNICATION

People send messages in verbal and nonverbal modes, which are closely bound together during interpersonal interaction. As we speak, we express ourselves through movements, tone of voice, facial expressions, and general appearance. These modes can convey the same or different messages. The nurse who learns skills of communication masters techniques of each mode.

## Metacommunication

Communication depends not only on the message but also on the relationship of the speaker to the other person. This is **metacommunication**. Satir (1983) defined metacommunication as "a comment on the literal content and nature of the relationship between the persons involved". It is a message within a message that conveys the sender's attitude towards the self and the message and the attitudes, feelings, and intentions towards the listener. Metacommunication can be verbal or nonverbal. Verbal metacommunication is usually an explicit statement on how to decode a message (for example, "That's an order" or "I was only kidding"). Nonverbal metacommunication is more implicit and therefore may show genuine feelings or may be an attempt to hide feelings (for example, smiling when angry).

## Verbal Communication

**Verbal communication** involves spoken or written words. Words are tools or symbols used to express ideas or feelings, arouse emotional responses, or describe objects, observations, memories, or inferences. They may also be used to convey hidden meanings, test the other's interest or degree of concern, or express hostility, or fear. *Language* is defined as words, their pronunciation, and the method of combining them that is used and understood by a community (Boyle and Andrews, 1989). Language is a code that conveys meaning. A single word can change the meaning of a phrase or sentence. Language is effective only when each person communicating understands the message clearly.

A nurse encounters people of various cultures who speak different languages. Also, some patients/clients speak the same language as the nurse but use subcultural variations of certain words. For example, the word *dinner* may mean a midday meal to one person and the last meal of the day to another. Dialects and subdialects may confuse the meaning. Consequently, a nurse may work with patients/clients who speak the same language but interpret messages differently from the way the nurse intended. To make a message clear, the nurse uses effective verbal communication techniques.

## Clarity and Brevity

Effective communication is usually simple, short, and direct. Because of the intrapersonal variables involved, human communication is imprecise in many ways, and vague phrases such as *you know* add little to the clarity of a message. Clarity is achieved by speaking slowly and enunciating clearly. Using examples may make an explanation easier to understand. For instance, teaching a patient/client with arthritis about self-care measures at home is more meaningful when the nurse provides specific examples, including demonstrations to reinforce the verbal message.

Repeating important parts of a message also makes communication clearer. The receiver should know the what, why,

**Learning Disabilities Nursing
Physical and psychological barriers
to communication**

A person with a learning disability may suffer physical or psychological alterations that impair communication. To speak spontaneously and clearly, the individual must have an intact respiratory system, normal oral and nasal cavities, and a functioning speech centre in the cerebral cortex. Normal reception of language requires an intact auditory system, as well as the cognitive ability to make sense of what is being heard.

For many people with learning disabilities, communication difficulties arise for psychological and emotional, rather than physiological, reasons. Sometimes this is due to the environment of care; for example, young children cared for in stimulus-deprived situations will become withdrawn, passive, and will fail to develop reciprocal vocalization. If individuals have lived for many years in institutions with other people who have poor verbal skills, and with staff who mainly communicated in the form of directives and rhetorical questions, there is little to stimulate communication skills, and little need to use them. This last point is becoming increasingly obvious as patients/clients who were considered to be non-verbal are transferring from large institutional settings into domestic environments and are demonstrating communication skills that they were not known to possess.

When working with profoundly disabled people who have no useful verbal communication skills, the nurse or carer should learn to discriminate between non-verbal cues such as facial expressions, posture, eye blinking and gestures, as well as autonomic responses, such as pulse rate, pupil size, respiration rate and muscle tone. As carers become more familiar with their patients/clients they are better able to determine that person's likes, dislikes, or responses to a new situation. This, in turn, enables even the most profoundly handicapped person to begin making choices about his or her life.

## TABLE 15-1 Relationships Between Verbal and Nonverbal Communication

| RELATIONSHIP | EXAMPLE |
|---|---|
| **Repeating**<br>verbal and nonverbal cues saying the same thing but in different ways | When a mother describes how tall her son is, she also holds her hands at a distance above the floor equal to the child's height. |
| **Contradicting**<br>verbal and nonverbal cues conveying different messages | The nurse tells the patient/client that obtaining a blood specimen "won't hurt a bit", but her sarcastic grin delivers a different message. |
| **Complementing**<br>nonverbal messages adding to verbal messages | A patient/client says she is afraid to be admitted to the hospital, and her anxious expression and trembling hands leave little doubt of her fear. |
| **Accenting**<br>nonverbal cues emphasizing verbal messages | A wave of the hand while saying hello accentuates the word spoken. |
| **Relating and regulating**<br>nonverbal cues indicating when to begin or stop talking | A patient/client who continually opens and closes her mouth briefly as her doctor is talking is seeking an opportunity to speak. |
| **Substituting**<br>a nonverbal cue being used instead of words | A person nods vigorously to show approval of another's decision. |

how, when, who, and where of ideas communicated.

Brevity is best achieved by using words that express an idea simply. "Tell me where your pain is" is better than "I would like you to describe for me the location of your discomfort". A simple, clear phrase communicates more effectively.

## Vocabulary

Communication is unsuccessful if the receiver is unable to translate the sender's words and phrases. In nursing and medicine, there are many technical terms and jargon. If the nurse uses these terms, the person may become confused and unable to follow instructions or learn important information. Rather than telling the patient/client, "Sit up while your lungs are auscultated," it might be better to say, "Sit up so that the doctor can listen to your lungs". The first statement might make the person feel anxious. A message spoken in terms that the individual understands makes communication more effective.

## Denotative and Connotative Meaning

A single word can have several meanings. A **denotative** meaning is one shared by individuals who use a common language. For example, the word *swimming* has the same meaning for all individuals who speak English. The denotative meaning is used to define a word so that it means the same to everyone.

The **connotative** meaning of a word is the thoughts, feelings, or ideas that people have about the word (Duldt *et al*, 1984). Using the word *serious* to describe a patient's/client's condition may suggest to some relatives that the patient/client is close to

death, but nurses may not consider him or her to be near death unless the word *critical* is used. Connotations are shades or interpretations of a word's meaning rather than different definitions.

When nurses communicate with patients/clients, they must carefully select words that cannot be easily misinterpreted. This is important when giving information or explaining conditions, therapies, or the purpose of therapies.

## Pacing

Verbal communication is more successful when expressed at an appropriate speed or pace. Talking rapidly, using awkward pauses, or speaking too slowly and deliberately can convey an unintended message.

In particular, long pauses and rapid shifts to another subject may give the impression that the truth is being hidden. Also, speed and pace of speech varies, depending on geographical location.

The speed with which a message is verbalized, in addition to the presence, absence, and length of pauses, can determine the degree to which communication satisfies the listener. The nurse should not talk so quickly that the words are unclear. Pauses should be used to accentuate or stress a particular point, giving the listener time to hear and comprehend the meaning of words. Proper pacing is achieved by thinking about what to say before saying it. Looking for nonverbal cues from the listener that might suggest confusion or misunderstanding is also useful. A person can also ask a listener if the pace is too fast or too slow or if the message needs repeating.

### Adult Nursing
### Using humour in nursing care

Humour can be a powerful tool in promoting well-being. The phrase 'laughter is the best medicine' applies when the nurse uses humour to help patients/clients adjust to stress imposed by illness. Dugan (1989) notes that laughter helps relieve stress-related tension and pain, increases the nurse's effectiveness in providing emotional support to patients/clients, and humanizes the experience of illness. Laughter serves as a psychological and physical release. Studies have shown that humour stimulates the production of catecholamines and hormones that enhance feelings of well-being, improve pain tolerance, reduce anxiety, facilitate respiratory relaxation, and enhance metabolism (Sullivan and Deane, 1988; Williams, 1986).

Nurses can appropriately use humour in conversations with patients/clients by telling jokes, sharing humorous incidents or situations, and using puns. A person who has become fearful or tense over events related to hospitalization can relax and may become more open to interaction as a result of humour. Sullivan and Deane (1988) have found patients/clients to be more self-disclosing and willing to share concerns of deeper significance.

However, humour is not always appropriate and nurses need to be particularly cautious in using humour to mask their own fears and discomforts, or their inability to communicate with patients/clients. Humour, therefore, should not become the only means of communication, but it can be an effective approach in helping patients/clients to interact more openly and honestly.

## Intonation

The tone of a speaker's voice can have a dramatic impact on a message's meaning. Depending on intonation, the simple question, "How are you?" can express enthusiasm, concern, indifference, and even annoyance. A person's emotions can directly influence tone of voice. Often this effect is unconscious, and the words send one message while the tone conveys the opposite. The nurse must be aware of emotions when interacting with patients/clients. Intention to convey sincere interest in an individual's welfare can be blocked if the nurse's tone of voice gives a different mood or meaning. Patients/clients may question credibility if a nurse's voice is not sincere and pleasing. Voice tone can be a cue to a person's emotional state. Fear, anger, and grief can be expressed through intonation and pitch. Similarly, tone may indicate a person's energy level. A rested, alert person usually has a voice full of variations and inflections in tone and rapidity, whereas a fatigued person may mumble and be unable to complete sentences (Duldt et al, 1984).

## Timing and Relevance

Timing is critical to the reception of a message. If a patient/client is distressed or crying, or in pain, it is the wrong time to give information or explanations, for example. Even though a message is clearly and concisely stated, poor timing can prevent it from being accurately received. Therefore, the nurse must be sensitive to the appropriate time for discussions. Often the best time for interaction is when a patient/client expresses an interest in communicating. By asking a simple question such as, "Would you like to talk about your operation?" the nurse can avoid wasting time and energy if the person does not.

A person is more likely to communicate when a message is important, for example, when an individual is facing surgery the next day, a discussion of the long-term risks of cigarette smoking has less relevance than a review of preoperative procedures. However, an explanation of the side effects of the contraceptive pill is relevant to the young woman who has received her first prescription of the medication. Verbal communication is more likely to have an impact when messages pertain to an individual's interests and needs.

## Nonverbal Communication

Actions often speak louder than words. **Nonverbal communication** is the transmission of messages without the use of words. It is one of the most powerful ways of conveying messages to others (Argyle, 1983). We continuously communicate nonverbally in every face-to-face encounter. Gestures impart meanings that are more significant than words. Ekman (1965) describes the ways in which nonverbal communication and verbal communication are interrelated. Nonverbal cues add meaning to the verbal message (Table 15-1).

A nurse needs to be aware of verbal and nonverbal messages sent to patients/clients. Even the phrase, "Good morning, how are you?" can convey a number of meanings. A verbal message should be reinforced or complemented by **nonverbal cues**. Patients/clients may sense a lack of trust or anxiety when a mismatch exists between a nurse's verbal and nonverbal messages.

During assessment, the nurse observes patients'/clients' verbal and nonverbal messages. Patients/clients who say that they feel fine but grimace at the same time are communicating two different messages. Becoming a good observer of nonverbal behaviour requires time and practice. The nurse who is aware of nonverbal messages is better able to understand patients/clients, detect changes in conditions, and determine nursing care needs.

## Personal Appearance

The general impression formed of another person influences the response to that person (Zunin, 1988). A person's appearance is one of the first things noticed during an interpersonal encounter. People form an impression about another person within 20 seconds to 4 minutes. This impression is based 84% on appearance (Lalli-Ascosi, 1990). Physical characteristics, dress, grooming, and the presence of jewellery and adornment provide clues to the person's physical well-being, personality, social status, occupation, religion, culture, and self-concept. Paying attention to one's appearance can contribute to positive self-image and professional image.

Clothing, cosmetics, and jewellery that are not part of a professional uniform represent a personal choice and are taken as clues to the way people want others to respond to them. The way a person dresses can also influence behaviour. Knapp (1978) notes that clothes fulfil functions of decoration, protection (psychological and physical), sexual attraction, self-assertion, group identity, and role display.

Nurses can help patients/clients maintain a sense of worth by helping them to wear their own clothes where possible. Personal clothes give a sense of identity, physical recovery and mental alertness.

Physical characteristics, such as the condition of hair, skin tone, weight, and energy level, may also communicate information about the level of health. There are no established standards for physical characteristics that demonstrate good health. Each individual displays combinations of physical characteristics. The nurse remains alert for changes in physical appearance because they can be indicators of well-being or of disease.

Physical appearance often leads to impressions about personality and self-concept. Unfortunately, stereotyped views regarding the 'perfect body' also influence the image of a person's body. Nurses should assess the importance of physical appearance to a patient/client threatened with loss of body parts or function. They also need to consider their own views and values about body image, since these can significantly influence an interaction.

The nurse's physical appearance influences the patient's/client's perception of care received. Each person has a preconceived image of a nurse. The traditional uniform can be a symbol of authority and competence. Although the uniform is not a reflection of abilities, some patients/clients may find it more difficult to establish a sense of trust and reliability if the nurse fails to meet the patient's/client's image. Today, nurses wear their own clothes, as well as varying uniforms when carrying out their work. Generally a neat look conveys the message of a competent professional. Conversely, a nurse who has bad breath or cigarette breath, 'messy' hair, poorly manicured nails, or dirty shoes, for example, may be considered unprofessional and may be taken less seriously than a nurse who has paid attention to these details of personal appearance.

## Facial Expression

The face is rich in communication potential. A mutual glance or meeting of eyes between two people may set the tone for an interpersonal encounter. The face and eyes send overt and subtle cues that assist in interpretation of messages. Studies show that the face reveals six primary emotions: surprise, fear, anger, disgust, happiness, and sadness (Knapp, 1978). Facial expressions often become the basis for important interpersonal judgements. Owing to the diversity of facial expressions, their meanings may be difficult to judge. The face may reveal genuine emotions or contradict true emotions, or facial expressions may be suppressed. Often people are unaware of the messages that their expressions convey. Providing clear feedback helps lessen confusion created by conflicting messages and expressions. When facial expressions fail to reveal clear messages, the receiver should seek verbal feedback to be sure of the speaker's intent.

For example, nurses are frequently watched by patients/clients. Consider the impact of a nurse's facial expression on a patient/client who asks, "Am I going to die?". The slightest change of expression can reveal the nurse's true feelings. It is difficult to control all facial expressions, but the nurse learns to be aware of what they can reveal. This is true also when caring, for example, for a debilitated or disabled person, when the nurse must consider the impact of his or her facial expression to avoid conveying signs of disgust.

**Eye contact** is an important facial expression. When two people meet each other, eye contact often prefaces a message. Wide eyes are associated with frankness, terror, and naiveté; downward glances reflect modesty or shyness. Raised eyebrows reveal displeasure, and a stare is often associated with hatred and coldness. However, initiating eye contact shows a willingness to communicate. People who maintain eye contact during a conversation are perceived as believable, and maintaining eye contact allows a person to become a good observer. It has been suggested that the level at which eye contact occurs significantly influences communication. The nurse should avoid looking down at a patient/client during a discussion; one way to avoid this is to sit down. The nurse appears less dominant and threatening sitting near the person at the same eye level.

## Posture and Gait

The way that people stand and move is a visible form of self-expression. Posture and gait reflect attitudes, emotions, self-concept, and physical well-being. Leaning forwards or towards a person conveys attention to that person. Leaning backwards in a more relaxed manner suggests less interest and caution.

An erect posture and a quick, purposeful gait communicate a sense of well-being and assuredness. A slumped posture and a slow, shuffling gait may indicate depression or discomfort. A bent-over posture may be a protective response to physical disease and injury. Nurses can collect useful information by observing an individual's posture and gait. Specific illnesses cause identifiable gaits such as the shuffle of Parkinsonism. Gait may be altered by many physical factors such as pain, drugs, or fractures.

## Gestures

A wave of the hand, a salute, and shifting of feet are gestures. They are visual italics, which emphasize, punctuate, and clarify the spoken word. Duldt *et al* (1984) identify three functions of gestures: illustrating an idea, expressing an emotional state, and signalling by use of a sign. Gestures alone may reveal specific meanings, or with other communication cues, they may send messages.

Gestures are used to illustrate an idea that is difficult or inconvenient to describe in words. Pointing to an area of pain may be more accurate than describing the pain's location. Gestures may be used to convey emotions about oneself or others. Covering the eyes, touching a part of the face, or pointing an accusing finger can reveal inner feelings.

## Touch

Touch is a personal form of nonverbal communication. People engaged in communication must be close to each other when touch is used. Since touch is more spontaneous than verbal communication, it generally seems more authentic. Various messages, such as affection, emotional support, encouragement, tenderness, and personal attention, are conveyed through touch. Touch is an important part of the relationship between the nurse and the patient/client, but it must be used very cautiously because strong social norms govern its use. Who, when, why, and where people touch are determined by unwritten sociocultural guidelines.

Nurses rely on touch when carrying out interventions. Nurses will touch patients/clients while performing physical assessments, giving baths, and assisting with dressing. The nurse who is unaccustomed to touching or being touched may feel uncomfortable when performing interventions. When performing specific interventions, the nurse should verbalize generally his or her actions (for example, "I'm going to put some cream on your back") so the patient/client does not misunderstand the action or its purpose (see Informed Consent, Chapter 13).

Similarly, people who are ill must permit closer physical contact than they normally tolerate. Illness places people in dependent roles that call for the nurse to initiate and maintain closer interpersonal contact. It is important to be sensitive to an individual's disposition towards touching. If a patient/client shies away from the nurse's touch he or she may be uncomfortable with being touched. Finally, touch can be a useful therapeutic tool. Holding the hand of grieving patients/clients can often convey understanding better than words or other gestures. A nurse must be sure to use touch purposefully during interactions and although touch can be helpful to patients/clients, its use must be clearly understood and accepted (Vortherms, 1991).

## FACTORS INFLUENCING COMMUNICATION

Perceptions, values, cultural background, knowledge, past experiences, roles, and the setting of the interaction can influence the content of a message and the manner in which it is shared. Interpersonal communication is made more complex because each person is influenced differently by these intrapersonal variables and they make each interpersonal communication unique. As a result each person makes different associations and interprets messages differently. A knowledge of these factors helps the nurse to understand that a patient/client may have difficulty communicating and he or she may then choose appropriate strategies to help.

### Development
Children are born with the physical mechanisms and capacity to develop speech and language skills. The rate of speech development varies and is directly related to neurological competence and intellectual development (Wong, 1995). A child's environment must also offer stimulation for normal development. The environment provided by parents also affects the ability to communicate. The nurse uses special techniques to communicate with children at different developmental stages.

To communicate effectively with children, the nurse must understand the influence of development on language and thought processes. Both affect the way children communicate and also the manner in which the nurse can successfully interact with them.

### Perceptions
Each person senses, interprets, and understands events differently. **Perception** is the personal view of events. A nurse might state, "I've noticed you have been quiet since your family left. Would you like to talk?". The patient's/client's perception of the nurse's intent will affect the willingness to talk. Perceptions are formed by expectations and experiences. Differences in perceptions between people who are interacting can be a barrier to communication.

### Values
Values are standards that influence behaviour (see Chapter 12). They are what a person considers important in life and thus influence expression of thoughts and ideas. Values also affect interpretation of messages. Since values are a general guide to behaviour, it is important for a nurse to develop an awareness of them. Some values may be identified easily and without conflict (for example, confidentiality or good skin care for an immobile patient/client); others may lead to a high level of conflict and be difficult to articulate (for example, values about death or the right to die). Knowing and clarifying values is important to decision making and interaction. Judgemental attitudes destroy trust and can be detrimental to effective communication.

### Emotions
Emotions are a person's subjective feelings about events. The way a person relates or communicates with others is influenced by emotions. A patient/client who is angry may react to the nurse's instructions differently than one who is frightened. Emotions influence the ability to successfully receive a message. Emotions can also cause a person to misinterpret or not hear a message (see box). Nurses should not take it personally if patients/clients use them to ventilate their emotions. Nurses can assess an individual's emotions by observing them interact with others, for example family, medical staff, or other patients/clients or nurses.

When nurses care for patients/clients, they must be aware of their own emotions. It is difficult to hide emotions. Patients/clients are perceptive and can sense anger, frustration, or sadness. It is usually inappropriate to discuss personal emotions with patients/clients. A social support system of colleagues may be a more useful way of allowing nurses to express their emotions.

### Sociocultural Background
Culture is the sum total of the learned ways of doing, feeling, and thinking; it is a form of conditioning that shows itself through behaviour (see Chapter 8). Language, gestures, values, and attitudes reflect cultural origin. Differences between culture and race may therefore impede effective communication (Foong, 1992).

Culture also influences methods of communicating symptoms or distress to others (Boyle and Andrews, 1989). Differences exist in **self-disclosure** or the willingness to convey emotions and psychological information to others. For many ethnic or racial

### Mental Health Nursing Communication Skills to Manage Aggression and Violence

Predicting, preventing and managing violence demand the highest levels of nursing perceptions and communication skills. In order to help prevent violence, nurses can make full and detailed assessment of the patient's/client's history, particularly of any previous violence. Nurses need to carefully listen for cues in what the person says, and also to what he/she omits to say. However, there should be caution in interpreting the meaning of what is said. Nurses can observe verbal and non-verbal behaviour, particularly during interactions, in order to build up a picture of the person's reality, his/her thoughts, feelings, needs and wants.

Enabling patients/clients to talk about what is troubling them can be helpful, but nurses should be cautious about reinforcing behaviour which induces fear, or in encouraging the person to express emotion, even if this is aimed to be cathartic (such as pillow-punching).

It can be helpful to identify physiological triggers to violence such as drugs, alcohol, metabolic disturbance (such as in diabetes mellitus) or toxic conditions (such as infection). Environments, particularly drab, neglected or impersonal settings, can also promote feelings which contribute to aggression.

Nurses can work with individual patients/clients towards medium and long term goals in developing strategies which will lead to personal satisfaction, and thus help to avoid the build-up of aggression. Other preventative measures include helping the person to develop communication skills and decision-making skills, which may help enhance feelings of self-control and self-esteem. Close multidisciplinary cooperation, individualized care planning, and continuity in care provision (such as a primary nursing team) can also contribute towards a reduction in violence.

For further details see Ritter: *Manual of clinical psychiatric nursing, principles and procedures*, Ch 13, 14, pp 82–97, London, 1989, Harper and Row.

behaviours and the way that they influence interaction. Sayers (1988) surveyed studies that revealed that certain speaker and listener behaviours support sex-linked deference and dominance patterns (that is, behaviours that show men dominating conversations by controlling the opportunity to speak and women providing support for this pattern of interaction). Tannen (1990), however, shows that women and men have different communication styles. From the age of three years old, girls play with a best friend or in a small group and use language to seek confirmation, minimize differences, and establish or reinforce intimacy. Boys, on the other hand, use language to establish independence and negotiate status activities in large groups; even when they want to make friends, they are likely to do it by playfully butting heads. Carrying these styles into adulthood, women and men have completely different impressions of the same conversation. Tannen claims that the frictions between the sexes arise because girls and boys grow up in essentially different cultures, so conversation between them is, in effect, cross-cultural. This approach differs from the deference-dominance theories and focuses instead on a predominate **female pattern** of seeking relationships and connection with others and a predominate **male pattern** of accomplishing tasks and seeking independence and status. Although such an approach does not explain all problems that arise in relationships between women and men, it makes it possible to explain dissatisfactions without blame and without discarding the relationship.

Certainly, nurses need to be aware of these differences when working with patients/clients or other health team members of the opposite sex. Active listening and seeking clarification will help prevent misperceptions and misunderstandings.

### Knowledge

Communication can be difficult when the people communicating have different levels of knowledge. A message will not be clear if the words or phrases are not part of the listener's vocabulary. "The incision is well approximated without drainage" means the same as "The incision is clean and healing well", but the latter is more easily understood.

Nurses communicate with patients/clients and professionals, both of whom have different levels of knowledge. A common language is essential when communicating across different knowledge levels. Through observation, the nurse can assess a patient's/client's knowledge, for example, by taking note of his or her ability to discuss health problems and to ask and answer questions. After assessment, nurses use terms and phrases that patients/clients understand to promote attention and interest.

### Roles and Relationships

People communicate in a style appropriate to their roles and relationships. Students talk with friends in different ways than with teachers, doctors or ministers. Words, facial expressions, tone of voice, and gestures depend on the person receiving the communication.

In contrast to everyday conversations with colleagues, for example sharing amusing stories, a nurse will find communicating with a patient/client (for example, a person entering a clinic for

groups, an inhibited silence occurs only in the presence of strangers or professionals of the dominant culture; sometimes this is due to historical mistrust based on discrimination. At other times, it can be attributed to family loyalties and an agreement not to share problems outside of the family.

Language differences can also hamper communication and relationships. When a nurse cares for a patient/client who speaks another language, an interpreter may be necessary. Hospital interpreters generally understand medical terminology and can convey hospital policies and procedures. If a family member serves as an interpreter, it may be easier for the nurse to devise ways to communicate with the patient/client. It is helpful if the nurse learns key words such as *water, pain*, or *lavatory* to ensure that the person's basic needs are assessed and understood.

### Gender

Lakoff (1975) pioneered linguistic research on language and gender that focused on sex differences in communication the first time) requires a different role. In case the person is feeling apprehensive, the nurse will convey respect by using the person's surname and will avoid being too jocular until it is possible to determine the individual's reaction to this. The patient/client is probably looking for support rather than funny stories. Subsequently, when the relationship between the nurse and patient/client is stronger, casual conversation and addressing the patient/client on a first-name basis may be appropriate.

People feel more comfortable when expressing ideas to individuals with whom they have developed positive, satisfying relationships. As a nurse-patient/client relationship develops, the nurse and patient/client gain confidence in relating ideas and feelings. Communication is more effective when the participants remain aware of their roles in a relationship.

### Environment

People tend to communicate better in a comfortable environment. A warm room, free of noise and distractions, is best. Noise and lack of privacy or space may create confusion, tension, or discomfort. For example, a person fearful of a particular diagnosis might hesitate to discuss their illness in a busy, crowded waiting room. Environmental distractions can also distort the messages sent between two people.

The nurse has some control when selecting the setting for communicating with patients/clients. A quiet room or office is ideal. When the person is visited at home, a bedroom may be best. The nurse's efforts to convey information must not be blocked by environmental distractions.

### Space and Territory

Territory is important because it provides people with a sense of identity, security, and control. In other words, individuals feel threatened when others invade their territory because it disrupts **psychological homeostasis**, creates anxiety, and produces feelings of loss of control. Hall (1969) coined the term *proxemics*, which means the use of space in interpersonal relationships or the distance between communicators. During social interaction, people consciously maintain a distance between themselves. Personal space is an invisible 'bubble', and it is mobile — it goes with a person. Territory can be separated and made visible to others, such as a fenced-in yard, towel on the beach, or hospital bed. When personal space is threatened by intrusion, a defensive response occurs, preventing effective communication. Nurses often work with patients/clients in situations in which space and territory are important. As with touch, the distance separating nurses from patients/clients must be judged by the situation and culture. Physically comforting patients/clients in distress, giving mouth-to-mouth resuscitation, holding crying infants, or facilitating the elimination functions of some patients/clients require invasion of intimate space. Intimate distance or space includes an area in which people are able to touch one another or make physical contact to an area of 50 cm. Patients/clients are sensitive about how nurses use distance. Nurses must convey confidence and gentleness.

As the distance becomes greater, the patient/client and nurse feel more at ease. Greater flexibility is afforded when intimate contact is not required. Sitting with a person to conduct an interview, discuss personal feelings or thoughts, or teach are examples of personal distance (50cm to 1.2 m). Increasing the physical distance makes it easier for the patient/client and nurse to communicate because the nurse becomes less imposing. Social distance (1.2m to 3.6m) is needed when dealing with groups. Clinical rounds or discussions are examples of group interaction. Communication at a social distance is less threatening than communication in a personal space since intimate sharing of thoughts and feelings is less likely to occur. Public distance (greater than 1.2m) is the distance maintained for formal speaking; a community health nurse presenting a health education talk to a group of older adults or a teacher lecturing to a class are some examples.

## THERAPEUTIC COMMUNICATION

Nursing students are often told to "get to know your patients/clients" as they establish interpersonal relationships with them. This is not easy, and sometimes it becomes the only barrier to an effective relationship. Nurses cannot *get to know patients/clients* without being able to appreciate their uniqueness. Without knowing this, nurses are unable to help individuals cope with health issues or problems. **Therapeutic communication** helps nurses form working relationships with patients/clients and fulfils the purposes of the nursing process.

Therapeutic communication is not casual. Instead, it is a planned, deliberate, professional act. However, preoccupation with the techniques of communication can cause the nurse to forget the patient/client as a person. When therapeutic communication techniques are first used, the communication process may seem artificial and contrived. It is more helpful to perceive each patient/client interaction as an opportunity to achieve a positive relationship that results in attainment of mutual care goals.

### Social Interaction

The first attempt at communicating with a patient/client usually consists of a brief social interaction. The messages conveyed are superficial in that neither the nurse nor patient/client discusses deeply personal matters of concern. Interpersonal exchange tends to be based on intuitive, unthinking, and automatic responses. Superficial interaction makes participants feel safe because the discussion has no hidden intent for personal disclosures.

A nurse often uses superficial social interaction at the beginning of a conversation to lay a foundation for a closer relationship. For example, the nurse might greet a patient/client by saying, "Good morning, Mrs Sears, it's nice to see you today", or "Hi, Mr Simpson, how do you like the weather we're having?"

The skilful nurse does not allow social interaction to dominate a conversation but does maintain a congenial and warm style to build up the patient's/client's trust. The goal is to help the person feel comfortable in sharing attitudes and feelings.

### Caring and Methods of Effective Communication

The nurse uses communication skills while establishing a

therapeutic relationship. There is no formula for forming a relationship with a patient/client. Each person communicates uniquely; consequently different communication techniques will be required for each individual. The nurse should be flexible with regard to the techniques used to foster communication with each patient/client.

## Listening Attentively

Listening is one of the most effective therapeutic communication techniques. It conveys a nonverbal interest in the person's needs, concerns, and problems. It requires complete attention. Attentive listening involves an attempt to understand the entire verbal and nonverbal message that a person is communicating. Although hearing is a passive, neurological process of receiving information, listening is an active, learned process.

Listening effectively may at first seem awkward and time consuming; however, as with any skill, it requires practice. An effective listener can develop an understanding of the patient's/client's deeper health concerns. To be an attentive listener, the nurse uses the following skills:

1. Face patients/clients while they speak.
2. Maintain natural eye contact to show willingness to listen.
3. Assume an attentive posture. Avoid crossing legs and arms because this may convey a defensive posture.
4. Avoid distracting body movements, such as wringing hands, tapping feet, or fidgeting with an object.
5. Nod in acknowledgement when patients/clients talk about important points or looks for feedback.
6. Lean towards the person to indicate involvement.

The nurse must appear natural while listening to patients/clients. Nonverbal cues, such as leaning towards the speaker, should not become overbearing or threaten personal space. Listening skilfully during a nursing procedure is beneficial and is an efficient use of time. For example, much can be learnt by a nurse who listens while helping a person with washing and dressing — patients/clients, not the bathing procedures, become the centre of attention.

## Conveying Acceptance

Showing **acceptance** means not judging another person as well as demonstrating a willingness to listen to the person's beliefs, values, and practices. This can be difficult at times because a nurse meets individuals from diverse backgrounds. Acceptance, however, is not the same as agreement. Acceptance is a willingness to hear the person without conveying doubt or disbelief.

Certainly, a nurse may not accept all aspects of a person's behaviour or illness, but will work to bring about change that improves a person's level of health. Acceptance is tolerance towards others that fosters a relationship between the nurse and patient/client.

To show acceptance the nurse should remain aware of personal nonverbal expressions and avoid facial expressions and gestures that suggest disapproval, such as frowning, rolling the eyes upwards, or shaking the head in disbelief. The following

demonstrates that the nurse accepts what a patient/client has to say:

1. Listening without interrupting.
2. Providing verbal feedback that demonstrates an understanding.
3. Being sure that nonverbal cues match verbal communication.
4. Avoiding arguments, expressing doubts, or attempting to change the person's mind.

## Asking Related Questions

Questioning is a direct method of communicating. The nurse's aim is to gain specific information concerning the patient/client. Questions used during a conversation set the tone of the verbal interaction and control its direction. Questions are most effective when they relate to the topic or subject being discussed and use words and word patterns in the person's normal sociocultural context. During assessment of the person's health status, questions follow a logical sequence. The following example demonstrates this technique:

| | |
|---|---|
| *Nurse:* | *Mr James, can you tell me where you are having pain?* |
| *Patient/client:* | *Well, it seems to be in my back.* |
| *Nurse:* | *What part of your back?* |
| *Patient/client:* | *Here, in the lower part.* |
| *Nurse:* | *How would you describe the pain?* |
| *Patient/client:* | *It feels like a knife went through me.* |

The nurse's line of questioning helps the person tell a story. Each question focuses on a specific aspect of the story. The nurse is careful not to ask more than one question at a time or move on to another subject until the current topic is adequately explored. The nurse selects a question on the basis of the person's previous response so that information flows logically.

If the nurse wants the patient/client to elaborate, **open-ended questions** are most effective. They give a patient/client a chance to talk more completely about problems or concerns. Such questions cannot be answered with *yes* or *no*. Examples of open-ended questions include the following:

1. "How would you describe the pain you have been feeling?"
2. "What seems to be the problem?"
3. "How does your family feel about your illness?"

Asking the patient/client open-ended questions allows the nurse to assess a number of factors, for example, the person's verbal and nonverbal responses can reveal emotions. The nurse may be able to judge the level of the patient's/client's vocabulary and understanding of health by the response. Often the nurse seeks details of physical signs and symptoms, and the open-ended question elicits more accurate and detailed descriptions. Because an open-ended question prompts a lengthy response, the nurse can assess gaps or discrepancies.

## Paraphrasing

**Paraphrasing** is restating patients'/clients' messages in the nurse's own words. Usually a paraphrased statement uses fewer words than the original statement. Through paraphrasing, the nurse sends feedback that lets patients/clients know whether their messages were understood and prompts further communication. The following example illustrates this point:

| | |
|---|---|
| *Patient/client:* | *I've had it. My doctor won't tell me what's going on. He doesn't seem to care what I think.* |
| *Nurse:* | *It sounds as though you're frustrated because you and your doctor haven't talked about your diagnosis?* |
| *Patient/client:* | *Yes, he obviously doesn't know what it's like to be sick.* |

Practice is required to paraphrase accurately. If the meaning of a message is changed or distorted through paraphrasing, communication may become ineffective. For example, a patient/client may say, "I've been overweight all my life and never had any problems. I can't understand why I need to be on a diet". Paraphrasing this statement by saying, "You mean you don't care if you're overweight or not?" is incorrect. "It seems that you're not convinced that you need a diet because you've remained healthy", is a more appropriate way of paraphrasing the statement.

## Clarifying

Despite efforts at paraphrasing, the nurse may not understand the patient's/client's message. When a misunderstanding occurs, the nurse momentarily stops the discussion to **clarify** the meaning. Without clarification, valuable information can be lost. Information critical to the person's care plan can be incomplete unless confusing or conflicting data are clarified. The nurse can attempt to repeat the message or admit confusion and ask the patient/client to restate the message. For example:

| | |
|---|---|
| *Patient/client:* | *I knew I might have a problem. It seems to be in my family. The last time I was here, though, it wasn't bad, so I didn't mention it.* |
| *Nurse:* | *Excuse me, Mr Brewer, can you tell me what type of problem you're having?* |

The nurse must also clarify messages. Examples can be used to clarify a vague, abstract idea. When using examples, the nurse describes ideas or situations to which the patient/client can easily relate. In the following dialogue, a nurse is explaining activity restrictions to a person who has had eye surgery:

| | |
|---|---|
| *Nurse:* | *Now, Mr Lee, once you go home you should not put your eye under any stress.* |
| *Patient/client:* | *I'm not sure I know what you mean.* |
| *Nurse:* | *Well, you should not stoop or bend over with your head down. For example, if you want to pick something up off the floor don't bend over. Instead, bend your knees and keep your head up.* |
| *Patient/client:* | *I have a dog at home. I suppose that means I can't bend over to pick him up?* |
| *Nurse:* | *That's right. But you can bend your knees to lower yourself down if you want to pick up your dog.* |

The more specific a clarifying message, the more likely it will be understood. Patients/clients who are easily confused by the complex terms and jargon of medicine appreciate a simple, down-to-earth explanation that uses familiar examples.

## Focusing

**Focusing** eliminates vagueness in communication by limiting the area of discussion. As patients/clients discuss topics related to health, their messages often become vague. For example, a person might say to the nurse, "Well, I've just been feeling funny lately. It doesn't really bother me that much. It's just this feeling I'm having in my head". This description conveys very little information except that the patient/client does not feel well. If the nurse does not help focus specifically on the physical complaint, the person will probably continue to use vague descriptions.

To focus the discussion, the nurse might respond to the patient/client by saying, "You said you've been feeling funny lately. Tell me when this feeling first started", or "Describe the feeling in your head". As in clarifying, the nurse seeks the meaning in the person's message. In the case of focusing, however, the nurse understands the patient's/client's message but realizes that it is nonspecific or vague.

The nurse does not use focusing if it means interrupting the patient/client while he or she is discussing an important issue. If the conversation continues without any new information being disclosed or the patient/client begins to repeat the same information again, focusing is useful.

## Summarizing

**Summarizing** is a concise review of the main ideas that have been discussed. It sets the tone for further interactions between the nurse and patient/client. Beginning a new interaction by summarizing a previous one helps the person recall topics discussed and shows him or her that the nurse has analysed their communication. The following example concerns a nurse, who over the last few days has been talking to Mrs Ramos, the patient/client, about diabetes:

*The nurse enters the patient's/client's room and says, "Good morning Mrs Ramos, I've come to talk with you some more about your diabetes. If you recall, yesterday we discussed the purpose of insulin, its side effects, and how to give an injection".*

Summarizing helps the nurse review key aspects of an interaction. Further communication can then focus on relevant issues. Patients/clients will be able to sense whether the nurse understood their part of the message. With a summary the person is able to review information and make additions or corrections.

## Stating Observations

When communicating, people are often unaware of the way that their messages are received. Feedback from others tells them whether they have communicated the intended message. One way that the nurse can provide feedback is by sharing with patients/clients observations of their behaviour during communication. The nurse describes the impressions created by the nonverbal cues. The following example tries to illustrate this point:

*Mrs Patel is sitting in the waiting room of her GP's surgery. She is slumped in the chair, her body movements are slow, and she yawns while speaking with the nurse. The nurse says, "Mrs Patel, you seem to be quite tired".*

If the patient's/client's verbal response conflicts with nonverbal cues, the nurse's observation may help convey a clearer message. Stating observations often leads the patient/client to communicate more clearly without the need for extensive questioning, focusing, or clarification.

The nurse does not state observations that might embarrass or anger the person. The nurse in the preceding example would not say, "Mrs Patel, you look a mess". Even if such an observation is made with humour, the patient/client can, not surprisingly, become resentful.

## Offering Information

When two people communicate, the process is rarely one sided. In an interaction with a patient/client, the nurse frequently offers information that gives the person additional data or insight. The patient/client in the following dialogue is scheduled to have surgery the next day for the removal of gallstones:

| | |
|---|---|
| *Patient/client:* | *The doctor has told me that I'm first on the operating list for tomorrow.* |
| *Nurse:* | *Yes, we'll be awakening you at about 7 AM.* |
| *Patient/client:* | *My husband wants to come in to see me after the operation.* |
| *Nurse:* | *That's no problem. If he rings the ward in the afternoon, say, after midday we can let him know how you are and together we can decide on a good time for him to come and see you.* |

Providing the patient/client with additional information encourages further response. Offering information on an ongoing, timely basis not only facilitates communication but also promotes health teaching.

It is usually not helpful to withhold information from patients/clients, particularly when they seek it. If the nurse avoids sharing information or gives only partial information, the patient/client may lose trust in the nurse. If doctors chose to withhold information, the nurse will need to clarify the reasons with them. However, there is a wide range of information the nurse can share (see Chapter 16). The nurse must avoid advising a patient/client when giving information. *Information can facilitate a person's decision making, but the nurse does not make the decision.*

## Maintaining Silence

Silence allows the nurse and patient/client to organize thoughts. The use of silence can be effective but is difficult because pauses in conversation that last several seconds or minutes can cause unease. Student nurses may need to practice this technique before feeling comfortable.

The use of silence requires skill and timing. Silence allows the patient/client an opportunity to communicate intrapersonally, organize thoughts, and process information. It gives patients/clients time to search for words or feelings. Silence is particularly useful when individuals are confronted with difficult decisions that they are not sure how to share with the nurse. For example, silence may help patients/clients gain the confidence needed to share the decision to refuse medical treatment.

Silence also allows the nurse to observe the patient/client. The nurse should pay particular attention to nonverbal messages, such as worried expressions or loss of eye contact. Remaining silent demonstrates the nurse's willingness to wait for a response. Often the nurse has many questions, but some patients/clients, especially older adults, are unable to reply quickly. Any impatience expressed by the nurse may frustrate the patient's/client's efforts at communication. Silence can show that the nurse is interested and will accept any response that the person can express.

When patients/clients become emotionally upset, silence helps them gather thoughts. A quiet period may diffuse an emotionally tense situation. A nurse's silence acknowledges the person's need for a few moments of privacy. When the person is ready to talk again, he or she will probably express his or her feelings more clearly.

## Using Assertiveness

**Assertiveness** is standing up for one's rights without violating those of others (Lidenfield and Adams, 1984). Through assertive techniques, people can express feelings and emotions confidently, spontaneously, and honestly. Assertive people make choices and decisions and are able to control their lives more effectively than non assertive individuals. Nurses can teach patients/clients assertiveness skills and enable them to use these to promote their health.

Examples of assertiveness skills include speaking clearly, dealing with manipulation, and protecting oneself against criticism.

To avoid being manipulated, nurses must acquire skills to protect themselves from others who consciously or unconsciously attempt to use them. Learning to say *no* and resisting guilt imposed by others are two helpful techniques. Learning to say *no* is illustrated as follows:

| | |
|---|---|
| *Staff member:* | *Listen, I'm really in a rush. Can you help me get this report completed before lunch?* |
| *Nurse:* | *No, I've planned a home visit this morning. But I can give you an hour this afternoon.* |

Constructive valid criticism can promote growth, but manipulative criticism makes people vulnerable (Bond, 1986). The following example illustrates a method of protecting oneself against criticism:

| | |
|---|---|
| *Supervisor* | *Nancy, I'm becoming concerned about your documentation.* |
| *Student Nurse:* | *What are your concerns?* |
| *Supervisor:* | *Well, four times this week the evaluation sheets of your care plans have not been completed for the end of your duty.* |

*Student Nurse:*     *I'm having difficulties with planning my work.*
*Can you suggest ways that will help me prioritize?*

**Negative inquiry** is a skill that involves asking for more information when a criticism has been made. The person remains unemotional and low-key when asking for information and avoids sounding angry or sarcastic. Using criticism for growth can help nurses feel better about themselves.

## Interpersonal Barriers to Effective Communication

Some communication techniques or styles result in interpersonal interactions that are not therapeutic. These barriers can be damaging when a nurse is building a patient/client relationship. Many techniques that normally promote effective communication can be harmful if used inappropriately.

## Giving an Opinion

Giving an opinion takes decision making away from the patient/client. It inhibits spontaneity, stalls problem solving, and creates doubt. The following example demonstrates how giving an opinion can be harmful:

*Nurse:*     *Mr Rosenberg, you look like you're deep in thought.*
*Patient/client:*     *Oh, no, not really. I was just thinking about whether my daughter is coming to see me.*
*Nurse:*     *Well, if you ask me, she should have been here before now. It would mean so much to you.*

Often the person simply needs an opportunity to express feelings. Giving an opinion prevents the patient/client from developing solutions to problems.

At times, an individual may require suggestions. For example, when a patient/client is selecting a special diet, the nurse's help may be needed to choose the right food. Suggestions are presented as options, however, the final decision rests with the patient/client.

## Offering False Reassurance

When a patient/client is seriously ill, the nurse is tempted to offer hope to the person with statements such as "You'll be fine" or "There's nothing to worry about". When a patient/client is reaching out for understanding, false reassurance from the nurse may discourage open communication.

Genuine, truthful reassurance, however, is important and helps validate a person's self-worth and sense of hope. Bradley and Edinberg (1990) have identified six basic conditions in which verbal reassurance can be given; a patient/client can be reassured:
1. That there is hope.
2. That the nurse is listening.
3. That care is available.
4. That certain undesirable changes can be expected (for example, loss of hair from chemotherapy).
5. That the patient/client will be treated like a person.
6. That the patient's/client's problem is understood.

## Being Defensive

Defensiveness in response to criticism suggests that the patient/client has no right to an opinion. When a nurse becomes defensive the person's concerns are often ignored. The following example illustrates this point:

*Mr Maguire has been a regular visitor to the health clinic for several years. The last time he visited the clinic, he had symptoms that resulted in his hospitalization. He is returning to the clinic for a check-up 1 week after discharge from the hospital.*

*Mr Maguire:*     *Well, I hope I don't have to see Dr Warren today.*
*Nurse:*     *I don't understand, Mr Maguire, is something wrong? Dr Warren has been your doctor here for some time.*
*Mr Maguire:*     *I don't care. He was the one who put me in the hospital, and that was a waste of time.*
*Nurse:*     *That's silly. Dr Warren is an excellent doctor.*
*Mr Maguire:*     *You think so, huh? He hasn't put you in the hospital for no reason.*
*Nurse:*     *You were very ill, Mr Maguire. I know Dr Warren made the right decision.*

The nurse has threatened the relationship with Mr Maguire; he may no longer trust the nurse sufficiently to divulge his concerns, while she has ignored his feelings and will probably not take any action to remedy the problem.

When patients/clients express criticism, the nurse should listen to what is being said. Listening does not imply agreement. To learn the reasons behind criticism, the nurse must avoid becoming defensive. There are two sides to any story, and the nurse should attempt to find out why patients/clients have become angry or dissatisfied. The following is an example of an alternative conversation:

*Mr Maguire:*     *Well, I hope I don't have to see Dr Warren today.*
*Nurse:*     *You seem upset, would you like to talk about it?*
*Mr Maguire:*     *I don't think he should have put me in the hospital.*
*Nurse:*     *You believe hospitalization was unnecessary?*
*Mr Maguire:*     *Yes, they really didn't do much of anything. They took a few tests and did some x-rays.*
*Nurse:*     *Mr Maguire, did your doctors tell you what the tests showed?*
*Mr Maguire:*     *No, not really. That's why I'm, so angry.*

The nurse's patience led to an identification of the person's real concern, not knowing the results of his investigations. By avoiding defensiveness the nurse defused Mr Maguire's anger so that he could describe his concerns.

## Showing Approval or Disapproval

Expressing excessive approval can be as harmful to a nurse-patient/client relationship as stating disapproval. Offering excessive praise implies that the behaviour being praised is the only acceptable one. Often the patient/client shares a decision with the nurse, not in an effort to seek approval but to provide a means to discuss feelings. The following example illustrates this point:

| | |
|---|---|
| *Patient/client:* | *I've decided that when I leave the hospital I'll stay with my son. He doesn't want me to go home and be alone.* |
| *Nurse:* | *Oh, I'm so glad to hear that. I think you definitely made the right decision. It's best for you to be with your son.* |

This nurse's comment will probably end further discussion of the topic. The person may perceive that the nurse agrees with the son. Perhaps the patient/client would be better off with his or her son, on the other hand, the person may have a strong desire to remain independent, and now that has been discouraged. The nurse's excessive approval did not allow the person to think or act freely and inhibited the potential for decision making. A better response by the nurse might be, "How do you feel about that?"

On the other hand, disapproval implies that the patient/client must meet the nurse's expectations or standards. In the following example, the nurse's response may hinder the person's positive attitude and recovery:

| | |
|---|---|
| *Patient/client:* | *Oh, I've had a great day today, I was able to get up in the chair once today.* |
| *Nurse:* | *Only once? You're going to have to get up more often than that!* |

It might have been better for the nurse to say, "You're making good progress, and the team would like you to try to be up at least three times today. Would you like to get up again for your meal?" A disapproving statement causes the person to feel rejected. The patient/client may avoid further interaction with the nurse, thus potentially slowing recovery.

## Stereotyping

Everyone is unique. However, stereotyped responses inhibit uniqueness and oversimplify the situation. **Stereotypes** are generalized beliefs held about people. The use of stereotypes inhibits communication and can threaten a nurse-patient/client relationship. Stereotyping statements, such as "old people are always confused" or "people with back problems cannot tolerate pain", seriously impair interpersonal communication.

Another nontherapeutic communication is the use of meaningless, stereotyped responses. Their use minimizes the importance of a person's message. The following example illustrates this point:

| | |
|---|---|
| *Patient/client:* | *I didn't sleep well last night. My wound seemed to be pulling.* |
| *Nurse:* | *You can't win them all. At least the wound is healing well.* |

## Asking Why

When people disagree with or fail to understand others, they are tempted to ask why the others believe or have acted in such a way. Individuals frequently interpret 'why' questions as accusations. They may also think that the nurse knows the reasons and is simply testing them. Regardless of the patient's/client's perceptions of the nurse's motivation, 'why' questions can cause resentment, insecurity, and mistrust.

If the nurse wants additional information, there are more effective ways of phrasing questions. For example, rather than asking, "Why didn't you do your exercises?", the nurse could say, "You didn't do your exercises. Is something wrong?". Rather than asking, "Why are you anxious?", the nurse could say, "You appear upset. Is there anything bothering you?"

## Changing the Subject Inappropriately

A nurse might inadvertently stop a patient/client from discussing a subject of importance by changing the subject. Abruptly interrupting conversation is rude and shows a lack of empathy, as the following example shows:

| | |
|---|---|
| *Nurse:* | *Good morning, Mr Olegbe. How are you feeling?* |
| *Mr Olegbe:* | *(facial expression shows discomfort) Oh, not so good. My wound is rather sore.* |
| *Nurse:* | *Well, let's get you up in a chair. We need to discuss your discharge.* |

The nurse's comment shows an unwillingness to discuss Mr Olegbe's discomfort. The chance for a therapeutic assessment of his discomfort is lost. In this example, changing the subject was not therapeutic because the nurse ignored a potentially serious problem.

Changing the subject stalls progress of a therapeutic communication. The person's thoughts and spontaneity are interrupted, ideas become tangled, and as a result, the information provided may be inadequate. It is particularly important to avoid changing the subject during assessment. If the patient/client has the opportunity to complete a message, the information will be more thorough and useful.

## Physical and Psychological Barriers to Communication

Review of medical history and physiological assessment provide clues to the person's physical ability to communicate. Physical barriers cause loss of speech, impaired articulation, or inability to find or name words.

The nurse should also consider whether patients/clients are taking medication that impairs speech. Some medications, such as antidepressants, neuroleptics, or sedatives, may cause a patient/client to slur words or use incomplete sentences. The nurse should be familiar with common side effects of such medications.

Some psychological illnesses such as psychosis or depression influence the ability to communicate. The person may demonstrate flight of ideas, constant verbalization of the same words or phrases, or a loose association of ideas. The nurse must isolate psychological causes of speech problems from possible neurological causes.

The inability to communicate effectively influences a person's ability to express needs or react to the environment or other people.

## HELPING RELATIONSHIPS

The nurse-patient/client relationship is more than a mutual partnership. It is a process in which the helper is asked to intervene in the life of the patient/client to help the person engage in more effective behaviour. Travelbee (1971) calls it a *human-to-human relationship*. King (1971) says that the nurse-patient/client relationship is a "learning experience whereby two people interact to face an immediate health problem, to share, if possible, in resolving it and to discover ways to adapt to the situation".

The nurse uses skills of interpersonal communication to develop a relationship with the patient/client that allows understanding of him or her as a whole person. This helping relationship is therapeutic, promoting a psychological climate that brings positive patient/client change and growth. The relationship also focuses on meeting the person's needs. Although the nurse may gain considerable satisfaction from the relationship, patients/clients should be the primary recipients and determiners of benefits.

Creation of a therapeutic environment rests on the nurse's ability to provide physical and psychosocial comfort to the patient/client. The nurse ensures that the person's physiological needs are satisfied. For example, the nurse positions the patient/client so that breathing is normal for comfortable sleep. The nurse's actions consider the individual's preferences. Together the nurse and patient/client determine how needs are to be met. In the following example, the nurse involves the patient/client in her own care:

> *Mrs Greer is a 63-year-old widow who is hospitalized for lung cancer. She makes frequent requests for pain medication before a dose is due. When a nurse delivers the medication, Mrs Greer criticizes her for being late. Nothing the nurses do seems to satisfy Mrs Greer.*

Nurse Edwards has cared for Mrs Greer for the past 2 days. Nurse Edwards enters her patient's/client's room and begins to straighten out the bed linen. Nurse Edwards asks, "Are you comfortable in that position, Mrs Greer? Can I change your position or would you like an injection for the pain?". Mrs Greer accepts the offer and begins to relax in Nurse Edwards' presence. The nurse helps Mrs Greer assume a more comfortable position on her side.

Once the patient's/client's pain has diminished, Ms Edwards sits by her bed and says, "I know you've been experiencing a lot of discomfort recently. Over the past few days we have not always been able to help you feel better. Can you help me to know the best way to make you feel comfortable?".

Efforts at improving Mrs Greer's comfort may make her more willing to discuss problems. The nurse may soon learn of Mrs Greer's fear of death. She has made frequent requests to the nurses to avoid feeling lonely. By unlocking Mrs Greer's fears, the nurse and patient/client are more able to find ways to minimize her loneliness.

A helping relationship between the nurse and patient/client does not just happen. It is built with care as the nurse uses therapeutic communication techniques.

## Dimensions of Helping Relationships

Characteristics of any helping relationship are trust, empathy, caring, autonomy, and mutuality (Sundeen *et al*, 1989). They are essential if the nurse wants to establish a positive and supportive relationship with the patient/client.

### Trust

With respect to helping relationships, Travelbee (1971) defines trust as "the assured belief that other individuals are capable of assisting in times of distress and will probably do so". Unless patients/clients believe that a nurse wishes to care for their needs, a trusting relationship cannot develop. Trust fosters open, therapeutic communication. Previous experiences may affect a person's willingness to trust a nurse. Lack of previous health care experience or traumatic experiences may cause the patient/client to hesitate with regard to trusting care givers. To foster trust, the nurse must act consistently, reliably, and competently. Honesty in sharing information with the person also builds trust. Without trust, a nurse-patient/client relationship does not progress beyond social interaction and tending to superficial needs only.

### Empathy and Sympathy

Empathy is widely accepted as a clinical component of the helping relationship, and within nursing it is considered an essential part of the nurse-patient/client relationship. Definitions of empathy reflect the influence of psychotherapist Carl Rogers, who is well known for his work in identifying and describing the characteristics of a helping relationship. Empathy is the ability to enter into the life of another and accurately perceive feelings and meaning (Sundeen *et al*, 1989). **Empathy** is sensing, comprehending, and sharing the person's frame of reference, beginning with the problem as the patient/client recognizes it. It is a fair, sensitive, and objective look at what another person experiences.

Empathy helps patients/clients explain and explore their feelings so that problem solving may occur. It takes time for empathy to develop in a relationship. A nurse cannot automatically understand a patient's/client's feelings or experiences.

In contrast to empathy, sympathy is the expression of one's own feelings about another's predicament. It is the concern, sorrow, or pity shown by the nurse for the patient/client in which the needs of the person are seen as the nurse's needs. Sympathy has a place in human relationships; sharing with another person feels good, creates an alliance, and minimizes differences. Sundeen *et al* (1989) claim that this poses a difficulty in the helping relationship however; helpers who share the needs of the patient/client may be unable to help the person identify realistic alternatives and problem solve.

Social scientists and nurse researchers are rethinking, reviewing, and reinvestigating the role of empathy in the nurse-patient/client relationship and the way that it is operationalized in nursing practice. The concept of empathy is not without controversy.

## Caring

Caring is having a positive regard for another person. It is basic to a helping relationship. Most individuals directly or indirectly express a need to be cared for at some time. Nurses show caring by accepting patients/clients for who they are and respecting them as individuals. When a person feels cared for, he or she will feel secure in threatening or anxiety-producing situations. Caring also promotes trust and decreases anxiety. Diminished anxiety and stress increase the body's defence and helps promote healing. As already discussed, the use of touch may be an effective way for nurses to communicate caring.

## Autonomy and Mutuality

**Autonomy** is an ability to be self-directed. **Mutuality** involves sharing with another. These are important in any helping relationship. The nurse and patient/client work in partnership, participating in care. The nurse offers opportunities to make decisions, even if it is as simple as choosing a bath time. As a patient/client becomes more independent, the nurse offers more opportunities for decision making. The nurse also acts as an advocate to keep the person informed of health care alternatives and gives support in decision making.

## Phases of a Helping Relationship

The **helping relationship** is established and maintained by the nurse and consists of pre-interaction, orientation, working, and termination phases. Ideally, the relationship is reciprocal; nurse and patient/client relate to each other as they progress to therapeutic rapport. A helping relationship progresses over time as the nurse and patient/client interact, but the helping relationship is not the same as the nursing process. The nursing process is a series of steps taken to manage a patient's/client's health problems. A helping relationship is a bond that allows the nurse to be more effective in carrying out the nursing process. The nurse is responsible for directing the patient/client through the helping relationship to ensure that the person's needs are met.

Chapter 3 discusses the interview as a method for obtaining a nursing health history and identifying changes in the person's level of wellness and living patterns. Although the phases of an interview and of a helping relationship are the same, communication patterns are different. The interview can initiate a nurse-patient/client relationship because it may be the first encounter. However, the interview is not the mechanism for maintaining a long-term therapeutic relationship. A helping relationship goes beyond the scope of an interview to establish rapport that is the basis for an ongoing resolution of the person's health problems.

## Pre-interaction Phase

Before the first meeting with a patient/client, the nurse reviews relevant information pertaining to that person. Such information may include the medical or nursing history, an entry in the nurse's notes of the medical record, or a discussion with another nurse who cared for the patient/client. During this review, the nurse thinks about concerns that may develop. For example, before entering a relationship with a young cancer patient/client, the nurse should consider how the person is adjusting and whether issues concerning death may arise in the discussion. The *pre-interaction phase* is a time when the nurse plans an approach. This process helps avoid stereotyping patients/clients and allows the nurse to think about personal values or feelings. Although the nurse may feel anxious about a patient/client, this sharpens mental processes and helps planning. A new student nurse should seek help from teachers if anxiety becomes intense.

A final step of the pre-interaction phase is to choose a location and setting for the first meeting with a patient/client. A comfortable, private, and attractive setting fosters interpersonal interaction. The nurse must also plan sufficient time for discussion.

## Orientation

The *orientation phase* begins when the nurse and the patient/client first meet. It sets the tone for the rest of the nurse-patient/client relationship. The orientation phase is superficial and is often marked by uncertainty and exploration.

During any initial encounter, both participants closely observe each other. The nurse and patient/client make inferences and form judgements about each other. Therapeutic communication will be more effective if the nurse is genuine, empathetic, and caring.

The nurse and patient/client meet and identify each other by name. It is wise to address the patient/client formally by using his or her surname; for example, the nurse might say, "Good morning, Mr Spencer. My name is Helen Tucker. I am a student nurse and I will be involved in looking after you today". As the therapeutic relationship develops, a patient/client may ask the nurse to be more informal. Failure to identify oneself can create uncertainty because the person often encounters many personnel when seeking health care.

At the beginning of the relationship, neither individual is able to perceive the other's uniqueness. The nurse perceives a person who has a health-related problem. The patient/client perceives the nurse as one of many health care professionals whose job is to help. Engaging in a social interaction initially helps the nurse and patient/client become relaxed. The following conversation demonstrates communication which aims to place a patient/client at ease:

| | |
|---|---|
| *Nurse:* | *It certainly is a lovely day, Mrs Samuel.* |
| *Patient/client:* | *Yes, isn't it? If I were home and feeling better, I'd be planting my garden.* |
| *Nurse:* | *You're a gardener? What types of plants do you enjoy growing?* |
| *Patient/client:* | *Oh, a little of everything. I like some tomatoes, lettuce, radishes, but flowers too.* |

The nurse directs the conversation so that she and Mrs Samuel feel at ease. Rushing into a therapeutically oriented discussion when the person feels uncomfortable serves no purpose. The nurse and Mrs Samuel can get to know each other better and begin to develop a meaningful relationship if the social interaction is properly directed.

## TESTING

The patient/client often tests the nurse during the orientation phase; this springs from difficulties in acknowledging a need for help, fear of expressing true feelings, and anxiety over the need to change. The nurse who is aware of the person's concerns attempts to display confidence and competence. The nurse should not be defensive during testing but should be open and interested in the person's concerns. The patient/client may use silence to avoid communicating. The nurse can show a desire to help by explaining the actions taken and performing care smoothly. The following case study shows communication involving testing:

*Mr Miles is a 52-year-old businessman who has been hospitalized for treatment of a bleeding stomach ulcer. He is very independent, and he is accustomed to making decisions for himself. Munju Gopal, the nurse, enters his room.*

| | |
|---|---|
| *Nurse Gopal:* | *Good morning, Mr Miles. My name is Munju Gopal, and I will be caring for you today.* |
| *Mr Miles:* | *You will, huh? Tell me, how long have you been a nurse?* |
| *Nurse Gopal:* | *About 2 years. I have worked in this hospital since I qualified.* |
| *Mr Miles:* | *Well, you won't have to worry about me. I can take care of myself.* |
| *Nurse Gopal:* | *I can imagine it's frustrating to be very independent one minute and then suddenly become ill and feel as though everyone is telling you what to do.* |
| *Mr Miles:* | *You can say that again. I'm just not used to needing help.* |
| *Nurse Gopal:* | *Mr Miles, I'm not here to take away your independence. There are a number of things that I need to do for you, but there are also many things I want you to be able to do for yourself. Let me explain some of the ones that I will be doing.* |
| *Mr Miles:* | *OK, I appreciate that.* |

Nurse Gopal recognizes Mr Miles' attempt to test her competence. Mr Miles is fearful of losing his independence. If Nurse Gopal only had minimal experience in developing relationships with patients/clients, she may have felt the need to remain superficial and nondirective. The patient/client will sense the nurse's superficiality during testing and avoid a meaningful discussion. In this case, Nurse Gopal acknowledges concerns and acts to minimize Mr Miles' fears.

## BUILDING TRUST

Trust is relying on someone without doubt or question. Confidence, dependability, confidentiality, and credibility result in a trusting relationship. It is not easy for a patient/client to perceive the need for help or to ask for it. Often an individual trusts the nurse but is incapable of asking for assistance. Trust provides the foundation for effective communication as an individual becomes more open in expressing feelings and thoughts.

Trusting another person involves risk. As a person begins to share feelings and attitudes with the nurse, he or she then becomes vulnerable. Patients/clients must feel comfortable when revealing personal information. The nurse who feels insecure with a patient/client may choose superficial methods to build trust: sharing secrets, telling private jokes, or encouraging the person to establish the relationship on a first-name basis. Some patients/clients accept such behaviours, but others may resent being treated differently. Instead of enjoying the nurse's extra attention, they become distrustful.

Genuine caring is a powerful method for acquiring trust. The nurse shows sensitivity and understanding of the person's needs. Expressing concern is one way to establish trust. Displaying concern encourages the patient's/client's growth and progress. The following example demonstrates communication to build trust:

| | |
|---|---|
| *Mr Squires:* | *I've been home now for 4 days, and I just don't know what to do.* |
| *Nurse Ramsey:* | *You seem upset. Tell me what is wrong. I'd like to help.* |
| *Mr Squires:* | *The doctor put me on that new diet. It seemed easy in the hospital, but I'm afraid I'm not eating right.* |
| *Nurse Ramsey:* | *You've improved so much since you were in hospital. Let's sit down together and see what kinds of foods you should eat. Then we'll look at the types of foods you like that are allowed in your new diet.* |

*Mr Squires begins to trust Nurse Ramsey, who shows a willingness to help, not out of duty but out of a desire to meet his needs.*

*Another element that aids establishment of trust is recognizing Mr Squires' individuality. He realizes that Nurse Ramsey respects him as a unique person.*

| | |
|---|---|
| *Mr Squires:* | *The doctor said I should eat more vegetables and fruits. I really don't like that many vegetables.* |
| *Nurse Ramsey:* | *Well, let's make a list of what you do like. You know there are different ways to prepare the same kinds of foods. If you're able to eat the things you like, you'll be able to follow the diet more easily.* |
| *Mr Squires:* | *That sounds good. Before I left the hospital, I didn't think I would have much choice in what I ate.* |
| *Nurse Ramsey:* | *Of course you do. I'll show you that you can have a lot of variety in your diet and even enjoy it. It's important that the diet be planned for you and not someone else.* |

*Trust develops on a foundation of caring. Nurse Ramsey's time, patience, and conscientiousness show her concern for Mr Squires' welfare.*

## IDENTIFYING PROBLEMS AND GOALS

During the initial encounter, the nurse begins to assess the patient's/client's health status. Through observations and interaction the nurse begins to make diagnostic conclusions. The individual's health goals may be simple, such as moving without discomfort, choosing foods that will be easily tolerated, or getting out of bed safely. The relationship with the patient/client is strengthened if the nurse identifies important problems. Also, the patient/client may not be able to recognize problems. During the orientation phase, the nurse uses communication techniques to direct the patient/client towards an awareness of problems, focus on the nature of the problems, and explore potential solutions. As problems are identified, the nurse and patient/client mutually set goals. When the person is able to participate in goal setting and see the desired benefits, nursing interventions are more effective.

Sometimes the aim of the interaction is a mutual sharing of information, thoughts, and feelings rather than identification of or addressing of problems. The nurse may find that the person is recovering without difficulty or coping well with the situation.

Identification of problems requires attentive listening, open-ended questioning, paraphrasing, and clarifying. Initially, the nurse avoids identifying a large number of actual or potential problems. Bombarding the patient/client with too many questions can result in emotional and physical fatigue. Also, it makes the person less trusting and more suspicious of the nurse's intentions. Limiting problem identification facilitates the person's understanding of the patient's/client's and nurse's roles. The following case study demonstrates communication to identify problems and goals:

*Mr Sachs is a 58-year-old man who has suffered a partial paralysis of his right side. Mr Sachs needs to regain function in his right hand to retain his job as a telephone repairman. He is also fearful of damage to his self-image. He feels deformed and unable to live normally again.*

| | |
|---|---|
| **Mr Sachs:** | *So much has happened to me. I know that I may never be able to do the things I once enjoyed.* |
| **Nurse:** | *I know it's a difficult time for you now, but there are many things we can do to help you regain normal function.* |
| **Mr Sachs:** | *But there are so many things wrong with me.* |
| **Nurse:** | *Let's take one at a time. What is most important to you?* |
| **Mr Sachs:** | *If only I could use my hand.* |
| **Nurse:** | *The physiotherapist has recommended some exercises to increase the strength in your hand. I'll help you to do each one. Shall we try them?* |
| **Mr Sachs:** | *Alright. If only I could use my hand again to work.* |
| **Nurse:** | *Well let's start with some simple goals. First we'll help you gain strength in your fingers so you can grasp cutlery or cups or a comb, or a razor. After that we'll try some more strenuous exercises.* |
| **Mr Sachs:** | *OK, that sounds reasonable. Show me again what I need to do.* |

### CLARIFYING ROLES.

After a helping relationship is initiated, roles must be clarified. This occurs through a sharing of information, including the person's immediate needs, perception of those needs, nursing care measures to be instituted, and steps for ensuring patient/client participation in care. The helping relationship requires participation from both parties, but the nurse assumes the leadership role. Leadership does not mean control in the manipulative sense. Instead, the nurse takes the initiative in determining the person's point of view. The patient/client assumes a role as receiver of care but also assumes an ongoing role as a participant in care.

### Working Phase

During the *working phase* of a helping relationship, the nurse strives to meet goals set during the orientation phase. The nurse and patient/client work together. The relationship broadens and becomes more flexible as the nurse and patient/client are more willing to share feelings and discuss problems.

The nurse encourages the open expression of feelings. This may be successfully achieved by listening. If a patient/client is unaccustomed to sharing feelings, the nurse must be patient and understanding. The nurse's empathy and respect will help to explore the person's true thoughts and feelings.

As the relationship progresses, patients/clients participate in more self-exploration and are better able to discuss relevant issues. The nurse helps the person to understand his or her feelings so that change can occur when necessary.

If the working phase is successful, the person is then able to act on ideas and feelings. This is often risky, and the nurse must remain supportive. The patient/client must be able to deal with both successes and failures as he or she makes decisions and attempts to resolve problems. Any attempt at change should be within patients'/clients' abilities. Change becomes less of a threat when patients/clients express feelings about change and accept temporary setbacks. The nurse should encourage even the slightest progress.

## INTEGRATING COMMUNICATION WITH NURSING ACTIONS

Nursing actions can generally be divided into four groups: physical, psychological, spiritual, and socioeconomic. Bradley and Edinberg (1990) categorize these groups by their visibility. Physical actions that attend to a person's physical needs, such as nutrition, elimination, and comfort, have high visibility. Most physical actions are nonverbal and routinely performed. Traditionally, emphasis has been placed on a nurse's ability to perform physical actions. Their high visibility allows the patient/client to recognize the nurse as a good practitioner.

In contrast, psychological, socioeconomic, and spiritual nursing actions have low visibility. Psychological actions serve emotional needs. Socioeconomic actions, such as referring patients/clients to community health agencies, assist them in adapting to an environment. Spiritual actions help patients/clients gain support from their belief systems. Low-visibility tasks are not readily observed or measured by others. Psychological, socioeconomic, and spiritual actions require cognitive and affective skills that are not routine and have traditionally proved to be less rewarding for the nurse.

Communication is important in performing both high- and low-visibility tasks. Providing emotional support or educating the person's family obviously require effective communication, but fundamental nursing care activities do as well. The following example shows how the nurse can integrate communication with nursing actions.

*The nurse, Jean Thomas, silently enters Mr Richards' room. She tells him, "It's time for your injection". He is mildly startled and grimaces as he turns to see Nurse Thomas. As Mr Richards starts to ask a question, she quickly turns back the bedclothes and prepares to administer the injection.*

*In contrast, later a second nurse, Mary Ives, enters Mr Richards' room and says, "I have that pain medication you asked for. Are you still feeling uncomfortable?". He turns and replies, "Yes, my back feels like a knife went through it. Will the pain ever go away?". Nurse Ives puts the equipment down, sits down next to Mr Richards, and says, "It's normal to have pain for the first few days after surgery. Let me give you the injection, and then I can show you how to move more carefully in bed to avoid making the pain worse".*

Through communication, a nurse can convey the confidence, credibility, and knowledge that patients/clients expect. In this example a few words of concern and reassurance (low-visibility communication skills) make receiving an injection more acceptable and encourage Mr Richards to express his feelings.

Communication facilitates all nursing care measures. Integrating high- and low-visibility tasks allows Nurse Ives to accomplish several goals simultaneously. She quickly and efficiently assesses Mr Richards' pain, provides a reassuring explanation, and demonstrates an alternative way of relieving pain. Therapeutic communication during high-visibility tasks increases the person's acceptance and understanding of procedures, lessens anxiety, and improves his or her willingness to cooperate. In any helping relationship, however, it is essential that the nurse be aware of his or her own limitations. This will ensure that more skilled help is requested as necessary.

### Termination

During the orientation phase, the nurse tells the patient/client when to expect the relationship to end. When *termination* occurs, the patient/client should not be surprised. By remaining aware of the goals of the relationship, the person should be prepared to function effectively without the nurse's support. Termination can nonetheless be difficult and painful for the patient/client. The primary objective at the end of any helping relationship is termination in a planned and satisfying manner. Summarizing accomplishments and reviewing any unmet needs or follow-up care are helpful.

### EVALUATION OF GOAL ACHIEVEMENT

Vital to termination is evaluation of goals. The nurse encourages assessment of the appropriateness and outcome of goals established. The following shows communication to evaluate goals.

*Nurse Garner has worked with Mr Spiro during his 4-week stay in the hospital. Mr Spiro had surgery for repair of a fractured leg. Together, Nurse Garner and Mr Spiro set goals for his physical rehabilitation and return home.*

| | |
|---|---|
| *Nurse Garner:* | *Well, Mr Spiro, you are going home tomorrow. How do you feel about that?* |

| | |
|---|---|
| *Mr Spiro:* | *Oh, I'll be glad to get out of here. My leg feels pretty good.* |
| *Nurse Garner:* | *How do you feel walking with the crutches?* |
| *Mr Spiro:* | *Not too bad. I have practised climbing stairs quite a bit in the gym. As you know, I have five stairs to climb up to my front door. I can climb them now without losing my balance.* |
| *Nurse Garner:* | *You've also worked hard on learning to transfer from the bed and chair to a standing position with the crutches.* |
| *Mr Spiro:* | *It's a lot easier now. All the practice the physiotherapist suggested helped. Since I've had all of the right ways to hold the crutches explained they feel more like a part of me now. I hope I can get rid of them soon though.* |
| *Nurse Garner:* | *Well, it sounds as if you're ready to leave. Continue your leg exercises as you've done them here, and soon you won't need those crutches.* |
| *Mr Spiro:* | *Thanks again for your encouragement. I didn't think I'd ever be able to walk with these things, but now the crutches are no problem.* |

Both Nurse Garner and Mr Spiro experience satisfaction in meeting goals, particularly because the goals are mutually set. If goals are left unaccomplished, the reasons are examined, and plans are made for attainment in the future. Mr Spiro has not achieved the ability to walk without his crutches. Nurse Garner encourages him to continue his exercise regimen so that he will become strong enough to walk independently.

### SEPARATION

Depending on the relationship between nurse and patient/client, the person may have feelings of anxiety or ambivalence as termination nears. Ideally, the person expresses feelings regarding termination. The nurse should try to plan time to allow the patient/client to share concerns or fears.

If the individual remains in the health care setting and the nurse is the one leaving as a result of a scheduled day off or holiday, the patient/client may feel abandoned. The nurse must ensure that the patient's/client's care is uninterrupted by introducing the new nurse or communicating the person's needs within a written care plan. The nurse shares information that might foster the development of a helping relationship between other nurses and the patient/client.

### Developing Social Skills

If ineffective coping or impaired social interaction is present, the nurse's interventions focus on helping the person to do the following:

1. Express feelings and needs.
2. Develop conversational skills.
3. Communicate thoughts and feelings clearly (verbally and nonverbally).
4. Demonstrate assertiveness.
5. Solve problems.
6. Facilitate conversation with peers and staff.

A nurse who has much more experience with communication skills and interpersonal dynamics may assist patients/clients through role playing; this allows the person to practise situations in which they usually have difficulty in communicating. The following simple interventions can also be used to reinforce attempts at interaction:

1. Encourage participation in normal social activities.
2. Discuss neutral topics or subjects in which patients/clients have interests.
3. Give positive reinforcement for acceptable social interactions.
4. Help patients/clients identify people with whom they feel comfortable and encourage activities with them.
5. Change beds or room to encourage friendships or associates with same interests.

## Communicating with Patient/Clients Who Have Special Needs

At times, it is necessary for nurses to use special communication techniques for successful nurse-patient/client interactions. Patients/clients with sensory and motor impairments, as well as children and older adults, require individualized approaches to communication.

## PROVIDING ALTERNATIVE COMMUNICATION METHODS

Patients/clients with physical communication barriers (for example, a patient/client with a laryngectomy or endotracheal tube) may be unable to speak, or clarity of speech is so poor that alternative methods of communication are needed (see box). For these patients/clients the nurse provides methods that are simple to use. Anything complicated can be frustrating and make communication more difficult. The nurse must be patient as the person tries to communicate. The person must be able to physically use the method that the nurse provides. Patients/clients must have the communication board or pencil and pad nearby. An individual who is unable to speak can be at risk of injury unless personal needs can be quickly communicated.

## EVALUATING COMMUNICATION

Evaluating whether or not communication has been therapeutic helps a patient/client in improving communication, and it improves the nurse-patient/client relationship. The nurse evaluates nursing interventions based on the previously established patient/client goals to determine whether strategies or interventions were effective and what patient/client changes have resulted because of the interventions.

Successful communication is evaluated by the nurse's observations of patient/client interactions. The nurse not only determines that communication exists, but also that the patient/client appears satisfied that the message was received. For example, the nurse might ask himself or herself the following questions:

1. Does the patient/client appear more physically comfortable?

**Children's Nursing**
**Techniques for communicating with children**

INFANT
- The child communicates primarily nonverbally (e.g. coos, smiles, cries) and seeks comfort.
- The nurse should avoid loud, harsh sounds and sudden movements.
- Gentle, close physical contact along with a quiet, low voice help a child to become quiet.
- The nurse keeps the mother in view while holding and interacting with the child.
- A newborn infant can focus up to 15 cm; this is particularly important to remember, since activities such as feeding are valuable opportunities for the nurse to engage in active communication with the infant.

TODDLER OR PRESCHOOL
- The child communicates verbally and nonverbally.
- The child is egocentric with all activities focused on the self.
- Speech and thought processes are concrete.
- The nurse should focus discussion on the child's personal needs and concerns.
- The child is told specifically what he or she can do and how he or she will feel.
- The child should be allowed to explore the environment (e.g. handle a stethoscope, play with a spatula).
- The nurse uses simple, short sentences, familiar words, and concrete explanations and avoids ambiguous phrases that the child can not interpret (e.g. "you will feel a little prick" or "take this medicine for your tummy ache").
- A child will concentrate on what he or she can see, sometimes to the detriment of what he or she may hear; for example, a child about to have a dressing changed will focus on the equipment, rather than the nurse saying "it won't hurt".

SCHOOL-AGED CHILD
- Communication is primarily verbal.
- The child seeks explanations of the world and is interested in functional aspects of objects and events.
- The child is concerned about body integrity.
- The nurse should give simple explanations, demonstrate how equipment works, and allow the child to manipulate equipment (e.g. hold a percussion hammer, wear a stethoscope).
- The child should be allowed to express fears or concerns.

ADOLESCENT
- An adolescent thinks more abstractly, fluctuates between childish and adult thinking behaviour, and likes talking with adults outside of the family.
- The nurse should avoid imposing values or judgements.
- The nurse allows the adolescent to talk, is attentive, and avoids interrupting or showing gestures of disapproval.
- The nurse avoids embarrassing questions or the impulse to give advice.
- Adolescents frequently use a language of their own; the nurse should clarify unfamiliar terms.
- Be careful not to 'take sides' between the adolescent and his or her family; confidentiality must always be maintained unless it is detrimental to do so.

2. Does the person talk about feelings, reactions, and thoughts, or was conversation superficial?
3. Were the appropriate team members consulted?

Nurses compare actual outcomes with expected outcomes when determining the success or effect of interventions. It is also useful for nurses to frequently reflect on and evaluate the effectiveness of their own communication styles and techniques and to make periodic written "process recordings" of the verbal and nonverbal interactions between them and the patient/client. Interactions and responses can then be examined by nurses, other designated nurses, or communication specialists. Some questions that could be asked during such examinations follow:

1. Did nurses encourage openness and allow the patient/client to express thoughts and tell the story?
2. Did responses block the patient's/client's efforts? If so, how?
3. Were responses supportive or critical, opinionated, or trite?
4. Were open-ended or closed questions used? Were they used appropriately?
5. How could the communication have been more effective?

If expected outcomes are not met or progress is not satisfactory according to the patient/client, the nurse needs to reassess and modify the care plan.

## SUMMARY

Communication is one of the most important nursing skills. It allows nurses to improve their understanding of patients'/clients' needs and to develop relationships that will help patients/clients attain healthy behaviours. Nurses' competence depends on their ability to send timely and intelligent messages as patients'/clients' needs dictate and on their ability to understand the person's communications. Communication is affected by many factors and is a complex process that includes verbal and nonverbal messages.

Therapeutic communication with the patient/client involves planned, deliberate interactions that foster a helping relationship. Throughout the relationship the nurse uses skills that promote communication and avoids words and actions that inhibit it. Through effective communication the nurse helps the patient/client adapt to changes resulting from health alterations. The nurse helps patients/clients with special communication problems communicate effectively in spite of physical, emotional, or developmental limitations.

## CHAPTER 15 REVIEW

### Key Concepts
- Effective communication skills help generate trust between the nurse and patients/clients and are a means for bringing about change that promotes patients'/client's well-being.
- The most effective message is clear and organized and expressed in a manner familiar to the person receiving it.
- Elements which are essential to good verbal communication are clarity and brevity, choice of words, pacing, tone, timing and relevance.

**Mental Health Nursing
Communicating with people who have hallucinations**

Hallucinations are common psychiatric symptoms and individuals suffering from hallucinations present nurses with a major challenge in communicating with him or her.

Nursing Assessment:

1. Identification of all sensory modes involved.
2. Determination of the length of time the hallucinations have been experienced.
3. The extent to which the person is experiencing the hallucinations as real, as well as the extent to which the person is able to recognize what is real or otherwise.
4. Identification of major content themes and underlying feelings.
5. Determination of whether command hallucinations are being experienced; whether the person follows the commands and their potential destructiveness.
6. The time of day or situations when hallucinations are most likely to occur.
7. The person's emotional response to hallucinations.
8. Any strategies that the person has tried to use in order to cope.
9. If the person denies hallucinations but gives non-verbal indications which suggest hallucinations, explore whether 'voices' may be asking the person not to talk about them.

*Adapted from William CA: Perspectives in the hallucinating process, 1989, University of South Carolina.*

**Adult Nursing
Communicating with an unconscious patient/client**

Even when persons are unconscious or nonresponsive, they may be able to receive stimuli. Hearing is thought to be the last sensation lost with unconsciousness and the first to be regained with consciousness. Consequently, nurses should be careful not to say anything to unconscious patients/clients or within their hearing range that they would not say to fully conscious individuals. Other important nursing interventions include talking to the patient/client while providing care; explaining procedures; providing orientation information, such as the nurse's name, place, date, and time of day; and avoiding bedside conversations with others about the patient/client.

- Elements which are essential to good nonverbal communication are personal appearance, facial expression, posture and gait, gestures and touch.
- Skills which promote positive communication include listening attentively, conveying acceptance, asking related questions, paraphrasing, clarifying, focusing and summarizing.
- Interpersonal barriers to effective communication include giving an opinion, offering false reassurance, being defensive,

## Communication Aids

- Pad and felt-tipped pen
- Communication board with words, letters, or pictures denoting basic needs (e.g. water, bedpan, pain medication)
- Call bells or alarms
- Sign language
- Use of eye blinks or movement of fingers for simple responses (e.g. yes or no)
- Flash cards with common words or phrases the patient/client may use
- Language cards for patients/clients who do not speak the dominant language

## Key Terms

Acceptance, p. 285
Assertiveness, p. 287
Communication, p. 275
Empathy, p. 291
Eye contact, p. 281
Feedback, p. 278
Female communication patterns, p. 283
Focusing, p. 286
Helping relationship, p. 291
Interpersonal communication, p. 276
Intrapersonal communication, p. 276
Male communication patterns, p. 283
Mutality, p. 291
Nonverbal communication, p. 280
Nonverbal cues, p. 280
Perception, p. 282
Psychological homeostasis, p. 284
Stereotypes, p. 289
Therapeutic communication, p. 284
Verbal communication, p. 286

showing approval or disapproval, stereotyping, asking why and changing the subject inappropriately.

- The way a person receives a message depends on perceptions, values, knowledge, roles, sociocultural factors, past experiences, sensory function, and personal expectations.
- The nurse should be flexible with regard to the techniques used to foster communication with each patient/client.
- The orientation phase of a helping relationship allows trust to be built and allows problems and goals to be identified.
- Trust, empathy, caring, autonomy, and mutuality are basic dimensions of a helping nurse-patient/client relationship.
- The working phase of a helping relationship involves the nurse and patient/client working together so that the person can express thoughts and feelings freely and constructively.
- Patients/clients with ineffective coping or impaired social skills may benefit from positive reinforcement and encouragement to participate in interactions.
- It is useful for nurses to frequently reflect on and evaluate the effectiveness of their own communication styles and techniques and to continue to develop these skills.

## CRITICAL THINKING EXERCISES

1. You are working in the neurological unit and are involved in caring for Tony, an 18-year-old boy who was hit by a car while riding his bicycle. He is unconscious as a result of a head injury. His mother is at the bedside. As you enter the room you notice her holding Tony's hand and crying.
a. Identify at least two ways you might respond to Tony's mother.
b. What factors that influence communication would you need to consider before developing a plan to help you respond to Tony's mother as she deals with this traumatic event? What additional information would you need?
2. Identify a habit that you have which conveys an obstructive message (for example, holding arms across the chest) that you would sincerely like to break.
a. Sensitize yourself to this habit by developing an exercise in which you use this message to excess.
b. Now pick alternative messages from the list of caring or confirming techniques identified in the chapter, substitute it for the obstructive message in the exercise above, and practise using it over and over again.

## REFERENCES

Argyle M: *The psychology of interpersonal behaviour*, Harmondsworth, 1983, Penguin.

Bond: *Stress and self awareness: a guide for nurses*, London, 1986, Heinemann.

Boyle JS, Andrews MA: *Transcultural concepts in nursing care*, Glenview, Ill, 1989, Scott, Foresman.

Bradley J, Edinberg MA: *Communication in the nursing context*, ed 3, Norwalk, Conn, 1990, Appleton & Lange.

Cartwright A, Bowling A: *Life after death: a study of the elderly widowed*, London, 1982, Routledge & Kegan Paul.

Dreher BB: *Communication skills for working with elders*, New York, 1987, Springer.

Dugan DO: Laughter and tears: best medicine for stress, *Nurs Forum* 24(1):18, 1989.

Duldt BW et al:: *Interpersonal communication in nursing*, Philadelphia, 1984, Davis.

Ekman P. Communication through nonverbal behavior: a source of information about an interpersonal relationship. In Tomkins SS, Izard CE, (editors): *Affect, cognition, and personality*, New York, 1965, Springer.

Foong A: Challenging the tower of babel , *Nursing*, 5 (5): 8-9, 1992.

Fritz P et al: *Intrapersonal communication in nursing: an interactionist approach*, East Norwalk, Conn, 1984, Appleton & Lange.

Hall ET: *The hidden dimension*, New York, 1969, Doubleday.

King I: *Toward a theory for nursing*, New York, 1971, John Wiley & Sons.

Knapp M: *Nonverbal communication in human interaction*, New York, 1978, Holt, Rinehart & Winston.

Knaus WA et al: An evaluation of outcome from intensive care in major medical centers, *Ann Intern Med* 104(3):410, 1986.

Lakoff R: *Language and woman's place*, New York, 1975, Harper & Row.

Lalli-Ascosi S: Polishing your self-image, *Health Trends Transition* 1(2):15, 1990.

Lindenfield G, Adams R: *Problem solving through self help groups*, Ilkley, 1984, Self Help Association.

Peplau HE: *Interpersonal relations in nursing*, New York, 1952, Putnam.

Ritter S: *Manual of clinical psychiatric nursing, principles and procedures*, London, 1989, Harper & Row.

Roper N, Tierney A, Logan W: *The elements of nursing*, ed 3, Edingburgh, 1990 Churchill Livingstone.

Sarvimaki A: Nursing care as moral, practical, communicative and creativity activity, *Journal of Advanced Nursing*, 13: 462, 1988.

Satir V: *Conjoint family therapy*, ed 3, Palo Alto, Calif, 1983, Science & Behavior Books.

Sayers F. Sex, sex-role and conversation: review of the literature and rationale. In Valentine CA, Hoar N, (editors): *Women and communication power: theory, research, and practice*, Annandale, Va, 1988, Speech Communication Association.

Stevens M: *Personal and vocational relationships of the practical nurse*, Philadelphia, 1975, WB Saunders.

Sullivan JL, Deane DM: Humor and health, *J Gerontol Nurs* 14(1):20, 1988.

Sundeen SJ *et al*: *Nurse-client interaction: implementing the nursing process*, ed 5, St Louis, 1994, Mosby.

Tannen D: *You just don't understand: women and men in conversation*, New York, 1990, Morrow.

Travelbee J: *Interpersonal aspects of nursing*, ed 2, Philadelphia, 1971, Davis.

Vortherms RC: Clinically improving communication through touch, *J Gerontol Nurs* 17(5):6, 1991.

Wong DL: *Nursing care of infants and children*, ed 5, St Louis, 1995, Mosby.

Williams H: Humor and healing: therapeutic effects in geriatrics, *Gerontologist* 1(3):14, 1986.

Zunin L: *Contact: the first four minutes*, New York, 1988, Ballantine.

## FURTHER READING

### Adult Nursing

Audit Commission: *What seems to be the matter: communication between hospitals and patients*. London, 1993, HMSO.

Bird B: *Talking with patients*, Philadelphia, 1973, Lippincott.

Cameron JE: Giant leap forward begins with the nursing interview, *Aust Nurses J* 12(2):47, 1982.

Chenevert M: *STAT: special techniques in assertiveness training for women in the health professions*, ed 3, St Louis, 1988, Mosby.

Coad-Denton A. Therapeutic superficiality and intimacy. In Longo D, Williams R: *Clinical practice in psychosocial nursing: assessment and intervention*, ed 2, New York, 1986, Appleton & Lange.

Ebersole P, Hess P: *Toward healthy aging*, ed 3, St Louis, 1990, Mosby.

Enelow A, Swisher SS (editors): *Interviewing and patient care*, ed 3, New York, 1985, Oxford University Press.

Horne E, Cowan T (editors): *Effective communication: some nursing perspectives* ed 2. London, 1992, Mosby–Wolfe.

Knowles RD: Building rapport through neuro-linguistic programming, *Am J Nurs* 83:1011, 1983.

Marchione J, Stearns SJ: Ethnic power perspectives for nursing, *Nurs Health Care* 11(6):229, 1989.

Marsden, C: Ethics of the "doctor-nurse game," *Heart Lung* 19:422, 1990.

Morath J: Empathy training: development of sensitivity and caring in hospitals, *Nurs Manage* 20(3):60, 1989.

Olson JK, Iwasiw CL: Effects of a training model on active listening skills of post-RN students, *J Nurs Educ* 26(3):104, 1987.

Pike AW: On the nature and place of empathy in clinical nursing practice, *J Prof Nurs* 6:235, 1990.

Podrasky DL, Sexton DL: Nurses' reaction to difficult patients, *Image J Nurs Sch* 20(1):16, 1988.

Rogers CR: *On becoming a person*, Boston, 1972, Houghton Mifflin.

Rothenberger RL: Transcultural nursing: overcoming obstacles to effective communication, *AORN J* 51:1357, 1990.

### Children's Nursing

Crompton M: *Children and counselling*, London, 1989, Edward Arnold.

Denehy T. Communicating with children through drawings. In *Nursing interventions for infants and children*, Philadelphia, 1990, WB Saunders.

Kanneh A: The need to communicate, *Nurs Stand* 5(5):19, 1990.

McConkey R, Price P: *Let's talk*, London, 1986, Souvenir Press.

Petrie P: *Communicating with children and adults*, London, 1989, Edward Arnold

### Learning Disabilities Nursing

Brudenell P: *The other side of profound handicap*, London, 1986, Macmillan.

Felce D, Toogood S. In Brechin A, Walmsley J (editors): *Making connections*. London, 1989, Hodder & Stoughton.

Orlowska D, McGill P, Mansell J: Staff-staff and staff-resident verbal interactions in a community-based group home for people with moderate and severe mental handicaps, *Ment Handicap Res* 4(1):3, 1991.

Sinason V In Brechin A, Walmsley J (editors): *Making connections*, London, 1989, Hodder & Stoughton.

### Mental Health Nursing

Kagan C, Evans J, Kay B: *Interpersonal skills in nursing: an experiential approach*, London, 1986, Harper & Row.

Skidmore D: *Communication*. In Brooking, Ritter and Thomas: A textbook of psychiatric and mental health nursing, Edinburgh, 1992, Churchill Livingstone.

# Teaching and Learning

## LEARNING OUTCOMES

After studying this chapter, you should be able to:
- *Define the key terms listed.*
- *Identify the purposes of patient/client education.*
- *Describe the similarities and differences between teaching and learning.*
- *Describe how to incorporate communication principles into the teaching-learning process.*
- *Describe the three domains of learning.*
- *Differentiate factors that determine motivation to learn from those that determine ability to learn.*
- *List the factors involved in patient/client assessment prior to formulation of a teaching plan.*
- *Write learning objectives for an organized and effective teaching plan.*
- *Discuss the different teaching approaches and suggest circumstances appropriate to each.*
- *Describe teaching methods which facilitate optimum learning.*
- *Identify different teaching approaches to use for patients/clients with specific learning needs.*
- *Identify methods for incorporating teaching into nursing care and evaluating patient/client learning.*

Patient/client education has become one of the more important roles for nurses working in every type of health care setting. Teaching healthy mothers in a general practitioner's surgery about prenatal care, teaching parents visiting a clinic about immunization of children, teaching heart attack victims about newly prescribed medications, and teaching people with diabetes about self-care are examples of patient/client education. Patients/clients and family members have the right to health education so that they can make informed decisions about their health and lifestyle. Many individuals who previously received treatments in hospitals now receive them in the community or on an outpatient basis. If they are hospitalized, they are discharged soon after treatment (Kruger, 1991; Webb, 1983). Effective health education is essential if nurses are to care for increasing numbers of patients/clients in the community and if the effects of preventable disease are to be minimized (Noble, 1991).

Increased demands on nurses' time and the need to give seriously ill people concise and meaningful information as soon as possible emphasize the importance of quality patient/client education. As nurses try to find the best ways to educate patients/clients, the general public has become more assertive in seeking knowledge and understanding of personal health and the resources available within the health care system (Parker, 1983; Kruger, 1991). Providing individuals with needed information about health care is necessary to ensure continuity of care from the home to the hospital to the home. A well-designed, comprehensive teaching plan that fits the individual's learning needs can reduce health care costs, improve the quality of care, and help the individual gain more independence.

The significance of patient/client education is enhanced

because of the individual's right to know and be informed about his or her diagnoses, prognoses, treatments, and risks. Information provided should be readily understandable. It is negligent to assume that patients/clients will learn on their own. Accurate and timely information is needed for patients/clients to make decisions about their health. More attention is being paid in courts of law as to whether patients/clients are adequately informed about ways to manage their health. Competent professional nursing practice includes patient/client education. Virginia Henderson (1966) stated that part of the nurse's role is to improve the patient's level of understanding and thus promote their health. In the 1983 Statutory Instrument Rule 18, one of the two stated competencies for nurses, midwives and health visitors is to "advise on the promotion of health and the prevention of illness" (HMSO, 1983). The nurse can provide adequate education only by identifying patients'/clients' learning needs and by using the most appropriate teaching strategies.

## PURPOSES OF PATIENT/CLIENT EDUCATION

The public has become more health conscious in recent years. Participation in fitness clubs, diet programmes, regular exercise activities, and health-screening programmes are examples of ways that people pay more attention to their health.

The aim of health education and patient/client teaching is to equip people intellectually and emotionally for making sound decisions on matters affecting their health and welfare (Macleod, Clark and Webb, 1985:).

The nurse is a convenient resource for patients/clients who want to improve their physical and psychological well-being. There are three main objectives of health education depending on the parents/clients level of wellness:

- **Maintaining Health and Preventing Illness:** In the school, home, clinic, or workplace, the nurse provides information and skills that will allow patients/clients to assume healthier behaviours and prevent illness. For example, in antenatal classes, midwives teach expectant parents what to anticipate and do during pregnancy. After learning about normal childbearing the mother is more likely to eat healthy foods, get physical exercise, and avoid drugs or other substances that might harm the fetus. Promoting healthy behaviour through education increases patients'/clients' self-esteem by empowering them to assume more responsibility for their health. When patients/clients become more health conscious, they are more likely to seek early diagnosis of health problems.

- **Restoring Health**: People who are injured or ill need information and skills that will help them regain improved levels of health. People recovering from illness or injury and adapting to the associated limitations often seek information about their conditions. However, people who find it difficult to adapt to illness may seem uninterested

in learning. The nurse learns to identify individuals' willingness to acquire knowledge and institutes methods to motivate interest.

The family is often a vital part of a person's return to health. If the nurse excludes the family from a teaching plan, conflicts may arise. For example, if the family does not understand a patient's/client's need to regain independent function, their efforts may cause the person to become unnecessarily dependent and may consequently retard progress.

- **Coping with Impaired Functioning:** Some people must learn to cope with permanent health alterations. Knowledge and skills are often necessary for these people to continue activities of living.

In the case of serious disability the patient's/client's role within the family may change, making understanding and acceptance by family members necessary. The family's ability to provide support can be enhanced by education. Families of people with other kinds of alterations, such as alcohol misuse, a learning disability, or multiple sclerosis, learn to adapt to the emotional effects.

It is important to learn how to work with patients/clients at different levels of wellness. To do this, you must consider the patients'/clients' needs in relation to their ability to meet them. Learning occurs when information is practical and useful. Comparing patients'/clients' desired levels of health with the actual states enables you to plan meaningful teaching programmes.

## TEACHING AND LEARNING

It is impossible to separate teaching from learning. **Teaching** is an interactive process between a teacher and one or more learners (Redman, 1988). It consists of a deliberate set of actions that help individuals gain knowledge or perform new skills. A teacher provides information that prompts the learner to participate in or initiate activities that lead to desired cognitive or behavioural change.

**Learning** is dynamic and fluid and is a shared, lifelong event (Rendon *et al*, 1986). To *learn* is to acquire knowledge or skills through reinforced practice and experience. For example, a patient/client with diabetes demonstrates to a nurse the technique for preparing insulin in a syringe. A person with arthritis learns the best ways to perform self-care activities at home. Generally, teaching and learning begin when a person identifies a need for knowing or acquiring an ability to do something. According to Knowles (1970), learning is an internal process, and there are superior conditions of learning and principles of teaching. **Teaching is most effective when it responds to a learner's needs.** The teacher identifies these needs by asking questions and determining the learner's interests. Teaching relies on principles of interpersonal communication. In other words, the teacher must send messages of significance to the learner and receive the learner's feedback.

## Role of the Nurse in Teaching and Learning

Patients/clients often ask nurses for health information. Identifying the need for teaching is easy when patients/clients request information. Often, however, a patient's/client's need for teaching may be less obvious.

The nurse is frequently able to anticipate a patient's/client's needs for information. Although the doctor is ultimately responsible for providing information about a diagnosis, treatment, and prognosis, the nurse must help the person understand the responses to illness. A nurse clarifies information provided by doctors and becomes the primary source of information that helps the patients/clients adjust to the health problem.

To be an effective **educator**, the nurse must do more than just pass on facts; you must engage the individual in learning (Spicer, 1982). Nurses have numerous opportunities to pass on facts. However, there is no assurance that the patient/client learns from these facts. As an educator, you must carefully determine what the individual needs to know and find the time when they are ready to learn.

It is critical for nurses to perceive the role of educator as important. Over the past two decades research has provided evidence of the importance of educating patients/clients. Boore (1978) suggested that giving patients/clients information and a role in their recovery both pre- and postoperatively led to reduced levels of anxiety, reduced postoperative complications and enhanced recovery. Wilson-Barnett (1978) similarly found that providing specific information to patients/clients undergoing barium enema examination benefited the patients/clients and reduced their anxiety. Hayward (1975) also found that patients/clients who received relevant preoperative information received less analgesic drugs and reported reduced postoperative pain. However, more research is needed to demonstrate the relationship between patient/client education and favourable patient/client outcomes. A goal of patient/client education is to change patient/client behaviour and to maintain or improve the individual's health. When nurses value patient/client education and are able to implement it into practice, patients/clients will be better prepared for assuming their own health care responsibilities.

## Teaching as a Form of Communication

The teaching process closely parallels the communication process (see Chapter 15). Effective teaching depends in part on effective interpersonal communication. The steps of the teaching process can be compared with those of the communication process. In teaching, the **referent** represents the need to provide the patient/client with information. The patient/client may request information, or the nurse may perceive a need for it. The nurse then identifies specific learning objectives. A **learning objective** describes what the learner will be able to do after successful instruction.

The nurse as teacher is the **sender**, whose aim is to convey a message to the patient/client. The nurse promotes learning by communicating in a language recognizable to the learner. It is important to be aware of your patients's/clients' cultural

### Mental Health Nursing
### Teaching–learning process

Patient/client teaching in mental health is orientated towards increased self-directness and greater self-actualization. Many of the methods are rooted in activities of creativity; some carried out on a one-to-one basis and some in a group. Examples include:

- Art therapy – the use of art and other visual media in a therapeutic or treatment setting to increase about greater intra- and interpersonal learning.
- Social skills and assertion training – to assist individuals who have become increasingly deskilled socially as a result of mental illness, or who have a poorly developed repertoire of social skills which make them vulnerable to life's stressors.
- Occupational therapy – a wide range of approaches used to promote individual competence in a whole range of life skills.
- Psychotherapy – a diverse collection of therapies aimed at increasing intra- and interpersonal learning.
- Creative therapy – aimed at developing the individual's awareness of one's own creativity and to positively channel one's energies in self-expression and self-transcendence.

### Learning Disabilities
### The teaching-learning process

With the move away from institutionalized care, the process of re-orientating people with learning disabilities back into society is termed *normalization*. This process includes making available to all people with learning disabilities, patterns of life and conditions which are as close as possible to the regular circumstances and ways of life of society.

Nirje (1980) identifies eight areas where training and education should focus on reproducing the lifestyle experienced by a non-disabled person:

- the rhythm of the day — patterns of waking, dressing, eating, retiring
- the rhythm of the week — weekdays, weekends, and work and leisure activities
- the rhythm of the year — seasonal events, holiday
- progression through the stages of the life cycle — exposure to normal expectations of childhood, adolescence, adulthood
- self-determination
- the development of sexual relationships
- economic standards (access to benefits)
- environmental standards.

background, as their concept of health and illness may affect their interpretation and understanding of your message. In addition, many intrapersonal variables will influence style and approach. Your attitudes, values, emotions, and knowledge influence the way that messages are sent. Past experiences with teaching will help you choose the best way to present information.

The **message** or content to be taught is delivered clearly and precisely. Organize information to be taught in a logical sequence so that the patient/client will more easily understand skills or ideas. Present each 'lesson' as a meaningful progression from

## Table 16-1 Domains of Learning

| Domain of Learning | Behaviour | Definition | Example |
| --- | --- | --- | --- |
| COGNITIVE | Knowledge | Acquiring new facts and being able to learn them. | Patient/client learns about a new drug and is able to describe its purpose and potential side effects. |
| | Comprehension | The ability to understand the meaning of learned material. | Patient/client is able to explain specifically how the new medication will improve physical condition. |
| | Application | Using abstract, newly learned ideas in concrete situations. | Patient/client learns to self-administer the medication according to a meal schedule to minimize side effects. |
| | Analysis | Relating ideas in an organized way. It allows a person to distinguish important from unimportant information. | Patient/client is able to distinguish which side effects are more likely to be experienced from the medication and to compare them with the effects experienced by another person. |
| | Synthesis | The ability to recognize parts of information as a whole. | Patient/client experiences side effects from a medication and is able to take preventive steps. |
| | Evaluation | Judgement of the worth of a body of information for a given purpose. | Patient/client is able to recognize a symptom associated with the medication. |
| AFFECTIVE | Receiving | Being willing to attend to another person's words. | A woman shows willingness to listen to a nurse explain the surgical procedure for removal of a breast. |
| | Responding | Active participation through listening and reacting verbally and nonverbally. The person feels satisfied by the response. | Patient/client asks the nurse about the appearance of the incision that she will have. |
| | Valuing | Attaching worth to an object or behaviour. This is shown through the learner's behaviour. | Patient/client expresses a concern about the effect of surgery on her appearance. After surgery, the patient/client refuses to look at the incision and wears a gown with a high neck. |
| | Organizing | Developing a value system by identifying and organizing values and resolving conflicts. | Patient/client learns to accept changes created by surgery and is willing to participate in social activities. |
| | Characterizing | Acting and responding with a consistent value system. The person behaves consistently when values are tested or challenged. | Patient/client assumes a normal lifestyle after having breast surgery and is able to discuss with others her positive feelings about herself. |

(Cont'd)

simple to more complex skills or ideas.

You may use several **channels** to present teaching content. All of the senses are channels for presenting information. The auditory channel is the simplest, as in a lecture or discussion. However, the learning process becomes more stimulating when several sensory channels are used. For example, a patient/client with newly diagnosed heart disease will learn how to measure a pulse best by actually feeling the pulsation of an artery.

The **receiver** in the teaching-learning process is the learner.

A number of intrapersonal variables affect motivation and ability to learn. Patients/clients are ready to learn when they express a desire to do so and are more likely to receive the message when they understand the content. Attitudes, anxiety, and values are a few factors that influence the ability to comprehend a message. The ability to learn depends on factors such as emotional and physical health, education, stage of development, previous knowledge, language and culture. During the teaching process, you will use a variety of skills in order to meet a variety of

## Table 16-1 Domain of Learning (Cont'd)

| Domain of Learning | Behaviour | Definition | Example |
|---|---|---|---|
| PSYCHOMOTOR | Perception | Being aware of objects and of qualities through the use of sense organs. A person associates a sensory cue with the task to perform. | After hearing the siren of an ambulance a person considers driving to the curb to avoid a collision. |
| | Set | A readiness to take a particular action. There are three sets: mental, physical, and emotional. | A patient/client might make the commitment (emotional set) to regularly perform exercises. A person uses judgement to determine the best way to perform a motor act (mental readiness). Before performing the act, such as rising from a wheelchair, the person aligns and postures properly (physical readiness). |
| | Guided Response | The performance of an act under the guidance of a teacher. Involves imitation of a demonstrated act. | Patient/client prepares an insulin injection after watching a nurse's demonstration. The nurse provides immediate reinforcement after the patient/client correctly performs the act. |
| | Mechanism | A higher level of behaviour whereby a person has gained confidence and skill in performing the behaviour. Usually the skill is more complex or involves several more steps than a guided response. | Patient/client is able to fill the insulin syringe for different insulin doses. |
| | Complex Overt Response | Performing a motor skill involving a complex movement pattern. Person performs the skill smoothly and accurately without hesitation. | Patient/client is able to self-administer an insulin injection using several sites. |
| | Adaptation | When a person is able to change a motor response when unexpected problems arise. | As a nurse administers an injection, the appearance of blood during aspiration results in changing the way that the syringe is handled. |
| | Origination | A highly complex motor act that involves creating new movement patterns. A person acts on the basis of existing psychomotor skills. | A nurse uses a different method of venepuncture on a patient/client whose arm is swollen. |

patient/client needs. There are now many teaching materials in various forms and languages to help you meet these individual needs (see Table 16.3).

An effective teacher provides a mechanism for evaluating the success of a teaching plan. Having a patient/client demonstrate a newly learned skill or asking the individual to describe the correct dosage schedule for a medication are ways to gather feedback. Feedback must show the success of the learner in achieving objectives; that is, the learner restates information or provides a return demonstration of skills learned.

## DOMAINS OF LEARNING

Learning occurs in three areas or domains (Table 16.1): **cognitive** (understandings), **affective** (attitudes), and **psychomotor** (motor skills) (Bloom, 1956). Any topic to be learned may involve all domains or only one. For example, patients/clients learn to understand about diabetes, the way that it affects the body, and ways to control blood sugar levels for healthier lifestyles (cognitive domain). In addition, patients/clients learn to accept the long-term nature of the disease (affective domain). Many diabetic people must also learn to administer insulin injections on a daily basis (psychomotor domain). The characteristics of learning within each domain affect the teaching and evaluation methods used. Understanding each learning domain prepares you to select proper teaching techniques. However, you also need to be able to apply the basic principles of learning to any teaching method (see later section).

## Cognitive Learning

The **cognitive learning** domain involves intellectual behaviours. Bloom (1956) classifies cognitive behaviours in an ordered hierarchy. The simplest behaviour is acquiring knowledge, whereas the most complex is evaluation.

## Affective Learning

**Affective learning** deals with expression of feelings and acceptance of attitudes, opinions, or values. Values clarification (see Chapter 12) is an example of affective learning. The simplest behaviour in the hierarchy is receiving, and the most complex is characterizing (Krathwohl *et al*, 1964).

## Psychomotor Learning

The **psychomotor learning** domain involves acquiring skills that require the integration of mental and muscular activity such as the ability to walk or to use an eating utensil. The simplest behaviour in the hierarchy is perception, whereas the most complex is origination (Simpson, 1972).

## BASIC LEARNING PRINCIPLES

To teach effectively, you must first understand the ways people learn. Learning depends on three conditions:

- **willingness** or motivation to learn – the patient's/client's willingness to become involved in learning influences a nurse's teaching approach. Previous knowledge, attitudes, and sociocultural factors influence motivation. Motivation addresses a person's willingness to put effort into learning (Redman, 1988).
- **ability to learn** – the ability to learn depends on physical and cognitive attributes. Developmental level, physical wellness, and intellectual thought processes determine a person's ability to learn. If a person's learning ability is impaired, a teacher may postpone teaching activities or modify strategies to better meet the learner's needs.
- **learning environment** – the environment has a significant impact on the ability to learn. One of the teacher's major tasks is to manipulate environmental conditions to facilitate learning. This can be particularly challenging for a nurse in a busy health care setting.

## Willingness to Learn
### Attentional Set

People's minds generally function with mental pictures. For example, as a teacher explains how to give support to a dying patient/client, students might envision grasping the fragile hand of a person taking a last breath. Before individuals can learn, they must give attention to, or concentrate on, information to be learned. An **attentional set** is the mental state that allows the learner to focus and comprehend the material. A number of factors influence this ability to attend, including physical discomfort, anxiety, and environmental distractions.

Any physical condition that impairs the ability to concentrate interferes with learning. Pain, fatigue, hunger, thirst, and even the urge to urinate or defecate create barriers to learning.

Anxiety may increase or decrease the ability of a person to learn. Anxiety is uneasiness from anticipation of threat or danger. When faced with change or the need to act differently, a person feels anxiety. Learning requires a change in behaviour and thus produces anxiety. A mild level of anxiety may motivate learning. However, a high level of anxiety prevents learning; it incapacitates a person, creating an inability to attend to anything other than its immediate relief.

Environmental distractions (discussed in a later section) interfere with the ability to attend to a teacher and learning activities. Unplanned interruptions or an uncomfortable environment are not conducive to learning.

### Motivation

**Motivation** is an internal impulse that causes a person to take action; it is the desire to learn. It implies that at some point in time a person is receptive to learning. A person may become motivated to learn by an idea, emotion, or physical need. If an individual does not want to learn, it is unlikely that learning will occur.

The social, task mastery, and physical motives stimulate a person to learn. *Social motives* are a need for affiliation, social approval, or self-esteem. People normally seek out others with whom to compare opinions, abilities, and emotions. For example, a student often works hard to win praise from a teacher or the admiration of peers.

*Task mastery motives* are based on needs such as achievement and competence. A student nurse repeatedly works to learn the technique for giving an injection, because of the motivation to master the task or skill. After a success, there is usually greater motivation to achieve more.

Often the motives of a patient/client are *physical*. If the individual suffers a physical change in function, that change may become a motivator for learning. According to Tanner (1989), knowledge that is necessary for survival creates a stronger stimulus for learning than knowledge that merely promotes health. For example, when a patient/client experiences a loss in strength of a body part, there is motivation to learn exercises that will rehabilitate and restore normal strength.

### Psychosocial Adaptation to Illness

Loss of health, whether temporary or permanent, is difficult for people to accept. The process of grieving gives them time to adapt psychologically to the emotional and physical implications of illness. The stages of grieving (see Chapter 11) are a series of responses that patients/clients experience during illness. People experience these stages at different rates and sequences, depending on their self-concepts before illness, the severity of illness, and the changes in lifestyle that the illness creates. Effective supportive care guides patients/clients through the grieving process.

Readiness to learn is significantly related to the stage of grieving (Table 16-2). When unable to accept the reality of illness, patients/clients cannot learn. However, when properly timed, teaching can facilitate adjustment to illness or disability.

## Active Participation

A patient's/client's involvement in learning implies an eagerness to acquire knowledge or skills. It also improves the opportunity for the patient/client to make decisions during teaching sessions. For example, a person diagnosed with diabetes learns to monitor blood glucose levels to gain control of the disease. Through participation with the nurse, the patient/client learns to adapt a monitoring system and schedule to personal lifestyle. The patient/client helps decide the type of glucose meter that will be easiest to use.

## Ability to Learn
### Developmental Capability

Cognitive level of development influences a person's ability to learn. A nurse can be a competent teacher, but teaching will be unsuccessful if the patient's/client's intellectual abilities are not considered. For example, a teaching booklet is not useful if a patient/client cannot read, and a patient/client who is unable to perform simple mathematical calculations will have difficulty learning to calculate medication doses.

Learning, like developmental growth, is an evolving process. The nurse should know patients'/clients' levels of knowledge before beginning teaching plans. In addition, learning occurs more readily when new information complements existing knowledge.

## AGE GROUP

Age reflects the developmental capability for learning and the type of learning behaviour that can be acquired. Without proper biological, motor, language, and personal-social development, many types of learning cannot take place. Learning occurs when behaviour changes as a result of experience or growth (Wong, 1995).

## Physical Capability

The ability to learn often depends on the level of physical development and overall physical health. To learn psychomotor skills, a patient/client must possess the necessary level of strength, coordination, and sensory acuity. For example, it is useless to teach a patient/client to transfer from a bed to a wheelchair if the individual has insufficient upper body strength. An older person cannot learn to apply an elastic bandage if arthritis in his or her fingers prevents him or her from grasping the bandage tightly.

Therefore the nurse should not overestimate the individual's physical capabilities.

Any condition that depletes a person's energy (for example, pain) will also impair the ability to learn. A patient/client who spends a morning undergoing diagnostic studies will possibly not be capable of a learning discussion in the afternoon. When an illness becomes aggravated by complications, such as a high fever or respiratory difficulty, teaching should be postponed. You can assess energy level by noting a patient's/client's willingness to communicate, amount of activity initiated, and responsiveness to questions. Halt teaching temporarily if the individual needs rest. You will achieve greater teaching success when the patient/client is an active participant in learning.

## Learning Environment

The physical environment where teaching takes place makes learning pleasant or difficult. Choose a setting that helps the patient/client focus on the learning task. The following factors are important when choosing the setting:
*   number of people being taught
*   need for privacy
*   temperature
*   lighting
*   noise
*   ventilation
*   furniture.

The ideal environment for learning is a room with good lighting, good ventilation, appropriate furniture, and a comfortable temperature. A darkened room interferes with the patient's/client's ability to see, especially during demonstrations and use of visual aids. A room that is cold, hot, or humid and stuffy makes the patient/client too uncomfortable to pay attention to the nurse's activities. Comfortable furniture helps eliminate distractions, such as the need to continually change position or shift body weight. A businesslike, yet warm and accepting atmosphere promotes learning in children and adults (Klausmeier, 1985; Redman, 1988). Posters, displays, or equipment for practising skills motivates a learner by stimulating curiosity. It is also important to choose a quiet setting to minimize distractions.

When working with only one patient/client, the best setting for learning is one that is quiet and offers privacy. You can provide privacy even in a busy hospital by closing cubicle curtains or taking the person to a quiet spot. In a home, a bedroom might separate the patient/client from household activities. If the individual desires, family members might share in discussions. However, some people are reluctant to discuss their illnesses when others, even close family members, are in the room.

Teaching a group of patients/clients requires a room that allows everyone to be seated comfortably and within hearing distance of the teacher. The size of the room should not overwhelm the group, tempting participants to sit outside the group along the room's perimeter. Arranging the group to allow participants to observe one another further enhances learning. More effective communication occurs as learners observe others' verbal and nonverbal interactions.

**TABLE 16-2 Relationship Between Psychosocial Adaptation to Illness and Learning**

| Stage | Patient's/Client's Behaviour | Learning Implications | Rationale |
|---|---|---|---|
| Denial or disbelief | Patient/client avoids discussion of illness ("There's nothing wrong with me"), withdraws from others, and disregards physical restrictions. Patient/client suppresses and distorts information that has not been presented clearly. | Provide support, empathy, and careful explanations of all procedures while they are being done. Let patient/client know you are available for discussion. Explain situation to family. Teach in present tense (e.g., explain current therapy). | Any attempt to convince or tell patient/client about illness will result in further anger or withdrawal. (Patient/client is not prepared to deal with problem.) Provide only information patient/client pursues or absolutely requires. |
| Anger | Patient/client blames and complains and often directs anger towards the nurse. | Do not argue with patient/client, but listen to concerns. Teach in present tense. Reassure family of patient's/client's normality. | Patient/client needs opportunity to express feelings and anger; patient/client is still not prepared to face future. |
| Bargaining | Patient/client offers to live a better life for promise of better health ("if God lets me live, I promise to be more careful".) | Continue to introduce only reality. Teach only in the present tense. | Patient/client may be unwilling to accept limitations. |
| Resolution | Patient/client begins to express emotions openly, realizes that illness has created changes, and begins to ask questions. | Encourage expression of feelings. Begin to share information needed for future, and set aside formal times for discussion. | Patient/client begins to perceive need for assistance and is ready to accept responsibility for learning. |
| Acceptance | Patient/client recognizes reality of condition, actively pursues information, and strives for independence. | Focus teaching on future skills and knowledge required. Continue to teach about present occurrences. Involve family in teaching information for discharge. | Patient/client is more easily motivated to learn. Acceptance of illness reflects willingness to deal with its implications. |

## INTEGRATING THE NURSING AND TEACHING PROCESSES

A relationship exists between the nursing and teaching processes. With the nursing process, a thorough assessment reveals the patient's/client's health care needs. The health care needs identified are unique to the patient's/client's situation. A care plan is individualized, prescribing nursing therapies designed to improve or maintain the individual's level of health. Evaluation determines the level of success in meeting goals.

While assessing an individual's health care problems, the nurse may also identify the need for education. When education becomes a part of the care plan, the teaching process begins. Like the nursing process, the teaching process requires a thorough assessment; in this case analysing the patient's/client's need, motivation, and ability to learn. When establishing a teaching plan, you will establish specific learning objectives. The implementation of a teaching plan involves the use of learning and teaching principles to ensure that the patient/client acquires knowledge and skills. Finally, the teaching process requires an evaluation of learning based on learning objectives. If objectives are unmet, additional teaching is provided.

The nursing and teaching processes are not the same. The nursing process requires an assessment of all sources of data to determine a patient'/client's total health care needs. The teaching process focuses primarily on the patient's/client's learning needs and the willingness and capability to learn.

## TEACHING AND LEARNING IN NURSING CARE

### Assessing

The nurse must assess the skills and knowledge that the patient/client may require, the patient's/client's motivation and ability to learn, and methods and resources for instruction. The patient/client, family members, and the health care team are resources for this assessment.

### Learning Needs

Determine the information that is critical for the patient/client to learn. The patient's/client's **learning needs** determine the choice of teaching content. Learning needs can change from the time a patient/client requires health care to the time of discharge and after the patient/client resumes self-care at home. You must therefore conduct an ongoing assessment of potential learning needs. An effective assessment should be the basis by which teaching can be individualized to a person's lifestyle and perceived needs (Redman, 1988).

## Terms Used for Objectives

### Terms with Many Interpretations

- To know
- To understand
- To realize
- To value
- To feel

### Terms with Few Interpretations

- To identify
- To describe
- To label
- To classify
- To demonstrate
- To select

## Motivation to Learn

Ask questions that will help define motivation. Even though the individual may have a variety of learning needs, a lack of motivation seriously threatens the success of the teaching plan.

## Ability to Learn

Determine the patient's/client's physical and cognitive capabilities to learn. A variety of factors can impair cognition, including body temperature, electrolyte levels, oxygenation status, and blood glucose level. In an acute care setting, several of these factors may influence a patient/client at one time.

## Teaching Environment

The environment for a teaching session must be conducive to learning. Assess the following factors when seeking a place to teach patients/clients:

- distractions or persistent noise; a quiet area should be set aside for teaching.
- comfort of the room, including ventilation, temperature, lighting, and furniture.
- room facilities and available equipment.

## Resources for Learning

A patient/client may require the support of family members or significant others. In this case, assess the readiness and ability of family and friends to learn the information necessary for the care of the patient/client. You must also understand the home environment. Assessment of resources also includes a review of any teaching tools available.

## Planning

After determining the patient's/client's learning needs, develop a **teaching plan** to promote cognitive, affective, and psychomotor learning. The teaching plan incorporates the information learned about the patient/client into individualized learning strategies. The patient/client should be an active participant in the teaching plan. For example, the person should agree to the plan, and help choose learning methods, and times, for the teaching sessions.

## Developing Learning Objectives

The first step in forming a teaching plan is developing learning objectives. The **learning objectives** of health teaching are the behaviours desired as a result of the learning process (Redman,

1988). A learning objective identifies the expected outcome of a **planned learning experience** and helps establish priorities for learning. Despite all planning, however, a particular teaching session may lead to unanticipated learning. It may be difficult to anticipate all objectives for a teaching session. However, objectives can help a teacher to plan sessions so that time is maximized and the best resources are available for learning.

Objectives are either short or long term. Short-term objectives relate to the patient's/client's immediate learning needs, such as knowing the nature of gallbladder disease to understand a diagnostic test. Long-term objectives relate to acquisition of the knowledge and skills that are needed to permanently adapt to a health problem (for example, learning to plan a diet within restrictions caused by gallbladder disease). Like a goal of care, a long-term objective is usually all encompassing. Short-term objectives can be compared with the steps taken to achieve long-term goals.

The objectives established by the nurse and patient/client guide the teaching plan. Poorly determined objectives can create confusion throughout the teaching-learning process. Thus, a learning objective includes the same criteria as goals or outcomes in a nursing care plan (see Chapter 3), such as the following:

- singular behaviours
- observable or measurable content
- timing or conditions under which the objective is measured
- goals mutually set between the nurse and patient/client.

Each objective is a statement of a singular behaviour that identifies the learner's ability to do something after a learning experience. A *behavioural objective* contains an active verb describing what the learner will do after the objective is met, such as *to administer* an injection (Bloom, 1956). The verb should have few interpretations and be stated in terms of what the learner is to learn rather than what the teacher is to teach (Redman, 1988) (see box). Singular behaviours are easier to evaluate at the end of instruction.

Behavioural objectives are measurable and observable, indicating content to be learned (for example, 'to prepare a meal which contains 200 grams of carbohydrate'). The objective describes precise behaviours and content. An example of a vague or nonspecific objective might be 'to understand about diabetes'. This example does not explain what the learner is to do, and it raises questions about how the behaviour can be measured. Observe for measurable behavioural changes in the patient/client after teaching. Thus, objectives should specify singular areas of content.

An objective is more precise when it describes the conditions or timing under which the behaviour occurs. Conditions or time frames should be realistic and designed for the learner's needs. It also helps to consider conditions under which the patient/client or family will typically perform the learning behaviour (for example, 'to walk from bedroom to bath using crutches'). The conditions for acceptable performance set a standard by which achievement of objectives is measured. A teacher sets *conditions* on the basis of a desired level of accuracy, success, or satisfaction. For example, a patient/client undergoing rehabilitation following a fractured femur will walk on crutches to the end of the hall within 7 days. Conditions are more acceptable when established by the learner and teacher. However, the nurse serves as a resource in setting the minimal conditions for success. Mutually agreed conditions help define expected behaviours and quality of performance. The patient/client uses the conditions as a form of self-evaluation, which is a powerful motivator of behaviour.

### Integrating Basic Teaching Principles

Teaching is the process of helping someone to learn. When developing a teaching plan, consider the principles that improve its effectiveness. The realm of teaching deals with teachers' behaviour, reasons why they behave the way they do, and effects of their behaviour on students. There is no single way to teach correctly. The best way to teach is determined by each learning situation. The principles of teaching are basically techniques for supporting the principles of learning.

### SET PRIORITIES

Priorities for teaching are based on nursing assessment and the learning objectives established with the patient/client. A patient's/client's learning needs must be set in order of priority to conserve the time and energy of the patient/client and nurse. For example, a patient/client who suffers a permanent leg injury has a knowledge deficit regarding the nature of the injury, its implications, and the types of skills needed to resume a normal life. The patient/client will benefit most from first learning about the injury and the resultant physical changes before learning how to cope with the disability.

### DETERMINE TIMING

Determine the right time to teach, whether it is before patients/clients enter hospitals, during admission for health care, or at discharge. Each of these times may be appropriate because patients/clients need to learn as long as they stay in the health care system. **Teaching must be timed to coincide with readiness to learn.**

Timing can be difficult in acute care settings because emphasis is placed on early discharge. For example, after surgery, it may take several days for a patient/client to become free of discomfort. A variety of medications can cause the individual to be drowsy and unable to attend to learning. By the time he or she feels ready to learn, discharge may already be scheduled. Many hospitals are providing information to patients/clients before their admission and after they return home. The patient's/client's activities should be organized to provide time for rest teaching-

learning interactions.

The length of teaching sessions also influences learning ability. Prolonged sessions cause decreased concentration and attentiveness. Frequent sessions lasting 20 to 30 minutes are more easily tolerated and retain the patient's/client's interest. You can assess for decreased concentration by observing for nonverbal cues, such as poor eye contact or slumped posture. If decreased concentration is noted, the session should be stopped. However, teaching sessions should not be too brief. The patient/client needs time during each session to comprehend the information and to give feedback.

The frequency of teaching sessions will depend on the speed of learning and the complexity of the material. Intervals between teaching sessions should not be so long that the patient/client might forget information. For a patient/client discharged early, community nurses should reinforce learning.

### ORGANIZE TEACHING MATERIAL

A good teacher carefully plans the order in which to present information. An outline helps organize information into a logical sequence. Material should progress from simple to complex ideas because a person must learn the basics before making associations or complex interpretations of ideas. For example, to teach a patient/client to calculate a 1200-calorie diet, the nurse should first ensure that the person understands calories, and then use simple maths to help the individual learn to calculate amounts.

Begin teaching sessions with essential content and then completes a teaching session with informative but less essential content. Patients/clients are more likely to remember information that is taught during the first third of a teaching session (Miller, 1985). Finally, a summary of the most important points covered during the session is very useful as it helps the learner know the most important information and reinforces learning.

### PROMOTE LEARNER ATTENTION AND PARTICIPATION

**Active participation** is a key learning principle. However, it is the teacher's responsibility to find ways to keep learners interested and involved. Learning is improved when more than one of the body's senses are stimulated. Audiovisual aids, drawings, and group participation are ways to stimulate learner attention. Several approaches can be used to promote participation, particularly when teaching sessions are lengthy.

When conducting a discussion with a patient/client, the teacher should stay active by changing tone and intensity of voice, making eye contact, and using gestures that accentuate key points. An effective teacher often uses as much energy as the learner, talking and moving among a group rather than remaining stationary behind a lectern or table. A patient/client remains interested when the teacher is enthusiastic.

### BUILD ON EXISTING KNOWLEDGE

A patient/client learns best on the basis of pre-existing cognitive abilities and knowledge. Thus, a teacher can be more effective by building on a learner's knowledge. To successfully build on a knowledge base, the nurse must conduct a thorough assessment of the learner's knowledge about the topic. A teaching plan must be individualized based on the patient's/client's learning needs. A patient/client quickly loses interest if a nurse begins with familiar information.

## SELECT APPROPRIATE TEACHING METHODS

During planning, choose appropriate teaching methods and encourage the patient/client to offer suggestions. A **teaching method** is the way that the teacher delivers information and is based on the individual's learning needs (see box). For example, a patient/client with a psychomotor deficit learns best through demonstrations and supervised practice. The person masters skills

by manipulating equipment and practising manual skills. Discussions, question-and-answer sessions, and formal lectures are effective for promoting cognitive learning. More than one method may be used for a teaching session.

## Writing Teaching Plans

In all health care settings, nurses can develop written teaching plans for use by colleagues.

**Teaching plans** might include topics for discussion, optional resources (for example, equipment or teaching booklets), recommendations for involving family, and objectives of the teaching plan.

The setting influences the complexity of any teaching plan. In

---

## Teaching Methods

### COGNITIVE
#### Discussion (one-to-one or group)
- May involve nurse and patient/client or nurse with several different patients/clients
- Promotes active participation and focuses on topics of interest to patient/client
- Allows peer support
- Enhances application and analysis of new information

#### Lecture
- Is a more formal method of instruction because it is controlled by the teacher
- Helps the learner acquire new knowledge and gain comprehension

#### Question-and-answer session
- Is designed specifically to address patient's/client's concerns
- Assists patient/client in applying knowledge

#### Role play, discovery
- Allows patient/client to actively apply knowledge in a controlled situation
- Promotes synthesis of information and problem solving

#### Independent project (computer-assisted learning), field experience
- Allows the patient/client to assume responsibility for completing learning activities at own pace
- Promotes analysis, synthesis, and evaluation of new information and skills

### AFFECTIVE
#### Role play
- Allows expression of values, feelings, and attitudes.

#### Discussion (group)
- Allows the patient/client to acquire support from others in group
- Permits the patient/client to learn from other experiences
- Promotes responding, valuing and organization

#### Discussion (one-to-one)
- Allows discussion of personal, sensitive topics of interest or concern

### PSYCHOMOTOR
#### Demonstration
- Provides for presentation of procedures or skills by the nurse
- Permits the patient/client to incorporate modelling of nurse's behaviour
- Allows the nurse to control questioning during demonstration

#### Practice
- Gives the patient/client opportunity to perform the skills using equipment
- Provides repetition

#### Return demonstration
- Permits the patient/client to perform a skill as the nurse observes
- Is an excellent source of feedback and reinforcement

#### Independent projects, games
- Requires a teaching method that promotes adaptation and origination of psychomotor learning
- Permits the learner to use new skills

an acute care setting, plans are concise and focused on the primary learning needs of the patient/client because there is limited time for teaching. A home care teaching plan may be more involved because nurses often have a longer period over which to work with patients/clients.

A plan should provide continuity of learning, particularly when several nurses are involved in caring for the patient/client. The more specific the plan, the easier it is for nurses to follow through. A step-by-step description of content areas to be covered is useful if several teaching sessions are needed. To avoid duplication, you should know the point at which the last teaching session ended.

## Implementing

Implementing a teaching plan involves application of all teaching and learning principles, including the following:
1. Know the patient's/client's learning needs.
2. Select a time that coincides with the patient's/client's readiness and ability to learn.
3. Know the patient's/client's ability to comprehend (Streiff, 1986).
4. Select a teaching method that fits the learning domain for the patient's/client's learning need.
5. Select and establish priorities for content.
6. Actively involve the patient/client and family in the teaching plan.
7. Be aware of personal teaching abilities (know content, be interested in the learner, and be aware of personal motives).
8. Use appropriate teaching aids and resources.
9. Control the environment so that it is conducive to learning.
10. Use repetition and reinforcement appropriately.
11. Give the patient/client feedback.

Implementation involves viewing each interaction with a patient/client as an opportunity to teach. The nurse maximizes opportunities for effective learning and uses a diversified approach to create an active learner-teacher exchange of ideas.

## Teaching Approaches

A nurse's approach in teaching is different from teaching methodologies. Approach involves the nurse's task and relationship behaviours (Paulish, 1987). Some situations require a teacher to be directive, whereas others require a nondirective approach. An effective teacher concentrates on the task and recognizes that the approach may change based on the learner's response and the relationship with the patient/client. A patient's/client's needs and motives can change over time. Thus, you must always be aware of the need to modify teaching approaches. Paulish (1987) suggests a model for teaching approaches based on the situational leadership theory.

## TELLING

This approach (high task–low relationship behaviour) is appropriate when limited information or instructions must be taught. For example, preparing an individual for an emergency diagnostic procedure. If a patient/client is highly anxious but it is vital for information to be given, telling can be effective. Paulish (1987) warns that telling may not be effective, especially when patient/client participation is desirable. When using telling, outline the task (cognitive or psychomotor) to be done by the patient/client and give explicit instructions. There is no opportunity for feedback from the individual concerned.

## SELLING

Although the nurse still provides structure and instruction in this approach (high task–high relationship behaviours), two-way communication is used. Pace teaching on the basis of patient/client response. Specific feedback is given to the patient/client who shows success at learning. For example, a patient/client learns the step-by-step procedure for a dressing change. Use the patient's/client's feelings about performing the procedure to adapt the teaching approach.

## PARTICIPATING

This approach (high relationship–low task behaviours) involves the nurse and patient/client setting objectives and participating in the learning process together. The patient/client helps decide content, and the nurse guides the individual with pertinent information. For example, a patient/client with diabetes must learn about diet, exercise, and possible complications of the disease. Learning activities must be adapted to incorporate elements of the home environment. There is opportunity for discussion, feedback, and revision of the teaching plan during participation.

## ENTRUSTING

With this approach (low relationship–low task behaviours) the patient/client shows the ability to manage self-care. Responsibilities are accepted, and tasks are performed well. The nurse observes the patient's/client's progress and remains available to assist without introducing a lot of new information. For example, a diabetic patient/client has been self-administering insulin for over 3 months. Injections are performed correctly, and the patient/client can explain signs and symptoms of low blood glucose levels. The nurse then teaches the patient/client about a new prescribed dose of medication.

## REINFORCING

The principle of reinforcement applies to the process of learning; however, the teacher must often be the source of reinforcement. **Reinforcement** is using a stimulus that increases the probability of a response. A learner who receives reinforcement before or after a desired learning behaviour will probably repeat the behaviour. Feedback is a common form of reinforcement.

Reinforcers are positive or negative. *Positive reinforcement*, such as a smile or approval, produces the desired responses. A reinforcement is negative if its removal after a learner's response produces the desired behaviour. Threatening, complaining, and criticizing are examples of negative reinforcers. People usually respond better to positive reinforcement. The effects of negative reinforcement are less predictable and often undesirable. There are three types of reinforcers:
- **social** – when a nurse works with patients/clients, most

reinforcers are social (for example, smiles, compliments, words of encouragement, or physical contact). A nurse uses verbal and nonverbal communication when acknowledging that a skill has been learned well.

- **material** – these include food, toys, and music, and work best with young children.
- **activity** – these rely on the principal that people are motivated to engage in activities if promised that, after its completion, they will be able to do something else they like better.

Choosing an appropriate reinforcer involves careful thought and attention to preferences. Observing behaviour often helps reveal the best reinforcer to use. Reinforcers should never be used as threats, and reinforcement is not always effective with every patient/client. A young child responds more to social reinforcers than do older children or adults. An adult with whom you have a good relationship is more effectively reinforced than an adult with whom you have a poor relationship.

## Incorporating Teaching with Nursing Care

Many nurses find that they can teach more effectively while delivering nursing care. For example, while bathing a diabetic patient/client the nurse discusses foot care, or while administering drugs the nurse may explain a medication's side effects. An informal, unstructured style relies on the positive therapeutic relationship between nurse and patient/client, which fosters spontaneity in the teaching-learning process. This does not suggest that teaching should occur without a formal plan. When you follow a teaching plan in an informal way, the patient/client feels less pressure to perform, and learning becomes more of a shared activity. In addition, teaching during daily care is very efficient and cost effective.

## Teaching Methods

The teaching methods you choose depend on the patient's/client's learning needs (domain of learning), the time available for teaching, the setting, the resources available, and the nurse's own comfort level with teaching. Redman (1988) notes that teachers who are less knowledgeable and skilled in teaching often give information that they think is needed. More skilled teachers are flexible in altering teaching methods according to the learner's responses. An experienced teacher uses more techniques and teaching aids. Don't expect to be an expert educator when first entering nursing practice. Learning to become an effective educator takes time and practice.

When first starting to teach patients/clients, it helps to remember that people usually perceive the nurse as an expert. However, this does not mean that you must have all of the answers. It simply means that patients/clients expect you will keep them appropriately informed. A variety of teaching methods can be used, and a variety of teaching aids is usually available.

## ONE-TO-ONE DISCUSSION

Perhaps the most common method of teaching used by nurses is one-to-one discussion. By teaching patients/clients at the bedside, in an office, or in the home, you share information directly with them. Various teaching aids can be used during discussions, depending on the learning needs of the individual. Information is usually given in an informal manner, allowing patients/clients to ask questions or share concerns. Use unstructured and informal discussion when helping patients/clients understand the implications of illness and ways to cope with health stressors.

### Adult Nursing
### Special needs of older adults

Older adults experience numerous physical changes as a result of ageing. Unless nurses understand these changes they can create barriers to learning unless adjustments are made in nursing interventions. Sensory changes such as visual and hearing deficits require techniques that enhance older adults' functioning senses (see Chapter 26). For example, the nurse sits to face patients/clients with hearing problems and speaks in a low tone of voice during discussions. Individuals with visual problems can benefit from the use of printed materials containing large print.

Research shows that the ability of older adults to learn and remember is virtually as good as ever, especially if specific care is taken with the pace, the relevance of material, and the appropriateness of feedback (Hesse, 1984; Whitman, 1986). When teaching older people, the nurse should include family members who may be assuming partial care for a dependent patient/client.

## GROUP TEACHING

You can use group teaching with patients/clients or families for either of the following reasons (Redman, 1988):

1. Groups are an economical way to teach a number of patients/clients at one time.
2. Being part of a group may help patients/clients to meet learning needs by enhancing their feelings of being supported by others undergoing similar experiences.

Group teaching can often involve lecture and discussion. Lectures are highly structured and are efficient in helping groups of people learn standard content about a subject. For example, a nurse might teach a group about the health risks of smoking. A lecture does not ensure that learners are actively thinking about the material presented, and thus discussion and practice sessions are essential (Redman, 1988).

After hearing information from a lecture, learners need the opportunity to share ideas and seek clarification. Group discussions allow patients/clients and families to learn from each other as they review common experiences. To be an effective group leader, you must be able to facilitate participation. Acknowledging a look of interest, asking questions, and summarizing key issues foster group involvement. However, not all patients/clients benefit from group discussions, and sometimes reduced physical or emotional levels of wellness may prohibit participation.

## PREPARATORY TEACHING

Frequently, patients/clients face unfamiliar tests or procedures that create significant anxiety. Providing information about procedures helps individuals form realistic images of what to anticipate. This is a common expectation of patients/clients in acute care settings, because information helps to give them a sense of control. When an experience matches expectations, the individual is more likely to attend to the nurse's future explanations. You can use the following guidelines for preparatory explanations:

1. Physical sensations during the procedure are described but not evaluated. For example, Mr. Reynolds is to have blood drawn as a routine admission test. Explain that he will feel a pricking sensation as the needle punctures the skin. Do *not* say, "It won't hurt very much".

2. Patients/clients are prepared only for aspects of the experience that have commonly been noticed by other patients/clients. For example, explain that, while blood is being drawn, the tight tourniquet often causes the hand to tingle and feel numb.

The patient/client finds comfort in knowing what to expect. The known is less threatening than the unknown. When the nurse's descriptions are accurate, the patient/client copes more effectively with stress of procedures and therapies.

## DEMONSTRATIONS

A demonstration is an acting out for a learner and includes the teacher showing a particular skill. The patient/client is able to observe a skill before practising it. Demonstrations are most effective when learners first observe the teacher and then practice the skill in mock or real situations (return demonstrations). Nurses commonly use demonstrations for teaching motor skills; however motor skills are not necessarily learned separately from attitudes and factual knowledge (Redman, 1988). A demonstration should be combined with discussion to clarify concepts and feelings. Before a demonstration of a motor skill, follow these steps:

1. Be sure the learner can easily see the demonstration. Position the learner to provide a clear view of the skill being performed.
2. Review the rationale and steps of the procedure.
3. Assemble and organize equipment. Be sure all equipment works.
4. Prepare to perform each step in sequence while analysing knowledge and skills involved.
5. Determine at what step explanations are to be given, considering the patient's/client's learning needs.
6. Judge proper speed and timing of the demonstration, based on the patient's/client's cognitive abilities and anxiety level.

Demonstrate a skill in the same order in which the patient/client will perform it. The demonstration involves the following:

1. Performing each step slowly and accurately.
2. Encouraging the patient/client to ask questions so that each step is understood.
3. Explaining the rationale for each step.
4. Allowing the patient/client to observe each step.
5. Avoiding a hurried approach.
6. Allowing the patient/client to handle equipment and practice the skill under supervision.

The patient/client demonstrates the procedure to ensure that learning has occurred. The independent demonstration should occur under the same conditions found at home or place where the skill is to be performed. For example, if a person is learning to walk with crutches, the nurse simulates the home environment. If short, narrow steps lead to the person's bedroom, the individual should learn to climb similar stairs in the hospital.

## ANALOGIES

Learning occurs when a teacher translates complex language or ideas into words or concepts that the patient/client understands. In addition, the patient/client benefits by integrating new information into daily routines. Analogies supplement verbal instruction with familiar images that make complex information more real and understandable (Elsberry and Sorensen, 1986). For example, when explaining intestinal peristalsis to a patient/client, an analogy would be the movement of an earthworm as the wave moves down the length of the worm. Another is comparing arterial blood pressure to the flow of water through a hose. To use analogies the nurse follows the following general principles:

1. Be familiar with the concept.
2. Know the patient's/client's background, experience, and culture.
3. Keep the analogy simple and clear.

## ROLE PLAYING

A nurse can use role play for teaching ideas and attitudes. For example, you may teach parents to respond to a child's behaviour, or assist families in communicating with dying relatives. During role play, people are asked to play themselves or someone else. The technique involves rehearsing a desired behaviour. As a result of role play, patients/clients are taught the skills required and feel more confident in being able to perform independently.

## DISCOVERY

Discovery is a useful technique for teaching patients/clients problem solving, application, and independent thinking. During individual or group discussion a nurse may pose a problem or situation for patients/clients to solve. The problem pertains to the patients'/clients' learning needs. For example, people with heart disease may be asked to plan a meal low in cholesterol. The individuals in the group work together to decide which foods would be appropriate in the diet. The nurse asks the group members to present their diet, providing an opportunity to identify mistakes and reinforce correct information and rectify misunderstandings.

### Speaking the Patient's/Client's Language

It is important to use words that patients/clients can understand. Define unfamiliar medical or nursing terms and use them consistently throughout a teaching session. Medical jargon can be confusing. Byrne and Edeani (1984) found that patients/clients understand fewer medical words than health professionals predict. Frequently asking individuals for feedback determines whether they comprehend the terms used.

## Using Teaching Aids and Equipment

Many aids are available for nurses to use when teaching a patient/client. Selection of the right aid depends on the teaching method chosen, the individual's learning needs, and his or her ability to learn (Table 16-3). For example, a printed pamphlet may not be the best aid to use for a patient/client with poor reading comprehension and an audiotape may be the best choice for a patient/client with visual impairment.

There are many specialist nurses in a variety of fields such as stoma care, pain control, diabetic care, palliative care and many others. These nurses have specialist knowledge in their field and are a valuable resource for patient/client teaching. The specialist nurse can be directly involved in patient/client teaching or can act as an adviser and educator to those providing nursing care and education. The specialist nurse is also able to advise on up-to-date teaching tools such as equipment (for example stoma appliances), audiovisual aids and written material, as well as providing current research references to the nursing staff.

## Evaluation, Teaching and Learning

Patient/client education is not complete until the nurse evaluates outcomes of the teaching-learning process and determines whether patients/clients have learned the material. **Evaluation** reinforces learners' appropriate behaviour, helps learners realize how they should change inappropriate behaviour, and helps the teacher determine adequacy of teaching (Cronbach, 1977). The nurse evaluates patients'/clients' success at meeting each learning objective by measuring performance of each expected behaviour under the desired conditions. Success depends on

---

### Children's Nursing
### Needs of children

A nurse's selection of teaching methods and application of teaching-learning principles may be based on the patient's/client's age. Children, adults, and older adults learn in different ways because of developmental differences. The nurse uses teaching strategies that maximize strengths and minimize the deficits that children and older adults bring to a learning experience.

Children pass through several developmental stages before adolescence (see Chapter 6). In each developmental stage, children acquire new cognitive abilities that foster different types of learning. For example, a nurse can teach school-aged children about health as they acquire the ability to see things through the point of view of others. Dental hygiene, nutrition, safety measures, and sex education are examples of topics that may be presented to school children of varying ages. Parental input is incorporated in planning health education for children.

---

patients'/clients' abilities to meet established performance criteria within the time frames identified within each objective.

**Direct observation of behaviour** is useful when determining how a person will act in the future. Watching a patient/client demonstrate a skill helps you to know if the correct technique is being used. However, an individual may choose to behave differently later. The most difficult measurement of behaviour occurs with the affective domain because an individual can easily control the expression of feelings (Redman, 1988). Observation works best in a situation when a patient/client is unaware of being watched.

**Oral and written questioning** are other useful evaluation methods. A patient's/client's success in cognitive learning can be measured verbally by answering questions about a specific topic that was taught. Questions measure behaviours that are not easily observed. The nurse should carefully phrase questions to be sure that the learner understands them and that objectives are truly measured.

Another form of evaluation includes **self-reports** (oral and written) and **self-monitoring** (written). This involves patients/clients or family members providing information independently. An example might include a patient's/client's report of the foods eaten during a specific week, matched against a newly prescribed diet. The nurse relies on the person's honesty and memory in self-reporting.

During evaluation, ask the patient/client to demonstrate the behaviours described in the learning objectives. If the evaluation process indicates a knowledge or skill deficit, repeat or modify the teaching plan. Evaluation may reveal new learning needs or existence of new factors that may interfere with the person's ability to learn. Alternative teaching methods often help clarify information or skills that the patient/client was unable to comprehend or perform originally. When an individual has difficulty in an acute care setting the nurse may make a referral to resources such as home health care for further education and evaluation. Like the nursing process, the teaching-learning process is continuous and changing.

## Documenting Patient/Client Teaching

Because patient/client teaching often occurs informally between the nurse and patient/client (for example, during medication administration or assistance with hygiene) consistent documentation may be difficult. However, because a nurse is legally responsible for providing accurate and timely information to patients/clients, it is essential to document the outcomes of teaching. Barron (1987) suggests the following procedure for documenting patient/client education:

1. *Specific content.* Specifically describe the material taught so that other nurses can follow up and reinforce teaching (for example, "Insulin injection demonstrated" or "Explained effects of insulin"). Avoid generalizations, such as "medications taught", that leave staff confused.

2. *Evaluation of learning.* Document evidence of the outcomes of the patient's/client's learning (for example, a return demonstration or the ability to describe a medication). This informs the health care team about the patient's/client's progress and determines information that still needs to be taught.

**TABLE 16-3 Teaching Tools**

| Description | Learning Implications |
|---|---|
| **PRINTED MATERIAL** | |
| Written teaching tools available as pamphlets, booklets, brochures. | Must be in understandable language. Information must be accurate, culture-sensitive and current. Method is ideal for understanding complex concepts and relationships. |
| **PROGRAMMED TEACHING** | |
| Written sequential presentation of learning steps requiring that learners answer questions and that teachers tell them where they are right or wrong. | Teaching is primarily verbal, but the teacher may use pictures or diagrams Method requires active learning, giving immediate feedback, correcting wrong answers, and reinforcing right answers. Learner works at own pace. |
| **COMPUTER** | |
| Use of programmed instruction format in which computers store response patterns for learners and select further lessons on the basis of these patterns (programs can be individualized.) | There is currently limited availability for health care patients/clients. Method requires reading comprehension, psychomotor skills, and familiarity with computer. |
| **NONPRINT MATERIALS** | |
| **Diagrams** | |
| Illustrations that show interrelationships by means of lines and symbols. | Method demonstrates key ideas, summarizes, and clarifies key concepts. |
| Graphs (bar, circle, or line). Visual presentations of numerical data. | Graphs help the learner to grasp information quickly about a single concept. |
| **Charts** | |
| Highly condensed visual summary of ideas and facts that may highlight series of ideas, steps, or events. | Charts demonstrate relationship of several ideas or concepts. Method helps learners know what to do. |
| **Physical objects** | |
| Use of actual equipment, objects, or models to teach concepts or skills. | Models are useful when real objects are too small, large, or complicated, or are unavailable. Learners can manipulate objects that are to be used later. |
| **Other audiovisual materials** | |
| Slides, audiotapes, television and videotapes used with printed material or discussion. | Material useful for patients/clients with reading comprehension problems and visual aids. |

3. *Method of teaching.* Describe teaching methods. Knowing the methods used in teaching (for example, demonstrations or discussion) helps nurses follow up more efficiently or offer alternative teaching methods if learning does not occur. When resources such as pamphlets or audiovisual materials are used the nurse documents this in the patient's/client's record. Many institutions have special forms that allow easy documentation.

## SUMMARY

More than ever, a goal in health care is to engage patients/clients and families in maintaining health and managing health problems. During interactions with patients/clients the nurse has an opportunity to teach the knowledge and skills needed to maintain health or gain an improved level of function. Patient/client education focuses on the individual's unique needs and capacity for learning. The nurse and patient/client work together to define information and skills that the person needs to learn.

Use of the teaching process allows you to first define a patient's/client's learning needs. Then the application of the teaching process ensures an individualized teaching plan. The nurse assesses a patient's/client's learning needs, readiness, and ability to learn; the teaching environment; and resources for learning. The teaching plan involves the nurse and patient/client in a collaborative effort, setting realistic learning objectives. The teaching approaches and methods are then selected on the basis of the person's learning needs and priorities.

A good teacher uses basic teaching principles to promote participation in learning. Teaching begins when the learner is most receptive. The teacher organizes teaching material in a format that progresses from simple to more complex ideas. The teacher's actions and use of teaching aids help stimulate interest in learning. To determine whether a patient/client has gained the necessary knowledge or skills, evaluate the success of the teaching plan on the basis of expected learning outcomes or objectives.

## CHAPTER 16 REVIEW

### Key Concepts

- In the health care system today, there is greater emphasis in providing quality health education.
- The nurse must ensure that patients/clients and families receive information needed to maintain optimal health.
- Patient/client education is aimed at the promotion, restoration, and maintenance of health.
- Teaching is a form of interpersonal communication; teacher and student are actively involved in a process that increases the student's knowledge and skills.
- Teaching a patient/client a specific behaviour can involve incorporation of behaviours from all three learning domains.
- The ability to learn depends on a person's physical and cognitive attributes.
- The ability to attend to the learning process depends on physical comfort, low anxiety, and the lack of environmental distractions.
- If a nurse can modify a patient's/client's perception of the severity of an illness and the individual's susceptibility to disease, the patient/client may become more receptive to learning.
- Teaching must be timed to coincide with the patient's/client's readiness to learn.
- Patients/clients of different ages require different teaching strategies as a result of developmental capabilities.
- When education becomes a part of the nurse's plan of care the teaching process begins.
- The patient/client should be an active participant in a teaching plan, agreeing to the plan, helping choose teaching methods, and recommending times for instruction.
- Learning objectives describe measurable, singular behaviours performed under set conditions and time frames.
- Presentation of teaching content should begin with essential information and progress to more complex ideas.
- A combination of teaching methods improves the learner's attentiveness and involvement.
- A teacher is more effective when presenting information that builds on a learner's existing knowledge.
- A teacher who uses reinforcers such as praise or encouragement for a behaviour is trying to increase the probability of the behaviour recurring.
- The older adult learns most effectively when information is presented in small amounts and at a slower pace.
- A nurse evaluates a patient's/client's learning by observing performance of expected learning behaviours under desired conditions.

## CRITICAL THINKING EXERCISES

1. Mrs Lee is a 40-year-old woman who is married and has three children. She is employed as an insurance agent for one of the top companies in the city. After an annual check-up, Mrs Lee learns that she has diabetes. No one in her family has had the disease. The doctor has prescribed daily insulin injections and a diabetic diet. What factors, if any, do you think may influence Mrs Lee's ability to learn and describe what methods you would use for teaching her.

2. John Stein underwent an amputation of his left lower leg as a result of a traumatic injury. It has been about 3 weeks since the injury. John comes to the outpatients clinic and usually becomes angry with the nurses and doctor. He openly complains about the outpatient facilities. How would you as the nurse approach teaching Mr. Stein?

3. Mr Taylor, 42 years old, has a right leg cast after repair of a fractured ankle. He is to begin crutch walking tomorrow and must learn about cast care. He is to be discharged in 2 days. What should the nurse assess regarding Mr Taylor's ability to learn? Develop two learning objectives for Mr Taylor.

### Key Terms

Active participation, p. 308
Affective learning, p. 304
Attentional set, p. 304
Cognitive learning, p. 304
Educator, p. 301
Evaluation, p. 313
Learning ability, p. 305
Learning environment, p. 305
Learning needs, p. 306
Learning objective, p. 301
Learning, p. 300
Motivation, p. 304
Planned learning experience, p. 307
Psychomotor learning, p. 304
Reinforcement, p. 310
Teaching method, p. 309
Teaching plan, p. 307, 309
Teaching process, p. 306
Teaching, p. 300

## REFERENCES

Barron S: Documentation of patient education, *Patient Educ Couns* 9:81, 1987.

Bloom BS, editor: *Taxonomy of educational objectives, vol 1, Cognitive domain*, New York, 1956, Longman.

Boore J: *Prescription for recovery*, London, 1978, Royal College of Nursing.

Byrne TJ, Edeani D: Knowledge of medical terminology among hospitalized patients, *Nurs Res* 33:178, 1984.

Cronbach LJ: *Educational psychology*, ed 3, New York, 1977, Harcourt Brace Jovanovich.

Elsberry NL, Sorensen ME: Using analogies in patient teaching, *Am J Nurs* 86:1171, 1986.

Hayward J: *Information: a prescription against pain*, London, 1975, Royal College of Nursing.

Henderson V: *The nature of nursing: a definition and its implication for practice, research, and education*, New York, 1966, McMillan.

Hesse H: How elders view learning, *Geriatr Nurs* 5(1):37, 1984.

HMSO: *Statutory instruments no. 873 for nurses, midwives and health visitors*, London, 1983, HMSO.

Klausmeier HJ: *Educational psychology*, ed 5, Philadelphia, 1985, Harper & Row.

Knowles M: *The modern practice of adult education*, Cleveland, 1970, Follett.

Krathwohl DR et al: *Taxonomy of educational objectives: the classification of educational goals, handbook II: Affective domain*, New York, 1964, David McKay.

Kruger S: The patient educator role in nursing, *Appl Nurs Res* 4(1):19, 1991.

Macleod Clark J, Webb P: Health education — a basis for professional nursing practice *Nurse EducToday* 5(5): 210, 1985.

Miller A: When is the time ripe for teaching? *Am J Nurs* 85:801, 1985.

Nirje B: The normalization principle. In Flynn RJ, Nitsch KE (editors): *Normalization, social integration and community service*, Baltimore, 1980, University Park Press.

Noble C: Are nurses good patient educators? *J Adv Nurs* 16:1185, 1991.

Parker MC et al: A nursing inservice curriculum for patient education. *Nurs Health Care*, 4(3), 1983.

Paulish C: A model for situational patient teaching, *J Contin Educ Nurs* 18:163, 1987.

Redman BK: *The process of patient education*, ed 6, St Louis, 1988, Mosby.

Rendon DC et al: The right to know, the right to be taught, *J Gerontol Nurs* (12):33, 1986.

Simpson EJ: The classification of educational objectives in the psychomotor domain. In *Contributions of behavioral science to instructional technology: the psychomotor domain*, Mt Rainer, Md, 1972, Gryphon Press.

Spicer J: Teaching the patient, *Nurs Mirror* 55:51, 1982.

Squires AJ: *Multicultural health care and rehabilitation of older people*, London, 1991, Edward Arnold.

Streiff LD: Can clients understand our instructions? *Image J Nurs Sch* 18(2):48, 1986.

Tanner G: A need to know, *Nurs Times* 85(31):54, 1989.

Webb C: Teaching for recovery from surgery. In Wilson-Barnett J editor: *Patient teaching — recent advances in nursing* ed 6, Edingburgh, 1983, Churchill Livingstone.

Whitman NI: Age-related factors influencing selection of teaching strategies. In Whitman NI et al, editors: *Teaching in nursing practice: a professional approach*, Norwalk, Conn, 1986, Appleton- Century-Croft.

Wilson-Barnett J: Patients' emotional response to barium x-rays *J Adv Nurs* 3, 1978.

Wong D: *Nursing care of infants and children ed 5*, St Louis, 1995, Mosby.

## FURTHER READING
### Adult Nursing

Bartlett EE: Advocacy skills and strategies for patient education managers, *Patient Educ Couns* 8:397, 1986.

Berg BK, Leisner B: Developing a geriatric patient education program, *Patient Educ Couns* 8:201, 1986.

Boyd CW: Patient education promotes transition from hospital to home, *Patient Educ Couns* 8:295, 1986.

Bradshaw P, editor: *Teaching and assessing in clinical nursing practice*, London, 1990, Prentice Hall.

Curzon LB: *Teaching in further education*, London, 1985, Holt, Reinhart & Winston.

Cushing M: Legal lessons on patient teaching, *Am J Nurs* 84:721, 1984.

Hansen SL, Pichest JW: Patient education: the importance of instructional time and active patient involvement *Medical Teacher* 7(3-4), 1985.

Kenworthy N, Nicklin P: *Teaching and assessing in nursing practice — an experiential approach*, London, 1984, Scutari Press.

Latter S et al: Perceptions and practice of health education and health promotion in acute care settings. *Nursing Times*, occasional paper 89(21), 1993.

Nielsen E, Sheppard MA: Television as a patient education tool: a review of its effectiveness, *Patient Educ Couns*, 11(1):3, 1988.

Quinn FM: *Principles and practice of nurse education*, ed 2, London, 1989, Chapman & Hall.

Turner PAC: Patient education *Senior Nurse*, 2(2), 1985.

Wilson-Barnett J: *Patient teaching — recent advances in nursing*, Edinburgh, 1988, Churchill Livingstone.

### Children's Nursing
Claxton G: *Live and learn*. Milton Keynes, 1984, Open University Press.

Dixon H, Mullingar G: *Taught, not caught: strategies for sex education ed 3*, London, 1987, Ebenezer, Baylis & Sons.

Meredith S: *What's inside you?* London, 1991, Osborne Books.

### Learning Disabilities Nursing
Brechin A, Walmsley J: *Making connections — reflecting on the lives and experiences of people with learning difficulties*, London, 1989, The Open University: Hodder & Stoughton Educational.

Flynn MC: *Independent living for adults with mental handicap — a place of my own*, London, 1989, Cassell Educational.

Tomlinson S: *Educational subnormality — a study in decision making*, London, 1981, Routledge & Kegan Paul.

United Nations: *Declaration on the rights of the mentally retarded persons*, Geneva, 1971, United Nations.

Wolfensburger W: *The principle of normalisation in human services*. Toronto, 1992, National Institute in Mental Retardation.

Wolfensburger W: Social role in valorisation: a proposed new term for the principle of normalisation, *Mental Retardation* 21(6): 234, 1983.

### Mental Health Nursing
Dalley T, editor: *Art as therapy*, London, 1984, Tavistock.

Holmes J, Lindley R: *The values of psychotherapy*, Oxford, 1989, Oxford University Press.

Jennings S: *Creative therapy*, Oxford, 1983, Kemble Press.

Priestley P, McGuire J: *Learning to help – basic exercises*, London, 1989, Tavistock/Routledge.

Priestley P, McGuire J, Flegg D et al: *Social skills and personal problem solving*, London, 1978, Tavistock.

# unit 4

# Human Needs and Nursing Practice

# Oxygenation

## LEARNING OUTCOMES

After studying this chapter, you should be able to:
- *Define the key terms listed.*
- *Describe the gross structure and function of the cardiopulmonary system.*
- *Identify physiological processes in maintaining cardiac output, myocardial blood flow, and coronary artery circulation.*
- *Describe the electrical conduction system of the heart.*
- *Describe how cardiac output can be altered by preload, afterload, contractility, and heart rate.*
- *Identify physiological processes involved in ventilation, exchange of respiratory gases and the neural and chemical regulation of respiration.*
- *Identify some of the factors causing alteration in cardiac and respiratory functioning.*
- *Identify the effects of alterations in cardiac and respiratory functions and perform a nursing assessment of the cardiopulmonary system.*
- *Describe nursing interventions to increase activity tolerance, maintain or promote lung expansion, promote mobilization of pulmonary secretions, maintain a patent airway, promote oxygenation, and restore cardiopulmonary function.*
- *Develop evaluation criteria for the nursing care plan for the patient/client with altered oxygenation.*

Oxygen is a basic human need and is required to sustain life. The nurse often encounters patients/clients who are unable to meet oxygen needs independently. To help these people meet their oxygen needs, the nurse must understand cardiac and respiratory physiology.

**Cardiac physiology** involves the delivery of oxygenated blood to the tissues and the delivery of deoxygenated blood to the pulmonary system. When blood is delivered to the pulmonary circulation, the lungs oxygenate the blood. This oxygenated blood is returned to the left side of the heart and then delivered to the tissues (Fig. 17-1).

**Respiratory physiology** involves oxygenation of the body through the mechanisms of ventilation, perfusion, and transport of respiratory gases. In addition, neural and chemical regulators control fluctuations in respiratory rate and depth to meet tissue oxygen demands. Together, the cardiac and respiratory systems function to supply the body's oxygen demands. (For a detailed description of these systems and their functions, please refer to a comprehensive anatomy and physiology textbook.)

## CARDIOVASCULAR SYSTEM

### Structure and Function

The heart pumps blood through the pulmonary circulation by way of the right ventricle and through the systemic circulation by way of the left ventricle (see Fig. 17-1, overleaf). The circulatory system is the route for the exchange of respiratory gases, nutrients, and waste products between the blood and the tissues.

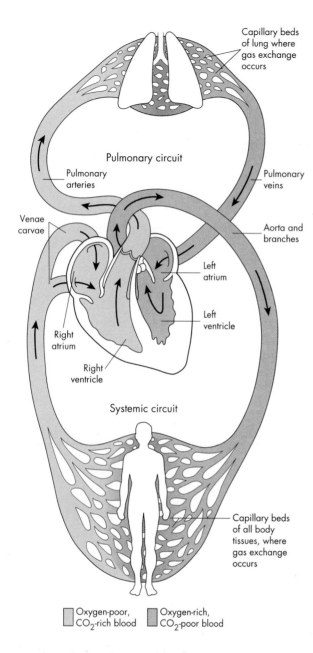

Capillary beds of lung where gas exchange occurs

Pulmonary circuit

Pulmonary arteries

Pulmonary veins

Venae cavae

Aorta and branches

Left atrium

Left ventricle

Right atrium

Right ventricle

Systemic circuit

Capillary beds of all body tissues, where gas exchange occurs

☐ Oxygen-poor, $CO_2$-rich blood  ☐ Oxygen-rich, $CO_2$-poor blood

**Fig. 17-1** The systemic and pulmonary circuits. From Marieb E: *Human anatomy and physiology*, ed 2, Redwood City, Calif, 1992, Benjamin Cummings.

## Cardiac Pump

The pumping action of the heart is essential to maintain oxygen delivery. Diseases that decrease the pumping effectiveness of the heart, such as coronary artery disease and cardiomyopathic conditions, decrease the volume of blood ejected from the ventricles. Similar conditions that affect circulating blood volume (for example, haemorrhage and dehydration) decrease the available blood for the heart to eject from the ventricles.

The chambers of the heart fill during **diastole** and empty during **systole**. A person's blood pressure reading helps determine the effectiveness of the diastolic and systolic events of the cardiac cycle (see Chapter 4).

The myocardial fibres have contractile properties that enable the heart muscle to stretch during filling. In a healthy heart, this stretch is proportionally related to the strength of contraction. That is, as the myocardium stretches, the strength of the subsequent contraction also increases. This response is the Frank–Starling (Starling's) law of the heart.

In the diseased heart, Starling's law does not apply because the stretch of the myocardium is beyond physiological limits. The heart stretches or dilates, but the subsequent contractile response results in insufficient ventricular ejection (volume). The heart loses its ability to pump the blood forward, and blood begins to 'back-up' in the pulmonary circulation (left heart failure) or systemic circulation (right heart failure).

The action of the four heart valves ensures a one-way flow of blood through the heart (Fig. 17-2). During ventricular diastole, the atrioventricular valves (mitral and tricuspid) open and blood flows from the higher pressure atria into the relaxed ventricles. After the ventricles fill, the systolic phase begins. As the systolic intraventricular pressure rises, the atrioventricular valves close, preventing the back flow of blood into the atria, and ventricular contraction begins.

As the ventricles begin the systolic phase, ventricular pressure rises, causing the semilunar valves (aortic and pulmonary) to open. As the ventricles eject blood past these open valves, the intraventricular pressure falls and the semilunar valves close, thus preventing the back flow of blood into the ventricles.

Patients/clients who have valvular diseases may have back flow or regurgitation of blood through the incompetent valve. This regurgitation causes a murmur that is heard on auscultation over the specific auscultation areas for each valve.

### Myocardial Blood Flow — Coronary Circulation

To maintain adequate blood flow to the pulmonary and systemic circulations, myocardial blood flow must sufficiently supply oxygen and nutrients to the myocardium itself.

Blood flow through the atria and ventricles does not supply oxygen and nutrients to the myocardium itself. It is the **coronary circulation**, a branch of the systemic circulation, that supplies oxygen and nutrients to, and removes waste from, the myocardium. The right coronary artery, left coronary artery and the circumflex arise from the aorta just above and behind the aortic valve (see Fig. 17-3 on p. 320). The most abundant blood supply feeds the left ventricular myocardium, which is more muscular and does most of the heart's work. The coronary arteries fill during ventricular diastole supplying the myocardium with oxygen. Venous blood returns via the anterior cardiac veins and the coronary sinus, into the right atrium.

### Systemic Circulation

The arteries and veins of the **systemic circulation** deliver nutrients and oxygen to, and remove waste from, the tissues. Oxygenated blood flows from the left ventricle by way of the aorta and into large systemic arteries. These arteries branch into smaller arteries and finally into arterioles. The arterioles branch further into the smallest vessels, the capillaries. At the capillary

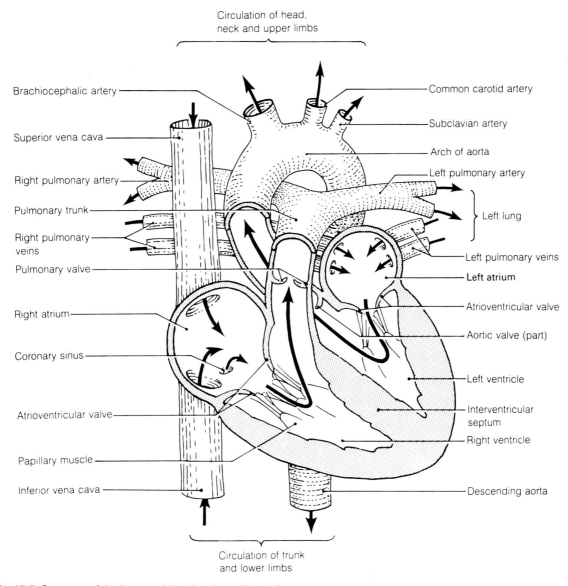

**Fig. 17-2** Structure of the heart and the direction of blood flow. From Hinchcliff S and Montague S, *Physiology for Nursing Practice*, London, 1988, Ballière Tindall.

level, the exchange of respiratory gases, nutrients, and wastes occurs; the tissues are oxygenated; and nutrients are received. The waste products exit the capillary network by way of the venules that join to form veins. These veins form larger veins, which carry deoxygenated blood to the right side of the heart to be returned to pulmonary circulation.

## Cardiac Output, Stroke Volume and Heart Rate

The amount of blood ejected by each ventricle each minute is the **cardiac output.** For a healthy 70 kg adult at rest, the cardiac output is approximately 5250 ml/min or 5.25 L/min:

Cardiac output (CO) = Stroke volume (SV) x Heart rate (HR)

**Stroke volume** is the amount of blood ejected from each ventricle with each contraction. Stroke volume and the heart rate

can be affected by the amount of blood in the ventricle at the end of diastole (preload), the resistance to ventricular ejection (afterload), and myocardial contractility.

**Preload** is essentially the end diastolic volume. As the ventricles fill, they stretch. According to the principles of the Frank-Starling law, the greater the stretch on the ventricle, the greater the contraction and the greater the stroke volume. In clinical situations, the preload and subsequent stroke volume can be manipulated by changing the amount of circulating blood volume. For example, in a patient/client with haemorrhagic shock, fluid therapy and replacement of blood volume increases volume, thus increasing the preload and subsequent cardiac output. If volume is not replaced, preload decreases, as does subsequent cardiac output, and ultimately the venous return to the right atrium decreases. This decreased venous return further decreases preload and cardiac output.

**Afterload** is the resistance to left ventricular ejection. For the

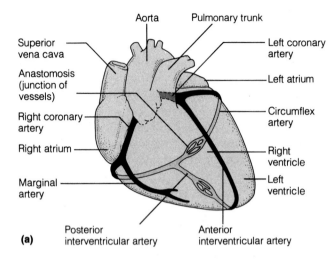

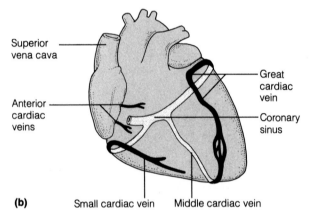

Fig. **17-3** Coronary circulation. From Marieb E: *Human anatomy and physiology, ed 2*, Redwood City, Calif 1992 Benjamin Cummings.

left side of the heart, afterload is the work the heart must overcome to fully eject blood from the left ventricle. The diastolic aortic pressure is a good clinical measure of afterload. In a person with an acute hypertensive crisis, the afterload is increased and the cardiac workload also increases. Afterload in this situation can be manipulated by decreasing systemic blood pressure.

**Myocardial contractility** also affects stroke volume and

cardiac output. Poor contraction decreases the amount of blood ejected by the ventricles during each contraction. Myocardial contractility can be increased by drugs that increase the force of contraction, such as digitalis preparations, adrenaline, and sympathomimetic drugs (drugs that mimic the effects of the sympathetic nervous system).

Heart rate affects blood flow because of the interaction between rate and diastolic filling time. With a faster heart rate, particularly sustained rates greater than 160 beats/min, diastolic filling time decreases. As filling time decreases, stroke volume and cardiac output decrease. Coronary artery filling time is also shortened, reducing oxygen supply to the myocardium at a time when it needs more (Sutcliffe, 1993).

### Conduction System

The rhythmic relaxation and contraction of the atria and ventricles depend on continuous, organized transmission of electrical impulses. These impulses are generated and transmitted by way of the **conduction system** (Fig. 17-4).

The heart's conduction system generates the necessary action potentials that conduct the impulses required to initiate the electrical chain of events resulting in the heart beat. The autonomic nervous system influences the rate of impulse generation as well as the speed of transmission through the conductive pathway and the strength of atrial and ventricular contractions. Sympathetic nerve fibres, which increase the rate of impulse generation and the speed of impulse transmission, innervate all parts of the atria and ventricles. Parasympathetic fibres from the vagus nerve, which decrease this rate, also innervate these parts, as well as the sinoatrial and atrioventricular nodes (Levick, 1991).

The conduction system originates with the **sinoatrial (SA) node**, which is the 'pacemaker' of the heart. The SA node is in the right atrium next to the entrance of the superior vena cava (Levick, 1991). Impulses are initiated at the SA node at an intrinsic rate of 60 to 100 beats/min. The resting adult rate is approximately 75 beats/min.

The electrical impulses are then transmitted through the atria to the **atrioventricular (AV) node**. The AV node mediates

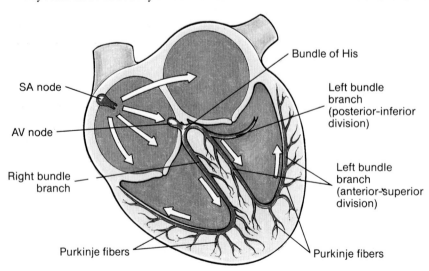

Fig. **17-4** Electrical conduction system. From Cannobio MM: *Cardiovascular disorders*, St Louis, 1990, Mosby.

impulses between the atria and the ventricles. It assists atrial emptying by delaying the impulse before transmitting it through the **bundle of His** and the ventricular **Purkinje network**.

The electrical activity of the conduction system is reflected by an **electrocardiogram (ECG)**. An ECG monitors the regularity and path of the electrical impulse through the conduction system. The normal sequence on the ECG is called **normal sinus rhythm (NSR)** (Fig. 17-5).

A finding of NSR means that the impulse originated at the SA node and followed the normal sequence through the conduction system. The P-wave on the ECG indicates that the atria have received an electrical impulse. Normally, atrial contraction follows the P-wave. The PR interval provides information about the delay in transmission of the impulse through the AV node. The normal length for the PR interval is 0.12 to 0.20 seconds. An increase in the time indicates that there is a block in the impulse transmission though the AV node, whereas a decrease indicates the initiation of the electrical impulse from a source other than the SA node. The QRS complex is a sign that the electrical impulse has travelled through the ventricles, and normally the ventricles contract following the QRS complex.

## RESPIRATORY SYSTEM

### Structure and Function

The respiratory system includes the respiratory airways that lead into the lungs, the lungs, and the structures of the thorax involved in producing movement of air through the airways into and out of the lungs. These main structures are represented in Fig. 17-6.

The major function of the respiratory system is to supply the body with oxygen and to dispose of carbon dioxide. There are four major steps in this process: pulmonary ventilation, gas exchange between the alveoli and blood, gas transport, and gas exchange between the blood and the tissue cells.

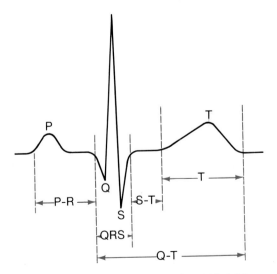

**Fig. 17-5** Normal ECG waveform. From Canobbio MM: *Cardiovascular disorders*, St. Louis, 1990, Mosby.

### Pulmonary Ventilation

**Pulmonary ventilation** is a mechanical process that depends on volume changes occurring in the thoracic cavity. Volume changes lead to pressure changes which result in the flow of gases. Boyle's law states that under conditions of constant temperature, the pressure in a gas varies inversely with its volume. Therefore, if the volume of the thorax increases, the pressure will decrease. The pressure in the lungs is now less than that of the atmosphere and air flows in down the pressure gradient.

During inspiration the volume of the thorax is increased by the contraction and descent of the diaphragm, increasing the vertical dimension of the lungs. This is accompanied by the contraction of the external intercostal muscles which results in the elevation of the rib cage and an increase anterior-posterior dimension of the thorax. Because the lungs adhere tightly to the thoracic wall via the pleural membranes, the intrapulmonary volume also increases. The increase in the intrapulmonary volume of the thorax leads to a decrease in the intrapulmonary pressure, and air moves into the lungs along the pressure gradient until the intrapulmonary and atmospheric pressures become equal.

Individuals with obstructive airway diseases, such as asthma, emphysema, or chronic bronchitis may use additional muscle groups to elevate the ribs further when inspiring in an attempt to increase their lung volume. These muscles are known as the **accessory muscles of inspiration** and include the anterior and medial scalenes, the sternocleidomastoid muscles of the neck, and the pectoral muscles in the chest. The nurse should observe for the use of accessory muscles during inspiration, and note if any sucking of the skin and muscles in between the ribs (intercostal retractions) occurs during inspiration. If this is observed it usually indicates that the patient/client is making a larger effort at inspiration than normal, often because the lungs are less compliant (less flexible).

In healthy individuals, expiration is mainly a passive process and depends on the natural elasticity of the lungs rather than on muscular contraction. The inspiratory muscles and the diaphragm relax and the lungs recoil, decreasing both the intrathoracic and intrapulmonary volumes. Consequently, the intrapulmonary pressure rises, which causes air to flow from the lungs to the atmosphere.

**Forced expiration** is an active process which involves the contraction of muscles in the abdominal wall (mainly the oblique and transverse muscles).

### Pulmonary Circulation

Pulmonary circulation begins at the pulmonary artery, which receives mixed (poorly oxygenated) venous blood from the right ventricle. Blood flow through this system depends on the pumping ability of the right ventricle, which has an output of approximately 5 to 6 L/min. The flow continues from the pulmonary artery through the pulmonary arterioles to the pulmonary capillaries. At the capillary level, blood comes in contact with the alveolar-capillary membrane and the exchange of respiratory gases occurs. The oxygen-rich blood then circulates through the pulmonary venules and pulmonary veins and returns to the left atrium.

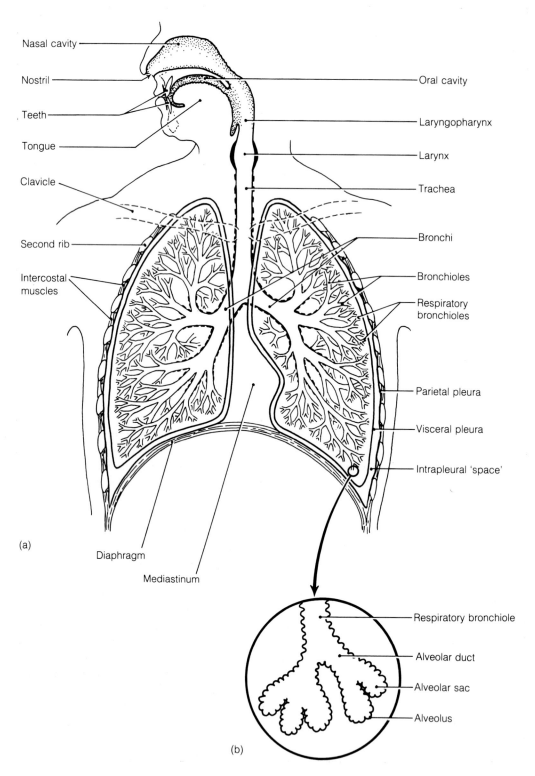

**Fig. 17-6**
Organization of the
respiratory system.
From Hinchliff S and
Montague S: *Physiology
of Nursing Practice,*
London, 1988, Ballière
Trindall.

## Exchange of Respiratory Gases

Respiratory gases are exchanged in the alveoli of the lungs and the capillaries of the body tissues. Oxygen is transferred from the lungs to the blood, and carbon dioxide is transferred from the blood to the alveoli to be exhaled as a waste product. At the tissue level, oxygen is transferred from the blood to tissues, and carbon dioxide is transferred from tissues to the blood to return to the alveoli and be exhaled. Exchange of gases occurs by diffusion down **partial pressure gradients**.

## Diffusion

**Diffusion** is the movement of molecules from an area of higher concentration to an area of lower concentration. Diffusion of respiratory gases occurs at the alveolar-capillary membrane, and

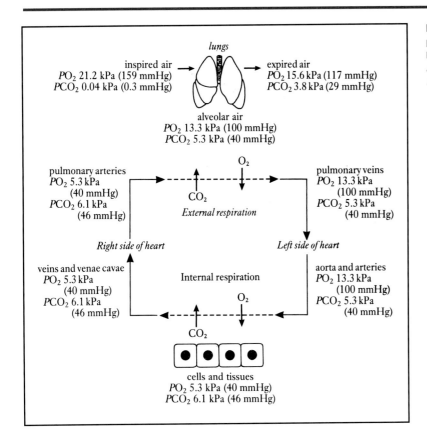

**Fig. 17-7** Gaseous exchange and partial pressure gradients — lungs and tissues. From Brooker C: *Human structure and function - nursing applications in clinical practice*, London, 1993, Mosby.

the rate of diffusion can be affected by thickness of the membrane.

Increased thickness of the membrane impedes diffusion because respiratory gases take longer to transfer across the thickened space. In patients/clients with pulmonary oedema, thickness of the respiratory membrane is increased. As a result, diffusion is slowed and the exchange of respiratory gases and subsequent delivery of oxygen to tissues are impaired.

The surface area of the alveolar-capillary membrane can be altered as a result of a chronic disease (such as emphysema), an acute disease (such as a pneumothorax), or a surgical process (such as a lobectomy). When fewer alveoli are functioning, the surface area is decreased.

## Partial Pressures

The pressure exerted by a particular gas is directly proportional to the percentage of that gas in the total air mixture. For example:

| Atmospheric air (approximate values) | | Partial pressure (mmHg) | |
|---|---|---|---|
| Nitrogen | 80% | $\dfrac{80 \times 760}{100}$ | = 608 |
| Oxygen | 20% | $\dfrac{20 \times 260}{100}$ | = 152 |

Fig. 17-7 shows the partial pressure gradients promoting $O_2$ and $CO_2$ exchange both at the respiratory membrane in the lungs and at the capillary membrane in the body tissues.

## Respiratory Transort of Gases
## Oxygen Transport

The oxygen transport system consists of the lungs and cardiovascular system. Delivery depends on the amount of oxygen entering the lungs **(ventilation)**, blood flow to the lungs and tissues **(perfusion)**, adequacy of diffusion, and capacity of the blood to carry oxygen. Capacity to carry oxygen is influenced by the amount of dissolved oxygen in the plasma, amount of haemoglobin, and tendency of haemoglobin to bind with oxygen (Ahrens 1987, 1990).

Only a relatively small amount of required oxygen, about 3%, is dissolved in the plasma. Most oxygen is transported by **haemoglobin**, which serves as a carrier for oxygen and carbon dioxide. The haemoglobin molecule combines with oxygen to form oxyhaemoglobin. Oxyhaemoglobin is easily reversible; haemoglobin and oxygen can dissociate, which frees oxygen to enter the tissues.

## Carbon Dioxide Transport

The transport of respiratory gases includes movement of carbon dioxide. Carbon dioxide diffuses into erythrocytes and is rapidly hydrated into carbonic acid ($H_2CO_3$) by the enzyme carbonic anhydrase. The carbonic acid then dissociates into hydrogen ($H^+$) and bicarbonate ($HCO_3^-$) ions. The hydrogen ion is buffered by haemoglobin, and the bicarbonate ion diffuses into the plasma. In addition, some of the carbon dioxide in erythrocytes reacts with

### Children's Nursing
### Developmental factors that affect respiration

Premature infants are at risk for hyaline membrane disease, which is thought to be caused by a surfactant deficiency. The surfactant-synthesizing ability of the lungs develops late in pregnancy and may therefore be lacking in preterm infants (Gröer and Shekleton, 1989).

Respiratory disease is the most common cause of acute illness in children and accounts for 50% of visits to the GP in children under 5 years old. Asthma is the most common chronic disease in children and is a common cause of admission to hospital.

Infants and toddlers are at risk for upper respiratory tract infections as a result of frequent exposure to other children. In addition, during the teething process some infants develop nasal congestion, which encourages bacterial growth and increases the potential for respiratory tract infection. Upper respiratory tract infections are usually not dangerous, and infants or toddlers recover with little difficulty. However, airway obstructions are nasopharyngitis (for example, rhinoviruses, respiratory syncytial virus, and adenovirus), pharyngitis (for example, viral and beta haemolytic streptococci), influenza, and tonsillitis. In addition, obstruction can occur with aspirated foreign objects, such as food, buttons, and sweets.

School-aged children and adolescents are exposed to respiratory infections and respiratory risk factors such as smoking. A healthy child usually does not have adverse pulmonary effects from respiratory infections. A person who starts smoking in adolescence and continues to smoke into middle age, however, has an increased risk for cardiopulmonary disease (see Chapter 7).

### Mental Health Nursing
### Medications that can affect heart function

Some medications used to alleviate the symptoms of mental distress and mental illness can affect the cardiopulmonary system. For example, antidepressants (used to alleviate depression) can affect the conduction system of the heart. Particular care must be taken to establish the patient's/client's medical history before such medication is prescribed.

Almost all tranquillizers, used to manage symptoms of mental illnesses, can drastically lower blood pressure. This is particularly significant if the patient/client is receiving the medication in injectable form. It is imperative to ensure the patient's/client's blood pressure is healthy before each injection of this medication.

## Regulation of Respiration

The main purpose of respiratory regulation is to supply sufficient oxygen to meet the body's demands, such as during exercise, infection, or pregnancy. In addition, respiratory regulation promotes exhalation of metabolically produced carbon dioxide, which is a determinant of acid-base status (see Chapter 18).

There are two respiratory regulators: neural and chemical. **Neural regulation** includes the central nervous system control of respiratory rate, depth, and rhythm. **Chemical regulation** involves the influence of chemicals such as carbon dioxide, oxygen and hydrogen ions on the rate and depth of respiration. In normal circumstances, an increasing level of $CO_2$ is the most powerful respiratory stimulus. Low levels of $CO_2$ (hypocapnia) depress respiration.

Arterial levels of oxygen below 60 mmHg constitute the **hypoxic drive** and stimulate respiration.

In some people with chronic lung diseases where $CO_2$ is retained (for example chronic bronchitis), arterial $PCO_2$ is chronically elevated and the chemorecepters become unresponsive to this chemical stimulus. In these individuals it is the *declining* $PO_2$ levels that provide the respiratory stimulus (hypoxic drive). If high levels of $O_2$ were given to these patients/clients [greater than 24–28% (1–3 L/min)], they might stop breathing because their respiratory stimulus would be removed.

## FACTORS AFFECTING OXYGENATION

The goal of ventilation is to produce a normal arterial carbon dioxide tension ($PaCO_2$) and maintain normal arterial oxygen tension ($PaO_2$). *Hyperventilation* and *hypoventilation* refer to alveolar ventilation and not to the patient's/client's respiratory rate.

### Hyperventilation

**Hyperventilation** is a state of ventilation in excess of that required to eliminate the normal venous carbon dioxide produced by cellular metabolism. Hyperventilation can be induced by:
* **anxiety** – acute anxiety can lead to hyperventilation and result in loss of consciousness.

amino acid groups, forming carbamino compounds. This reaction can occur rapidly without the presence of an enzyme. Since reduced haemoglobin (deoxyhaemoglobin) can combine with carbon dioxide more easily than oxyhaemoglobin, the venous blood transports the majority of carbon dioxide.

### Mental Health Nursing
### The effects of anxiety on respiration

A continuous state of severe anxiety increases the body's metabolic rate and demand for oxygen (hyperventilation). The body responds to anxiety and other stresses by increasing the rate and depth of respiration. Most people can adapt to this, but some people, particularly those with chronic illnesses or acute, life-threatening illnesses such as myocardial infarction, cannot tolerate the oxygen demands associated with anxiety.

Particular care must be taken to establish whether there are physical causes for the hyperventilation, rather than assuming the symptom is solely psychological in nature. Even when the cause is primarily psychological, the patient's/client's behaviour is nevertheless indicative of some need which nurses should attempt to meet.

## Signs and Symptoms of Alveolar Hyperventilation

- Tachycardia
- Shortness of breath
- Chest pain
- Dizziness
- Lightheadedness
- Decreased concentration
- Paraesthesia
- Numbness (extremities, circumoral)
- Tinnitus
- Blurred vision
- Disorientation
- Tetany (carpopedal spasm)

## Signs and Symptoms of Alveolar Hypoventilation

- Dizziness
- Headache (may be occipital only on awakening)
- Lethargy
- Disorientation
- Decreased ability to follow instruction
- Cardiac dysrhythmias
- Electrolyte imbalances
- Convulsions
- Coma
- Cardiac arrest

- **infections** – fever can occur in hyperventilation because of compensatory mechanisms within the body. For each degree centigrade increase in body temperature, there is a 7% increase in the metabolic rate (Gröer and Shekleton, 1989).
- **hypoxia** – higher metabolic rates increase carbon dioxide production. This state leads to an increased respiratory rate and depth in patients/clients without chronic obstructive pulmonary disease.
- **drugs** – salicylate poisoning causes excessive stimulation of the respiratory centre because of the body's attempt to compensate for carbon dioxide excess. Amphetamines also increase ventilation, primarily by raising carbon dioxide production.
- **acid-base imbalance** – hyperventilation can also occur as the body tries to compensate for metabolic acidosis. Ventilation increases to reduce the amount of carbon dioxide available to form carbonic acid (see Chapter 18).

Alveolar hyperventilation produces many signs and symptoms that can be assessed (see box above). Haemoglobin does not release oxygen to tissues as readily, and tissue hypoxia results. As symptoms worsen, the client may become more agitated, which further increases the respiratory rate and can result in respiratory alkalosis.

## Hypoventilation

**Hypoventilation** occurs when alveolar ventilation is inadequate to meet the body's oxygen demand or to eliminate sufficient carbon dioxide. As alveolar ventilation decreases, $PaCO_2$ is elevated. Severe atelectasis can produce hypoventilation. **Atelectasis** is a collapse of the alveoli that prevents normal respiratory exchange of oxygen and carbon dioxide. As alveoli collapse, less of the lung can be ventilated and hypoventilation occurs.

Hypoventilation may cause many signs and symptoms revealed through physical assessment (see box, above right). If untreated, the person's status can rapidly decline. Convulsions, unconsciousness, and death can result.

The goals of treatment for hyperventilation and hypoventilation are to first treat the underlying cause while simultaneously restoring optimal ventilatory function, improving tissue oxygenation, and achieving acid-base balance (Gröer and Shekleton, 1989).

### Hypoxia

**Hypoxia** is inadequate cellular oxygenation that results from a deficiency in the delivery or use of oxygen at the cellular level (Gröer and Shekleton, 1989). Hypoxia can be caused by (1) a decreased haemoglobin level and lowered oxygen-carrying capacity of the blood, (2) a diminished concentration of inspired oxygen such as may occur at high altitudes, (3) the inability of the tissues to extract oxygen from the blood such as with cyanide poisoning, (4) decreased diffusion of oxygen from the alveoli to the blood such as with pneumonia, (5) poor tissue perfusion with oxygenated blood such as with shock, and (6) impaired ventilation.

The clinical signs and symptoms of hypoxia include apprehension, restlessness, inability to concentrate, declining level of consciousness, dizziness, and behavioural changes (see box below). A person with hypoxia is unable to lie down and appears fatigued and agitated. Changes in vital signs include an increased pulse rate and increased rate and depth of respiration. However, as the hypoxia worsens, the respiratory rate may decline as a result of fatigue. During early stages of hypoxia the blood pressure is elevated unless the condition is caused by shock. **Cyanosis**, a blue discolouration of the skin and mucous membranes caused by the presence of desaturated haemoglobin in capillaries, is a late sign of hypoxia. Central cyanosis observed in the tongue and soft palate, where blood flow is high, indicates hypoxaemia. Peripheral cyanosis, as observed in the fingernail beds, may merely reflect stagnant blood flow (Luce *et al*, 1984). The nurse should observe other areas of the body, in addition to the skin, for signs of

## Signs and Symptoms of Hypoxia

- Restlessness
- Apprehension, anxiety
- Decreased ability to concentrate
- Decreased level of consciousness
- Increased fatigue
- Dizziness
- Behavioural changes
- Increased pulse rate
- Increased rate and depth of respiration
- Elevated blood pressure
- Cardiac dysrhythmias
- Pallor
- Cyanosis
- Clubbing
- Dyspnoea

cyanosis, such as the conjunctivae, mouth, nail beds, and extremities. The presence or absence of cyanosis is not an absolute measure of oxygenation status.

## Dyspnoea

**Dyspnoea** is another clinical sign of hypoxia and manifests as shortness of breath or difficulty in breathing. It is the subjective sensation of difficult or uncomfortable breathing (Carrieri *et al*, 1991). Pathological dyspnoea must be differentiated from physiological dyspnoea, which is shortness of breath after exercise or excitement. Pathological breathlessness is a distressing sensation of not being able to catch a breath (Gröer and Shekleton, 1989).

Hypoxia is a life-threatening condition. Untreated, it can produce cardiac dysrhythmias that result in death. Hypoxia is managed by administration of oxygen and by treatment of the underlying cause, such as shock or pneumonia.

## CONDITIONS AFFECTING CARDIO-VASCULAR FUNCTIONING

Conditions that affect cardiovascular functioning directly affect the body's ability to meet oxygen demands. Alterations in cardiac functioning are caused by illnesses and conditions that affect cardiac rhythm, strength of contraction, blood flow through the chambers, myocardial blood flow, and peripheral circulation.

### Disturbances in Conduction

Some disturbances in conduction are the result of electrical impulses that do not originate from the sinoatrial (SA) node. These rhythm disturbances are called **dysrhythmias**, meaning a deviation from the normal sinus heart rhythm. Dysrhythmias may occur as a primary conduction disturbance; as a response to ischaemia, valvular abnormality, anxiety, and drug toxicity; as a result of caffeine, alcohol, or tobacco use; or as a complication of acid-base or electrolyte imbalance (see Chapter 18).

Dysrhythmias are classified by cardiac response and site of impulse origin. Cardiac response can be either tachycardic (greater than 100 beats/min), bradycardic (less than 60 beats/min), premature (early beat), or blocked (delayed or absent beat).

### Altered Cardiac Output

Failure of the myocardium to eject sufficient volume to the systemic and pulmonary circulations can result in decreased cardiac output and heart failure. Failure of the myocardial pump results from primary coronary artery disease, cardiomyopathic conditions, valvular disorders, and pulmonary disease.

**Left-sided heart failure** is an abnormal condition characterized by impaired functioning of the heart's left side and by elevated pressure and congestion in pulmonary veins and capillaries. If failure of the left ventricle is significant, the amount of blood ejected from the left ventricle drops greatly. As a result, cardiac output also falls. Decreases in cardiac output can cause tissue hypoxia, which may result in decreased activity tolerance, breathlessness, dizziness, and confusion. As the left ventricle continues to fail, blood begins to 'back up' in the pulmonary

circulation, eventually causing pulmonary congestion. This results in crackles, hypoxia, dyspnoea, cough, and paroxysmal nocturnal dyspnoea (Canobbio, 1990).

**Right-sided heart failure** results from impaired functioning of the right ventricle, characterized by venous congestion in the systemic circulation. Right-sided heart failure more commonly results from pulmonary disease or as a sequelae to left-sided failure. The primary pathological factor in right-sided failure is elevated pulmonary vascular resistance (PVR). As the PVR continues to rise, the right ventricle must generate more work, and the oxygen demand of the heart increases with the workload. As the failure continues, the amount of blood ejected from the right ventricle declines, and blood begins to 'back up' in the systemic circulation. Clinically, the patient/client has weight gain, distended neck veins, abdominal organ distension (for example, hepatomegaly and splenomegaly), and dependent peripheral oedema.

### Impaired Valvular Function

**Valvular heart disease** is an acquired or congenital disorder of a cardiac valve characterized by stenosis and obstructed blood flow or valvular degeneration and regurgitation of blood (Canobbio, 1990).

When stenosis occurs in the semilunar valves (aortic and pulmonic valves), the adjacent ventricles must work harder to move the ventricular volume beyond the stenotic valve. Over time, the stenosis can cause the ventricle to hypertrophy (enlarge), and if the condition is untreated, left- or right-sided heart failure can occur. If stenosis occurs in the atrioventricular valves (mitral and tricuspid valves), the atrial pressure rises, causing the atria to hypertrophy.

When regurgitation occurs, there is a back flow of blood into an adjacent chamber. For example, in mitral regurgitation the mitral valves do not close completely. When the ventricle contracts, blood escapes back into the atria, causing a murmur, a 'whooshing' sound (see Chapter 4).

### Myocardial Ischaemia

**Myocardial ischaemia** results when the supply of blood to the myocardium from the coronary arteries is insufficient to meet the oxygen demands of the organ. Two common manifestations of this ischaemia are angina pectoris and myocardial infarction.

**Angina pectoris** is usually a transient imbalance between myocardial oxygen supply and demand. The condition results in chest pain. Anginal chest pain can be aching, sharp, tingling, burning, or feel like pressure. The location of the pain may be on either the left side or substernal and may radiate to the left or both arms, jaw, neck, and back. In some individuals, anginal pain may not radiate. The pain lasts from 3 to 15 minutes. Patients/clients sometimes report that pain is precipitated by activities that increase myocardial oxygen demand (for example, exercise, anxiety, and stress). The pain is relieved with rest and coronary vasodilators, the most common being a nitroglycerine preparation.

**Myocardial infarction** results from sudden decreases in coronary blood flow or from an increase in myocardial oxygen

## Mother and Child Nursing
## How does pregnancy affect respiration?

During pregnancy, ventilation increases up to 40%. This is achieved by increasing the tidal volume, rather than the respiratory rate (Dewhurst *et al*, 1986). However, total lung capacity decreases by 200 ml as the fetus grows and the increasing size of the uterus pushes abdominal contents upward against the diaphragm. During the last trimester, therefore, the inspiratory capacity of the pregnant woman declines. She may experience shortness of breath during exertion, and may become easily fatigued.

demand without adequate coronary perfusion. Infarction occurs because of ischaemia and necrosis of myocardial tissue. It is not reversible (Canobbio, 1990).

Chest pain associated with myocardial infarction is described as crushing, squeezing, or stabbing. The pain may be retrosternal and left precordial. If the pain radiates, it may move down the left

## Adult Nursing
## The effects of obesity on respiration

Obese people often have a heavy lower thorax and abdomen, which reduces lung volumes, particularly in the recumbent and supine positions. In some individuals an obesity-hypoventilation syndrome develops in which oxygenation is decreased and carbon dioxide is retained, resulting in daytime sleepiness. The obese patient/client is also susceptible to pneumonia after an upper respiratory tract infection, because the lungs cannot fully expand and pulmonary secretions are not mobilized in the lower lobes.

arm and to the neck, jaws, teeth, epigastric area, and back. The pain occurs at rest or exertion. The pain lasts more than 30 minutes. It is unrelieved by rest, position change, or sublingual nitroglycerine administration.

## CONDITIONS AFFECTING RESPIRATORY FUNCTIONING

Conditions affecting the lung may be classified as obstructive, restrictive, vascular or environmental (West, 1992).

### Obstructive Diseases

Airway obstruction may be caused by a) increased resistance to flow inside the lumen of the airway, for example, if it is partially blocked by excessive secretions, as in chronic bronchitis, or by the inhalation of foreign bodies (more common in childhood); b) contraction of the airway walls, as in asthma; or c) destruction of the tissue outside the airways which causes loss of radial traction, as in emphysema.

Obstructive airway limitation is common in the UK. It is a major cause of disability and an increasingly important cause of mortality.

### Restrictive Diseases

These are diseases where the expansion of the lung is restricted, due to either a) alterations in the lung tissue such as pulmonary fibrosis, or b) diseases of the pleura (pneumothorax) or chestwall (scoliosis), or nerves supplying the respiratory muscle (Guillain-Barre Syndrome).

### Vascular Diseases

Vascular diseases can result in pulmonary oedema, pulmonary embolism, and pulmonary hypertension.

### Environmental Diseases

Environmental diseases are caused by inhaled dusts and atmosphere pollutants. Many occupational and industrial diseases fall into these categories. A more detailed discussion of pulmonary pathophysiology can be found in West (1992b).

## NURSING PROCESS AND OXYGENATION

 ASSESSMENT

Assessment of a patient's/client's cardiopulmonary functioning should include data collected from the following areas:
1. Nursing history of the patient's/client's normal and present cardiopulmonary function, past impairments in circulatory or respiratory functioning, and measures the patient/client may use to optimize oxygenation.
2. Nursing observations.
3. Specimens for laboratory and diagnostic tests.

### Nursing History

The nursing history should focus on the individual's ability to meet oxygen needs. The nursing history for cardiac function includes pain and characteristics of pain, dyspnoea, fatigue, peripheral circulation, cardiac risk factors, and the presence of past or concurrent cardiac conditions (Table 17-1). The nursing history for respiratory function includes presence of a cough, shortness of breath, wheezing, pain, environmental exposures, frequency of respiratory tract infections, pulmonary risk factors, past respiratory problems, and current medication use (Tables 17-2, 17-3).

### FATIGUE

Fatigue is a subjective sensation in which the patient/client reports a loss of endurance. Fatigue in the person with cardiopulmonary alterations is often an early sign of a worsening of the chronic underlying process. To provide an objective measure of fatigue, ask the patient/client to rate the fatigue on a visual analogue scale of 1 to 10, with 10 correlating with the worst level of fatigue and 1 representing no fatigue.

## TABLE 17-1 Inspection of Cardiopulmonary Status

| Abnormality | Cause |
|---|---|
| **EYES** | |
| Xanthelasma (yellow lipid lesions on eyelids) | Associated with hyperlipidaemia |
| Corneal arcus (whitish opaque ring around junction of cornea and sclera) | Abnormal finding in young to middle adults associated with hyperlipidaemia (normal finding in older adults with arcus senilius) |
| Pale conjunctivae | Associated with anaemia |
| Cyanotic conjunctivae | Associated with hypoxaemia |
| Petechiae on conjunctivae | Associated with fat embolus or bacterial endocarditis |
| **SKIN** | |
| Peripheral cyanosis | Vasoconstriction and diminished blood flow |
| Central cyanosis | Hypoxaemia |
| Decreased skin turgor | Dehydration (normal finding in older adults as a result of decreased skin elasticity) |
| Dependent oedema | Associated with right- and left-sided heart failure |
| Periorbital oedema | Associated with kidney disease |
| **FINGERTIPS AND NAIL BEDS** | |
| Cyanosis | Decreased cardiac output or hypoxia |
| | Bacterial endocarditis |
| **MOUTH AND LIPS** | Chronic hypoxaemia |
| Cyanotic mucous membranes | Decreased oxygenation (hypoxia) |
| Pursed-lip breathing | Associated with chronic lung disease |
| **NECK VEINS** | |
| Distension | Associated with right-sided heart failure |
| **NOSE** | |
| Flaring nares | Air hunger, dyspnoea |
| **CHEST** | |
| Retractions | Increased work of breathing, dyspnoea |
| Asymmetry | Chest wall injury |

## DYSPNOEA

The sensation of dyspnoea can occur with other objective findings, for example, exaggerated respiratory effort, use of the accessory muscles during respiration, flaring of the nares, and an extreme increase in the rate and depth of respirations (Gröer and Shekleton, 1989). To attempt to provide an objective measure of dyspnoea, ask the patient/client to use a visual analogue scale. This objective measure allows the nurse and patient/client to determine if specific nursing interventions are having an effect on the dyspnoea. The visual analogue scale is a 100 mm vertical line with 0 equated with no dyspnoea, and 100 mm equated with severe breathlessness. The use of a visual analogue scale to evaluate a patient's/client's dyspnoea in the clinical setting is valid and reliable (Gift et al, 1986; Gift, 1989).

The nursing history of dyspnoea includes the circumstances under which it occurred, such as with exertion, stress, or respiratory tract infection. The nurse also determines whether the person's perception of dyspnoea affects the ability to lie flat. **Orthopnoea** is an abnormal condition in which the person must use multiple pillows when lying down or must sit to breathe. The presence of orthopnoea is usually quantified, such as two- or three-pillow orthopnoea. This means that the person perceives shortness of breath unless two or three pillows are used for sleeping.

## COUGH

Cough is a sudden, audible expulsion of air from the lungs. The person breathes in, the glottis is partially closed, and the accessory muscles of expiration contract to expel the air forcibly. Coughing is a protective reflex to clear the trachea, bronchi, and lungs of irritants and secretions.

A cough is difficult to evaluate. Almost everyone has periods

## TABLE 17-2 Assessment of Breathing Patterns

| Pattern | Cause |
| --- | --- |
| Eupnoea — normal respiratory rate; adult range of 12-20 breaths/min; normal tidal volume of 5-7 ml/kg body weight* | |
| Tachypnoea — increased respiratory rate above client's normal rate; shallow respirations | Exercise, pregnancy, fever, pulmonary diseases, anxiety, neurological conditions, airway obstruction |
| Bradypnoea — decreased respiratory rate below client's normal rate | Drug overdose, central nervous system dysfunction, airway obstruction |
| Kussmaul respiration — abnormally deep, very rapid sighing type of respiration; increased tidal volume and rate | Diabetic ketacidosis |
| Ataxic respirations — uncoordinated rate or depth of respiration | Central nervous system disorders |
| Cheyne-Stokes respiration — breathing pattern characterized by alternating periods of apnoea and deep rapid breathing; cycle beginning with slow, shallow breaths that gradually increase to abnormal depth and rate; respiration gradually subsiding as breathing slows and becomes shallow | Congestive heart failure, bronchopneumonia, drug overdose, sleep, central nervous system damage |

*From Luce JM, Tyler ML, Pierson DJ: Intensive respiratory care, Philadelphia, 1984, Saunders.*

## TABLE 17-3 Assessment of Abnormal Chest Wall Movement

| Abnormality | Cause |
| --- | --- |
| Retraction — visible shrinking in soft tissues of chest between and around firmer tissue and cartilaginous and bony ribs; retractions having specific beginning point and worsening with need for increased inspiratory effort; possibly found at intercostal space, intraclavicular space, trachea, and substernally* | Any condition that causes increased inspiratory effort (e.g., airway obstruction, asthma, tracheobronchitis) |
| Paradoxical breathing — asynchronous breathing; chest contraction during inspiration and expansion during expiration | Flail chest |
| Increased anteroposterior diameter | Emphysema or chronic obstructive pulmonary disease |

*Infants can experience sternal and substernal retractions with only slight inspiratory effort because of chest pliability.*

of coughing. Moreover, people with a chronic cough tend to deny, underestimate, or minimize their coughing, often because they are so accustomed to it that they are unaware of how frequently it occurs.

Once the nurse determines that the patient/client has a cough, it must be identified as *productive* or *nonproductive* and its frequency must be assessed. A **productive cough** results in sputum. Sputum is material coughed up from the lungs that may be swallowed or expectorated through the mouth. It contains mucus, cellular debris, and microorganisms, and it may contain pus or blood. The nurse must collect data about the type and quantity of sputum. The patient/client should try to produce some sputum so that the nurse can inspect it for colour, consistency, odour, and amount.

If **haemoptysis** (bloody sputum) is reported, the nurse should

be certain that it is associated with coughing and bleeding from the upper respiratory tract or from the gastrointestinal tract **(haematemesis)**. In addition, the haemoptysis should be described according to amount, colour, and duration and whether it is mixed with sputum. When a patient/client reports bloody or blood-tinged sputum, diagnostic tests, such as examination of sputum specimens, chest x-ray examinations, bronchoscopy, and other x-ray studies, should be performed.

Coughing is classified according to the time when the patient/client most frequently coughs. People with chronic sinusitis may cough only in the early morning or immediately after rising from sleep. This clears the airway of mucus resulting from sinus drainage. Individuals with chronic bronchitis generally produce sputum all day, although greater amounts are produced after rising from a semi-recumbent or flat position. This is the result of the dependent accumulation of sputum in the airways and is associated with reduced mobility (see Chapter 24).

## WHEEZING

Wheezing is characterized by a high-pitched musical sound. It is caused by high-velocity movement of air through a narrowed airway. Wheezing may be associated with asthma and acute bronchitis. It can be a frightening, as well as an unpleasant, experience. Patients/clients can usually describe when they wheeze and whether wheezing is present on inspiration or expiration. The nurse should also obtain information about any precipitating factors such as a respiratory infection, allergens, exercise, and stress.

## PAIN

The presence of chest pain should be thoroughly evaluated with regard to location, duration, radiation, and frequency. Cardiac pain does not occur with respiratory variations. It is most often on the left side of the chest and may radiate. Pericardial pain resulting from inflammation of the pericardial sac is usually nonradiating and may occur with inspiration.

**Pleuritic chest pain** is peripheral and may radiate to the scapular regions. It is worsened by inspiratory manoeuvres, such as coughing, yawning, and sighing. Pleuritic pain is often caused by an inflammation or infection in the pleural space. Patients/clients often describe pleuritic pain as knifelike. It lasts from a minute to hours and is always associated with inspiration.

**Musculoskeletal pain** may be present following exercise, rib trauma, and prolonged coughing episodes. This pain is also aggravated by inspiratory movements and may easily be confused with pleuritic chest pain.

## ENVIRONMENTAL OR GEOGRAPHICAL EXPOSURES

Environmental exposure to many inhaled substances is closely linked with respiratory disease. The nurse should investigate exposures in the patient's/client's home and workplace. The most common environmental exposure in the home is cigarette smoke. The nurse should determine whether a patient/client who is a nonsmoker is passively exposed to smoke. Another hazard is radon gas, a radioactive substance, which enters homes through the ground. When homes are overinsulated, this gas is not able to escape into the atmosphere, and becomes trapped in the home.

An employment history should be obtained to assess exposure to substances such as asbestos, coal, cotton fibres, fumes, or chemical inhalants. This is particularly important with middle-aged and older adults who may have worked in places before regulations to protect workers from carcinogens.

Exposure to substances may occur during travel. For example, schistosomiasis infection can be acquired in Asia, Africa, the Caribbean, and South America.

## RESPIRATORY INFECTIONS

A nursing history should contain information about the patient's/client's frequency and duration of respiratory tract infections. Although everyone occasionally experiences a cold, for

some people it can result in bronchitis or pneumonia. The nurse also asks about any known exposure to tuberculosis and about the results of the tuberculin skin test.

Because the acquired immunodeficiency syndrome (AIDS) may initially be diagnosed after *Pneumocystis carinii* or *Mycobacterium pneumonia* infection is found, the nurse needs to assess the patient/client for high-risk factors related to AIDS. Some of these risks include exposure to intravenous drug use, multiple heterosexual and homosexual contacts (Bennett, 1986) or blood transfusions before HIV screening was introduced.

## RISK FACTORS

The nurse must also investigate familial risk factors. A family history of cancer, particularly lung cancer, or cardiovascular diseases should be noted. If the person's family has such a history, it is necessary to document which blood relatives have had the disease and their present level of health or age at time of death. Other family risk factors include the presence of infectious diseases, particularly tuberculosis. The nurse should determine who in the patient's/client's household has been infected and the status of treatment.

## MEDICATIONS

The last component of the nursing history should describe medications the patient/client is using. These include prescribed, over-the-counter, and illicit drugs and substances. Such medications may have adverse effects by themselves or because of interactions with other drugs.

As with all medication, the nurse assesses the patients'/clients' knowledge and ability to use his or her medication. Of particular importance is the nurse's assessment of the individual's understanding of potential side effects of the medications.

### Diagnostic Tests

## TESTS TO DETERMINE ADEQUACY OF THE CARDIAC CONDUCTION SYSTEM

Tests used to determine the adequacy of the cardiac conduction system include electrocardiogram, portable cardiac monitor, exercise stress test, and electrophysiological studies.

**Electrocardiogram** The electrocardiogram (ECG) produces a graphic recording of the heart's electrical activity. The ECG commonly detects the abnormal transmission of impulses and the electrical position of the heart (the axis).

**Portable Cardiac Monitor** A portable cardiac monitor records the heart's electrical activity and produces a continuous ECG over a specified period, such as 24 hours. The monitor allows patients/clients to continue their normal activities as it records the heart's electrical activity. This device enables clinicians to determine if activities, such as walking or straining at stool, are associated with abnormal electrical activity.

**Exercise Stress Test** The exercise stress test is used to evaluate the cardiac response to physical stress. It provides information on myocardial response to increased oxygen requirements and determines the adequacy of coronary blood flow. Heart rate, electrical activity, and cardiac recovery time are reflected in the ECG tracing (Canobbio, 1990). In addition, data about the patient's/client's blood pressure, presence of chest pain, changes in respiration, and colour are monitored.

## TESTS TO DETERMINE MYOCARDIAL CONTRACTION AND BLOOD FLOW

Echocardiography, scintigraphy, cardiac catheterization and angiography are used to determine myocardial contraction and blood flow.

**Echocardiography** Echocardiography is a noninvasive measure to evaluate the internal structures of the heart and heart wall motion. Sonar (radar) technology is used to measure ultrasonic waves and translate these into formed images. The echocardiogram graphically demonstrates overall cardiac performance.

**Radionuclide Angiography** Radionuclide **angiography**, is a noninvasive imaging technique that uses radioisotopes to evaluate cardiac structures, myocardial perfusion, and contractility (Canobbio, 1990).

**Cardiac Catheterization and Angiography** Cardiac catheterization and angiography is an invasive procedure used to visualize cardiac chambers, valves, the great vessels, and coronary arteries. Pressure and volume determinants within the four chambers are also measured. This procedure requires the insertion of a catheter into the heart via a percutaneous venous puncture. A contrast material is injected through the catheter, and fluoroscopic pictures are obtained of the vessels. Both right- and left-sided catheterizations can be performed.

## TESTS TO MEASURE ADEQUACY OF VENTILATION AND OXYGENATION

Pulmonary function tests, peak expiratory flow rates, arterial blood gas tests, oximetry, and complete blood counts are used to assess the adequacy of ventilation and oxygenation.

**Lung Function Tests** For descriptive purposes, the total volume of air in the lungs is divided into volumes and capacities (Fig. 17-8). A capacity is composed of two or more volumes (Kendrick and Smith, 1992).

The most commonly used method to assess lung volumes is the spirometer. This is frequently a wedge-bellows spirometer (Fig. 17-9).

All of the volumes and capacities in Fig. 17-8 can be measured using basic spirometry, with the exception of the residual volume, functional residual capacity and total lung capacity. More complex tests are used to assess these (see West, 1992).

The spirometer is used to measure:
- the forced vital capacity (FVC) – where the subject exhales forcibly from TLC to RV

- the vital capacity (VC) – where the subject exhales from TLC to RV in his/her own time

The spirometer allows a volume-time trace to be obtained (Fig. 17-10 A-C) in addition to static measurements of lung volume.

Obstruction is represented by reduced flow rates (Fig. 17-10 B). This can be seen if the forced expiratory volume in one second (FEV$_1$) is considered as a proportion of the Forced Vital Capacity (FVC), (the FEV$_1$/FVC ratio). In general the FVC is only slightly reduced but the FEV$_1$/FVC ratio is reduced indicating reduced flow rate.

Restriction (Fig. 17-10 C) is represented by reduced lung volumes. The FEV$_1$/FVC ratio is generally unchanged, but the FVC is reduced.

These tests are usually performed in a Lung Function Laboratory. To standardize the procedure tests are usually performed with the patient/client seated and a nose-clip *in situ*.

The nurse must be familiar with the commonly used procedures so that the patient/client can be adequately prepared

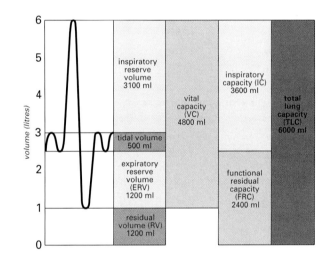

**Fig. 17-8** Lung volumes and capacities. From Brooker C: *Human structure and function - nursing applications in clinical practice*, London, 1993, Mosby.

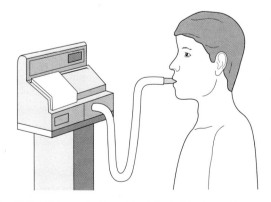

**Fig. 17-9** Vitalograph. From Hinchliff S, Montague S: *Physiology for nursing practice*, ed 2. London, 1988, Ballière Tindall.

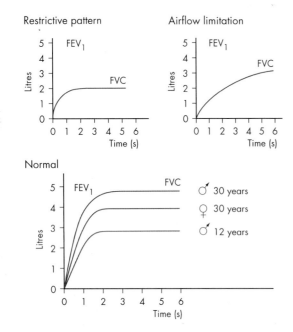

Fig. 17-10 Volume time curves a) normal, b) obstructive, c) restrictive. From Hinchliff S, Montague S: *Physiology for nursing practice*, ed 2, London, 1989, Ballière Tindall.

for the assessment. (A more detailed account of the procedure can be found in Kendrick and Smith, 1992b.)

**Peak Expiratory Flow Rates** The **peak expiratory flow rate (PEF)** is the maximum flow during a forced expiration from TLC. It has a duration of 30 ms and is effort-dependent (Kendrick and Smith, 1992b).

The most frequently used methods to measure PEF are the Wright and Mini-Wright peak flow meters (Fig. 17-11A, B). The Wright meter is more robust and is frequently used in lung function laboratories, and on wards. The mini-Wright is less robust and cheaper and is used at home by patients/clients to assess PEF. For people with asthma, home self-monitoring of PEF provides a good indicator of how well controlled the asthma is. In poorly controlled asthma, a diurnal valve is seen with a dip in the morning. Based on their PEF and their symptoms, patients/clients can agree, in conjunction with their practitioner and nurse, an appropriate treatment plan (Kendrick and Smith, 1992a).

**Arterial Blood Gas Tests** Arterial blood gas measurement is performed in conjunction with pulmonary function tests to determine the hydrogen ion concentration, partial pressure of carbon dioxide and oxygen concentration, and oxyhaemoglobin saturation. Arterial blood gas tests provide information about diffusion of gas across the alveolar-capillary membrane and adequacy of tissue oxygenation .

**Oximetry** Continuous measurements of capillary oxygen saturation are available with cutaneous **oximetry**. Oxygen saturation ($O_2$ sat) is the percentage of haemoglobin saturated with oxygen. One of the most common is a finger oximeter. The nurse attaches a noninvasive sensor to the patient's/client's finger.

The sensor monitors capillary blood oxygen saturation. Continuous monitoring of oxygen saturation is useful in assessing sleep disorders, exercise tolerance, and transient decreases in oxygen saturation.

Transcutaneous oximeter measurements are easy to use, noninvasive, and readily available (Whitney, 1990). Individuals with poor tissue perfusion, such as with shock, hypothermia, and peripheral vascular diseases, may not have reliable oximetry measures. The reader is referred to articles by Coull (1992) and Dobson (1993) for more detailed information on pulse oximeters.

**Full Blood Count** A full blood count determines the number and type of erythrocytes and leucocytes per $mm^3$ of blood. A venous blood sample is obtained by using the venepuncture technique. Blood is usually taken from the ante-cubital fossa region (front of the elbow). Normal values for a complete blood count vary with age and gender.

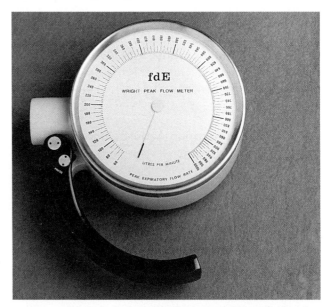

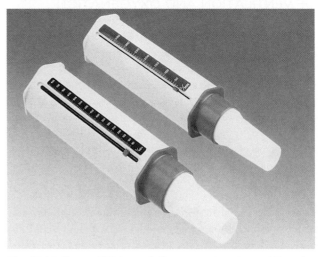

Fig. 17-11 Upper, Wright peak flow meter (courtesy of Ferraris Development & Engineering Co Ltd, London). Lower, Mini-Wright peak flow meter (courtesy of Clement Clarke International Ltd, Harlow, Essex).

The full blood count also measures the haemoglobin level. Haemoglobin is contained within the erythrocytes. A deficiency in red blood cells decreases the blood's oxygen-carrying capacity, because there are fewer haemoglobin molecules available to carry oxygen to tissues.

When the number of erythrocytes is increased, such as with polycythaemia in chronic lung conditions and cyanotic heart conditions, the oxygen-carrying capacity of the blood is increased. However, increased erythrocytes increase blood viscosity and the patient's/client's risk for thrombus formation.

## TESTS TO VISUALIZE STRUCTURES OF THE RESPIRATORY SYSTEM

Chest x-ray examination, bronchoscopy, and lung scan are used to visualize structures of the respiratory system.

**Chest X-ray Examination** A chest x-ray examination consists of a radiograph of the thorax that allows the doctor and nurse to observe the lung fields for fluid (such as in pneumonia), masses (as with lung cancer), fractures (as with rib and clavicular fractures), and other abnormal processes (such as tuberculosis). A brief step-by-step guide on how to interpret the normal chest x-ray is provided by Desai and Chan (1992).

**Bronchoscopy** Bronchoscopy is the visual examination of the trachea and bronchial tree. A narrow, flexible fibreoptic bronchoscope is used. Bronchoscopy is performed to obtain biopsy and fluid or sputum samples for examination. It can also be used to remove mucus plugs or foreign bodies that have become lodged in the airways.

Before bronchoscopy, the patient/client is maintained in a fasting state. The nurse also administers medications before the procedure. A sedative is usually administered, and atropine may be used occasionally to reduce oral secretions. The nurse continues to observe the patient/client after the procedure for signs and symptoms of respiratory distress or hypoxia. Assessment of the individual's gag/swallow reflex is obtained before beginning oral fluids.

**Lung Scan** The most common lung scan is the computed tomogram (CT) scan. CT scanning combines x-ray and computer technology. X-ray beams pass through a section or plane of the thorax from different angles, and the computer calculates tissue absorption and displays a printout and scan picture of the tissues showing densities of various intrathoracic structures. A CT scan can identify abnormal masses by size and location, but cannot identify tissue types, which requires a biopsy.

## TESTS TO DETERMINE ABNORMAL CELLS OR INFECTION IN THE RESPIRATORY TRACT

Tests to determine whether there are abnormal cells or infection in the respiratory tract include throat cultures, sputum specimens, skin testing, and thoracentesis.

**Throat Cultures** A throat culture sample is obtained by swabbing the oropharynx and tonsillar regions with a sterile swab. The throat culture determines the presence of pathogenic microorganisms and the antibiotics to which they are most sensitive.

When obtaining a throat culture, the nurse inserts the swab into the pharyngeal region and passes it along reddened areas, and areas of exudate. Some patients/clients have an active gag reflex, making it difficult to obtain the specimen. The reflex may be less active if the person is sitting straight and leaning forward slightly. In addition, the person may be able to control gagging if informed that the procedure will take only a few seconds.

**Sputum Specimens** Sputum specimens identify a specific microorganism and its drug resistance and sensitivities. This specimen is referred to as *sputum for culture and sensitivity* (C and S). A sputum specimen may also be obtained to identify the presence of the tubercle bacillus (TB). This sputum specimen is called *sputum for acid-fast bacillus* (AFB). The AFB specimen is obtained on each of three consecutive days in the early morning. Finally, sputum specimens are obtained to identify abnormal cells. This is called *sputum for cytology* and involves a serial collection of three early morning sputum specimens. Cytological sputum examination is performed to identify lung cancers by cell type.

When sputum specimens are obtained, the nurse must ensure that the specimen consists of mucus deep from the bronchus and not saliva. The nurse should record the colour, consistency, amount, and odour of the sputum, and should document that the specimen was sent to a specific laboratory for analysis on a specific date and time.

**Skin Testing** Skin testing enables the clinician to determine the presence of bacterial, fungal, or viral pulmonary diseases. The antigen is injected intradermally. The antigen should be properly injected, the injection site should be circled, and the patient/client should be instructed not to wash off the circle. This procedure enables the clinician to evaluate the response.

Positive results are based on the size of the induration. An induration is a palpable, elevated, hardened area around the patient's/client's injection site. It is caused by oedema and inflammation from the antigen/antibody reaction. If induration is present, it is measured in millimetres. Reddened flat areas are not positive reactions and thus should not be measured.

**Thoracocentesis** Thoracocentesis is surgical perforation of the chest wall and pleural space with a needle to aspirate fluid for diagnostic or therapeutic purposes or to remove a specimen for biopsy. The procedure is performed with aseptic technique using a local anaesthetic. The patient/client usually sits upright with the anterior thorax supported by pillows or an over-the-bed table (Fig. 17-12).

Whether this procedure is painful depends, in part, on the person's tolerance to pain (see Chapter 27). The nurse can reduce the patient's/client's anxiety by explaining the procedure and telling the person what to expect. The patient/client must understand the importance of holding his or her breath as requested and of not coughing during the procedure. Sudden movements of the thorax may result in the lung being punctured by the thoracocentesis needle. The patient/client is instructed to notify the doctor before coughing or sneezing so that the needle can be withdrawn. After the procedure the nurse monitors the patient/client for signs of pneumothorax.

 **PLANNING**

Patients/clients with impaired oxygenation require a nursing care plan directed towards meeting the actual or potential oxygenation needs of the patient/client. The plan includes one or more of the following patient-client-centred goals:
- patient/client achieves improved activity tolerance
- patient/client continues maintenance and promotion of lung expansion
- patient/client maintains mobilization of pulmonary secretions
- patient/client has a patent airway
- patient/client tissue oxygenation is maintained or promoted
- patient's/client's cardiopulmonary function is restored

The patient's/client's level of health, age, lifestyle, and environmental risks affect the level of tissue oxygenation. Individuals with severe impairments in oxygenation frequently require nursing interventions directed towards all six goals.

 **IMPLEMENTATION**

Nursing interventions for promoting and maintaining adequate oxygenation include independent nursing actions (such as positioning, coughing techniques, and preventive health behaviours) and interdependent or dependent interventions (such as oxygen therapy, lung inflation techniques, hydration, medications, and in assisting in the use of chest physiotherapy).

### Improved Activity Tolerance

Nursing interventions for improving activity tolerance primarily include measures such as management of dyspnoea, cardiopulmonary reconditioning, and respiratory muscle training.

### DYSPNOEA MANAGEMENT

Dyspnoea is difficult to quantify and to treat. Treatment methods need to be individualized for each person, and more than one therapy is usually implemented.

Ideally, the underlying process that causes or worsens dyspnoea must be treated. After this initial phase, there are four additional therapies: pharmacological measures, oxygen therapy, physical techniques, and psychosocial techniques (Gift, 1990). Pharmacological agents may include bronchodilators, steroids, mucolytics, and antianxiety medications. Oxygen therapy can reduce dyspnoea associated with exercise. Physical techniques, such as cardiopulmonary reconditioning, breathing techniques, and cough control, can help to reduce dyspnoea (DeVito, 1990). Relaxation

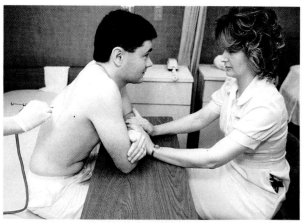

**Fig. 17-12** Position for thoracentesis. From Wilson SF, Thompson JM: *Respiratory disorders*, St Louis, 1990, Mosby.

techniques, biofeedback, and meditation are psychosocial measures that can lessen the sensation of dyspnoea (Gift, 1990).

### CARDIOPULMONARY RECONDITIONING

The major method of cardiopulmonary reconditioning is a structured rehabilitation programme. **Cardiopulmonary rehabilitation** is actively assisting the client to achieve and maintain an optimal level of health through controlled physical exercise, nutrition counselling, relaxation and stress management techniques, prescribed medications and oxygen, and adherence to the programme. Goals of rehabilitation are defined by the patient/client and the rehabilitation team.

As physical reconditioning occurs, the patient's/client's complaints of dyspnoea, chest pain, fatigue, and activity intolerance should decrease. Researchers noted the amount of anxiety, depression, and somatic concerns decreased as individuals participated in cardiopulmonary rehabilitation. This occurred whether or not there was clinical improvement in the cardiopulmonary disease itself (Shenkman, 1985; Agle *et al*, 1973).

### Maintenance or Promotion of Lung Expansion

Nursing interventions to maintain or promote lung expansion include noninvasive techniques, such as positioning and breathing exercises. Lung expansion may also be promoted by procedures using equipment such as incentive spirometers. In cases of pneumothorax and pleural effusions, re-expansion can also be achieved by invasive procedures such as insertion of a chest tube.

### POSITIONING

In the healthy, completely mobile person, adequate ventilation and oxygenation are maintained by frequent changes of position during the activities of living. However, when a person's mobility is restricted as a result of illness or injury, there is a risk for respiratory impairment. Frequent changes of position are simple and cost-effective methods for reducing the risks of pulmonary complications such as stasis of pulmonary secretions and decreased chest wall expansion (see Chapter 24).

The most effective position for people with cardiopulmonary diseases is high-Fowler's position (see Fig. 24-9). This position

### Children's Nursing
### Oxygen therapy in infants

It is very important when caring for infants undergoing oxygen therapy that the oxygen does not blow directly onto the infant's face, because this will stimulate receptors which cause a diving reflex. This results in bradycardia and shunting of blood from peripheral to central circulation.

The concentration must be monitored. High oxygen concentrations can cause blindness in young babies.

uses gravity to assist in lung expansion and to reduce pressure from the abdomen on the diaphragm. When the patient/client uses this position, the nurse should ensure that the individual does not slide down in the bed, which could reduce lung expansion.

## BREATHING EXERCISES

Breathing exercises include techniques to improve ventilation and oxygenation. The three basic techniques are deep breathing and coughing exercises, pursed-lip breathing, and diaphragmatic breathing. Deep breathing and coughing exercises are routine interventions for postoperative patients/clients (see Chapter 29).

**Pursed-lip breathing** involves deep inspiration and prolonged expiration through pursed lips. This exercise keeps the alveoli from collapsing. While sitting up, the patient/client is instructed to take a deep breath and to exhale slowly through pursed lips. Patients/clients need to gain control of the exhalation phase so that exhalation is longer than inhalation (Dettenmeier, 1992). The person is usually able to perfect this technique by counting inhalation time and gradually increasing the count during exhalation.

**Diaphragmatic breathing** is more difficult and requires the patient/client to relax intercostal and accessory respiratory muscles while taking deep inspirations. The individual is taught to place one hand flat below the breastbone above the waist and the other hand 2 to 3 cm below the first hand. The patient/client is asked to sniff, and with the sniff, the diaphragm will expand outward, causing his or her hand to move. Second, the patient/client concentrates on expanding the diaphragm during controlled inspiration. The lower hand should move outward during expiration. The patient/client observes for inward movement as the diaphragm ascends. These exercises are initially taught with the person in the supine position and are then practised while the person sits and stands. The exercise is often used with the pursed-lip breathing technique.

The pulmonary results of these exercise patterns include decreased air trapping and reduced work of breathing (Luce *et al*, 1984). Diaphragmatic breathing is also useful for people with pulmonary disease, for postoperative patients/clients, and for women in labour to promote relaxation and provide pain control.

## INCENTIVE SPIROMETRY

**Incentive spirometry** is a method of encouraging voluntary deep breathing by providing visual feedback to patients/clients about inspiratory volume. Incentive spirometry is used to prevent or treat atelectasis and is particularly useful for postoperative patients/clients (Luce *et al*, 1984). Postoperative complications are prevented by reinflating collapsed alveoli and removing secretions.

Flow-oriented incentive spirometers consist of one or more plastic chambers that contain freely moving coloured balls. The person inhales briskly to elevate the balls and to keep them floating as long as possible. The goal is to keep the balls elevated for as long as possible to ensure a maximally sustained inhalation. Even if a very slow inspiration does not elevate the balls, this breathing pattern alone may achieve greater lung expansion (Luce *et al*, 1984).

Volume-oriented incentive spirometry devices have bellows that are raised to a predetermined volume by an inhaled breath. An achievement light or counter is used in some devices. Some devices are constructed so that the light will not turn on unless the bellows are held at a minimum desired volume for a specified period to enhance lung expansion.

Incentive spirometry encourages patients/clients to breathe to their normal inspiratory capacities. Because of postoperative pain, a postoperative inspiratory capacity one-half to three-quarters of the preoperative volume is acceptable (Luce *et al*, 1984).

## CHEST TUBES

Chest tubes are inserted to remove air and fluids from the pleural space, to prevent air or fluid from re-entering the pleural space, and to re-establish normal intrapleural and intrapulmonic pressures (Dettenmeier, 1992). A **chest tube** is a catheter inserted through the thorax to remove fluid or air and thus promote lung re-expansion. Chest tubes are used after chest surgery and chest trauma and for pneumothorax or haemothorax. Further detail on chest drainage can be found in articles by Walsh (1989), Campbell (1993) and Welch (1993).

A **pneumothorax** is a collection of air or other gas in the pleural space. The gas causes the lung to collapse because it obliterates the negative intrapleural pressure and a counterpressure is exerted against the lung, which is then unable to expand. There are a variety of mechanisms for a pneumothorax. It may occur spontaneously or from chest trauma, such as a stabbing or road traffic accident; from the rupture of an emphysematous vesicle on the surface of the lung; or from an invasive procedure, such as a thoracocentesis or insertion of a subclavian intravenous line.

A patient/client with a pneumothorax usually feels pain as atmospheric air irritates the parietal pleura. The pain may be sharp and pleuritic. Dyspnoea is common and worsens as the size of the pneumothorax increases.

**Haemothorax** is an accumulation of blood and fluid in the pleural cavity between the parietal and visceral pleurae, usually as the result of trauma. It produces a counterpressure and prevents the lung from full expansion. A haemothorax can also be caused by rupture of small blood vessels from inflammatory processes, such as with pneumonia or tuberculosis. In addition to pain and dyspnoea, signs and symptoms of shock can develop if blood loss is severe.

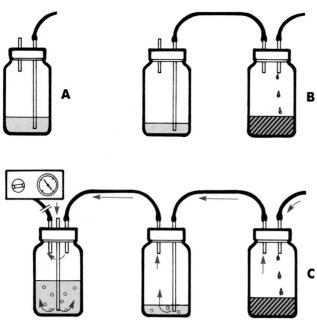

**Fig. 17-13** Chest tube drainage. **A,** One-bottle system. **B,** Two-bottle system. **C,** Three-bottle system with suction.

The one-bottle system is the simplest closed drainage system because the single bottle serves as a collector and a water seal (Fig. 17-13, A). During normal respiration, fluctuations in the water-seal tube are expected. The fluid should ascend with inspiration. A two-bottle system permits the liquid to flow into the collection bottle and air flows into the water-seal bottle (Fig. 17-13, B). Fluctuations in the water-seal tube are still anticipated. The advantage of the two-bottle system is that it permits more accurate measurement and observation of chest drainage (Erikson, 1981a).

A three-bottle system is used to evacuate any volume of air or fluid with controlled suction (Fig. 17-13, C). The suction-control bottle contains a long tube, submerged under water, and two short tubes. The longer tube is submerged in water and vented to the atmosphere. One short tube connects bottles two and three. The second short tube is connected to an external suction source at a pressure that causes gentle, continuous bubbling in bottle three. Suction pressure, measured in centimetres of water, is equated with length of submersion in water of the long tube, as measured in centimetres. Usually -15 to -20 cm water, which requires the long tube to be submerged in 15 to 20 centimetres of water, is used for adults and a lesser amount for children (Erikson, 1981a). The disposable systems are a one-piece moulded plastic unit that duplicates the three-bottle system. The disposable units appear to be the system of choice because they are cost effective and some facilitate autotransfusion, a common practice in open-heart surgeries. General knowledge of chest tube management and troubleshooting manoeuvres reduces the patient's/client's side effects.

**Special Considerations** Clamping chest tubes is contraindicated when a person is ambulating. The nurse should handle the bottles carefully and maintain the drainage device

below the patient's/client's chest. If the tubing disconnects from the bottles, the nurse should instruct the patient/client to exhale as much as possible and to cough. This manoeuvre rids the pleural space of as much air as possible. The nurse should cleanse the tips of the tubing and reconnect them to the bottles.

Removal of chest tubes requires patient/client preparation. A recent study investigated patient's/client's reported sensations during chest tube removal. The most frequent sensations reported included burning, pain, and a pulling sensation (Gift *et al*, 1991).

## Mobilization of Pulmonary Secretions

The ability of a patient/client to mobilize pulmonary secretions may make the difference between a short-term illness and a long period of recovery involving complications. Nursing interventions that promote mobilization of pulmonary secretions include hydration, humidification, nebulization, and chest physiotherapy.

### HYDRATION

Maintenance of adequate systemic hydration keeps mucociliary clearance normal. In individuals with adequate hydration, pulmonary secretions are thin, white, watery, and easily removable with minimal coughing. Excessive coughing required to clear thick, tenacious secretions is fatiguing and leaves the patient/client with little energy (Feldman, 1982). Unless contraindicated, most clinicians recommend a fluid intake of 1500 to 2000 ml per day (Luce *et al*, 1984). Adequacy of hydration can be determined by the colour, consistency, and ease of secretion expectoration.

### HUMIDIFICATION

**Humidification** is the process of adding water to gas. Temperature is the most important factor affecting the amount of water vapour a gas can hold. The percentage of water in the gas in relation to the gas' capacity for water is the *relative humidity*. Air or oxygen with a high relative humidity keeps the airways moist and loosens and mobilizes pulmonary secretions.

Humidification is necessary for people receiving oxygen therapy. Oxygen delivered to the upper airways, as with a nasal catheter, nasal cannula, or face mask, can be humidified by bubbling it through water. Generally, humidification is added when oxygen flow rates exceed 5 L/min.

Heating of humidifiers is impractical because condensed moisture fills the narrow tubing. Therefore, the relative humidity of oxygen delivered to the upper airways is only 30% (Luce *et al*, 1984).

When humidity is needed, the nurse needs to ensure that the right solution is used for humidification and that the solution is changed according to agency procedures. Excess humidification and reservoirs used for humidity solutions are environments that support the growth of pathogens. Thus, humidification can be a source for nosocomial infections in patients/clients.

### NEBULIZATION

**Nebulization** is a process of adding moisture or medications to inspired air by mixing particles of varying sizes with the air. A nebulizer uses the aerosol principle to suspend a maximum

### Children's Nursing
### Humidification for children

A humidity tent is used for infants and children with illnesses such as croup and tracheitis, if the condition requires high humidity, but not oxygen. Children with these disorders require high humidity to liquify secretions and help reduce fever. The nebulizer at the top of the humidity tent must remain filled with water to prevent nonhumidified air or oxygen from entering the tent. Air in the humidity tent can become cool and fall below 20° C (68° F), causing the child to become chilled. Therefore the nurse monitors the child's body temperature as well as respiratory status. Children in humidity tents require frequent changes of clothing and bed linen to remain warm and dry.

Condensation on the canopy may make it difficult to observe the child, so the inside of the canopy must be wiped frequently. The mist may also cause maceration of the skin, so the child should be removed from the mist periodically (if possible) and the mist delivered via nebulizer tubing or a mask. During these periods, observe the child for overhydration, which can result from intensive care of a nebulizer.

number of water drops or particles of the desired size in inspired air. The moisture added to the respiratory system through nebulization improves clearance of pulmonary secretions.

When the thin layer of fluid that supports the mucus layer over the cilia is allowed to dry, the cilia are damaged and cannot adequately clear the airway. Humidification through nebulization enhances mucociliary clearance, the body's natural mechanism for removing mucus and cellular debris from the respiratory tract. Therefore, nebulization is often used for administration of bronchodilators and mucolytic agents.

The major types of nebulizers are the jet-aerosol nebulizer and the ultrasonic nebulizer. A jet-aerosol nebulizer uses gas under pressure, and the ultrasonic nebulizer uses high-frequency vibrations to break up the water or medication into fine drops or particles. When inspired with air or administered oxygen, the drops of particles are deposited throughout the tracheobronchial tree.

### CHEST PHYSIOTHERAPY

**Chest physiotherapy (CP)** is a group of therapies used in combination to mobilize pulmonary secretions. These therapies include postural drainage, chest percussion, and vibration. Chest physiotherapy should be followed by productive coughing. Suctioning is used if the patient's/client's ability to cough is inadequate. CP also has multiple implications for a variety of lung diseases. Eid *et al* (1991) present a practical clinical synopsis of CP manoeuvres for a variety of clinical problems. The nurse may be involved in assisting the physiotherapist with the following procedures.

**Chest percussion** involves striking the chest wall over the area being drained. The hand is positioned so that the fingers and thumb touch and the hand is cupped. Percussion on the surface of the chest wall sends waves of varying amplitude and frequency

through the chest. The force of these waves can change the consistency of the sputum or dislodge it from airway walls (Luce *et al*, 1984). Chest percussion is performed by alternating hand motion against the chest wall. Percussion is performed over a single layer of clothing and not over buttons, or zips. The single layer of clothing prevents slapping the individual's skin. Thicker material dampens the vibrations from percussion.

Percussion is contraindicated in people with bleeding disorders, osteoporosis, or fractured ribs. Caution should be taken to percuss the lung fields and not the scapular regions, or trauma may occur to the skin and underlying musculoskeletal structures.

**Vibration** is a fine, shaking pressure applied to the chest wall only during exhalation. This technique is thought to increase the velocity and turbulence of exhaled air, facilitating secretion removal (Dettenmeier, 1992). Vibration increases the exhalation of trapped air and may shake mucus loose and induce a cough. Vibration is not recommended in infants and young children.

**Postural drainage** is the use of positioning techniques that draw secretions from specific segments of the lungs and bronchi into the trachea. Coughing or suctioning normally removes secretions from the trachea. The procedure for postural drainage can include most lung segments. Because patients/clients may not require postural drainage of all lung segments, the procedure is based on clinical assessment findings. For example, individuals with left lower lobe atelectasis may require postural drainage of only the affected region, whereas a child with cystic fibrosis may require postural drainage of all lung segments.

### Maintenance of a Patent Airway

The airway is patent when the trachea, bronchi, and large airways are free from obstructions. Three types of interventions are used to maintain a patent airway: coughing techniques, suctioning, and insertion of an artificial airway.

### COUGHING TECHNIQUES

Coughing is effective for maintaining a patent airway. Coughing permits the patient/client to remove secretions from both the upper and lower airways. The normal series of events in the cough mechanisms are deep inhalation, closure of the glottis, active contraction of the expiratory muscles, and glottis opening. Deep inhalation increases lung volume and airway diameter. Thus, air can pass to partially obstructing mucus plugs or other foreign matter. Contraction of the expiratory muscles against the closed glottis allows a high intrathoracic pressure to develop. As a result, when the glottis is opened, a large flow of air is expelled at a high speed, providing momentum for mucus to move to the upper airway. After the cough the mucus can be expectorated or swallowed (Traver, 1982).

Various coughing techniques can be taught to different patients/clients. (Chapter 29 details the technique of deep breathing and coughing for the postoperative person.) Other cough techniques are cascade, huff, and quad coughing.

**Cascade cough:** the patient/client takes a slow, deep breath and holds it for 2 seconds, while contracting expiratory muscles. Then the patient/client opens the mouth and performs a series of coughs throughout exhalation, thereby coughing at progressively lowered lung volumes. This technique promotes airway clearance and a patent airway in patients/clients with large volumes of sputum.

**Huff cough:** the patient/client, while exhaling, opens the glottis by saying the word 'huff'. The huff cough stimulates a natural cough reflex. This is generally effective only for clearing central airways, but with practice the individual inhales more air and may be able to progress to the cascade cough.

**Quad cough:** this is used for people without abdominal muscle control, such as those with spinal cord injuries. The patient/client or nurse pushes inward and upward on the abdominal muscles towards the diaphragm while the patient/client breathes with maximal expiratory effort, causing the cough (Luce *et al*, 1984).

The effectiveness of coughing is evaluated by sputum expectoration, the patient's/client's report of swallowed sputum, or clearing of adventitious sounds on auscultation. People with chronic pulmonary diseases, upper respiratory tract infections, and lower respiratory tract infections should be encouraged to cough at least every 2 hours when awake. People with a large amount of sputum should be encouraged to cough every hour while awake and every 2 to 3 hours while asleep until the acute phase of mucus production has ended. Further detail on the management of sputum retention can be found in Hough (1992).

## SUCTIONING TECHNIQUES

When a patient/client is unable to clear respiratory tract secretions with coughing, the nurse must use suctioning to clear the airways. The three primary suctioning techniques are oropharyngeal and nasopharyngeal suctioning, orotracheal and nasotracheal suctioning, and suctioning an artificial airway.

These techniques are based on common principles. Because the oropharynx and trachea are considered sterile, sterile technique is required for suctioning. The mouth is considered clean, and therefore the suctioning of oral secretions should be performed after suctioning of the oropharynx and trachea. Each type of suctioning requires the use of a beaded-tip catheter with a ring of holes along the side of the catheter at the distal end. Frequency of suctioning is determined by continued patient/client assessment. If secretions are identified by inspection or auscultation techniques, suctioning is required. Sputum is not produced continuously or every 1–2 hours, but occurs as a response to a pathological condition. Therefore, there is no rationale for routine suctioning of all patients/clients every 1–2 hours.

### Oropharyngeal and Nasopharyngeal Suctioning

The oropharynx extends behind the mouth from the soft palate above the level of the hyoid bone and contains the tonsils. The nasopharynx is located behind the nose and extends to the level of the soft palate. Oropharyngeal or nasopharyngeal suctioning is used when the patient/client is able to cough effectively but is unable to clear secretions by expectorating or swallowing. The suction procedure is used after the individual has coughed (Procedure 17-1). As the amount of pulmonary secretions is reduced and the person is less fatigued, the patient/client may be able to expectorate or swallow the mucus. This type of suctioning is then no longer required.

### Orotracheal and Nasotracheal Suctioning

Orotracheal or nasotracheal suctioning is necessary when the person with pulmonary secretions is unable to cough and does not have an artificial airway present (see Procedure 17-1). A catheter is passed through the mouth or nose into the trachea. The nose is the preferred route because stimulation of the gag reflex is minimal. The procedure is similar to nasopharyngeal suctioning, but the catheter tip is moved farther into the patient/client to suction the trachea. The entire procedure from catheter passage to its removal cannot take more than 15 seconds because oxygen does not reach the lungs during suctioning. Unless in respiratory distress, the patient/client should be allowed to rest between passes of the catheter. If the patient/client is using supplemental oxygen, the oxygen cannula or mask should be replaced during rest periods.

**Artificial Airway** An artificial airway is an oral airway or an endotracheal, nasotracheal, or tracheotomy tube. Indications for an artificial airway include decreased level of consciousness, airway obstruction, mechanical ventilation, and removal of tracheal secretions.

*Oral Airway* The oral airway, the simplest type of artificial airway, prevents obstruction of the trachea by displacement of the tongue into the oropharynx in the unconscious patient/client (Fig. 17-14). The oral airway extends from the teeth to the oropharynx, maintaining the tongue in the normal position. The correct size airway must be used. If the airway is too small, the tongue is not held in the anterior portion of the mouth. If it is too large, it may force the tongue towards the epiglottis and obstruct the airway.

The artificial oral airway is inserted by turning the curve of the airway towards the cheek and placing it over the tongue into the oropharynx. When the airway is in the oropharynx, the nurse turns it so that the opening points downwards. The correctly

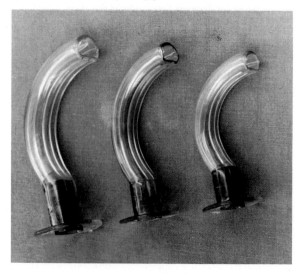

**Fig. 17-14** Artificial oral airways.

placed airway moves the tongue forward away from the oropharynx. The flange, the flat portion of the airway, should rest against the patient's/client's teeth.

If the nurse attempts to insert the oral airway with a curve towards the tongue, the patient's/client's natural airway can be further obstructed. Incorrect insertion merely forces the tongue back into the oropharynx.

*Tracheal Airway* Artificial tracheal airways include endotracheal, nasotracheal, and tracheal tubes. These allow easy access to the patient's/client's trachea for deep tracheal suctioning. Because of the presence of the artificial airway, the patient/client no longer has normal humidification of the tracheal mucosa. The nurse should ensure that humidity is being supplied to the airway through nebulization or with the oxygen-delivery system. This humidification is protective and helps removal of tracheal secretions. Removal of tracheal secretions must be aseptic, atraumatic, and effective.

Asepsis involves using a freshly opened sterile suction catheter that is handled with a sterile glove. Secretion removal should be as atraumatic as possible. To avoid trauma, suction should never be applied during insertion of the catheter but only during its withdrawal. The catheter is rotated and suction is applied intermittently during withdrawal.

## Maintenance and Promotion of Oxygenation

Promotion of lung expansion, mobilization of secretions, and maintenance of a patent airway assist the patient/client in meeting oxygenation needs. However, some individuals also require **oxygen therapy** to keep a healthy level of tissue oxygenation.

### GOAL OF OXYGEN THERAPY

The goal of oxygen therapy is to prevent or relieve hypoxia. Any person with impaired tissue oxygenation can benefit from controlled oxygen administration. Oxygen is not a substitute for other treatment, however, and should be used only when indicated. Oxygen should be treated as a drug. It is expensive and has dangerous side effects. As with any drug, the dosage or concentration of oxygen should be continuously monitored. The nurse should routinely check the doctor's orders to verify that the patient/client is receiving the prescribed oxygen concentration.

### SAFETY PRECAUTIONS WITH OXYGEN THERAPY

Oxygen is a highly combustible gas. Although it will not spontaneously burn or cause an explosion, it can easily cause a fire to ignite if it contacts a spark, such as from a cigarette or electrical equipment. Oxygen in high concentrations has a great combustion potential and fuels fire readily.

With increasing use of home oxygen therapy, patients/clients and health care professionals must be aware of the dangerous combustible effects.

The nurse should promote safety by using the following measures:
1. 'No smoking' signs should be placed on the person's room door and over the bed. The patient/client, visitors and all personnel should be informed that smoking is not permitted in areas where oxygen is in use.
2. The nurse determines that all electrical equipment in the room is functioning correctly and is properly earthed. An electrical spark in the presence of oxygen can result in a serious fire.
3. The nurse should know the fire procedures and the location of the nearest fire extinguisher.

### SUPPLY OF OXYGEN

Oxygen is supplied to the patient's/client's bedside either by oxygen cylinders or through a permanent wall-piped system. Oxygen cylinders are transported on wide-based carriers that allow the tank to be placed upright at the person's bedside. Regulators are used to control the amount of oxygen delivered. One common type is an upright flow meter with a flow-adjustment valve at the top. A second type is a cylinder indicator with a flow-adjustment handle.

In the hospital or home, oxygen cylinders are delivered with the regulator in place. In the hospital, connecting the regulator is usually done prior to the oxygen cylinders being delivered to the ward. Most hospitals now have piped oxygen and use cylinders only when transporting patients.

### METHODS OF OXYGEN DELIVERY

Oxygen can be delivered to the patient/client by nasal cannula, nasal catheter, face mask, or mechanical ventilator.

**Nasal Cannula** A nasal cannula (Fig. 17-15) is a simple, comfortable device (Procedure 17-2). The two cannulae, about 1.5 cm long, protrude from the centre of a disposable tube and are inserted into the nares. Oxygen is delivered via the cannulae with a flow rate of up to 4 L/min. Higher flow rates dry airway mucosa and do not further increase inspired oxygen concentrations (Luce *et al*, 1984). The nurse must know what flow rate produces a given percentage of inspired oxygen concentration ($Fio_2$).

**Nasal Catheter** Nasal catheters are used less frequently than nasal cannulae, but they are not obsolete. The procedure involves inserting an oxygen catheter into the nose to the nasopharynx. Because securing the catheter can cause pressure on the nostril, the catheter must be changed at least every 8 hours and inserted into the other nostril. For this reason the nasal catheter is often a less desirable method because the patient/client may have pain when the catheter is passed into the nasopharynx and because trauma can occur to the nasal mucosa.

**Oxygen Masks** An oxygen mask is a device used to administer oxygen, humidity, or heated humidity. It is shaped to fit snugly over the mouth and nose and is secured in place with a strap. There are two primary types of oxygen masks: high and low concentration.

A plastic face mask with a reservoir bag (Fig. 17-16) and a Venturi mask (Fig. 17-17) are capable of delivering higher concentrations of oxygen. When used as a nonrebreather, the plastic face mask with a reservoir bag can deliver from 80% to 90% oxygen (70% when used as a rebreather) with a flow rate of

### Children's Nursing
### Endotracheal suctioning in
### children: special considerations

There are many potential hazards of endotracheal suctioning procedures; for example, dysrhythmias, laryngospasm, trauma, hypoxaemia and sepsis (Knox, 1993). Suctioning should be undertaken only by skilled personnel using correct procedures and observation. For example, children should be monitored for shock and signs of decreased cardiac output, and the catheter should be inserted only as far as necessary to minimize the risk of direct vagal stimulation (Klieber, 1986; Shorten, 1989). The priority should be to minimize trauma and to minimize the levels of negative pressure applied.

Deep suctioning should include gentle advancement of the catheter tip until resistance can be felt. The catheter should then be withdrawn 1 cm prior to applying negative pressure, to reduce the risk of mucosal trauma (Knox, 1993).

Suction should also be preceded by hyperoxygenation and hyperventilation to prevent hypoxia during the procedure. The technique should be scrupulously clean. Sputum specimens should be sent for microscopy, culture and sensitivity at least twice weekly, and equipment changed as per unit policy (Knox, 1993).

10 L/min. This oxygen mask maintains a high-concentration oxygen supply in the reservoir bag. The nurse should frequently inspect the bag to make sure it is inflated. If it is deflated, the patient/client may be breathing large amounts of exhaled carbon dioxide.

The Venturi mask can be used to deliver oxygen concentrations of 24% to 28%, 30%, 35%, 40%, 45%, 55% with oxygen flow rates of 2 to 3, 4, 6, 8, 14 L/min, respectively, depending on which flow control meter is selected (Dettenmeier, 1992).

The simple face mask (Fig. 17-18) is used for short-term oxygen therapy. It fits loosely and delivers oxygen

### Adult Nursing
### Use of oxygen at home

When home oxygen is required, it is usually delivered by nasal cannula. When a person has a permanent tracheotomy, however, a T-tube or tracheotomy collar is necessary.

Individuals requiring home oxygen need extensive teaching so that they are able to continue oxygen therapy efficiently and safely. For this preparation, the nurse must liaise with community nursing services and the home oxygen equipment supplier. Sufficient time must be allowed for teaching so that the person and family care are is confident in maintaining the oxygen-delivery system. This procedure is part of good discharge planning.

Fire safety is important when oxygen is used in the home. Clients, carers and visiting staff should be aware of the risks.

concentrations from 30% to 60%. The mask is contraindicated for individuals with carbon dioxide retention because retention can be worsened. More detailed descriptions of oxygen delivery systems can be found in Allen (1989), Foss (1990) and Bambridge (1993).

## Restoration of Cardiopulmonary Functioning

If a patient's/client's hypoxia is severe and prolonged, cardiac arrest may result. A **cardiac arrest** is a sudden cessation of cardiac output and circulation. When this occurs, oxygen is not delivered to tissues, carbon dioxide is not transported from tissues, tissue metabolism becomes anaerobic, and metabolic and respiratory acidosis occur. Permanent heart, brain, and other tissue damage occurs within 5 minutes.

### CARDIOPULMONARY RESUSCITATION

Cardiac arrest is characterized by an absence of pulse and respiration and by dilated pupils. If the nurse determines that a person has cardiac arrest, **cardiopulmonary resuscitation (CPR)** must be initiated. CPR is a basic emergency procedure of artificial respiration and manual external cardiac massage (Procedure 17-3). CPR has three main goals – the ABCs of cardiopulmonary resuscitation: to establish an airway, initiate breathing, and maintain circulation. An outline of the European Resuscitation Council's new guidelines can be found in Wynne (1993).

 **EVALUATION**

Nursing interventions are evaluated by comparing the patient's/client's progress as a result of nursing therapies to the goals and desired outcomes of the nursing care plan. Each goal and category of interventions has objective evaluation criteria (see evaluation box).

When nursing measures directed to improve oxygenation are unsuccessful, the nurse must immediately modify the nursing care plan. New interventions are then developed. The nurse should not hesitate to notify the doctor about a patient's/client's deteriorating oxygenation status. Prompt notification can avoid an emergency situation or even the need for cardiopulmonary resuscitation.

## SUMMARY

People with impaired oxygenation require planned nursing care that focuses on returning the person to a maximal level of wellness. Many nursing interventions can be used to promote lung expansion, mobilize secretions, maintain a patent airway, promote oxygenation, and restore cardiopulmonary functioning.

Nursing interventions are individualized to the patient's/client's level of health, age, lifestyle, and needs. Many nursing skills are used to help the individual achieve a maximal level of oxygenation.

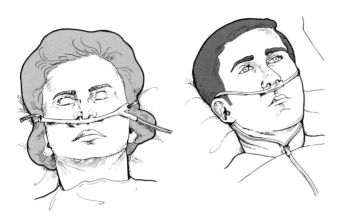

**Fig. 17-15** Nasal cannula. From Wade JF: *Comprehensive respiratory care*, ed 3, St Louis, 1983, Mosby–Year Book.

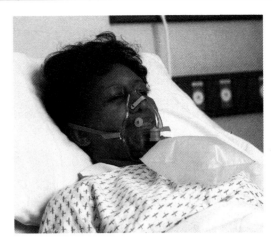

**Fig. 17-16** Plastic face mask with reservoir bag.

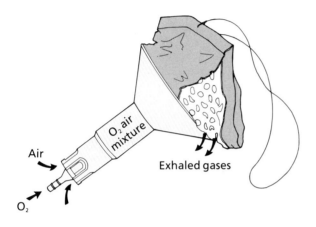

**Fig. 17-17** Venturi mask. Courtesy of Puritan-Bennett Corp, Overland Park, Kansas.

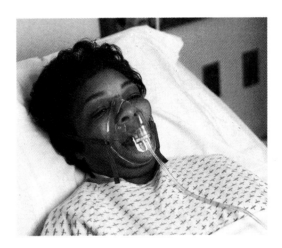

**Fig. 17-18** Simple face mask.

## Sample Evaluation of Interventions for Ineffective Airway Clearance

| Goals | Evaluative Measures | Expected Outcomes |
|---|---|---|
| Pulmonary secretions will be removed. | Auscultate all lung fields after coughing and postural drainage manoeuvres. | Adventitious lung sounds will be absent with 48 hr. |
| | Observe patient/client while coughing for amount of secretions, fatigue, dyspnoea. | Patient/client will maintain productive cough. |
| | Inspect sputum after cough and/or after suctioning. | Sputum will be clear, white, and frothy within 48 hr. |
| Lung expansion will be improved. | Auscultate all lung fields after position change and coughing/suctioning. | Breath sounds will improve and adventitious lung sounds will be absent. |
| | Observe chest wall motion. Chest wall motion will be symmetrical. | Observe for dyspnoea. There will be no nasal flaring or use of accessory muscles. |

## PROCEDURE 17-1 Cardiopulmonary Resuscitation

| SEQUENCE OF ACTIONS | RATIONALE |
|---|---|

### ONE NURSE

| | |
|---|---|
| 1. Assess for unresponsiveness, observe for spontaneous respirations, palpate carotid pulse; ask victim, "Are you alright?" | Prevents injury from attempted resuscitation of person who has not suffered a cardiac or respiratory arrest. |
| 2. Call for help: in hospital setting, call a "code"; in community setting, call emergency phone number. | Activates mechanism for additional personnel. |
| 3. Place victim supine on firm, flat surface or use backboard. | Facilitates external compression of heart. Heart is compressed between sternum and hard surface. |
| 4. Kneel at victim's side. | Allows performance of rescue breathing and chest compressions without moving knees. |
| 5. Open victim's airway:<br><br>a. Head-tilt/chin-lift manoeuvre (adults and children):<br>Place one hand on victim's forehead and apply firm, backward pressure with palm to tilt head back. Place fingers of other hand under bony part of lower jaw near chin and lift to bring chin forward and teeth almost to occlusion, thus supporting jaw and helping to tilt head back (see illustration). The fingers must not press deeply into the soft tissue under the chin. Thumb should not be used to lift chin. | This manoeuvre is more effective in opening airway than previously recommended head-tilt/neck-lift.<br>Removes tongue from epiglottis as airway obstruction. |
| b. Jaw thrust manoeuvre (adults and children):<br>Grasp angles of victim's lower jaw and lift with both hands, one on each side, displacing mandible forward while tilting head backward. | This technique, without head-tilt, is the safest first approach to opening airway of victim with suspected neck injury because it can usually be accomplished without extending neck. |
| 6. Prepare for artificial respiration:<br><br>a. For mouth-to-mouth resuscitation of adult, pinch victim's nose and occlude mouth. For infant, place your mouth over infant's nose and mouth. | Forms airtight seal and prevents air from escaping from nose. |
| b. For Ambu bag resuscitation, use proper size face mask and apply it over victim's mouth and nose. | Forms airtight seal as bag is compressed and oxygen enters patient/client. |
| 7. Administer artificial respiration:<br><br>a. For mouth-to-mouth resuscitation of adult, take a deep breath and seal lips around victim's mouth, creating air-tight seal. Give two slow breaths, followed by 10 to 12 breaths per min. | In most adults this volume of air is 800 ml and is sufficient to make chest rise. Adequate ventilation is indicated by observing chest rise and fall and hearing air escape during exhalation. Excess, rapid volume causes pharyngeal pressures to exceed oesophageal opening pressures, allowing air to enter stomach. |

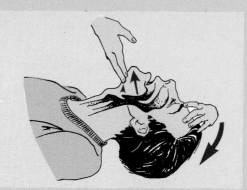

**PROCEDURE 17-1 Cardiopulmonary Resuscitation (Cont'd)**     **ONE NURSE**

SEQUENCE OF ACTIONS

RATIONALE

b.  For mouth-to-mouth resuscitation of infant or child, administer two slow breaths, 1-1½ seconds per breath with pause between for rescuer to take a breath, followed by 20 breaths per min.

Since an infant's air passages are smaller, with resistance to flow quite high, it is difficult to make recommendations about the force or volume of the rescue breaths. However, three factors should be remembered: (1) rescue breaths are the single most important manoeuvre in assisting a nonbreathing child, (2) an appropriate volume is one that makes the chest rise and fall, and (3) slow breaths provide an adequate volume at the lowest possible pressure, thereby reducing the risk of gastric distension.

c.  For artificial respiration with an Ambu bag in an adult, compress the bag fully for two breaths.

d.  For Ambu bag resuscitation in a child, use two small compressions of bag.

Prevents overinflation of child's lungs.

8.  Observe for rise and fall of chest wall with each respiration. If lungs do not inflate, reposition head and neck and check for visible airway obstruction, such as vomitus.

Ensures artificial respirations are entering lungs.

9.  Suction any secretions from airway. If suction is unavailable, turn victim's head to one side.

Prevents airway obstruction. Allows gravity to drain secretions.

10. Assess for presence of carotid pulse; pulse check should take 5-10 sec.

Carotid artery pulse will persist when more peripheral pulses are no longer palpable. Performing external cardiac compressions on a victim who has a pulse may result in serious medical complications.

a.  Carotid pulse is most central and accessible artery in children over 1 yr. However, in an infant the short, stubby neck makes carotid difficult to palpate; brachial artery is recommended instead.

11. If victim is pulseless, begin external cardiac compression.

Properly performed external chest compressions can provide systolic blood pressure peaks of more than 100 mmHg, but diastolic pressure is low, with mean blood pressure in carotid arteries seldom exceeding 40 mmHg. Blood flow through carotid artery is only one fourth to one third of normal.

Adult

a.  Proper hand position (see illustration)
    (i)  Rescuer's hand locates lower margin of victim's rib cage on side next to rescuer.

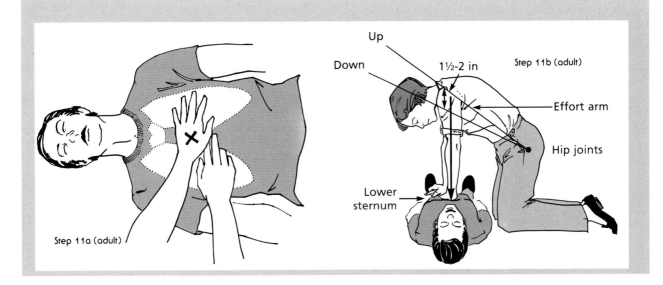

Step 11a (adult)

Up

Down

Down

1½-2 in

Step 11b (adult)

Effort arm

Hip joints

Lower sternum

**PROCEDURE 17-1 Cardiopulmonary Resuscitation (Cont'd)**     **ONE NURSE**

| SEQUENCE OF ACTIONS | RATIONALE |
|---|---|
| (ii) Fingers are moved up rib cage to notch where ribs meet the lower sternum in centre of lower part of chest. | Results in maximum compression of heart between sternum and vertebrae. If compressions occur over xiphoid process, victim's liver can be lacerated. |
| (iii) Place heel of hand on lower half of sternum and place other hand on top of hand on sternum so that hands are parallel. | |
| (iv) Fingers may be extended or interlaced but should be kept off chest. | Reduces risk of rib fracture during compression. |
| b. Lock elbows, maintain arms straight and shoulders directly over hands on victim's sternum (see illustration): | Thrust for each compression is straight down on sternum. |
| (i) Compress chest 3.8-5.0 cm | |
| (ii) Compress chest 80-100 times/min. Perform 15 external compressions with mnemonic "one and, two and, three and..." to 15. | Increases blood flow with increased flow to brain and heart. Allows pause for ventilation in two-rescuer CPR. |
| c. Ventilate lungs with two slow rescue breaths as in Step 7a. | |
| d. Reassess victim after four complete cycles (15 compressions, 2 ventilations each cycle). | Determines return of pulse and respiration and need to continue CPR. |

**Infant (1-12 months)**

| | |
|---|---|
| a. Proper hand position: | Results in maximum compression. |
| (i) Draw imagery line between nipples over breast bone (sternum). | |
| (ii) Place index finger of hand farthest from infant's head just under inframammary line where it intersects sternum. | Area of compression is one finger's width below this intersection at the location of middle and ring fingers. |
| b. Using two or three fingers, compress 1.3-2.5 cm at least 100 times/min. | Promotes adequate cardiac output. |
| c. At the end of every fifth compression, allow a pause for ventilation (1.5 seconds). | At end of every fifth compression, allow a pause for ventilation (1.5 seconds). |
| d. Reassess victim after ten cycles (5 compressions, 1 ventilation each cycle). | Determines return of pulse and respiration and need to continue CPR. |

**Child (1-7 yr)**

| | |
|---|---|
| a. Proper hand position: | Results in maximum compressions. |
| (i) Locate lower margin of victim's rib cage on side next to rescuer with middle and index fingers. | |
| (ii) Follow margin of rib cage with middle finger to notch where ribs and sternum meet. | |
| (iii) Place index finger next to middle finger. | |
| (iv) Place heel of hand next to point where index finger was located, with long axis of heel parallel to sternum. | |
| (v) Rescuer's other hand maintains child's head position. | |
| b. Compress sternum with one hand 2.5-3.8 cm at rate of 100 times/min. | Promotes adequate cardiac output. |
| c. At end of every fifth compression, allow a pause for a ventilation (1-1.5 seconds). | Promotes adequate ventilation during CPR. |
| d. Reassess victim after 10 cycles (5 compressions, 1 ventilation each cycle). | Determines return of pulse and respiration and need to continue CPR. |

(Cont'd)

**PROCEDURE 17-1 Cardiopulmonary Resuscitation (Cont'd)**

SEQUENCE OF ACTIONS                    RATIONALE

**TWO NURSES**

12. One person is positioned at victim's side and performs external cardiac compression, while other remains at victim's head, maintains an open airway, and monitors carotid pulse. Compression rate is 80-100/min. The compression-ventilation ratio is 5:1 with a pause for slow rescue breath (1-1½ seconds). When compressor becomes fatigued, rescuers should exchange positions as soon as possible.

Data from Emergency Cardiac Care Committee and Subcommittee, American Heart Association: Guideline for cardiopulmonary resuscitation and emergency cardiac care, *JAMA* 268: 2171, 1992. Procedure complies with 1993 European Resuscitation Council guidelines.

## CHAPTER 17 REVIEW

### Key Concepts

- The primary function of the heart is to deliver deoxygenated blood to the lungs for oxygenation and to deliver oxygen and nutrients to the tissues.
- Cardiac output is altered by preload, afterload, contractility, and heart rate.
- The primary function of the lungs is to transfer oxygen from the atmosphere into the alveoli and to transfer carbon dioxide out of the body as a waste product.
- Ventilation is the process of providing adequate oxygenation from the alveoli to the blood.
- The ability of the lungs to expand and contract depends on the function of musculoskeletal and neurological systems and on other physiological factors.
- The process of inspiration (active process) and expiration (passive process) is achieved by changes in volume and pressure.
- Respiration is controlled by the central nervous system and by chemicals within the blood.
- Any condition that affects cardiopulmonary functioning directly affects the body's ability to meet oxygen demands.
- Hyperventilation is a respiratory rate greater than that required to maintain normal levels of carbon dioxide.
- Hypoventilation causes carbon dioxide retention.
- Hypoxia occurs if the amount of oxygen delivered to tissues is too low.
- The nursing assessment includes information about the patient's/client's cough, dyspnoea, fatigue, wheezing, chest pain, environmental exposures, respiratory infection, cardiopulmonary risk factors, use of medications, and physical functioning.
- Diagnostic and laboratory tests may be needed to complete the database for a patient/client with decreased oxygenation.
- Breathing exercises improve ventilation, oxygenation, and sensations of dyspnoea.
- Nebulization delivers small drops of water or particles of medication to the airways.
- Chest physiotherapy includes postural drainage, percussion, and vibration to mobilize pulmonary secretions.
- Coughing and suctioning techniques are used to maintain a patent airway.
- Oxygen therapy is used to improve levels of tissue oxygenation and is delivered by nasal cannula, nasal catheter, or oxygen mask.
- Cardiac arrest requires the use of cardiopulmonary resuscitation.

### CRITICAL THINKING EXERCISES

1. Mr Havens is 65 years old and has a history of congestive heart failure. In addition, he mentions poor activity tolerance. What data are important in determining the cardiac response to exercise? What criteria are used to determine when the exercise demand has exceeded cardiac workload capacity?

2. Your patient/client experiences chest pain. State how you assess this pain. What are three important interventions for a person with chest pain?

3. You are caring for a patient who had abdominal surgery 24 hours ago. This patient has a 10-year history of chronic obstructive pulmonary disease. What are the important aspects of assessment and intervention necessary to maintain a patent airway?

4. You are working on your mental health care placement, where a 56-year-old male patient has been admitted in a very excitable state. The multidiscplinary team plans to sedate him. Consider the effects on his cardiopulmonary system of the combined effects of his hyperactivity and sedation with major tranquillizers.

## Key Terms

Angina pectoris, p. 326
Cardiac arrest, p. 340
Cardiac physiology, p. 317
Cardiopulmonary resuscitation (CPR), p. 340
Coronary circulation, p. 318
Cyanosis, p. 325
Dyspnoea, p.326
Dysrhythmias, p.326
Electrocardiogram (ECG), p.321
Exercise stress test, p. 330
Haemoglobin, p. 323
Hypoxia, p. 325
Myocardial infarction, p.326
Myocardial ischaemia, p.326
Normal sinus rhythm (NSR), p.321
Orthopnoea, p. 328
Oxygen therapy, p. 339
Peak expiratory flow rate (PEF), p.332
Pulmonary ventilation, p. 321
Respiratory physiology, p. 317
Systemic circulation, p. 318
Ventilation, p. 323

## REFERENCES

Agle DP *et al*: Multidiscipline treatment of chronic pulmonary insufficiency, *Psychosom Med* 35:41, 1973.

Ahrens TS: Concepts in the assessment of oxygenation, *Focus Crit Care* 14(1):36, 1987.

Ahrens TS: Monitoring: is it being used appropriately? *Crit Care Nurs* 10(7):70, 1990.

Alan D: Making sense of oxygen delivery, *Nurs Times* 85(18):40, 1989.

Bambridge AD: An audit of comfort and convenience; a comparison of oxygen mask and nasal catheter provision of postoperative oxygen therapy, *Prof Nurs*: 8(8):513, 1993.

Bennett JA: What we know about AIDS, *Am J Nurs* 86:1016, 1986.

Campbell J: Making sense of underwater sealed drainage, *Nurs Times* 89(9):34, 1993.

Canobbio MM: *Cardiovascular disorders*, St Louis, 1990, Mosby.

Carrieri VK *et al*: The sensation of pulmonary dyspnoea on school age children, *Nurs Res* 40:81, 1991.

Coull A: Making sense of pulse oximetry, *Nurs Times* 88(32):42, 1992.

Desai S, Chan O: Interpretation of the normal chest x-ray, *Nurs Stand* 17(7):38, 1992.

Dettenmeier PA: *Pulmonary nursing care*, St Louis, 1992, Mosby.

DeVito AJ: Dyspnea during hospitalizations for acute phase of illness as recalled by patients with chronic obstructive pulmonary disease, *Heart-Lung* 19(2):186, 1990.

Dobson F, Dobson MJ: Shedding light on pulse oximetry, *Nurs Stand* 7(46):4, 1993.

Eid N *et al*: Chest physiotherapy in review, *Resp Care* 36(4):270, 1991.

Emergency Cardiac Care Committee and Subcommittee, American Heart Association: Guidelines for cardiopulmonary resuscitation and emergency cardiac care, *JAMA* 268:2171, 1992.

Erickson R: Chest tubes: they're really not that complicated, *Nurs 81* 11(5):34, 1981a.

Erickson R: Solving chest tube problems, *Nurs 81* 11(6):62, 1981b.

Farley J: About chest tubes, *Nurs 88* 18(6):16, 1988.

Feldman J: Chronic obstructive pulmonary disease. In Traver GA, editor: *Respiratory nursing: the science and the art*, New York, 1982, John Wiley & Sons.

Foss MA: Oxygen therapy, *Prof Nurs* 5(4):188, 1990.

Gift AG: Validation of a vertical visual analog scale as a measure of clinical dyspnea, *Rehab Nurs* 14:323, 1989.

Gift AG: Dyspnea, *Nurs Clin North Am* 25(4):955, 1990.

Gift AG, Bolgiano CS, Cunningham J: Sensations during chest tube removal, *Heart Lung* 20(2):131, 1991.

Gift AG, Plaut SM, Jacox AK: Psychologic and physiologic factors related to dyspnea in subjects with chronic obstructive pulmonary disease, *Heart Lung* 15:595, 1986.

Gröer MW, Shekleton MS: *Basic pathophysiology: a holistic approach*, St Louis, 1989, Mosby.

Herrick TW, Yeager H: Home oxygen therapy, *Ann Fam Pract* 32(2):157, 1989.

Hough A: Making sense of sputum retention, *Nurs Times* 88(36):33, 1992.

Kendrick AH, Smith EC: Simple measurements of lung function, *Prof Nurs* 7(6):395, 1992a.

Kendrick AH, Smith EC: Respiratory measurements 2: interpreting simple measurements of lung function, *Prof Nurs* 7(11):748, 1992b.

Klieber C: Clinical implication of deep and shallow suctioning in neonatal patients, *Focus Crit Care* 13(4):36, 1986.

Knox A: Performing endotracheal suction on children: a literature review and implications for practice, *Intensive Crit Care Nurs* 9:48, 1993.

Levick JR: *An introduction to cardiovascular physiology*, London, 1991, Butterworth & Co Publishers.

Luce JM, Tyler ML, Pierson DJ: *Intensive respiratory care*, Philadelphia, 1984, Saunders.

O'Connors: *The cardiac patient*, London, 1985, Mosby.

Shenkman B: Factors contributing to attrition rates in a pulmonary rehabilitation program, *Heart Lung* 14(1):53, 1985.

Shorten D: Effects of tracheal suctioning on neonates: a review of the literature, *Intensive Care Nurs* 5:167, 1989.

Sutcliffe L: RCN nursing update, *Nurs Stand* 8(6):3, 1993.

Traver GA: *Respiratory nursing: the science and the art,* New York, 1982, John Wiley & Sons.

Walsh M: Making sense of chest drainage, *Nurs Times* 85(24):40, 1989.

Welch J: Chest drains; chest tubes and pleural drainage, *Surg Nurs*, 7:7, 1993.

West JB: *Respiratory physiology, the essentials*, ed 3, Baltimore, 1992, Williams & Wilkins.

Whitney JD: The measurement of oxygen tension in tissues, *Nurs Res* 39(4):203, 1990.

Wynne G: Revival techniques, *Nurs Times* 89(11):26, 1993.

## FURTHER READING

### Adult Nursing

Smith JJ, Kampine JP: *Circulatory physiology — the essentials*, Baltimore, 1990, Williams & Wilkins.

Weilitz P: *Pocket guide to respiratory care*, St Louis, 1991, Mosby–Year Book.

Widdicombe J, Davies A: Respiratory physiology, London, 1991, Edward Arnold.

### Children's Nursing

D Hull, D Johnson: *Essential paediatrics*, ed 3, Edinburgh, 1993, Churchill Livingstone.

Hurrell E: Choosing inhaler devices for children with asthma, *Paed Nurs* 5(7):22, 1993.

Jenning P: Caring for a child with a tracheostomy, *Nurs Stand* 4(32), 1990.

Morkey C *et al*: Respiratory rated severity of illness in babies under 6 months old,

*Arch Dis Child* 65:834, 1990.

Ramsay J: *Nursing the child with respiratory problems*, London, 1989, Chapman & Hall.

Roberts A: Systems of life, *Nurs Times* 87(7):53, 1991.

Wooler E: Continuing education asthma, *Paed Nurs* 5(6):22, 1993.

## Learning Disabilities Nursing

Blackman JA: The relationship between inadequate oxygenation of the brain at birth and developmental outcome, Topics in Early Childhood Special Education, 9 (1):1-13, 1989.

## Mental Health Nursing

Bachman S, Master JD, editors: *Panic — psychological perspectives*, New Jersey, 1988, Lawrence Erlbaum.

Garland A: In a panic, *Nurs Times* 88(52), 1992.

Lazarus R, Folkman S: *Stress, appraisal and coping,* New York, 1984, Springer.

Powell TJ, Enright SJ: *Anxiety and stress management*, London, 1990, Routledge.

Snell V: Stressing natural harmony, *Nurs Mirror*- Nov 22, 1979.

Trower P, Casey A, Dryden W: *Cognitive behavioural counselling in action*, London, 1988, Sage Publications Ltd.

# Fluid, Electrolyte and Acid-Base Balances

## CHAPTER OUTLINE

**Fluid and Electrolyte Balances**

*Distribution of body fluids*
*Composition of body fluids*
*Movement of body fluids*
*Regulation of body fluids*
*Regulation of electrolytes*

**Acid-Base Balance**

*Chemical regulation*
*Biological regulation*
*Physiological regulation*

**Disturbances in Fluid, Electrolyte, and Acid-Base Balances**

*Fluid disturbances*
*Electrolyte imbalances*
*Acid-base imbalances*

**Variables Affecting Fluid, Electrolyte, and Acid-Base Balances**

*Age*
*Body size*
*Environmental temperature*
*Lifestyle*
*Level of health*

**Nursing Process and Fluid, Electrolyte, and Acid-Base Imbalances**

*Assessment*
*Planning*
*Implementation*
*Evaluation*

## LEARNING OUTCOMES

After studying this chapter, you should be able to:
- *Define the key terms listed.*
- *Describe variables affecting body water content percentages.*
- *Differentiate between extra- and intracellular fluids and describe body fluid composition and movement.*
- *Describe the regulation of sodium, potassium, calcium, magnesium, chloride, bicarbonate and phosphate.*
- *Describe the three buffer systems of the body which regulate acid-base balance..*
- *Describe fluid volume excess and fluid volume deficit.*
- *Discuss the alterations in osmolality caused by water excess and deficit.*
- *Discuss the variables affecting fluid, electrolyte, and acid-base balances.*
- *Describe laboratory studies associated with fluid, electrolyte, and acid-base imbalances.*
- *Carry out a nursing assessment and develop a nursing care plan for patients/clients with fluid, electrolyte, and acid-base imbalances.*
- *Discuss the purpose of intravenous therapy.*
- *Discuss the procedure for maintaining an intravenous line and calculating intravenous flow rate.*
- *Describe how to change intravenous solutions, tubing, and dressings and discontinue an infusion.*
- *Discuss the procedure for administering a blood transfusion and nursing actions for a transfusion reaction.*

Fluid, electrolyte, and acid-base balances within the body are necessary to maintain health and function of all systems. These balances are maintained by the intake and output of water and electrolytes, their distribution in the body, and the regulation of renal and pulmonary function. Imbalances may result from many factors, and are associated with illnesses. Therefore, nursing care for many patients/clients includes assessment and correction of imbalances or maintenance of balance (homeostasis). Acid-base balance is necessary for physiological processes, and imbalances can alter respiration, metabolism, and central nervous system function.

A healthy, mobile, well-orientated adult can usually maintain normal fluid, electrolyte, and acid-base balances because of the body's adaptive mechanisms. However, the infant, the severely ill adult, the older adult and the disorientated or immobile patient/client are frequently unable to respond independently and, after time, the body's adaptive capacities can no longer maintain balance.

## FLUID AND ELECTROLYTE BALANCES

### Distribution of Body Fluids

Body water content is dependent on weight, age, sex and the relative amount of body fat. Thus, the percentage of water in terms of body weight will differ across the age spectrum (Fig. 18-1).

The figures cited in this chapter are for those of a young male adult, where 60% of body weight is equivalent to 45 litres of fluid.

Body fluids are distributed in two distinct compartments, one containing extracellular fluids and the other containing intracellular fluids.

**Extracellular fluids** include:

- **Interstitial fluid** which fills the spaces between most cells of the body and provides a substantial portion of the body's liquid environment. About 15% (12 L) of body weight consists of interstitial fluids.

- **Plasma** is the watery, colourless, fluid portion of the lymph and blood in which the leucocytes, erythrocytes, and platelets are suspended. Plasma composes 5% (3 L) of body weight.

**Intracellular fluids** are liquids within cell membranes containing dissolved substances or solutes essential to fluid and electrolyte balance and metabolism. Intracellular fluids constitute 40% (30 L) of body weight. Many of the solutes in the intracellular fluid compartment are the same as those located in the extracellular fluid space. However, the proportion of the substances is different. For example, a larger proportion of potassium exists in intracellular fluids than in extracellular fluids.

## Composition of Body Fluids

The fluids circulating throughout the body in extracellular and intracellular fluid spaces contain electrolytes, minerals, and cells.

An **electrolyte** is an element or compound that, when melted or dissolved in water or another solvent, dissociates into **ions** and is able to carry an electric current. Electrolytes which carry a

### Children's Nursing
### Fluid balance in infants

The proportion of body water in a newborn infant declines rapidly during the neonatal period and then more slowly throughout infancy. It reaches the adult value (60%) when the infant is approximately 2 years old.

Infants have proportionately more water in their extracellular compartment compared to adults; infants are therefore more vulnerable to fluid volume deficit than adults.

Infants exchange a greater proportion of extracelluar fluid (50%) than adults (17%), and thus have less reserve of body water than adults. The fluid exchange range in infants is greater because their basal metabolic rate is twice as high as adults per unit of body weight. Therefore, infants produce a large volume of urine daily.

Infants have immature kidneys which are unable to concentrate the urine effectively. Since infants have a proportionally larger surface area (preterm baby x5, newborn x3) in relation to weight, there is a relatively greater fluid loss through the skin.

Any problem which causes a pronounced decrease in intake or increase in output of fluids and electrolytes threatens the fluid economy of the infant. An infant can live only 3–4 days without water, compared to an adult who may survive 10 days.

positive charge are called **cations**, those carrying a negative charge are **anions**. The concentration of each electrolyte differs in extracellular and intracellular fluids. However, the total number of anions and cations in each fluid compartment should be the same (Fig. 18-2).

Electrolytes are commonly measured in millimols per litre (mmol/L). Electrolytes are vital to many body functions: for example, neuromuscular function and acid-base balance.

Minerals are constituents of all body tissues and fluids, and are important in maintaining physiological processes. Examples of minerals include iron and zinc.

Cells, which are also located in body fluids, are the basic functional units of all living tissue. Examples of cells within body fluids are the erythrocyte (red blood cell, RBC) and the leucocyte (white blood cell, WBC).

## Movement of Body Fluids

Body fluids are not static. Fluids and electrolytes shift from compartment to compartment, to meet metabolic needs such as tissue oxygenation, response to illness, acid-base disturbances, and response to drug therapies. Body fluid and electrolyte movement occur by diffusion, osmosis, active transport, or filtration. In addition, movement of fluid components depends on cell membrane permeability (the ability of the membrane to allow fluids and electrolytes to pass through it).

## Diffusion

**Diffusion** is a process in which solid, particulate matter, such as sugar in a fluid, moves from an area of higher concentration to an area of lower concentration This results in an even distribution of

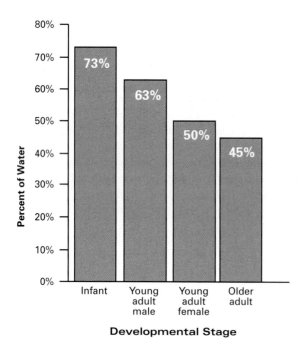

**Fig. 18-1** Percentage of body weight from water varies with age.

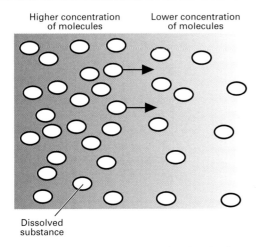

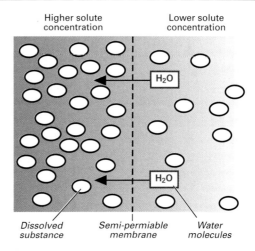

**Fig. 18-3** Diffusion is the movement of molecules from an area of higher concentration to an area of lower concentration (along its concentration gradient).

**Fig. 18-4** In osmosis, water molecules move from the less concentrated area to the more concentrated area in an effort to equalize the concentration of solutions on two sides of a membrane.

the particles in the fluid or across a cell membrane permeable to that substance (Fig. 18-3). For example, the movement of oxygen across the alveolar membrane in the lungs. Substances that are diffusing move down their concentration gradients until equilibrium is achieved.

## Osmosis

**Osmosis** is the movement of a pure solvent, such as water, through a semipermeable membrane from a solution that has a lower solute concentration to one that has a higher solute concentration (Fig. 18-4). *The membrane is permeable to the*

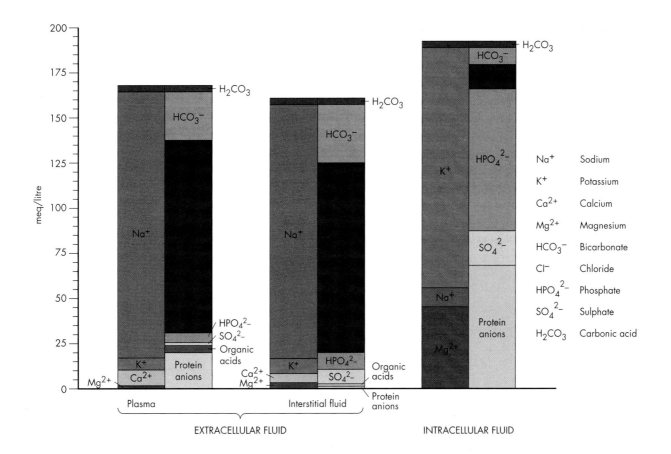

**Fig. 18-2** Comparison of electrolyte concentrations. From Tortora GR and Anagnostakos NP: *Principles of anatomy and physiology, ed 6*, New York, HarperCollins, 1990.

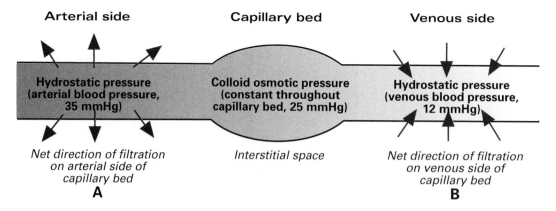

**Fig. 18-5** An example of filtration pressure changes within a capillary bed. **A,** Arterial blood pressure exceeds colloid osmotic pressure, resulting in the movement of water and dissolved substances out of the capillary into the interstitial space. **B,** Venous blood pressure is less than colloid osmotic pressure, resulting in the movement of water and dissolved substances into the capillary.

*solvent, but it is impermeable to the solute.* The rate of osmosis depends on the concentrations of the solutes in the solutions, the temperature of the solutions, the electrical charges of the solutes, and the differences between the osmotic pressures exerted by the solutions. The concentration of a solution is measured in osmoles, which reflect the amount of a substance in solution in the form of molecules, ions, or both, and thus its ability to cause osmosis.

**Osmotic pressure** is the drawing power for water and depends on the number of molecules in the solution. A solution with a high solute concentration has a high osmotic pressure and draws water into itself. Osmotic pressure is exerted through a semipermeable membrane and depends on the activity of the solute separated by the membrane. If the concentration of the solute is greater on one side of the semipermeable membrane, the rate of osmosis is quicker, and a more rapid transfer of solvent across the membrane occurs. This continues until equilibrium is reached. The osmotic pressure of a solution is also called its *osmolality*.

A solution with the same osmolality as blood plasma is called *isotonic*. The intravenous (IV) administration of an isotonic solution prevents shifting of fluid and electrolytes from intracellular compartments. A **hypotonic** solution, that has a lesser concentration of solutes than is normal in body fluids, may be administered to a patient/client to help promote movement of water into the cells.

Conversely, a **hypertonic** solution has a greater concentration of solutes than is normal in body fluids. Intravenous administration of a hypertonic solution results in movement of water out of cells.

The osmotic pressure of the blood is affected by **plasma proteins**, especially albumin, a serum protein naturally produced by the body. Albumin exerts colloid osmotic or **oncotic pressure**, which tends to keep fluid in the capillaries.

### Filtration

**Filtration** is the process by which water and diffusible substances move together in response to fluid pressure. This process is active in capillary beds, where pressure differences determine the movement of water, electrolytes, and other dissolved substances

between the capillaries and interstitial fluid.

**Hydrostatic pressure** is the pressure exerted by a liquid in a column. In the body, this is the force exerted by a fluid pressing against the vessel wall. The pumping of the heart maintains a hydrostatic pressure within the blood. Blood and fluid entering the capillaries do so at a pressure greater than interstitial pressure, so fluid and solutes move out of the capillaries. At the venous end of the capillary bed, hydrostatic pressure is less than interstitial pressure, so fluid and waste products move back into the capillaries (Fig. 18-5).

### Active Transport

**Active transport** is the movement of materials across the cell membrane by chemical activity or by energy expenditure. This enables the cell to admit larger molecules than it would otherwise be able to admit or to move molecules from areas of lesser concentration to areas of greater concentration. Unlike diffusion and osmosis, active transport requires metabolic activity and energy expenditure. An example of active transport in the body is the sodium–potassium pump (Fig. 18-6). Sodium is pumped out of the cell, while potassium is pumped in, against a concentration gradient.

### Regulation of Body Fluids
### Fluid Intake

Fluid intake is regulated primarily through the **thirst mechanism**. The thirst-control centre is located within the hypothalamus in the brain. A combination of psychological factors, dry pharyngeal mucous membranes, and angiotensin I create the sensation of thirst (Gröer and Shekleton, 1989) (Fig. 18-7). Major physiological stimuli to the thirst centre are increased plasma concentration and decreased blood volume. Receptor cells called **osmoreceptors** continually monitor osmolality. When too much fluid is lost, the osmoreceptors detect the loss and activate the thirst centre. Consequently, the person feels thirsty and seeks water.

Water is also acquired from food intake, such as fruits, vegetables, and meat, and from the oxidation of food substances during digestion. Water is also one of the end products of the metabolism of carbohydrates, proteins, and fats. This quantity ranges between 150 and 250 ml/day, depending on a person's rate of metabolism (Guyton, 1986). Oral fluid intake requires an alert state. Infants, individuals with neurological or psychological impairments, some older adults, and patients/clients who are restrained, are unable to perceive or respond to their thirst mechanisms. As a result, they are at risk for dehydration.

## Fluid Output

Fluid output occurs through the kidneys, skin, lungs and the gastrointestinal tract. Average daily fluid losses are summarized in Table 18-1.

The kidneys are the major regulatory organs of fluid balance. They receive about 170 L of plasma to filter each day and in the adult produce 1.5 L of urine to be excreted. The amount of urine produced by the kidneys is influenced by **antidiuretic hormone (ADH)** and **aldosterone**. These hormones affect water and sodium excretion and are stimulated by changes in blood volume.

Water loss from the skin is regulated primarily by the sympathetic nervous system, which activates the sweat glands. Stimulation of the sweat glands can result from muscular exercise, elevated environmental temperature, and increased metabolic activity (for example, fever).

Water loss from the skin can be a sensible or insensible loss. **Insensible water loss** is continuous and is not perceived by the person. The average insensible water loss is 600 ml/day (Metheny, 1992). **Sensible water loss** occurs through excessive perspiration and is perceived by the person. The amount of sensible perspiration is directly related to the amount of exercise, environmental temperature, and metabolic activity. As these factors increase, so does the amount of sweat produced and water lost through the skin. Sensible water loss can range up to 1000 ml or more, depending on exercise, and external and body temperatures (Metheny, 1992).

The lungs also produce an insensible water loss by expiring approximately 400 ml of water daily. This loss may increase in response to changes in respiratory rate and depth (for example, increased exercise or fever). In addition, devices for oxygen administration can increase insensible water loss from the lungs.

The average fluid loss from the gastrointestinal tract is approximately 100 ml/day. Vomiting or diarrhoea increases fluid loss by preventing the normal absorption of water and electrolytes, which have been secreted for the digestive process.

## Hormones

The major hormones affecting fluid and electrolyte balance are ADH and aldosterone. The stimulus for ADH secretion is an increase in blood osmolarity (concentration of solute per litre of solution), which indicates a state of water deficit. The hormone itself is released by the posterior pituitary gland. ADH decreases the production of urine by increasing the reabsorption of water by the kidney tubules.

Aldosterone is produced by the adrenal cortex, and regulates sodium and potassium balance. The presence of aldosterone causes the kidney tubules to excrete potassium and reabsorb sodium. As a result, water is also reabsorbed and returned to the blood volume.

A third class of hormones, glucocorticoids, also affects water and electrolyte balance. Whereas normal glucocorticoid hormone secretion does not result in major fluid imbalances, excesses of the hormone in the circulation alter fluid and electrolyte balance. A person receiving steroid medications, such as cortisone or prednisone, retains sodium and water.

## Regulation of Electrolytes
## Cations

The major cations — sodium ($Na^+$), potassium ($K^+$), calcium ($Ca^{2+}$), and magnesium ($Mg^{2+}$) — are located in the extracellular and intracellular fluid. Their actions affect neurochemical and neuromuscular transmissions, which influence muscular function, cardiac rhythm and contractility, mood and behaviour, and gastrointestinal functioning, as well as other processes.

### SODIUM REGULATION

Sodium is the most abundant cation in the extracellular fluid. Sodium ions are involved in maintaining water balance,

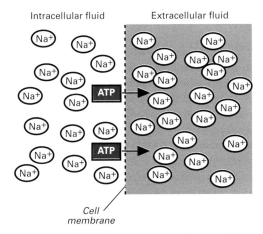

Intracellular fluid          Extracellular fluid

Cell membrane

**Fig. 18-6** An example of active transport. Energy ATP (adenosine triphosphate) is used to move sodium molecules across a semipermeable membrane against sodium's concentration gradient (that is, from an area of lesser concentration to an area of greater concentration).

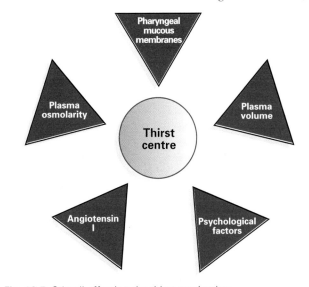

**Fig. 18-7** Stimuli affecting the thirst mechanism.

**TABLE 18-1 Average Daily Fluid Output in a 70-kg Adult**

| Organ or System | Amount (ml) |
|---|---|
| Kidneys | 1500 |
| Skin | |
|   Insensible loss | 600-900 |
|   Sensible loss | 0-5000 |
| Lungs | 400 |
| Gastrointestinal tract | 100 |
| **TOTAL*** | **2600-2900** |

* Excludes sensible loss.

transmitting nerve impulses, and contracting muscles. The normal extracellular concentration of sodium is 135 to 145 mmol/L.

In fluid and electrolyte balances water follows where sodium moves. For example, if the kidneys retain sodium, they retain water also. Conversely, if the kidneys excrete sodium, they excrete water. The action of many drugs (for example, diuretics) is based on this principle.

Sodium is regulated by salt intake, aldosterone, and urinary output. The major sources of sodium are table salt, processed meats, snack foods, and tinned vegetables. In individuals with normal renal function the excretion of urine sodium can be increased to keep the serum sodium level within normal limits. When sodium intake decreases or a person loses body fluids (for example, through burns or trauma), the body attempts to conserve sodium through the secretion of aldosterone. Aldosterone exerts its action on the kidney tubules to reabsorb sodium, thus returning sodium to the extracellular fluid.

## POTASSIUM REGULATION

Potassium is the predominant intracellular cation regulating neuromuscular excitability and muscle contraction. Potassium is needed for protein synthesis and correction of acid-base imbalances.

Potassium assists in regulating the acid-base balance because the potassium ion can be exchanged with the hydrogen ion ($H^+$) to correct acidosis. The opposite occurs in alkalosis.

Potassium is regulated primarily by the kidneys. Any condition that decreases urine output decreases potassium excretion. The normal range for serum potassium is 3.5 to 5.0 mmol/L.

## CALCIUM REGULATION

Calcium is the most abundant element in the body (Metheny, 1992). The body requires calcium for cell membrane integrity and structure, adequate cardiac conduction, blood coagulation, bone growth and formation, and muscle relaxation. The major portion of calcium is in bones and teeth.

Calcium in extracellular fluid is regulated through the actions of the parathyroid and thyroid glands. Parathyroid hormone (PTH) controls the balance among bone calcium, gastrointestinal

absorption of calcium, and kidney excretion of calcium. Calcitonin from the thyroid gland also has a minor role in determining serum calcium levels by inhibiting release of calcium from bones.

## MAGNESIUM REGULATION

Magnesium is the second most important cation of the intracellular fluids and is essential for enzyme activities, neurochemical activities, and muscular excitability.

### Anions

The major anions are chloride ($Cl^-$), bicarbonate ($HCO_3^-$), and phosphate ($PO_4^{3-}$). Like cations, they are found in the extracellular and intracellular spaces. Anions affect fluid, electrolyte, and acid-base balances and functions.

## CHLORIDE REGULATION

Chloride is found in extracellular and intracellular fluid. The chloride ion balances cations within the extracellular fluid. If a negatively charged ion leaves the extracellular fluid and enters the intracellular fluid, a chloride ion will be exchanged and enter the extracellular fluid. The ion exchange maintains electrical neutrality. The processes regulating sodium, chloride, and bicarbonate ions are related, and any factor that affects one can affect the others. Therefore, changes in serum chloride levels can affect fluid, electrolyte, and acid-base balances.

Chloride is regulated through the kidneys. The amount excreted is related to dietary intake.

## BICARBONATE REGULATION

Bicarbonate is the major chemical base buffer within the body. A **buffer** is a substance or group of substances that can absorb or release hydrogen ions to correct an acid-base imbalance. The bicarbonate ion is found in extracellular and intracellular fluid. The kidneys regulate bicarbonates. When the body needs to retain more base, the kidneys reabsorb greater quantities of bicarbonate and return it to the extracellular fluid. The bicarbonate ion is an essential component of the carbonic acid bicarbonate buffering system essential to acid-base balance.

## PHOSPHATE REGULATION

Phosphate is a buffer anion in intracellular and extracellular fluid. Phosphate and calcium help develop and maintain bones and teeth. Phosphate also promotes normal neuromuscular action, participates in carbohydrate metabolism, and assists in acid-base regulation.

Serum phosphate concentration is regulated by the kidneys, parathyroid hormone, and activated vitamin D (Gröer and Shekleton, 1989). Phosphate is normally absorbed through the gastrointestinal tract. Calcium and phosphate are inversely proportional. If one rises, the other falls.

## ACID-BASE BALANCE

**Acid-base balance** exists when the net rate at which the body produces acids or bases equals the rate at which acids or bases are excreted. This balance results in a stable concentration of hydrogen ions in body fluids. The concentration of hydrogen ions in a body fluid is expressed as the pH value. The **pH** is a scale for measuring the acidity or alkalinity of a fluid. A pH value of 7 is neutral. Below 7 is acid, and above 7 is alkaline. An increase in the number of hydrogen ions in the bloodstream increases the acid component, thereby lowering the pH. Normal arterial pH values range from 7.35 to 7.45.

The human body has regulatory mechanisms for maintaining the acid-base balance and for adapting to short-term changes in hydrogen ion concentration. Such changes occur during physical exercise, moderate anxiety states, and minor gastrointestinal upsets. The body can make adjustments (compensate) for transient changes in pH. However, with severe trauma, uncontrolled diabetes mellitus, or shock, the body's normal compensatory mechanisms are unable to maintain the pH within a physiological range. In such cases, medical intervention is required.

The types of acid-base regulators within the body are chemical, biological, and physiological buffering systems.

### Chemical Regulation

The largest chemical buffer in extracellular fluid is the carbonic acid bicarbonate buffer system. The carbonic acid bicarbonate buffer system responds immediately to acid-base imbalance, is an adaptive system, and has a relatively brief effect. This system can be expressed as the following equation:

$$CO_2 + H_2O \rightleftharpoons H_2CO_3 \rightleftharpoons H^+ + HCO_3^-$$

carbon dioxide    water    carbonic acid    hydrogen    bicarbonate

The carbonic acid bicarbonate buffer system is the first buffering system to react to change in the pH of extracellular fluid, and it reacts within seconds. The excretion of carbon dioxide resulting from metabolism is controlled primarily by the lungs. The excretion of hydrogen and bicarbonate ions is controlled by the kidneys. The reaction of these substances buffers a strong acid or base to maintain a relatively constant pH.

A second chemical buffering system involves the plasma proteins (albumin, fibrinogen, and prothrombin) and the gamma globulins, which constitute about 6 to 7% of blood plasma. These proteins can bind with or release hydrogen ions to correct acidosis or alkalosis. However, their capacity to maintain the acid-base balance of extracellular fluid is limited, and they cannot correct long-term imbalances.

### Biological Regulation

Biological buffering occurs when hydrogen ions are absorbed or released by body cells. The hydrogen ion has a positive charge and must be exchanged with another positively charged ion, frequently potassium. In conditions with excessive acid, a hydrogen ion enters the cell, and a potassium ion leaves the cell and enters the extracellular fluid. The extracellular fluid is thus less acidic because fewer hydrogen ions are present. After the acidosis is corrected, potassium re-enters the cells, and potassium levels return to normal. This biological buffering occurs after chemical buffering and takes 2 to 4 hours.

A second type of biological buffer is the haemoglobin-oxyhaemoglobin system. Carbon dioxide diffuses into the RBC and forms carbonic acid. The carbonic acid dissociates into hydrogen and bicarbonate ions. The hydrogen ions attach to the haemoglobin, and the bicarbonate ion becomes available for buffering by exchanging with extracellular chloride (Kokko and Tannen, 1990).

### Physiological Regulation
#### Lungs

The physiological buffers in the body are the lungs and the kidneys. The lungs can provide a rapid adaptation to an acid-base imbalance. In fact, they can act to return the pH to normal before the biological buffers can.

Ordinarily, hydrogen ions and carbon dioxide provide the stimulus for respiration. When the concentration of hydrogen ions is altered, the lungs react to correct the imbalance by altering the rate and depth of respiration. In alkalosis, the rate of respiration is reduced, and the person retains carbon dioxide. The carbon dioxide combines with water in the blood to form carbonic acid, which helps increase the acid component and balance the alkaline excess. If an excess in acid occurs, respiratory rate is increased, and the lungs excrete larger amounts of carbon dioxide (Gröer and Shekleton, 1989). Therefore less carbon dioxide is available to combine with water and create carbonic acid.

#### Kidneys

The kidneys can take from a few hours to several days to regulate acid-base abnormalities. They use three mechanisms to regulate hydrogen ion concentration. They can reabsorb bicarbonate during acid excess and excrete it during acid deficit. The kidneys use a phosphate ion, $PO_4^{3-}$, to carry hydrogen ions by excreting phosphoric acid ($H_3PO_4$) and forming an acid base. The kidneys also convert ammonia ($NH_3$) to ammonium ($NH_4^+$) by attaching a hydrogen ion to ammonia.

## DISTURBANCES IN FLUID, ELECTROLYTE, AND ACID-BASE BALANCES

Disturbances in fluid, electrolyte, and acid-base balances seldom occur alone and can disrupt normal body processes. A patient/client who loses body fluids through burns, illness, or trauma is at risk for electrolyte imbalances. In addition, untreated electrolyte imbalances (for example, potassium loss) result in acid-base disturbances.

### Fluid Disturbances

The basic types of fluid imbalances are isotonic and osmolar. Isotonic deficit and excess exist when water and electrolytes are gained or lost in equal proportions. In contrast, osmolar imbalances are losses or excesses of only water so that the concentration (osmolality) of the serum is affected.

**Children's Nursing
Acid-base regulation in newborns**

Newborn and preterm babies have less homeostatic buffering capacity than do older children. They have a tendency towards metabolic acidosis with slightly lower pH averages. The metabolic acidosis is thought to be related to high metabolic acid production and to renal immaturity.

## Isotonic Imbalances

**Fluid volume deficit (FVD)** results when water and electrolytes are lost in isotonic proportions. Unless other imbalances are present, serum electrolyte levels remain unchanged. Patients/clients at risk include those with gastrointestinal losses of fluid and electrolytes such as from vomiting, gastric suction, diarrhoea, or fistulae. A fistula is an abnormal opening from the gastrointestinal tract into the peritoneum, another organ, or the skin. The very young and old are quickly affected by these losses (Metheny, 1992). Other causes can include haemorrhage, diuretic administration, profuse sweating, fever, and decreased oral intake.

**Fluid volume excess (FVE)** results when water and sodium are retained in isotonic proportions, resulting in hypervolaemia with unchanged levels of serum electrolytes. Patients/clients at risk include those with congestive heart failure, cirrhosis, increased serum levels of aldosterone and glucocorticoids, and abnormal intake of salt (for example, in the too-rapid administration of IV fluids containing sodium) (Metheny, 1987).

## Osmolar Imbalances

Hyperosmolar imbalance **(dehydration)** occurs when there is a loss of water without a proportionate loss of electrolytes, especially sodium, or a gain in osmotically active substances. This results in an increased serum sodium level and osmolality (concentration), and intracellular dehydration.

Risk factors for dehydration include conditions that impair sufficient oral intake (for example, alterations in neurological function). Frail, infirm older patients/clients are at great risk for developing dehydration because there is a marked decrease in intracellular fluid, decrease in renal concentrating ability, decrease in responsiveness to thirst, and increase in proportion of body fat, which limits the older person's reserve in situations of water deficit (Aaronson and Seaman, 1989).

Hypo-osmolar imbalance (water excess) occurs when there is an excess intake of water or excess ADH secretion. Surgery or injury to the brain can cause a syndrome of inappropriate secretion of ADH. The overall effect is dilution of the extracellular fluid volume with osmotic movement of water into the cells (Gröer and Shekleton, 1989). Brain cells are particularly sensitive, which can cause decreased level of consciousness, coma, and even death.

## Electrolyte Imbalances
### Sodium Imbalances

Sodium excess and deficit share many characteristics with osmolar fluid disturbances. **Hyponatraemia** is a less-than-normal concentration of sodium in the blood, which can take place when a net sodium loss or net water excess occurs. Usually hyponatraemia results in a decrease in the osmolality of plasma and extracellular fluid (Gröer and Shekleton, 1989).

When a sodium loss occurs, the body initially adapts by reducing water excretion to maintain serum osmolality at near-normal levels. As sodium loss continues, the body attempts to preserve the blood volume. As a result, the proportion of sodium in the extracellular fluid lessens.

**Hypernatraemia** is a greater-than-normal concentration of sodium in the extracellular fluid, which can be caused by extreme water loss or overall sodium excess. If the cause of hypernatraemia is increased aldosterone secretion, sodium is retained and potassium is excreted. When hypernatraemia occurs, the body attempts to conserve as much water as possible through renal reabsorption. Interstitial osmotic pressure increases, and fluid shifts from the cells into the extracellular fluid, causing the cells to shrink and interrupting most of the physiological cellular processes.

## Potassium Imbalances

**Hypokalaemia** is a condition in which an inadequate amount of potassium circulates in the extracellular fluid. When severe, hypokalaemia can affect cardiac conduction causing dangerous irregularities. Because the normal amount of potassium is so small, there is little tolerance for fluctuations in serum potassium levels.

Hypokalaemia can result from several conditions. The most common cause is the use of potassium-wasting diuretics such as frusemide. Hypokalaemia is also observed in patients/clients who are recovering from massive cellular injuries such as burns, crushing injuries, or massive trauma.

**Hyperkalaemia** is a greater-than-normal amount of potassium in the blood. Severe hyperkalaemia produces marked cardiac conduction abnormalities such as ventricular dysrhythmia and cardiac arrest (Metheny, 1987). The primary cause of hyperkalaemia is renal failure, but other illnesses also result in increased potassium. Any decrease in renal function diminishes the amount of potassium the kidney can excrete.

**Children's Nursing
Diarrhoea, vomiting and fluid imbalance in children**

Children who have an actual or potential fluid imbalance present in similar fashion as adults; however, a small fluid and electrolyte imbalance may have greater consequences, as it can threaten the body fluid economy of the infant.

In assessing children with diarrhoea and vomiting, the children's nurse must consider the child's general condition; examine eyes for a potential sunken appearance and presence of tears; mouth for dryness (although children who are vomiting or drinking excessively may have a moist mouth); and assess whether the child is thirstier than normal. Assess skin turgor by pinching; if the skin goes back very slowly, it may indicate severe dehydration.

## Calcium Imbalances

**Hypocalcaemia** represents a drop in serum and ionized calcium levels, and can result from several illnesses, some of which directly affect the thyroid and parathyroid glands. **Hypercalcaemia** is an increase in the total serum concentration of calcium.

## Acid-Base Imbalances

The primary types of acid-base imbalance are respiratory acidosis, respiratory alkalosis, metabolic acidosis, and metabolic alkalosis.

## Respiratory Acidosis

**Respiratory acidosis** is marked by an increased partial pressure of carbon dioxide ($PaCO_2$), excess carbonic acid, and an increased hydrogen ion concentration (decreased pH). Respiratory acidosis is caused by hypoventilation or any condition that depresses ventilation, such as respiratory failure or drug overdose.

## Respiratory Alkalosis

**Respiratory alkalosis** is marked by decreased partial pressure of carbon dioxide ($PaCO_2$) and decreased hydrogen ion concentration (increased pH). Respiratory alkalosis results from excessive exhalation of carbon dioxide or hyperventilation. This can occur with anxiety or the initial phases of an acute asthma attack.

## Metabolic Acidosis

**Metabolic acidosis** results from a rise in hydrogen ion concentration (decreased pH) in the extracellular fluid, caused by an increase in hydrogen ion levels or a decrease in bicarbonate levels (Gröer, 1981). Metabolic acidosis is caused by many conditions; for example starvation or diabetic ketoacidosis.

## Metabolic Alkalosis

**Metabolic alkalosis** is marked by heavy loss of acid from the body or by increased levels of bicarbonate. The most common cause is vomiting.

# VARIABLES AFFECTING FLUID, ELECTROLYTE, AND ACID-BASE BALANCES

Fluid, electrolyte, and acid-base states are neither static nor single physiological entities. Many variables can change the distribution of body fluid and electrolytes. In some instances (for example, with normal changes during pregnancy and exercise), fluid and electrolyte alterations are a normal and expected response. In other situations, however, fluid, electrolyte, and acid-base imbalances can have severe consequences.

During assessment the nurse identifies altered fluid, electrolyte, and acid-base states. To assess patients/clients effectively, the nurse considers variables influencing fluid, electrolyte, and acid-base status, the way normal balance changes, and whether the change is a normal anticipated change or a consequence of a pathological process. The major factors that can affect fluid, electrolyte, and acid-base status include age, body size, environmental temperature, lifestyle, and level of health.

## Age

Age affects distribution of body fluids and electrolytes. The major differences are observed in infants, older adults, and pregnant women.

Fluid and electrolyte changes occur normally with developmental changes. However, when an illness is also present, the patient/client may be unable to adapt adequately to these changes. Therefore, the nurse needs to include the fluid changes associated with ageing and development in the nursing assessment.

## Infants

Infants' proportions of total body water are greater than those of school-aged children, adolescents, or adults. However, although infants have greater proportions of body water, they are not protected from fluid loss (for example, from diarrhoea) because they ingest and excrete a relatively greater daily water volume than adults (Riddle, 1992). In fact, infants are at greater risk for FVD or hyperosmolar imbalances because their water losses are proportionately greater per kilogram of body weight.

## Children

In childhood illnesses, the regulatory and compensatory responses to imbalances are less stable and tend to operate within a more narrow range with less tolerance for large changes in balance. Children frequently respond to illness with fevers of higher temperature or longer duration than those of adults. Fever in childhood can increase the rate of insensible water loss (Metheny, 1987).

## Adolescents

In adolescence, rapid and major changes occur in anatomical and physiological processes. The increased growth rate increases metabolism and, as a result, the amount of water produced as an end product of metabolism. Changes in fluid balance are greater in adolescent girls because of hormonal changes associated with the menstrual cycle.

## Pregnant Women

The pregnant woman experiences several changes in fluid and electrolyte balance. Aldosterone secretion and excretion increase as a result of changes in reproductive hormones and the renin-angiotension system (Methany, 1987). In some, the elevation can be 10 times the normal, which may result in fluid retention.

## Older Adults

The older patient's/client's risk of fluid and electrolyte imbalance may be closely associated with decreased renal function and a consequent lack of urine concentration. The older adult may also have chronic illness, such as diabetes mellitus, cardiovascular disorders, or cancer, that can impair fluid balance. Other risk factors that particularly affect the older adult are use of diuretics, often given for hypertension and congestive heart failure, and overuse of laxatives and enemas.

### Mental Health Nursing
### Psychotropic medications

Patients/clients who are taking psychotropic medication (medication used in the treatment of mental illnesses) will experience a very dry mouth, a common side effect of these medications. This can cause great discomfort and irritation for the patient/client and these people may require large amounts of fluids at regular intervals.

### Learning Disabilities Nursing
### Causes of fluid and electrolyte imbalances

Maintaining fluid and electrolyte balance in people with learning disabilities is rarely a problem, if the individual eats a balanced diet. However, there are situations where attention to these physiological needs is important. A study by MacDonald *et al* (1989) found that in one large institution, people with profound mental and physical handicaps were at high risk of life-threatening hypernatraemic dehydration due to a combination of factors, including:
• inability to indicate thirst or obtain fluids independently
• dependence on others for food and drink
• regular use of hypertonic enemas
• low staffing levels

A small minority of people with severe learning disability are treated for a unipolar or bipolar affective disorder, such as manic-depressive psychosis, using lithium salts. In these people, attention to thirst and excessive drinking (polydipsia) is vital, as it is an indicator of lithium toxicity. It is not unknown for staff to mistake this excessive drinking for aberrant or 'attention seeking' behaviour, particularly if independent access to drinking water is restricted and the person consequently resorts to drinking water from flower vases or toilets. Careful observation of the patient/client, as well as rigorous and diligent adherence to care management protocols, including regular assessment of blood lithium levels, are necessary if these situations are to be avoided.

### Adult Nursing
### Special considerations when assessing older people

Obtaining assessment data related to fluid and electrolyte disturbance requires modification when caring for an older patient/client. For example, skin turgor is best tested over the forehead or sternum because the skin maintains its elasticity in these areas. The older adult has decreased salivation, so mucous membrane moistness is assessed by inspecting the area under the tongue for a pool of saliva. Other elements of fluid balance assessment include using intake and output measurements and daily weight measurements so that trends can be detected despite the renal function changes.

## Body Size

Body size has an effect on total body water. Because fat contains no water, the obese person has proportionately less body water. Women have more fat deposits, such as the breasts and hips, than men. As a result, the total body water in women is less than in men of the same age.

## Environmental Temperature

Fluid and electrolyte imbalances are associated with extremes in environmental temperature and relative humidity. The overall body response to environmental temperatures exceeding 28°C is to increase sensible water loss by sweating, which cools the peripheral blood and helps reduce body temperature.

The healthy adult can sweat about 1 L/hr for 2 hours, losing about 5% of body weight without straining the cooling mechanism. However, after a body weight loss of 7% is exceeded, the cooling mechanism declines to conserve body water (Methany, 1987).

The relative humidity of the environmental temperature also affects body water loss and body temperature regulation. The evaporation of sweat decreases at 60% humidity and ceases at 75% (Methany, 1987).

The body responds with fluid changes to excessive environmental temperature. It increases peripheral vasodilatation, which allows more blood to come to the surface for cooling. Sweating increases body fluid loss, which results in loss of sodium and chloride ions. The body also increases cardiac output and pulse rate. Finally, increased aldosterone secretion occurs, resulting in sodium retention and potassium excretion by the kidneys (Methany, 1987). Each of these responses can affect overall fluid and electrolyte balance, and the nurse needs to assess the environment to determine actual or potential alterations in fluid and electrolyte balance.

## Lifestyle

Lifestyle can have a direct affect on fluid, electrolyte, and acid-base balance. Habits that can affect fluid balance include diet, exercise and stress (see Chapter 10).

## Diet

Dietary intake of fluids, potassium, calcium, magnesium, and necessary carbohydrates, fats, and proteins helps maintain normal fluid, electrolyte, and acid-base status. When nutritional intake is inadequate, the body tries to preserve its protein stores by breaking down glycogen and fat stores. When excess free fatty acids are released, metabolic acidosis can occur because the liver converts free fatty acids to ketones. However, after those resources are depleted, the body begins to destroy protein stores. When serum albumin levels drop below normal, **hypoalbuminaemia** results. In hypoalbuminaemia the serum colloid osmotic pressure is decreased, and fluid shifts from the circulating blood volume and enters the interstitial fluid spaces, resulting in oedema.

## Exercise

Exercise results in increased sensible water loss through sweat. The person who exercises can respond to the thirst mechanism

## Fasting and Fluid Balance

People from some religious groups, for example Muslims, Hindus or Jews, may wish to observe a total fast during which they will not take anything by mouth. During some festivals these people fast from sunrise to sunset, or from sunset on one day to sunrise on the next. Fluid restrictions can cause physiological problems for people whose fluid balance is sensitive. However, these individuals can gain great spiritual comfort from being able to follow the practices of their faith.

and help maintain fluid and electrolyte balance by increasing fluid intake. Athletes undergoing sustained vigorous exercise must have fluid loss replaced by a liquid that contains electrolytes.

## Level of Health

One of the most important nursing functions is to recognize patients/clients at risk for fluid and electrolyte disturbances. People with chronic illness, concomitant depression of the immune system, and decreases in nutritional intake are at a greater risk for fluid, electrolyte and acid-base imbalances than are healthier persons who have an acute gastrointestinal inflammation for 24 to 36 hours. In all cases the nurse must assess the actual or potential risk factors for fluid, electrolyte, and acid-base balances.

## Surgery

Surgical procedures result in changes in fluid balance because of the body's stress response to surgical trauma during the second to fifth days after surgery. The more extensive the surgery, the greater the response of the body. Postoperative fluid and electrolyte changes are normal and should be anticipated in surgical patients/clients.

## Burns

Individuals with severe, partial or full thickness burns lose body fluids. The greater the body surface burned, the greater the fluid loss. The burned patient/client loses body fluids in a number of ways. Plasma may leave the intravascular space and become trapped as oedema in interstitial fluid. Along with the shifting of fluid, serum proteins are lost from extracellular fluids. Also, water vapour and heat are lost because burned skin can no longer serve as a barrier against such losses. This loss increases in proportion to the amount of skin burned. Blood may also leak from damaged capillaries, contributing to an already decreased extracellular fluid volume.

## Cardiovascular Disorders

The failing heart has a diminished cardiac output. As a result, perfusion to the kidneys is decreased, and urinary output drops. The patient/client retains sodium and water, and oedema, circulatory overload, and pulmonary oedema may result.

Fluid and electrolyte imbalances associated with heart failure can be controlled for a time with drugs, such as diuretics, and fluid and sodium restrictions. The goal of fluid reduction is to reduce the work of the left ventricle by relieving the excess extracellular fluid volume.

## Renal Disorders

Failing kidneys alter fluid and electrolyte balance. There is an abnormal retention of sodium, chloride, potassium, and water in the extracellular fluid. The plasma levels of metabolic waste products such as urea and creatinine (from muscle metabolism) are elevated because the kidneys are unable to filter and excrete waste products.

Hydrogen ions are also retained when renal function is decreased, which results in metabolic acidosis. The usual renal compensatory mechanisms, such as bicarbonate reabsorption, are not available, so the body's ability to restore normal acid-base balance is limited.

The severity of fluid and electrolyte imbalance is proportional to the degree of renal failure. Occasionally, acute renal failure induced by shock or a decrease in extracellular fluid may be reversible. Although chronic renal failure is progressive, the patient/client may be treated successfully with dietary control of protein and salt intake, diuretic medications, and fluid restrictions. Many individuals with chronic renal failure eventually require dialysis to maintain fluid and electrolyte balance.

# NURSING PROCESS AND FLUID, ELECTROLYTE, AND ACID-BASE IMBALANCES

 ASSESSMENT

Full assessment is a fundamental component of care in all settings — hospital, home or community. During assessment the nurse identifies potential and actual fluid, electrolyte, and acid-base imbalances. In addition, assessment helps the nurse determine the effectiveness of interventions. For example, if a diuretic medication is prescribed for a patient/client with congestive heart failure, the nurse assessing the individual expects to note a decrease in weight, an increase in 24-hour urine output, and a decrease in or absence of dependent oedema.

The nurse also assesses fluid, electrolyte, and acid-base balances to detect adverse reactions to treatment. For example, if IV fluids are ordered for a person with progressive renal failure, the nurse may find, on the third day, that the 24-hour fluid intake exceeds renal output by four to one, that the individual's weight is increased, and that dependent oedema (such as around the ankles) is present.

Finally, fluid, electrolyte, and acid-base assessment helps the nurse anticipate needs for nursing care. For example, a patient/client with oedema who is placed on diuretic therapy should have a care plan to anticipate needs such as an increased use of the toilet, bedpan, or urinal.

## Nursing History

To collect data about fluid, electrolyte, and acid-base status the nurse must understand fluid and acid-base regulation, electrolyte and acid-base imbalances, and volume disturbances. In addition, the nurse needs to know why and how some diseases, treatments, drug therapies, and diet changes alter fluid balance. This information assists the nurse in identifying those at risk for fluid, electrolyte, and acid-base imbalances.

Patients/clients with cardiovascular and renal diseases or severe burns are at high risk for fluid, electrolyte, and acid-base disturbances. In addition, prolonged gastrointestinal upsets, particularly in the very young and very old, can result in these imbalances.

The nurse also collects the nursing history to identify risk factors increasing the chances of fluid, electrolyte, and acid-base imbalances. Eventually, all types of chronic diseases can cause these imbalances. Because the progression of these diseases is usually slow, imbalances can be controlled. When nurses care for individuals with chronic illnesses, however, they often find that the disease processes are no longer stabilized and that imbalances are present.

## Physical Examination

Because fluid, electrolyte, and acid-base disturbances can affect all systems, the nurse must systematically identify any abnormalities during the physical examination.

## Measuring Fluid Intake and Output

Measuring and recording all liquid intake and output during a 24-hour period helps complete the assessment data base for fluid, electrolyte, and acid-base balances. Intake includes all liquids taken orally (including soup and ice-cream), by feeding tube, and parenterally. Liquid output includes urine, diarrhoea, vomit and drainage from postsurgical tubes and drains.

These data are recorded on a fluid balance chart (Fig. 18-8). Taking fluid balance measurements is a procedure which requires help from the patient/client and family. Patients/clients may also be asked to measure and record their own output.

The nurse looks for trends over 24-, 48-, and 72-hour periods. An accurate fluid balance chart helps to maintain an ongoing evaluation of hydration status and to prevent severe imbalances.

## Laboratory Studies

Laboratory tests are performed to obtain further objective data about fluid, electrolyte, and acid-base balances. These tests include serum electrolyte levels, full blood count (FBC), haematocrit, blood urea and creatinine levels, and urine specific gravity. The nurse must be familiar with the normal values of common laboratory tests (see box).

Serum electrolyte levels are measured to determine the hydration status, the electrolyte concentration of the blood plasma, and the acid-base balance. Electrolytes frequently measured in venous blood include sodium, potassium, calcium, chloride, and bicarbonate ions. The severity of the illness usually determines the frequency of the electrolyte measurements.

Serum electrolytes are routinely measured when an individual is admitted to the hospital. This provides baseline data for electrolyte status.

The FBC is a determination of the number and type of

### Mental Health Nursing
### Refusal to take in fluids

There are times in individuals' lives when they have lost the will to live and, for whatever reason, the intrapsychic pain is so overwhelming that sometimes people consciously choose to not eat or take in any fluids. This can have serious repercussions for the individual's overall health. If health care professionals are unable to persuade the individual to accept food or fluids and there is concern for the individual's health, then the Mental Health Act of 1983 may be invoked to provide carers with the legal power to intervene to maintain life and health.

erythrocytes and leucocytes blood cells per cubic millimetre of blood. Changes in the FBC, especially in the haematocrit, occur in response to dehydration or overhydration. Serious alterations in the FBC, such as anaemia, can also affect oxygenation,

Blood creatinine levels are useful in measuring kidney function. Creatinine is a normal by-product of muscle metabolism and is excreted at fairly constant levels, regardless of factors such as fluid intake, diet, and exercise.

## PLANNING

Based on the assessment, the nurse develops a care plan (see care plan). The care plan is individualized according to the patient's/client's acute or chronic fluid, electrolyte, or acid-base imbalance. A person with a fluid, electrolyte, or acid-base imbalance requires a nursing care plan directed at meeting actual or potential fluid needs. The plan is based on one or more of the following goals:

1. Patient's/client's fluid, electrolyte, and acid-base balances are restored and maintained.
2. Causes of imbalance are identified and corrected.
3. Patient/client has no complications from therapies needed to restore balance.

It is particularly important to include the patient/client and family in this planning process. Fluid, electrolyte, and acid-base imbalances often result in subtle changes in behaviour, and only the family may be sufficiently familiar with the individual's usual behaviour to identify these changes early. The patient/client and family should understand preventive measures, signs and symptoms to report, and measures that can be implemented if the imbalance occurs. When medications, special diets, or oral or intravenous fluids are administered in the home, the patient/client and family need careful teaching so that these interventions are performed safely. In the hospital, the nurse anticipates these needs and initiates teaching before discharge so that the patient/client and family are ready for these procedures. The community nurse continues the teaching and evaluates the effectiveness of the home interventions. In the future, more

## Normal Laboratory Test Values

- Calcium levels: 2.2-2.65 mmol/L
- Carbon dioxide content (bicarbonate in venous blood): 24-30 mmol/L
- Chloride level: 100-106 mmol/L
- Magnesium level: 0.8-1.3 mmol/L
- Phosphate 0.8–1.5 mmol/L
- Potassium level: 3.5-5.0 mmol/L
- Sodium level: 135-145 mmol/L
- Serum osmolality: 280-295 mmol/L
- Urine specific gravity: 1.012-1.030
- Arterial blood gas levels
  - pH: 7.35-7.45
  - $PaCO_2$: 4.7-6.0 kPa
  - $PaO_2$: 10.0-13.3 kPa
  - $SaO_2$: 95-99%
- Bicarbonate level: 24-30 mmol/L

patients/clients with severe illness will be cared for at home, following early discharge. The role of the community nurse will be enlarged in this respect.

 IMPLEMENTATION

Prevention of fluid, electrolyte, and acid-base imbalances is important. When imbalances occur, the nurse removes or treats the cause of the imbalance if possible. Other nursing interventions aim to correct fluid and electrolyte imbalances.

When volume is depleted, fluids and electrolytes can be replaced orally, with intravenous administration of fluids and blood components, or through total parenteral nutrition if the fluid deficit is caused by malnutrition. For patients/clients with fluid excess, the nurse implements measures to reduce fluids, such as fluid intake restrictions, reduced sodium intake, and administration of prescribed diuretics.

## Correcting Fluid and Electrolyte Imbalances
### DAILY WEIGHING

All patients/clients with fluid and electrolyte disturbances should be weighed daily. In this way, fluid retention can be detected early because 2.5 to 4.5 kg of fluid is retained before oedema appears (Metheny, 1987). Weight should be determined at the same time each day, and the same scale should be used. If possible, the patient/client should also wear the same clothes.

### MEASURING FLUID INTAKE AND OUTPUT

In addition to providing assessment data, intake and output records provide current information about fluid balance. These measurements can indicate whether excess fluid is excreted in the urine. Likewise, they can show whether the excretion of fluids through the kidneys has diminished.

### RESTRICTION OF FLUIDS

Patients/clients who retain fluids and have fluid volume excess require restricted fluid intake. Fluid restriction is often difficult for patients/clients, particularly if they are taking medications that dry the oral mucous membranes. The nurse should explain the reason

## Laboratory Data for Fluid, Electrolyte, and Acid-Base Imbalances

### FLUID AND ELECTROLYTE IMBALANCES
- Altered concentrations of sodium, chloride, and bicarbonate ions
- Altered serum osmolality
- False elevation of RBC or WBC count because of haemoconcentration caused by dehydration
- False lowering of full blood count (FBC) values with fluid volume excess (FVE) or hypo-osmolar imbalance
- False elevation of the serum urea level when patient/client is dehydrated and extracellular fluid is haemoconcentrated
- False lowering of serum urea level because of FVE and hypo-osmolar imbalance
- Concentrated urine, causing higher specific gravity of urine
- FVE and hypo-osmolar imbalance, causing a fall in specific gravity of urine

### ACID-BASE IMBALANCES
Metabolic Alkalosis
- pH greater then 7.45
- $PaCO_2$ normal or greater than 6.0 kPa if lungs are compensated
- $PaO_2$ normal
- $SaO_2$ normal
- Bicarbonate level greater than 30 mmol/L
- Potassium level less than 3.5 mmol/L

Metabolic Acidosis
- pH less than 7.35
- $PaCO_2$ less than 4.7 kPa if lungs are compensating
- $PaO_2$ normal
- $SaO_2$ normal
- Bicarbonate level below 24 mmol/L
- Potassium level above 5.0 mmol/L

Respiratory Alkalosis
- pH 7.45 or greater
- $PaCO_2$ less than 4.7 kPa
- $PaO_2$ normal
- $SaO_2$ normal
- Bicarbonate level normal
- Potassium level below 3.5 mmol/L

Respiratory Acidosis
- pH less than 7.35
- $PaCO_2$ greater than 6.0 kPa (unless patient/client has chronic obstructive pulmonary disease)
- $PaO_2$ normal or below 10.0 kPa, depending on severity of underlying disease
- $SaO_2$ normal or below 95%, depending on severity of underlying disease
- Bicarbonate level normal in early respiratory acidosis or elevated if kidneys are compensating
- Potassium level above 5.0 mmol/L

that fluids are restricted. The patient/client should also know how much fluid is permitted and that ice cubes and ice cream are fluids.

Given this information, the patient/client should help decide the amount of fluid with each meal, between meals, before bed, and with medications.

The nurse should also ensure that patients/clients receive their preferred fluids (unless contraindicated).

**24 HOUR FLUID CHART** Name ______________ Ward ______________ Date ______________ WD41 U

| TIME | INTAKE | | | | | | DRUGS IN INFUSION | OUTPUT | | | | | | | |
|---|---|---|---|---|---|---|---|---|---|---|---|---|---|---|---|
| | MOUTH | INTRAVENOUS: Blood or Plasma | INTRAVENOUS: Normal Saline | INTRAVENOUS: Dextrose Saline | INTRAVENOUS: 5% Dextrose | OTHER | | GASTRIC CONTENTS | URINE | FAECES | OTHER | BLOOD PRESSURE | | | |
| 6.00 | | | | | | | | | | | | | | | |
| 7.00 | | | | | | | | | | | | | | | |
| 8.00 | | | | | | | | | | | | | | | |
| 9.00 | | | | | | | | | | | | | | | |
| 10.00 | | | | | | | | | | | | | | | |
| 11.00 | | | | | | | | | | | | | | | |
| 12 Noon | | | | | | | | | | | | | | | |
| 13.00 | | | | | | | | | | | | | | | |
| 14.00 | | | | | | | | | | | | | | | |
| 15.00 | | | | | | | | | | | | | | | |
| 16.00 | | | | | | | | | | | | | | | |
| 17.00 | | | | | | | | | | | | | | | |
| 18.00 | | | | | | | | | | | | | | | |
| TOTAL 12 HOURS | | | | | | | | | | | | | | | |
| 19.00 | | | | | | | | | | | | | | | |
| 20.00 | | | | | | | | | | | | | | | |
| 21.00 | | | | | | | | | | | | | | | |
| 22.00 | | | | | | | | | | | | | | | |
| 23.00 | | | | | | | | | | | | | | | |
| 24.00 Midnight | | | | | | | | | | | | | | | |
| 1.00 | | | | | | | | | | | | | | | |
| 2.00 | | | | | | | | | | | | | | | |
| 3.00 | | | | | | | | | | | | | | | |
| 4.00 | | | | | | | | | | | | | | | |
| 5.00 | | | | | | | | | | | | | | | |
| 6.00 | | | | | | | | | | | | | | | |
| TOTAL 12 HOURS | | | | | | | | | | | | | | | |

**Fig. 18-8** 24-hour fluid chart. *Courtesy of Royal London Hospitals NHS Trust.*

## ENTERAL REPLACEMENT OF FLUIDS

Fluids are replaced enterally via the oral route and tube feeding.

**Oral** Unless contraindicated, oral replacement of fluids and electrolytes is appropriate if the patient/client is not vomiting, not experiencing a profound fluid loss, or does not have a mechanical obstruction in the gastrointestinal tract. Individuals unable to tolerate solid foods may still be able to ingest fluids. Oral fluid replacement is easily implemented in the home and hospital. Mild illnesses such as viral diarrhoea and respiratory tract infections, as well as fevers, may cause fluid and electrolyte disturbances. In addition, patients/clients recovering from anaesthesia or gastrointestinal surgery usually receive clear liquids first and then advance to a solid diet if they tolerate the liquids. When replacing fluids by mouth, the nurse should choose fluids with adequate calories and electrolyte content, but if fluids are replaced through a feeding tube, the doctor usually prescribes a nutritional supplement (see Chapter 21).

**Tube Feedings** A feeding tube may be appropriate when the patient's/client's gastrointestinal tract is healthy but he or she cannot ingest fluids (for example, after oral surgery or with impaired swallowing). Fluids can be replaced through nasogastric, gastrostomy, or jejunostomy feeding tubes (see Chapter 21).

## PARENTERAL REPLACEMENT OF FLUID AND ELECTROLYTES

Fluid and electrolytes may be replaced by infusion directly into the blood rather than intake through the digestive system. Parenteral replacement includes total parenteral nutrition (TPN) IV fluid and electrolyte therapy, and blood replacement.

---

### Sample Nursing Care Plan for Fluid Volume Deficit

**Nursing Assessment:** Fluid volume deficit related to active loss of gastrointestinal fluid
**Definition:** Fluid volume deficit is the state in which an individual experiences vascular, cellular, or intracellular dehydration related to active loss (Kim *et al* 1991).

| Goals | Expected Outcomes | Interventions | Rationale |
|---|---|---|---|
| Fluid balance will return to normal values within 48 hr. | Weight will stabilize by 25/1<br>Urine output will increase (>70 ml/hr) by 24/1<br>Specific gravity will decrease (<1.030) by 24/1<br>Patient/client will have normal skin turgor by 24/1<br>Patient/client will experience no thirst or weakness by 25/1<br>Patient/client will have moist mucous membranes by 25/1<br>Patient/client will experience no vomiting by 26/1 | Encourage intake of small amount of fluids containing electrolytes.<br><br>Discourage intake of plain water. | Ingesting small volumes may prevent further vomiting. Presence of electrolytes prevents further depletion.<br><br>Ingestion of plain water causes sodium content in stomach to increase as body attempts to make water isotonic to allow absorption. |
| | | If vomiting occurs before absorption, more fluids and electrolytes are lost. | |
| | | Alter environment to lessen stimuli for vomiting (e.g. keep unpleasant odours to minimum). | This prevents triggering vomiting centre in brain. |
| | | Promote bed rest. | Sudden, quick movements may trigger vomiting. |
| | | Measure amount of vomitus. | This allows precise replacement of lost fluid and electrolytes. |
| | | Implement doctor's orders to provide parenteral fluids containing electrolytes during prolonged periods of vomiting. | These fluids will precisely replace losses. |

Adapted from Methany NM: *Fluid and electrolyte balance: nursing considerations,* Philadelphia, 1987, Lippincott.

With increasing risk to health care workers for transmission of the human immunodeficiency virus (HIV), the principles of body fluid substance isolation must be practised when administering parenteral fluids (see Chapter 28).

**Vascular Access Devices** **Vascular access devices** are catheters or cannulae designed for long-term repeated access to the vascular system. These devices are safer than peripherally placed catheters and have improved mechanisms for delivering long-term IV therapy. Recently, temporary central venous catheters (such as subclavian lines) have begun to be used for patients/clients with poor peripheral venous access who need infusion therapy for 1 week to 3 months (Silvestri and Masoorli, 1990).

**Total Parenteral Nutrition (TPN)** **TPN** is a nutritionally adequate hypertonic solution consisting of glucose and other nutrients and electrolytes, usually given through a central venous catheter.

**IV Therapy** The goal of IV fluid administration is to correct or prevent fluid and electrolyte disturbances.

When IV fluid administration is required, the nurse must know the correct solution, equipment needed, and procedures required to initiate an infusion, regulate the fluid infusion rate, maintain the system, identify and correct problems, and discontinue the infusion.

**Types of Solutions** Many prepared electrolyte solutions are available for use. Electrolyte solutions fall into the following categories: **isotonic**, **hypotonic**, and **hypertonic**.

In general, isotonic fluids are used for extracellular volume replacement (for example, 0.9% saline after prolonged vomiting). The decision to use a hypotonic or hypertonic solution is based on the specific electrolyte imbalance (Table 18-2).

Certain additives are frequently instilled into IV solutions, most commonly vitamins and potassium chloride (KCl).

**Equipment** Correct selection and preparation of equipment assists in safe and quick placement of an IV line. Because fluids are instilled into the bloodstream, aseptic technique is necessary, and therefore the nurse must have all the needed equipment organized and at the bedside. Standard equipment includes IV solution and tubing, needle or catheter, antiseptic, tourniquet, gloves, and dressing.

Infusion pumps and syringes are used with children, with individuals with renal or cardiac failure, with critically ill patients/clients and when potent drugs are being infused. (Additional information on volume control devices is presented in the section on regulating the infusion flow rate.)

**Initiating the Intravenous Line** A **venepuncture** is a technique in which a vein is punctured transcutaneously by a sharp, rigid stylet (for example, a butterfly needle or a metal needle) partially covered by a plastic catheter or by a needle attached to a syringe. The general purposes of venepuncture are to collect a blood specimen, instil a medication, start an IV

infusion, and inject a radio-opaque or radioactive tracer for special examinations.

Because very young and old people have fragile veins, the doctor should avoid sites that are easily moved or bumped. It is often difficult to insert IV lines in patients/clients who have had many venepunctures, because their veins may be sclerosed with scar tissue. Obese patients/clients present problems for venepuncture because of the difficulty in locating superficial veins. The veins of thin and emaciated patients/clients are also difficult to puncture. Although they may be visible, the veins are quite fragile, and as a result the needle may puncture through entire veins instead of being placed needles or catheters within them. When patients/clients are severely dehydrated or have decreased extracellular fluid, such as with shock, the veins may collapse. The collapse results from decreased circulating blood volume. Some hospitals have IV therapy teams whose members have special expertise in performing venepunctures and maintaining IV infusions.

Venepuncture is contraindicated in a site that has signs of infection, infiltration, or thrombosis (clotting). An infected site is red, tender, swollen, and possibly warm to the touch. Exudate may be present. An infected site is not used because of the danger of introducing bacteria from the skin surface into the bloodstream.

Common IV puncture sites include the hand and arm (Fig. 18-9A and B. However, the superficial veins of the foot can be used if the individual is not ambulatory. The use of the foot for an IV site is more common with children but is generally avoided in adults.

Large catheters placed into a central vein such as the subclavian vein or internal jugular vein; are used to monitor central venous pressure and to deliver large volumes of fluids and TPN.

**Regulating the Infusion Flow Rate** After the IV infusion is secured and the IV line is patent, the nurse must regulate the rate of infusion according to the doctor's prescription (Procedure 18-1). An infusion rate that is too slow can lead to further cardiovascular and circulatory collapse in a patient/client who is dehydrated, in shock, or critically ill. An infusion rate that is too rapid can result in fluid overload, which is particularly dangerous in some cardiovascular, renal, and neurological disorders.

**Infusion pumps** regulate the flow of IV fluids. They are designed to deliver a measured amount of fluid over a specified period of time or to deliver fluids based on the flow rate or drops per minute.

If the required number of drops or volume per minute is not achieved, an alarm will sound. The alarm can be sounded if the IV bag is empty, the infusion tubing is kinked, or the vein is clotted. If the alarm sounds, the nurse investigates and corrects the cause of the drip rate problem. IV flow rates can be affected by the patency of the IV needle or catheter, extravasation, a knot or kink in the tubing, the height of the solution, and the position of the patient's/client's extremity.

**Patency** of the IV needle or catheter means that there are no clots at the tip of the needle or catheter and that the catheter or

**TABLE 18-2 IV Fluids**

| Solution | Concentration | Contents | Indications | Contraindications | Comments |
|---|---|---|---|---|---|
| Dextrose | 5% | Water Glucose 50 mg/ml. | Fluid replacement. | 1. Hyperglycaemia. | Used where there is no significant electrolyte imbalance. |
| Saline | 0.9% | Water Sodium Chloride 50mmol/L Sodium 150mmol/L Chloride | Sodium depletion. | 1. Impaired renal function. 2. Cardiac failure. 3. Hypertension. 4. Peripheral and pulmonary oedema. | Used to correct sodium depletion, as isotonic saline provides the necessary ions in near physiological concentration. |
| Dextrose and Saline | 4% Dextrose 0.18% Sodium Chloride | Water Glucose Sodium Chloride 40g/L Glucose 30mmol/L Sodium 30mmol/L Chloride | Combined water and sodium depletion. | Be aware of contraindications for saline. | This solution allows water to enter body cells to correct dehydration, while sodium and a little water remains extracellular to correct sodium depletion. |
| Hartman's (Sodium Lactate Compound) | | Water Sodium (131mmol/L) Potassium(5mmol/L) Calcium (2mmol/L) Chloride (111mmol/L) Bicarbonate (29mmol/L) | Correction of multiple electrolyte imbalance. Diabetic coma. Diminished alkali reserve. | As the bicarbonate is in the form of lactate there is a risk of lactic acidosis in seriously ill patients with poor tissue perfusion or impaired hepatic function. | Used to correct multiple electrolyte imbalance ions in near physiological concentrations. |
| Sodium Bicarbonate | 1.26% 8.4% | Sodium (150mmol/L) Bicarbonate (15mmol/L) 8.4% = Sodium (1000mmol/l) Bicarbonate (1000mmol/L) | Metabolic acidosis. | 1. Hypokalaemia. 2. Over expansion of extracellular fluid. 3. Too much too quickly may produce tetany or convulsions. | 1.26% (isotonic). used to correct acidosis of any origin. 8.4% (hypertonic) used to correct severe metabolic acidosis in cardiac arrest. |
| Mannitol | 10% 20% 25% | | Cerebral oedema. To produce a forced diuresis. | 1. Congestive cardiac failure. 2. Pulmonary oedema. | A hypertonic solution. An osmotic diuretic. Not used in cardiac failure as they expand blood volume. |
| Dextran | 6% | Can be given either 0.9% Sodium Chloride or 5% Dextrose | Restoration and maintenance of circulating volume. | Risks: although rare anaphylactic reactions. May produce hypotension and bronchospasm. | Commonly used as a plasma expander. Can be used for this reason in prophylactic deep vein thrombosis therapy in gynaecology. Any blood required for cross-matching or electrolyte estimation must be taken prior to this infusion commencing. |

From Miller J: Intravenous therapy in fluid and electrolyte imbalance, *Prof Nurse*, 4(5): 237 1989.

## PROCEDURE 18-1  Regulating IV Flow Rates

**SEQUENCE OF ACTIONS**

1. Ensure patient/client is comfortable. Maximize your opportunities for communication.

2. Observe patency of IV line and needle. Open drip regulator and observe for rapid flow of fluid from IV solution into drip chamber, and then close drip regulator to prescribed rate.

3. Check IV drug chart for correct solution volume and additives. Chart also shows time over which fluid is to infuse.

4. Know drop factor in drops/ml of infusion set:
   Microdrip:            60/ml
   Macrodrip (blood)     15/ml
   (clear fluid)         20/ml

5. Formula for calculation of flow rate in drops per minute.

   $$ml/hr = \frac{total\ volume\ (ml)}{hours\ of\ infusion}$$

   $$\frac{ml/hr \times drop\ factor}{60\ min} = drops/min$$

6. If infusion pump or volume control device is used, place it at bedside.

7. Follow this procedure for infusion pump:
   a. Monitor infusion rates at least hourly.
   b. Assess patency of IV system when alarm sounds.

8. Observe patient/client hourly to determine response to IV therapy and restoration of fluid and electrolyte balance. Also check IV site for signs of extravasation inflammation, and phlebitis.

9. Record rate of infusion, drops/min and ml/hr, in patient's/client's chart as required by hospital/ward.

**RATIONALE**

For fluid to infuse at proper rate, IV line and needle must be free of kinks, knots and clots.
Rapid flow of fluid into drip chamber denotes patency of IV line. Closing drip to prescribed rate prevents fluid overload.

IV fluids are medications. Five rules are followed to decrease chance of medication error.

Microdroppers, also called *minidrip*, universally deliver 60 drops per ml. However, commercial parenteral administration sets for microdrip exist. The nurse should know which company's infusion set is being used.

After hourly rate has been determined, formula will give correct flow rate in drops/min.

Increases accuracy of fluid delivery rate.

Infusion pumps are not infallible and do not replace frequent, accurate assessments.

Signs and symptoms of dehydration or overhydration warrant changing rate of fluid infused. Signs of infiltration, inflammation, and phlebitis warrant changing IV site.

Documents that prescribed IV flow is being delivered to patient/client.

needle tip is not against the vein wall.

An **extravasation** may be present when the IV insertion site is cool, clammy, swollen, and in some cases painful. This occurs when the IV needle or catheter has become dislodged from the vein and is in the subcutaneous space. When this occurs, the IV line must be discontinued and a new line inserted.

A knot or kink in the tubing can decrease the flow rate. Occasionally, the tubing is kinked under the IV dressing, which requires the nurse to open the dressing to locate the problem. Frequently the flow rate resumes after the tubing is straightened. The patient/client may also occlude the tubing by lying or sitting on it. The height of the IV bag can also affect flow rates. Raising the bag may increase the rate, because of gravity.

The extremity position can decrease flow rates, particularly with IV sites at the wrist or elbow. Sometimes, it is more comfortable for the patient/client to have an infusion started in a new location rather than dealing with a site that causes problems.

These influences on IV flow rates can occur with any patient/client at any time. When caring for a person with an infusion, the nurse should assess the site and the infusion rate at least every hour.

Children, older adults, people with severe head trauma, and people susceptible to volume overload must be protected from sudden increases in infusion volumes. Sudden increases can occur accidentally. For example, a restless patient/client may, with a sudden movement, loosen the roller clamp and increase the flow rate, or the flow rate may be accidentally increased if the patient/client ambulates. A sudden increase in IV volume can result in serious illness or death. Volume control devices, such as buret, can prevent sudden increases in volume.

The volume control device is placed between the IV bag and insertion spike of the infusion set or may be part of the infusion set. Most control devices can hold 150 ml. If the nurse does not return to the patient/client in exactly 1 hour, the IV line does not

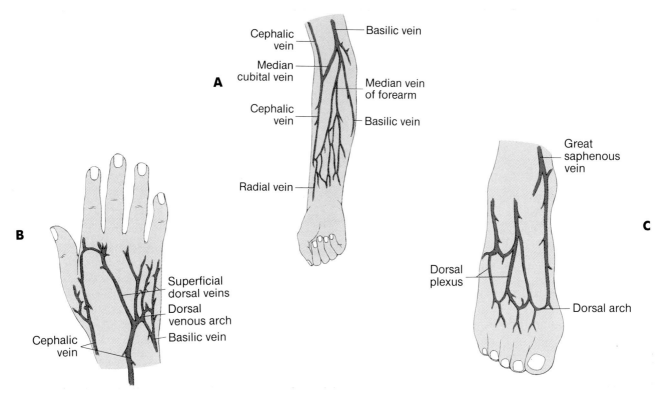

**Fig. 18-9** Possible IV sites. **A,** Inner arm. **B,** Dorsal surface of the hand. **C,** Dorsal surface of the foot.

run through. In addition, if an accidental increase in flow rate occurs, the patient/client receives at most only 1 hours' allotment of fluid instead of 500 or 1000 ml.

**Maintaining the system** After the IV line is in place and the flow rate is regulated, the nurse must maintain the system. The nurse provides comfort and assistance with hygiene measures, meals, and ambulation.

Because an individual with an infusion in the arm finds it difficult to meet hygiene needs, the nurse should help with bathing and changing clothes.

A new solution bag or bottle should be hung at least once every 24 hours, even if the old bag is not empty, because the sterility and stability of the solution cannot be guaranteed for longer than a day. When an IV solution container is changed, the nurse uses sterile technique and follows an organized procedure.

Technically, IV tubing can remain sterile for 48 hours. However, most clinical areas recommend that new sterile tubing be used every 24 hours. The procedure is much easier and more efficient if the nurse changes the infusion tubing when preparing to hang a new IV bag or bottle. To prevent entry of bacteria into the bloodstream, sterility must be maintained.

The dressing over the IV insertion site is changed according to hospital policy. Transparent dressings enable the nurse to continually assess venepuncture sites. Dressings should be changed only when soiling is visible. This practice is more cost effective and does not increase the risk of infection.

**Complications of IV Therapy** The major complications of IV therapy are extravasation, phlebitis, fluid overload, bleeding, and infection. Extravasation is manifested as swelling (from increased tissue fluid) and pallor (caused by decreased circulation) around the venepuncture site. Fluid may be flowing through the IV line at a decreased rate or may have stopped. Pain may also occur, usually resulting from oedema.

When extravasation occurs, infusion must be discontinued, and if necessary, the needle is resited. To reduce discomfort caused by extravasation, the nurse raises the extremity, which promotes venous drainage and helps decrease oedema.

**Phlebitis** is an inflammation of the vein caused by the catheter or by the chemical irritation of additives and drugs given intravenously. Signs and symptoms include pain, increased skin temperature over the vein, and in some instances redness travelling along the path of the vein. The IV line must be discontinued and a new line inserted in another vein. Phlebitis is potentially dangerous because blood clots (thrombophlebitis) can occur and in some cases may result in emboli.

Fluid overload occurs when the patient/client has received too-rapid administration of solutions. Assessment findings are similar to those of FVE. The nurse should slow the rate of infusion and notify the doctor. Prompt action is necessary to prevent worsening of the condition or even death.

Infusion-related infections are caused by contamination of the IV system, venepuncture site, or the solution itself (Messner and Gorse, 1987). Clinical manifestations of these infections include purulent thrombophlebitis, cellulitis, and site infections, as evidenced by erythema, swelling, and pain at the venepuncture site.

**Discontinuing IV Infusions** Discontinuing an infusion is necessary after the prescribed amount of fluids or drugs has been infused, when an extravasation occurs, if phlebitis is present, or if the infusion catheter or needle develops a clot at its tip. To discontinue an infusion the nurse:

1. Applies disposable gloves and removes the tape and dressing.
2. Moves the roller clamp to the *off* position to prevent spillage of IV fluid.
3. Places a gauze pad over the venepuncture site
4. Using the other hand, withdraws the catheter needle by pulling straight back from the puncture site if needed.
5. Applies pressure to the site for 1 to 2 minutes to control bleeding and prevent haematoma formation.
6. Applies a sterile dressing over the venepuncture site.
7. Records the amount of fluid infused and the time of the discontinuation.

**Blood Transfusion** Blood transfusion is the IV administration of whole blood or a component such as plasma, packed RBCs, or platelets. The following list includes objectives for blood transfusion:

- To increase circulating blood volume after surgery, trauma, or haemorrhage
- To increase the number of RBCs and to maintain haemoglobin levels in patients/clients with severe anaemia
- To provide selected cellular components as replacement therapy (for example, plasma-clotting factors to help control bleeding).

The most important grouping for blood transfusion is the ABO system, which includes the following groups: A, B, O, and AB. The determination of blood groups is based on the presence or absence of A and B red cell antigens. Individuals with A antigens, B antigens, or no antigens belong to groups A, B, and O, respectively. The person with A and B antigens has AB blood (Porth, 1986).

**Agglutinins**, or antibodies that work against the A and B antigens, are called *anti-A* and *anti-B agglutinins*. These agglutinins occur naturally in plasma (Patrick et al, 1986). Individuals with type A blood naturally produce anti-B agglutinins in their plasma. Similarly, type B individuals naturally produce anti-A agglutinins in their plasma. A type O individual naturally produces both agglutinins, which is why a person with type O blood is considered a universal donor. An AB type individual produces neither antibody, which is why type AB individuals can be universal recipients. If blood that is mismatched with the patient's/client's blood is transfused, a transfusion reaction occurs. The **transfusion reaction** is an antigen-antibody reaction and can range from a mild response to severe anaphylactic shock.

Another consideration when matching for blood transfusions is the **Rh factor**, an antigenic substance in the erythrocytes of most people. A person with the factor is Rh positive, whereas a person without it is Rh negative. If the blood given to an Rh-negative person is Rh positive, **haemolysis** (erythrocyte destruction) and anaemia occur. This is why a person with group

O Rh-negative blood is considered to be a universal donor. If a Rh-negative mother carries a Rh-positive fetus, the fetus may be exposed to antibodies in the mother's Rh-negative blood.

**Autotransfusion** is the collection, anticoagulation, filtration, and reinfusion of blood from an active bleeding site. Because the reinfused blood is the patient's/client's own, there are many advantages to autotransfusion. The risk of technical errors in blood typing and crossmatching is eliminated. Possible adverse effects associated with homologous blood transfusion are also eliminated. In addition, dependence on homologous blood banks is reduced, and possible exposure to serum hepatitis, HIV, and other blood-borne infections is eliminated.

When an elective surgical procedure is anticipated and transfusions are required, some individuals choose to give one or more units of their own blood in advance. This blood is stored and is available intraoperatively and postoperatively. This, too, is a type of autotransfusion.

The nurse is responsible for assessment *before* and *during* the transfusion and regulation of the transfusion (Procedure 18-2).

If the patient/client has an IV line in place, assess the venepuncture site for signs of infection or extravasation. The nurse should determine that the catheter is patent and functioning properly. Tubing for blood transfusion has an in-line filter and should be primed with 0.9% normal saline. Use of any other IV solution results in haemolysis.

**Pretransfusion assessment** also includes obtaining information from the patient/client. The nurse asks whether the patient/client knows the reason for the blood transfusion and whether he or she has ever had a transfusion or a transfusion reaction. A person who has had a transfusion reaction is usually at no greater risk for a reaction with a subsequent transfusion. However, the patient/client may be anxious about the transfusion, necessitating nursing intervention.

Pretransfusion assessment must include a baseline measurement of vital signs temparature, pulse, respiration, blood pressure. These values must be recorded before the nurse gives any blood products, because a change in vital signs can indicate a reaction.

When giving a transfusion, explain the procedure and ask the patient/client to report any side effects. The IV line is primed with 0.9% normal saline. The nurse then follows hospital procedure for obtaining blood products. With two nurses, one of whom is a registered nurse, the identity of the blood products, the patient/client, the hospital number, the blood group, the compatibility of the blood to be infused against the individual's blood and the expiry date are checked. The infusion is begun slowly. The infusion is maintained, side effects are monitored, and the transfusion is recorded.

During blood infusion the patient/client is at risk for a reaction, particularly during the first 15 minutes. Therefore, the nurse should remain with the individual and assess skin colour and vital signs (T, P, R, BP). Continue to monitor the patient/client and obtain vital signs periodically during the transfusion as directed by hospital policy (often every 15 minutes), and take vital signs when a reaction is suspected. The

## PROCEDURE 18-2 Administering a Blood Transfusion

| SEQUENCE OF ACTIONS | RATIONALE |
|---|---|
| 1. Explain procedure to patient/client. Determine if there have been prior transfusions and note reactions, if any. | Patients/clients who have had blood transfusion reactions in the past may have greater fear of transfusion. Past occurence of certain reactions may increase possibility of recurrence. |
| 2. Ask patient/client to report chills, headaches, itching, or rash immediately. | These are signs of transfusion reaction. Prompt reporting and discontinuation of transfusion can help minimize reaction. |
| 3. Be sure patient/client has given verbal consent. | |
| 4. Wash hands. Apply disposable gloves. | Reduces risk for transmission of HIV, hepatitis, and other blood-borne microorganisms. |
| 5. Establish IV line with large-gauge catheter. | Large-gauge catheters permit infusion of whole blood and prevent haemolysis. |
| 6. Use infusion tubing that has in-line filter. Tubing should also be Y-type administration (see illustration). | Filter removes debris and tiny clots from blood. Y-type set permits administration of additional products or volume expanders easily and permits immediate infusion of isotonic 0.9% sodium chloride solution after completion of isotonic infusion. |

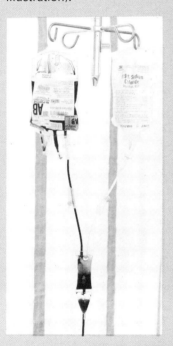

Step 6

| | |
|---|---|
| 7. Hang solution container of 0.9% normal saline to be administered after blood transfusion. | Prevents haemolysis of erythrocytes. |
| 8. Follow local protocol in obtaining blood products from blood bank. Request blood when you are ready to use it. | Whole blood or packed erythrocytes must remain in cold (1 to 6°C) environment. |
| 9. With another registered nurse, correctly identify blood product and patient/client: | |
| a. Check compatibility label attached to blood bag and information on bag itself. | One nurse reads out loud while other nurse listens and double-checks information. Reduces risk of error. |
| b. For whole blood, check ABO group and Rh type, which is on patient's/client's chart. | Verifies that ABO group, Rh type, and unit number match. |
| c. Double-check blood product with doctor's order. | Verifies that information matches that on compatibility tag and blood bag. |
| d. Check expiry date on bag. | Verifies correct blood component. |

(Cont'd)

**PROCEDURE 18-2 Administering a Blood Transfusion (Cont'd)**

| SEQUENCE OF ACTIONS | RATIONALE |
|---|---|
| e. Inspect blood for clots. | After 21 days, blood has only 70 to 80% of original number of cells and 23 mmol/L of potassium (Metheny and Snively, 1983). Anticoagulant citrate-phosphate-dextrose (CPD) is added to blood and permits preserved blood to be stored for 21 days. Another anticoagulant, citrate-phosphate-dextrose-adenine (CPD-A), allows storage for 35 days (Metheny and Snively, 1983). If clots are present, return blood to blood bank. |
| f. Ask patient's/client's name, and check arm band. | Verifies correct patient/client. Do not administer blood to patient/client without arm band. Identification name and number on wristband must be identical to those on blood compatibility tag. |
| 10. Obtain baseline vital signs. | Verifies pre-transfusion temperature, pulse rate, blood pressure, and respirations. |
| 11. Begin transfusion: | |
| a. Prime infusion line with 0.9% normal saline. | Isotonic saline prevents haemolysis. |
| b. Adjust rate to 2 ml/min for first 15 min, and remain with patient/client. If you suspect reaction, stop transfusion, flush line with normal saline, infuse normal saline slowly, and notify blood bank and doctor. | Allows detection of reaction while infusing smallest possible volume of blood product. Flushing line prevents further infusion of blood product. |
| 12. Monitor vital signs: | |
| a. Take vital signs every 5 min for first 15 min of transfusion and every hr thereafter. | Documents change in vital sign status that could indicate early warning of reaction. |
| b. Observe patient/client for flushing, itching, dyspnoea, hives, and rash. | May indicate early sign of reaction. |
| 13. Maintain prescribed infusion rate using infusion pumps, if necessary. | Infusion pumps maintain prescribed rate. |
| 14. Remove and dispose of gloves. Wash hands. | Reduces transmission of microorganisms. |
| 15. Continually observe for adverse reactions. | Adverse reactions can occur at any point during transfusion (Table 18-3). |
| 16. Record administration of blood or blood product. | Documents administration of blood component. |
| 17. When infusion is completed, return blood bag and tubing to blood bank. | Provides material for analysis if reaction is discovered later. |

rate of a transfusion is specified on the drug sheet.

Patients/clients with severe blood loss, such as with a haemorrhage, may receive rapid transfusions through a central venous pressure catheter. A blood-warming device is often necessary because the tip of the central venous pressure catheter lies in the superior vena cava, above the right atrium. Rapid administration of cold blood can result in cardiac dysrhythmias (LaRocca and Otto, 1989).

A **transfusion reaction** is a systemic response by the body to blood incompatible with that of the recipient. It is caused by erythrocyte incompatibility or allergic sensitivity to the leucocytes, platelets, or plasma protein components of the transfused blood or to the potassium or citrate preservative in the blood. Blood transfusion can also result in disease transmission.

Several types of reactions can result from blood transfusions.

General adverse reactions (Table 18-3) range from immediate onset of fever, chills, and skin rash to hypotension, shock, and a delayed reaction that may not occur until several days or weeks after the transfusion.

A second category of reactions includes diseases transmitted by blood donors who have no symptoms of problems. Diseases transmitted through transfusions include malaria, hepatitis and HIV infection. Because all units of collected blood must undergo serological testing and HIV screening, the risk of acquiring blood-borne infections from transfusions has now been reduced.

Correct administration of blood and blood products reduces the risk of transfusion reactions. The nurse is responsible for determining that the blood delivered to the ward corresponds to the individual's blood type listed on the request sheet. Two nurses should check the blood against the patient's/client's identification number, blood group, and complete name. If even a minor

### Children's Nursing
### IV therapy in children

Caring for a child undergoing IV therapy? Be prepared for potential complications! The child's size, age, weight and developmental stage have implications for special nursing. His or her increased Basal Metabolic Rate (BMR) make fluid volume and rate calculations more difficult. The child is more susceptible to fluid imbalance and particularly fluid overload. The small child is usually active and alert, and has small veins so the cannulae can dislodge very easily.

The main points to be aware of when administering IV therapy to children are:
- sites used
- greater accuracy required in giving small amounts of IV fluid
- the increased risk of overloading the child's circulating blood volume (300ml in newborn)
- restraint needed to keep cannula in position

## Blood Transfusion and Jehovah's Witnesses

Jehovah's Witnesses will not accept blood or blood products for themselves, their children or their next of kin. This can mean that decisions concerning major surgery or organ transplant can cause dilemmas for medical staff, and possibly for the patient's family.

Decisions concerning the treatment of children, for example those with leukaemia who require blood transfusion or bone marrow transplant, can be especially difficult. The parents may want to exercise their right to bring up their child within their beliefs as Witnesses. Medical staff will want to treat the child and, in order that treatment can be carried out, have sometimes intervened to make the child a ward of court.

These situations are difficult for all concerned and require sensitive handling.

discrepancy exists, the blood should not be given and the blood bank laboratory should be notified.

In addition to allergic reactions and the transmission of illnesses, certain risks (**hyperkalaemia, hypocalcaemia, and circulatory overload**) are associated with blood transfusions.

- **Hyperkalemia**: (excessive potassium in the blood) may be caused by stored blood. Blood that is 1 day old has a plasma potassium content of approximately 7 mmol/L, and blood stored for 21 days has a plasma potassium content of 23 mmol/L (Metheny and Snively, 1983). The increase in potassium is related to the destruction of erythrocytes. At the end of 21 days, 20 to 30% of cells are destroyed because the major intracellular cation, potassium, enters the plasma as cells are destroyed.

- **Hypocalcaemia**: (decreased calcium in the blood) can develop in patients/clients receiving massive transfusions because of the action of the citrated blood as it combines with ionized calcium (Metheny, 1987). The preservative often added to blood, citrate-phosphate-dextrose (CPD), contains more citrate than is needed to combine with calcium in the blood collected for the transfusion. Therefore, when transfused blood is infused into the bloodstream, the preservative combines with the ionized calcium, and tetany can result. The risk of hypocalcaemia increases with the number of blood transfusions the individual receives.

- **Circulatory overload** is a risk when a patient/client receives massive whole blood or packed erythrocyte transfusions for haemorrhagic shock, or when a person with normal blood volume receives whole blood. People particularly at risk for circulatory overload are older adults and those with cardiopulmonary and renal failure diseases.

Transfusion reactions are life threatening, but prompt nursing intervention can maintain the patient's/client's physiological stability. In the event of a suspected reaction, the nurse should do the following:

1. Stop the transfusion immediately.
2. Turn off the blood, change the giving set and turn on 0.9% normal saline. *Do not* put saline through the blood set because this will merely infuse the blood that is in the tubing into the patient/client. Even a small amount of mismatched blood can cause a major reaction.
3. Notify the doctor.
4. Remain with the patient/client, observe signs and symptoms, and monitor vital signs every 5 minutes.
5. Prepare to administer emergency drugs, such as antihistamines, vasopressors, fluids, and steroids.
6. Prepare for cardiopulmonary resuscitation.
7. Save the blood container and tubing for return to the laboratory.

Although anaphylactic transfusion reactions are relatively rare, they can occur with any patient/client. Correct administration of blood and blood products prevents reactions. **When an individual has a transfusion reaction, prompt nursing actions can decrease the severity of the response.**

### Correcting Acid-Base Imbalances

Nursing interventions to promote acid-base balance are performed to support prescribed medical therapies. Doctors often order a variety of drug therapies to correct acid-base imbalances. Because acid-base disturbances can be life threatening and require rapid correction, the nurse must maintain a functional IV line and frequently check the doctor's prescription on the drug chart for new medications or fluids. Prescribed drugs, such as insulin or sodium bicarbonate, and fluid and electrolyte replacement should be given promptly.

The nurse implements appropriate nursing measures to promote ventilation and oxygenation (see Chapter 17). This is particularly important for the patient/client with respiratory acidosis.

## TABLE 18-3 Adverse Reactions to Blood Transfusions

| Description | Cause | Onset | Signs and Symptoms | Nursing Actions |
|---|---|---|---|---|
| **FEBRILE NON HAEMOLYTIC** Is most common Usually occurs in previous transfusion recipients or multiparous patients/clients | Antigen-antibody reaction to leucocytes or platelets contained in blood product | Immediately or within 6 hr after transfusion | Fever (with or without chills), headache, nausea and vomiting, non-productive cough, hypotension, chest pain, dyspnoea | Stop transfusion Keep vein open Notify doctor and blood bank Take vital signs as necessary |
| **ALLERGIC URTICARIAL** Is generally innocuous | Allergic reaction to plasma-soluble antigen contained in blood product | Any time during transfusion or within 1 hr after transfusion | Skin rash | Slow transfusion to keep vein open Notify doctor and blood bank |
| **DELAYED HAEMOLYTIC** Is more common than acute haemolytic reaction Is frequently missed Occurs in previous transfusion recipients or multiparous patients/clients | Incompatibility of erythrocyte antigens other than ABO group | Days to weeks after transfusion | Decreasing haemoglobin level, possible persistent low-grade fever | Notify doctor and blood bank |
| **ACUTE HAEMOLYTIC** Can be life threatening | ABO group incompatibility | Usually during first 5 to 15 min, but any time during transfusion | *Mild form:* fever, chills, back pain, hypotension, nausea, vomiting, flushing, haematuria, oliguria *Severe form (in addition to above):* dyspnoea, chest pain, anuria, shock, disseminated intravascular coagulation | Stop transfusion Keep vein open Notify doctor and blood bank Take vital signs as necessary Assess for signs and symptoms of shock Monitor input and output Check for decreased urinary output Start resuscitative measurements as necessary |
| **ANAPHYLACTIC** Is extremely rare Can be life threatening | Idiosyncratic reaction in patients/clients with immunoglobulin A (IgA) deficiency, sensitized to IgA through previous transfusion or pregnancy | Immediately (after transfusion of only few millilitres of blood) | Severe respiratory and cardiovascular collapse (with dyspnoea, tachypnoea, tachycardia, hypotension, cyanosis); severe gastrointestinal disturbances (with nausea, vomiting, diarrhoea, cramping) | Stop transfusion Keep vein open Notify doctor and blood bank Take vital signs every 15 min (or as necessary) Start resuscitative measures as necessary |

From Querin JJ, Stahl LD: *Nurs 83* 13:34, 1983.

## ARTERIAL BLOOD GASES

Patients/clients with acid-base disturbances usually require repeated arterial blood gas analysis. This procedure requires the removal of blood from an artery to determine acid-base status and adequacy of ventilation and oxygenation. Arterial blood gas samples are drawn from an artery such as the radial or femoral artery.

 **EVALUATION**

The nurse evaluates the effectiveness of care provided to the patient/client with alterations in fluid, electrolyte, or acid-base imbalances, based on expected outcomes. Ongoing assessment enables the nurse to evaluate the response to therapy. Using evaluation data, the nurse determines if the care goals have been met or if the care plan requires modification.

Goals for patient/client care are developed using objective criteria to measure progress.

## SUMMARY

Patients/clients with altered fluid and electrolyte status require nursing care plans designed to assist in restoring normal fluid volume and electrolyte concentrations. The nurse restores fluid balance through oral fluid replacement, administration of IV fluids, and maintenance of fluid restrictions. Electrolytes can be given orally or parenterally. The nurse also treats underlying illnesses that may cause fluid and electrolyte imbalances.

Acid-base imbalances may result from a number of underlying illnesses. With minor imbalances, the body compensates by chemical, biological, and physiological regulatory mechanisms. With more severe imbalances, however, medical and nursing interventions are required, because acid-base imbalances are life threatening. Each type of imbalance creates clinical signs and symptoms assessed by the nurse. When providing care to patients/clients with altered fluid, electrolyte, or acid-base balances, the nurse continually monitors for changes in the individual status and uses all components of the nursing process to maintain and restore balance.

## CHAPTER 18 REVIEW

### Key Concepts
- Body fluids are distributed in extracellular and intracellular fluid compartments and are composed of electrolytes, minerals, cells, and water.
- Body fluids are regulated through fluid intake, output, and hormonal regulation.
- Acid-base balance depends on the hydrogen ion concentration in the blood.
- The body's chemical buffering system is the first system to respond to acid-base abnormalities.
- Biological buffering occurs when hydrogen ions are absorbed or released by the cells to compensate for acid-base imbalances.
- Physiological buffering involves compensatory responses in the lungs or kidneys.
- Volume disturbances include isotonic and osmolar fluid volume deficits and excesses.
- Chronic and severe acute illnesses increase the risk of fluid, electrolyte, and acid-base imbalances, and very young or old patients/clients are at risk.
- Assessment for fluid, electrolyte, and acid-base balances includes the nursing history, physical and behavioural assessment, measurements of intake and output, daily weighing, specific laboratory data such as complete blood count and measurement of serum electrolyte levels, specific gravity, and arterial blood gas levels.
- Fluid volume deficits can be corrected by oral or parenteral administration of fluid.
- Complications of intravenous therapy include extravasation, phlebitis, fluid overload, and bleeding at the infusion site.
- Blood transfusions replace fluid volume loss resulting from haemorrhage, treat anaemia, and replace coagulation factors.
- Administration of blood or blood products requires the nurse to follow specific guidelines to prevent transfusion reactions.
- The risks of transfusion include transfusion reactions, hyperkalaemia, hypocalcaemia, circulatory overload, and blood-borne infections.
- Respiratory acidosis is characterized by increased carbon dioxide concentration, excess carbonic acid, and increased hydrogen ion concentration.
- Respiratory alkalosis is characterized by decreased carbon dioxide and hydrogen ion concentrations.
- Metabolic acidosis is characterized by a rise in hydrogen ion concentration.
- Metabolic alkalosis is characterized by a decrease in hydrogen ion concentration.
- The goals of therapy for acid-base imbalances are treatment of the underlying illness and restoration of the arterial pH to normal.

### CRITICAL THINKING EXERCISES

1. Mrs. Jay, 76 years old, has been visited by the community psychiatric nurse on the request of Mrs Jay's General Practicioner. Since being widowed 2 months ago Mrs Jay has become increasingly withdrawn. Her daugher believes that Mrs Jay has not been eating properly or drinking adequately for the past 9 days or so. What are the immediate health concerns associated with fluid and electrolyte balance for Mrs Jay?

2. Mr. Mason is receiving intravenous fluids. He complains that his right arm hurts just above the IV insertion site. The nurse finds that the IV site is warmer than the surrounding skin and the vein is reddened. Based on these findings, which complication has Mr. Mason developed? What is the most appropriate nursing intervention?

3. After a blood transfusion is started, the patient/client complains of back and chest pain. His blood pressure has dropped from 130/80 mm Hg to 100/40 mm Hg. What should the nurse do?

## Key Terms

## REFERENCES

Aaronson L, Seaman L: Managing hypernatremia in fluid deficient elderly, *J Gerontol Nurs* 15(7):29, 1989.

Gröer, MW: *Physiology and pathophysiology of the body fluids,* St Louis, 1981, Mosby.

Gröer M, Shekleton M: *Basic pathophysiology: a holistic approach,* ed 3, St Louis, 1989, Mosby.

Guyton AC: *Textbook of medical physiology,* ed 7, Philadelphia, 1986, WB Saunders.

Kim MJ, McFarland GK, McLane AM: *Pocket guide to nursig diagnoses,* ed 4, St Louis, 1989, Mosby.

Kokko J, Tannen R: *Fluids and electrolytes,* ed 2, Philadelphia, 1990, WB Saunders.

LaRocca J, Otto S: *Pocket guide to intravenous therapy,* St Louis, 1989, Mosby.

MacDonald NJ et al: Hypernatraemic dehydration in patients in a large hospital for the mentally handicapped, *BMJ* 229:1426, 1989.

Messner RL, Gorse GJ: Nursing management of peripheral intravenous sites, *Focus Crit Care* 14(2):25, 1987.

Metheny NM, editor: *Fluid and electrolyte balance: nursing considerations,* Philadelphia, 1987, Lippincott.

Metheny NM, editor: *Fluid and electrolyte balance: nursing considerations,* ed 2, Philadelphia, 1992, Lippincott.

Metheny NM, Snively WD Jr: *Nurse's handbook of fluid balance,* ed 4, Philadelphia, 1983, Lippincott.

Millar J: Intravenous therapy in fluid and electrolyte imbalance, *Prof Nurs* 4(5):237, 1989.

Patrick ML *et al*: *Medical-surgical nursing: pathophysiological concepts,* Philadelphia, 1986, Lippincott

Porth CM: *Pathophysiology: concepts of altered health status,* Philadelphia, 1986, Lippincott.

Querin J, Stahl L: Twelve simple sensible steps for successful blood transfusions, *Nurse 83* 13:34, 1983.

Riddle I: Fluid balance in infants and children. In Metheney N: *Fluid and electrolyte balance: nursing considerations,* ed 2, Philadephia, 1992, Lippincott.

Silvestri A, Masoorli S: PICC lines: a new dimension in home health care, *J Home Health Care Practice* 2(4):1, 1990.

## FURTHER READING

### Adult Nursing

Dougherty L: Intravenous therapy, *Surg Nurs* 10, 1992.

Eisenberg P, Howard R, Gianino M: Improved long-term maintenance of central venous catheters with a new dressing technique, *J Intravenous Nurs* 13(5):279, 1990.

Feldstein A: Detect phlebitis and infiltration, *Nurs* 86(16):44, 1986.

Felver L, Pendarvis J: Electrolyte imbalances, *AORN J* 49(4):991, 1989.

Gatford JD: Nursing calculations, ed 2, Edinburgh, 1987, Churchill Livingstone.

Goodinson S: The risks of IV therapy, *Prof Nurs,* 5(5*):235*, 1990.

Hahn K: Monitoring a blood transfusion, *Nurs 89* 19:20, 1989.

Hecker J: Improved technique in IV therapy, *Nurs Times* 84(34):28-33,1988.

Hecker J: Potential for extending survival of peripheral intravenous infusions, *BMJ* 304: 619, 1992.

Horne M, Heitz U, Swearingen P: *Fluid, electrolyte, and acid-base balance: a case study approach,* St Louis, 1991, Mosby.

Klass K: Troubleshooting central line complications, *Nurs* 87(17):58, 1987.

Keenlyside D: Every little detail counts: infection control in IV therapy, *Prof Nurs,* 7(4): 226, 1992.

McLaughlin M, Kassirer J: Rational treatment of acid base disorders, *Drugs* 39(6):841, 1990.

McVicar A, Clancy, J: Which infusate do I need? Physiological basis of fluid therapy, *Prof Nurs,* 7(9): 586, 1992.

O'Neill P et al: Reduced survival with increasing plasma osmolality in elderly continuing-care patients, *Age Aging,* 19:68, 1990.

Sommers M: Rapid fluid resuscitation, *Nurs 90* 20(1): 52, 1990.

### Children's Nursing

Auroe S: Parental Involvement in intravenous therapy, *Nurs Times.* 85(9):42, 1989.

Ellis J: Let parents give the care: IV therapy at home in cystic fibrosis. In Glasper A, editor: *Child care ,* London, 1991, Wolfe Publishing.

Finberg L et al: *Water and electroytes in paediatrics,* Philadelphia, 1982, WB Saunders Co.

Leuine M, editor: *Jolly's disease of children,* London, 1991, Blackwell Scientific Publishers.

McClaren, Burman: *Textbook of paediatric nutrition,* Edinburgh, 1982, Churchill Livingstone.

Sacharin R: *Principles of paediatric nursing,* Edinburgh, 1986, Churchill Livingstone.

### Learning Disabilities Nursing

Kennedy M: Solving the nutritional problems of people with a mental handicap, *BDA Adviser,* Summer, 1990.

### Mental Health Nursing

Boyd MA *et al*: A target weight procedure for disordered water balance in long-term care facilities, *J Psychosocial Nurse Ment Health Serv,* 30 (12): 22, 1992.

Cosgray R *et al*: A program for water-intoxicated patients at a state hospital, *Clinical Nurse Specialist,* 7 (2): 55-61, 1993.

Davidhizar R, Kriesl R: Water intoxication: one nursing staff's response and intervention, *JAN,* 18 (12): 1975-80, 1993.

Field WE Jr: Physical causes of depression, *J Psychosocial Nurse Ment Health Serv,* 23 (10): 6-11, 1985.

Prim RG: Water intoxication and psychosis sydnrome... clinical cautions, *J Psychosocial Nurse Ment Health Serv,* 26 (11): 16-8, 1988.

# Safety and the Prevention of Accidents

## CHAPTER OUTLINE

**Environmental Safety**
*Basic needs*
*Reducing physical hazards*
*Reducing transmission of pathogens*
*Pollution control*

**Nursing Process, Safety and Accidents**
*Assessment*
*Planning*
*Implementation*
*Evaluation*

## LEARNING OUTCOMES

After studying this chapter, you should be able to:
- *Define the key terms listed.*
- *Describe how unmet basic physiological needs of oxygen, fluids, nutrition, and compatible temperature can threaten a patient's/client's safety.*
- *Discuss methods to reduce the risk of physical hazards and accidents in the health care setting and at home.*
- *Describe current methods to reduce the transmission of pathogens and parasites.*
- *Describe three types of pollutant and identify methods of pollution control.*
- *Discuss aspects of safety and accidents, and potential risk factors related to developmental age.*
- *Suggest methods of reducing the specific safety risks for patients/clients from each developmental age group.*
- *Give examples of risks in a health care setting and suggest preventive measures.*
- *Develop a care plan for patients/clients whose safety is threatened.*
- *Describe nursing interventions specific to the patient's/client's age for reducing the risk of falls, fires, poisonings and electrical hazards.*
- *Describe examples of the nurse's contribution to reducing accidents.*

Nursing care directed at the maintenance of health and the prevention of ill health involves promoting patient/client safety in the health care setting, at home and elsewhere in the community. It is just as essential as meeting other physiological and psychosocial needs. Safety and the prevention of accidents are basic to survival, and these needs continue throughout life. Prevention and reduction of accidents is an aim throughout the UK and this emphasis helps to reduce injury and death.

Defined broadly, an **environment** is all of the many physical and psychosocial factors that influence or affect the life and survival of the patient/client. A safe health care environment reduces the length of treatment or the length of stay in hospital, the frequency of treatment-related accidents, the number of work-related injuries to personnel, and the overall cost of health care services (Hobbs *et al*, 1979). In addition, a safe health care environment allows staff members to function at their optimal levels.

Safety in the home reduces the risk of accidents and illnesses and the subsequent need for health and social care service. Safety and accident prevention is positively correlated to health promotion.

## ENVIRONMENTAL SAFETY

A safe environment is one in which basic needs are achieved, hazards are reduced, transmission of disease carrying pathogens and parasites is reduced, hygiene is maintained, and pollution is controlled.

### Basic Needs
Meeting basic human needs is necessary for achieving safety (see Chapter 7). Frequently, certain physiological needs, including oxygen, temperature and nutrition, influence a person's safety.

### Oxygen
The nurse must be aware of factors in a patient's/client's environment that decrease the amount of available oxygen. One of the most common environmental hazards in the home is a faulty gas appliance such as a gas cooker, fire or central heating

## UK Health Targets
## Accidents

### England
Accidents are the most common cause of death in people under 30 and account for approximately 13% of all years of life lost under age 65 and 7% of NHS expenditure. Priorities for action in England include accidents in the home, at work, on the road, and those involving children (DOH, 1992).

### Scotland
More than 1,100 Scots die in accidents each year. Particular areas of concern are:
- Accidents in the home, which kill more people than road accidents.
- Fires in the home. Scotland's record is 80% higher than England and Wales.
- Road Accidents, which result in large numbers of people killed, as well as serious and minor injuries. (Scottish Office, 1992)

### Northern Ireland
Accidents, mainly caused by road traffic, are the major cause of death and long-term disability in the under 35s. Objectives and targets include:
- By 1997 the annual number of deaths from accidents should be reduced by 15%.
- A regional inter-agency group to promote and monitor accident prevention initiatives. Also a pilot study to monitor the incidence and causation of deaths from accidents.
- Alcohol consumption should be reduced. By 1997 the proportion of 12 -64 year olds drinking more than the recommended limits should be reduced from 33% to 25% for males, and from 11% to 7% for females. (Northern Ireland Office, 1992)

### Wales
Wales has identified injuries as a health priority area and earmarked 6.6% of its 1993/94 NHS expenditure for this category. Particular aims include:
- The achievement of ambulance response standards
- Road safety plans
- First aid training for NHS staff and the public (NHS Cymru Office, 1992).

system. A gas appliance that is not operating properly or is not properly vented introduces carbon monoxide into the environment. Carbon monoxide is a colourless, odourless, poisonous gas produced by the combustion of carbon or organic fuels. **Carbon monoxide** binds strongly with haemoglobin, preventing the formation of oxyhaemoglobin and thus reducing the supply of oxygen delivered to tissues (see Chapter 17). A person who moves to a new residence or who has an old gas appliance should be encouraged to have the system inspected. This inspection is usually performed free of charge or for a nominal fee by the Gas Board. Public buildings such as schools, hospitals, and businesses are required by legislative codes to have periodic appliance inspections to reduce the risk of carbon monoxide poisoning. There is currently pressure for compulsory inspections of all gas appliances in rented living accomodation.

## Temperature

The most comfortable environmental temperature varies among individuals, but the usual comfort range is between 18.3 and 23.9°C. Extremes of temperature, that frequently occur during the winter and summer, affect not only comfort and productivity but also safety.

Exposure to severe cold for prolonged periods causes frostbite and hypothermia. **Hypothermia** occurs when the core body temperature is 35°C or below. The person experiences confusion and a declining level of consciousness, which can result in a coma. Shivering is present in the early stages, and trembling may occur on one side of the body or in one extremity. Ultimately, the patient's/client's vital signs decline, and death ensues.

Older adults, neonates, young babies and patients/clients with spinal cord injuries and diseases of the nervous system (for example, paraplegia and multiple sclerosis) are at a higher risk for hypothermia. Chronic or acute illness increases susceptibility to hypothermia. Similarly, the ingestion of alcohol interferes with temperature regulation and increases the risk for hypothermia.

Exposure to extreme heat can result in **heat exhaustion** or **heatstroke**. In either case the body's electrolyte balance changes, the core body temperature rises, and brain damage results. With heat exhaustion a person has sudden changes in mental status, gastrointestinal distress, and an elevated rectal temperature up to 41.1°C. Heatstroke, the final stage of heat exhaustion, is a life-threatening condition that can lead to hyperpyrexia, coma, abnormal fluid and electrolyte status, hyperpyrexia, and death. The chronically ill, older adults, infants, and the poor are at greatest risk for injury from extreme heat.

## Nutrition

Meeting nutritional needs adequately and safely requires environmental controls and knowledge. In the home, ideally people need a refrigerator and a freezer compartment to keep perishable foods fresh. An adequate, clean water supply is needed to wash fresh produce and dishes. Provision for refuse collection is necessary to maintain hygienic conditions.

Foods that are inadequately prepared or stored increase a person's risk for **food poisoning** (an illness resulting from the ingestion of a food contaminated by toxic substances or by bacteria containing toxins). Symptoms of food poisoning can occur immediately or up to a week after ingestion of the toxic food (Donaldson, 1987). Assessments for suspected food poisoning include obtaining a patient's/client's history, gathering gastrointestinal and central nervous system data, observing for a fever, and analysing laboratory samples of faeces for leucocytes, blood, and *Vibrio* (comma-shaped) organisms. Accurate assessment data are crucial in isolating the type of organism present.

There is considerable legislation concerning the control of food poisoning. Most of it is enforced by local authorities, whose main officials are a Community Physician and the Chief Environmental Health Officer. All doctors have a legal duty under the Public Health Acts of 1936 and 1961 to notify the names and addresses of people recognized as, or suspected of, having certain types of food poisoning (Hobbs and Roberts, 1992).

## Reducing Physical Hazards

Physical hazards in the environment may threaten safety. These hazards can result in a physical injury. Injuries are the leading cause of death for individuals up to 45 years of age (ROSPA, 1989). Between 1981 and 1986, the rate of deaths and major injuries in manufacturing increased by 37%, in the chemical industry by 50.6% and in construction by 43% (DHSS, 1988). Many physical hazards can be minimized through adequate lighting, reduction of obstacles, control of bathroom hazards, and security measures.

## Ensuring Adequate Lighting

Adequate lighting reduces physical hazards by illuminating areas in which people move and work. Outside the home, lighting brightens walkways from the street to the house, from the garage to the house, and on the steps to the front or back door. Inside the house, the halls, staircases, and individual rooms should be adequately lit so that residents can safely carry out activities of daily living. Night-lights in dark halls and bathrooms help maintain safety by reducing the risk of falls. This may be particularly important for older people with age-related sight changes who may experience difficulty in seeing in the dark or in adapting from dark to brightly lit environments. A night-light helps to orientate individuals who may need to get up in the middle of the night. Adequate lighting also helps protect the home and its inhabitants from crime. Well-lit garages, pathways, and doorways discourage intruders from entering the premises or hiding in shadows.

## Decreasing Obstacles

Injuries in the home frequently result from objects on the stairs and floor, wet patches on the floor, and clutter on surfaces such as bedside tables, shelves, the top of the refrigerator, and bookshelves. The risk of injury from obstacles is greatest for older adults. Injury can result from an illness (for example, one that makes a person weak or disorientated), normal changes associated with ageing (due to decreased sensory ability), and medications (DHSS, 1988).

To reduce the risk of injury, all obstacles should be removed from halls and other heavily travelled areas. Necessary objects such as clocks, glasses, tissues, or medications should remain on bedside tables within reach of the patient/client but out of the reach of children. Tables and chairs should be secure and should have stable legs and feet.

Small mats and rugs should be secured with a nonslip pad or skid-resistant adhesive strips. Small rugs and runners should not be used on stairs. Any carpeting on the stairs should be secured with carpet tacks.

## Controlling Bathroom Hazards

Accidents happen frequently in the bathroom. These range from scalds and burns, to accidental poisoning. Care should be taken to lower the thermostat setting on water heaters to reduce the risk of burns and scalds. Secure, easily seen grab bars, and non-slip coloured adhesive tape are useful in reducing accidental falls in the bath (HEA, 1991). Medication in the medicine cabinet should be clearly marked and out of the reach of children, and excess or out-of-date medication should be discarded by returning to the local chemist for safe disposal.

## Security at Home

People should take precautions to secure their homes from intruders. When assessing a person's home for safety, the nurse should advise on the presence and quality of locks on doors and windows. Local police stations have crime prevention officers who are able to visit people at home and provide appropriate advice. Adequate exterior lighting can also reduce the risk of break-ins.

For the patient/client who is moving house, it might help to inquire about the crime rate in the proposed location. Statistics about crime rates can be obtained from the local police station, home insurance companies and local neighbourhood watch schemes. Local crime rates can have a significant impact upon the community, and nurses working with patients/clients in their own home need to be aware of such factors.

The safety of the patient/client and of the community nurse both need to be considered. Nurses visiting patients/clients at home and elsewhere in the community should always tell colleagues where they are going and when they can be expected to return to the work base.

## Reducing Transmission of Pathogens

A **pathogen** is any microorganism capable of producing an illness. A **parasite** is an organism living in or on another organism and obtaining nourishment from it. Pathogens and parasites can be found in water, food, humans and other animals, and insects.

In a health care setting, effective and efficient methods are used to control pathogen transmission, including medical and **surgical asepsis** (see Chapter 28). The transmission of pathogens from person to person can be reduced and in some cases prevented by immunization. **Immunization** is the process by which resistance to an infectious disease is produced or augmented. Immunity is acquired after the oral administration or injection of an **antigen**, which causes the production of an antibody within the body. The body is then immune to the effects of the intended pathogens (DOH, 1992a).

The rising number of cases of acquired immune deficiency syndrome (AIDS) and other sexually transmitted diseases is increasing the public's awareness of pathogen transmission. Safe sexual practices through the correct use of condoms and a decrease in casual sexual activities can reduce the risk of acquiring sexually transmitted diseases.

The human immune deficiency virus (HIV), the pathogen that causes acquired immune deficiency syndrome (AIDS), is also transmitted through intravenous (IV) drug abuse. Drug dependent individuals frequently share syringes and needles, which increases the risk of acquiring AIDS. HIV is blood borne and thus it is transmitted through contaminated syringes and needles. In the community, the risk factors for acquiring HIV and other blood-borne pathogens can be reduced or eliminated by modifying certain illness-causing behaviours. These include the provision of 'needle exchange schemes' (Scottish Office, 1992), providing opportunities and receptacles for the safe disposal and collection of sharps, and for universal precautions to be taken by all health care workers when handling blood and body fluids (DOE, HEA, 1991) (see Chapter 28).

## Food Hygiene

Improperly processed or contaminated food can cause illness and death through transmission of pathogens and parasites (Bassett, 1992). Commercially processed and packaged foods are subject to the Ministry of Agriculture Fisheries and Food (MAFF) regulations and usually contain a minimal amount of contaminants. MAFF is a Government agency responsible for the enforcement of regulations regarding the manufacture, processing, and distribution of food to protect consumers against the sale of impure or dangerous substances.

## Pest Control

Control of fleas and ticks on domestic animals and in the environment reduces the incidence of bites, skin irritations, and disease transmission. The common house fly (*Musca domestica*) and other flies feed on human and animal excreta, as well as on food. Other insects such as cockroaches and beetles are also of public health importance. Insects and flies can transfer pathogenic organisms to food, either mechanically on their feet, via their faeces or by regurgitation as part of their feeding process.

Rodents also transmit pathogens. The rat most frequently encountered in the United Kingdom is the brown rat (*Rattus norvegicus*), sometimes called the water or sewer rat. Rats and mice destroy animal and human foodstuffs and can spread disease. A rat or mouse may appear to be symptomless but may excrete types of salmonellae bacteria known to infect humans. Although these organisms are sensitive to penicillin, the best approach to controlling rat and mice infestation is prevention. This is achieved by eliminating the opportunity for rats and mice to access foodstuffs and waste, as well as controlling the rodent population through pesticides (Hobbs *et al*, 1992).

## Disposal of Human Waste

Transmission of pathogens is also controlled by adequate disposal of human waste through proper construction and repair of sewers and drains. Without a satisfactory sewer and waste system, the population is at risk for illnesses transmitted by human faeces (for example, typhoid fever and hepatitis).

## Pollution Control

A healthy environment is free of pollution. A **pollutant** is a harmful chemical or waste material discharged into the water or air. People commonly think of pollution only in terms of air or water pollution, but noise can also be a form of pollution that presents health risks (Ashton, 1993).

**Air pollution** is the contamination of the atmosphere. Prolonged exposure to air pollution increases the risk of pulmonary disease. In urban areas, industrial waste and vehicle exhaust are common contributors to air pollution. In the home, school, or workplace, cigarette smoke is the primary cause of air pollution. Environmental pollution can also be caused by improper disposal of radioactive and bioactive waste products such as dioxin.

**Water pollution** is the contamination of lakes, rivers, and streams, by industrial, agricultural or other pollutants. Water-treatment facilities filter harmful contaminants from the water, but these systems often contain flaws. If water exiting the treatment facility becomes contaminated, the public is notified to boil water used for drinking and cooking. Flooding can also damage water-treatment stations, thus requiring drinking and cooking water to be boiled.

**Noise pollution** occurs when the noise level becomes uncomfortable to the inhabitants of that environment. Noise levels are measured in units of sound intensity called **decibels**. Noise level tolerances vary from one individual to another and are influenced by health status. A high noise level can produce hearing loss over time. If the noise level is maintained or the person does not use earplugs, complete deafness can result.

A health care setting such as an intensive care unit can also be polluted by noise (Hinds, 1987). The sounds of machines, people talking, and intercoms can create increased noise levels. Even when the noise level is not high enough to affect hearing acuity, it may produce a syndrome called **sensory overload**. Sensory overload is a marked increase in the intensity of auditory and visual stimuli. It disrupts processing of information and problem-solving and can increase anxiety, paranoia, hallucinations, depression, and unrealistic feelings.

Pollution impairs the level of health of all those exposed to it. A nurse assessing a patient's/client's environment may be the first to recognize the potential threat to the individual and family.

## NURSING PROCESS, SAFETY AND ACCIDENTS

 ASSESSMENT

Nurses can help identify risks to an individual's safety, whether in the health care setting, at home or elsewhere in the community. Assessment of individual need can reveal clusters of data that indicate when a patient/client has an actual or potential risk of accidents.

Assessment also includes considering information that identifies the total population at risk. The Office of Population Census and Surveys provides national data on the morbidity and mortality rates caused by accidents. This data can then be used locally to target specific 'at-risk' groups. In addition, statistical information provides a basis for changing working practice so that it can more adequately reflect patients'/clients' needs.

## Risk Factors in Developmental Age Groups

Threats to safety within the community are influenced by developmental stage, lifestyle habits, mobility status, sensory impairments, and safety awareness. These have been outlined in the health targets for the four UK countries.

**Children's Nursing**
**Activities to preventing accidents in children of different ages**

**Babies and Infants in the First Year of Life**

- Practise safety in cars
- Practise safety on parents' bicycles
- Provide stair and fire guards in the home
- Remove sharp and dangerous items to places out of reach

**Children Aged 1 to 4 Years**

- Provide road safety training for children and parents
- Store medicines and poisonous substances safely, use child-resistant medicine containers
- Use child liaison services between hospital and community services
- Ensure playgrounds are a safe environment
- Educate parents about risks, such as plastic bags, inappropriate toys, baby walkers
- Install safety glass or film in patio doors
- Install smoke alarms in the home
- Use child-proof car door locks
- Use clothing reflectors

**School Children (5 to 14 Years)**

- Provide road safety and cycle training for unaccompanied children
- Ensure adequate coaching and training for sports and leisure activities
- Teach first aid and resuscitation skills
- Teach correct use of seat belts and cars
- Teach use of cycle helmets and clothing reflectors
- Encourage traffic clubs
- Teach daily living skills in kitchens and the use of appliances
- Provide safety education within the school curriculum
- Teach children to swim and teach 'water safety'
- Teach fire safety

  Useful addresses:
  Child Accident Prevention Trust
  Clark's Court
  18-20 Farringdon Lane
  London EC1R 3AU

  Royal Society for the Prevention of Accidents
  Cannon House
  The Priory
  Queensway
  Birmingham B4 6BS

*Adapted from Department of Health: The Health of the Nation: A Strategy for Health in England, HMSO, London, 1992.*

## CHILDREN UNDER 15 YEARS

Road traffic accidents, scalds and burns, drowning and suffocation are the major causes of death for this age group. Most fatal accidents to children up to the age of four occur in the home. Road traffic accidents account for most fatalities in children over five years of age, usually the child is a pedestrian. Nearly twice as many boys as girls die as a result of accidents (Avery, 1992).

Accidents involving children are largely preventable, but frequently parents need to be shown the specific dangers by nurses, health visitors, school nurses and other health care professionals. As the infant grows, accident potential increases. The newborn's **accident potential** is influenced by people or external agents, but growth and the acquisition of new motor skills place the active child at risk for injuries. Accident prevention thus requires health education for parents and removal of dangers whenever possible (see box).

When a child enters school, the environment expands to include the school, transportation to and from school, school friends, and after-school activities. Each of these is a potential threat to the child's safety. Injuries can be minor (falling and bruising the knee), or major (breaking an arm while playing football). Through discussions and examples, parents, teachers, and nurses can teach the child to cross the street safely, choose suitable foods to eat, brush his or her teeth, and perform other hygiene measures.

Since school-aged children participate in more activities outside their home, they are at greater risk of injury from strangers. Therefore, the child should be warned repeatedly not to accept sweets, food, gifts, or lifts from strangers. In addition, a child needs to know what to do if approached by a stranger. Nurses can work with schools or neighbourhoods to initiate health education and teaching in order to provide information both for parents and their children.

Sports safety is stressed in school sports, but parents and health professionals can reinforce these safety tips by insisting that children wear protective gear while participating in sports in the home. For example, schools should be encouraged to promote the use of helmets for cricket games, and parents should also provide this equipment when children are playing in their own homes and gardens.

Bicycle safety is an important issue for nurses and parents. Injury to the central nervous system (CNS) is the primary cause of death in 90% of childhood fatalities from bicycle or pedestrian collision with a motor vehicle. Recent studies have demonstrated that the risk of head injuries to bicyclists could be reduced by 80% if bicyclists wore proper safety helmets (Bartlett, 1991).

## YOUNG ADULTS AGED 15-24

As children enter adolescence, they develop greater independence and begin to develop a sense of identity and their own values. In addition, adolescents begin to separate emotionally from their families and become more influenced by peer groups.

The struggle towards identity may cause the teenager to experience shyness, fear, and anxiety, with resulting problems at home, school, or within the peer group. Substances, such as drugs and alcohol, may make the world more bearable for the troubled teenager, but put the adolescent at a high risk for continued alcohol or drug dependence.

Drowning is one of the largest categories of fatal leisure accidents. Swimming and water sports all play a significant role. Alcohol and drugs increase the frequency of these accidents due to the affect on the CNS (DHSS, 1988).

When adolescents learn to drive, their environment expands

and so does their potential for injury. The young driver must be taught to comply with the Highway Code. Road traffic accidents are the single largest cause of accidental death in young adults; nearly 50% of deaths in men and 30% of deaths in women in the 15-to-24 year age group are as a result of an accident. **Risk-taking behaviour,** combined with lack of experience, and the use of alcohol or drugs are significant factors in accident causation in this group (DOH, 1993a).

Since adolescence is a time when mature sexual physical characteristics develop, adolescents also begin to have physical relationships with other people. They need prompt, correct instruction about safe sexual practices and birth control. They also need counselling about peer pressure. Specifically, the nurse must determine how teenagers handle constant pressure to participate in sexual or drug-related activities. Many schools have education programmes for teenagers about sexual health and drug and alcohol misuse.

## ADULTS

The threats to an adult's safety are frequently related to **lifestyle habits**. For example, someone who uses alcohol excessively has a greater risk of having a car accident. A long-term smoker has a greater risk of cardiovascular or pulmonary disease from inhaling smoke into the lungs and from the effect of nicotine on the circulatory system. Similarly, an adult experiencing a high level of stress is more likely to have an accident or illnesses such as headaches, gastrointestinal disorders, and infections.

## PEOPLE AGED 65 YEARS AND OVER

Falls and road traffic accidents cause most of the accidental deaths in this age group. Although accidents are not a major cause of death compared to other causes in this age group, the death rate from accidents in people over 75 years is considerably greater than in any other age group. Accidents, such as falls, are an important cause of disability and the need for health and social services. In the over 75 years age group in England in 1991, falls were responsible for 67% of the female accidental deaths and 52% of the male accidental deaths (DOH, 1993a).

Accidents in people over 65 years old account for only 12.5% of all home accidents, but 64% of all fatalities are women. Falls, and their resulting injuries can have environmental, physiological and psychological repercussions, and these should be acknowledged as risk factors in the older person (Tideiksarr, 1989) (see box).

## OTHER RISK FACTORS

Other risk factors in the community include lifestyle, mobility, sensory impairments, and safety awareness.

**Lifestyle** Lifestyle can increase safety risks. At greater risk of injury are people who drive or operate machinery while under the influence of chemical substances, who work at inherently dangerous jobs, and who are risk-takers. In addition, people experiencing stress, anxiety, fatigue, alcohol, drug withdrawal or who are taking prescribed medications may be more accident prone. Because of these factors, individuals may be too

---

### Physiological Changes that Increase the Risk of Falls

- Arthritic changes affecting range of motion, balance, and weight bearing
- Decreased circulation in the brain, causing dizziness and fainting
- Mechanical obstruction of vertebral arteries to the brain, caused by crushed osteoporotic vertebrae
- Decreased auditory acuity
- Decreased night vision, colour vision, and visual acuity
- Orthostatic hypotension
- Loss of sense of position
- Diminished space perception
- Decreased muscle mass, strength, and coordination or hemiparesis or hemiparalysis
- Decreased ability to balance
- Osteoporosis and increased stress on weight-bearing areas, resulting in an unsteady gait and susceptibility to fractures
- Decreased muscle activity necessary for adequate venous return
- Decreased capacity of blood vessels
- Slowed nervous system response
- Changes in metabolism, which affect the rate of drug metabolism and the systemic effects of medications

*Modified from Tideiksarr R: Geriatr Nurs 116:280, 1989; and Witte NS: AM J Nurs 79:1950, 1979.*

---

preoccupied to notice the source of potential accidents, such as cluttered stairs or a stop sign.

**Mobility** An individual with impaired mobility has many kinds of safety risk. First, immobilization itself can predispose the person to other physiological and emotional hazards, which in turn can further restrict mobility and independence (see Chapter 24). A patient/client with impaired mobility is at risk for injury when entering motor vehicles and buildings that are not equipped for people with a disability.

**Sensory Impairment** Patients/clients with visual, hearing, or communication impairments, such as aphasia, learning difficulties, or language barriers, are at greater risk for injury in the community. Such patients/clients may not be aware of the potential danger of a situation or express the need for assistance (see Chapter 26).

**Safety Awareness** Some individuals are unaware of safety precautions, such as keeping medicine away from children or reading the expiry date on food products. A complete nursing assessment should help the nurse identify the patient's/client's level of knowledge regarding home safety, so deficiencies can be corrected with an individualized nursing care plan.

### Risks in the Health Care Environment

Institutions and formal health care settings are bound by legislation to ensure that a safe environment is maintained, to protect both the patient/client and the health care worker (HSE, 1974; COSHH, 1988). The basic types of risks to a person's safety within the health care environment are falls, procedure-

### Learning Disabilities Nursing
### The need to enable people to take risks

It was a characteristic of institutional care that people with a learning disability were so insulated from danger that any risk to them or the people who cared for them was regarded as unacceptable. Consequently, policies and procedures were established in these institutions which inhibited opportunities for individuals to learn and develop to their full potential, thereby increasing the impoverishment of their lives.

A distinction must be made between the sort of risk that it is sensible to expose people to and the sort of risk that is not sensible, due to the probability of injury being sustained. An example of unacceptable risk would be to allow an attractive but naive 19-year-old woman with a moderate learning disability to go out to a pub or night club alone. A calculated risk might be to allow a patient/client with well-managed epilepsy and good self-help skills to bath in privacy, so long as staff or carers are aware the patient/client is using the bathroom and check at regular intervals, by knocking on the door, that the patient/client is not in any difficulty.

**The assessment of acceptable risk**
In essence, 'risk management' implies the use of a process whereby risks are identified, categorized and addressed before any activities that engender potential risks are undertaken.

It is essential to remember that what is 'safe' for a person of average mental ability may be an undertaking of entirely different proportions for someone whose mental abilities are significantly less. Crossing a busy road safely, for example, requires the ability to process a complex range of cognitive, motor, and spatial information prior to taking action.

**Minimizing risks**
The skills involved in minimizing risk involve establishing the nature of that risk. If the risk results in serious injury to the individual (such as being hit by a car when crossing a road) our efforts are directed at reducing that risk, through patient/client education, systemic training and graduated exposure to potentially risky situations. In this example, begin by teaching the individual to cross quiet roads. The same principles apply in other practical situations, such as preparing and cooking food. Rather than trying to avoid exposing the individual to any risk, graduated exposure to the dangerous elements of the activity, such as working with sharp knives or hot liquids, provides an acceptable approach to balancing the patient's/client's needs with the nurse's responsibilities.

In all situations, a planned and thoughtful approach to risk is the one that is most efficacious. At each stage in the process of learning to manage and master activities of daily living, there needs to be built-in, fail-safe criteria to ensure that the person with a learning disability does not become exposed to unreasonable and foreseeable harm.

---

problem areas and to take steps to prevent or minimize accidents.

If an accident occurs in the health care environment an **incident report** must be filed. This is a confidential document that completely describes any patient/client accident occurring within the health care setting (see Chapter 13). It documents the accident, any reactions by or effects on the patient/client, and treatment performed for him or her. In addition to completing the incident report, the nurse must document the accident in the patient's/client's nursing notes and ensure that the patient/client is seen by a doctor. The Merseyside Accident Information Model (Troup *et al*, 1988) provides a framework for recording accidents in the work place.

## FALLS

Falls result from slipping or sliding, knees buckling under, fainting, or tripping over tubes, equipment, or furniture. A person can fall from the bed, wheelchair, toilet or commode, or can fall while walking. The occurrence of falls in the health care setting increases during the evening and night.

When delivering nursing care in the home, the nurse must also assess this environment for risk of falls. The assessment and subsequent prevention of falls reduces the chance of further physical impairment to the patient/client. In addition, family members and friends are also protected from injury. The prevention of injury to the primary care giver in the home also reduces the chance of future hospitalization of the patient/client.

## PROCEDURE-RELATED ACCIDENTS

A **procedure-related accident** occurs while care is being undertaken. They include medication and fluid administration errors, improper application of external devices, and accidents related to improper performance of procedures, such as dressing changes.

Nurses can prevent many procedure-related accidents. For example, correct administration of medications, following local policy will help to prevent medication errors (see Chapter 31). Also, injury from the introduction of pathogens is reduced when surgical asepsis is used for sterile dressing changes (see Chapter 29) or invasive procedures, such as insertion of a Foley catheter (see Chapter 22). Finally, correct use of body mechanics and transfer techniques reduces the risk of injuries from lifting and handling procedures (see Chapter 24).

## EQUIPMENT-RELATED ACCIDENTS

**Equipment-related accidents** result from the malfunction, disrepair or misuse of equipment, or from an electrical hazard. To avoid injury, the nurse should not operate monitoring or therapy equipment without instruction.

### Reducing Ill-Health, Disability and Death from Accidents

Accident prevention and reduction is one of the key strategies within in the UK Health Targets. The contribution of nurses, midwives and health visitors in reducing and preventing accidents is outlined and summarized here (see box).

---

related accidents, and equipment-related accidents. The nurse learns to recognize factors associated with these three potential

## Adult Nursing
### Assessing the environment to prevent falls in older adults

### Home Exterior

Are pavements and floors uneven?
Are steps in good repair?
Do stairs and steps have handrails?
Is there adequate lighting?

### Home Interior

Is there sufficient light?
Do rugs and mats have non-slip backings?
Are rooms free of obstacles?
Do chairs and stools provide sufficient support for sitting down and getting up?
Is the temperature within a comfortable range?
Are there any trailing leads or flexes.

### Stairs

Are stairways well lit?
Are steps and carpets in good repair?
Are step edges easy to see?
Are handrails available and in good repair?

### Kitchens

If there is a gas stove is it in good repair?
Are storage areas easily reached without stretching?
Are floors slippery?
Is there adequate light?

### Bathrooms

Is there a mat or skid-proof strip in the bath or shower?
Is the bath or shower easy to get in and out of?
Is the toilet easy to sit on or get off?
Are there handrails?
Is the medicine cabinet within reach without stretching?

### Bedrooms

Is there adequate lighting?
Are beds of an adequate height to allow for getting in and out of easily?
Are rugs and mats well anchored?
Are night lights available?
Are light switches accessible?

Modified from: Tideiksaar R: Home safe home: practical tips for fall-proofing, *Geriatr Nurs* 11(6):280, 1989.

## Children's Nursing
### Guidelines for A & E departments

Accidental injuries are a major cause of presentation to the Accident and Emergency department among children. The British Paediatric Association has set the following minimum requirements for children in A & E:

* separate waiting area with play facilities
* separate treatment area suitably decorated and equipped
* private room for distressed parents
* a consultant paediatrician to have responsibility with the consultant in A & E medicine concerning general arrangements for children
* a liaison health visitor to facilitate communication between the department and the community

It is also strongly recommended that there is a children's nurse among the staff, preferably one on each shift.

 PLANNING

The nurse plans therapeutic interventions for patients/clients with actual or potential risks to safety. Nursing care plans should to be written to meet the needs of the individuals according to his or her developmental stage, level of health, and home environment on discharge from the health care setting. Nursing activity should be planned in partnership with the patient/client and should reflect their need to maintain independence (see sample care plan).

 IMPLEMENTATION

Nursing interventions are directed at maintaining the patient's/client's safety in the health care setting, home and elsewhere in the community. Most nursing interventions are applicable in all environments and therefore should include developmental considerations and environmental protection.

The first category of interventions includes those specifically for reducing risks for each developmental age group. Environmental interventions are developed to modify the environment so that present or potential hazards are eliminated or minimized.

## Reducing Risks in Developmental Age Groups

### CHILDREN UNDER 15 YEARS

Infants and pre-school children depend upon adults to protect them from injury. Growing children are curious and completely trusting of their environment and do not perceive themselves to be in danger. Safety should be an important subject of discussion during home visits (HEA, 1991; Moore, 1992). Colver and Pearson (1985) also point out the need for families on a low income to have access to financial sources in order to purchase safety equipment, such as stair gates and cooker guards.

Nurses, midwives and health visitors working in the community can assess the home, show parents how to promote safety in the home, and teach the child and the parents about safety. Nurses working in parent craft classes and antenatal clinics can easily incorporate safety into the care plan of prospective parents.

School children increasingly explore their environment. They have friends outside their immediate neighbourhood, they may walk to school, and they become more active in school and community activities. All of these activities help the child develop social skills and independence, but they also increase the risk of injury, such as falls from playground equipment and sports injuries. Some children also die from drowning. The school-aged child may also begin to associate with activities undertaken by adults including parents, teachers, and often television heroes. This pattern of behaviour and activities is not necessarily a threat to the child, except when the child imitates adult behaviour that presents safety risks (for example, operating an electric saw).

Bicycle accidents and resultant head injuries are a major cause of death and disability in children. This is one example where

## Care Plan

Nursing Assessment: Mrs Jones, aged 75 years. Home assessment in relation to risk of falls.

| Assessment | Care Plan | Expected Outcome |
|---|---|---|
| **Medication** – verapamil – Risk of falls due to hypotension | 1. Ensure that Mrs Jones understands the effects and the possible side effects, such as postural hypotension | 1. Mrs Jones will understand the possible side effects of her medication |
| | 2. Teach her to stand up slowly and to ensure that she feels safe when standing | 2. Mrs Jones will get up slowly from a sitting or standing position |
| | 3. Discuss the need for a regular review of the medication and monitoring of blood pressure | 3. Mrs Jones will attend the GP for regular review of her medication |
| **Obstacles in the home:** Rugs and mats Trailing flexes | 1. Indicate to her where mats and rugs are at risk of slipping | 1. Rugs and mats will be secured where possible with non-slip under mat and/or velcro strips |
| | 2. Identify torn and frayed mats | 2. Worn and frayed mats and rugs will be removed and replaced |
| | 3. Show Mrs Jones where there are risks of falling over trailing flexes | 3. Trailing flexes will be re-routed around the outside of the room and away from traversed floors |
| | 4. Ask relatives to assist with removal and replacement | |
| **Lighting** | 1. Suggest lighting should be improved and brighter bulbs installed | Stairs and steps will be well lit with a 100 watt bulb |
| | 2. Arrange for a relative or neighbour to replace the bulbs | |
| **Eye sight** | 1. Remind Mrs Jones of the need for an annual eye test and help to arrange an appointment with a domiciliary optician | Mrs Jones will attend the optician yearly for eye checks and new glasses |
| **Footwear** – Loose-fitting, canvas shoes | 1. Advise Mrs Jones on the need for well-fitting, rubber soled shoes that support the foot and ankle | Mrs Jones will wear shoes that are well-fitting, support her ankle and have rubber or non-slip soles |
| **Reduced exercise due to poor mobility** | 1. Teach active leg and ankle movements to be undertaken when she is in bed or sitting down | Mrs Jones will undertake passive leg and ankle movement where possible |

## Adult Nursing
## Activities to prevent/reduce patient/client accidents at home

- Provide advice and training in avoiding hazards
- Review medication regularly and suggest its discontinuation unless absolutely necessary
- Assess and refer for specialist equipment and adaptations to the environment
- Notify appropriate agencies where pavements and roads may be hazardous or contain obstacles
- Encourage appropriate mobility and flexibility exercises
- Undertake home safety checks as part of health assessment
- Include home safety advice as part of health assessments
- Provide advice on financial benefits in order to ensure that claims are made towards heating and essential home safety needs

Modified From Department of Health: *The Health of the Nation: Key* Area Handbook — Accidents, London, HMSO, 1993.

nurses can identify trends and collaborate with parents, teachers, the police and other agencies to minimize the risk of accidents.

## YOUNG ADULTS AGED 15 TO 24 YEARS

Adolescents spend much of their time away from home and with their peer group. During adolescence, young people learn to drive. Risks to the adolescent's safety therefore involve many factors outside the home environment. Adults serve as role models for adolescents and, through example and education, can help adolescents minimize risks to their safety.

Adolescents' adjustment to responsibilities and changes in their bodies may result in mood swings, withdrawal, or depression. In addition, this age group has a high incidence of suicide because of depression, poor body image, or feelings of decreased self-worth (Bee and Mitchel, 1984). The UK health strategies (eg. DOH, 1992b) provide targets for reducing the number of deaths from suicide by approximately 15% by the year 2000.

Suicide has a devastating effect because family members are left with feelings of loss, anger, guilt, inadequacy, and pain. Nurses can provide emotional support to these families and refer them to counsellors and support groups.

## ADULTS

Risks to adults frequently result from **lifestyle factors** such as child rearing, high levels of stress, inadequate nutrition, excessive alcohol intake, and substance abuse. Adults need to be taught that their safety is threatened and as a result their lifestyle needs to be modified.

Stress-management (see Chapter 10) and health-promotion (see Chapter 9) are incorporated into many hospital and community service programmes. In addition, neighbourhood centres, community clinics, and outpatient clinics are equipped to assist the adult in modifying lifestyle habits that present risks to health (for example, smoking, overeating, lack of exercise, and alcohol and drug dependence). Provision is also made within the General Practitioner Contract legislation for GPs and practice nurses to undertake health promotion activities with specific groups of clients (Huntington, 1991; UKCC, 1990).

## The Nurse's Contribution to Reducing the Risk of Accidents

### Contribute to Changing Behaviour

- Identify the population at risk by examining national and local data as well as including accident prevention in individual patient/client assessments.
- Provide roadshows, health promotion leaflets and posters in public places, including day centres and nurseries, schools, youth clubs, luncheon clubs, social centres for older people, health centres, libraries and A & E departments.
- Design and develop better literature, including literature that is translated into different languages and use the media to communicate the message of accident prevention to a wide range of people.

### Contribute to Changing Practice

- Provide information to staff and colleagues on accident prevention.
- Become involved in research to determine what influences risk behaviour in relation to accidents.
- Evaluate the success of individual and group campaigns, use statistical information by auditing trends in accidents in different age groups, define the need for new services or adapt current services to meet local needs.
- Provide safety and first aid courses for local people.
- Appoint specialist nurses to identify the cause of accidents and address the need for prevention.

### Contribute to Changing the Environment

- Take a prominent role in multi-agency accident prevention strategies.
- Liaise with local agencies to highlight potential causes of accidents and the need for action.
- Increase awareness in the local population and empower action among local pressure groups, such as residents' associations.

Modified from: Department of Health: Health of the nation. *Targeting practice: the contribution of nurses, midwives and health visitors*, London, 1993 DOH.

## PEOPLE AGED 65 YEARS AND OVER

Most injuries to the older adult involve falls, car accidents, and burns. Advancing age and the concurrent physiological changes in vision, hearing, mobility, circulation, and the ability to make quick judgements may predispose some older adults to falls and other accidents. In addition, many medications make falls more likely (DHSS, 1988). Nursing interventions designed to reduce the risk of falls may compensate for the physiological changes of ageing.

Pedestrian accidents can also be reduced by persuading older adults to wear reflectors on garments when walking at night, to stand on the pavement and not in the road when waiting to cross, to cross with the traffic light and not against it, and to look right, left and right again before entering the road or pedestrian crossing.

Burns and scalds are also more likely to occur with older people as the sensation for heat may be reduced. Impaired visual acuity and sense of smell increase the danger that older people may not detect smoke or gas fumes (Cooper, 1981).

### Environmental Considerations

#### GENERAL PREVENTIVE MEASURES

Nurses can contribute to a safer environment by helping the patient/client meet basic physiological and psychosocial needs. Nurses use effective and efficient methods to control pathogen transmission. These include medical asepsis, the use of hand washing and environmental cleanliness to reduce the number of pathogens, and surgical asepsis, the removal or destruction of disease-causing organisms or infected material (see Chapter 28). Pathogen transmission from person to person can be reduced or prevented by immunization. In the home, awareness of methods of food handling helps reduce the risk of pathogen and parasite transmission through contaminated food.

#### SPECIFIC SAFETY CONCERNS

Specific safety concerns include falls, fires, poisoning, electrical hazards, and radiation.

**Falls** Modifications in the home or health care setting, as discussed earlier, can easily reduce the risk of falls. A heavy or debilitated patient/client in a bed or wheelchair or on a toilet should be properly secured or supported. Excess furniture and equipment should be removed, and patients/clients should wear rubber-soled shoes or slippers for walking or transferring from one device to another. Patients/clients need to be taught to inspect sticks, frames, and crutches to ensure that the rubber tip is intact.

**Fires** The home and hospital are always at risk for fires and there is currently a great deal of scope for a substantial reduction in the numbers that occur (Scottish Office, 1992). Accidental home fires typically result from smoking in bed, careless extinguishing of cigarettes, or electrical fires resulting from faulty wiring or appliances. Institutional fires typically result from a patient/client smoking in bed or from an electrical or anaesthetic gases-related fire (COI, 1987).

The following interventions are directed towards fires occurring in health care settings, but the same principles apply for fires in the home. It is important to have a plan of action in the event of fire. Local procedures will differ, but the general principles are presented below.

If a fire occurs in a health care setting, the nurse should:
- protect clients from injury
- report the location of the fire
- contain the fire
- discontinue oxygen (which is combustible and can fuel an existing fire) if a patient/client is receiving oxygen but not life support
- maintain the patient's/client's respiratory status manually with an Ambu bag ® (see Chapter 17) until the person is moved away from the threat of fire
- direct ambulatory patients/clients to walk by themselves to a safe area (some may be able to assist in moving individuals in wheelchairs)
- move bedridden patients/clients from the scene of a fire by a stretcher, their bed and fire mattress straps, or a wheelchair.

If none of these methods is appropriate, patients/clients must be carried from the area. If a person must be carried, the nurse should be careful not to overextend physical limits for lifting, because injury to the nurse can result in further injury to the patient/client. If the fire brigade are on the scene, they can help evacuate the patients/clients.

There are many types of fire extinguishers. Each uses a different process to extinguish different types of fires. Some manufacturers provide a colour-coded label, others colour the entire body of the extinguisher. Nurses should learn what types of extinguishers are provided in their working environment, where they are located, and how to use them properly.

**Poisoning** A **poison** is any substance that impairs health or destroys life when ingested, inhaled, or absorbed by the body. Specific antidotes or treatments are available for only some types of poisons. The capacity of body tissue to recover from the poison determines the reversibility of the effect. Poisons can impair the respiratory, circulatory, central nervous, hepatic, gastrointestinal, and renal systems of the body.

Accidental poisonings are a greater risk for the toddler, preschool child, and young school child. The nurse can help parents reduce the risk of accidental poisoning by storing medications in child-resistant containers and out of reach of children. Children's accidental poisonings have also been reduced by limiting the number of tablets in each container. Adolescents are at risk of poisoning if they take drugs or abuse solvents.

Older adults are also at risk for poisoning because diminished eyesight may cause an accidental ingestion of toxic substances. The impaired memory of some older adults may result in accidental overdose of prescribed medications.

Patients/clients with mental distress or severe mental illness are also at risk from self-induced poisoning. Safety with this particular group of individuals is an absolute priority. If in doubt, the nurse must err on the side of caution and request medical intervention for such patients/clients.

In the home the two major sources of poisons are plants and household cleaners. Experts recommend that, when poisoning is suspected, the nurse or family member calls the **Poisons Information Service**, a facility that provides information regarding all aspects of intoxication, treatment, and referrals. The nurse should teach parents that calling such a centre for information before attempting home remedies can save their child's life. A full list of the national centres and telephone numbers can be found in the *British National Formulary* (British Medical Association and The Pharmaceutical Press, 1993).

**Electrical Hazards** Much of the equipment used in health care settings is electrical and must be well maintained to prevent electrical hazards. Injury is the result of an electrical current passing through the body. The immediate effect may be extremely severe and cause irregular fibrillation or cessation of the heart muscle contraction.

If an individual receives an electrical shock, the nurse should immediately break the contact with the electricity by switching off the current and removing the plug before touching the person.

If the person has no pulse, cardiopulmonary resuscitation (CPR) should be initiated and emergency services should be called. If the patient/client has a pulse and remains alert and oriented, the nurse should quickly obtain vital signs and assess the skin for signs of burn injury.

If an electrical shock occurs in the home, the nurse follows the same procedure but suggests that the patient/client attends the accident and emergency department or notifies their general practitioner.

**Radiation** Radiation is a health hazard in the hospital environment and the community. In the hospital, particularly in large medical centres, radiation hazards can develop in the nuclear medicine departments and the research laboratories.

The community is also at risk for **radiation exposure** because of incorrect disposal and transportation of radioactive waste products.

*The Control of Substances Hazardous to Health Regulations* (COSHH, 1988) provides guidelines for preventing hazards in the work place. Hospitals and health centres have local guidelines on the care of patients/clients who have radioactive implants. The general principles include isolating patients/clients to one room, and encouraging nursing and medical staff to follow strict guidelines to reduce their own and other patients'/clients' risks of exposure by close monitoring of their exposure to radiation.

Researchers and laboratory workers must follow strict policies when using radioactive substances. Failure to follow these guidelines can result in loss of research funds, loss of research space, and loss of employment.

 **EVALUATION**

Nursing activity aimed at reducing the threat to a patient's/client's safety, as well as at reducing the risk of accidents, can be evaluated by comparing the responses to outcome criteria established during care planning. The optimal outcomes are the patient's/client's ability to maintain a safe environment, to have a safe environment created by families or nurses, and for the patient/client to remain uninjured.

The nurse also evaluates specific interventions designed to promote safety and to teach the patient/client and family how to reduce threats to safety. Using the nursing process, the nurse collects data relating to the patient's/client's safety, exposure to safety risks, and physical condition. Nursing interventions promote safety and provide support to patients/clients unable to independently maintain their own safety needs. The nurse also evaluates the patient's/client's and family's need for additional support services (for example, home health care, physiotherapy, and counselling) and initiates the referral.

## SUMMARY

A safe environment is essential to maintaining and restoring health. Nurses working in a health care or community based setting are the patient's/client's first line of defence against falls, environmental hazards, medication errors, poisoning, and other injuries.

Patients'/clients' risks for injury increase with declining health status, reduced functioning of special senses and decreased mobility. In addition, very young infants and older people have greater risks to their safety.

The nursing process is used to reduce the risk of injury through specific nursing assessment, care planning in partnership with patients/clients and through the evaluation of care activity and patient/client education. The nurse promotes a safe environment by removing threats to safety and by teaching patients/clients and families about hazards in their homes.

## CHAPTER 19 REVIEW

## KEY CONCEPTS

*   A safe health care environment reduces the length of treatment or hospitalization, frequency of treatment-related accidents, the number of work-related injuries to staff, and the overall cost of health and social services.
*   In the community a safe environment is one in which basic needs are achievable, physical hazards are reduced, transmission of pathogens and parasites are reduced, pollution is controlled, and hygiene is maintained.
*   Factors that reduce the amount of available atmospheric

oxygen include poorly maintained gas appliances and high carbon monoxide levels from car exhaust fumes and cigarette smoke.

- Prolonged exposure to extremely hot or cold environmental temperatures can reduce the individual's level of health or even cause death.
- Reduction of physical hazards in the environment includes providing adequate lighting, decreasing clutter, and ensuring a secure home.
- The transmission of pathogens and parasites is reduced through medical and surgical asepsis, immunization, food sanitation, insect and rodent control, and appropriate disposal of human wastes.
- Children under 5 years of age are at greatest risk for home accidents that may result in severe injury and death.
- School children are at risk for injury while at home and at school and while travelling to and from school.
- Adolescents are at risk for injury from car accidents and substance misuse.
- Threats to an adult's safety are frequently associated with poor lifestyle habits.
- Risks of injury for older patients/clients may be related to physiological changes as part of the ageing process.
- Risks to patient/client safety within a health care setting include falls, accidents related to nursing and medical procedures and accidents related to improper use of equipment, faulty or poorly maintained equipment.
- Nursing interventions for promoting safety need to take into account the health, lifestyle and environment of the individual.
- Nursing care plans to promote safety need to be continually evaluated to identify new or continued risks to the patient/client.

## CRITICAL THINKING EXERCISES

1. You are assigned to provide home visits to a person with Alzheimer's disease. During one of these visits, the patient's/client's wife mentions that her husband has been wandering around during the night on a more regular basis and that she is concerned for his safety. What measures are necessary in the home to promote this patient's/client's safety?

2. During a home visit for a family with twin 2-year-old boys, you notice that medications are placed in cabinets with the dishes and glasses and that the household cleaners are placed under the kitchen sink. How do you approach the parents about the potential threat of poisoning? What interventions are appropriate?

3. Consider some practical steps which community nurses may take to help reduce the incidences of accidental and intentional self-poisoning with medication in patients/clients.

## Key Terms

Accident potential, p. 379
Antigen, p. 377
Carbon monoxide, p. 376
Decibels, p. 378
Environment, p. 375
Equipment-related accident(s), p. 381
Food poisoning, p. 376
Hypothermia, p. 376
Immunization, p. 377
Incident report, p. 381
Lifestyle habits/factors, p. 380, 384
Parasite, p. 377
Pathogen, p. 377
Poison, p. 385
Pollutant, p. 378
Procedure-related accident, p. 381
Radiation exposure, p. 386
Risk factors, p. 380
Risk-taking behaviour, p. 380

## REFERENCES

Ashton, J: *Healthy cities.* Milton Keynes, Open University Press, 1993.

Avery JG, Jackson RH: *Children and their accidents.* London, Edward Arnold, 1992.

Bartlett GD: Preventing bicycling injuries. *Physician Assistant*, September, 15(9):51, 1991.

Bassett WH: *Environmental Health Procedures*, 3rd ed, London, Chapman & Hall, 1992.

Bee H, Mitchel S: *The Developing Person: A life-span approach*, 2nd ed, p. 100, 330-331, New York, Harper & Row 1984.

British Medical Association and Royal Pharmaceutical Society, British National Formulary, London, 1993.

Colver A, Pearson P: Safety in the Home: How are we doing? *Health Visitor.* 58:41-42, 1985.

Cooper S: *Common concern: accidents and older adults,* Geriatr Nurs 2:287, 1981.

COI: *How to choose and use fire extinguishers.* Produced for the Home Departments by the Central Office of Information. London, 1987, HMSO.

COSHH: *The Control of substances Hazardous to Health Regulations*, SI London, 1988, HMSO.

DOE, HEA *AIDS and the Workplace: A guide for employees.* Department of Employment and Central Office of Information, Bradford, 1991, HMSO.

DOH: *Immunisation against Infectious Diseases*, London, 1992a, HMSO.

DOH: *The Health of the Nation: A Strategy for Health in England*, London, 1992b, HMSO.

DOH: *The Health of the Nation: Key Area Handbook-Accidents.* January, Department of Health, London, 1993a, HMSO.

DOH: Health of the Nation. Targeting Practice: *The Contribution of Nurses, Midwives and Health Visitors.* London, 1993b, Department of Health.

DHSS: *Strategies for Accident Prevention.* Department of Health & Social Security, London, 1988, HMSO.

Donaldson RJ, Donaldson LJ: *Essential Community Medicine.* Lancaster, 1987, MTP Press Limited.

HEA: *Preventing Accidents to Children: a Training Resource for Health Visitors.* London, 1991, Health Education Authority.

Hinds CJ: *Intensive Care: A concise textbook.* London, 1987, Baillière Tindall.

Hobbs L, Grattan E, Hobbs J: *Classification of Injury by Length of Stay in Hospital.* TRL Laboratory Report No. 871, 1979.

Hobbs B, Roberts D: *Food Poisoning and Food Hygiene*, ed 6, London, 1992, Edward Arnold.

Huntington J, Killoran A: Winning at the primaries (The GP contract and health promotion), *Health Service Journal*, 101:24-25, 1991.

HSE: *The Health and Safety at Work Act 1974*, Sheffield, 1974, Health and Safety Executive Information Centre.

Moore J: Can they be prevented? *Community Outlook,* 78 (32)212-214, 1982.

NHS Cymru Wales: Caring for the future, 1992, Cardiff, 1992, Central Office of Information, The Welsh Office.

ROSPA: *Action on Accidents: The Unique Role of the Health service*, Birmingham, 1989, National Association of Health Authorities and Trusts/Royal Society for the Prevention of Accidents.

Scottish Office: Scotland's health: a challenge to you, Edinburgh, 1992, Scottish Office.

Tideiksaar R: Home safe home: practical tips for fall-proofing, *Geriatric Nursing* 11(6):280, 1989.

Troup D, Davies J, Manning P: A model for the investigation of back injuries and manual handling problems at work. *Journal of Occupational Accidents,* 10:107-109, 1988.

UKCC: *Statement on Practice Nurses. Aspects of the new GP Contract*, London, 1990, UKCC.

## FURTHER READING

### Adult Nursing

British Medical Association: *Cycling Towards Health and Safety*, Oxford, 1992, Open University Press.

Constantinides P: *The Management Response to childhood Accidents*. London, 1987, Kings Fund Centre.

DOH: *The Health of the Nation. Specification of National Indicators*, London, 1992, Department of Health.

NHSE: *First steps for the NHS: Recommendations of the Health of the Nation Focus Groups*, London, 1992, Department of Health, NHS executive.

NHSE: *A vision for the future: The Nursing, Midwifery and Health visiting contribution to Health and Health Care*, London, 1993, Department of Health, NHS Executive.

Northern Ireland Office: A regional strategy for the N. Ireland Health and Personal Social Services 1992-1997, Belfast, 1991, Nothern Ireland Office.

Burton R: Parental perception of accident and emergency, *Paed Nursing* Nov 19-20, 1989.

### Children's Nursing

Avery J, Jackson R: *Children and their accidents*, London, 1992, Edward Arnold.

CAPT: *Accidents to Children on Hospital Wards*. A study for the child accident prevention trust the RCN with help from SMA Nutrition, London, 1992, Child Accident Prevention Trust.

Cody A, Waine N: Preventing childhood accidents. *British Journal of Nursing* 2(21):1059-1064, 1993.

Colver A, Pearson P: Safety in the home. How are we doing? *Health Visitor* 58:41-4, 1985.

HEA: *Play it Safe. A guide to preventing children's accidents*. Health Education Authority, London, 1981.

Ingram S: Safe House. *Nursing Standard*. June 3, 23(3):46,1989.

Jackson R, editor: *Childhood, the Environment and Accidents*. Tunbridge Wells, 1977, Pitman Medicine.

Mead D, Sibert J: *The Injured Child – an Action Plan for Nurses. London*, 1991, Scutari.

### Learning Disabilities Nursing

Collins BC: A national survey of safety concerns for students with special needs, *Journal of Developmental and Physical Disabilities*, 4(3): 263-76, 1992.

Emberson J, Walker E: Self-injurious behaviour in people with a mental handicap, *Nursing Times*, 86(23): 43, 1990.

Heyman B, Huckle S: 'Normal' life in a hazardous world: how adults with moderate learning difficulties and their carers cope with risks and dangers, *Disability, Handicap & Society*, 8(2): 143-60, 1993.

Tymchuk AJ: Assessing home dangers and safety precautions: instruments for use, *Mental Handicap*, 19(1): 4-10, 1991.

Watson M *et al*: A preliminary study in teaching self-protective skills to children with moderate and severe mental retardation, *Journal of Special Education*, 26(2): 181-94, 1992.

### Mental Health Nursing

Sainsbury P, Jenkins J, Levey A. In Farmer R, Hirsh S: *The suicide syndrome*, Beckenham, 1982, Croom Helm.

Owens RG, Ashcroft JB: *Violence: a guide for the caring profession*, Beckenham, 1985, Croom Helm.

Breier A, Astrachan BM: Characterization of schizophrenia patients who commit suicide, *Am J Psych* 141(2): 206, 1984.

# Sleep and Rest

## CHAPTER OUTLINE

## LEARNING OUTCOMES

After studying this chapter, you should be able to:
- ■ *Define the key terms listed.*
- ■ *Compare the characteristics of sleep and rest.*
- ■ *Explain the effect the 24-hour sleep–wake cycle has on biological function.*
- ■ *Discuss mechanisms that regulate sleep.*
- ■ *Describe the stages of a normal sleep cycle.*
- ■ *Explain the functions of sleep.*
- ■ *Compare and contrast the sleep requirements of different age groups.*
- ■ *Identify factors that normally promote and disrupt sleep.*
- ■ *Discuss characteristics of common sleep disorders.*
- ■ *Conduct a sleep assessment for a patient/client.*
- ■ *Identify sleep problems with patients/clients.*
- ■ *Identify nursing interventions designed to promote normal sleep cycles for patients/clients of all ages.*
- ■ *Describe ways to evaluate sleep therapies.*

Individuals need and receive different amounts and qualities of sleep and rest. Physical and emotional health depend on the ability to fulfil these basic human needs. Without rest and sleep, the ability to concentrate, make judgements, and participate in daily activities decreases, and irritability increases.

The theory that sleep is associated with healing (Torrance, 1990) suggests that achieving optimum sleep quality is important for the recovery of all patients/clients. Nurses care for individuals who often have pre-existing sleep disturbances and for patients/clients who develop sleep problems as a result of illness or hospitalization. Sleep problems may cause individuals to seek health care, or problems may go unnoticed for years. Ill patients/clients often require more sleep and rest than healthy ones. However, the nature of illness may prevent patients/clients from gaining adequate rest and sleep. The environment of a hospital or long-term care facility and the activities of health care personnel may also make sleep difficult.

Identifying and treating sleep disturbances is an important goal for a nurse. To help an individual gain needed rest and sleep, a nurse must understand the nature of sleep, the factors influencing it, and the person's sleeping habits. Each person requires an individualized approach. Interventions can be effective in resolving short- and long-term sleep disturbances.

## SLEEP AND REST

Individuals at rest are in a state of decreased mental and physical activity that leaves them feeling refreshed, rejuvenated, and ready to resume the activities of the day. Rest does not imply inactivity; rest may be gained, for example, from reading a book, practising a relaxation exercise (see Chapter 27), or taking a long walk. Each person has his or her own way of attaining rest and can usually adjust to new environments or conditions that affect the ability to rest.

Nurses frequently care for patients/clients on **bed rest**. This treatment aims to reduce physical and psychological demands on the body by the patient/client remaining in bed. Such people are not necessarily rested. They still may have emotional worries that prevent complete relaxation. Depending on others for care may cause such individuals to feel stressed.

**Sleep** is a recurrent, altered state of consciousness that occurs for sustained periods, restoring energy and well-being. Sleep provides time for the repair and recovery of body systems for the next period of wakefulness. A sleeping person interacts less with the environment.

The rest and sleep habits of people entering a hospital or other health care facility can easily be changed by illness or hospital activities. The extent of change depends on their physiological and psychological states and environment. The nurse must always be aware of patients'/clients' needs for rest. The lack of rest for long periods can cause illness or worsening of existing illness. The nurse can help individuals learn the importance of rest and ways to promote it at home or in the health care environment.

## Promoting Rest

Many factors affect the ability to gain adequate rest. In the home the nurse helps individuals develop behaviours conducive to rest and relaxation. This may include controlling factors in the environment or changing certain lifestyle habits. For example, the community nurse frequently cares for individuals with chronic debilitating disease. A simple care plan might include asking patients/clients to set aside afternoons for rest. The nurse helps adjust medication schedules and suggests that patients/clients pass urine regularly before rest periods and ask friends not to telephone during a set time so that rest periods are uninterrupted.

### Conditions for Proper Rest

**Physical Comfort**
- Eliminate sources of physical irritation
- Control sources of pain
- Provide comfortable temperature
- Maintain hygiene
- Maintain proper anatomical alignment or positioning
- Remove environmental distractions
- Provide adequate ventilation

**Freedom From Worry**
- Make own decisions
- Participate in personal health care
- Have knowledge needed to understand health problems and implications
- Practise restful activities regularly
- Know that the environment is safe

**Sufficient Sleep**
- Obtain average hours of sleep needed to avoid fatigue
- Follow good sleep preparation habits

### Mother and child nursing
### Sleep disturbance in childbearing

During pregnancy and in the early weeks following birth, women often suffer from sleep disturbance. In early pregnancy frequency of micturition and early morning sickness may disrupt sleep; in late pregnancy discomfort due to the increased abdominal size, fetal movements and gastric acid reflux (heart burn) are additional causes of frequent awakening at night. The midwife can recommend simple remedies for some of these problems; for example, avoiding spicy foods and large meals, and elevating their sleeping position with extra pillows, to combat heart burn.

During the early weeks following birth, it is the baby's demand for attention that interferes with 'a good night's sleep'. Babies require round-the-clock attention and may take 2 or 3 months to settle into a diurnal rhythm for sleep and wakefulness. McKenna (1993) is examining the concept of mother-infant co-sleeping as a method of promoting normal psychological development and preventing some neonatal sudden deaths. Women are also advised to synchronize their sleep with the baby, if possible, by sleeping during the day.

Disturbances in maternal patterns of sleep other than those mentioned above, for example, insomnia or feeling tired after a good sleep, may be signs of psychiatric disorder or mood disturbance and midwives are vigilant in recognizing and reporting such symptoms to a doctor.

In a health care setting the nurse promotes rest by controlling patients'/clients' physical symptoms and altering stressful factors in the environment. This can be difficult on a busy ward or unit. Loud or unfamiliar noises, irritating lighting, loss of privacy, and frequency of therapeutic procedures can interfere with rest. For example, individuals who are hospitalized for extensive diagnostic testing often have difficulty resting because of the uncertainty about their future. A nurse can promote rest by allowing patients/clients to determine the timing and methods of delivery of all care measures. Providing information about the purpose of all procedures can also help. Providing individuals with control over their health care minimizes uncertainty and anxiety. The box (left) lists conditions needed to ensure proper rest.

## PHYSIOLOGY OF SLEEP

Sleep is a set of complete physiological processes. It involves a sequence of states maintained by highly integrated central nervous system (CNS) activity associated with changes in the peripheral nervous, endocrine, cardiovascular, respiratory, and muscular systems (Hoch and Reynolds, 1986; Closs, 1988). Each sequence can be identified by specific behaviours, physiological responses, and patterns of brain activity. Instruments such as the electroencephalogram (EEG), which measures electrical activity in the cerebral cortex, the electromyogram (EMG), which measures muscle tone, and the electrooculogram (EOG), which measures eye movements, provide information about the physiological aspects of sleep.

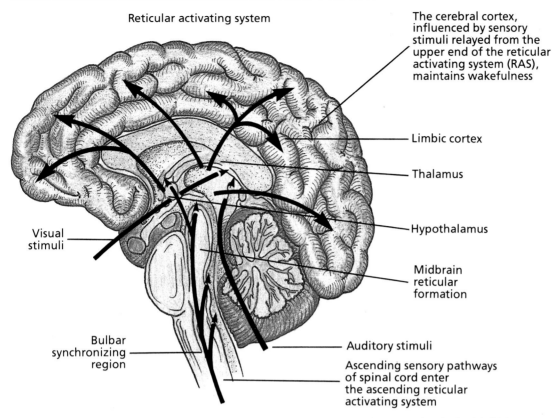

Reticular activating system

The cerebral cortex, influenced by sensory stimuli relayed from the upper end of the reticular activating system (RAS), maintains wakefulness

Limbic cortex

Thalamus

Hypothalamus

Midbrain reticular formation

Auditory stimuli

Ascending sensory pathways of spinal cord enter the ascending reticular activating system

Visual stimuli

Bulbar synchronizing region

**Fig. 20-1** RAS and BSR control sensory input, intermittently activating and suppressing the brain's higher centres to control sleep and wakefulness.

## Circadian Rhythms

Each person's life is a series of cyclical rhythms that influence and regulate physiological function and behavioural responses. The most familiar rhythm is the 24-hour, day-night cycle known as the *diurnal* or **circadian rhythm** (derived from Latin: *circa*, 'about', and *dies*, 'day'). Another rhythm is the woman's menstrual cycle, an **infradian rhythm** (longer than 24 hours). Biological cycles lasting less than 24 hours are called **ultradian rhythms**. Circadian rhythms influence the pattern of major biological and behavioural functions. The fluctuation and predictability of body temperature, heart rate, blood pressure, hormone and electrolyte secretions, sensory acuity, and mood depend on the 24-hour circadian cycle.

Circadian rhythms, including daily sleep-wake cycles, are most affected by light and temperature. However, these **biological clocks** are also influenced by external factors such as social activities and work routines. All persons have biological clocks that synchronize their sleep cycles. Some people can fall asleep at 8 PM, whereas others go to bed at midnight or early in the morning. Different people also function best at different times of the day.

Hospitals or long-term facilities may fail to adapt care to an individual's preference for sleep. If a person's **sleep-wake cycle** is altered significantly, a poor quality of sleep results. Reversals in the sleep-wake cycle such as sleeping during the day instead of the night (or vice versa for people who work nights) can indicate a serious illness. Anxiety, restlessness, irritability, and impaired judgement are common symptoms of reversal of the sleep cycle.

The biological rhythm of sleep frequently becomes synchronized with other body functions. Changes in body temperature, for example, correlate with sleep patterns. Normally, body temperature peaks in the afternoon, decreases gradually, and then drops sharply after a person falls asleep (see Chapter 4). When the sleep-wake cycle becomes disrupted (for example, by rotating job shifts), other physiological functions change as well. The integrity of the sleep-wake cycle can influence the person's overall health.

## Sleep Regulation

The control and regulation of sleep may depend on the interrelationship between two cerebral mechanisms that work against one another. Both intermittently activate and suppress the brain's higher centres to control sleep and wakefulness. One mechanism causes wakefulness, whereas the other causes sleep.

The **reticular activating system (RAS)** is located in the upper brainstem. It is believed to contain special cells that maintain alertness and wakefulness. The RAS receives visual sensory input and auditory pain and tactile stimuli. Activity from the cerebral cortex (for example, emotions or thought processes) also stimulates the RAS. Studies reported by Canavan (1984) and Chuman (1983) suggest that wakefulness results from neurons in the RAS releasing catecholamines such as noradrenaline.

Sleep may be produced by the release of serotonin from specialized cells in the raphe sleep system of the pons and medial forebrain. This area of the brain is also called the **bulbar synchronizing region (BSR)**. Whether a person remains awake or falls asleep depends on a balance of impulses received from higher centres (for example, thoughts), peripheral sensory receptors (for example, sound or light stimuli), and the limbic system (emotions) (Fig. 20-1).

## Stages of Sleep

### Stage 1: NREM

- Stage includes lightest level of sleep.
- Stage lasts a few minutes.
- Decreased physiological activity begins with gradual fall in vital signs and metabolism.
- Person is easily aroused by sensory stimuli such as noise.
- Awakened, person feels as though daydreaming has occurred.

### Stage 2: NREM

- Stage 2 is period of sound sleep.
- Relaxation progresses.
- Arousal is still easy.
- Stage lasts 10 to 20 minutes.
- Body functions continue to slow.

### Stage 3: NREM

- Stage 3 involves initial stages of deep sleep.
- Sleeper is difficult to arouse and rarely moves.
- Muscles are completely relaxed.
- Vital signs decline but remain regular.
- Stage lasts 15 to 30 minutes.

### Stage 4: NREM

- Stage 4 is deepest stage of sleep.
- It is very difficult to arouse sleeper.
- If sleep loss has occurred, sleeper will spend considerable portion of night in this stage.
- Stage is responsible for restoring and resting body.
- Vital signs are significantly lower than during waking hours.
- Stage lasts approximately 15 to 30 minutes.
- Sleepwalking and enuresis may occur.

### REM Sleep

- REM stage is a period of vivid, full-colour dreaming. (Less vivid dreaming may occur in other stages.)
- Stage usually begins every 50 to 90 minutes after sleep has begun.
- It is typified by autonomic response of rapidly moving eyes, fluctuating heart and respiratory rates, and increased or fluctuating blood pressure.
- Loss of skeletal muscle tone occurs.
- Gastric secretions increase.
- This stage is responsible for mental restoration.
- It is very difficult to arouse sleeper.
- Duration of REM sleep increases with each cycle and averages 20 minutes.

As people try to fall asleep, they close their eyes and assume relaxed positions. Stimuli to the RAS decline. If the room is dark and quiet, activation of the RAS further declines. At some point the BSR takes over, causing sleep.

## Stages of Sleep

Studies show different levels of brain activity indicating different stages of sleep. Sleep involves two phases: nonrapid eye movement **(NREM sleep)** and rapid eye movement **(REM**

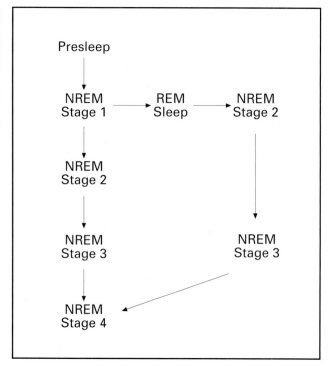

**Fig. 20-2** Adult sleep cycle.

**sleep)** (see box, left). During NREM a sleeper progresses through four stages during a typical sleep cycle. The quality of sleep from stage 1 through to stage 4 becomes increasingly deep. Light sleep is characteristic of stages 1 and 2, and a person is easily arousable. Stages 3 and 4 involve a deeper sleep called **slow-wave sleep**. REM sleep is the phase at the end of each sleep cycle. A person is usually difficult to arouse, and psychological restoration may occur at this time. The sleeping stages are highly individualized for each person. Many different factors promote or interfere with various stages of the sleep cycle. The nurse chooses therapies that foster sleep or attempts to eliminate factors that can disrupt it.

## Sleep Cycle

Normally, in an adult the routine **sleep pattern** begins with a presleep period during which the person is aware only of a gradually developing drowsiness. This period normally lasts 10 to 30 minutes, but if a person has difficulty falling asleep, it may last for an hour or more.

Once asleep, the person usually passes through four to six complete sleep cycles, each consisting of four stages of NREM sleep and a period of REM sleep. The cyclical pattern usually progresses from stage 1 through stage 4 of NREM, followed by a reversal from stage 4 to 3 to 2, ending with a period of REM sleep (Fig. 20-2). A person usually reaches REM sleep within 90 minutes.

With each successive cycle, stages 3 and 4 shorten, and the period of REM lengthens. REM sleep may last 30 to 60 minutes during the last sleep cycle. If a person awakens from sleep during any stage, sleep begins again at stage 1.

Not all people progress consistently through the stages of sleep. For example, a sleeper may fluctuate for short intervals between NREM stages 2, 3, and 4 before entering REM stage.

The amount of time spent in each stage varies. Shifts from stage to stage tend to accompany body movements, and shifts to light sleep tend to occur suddenly, whereas shifts to deep sleep tend to be gradual (Closs, 1988). The number of sleep cycles depends on the total amount of time spent asleep.

## FUNCTIONS OF SLEEP

Many functions of sleep have been proposed, and it is described as a restorative, protective, instinctive or ethnologically adaptive process (Hodgson, 1991), contributing to physiological and psychological restoration. Traditionally, sleep is viewed as a time of restoration and preparation for the next period of wakefulness. During NREM sleep, biological functions slow. A healthy adult's normal heart rate throughout the day averages 70 to 80 beats per minute or less if the individual is in excellent physical condition. However, during sleep the heart rate falls to 60 beats per minute or less. Clearly, then, restful sleep is beneficial in preserving cardiac function.

Sleep is needed to routinely restore biological processes. During deep slow-wave (NREM stage 4) sleep the body releases human growth hormone for the repair and renewal of epithelial and specialized cells such as brain cells (Chuman, 1983). Other studies have shown that protein synthesis and cell division for renewal of tissues such as the skin, bone marrow, gastric mucosa, or brain occur during rest and sleep (Fordham, 1988). Nonrapid eye movement sleep may be especially important in children, who experience more stage 4 sleep.

The body conserves energy during sleep. The skeletal muscles relax progressively, and the absence of muscular contraction preserves chemical energy for cellular processes. Lowering of the basal metabolic rate further conserves the body's energy supply.

REM sleep appears to be important for psychological restoration. REM sleep is associated with changes in cerebral blood flow, increased cortical activity, increased oxygen consumption, and adrenaline release. This association may assist with memory storage, learning, and emotional adaptation (Chase and Weitzman, 1983). The brain filters stored information of the day's activities.

## Dreams

**Dreams** occur during NREM and REM sleep. The dreams of REM sleep are more vivid and elaborate. REM dreams progress in content throughout the night from dreams about current events to emotional dreams of childhood or the past. Personality can influence the quality of dreams; for example, a creative person may have creative dreams, and a depressed person can dream of helplessness.

The dreams of REM sleep are believed to be functionally important. Freud believed that dreams were a product of unconscious desires and released psychological tensions. Thus, the nature and occurrence of dreams became a basis for psychoanalytic therapy.

Another theory suggests that dreams erase certain fantasies or nonsensical memories. Most dreams are forgotten. In fact, during REM sleep, consolidation of short-term memory is impaired. To remember a dream, a person must consciously think about it on awakening. People who recall dreams vividly usually awake just after a period of REM sleep.

## Normal Sleep Requirements and Patterns

Sleep duration and quality vary widely among people of all age groups. One person may gain adequate rest after 4 hours of sleep, whereas another may require 10 hours. Fig. 20-3 shows the change in the distribution of sleep stages during life.

### Neonates

A neonate averages 16 hours of sleep a day, with a range of 10 to 23 hours. For the first week of life the neonate sleeps almost constantly to recover from birth. Approximately 50% of this sleep is REM sleep, which stimulates the higher brain centres. This is essential for development because the neonate is not awake long enough for significant external stimulation. A newborn baby has five distinct states of sleep. The cycle of states varies based on the number of hours the newborn sleeps.

### Infants

Sleep patterns vary among infants. Active infants typically sleep less than quiet infants (Wong, 1995). Infants usually develop a night-time pattern of sleep by the age of 3 to 4 months. The infant may take several naps during the day but usually sleeps an average of 8 to 10 hours during the night. Awakening commonly occurs early in the morning, although it is not unusual for an infant to awaken during the night.

### Toddlers

By the age of 2, children usually sleep through the night and take daily naps. Total sleep averages 12 hours a day. Naps may be eliminated at 3 years. It is common for toddlers to awaken during the night. The percentage of REM sleep begins to fall because toddlers have access to a variety of meaningful external stimuli.

**Mental Health Nursing
The benefits of sleep on behaviour**

The benefits of sleep on behaviour often go unnoticed until a person develops a problem resulting from sleep deprivation. Aggression, irritability and antisocial feelings have been reported after 24–48 hour periods of sleep deprivation (McIntosh, 1989). Although no clear cause-and-effect relationship exists between sleep deprivation and a specific body dysfunction (Webster and Thompson, 1986), various body functions (for example, reflexes, memory, and equilibrium) can be altered when prolonged sleep deprivation occurs.

At various times in mental health, sleep has been used as a form of treatment; for example, sleep deprivation therapy for people with depression, and modified narcosis (sleep) therapy for people with severe elevation of mood. The exact means by which improvement occurs is unclear, but it is believed to be related to the variations in the brain amines which affect our mood.

## Preschool Children

An average preschool child sleeps about 12 hours a night and rarely takes naps (Wong, 1995). They may have difficulty relaxing or quietening down after long, active days. A preschool child also has problems with bedtime fears, waking during the night, or nightmares. Parents can be most successful in getting a preschool child to bed by establishing a consistent bedtime ritual.

## School-Aged Children

The amount of sleep needed during the school years is highly individualized because of varying states of activity and levels of health. The school-aged child usually does not require a nap. A 6-year-old averages 11 to 12 hours of sleep nightly, whereas an 11-year-old sleeps about 9 to 10 hours (Wong, 1995). The 6- or 7-year-old can usually be persuaded to go to bed by encouraging quiet activities. The older child often resists going to sleep due to a lack of awareness of fatigue or a need to be independent.

## Adolescents

An adolescent's day is usually active and mentally and physically exhausting. Often the desire to spend time with peers prevents adolescents from realizing their need for sleep. Once bedtime approaches, however, the adolescent offers little resistance to sleep. An adolescent averages 8 to 9 hours of sleep a night. Owing to staying up late, an adolescent frequently sleeps late in the mornings.

## Young Adults

Healthy young adults require rest and sleep to participate in the busy activities that fill their days. However, it is common for busy lifestyles to interrupt sleep patterns. Most young adults average 6 to 8 hours of sleep a night, but this can vary. It is unusual for young adults to take regular naps. Approximately 20% of sleep time is spent in REM sleep, which remains consistent throughout life.

## Middle Adults

During adulthood the total time spent sleeping at night begins to decline. Also the amount of stage 4 sleep begins to fall, continuing throughout older age. Sleep disturbances are common; insomnia is particularly common because of the changes and stresses of middle age. Sleep disturbances can be caused by anxiety, depression, or certain physical ailments.

## Older Adults

The total amount of sleep does not change as age increases. **Quality of sleep** deteriorates and there is a progressive decrease in stages 3 and 4 NREM, and an older adult has almost no stage 4 sleep (Clapin-French, 1986). An older adult awakens more often during the night, and total wake time increases.

Hayter (1983) studied the sleeping habits of 212 older people ranging from 65 to 93 years and found considerable variability among the sleep behaviours of different subjects. The total time asleep for naps seems to increase progressively with age. By the age of 75 years, there was a definite increase in the amount of time spent in bed, both when nap time is included and excluded.

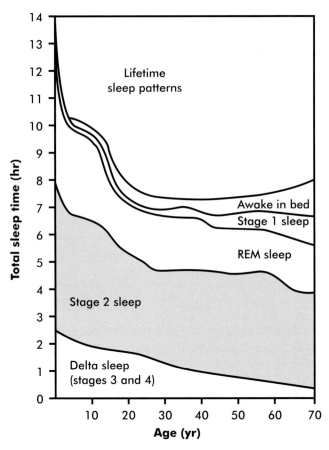

**Fig. 20-3** Distribution of sleep stages over the life span. From Berman TM, Nino-Murcia G, Roehrs T: *Patient Care* 24:85, 1990.

Hayter (1983) also found a pattern of a gradually increasing need for rest and sleep with advancing age. The need for increased rest occurs earlier than the need for increased sleep.

The changes in an older person's sleep pattern are due to changes in the CNS that affect the regulation of sleep. Sensory impairment, common with ageing, may reduce sensitivity to time cues that maintain circadian rhythms. An older adult's chronic illnesses may also impair the quality of sleep.

## FACTORS AFFECTING SLEEP

Factors that promote sleep in one person may hinder sleep in another. A single factor may not be the only cause for a sleep problem. Physiological, psychological, and environmental factors can alter the quality and quantity of sleep.

### Physical Illness

Physical pathology can be associated with many sleep abnormalities (Hodgson, 1991). Conditions which alter CNS physiology or increase intracranial pressure often adversely affect sleep. Any illness that causes pain, physical discomfort (such as difficulty swallowing), anxiety, or depression can result in sleep problems. People with such alterations may have trouble falling asleep or staying asleep. Illnesses also force individuals to sleep in positions to which they are unaccustomed. Assuming an awkward

## Learning Disabilities Nursing
## Misconceptions about sleep

Sleep requirements for people with learning disabilities are no different from other patients/clients. However, sometimes those who care for people with learning disabilities overestimate the amount of sleep required, because they view the patient/client as 'sick' or 'frail'. Allowing the patient/client to spend time in bed, rather than engaging him or her in more physical activities, deprives the patient/client of opportunities for physical, social and emotional development.

Some parents of children with learning disabilities allow the child to share the parental bedroom for far longer than usual — sometimes into adult life. There are various reasons for this, but it is often due to anxieties about the child having seizures during the night or waking and wandering about without being heard.

Disrupted sleep patterns, repeated waking, and nocturnal enuresis are also common in people with learning disabilities, and can be difficult behaviours to eradicate, particularly if the family believes that these behaviours are an inevitable consequence of the child's learning disability. In these situations, the parents (or carers) may require education about 'normal' sleep patterns and assistance in adopting systematic approaches to eradicating disruptive nocturnal behaviours, rather than resorting to night sedation.

As with other patients/clients, changes in sleep patterns may indicate changes in the person's physical or mental health status.

## Mental Health Nursing
## Drugs and their effects on sleep

HYPNOTICS
- Interfere with reaching deeper sleep stages
- Provide only temporary (1 week) increase in quantity of sleep
- Eventually cause 'hangover' during day: excess drowsiness, confusion, decreased energy
- May worsen sleep apnoea in older adults

DIURETICS
- Cause nocturia

ANTIDEPRESSANTS AND STIMULANTS
- Suppress REM sleep

ALCOHOL
- Speeds onset of sleep
- Disrupts REM sleep
- Awakens person during night and causes difficulty in returning to sleep

CAFFEINE
- Prevents person from falling asleep
- May cause person to awaken during night

DIGOXIN
- Causes nightmares

BETA-BLOCKER
- Causes nightmares
- Causes insomnia
- Causes awakening from sleep

VALIUM
- Decreases stages 2, 4, and REM sleep
- Decreases awakenings

NARCOTICS (MORPHINE)
- Suppress REM sleep
- If discontinued quickly, can increase risk of cardiac dysrhythmias because of 'rebound' REM periods
- Cause increased awakenings and drowsiness

position while in traction, for example, can interfere with sleep.

In conditions where cardiac or respiratory function is affected by day, further problems can occur at night. Patients/clients with chronic lung disease such as emphysema are short of breath and frequently cannot sleep without two or three pillows to raise their heads. Asthma, bronchitis, and allergic rhinitis alter the rhythm of breathing and disturb sleep. A person with a common cold has nasal congestion, sinus drainage, and a sore throat, which impair breathing and the ability to relax.

Coronary heart disease is characterized by episodes of sudden chest pain and irregular heart rates. Patients/clients with this disease are often afraid to go to sleep because of the fear of a heart attack at night.

Hypertension often causes early morning awakening and fatigue. Hypothyroidism decreases stage 4 sleep, whereas hyperthyroidism causes people to take more time to fall asleep.

Individuals with peptic ulcers often awaken in the middle of the night. Gastric acid levels reach a peak in the stomach around 1 to 3 AM (McNeil *et al*, 1986), causing stomach pain.

**Nocturia**, or urination during the night, disrupts sleep and the sleep cycle. After a person awakens to urinate, returning to sleep may be difficult.

## Drugs and Substances

Various types of drugs affect the pattern and quality of sleep (see box). Medications prescribed for sleep can cause more problems than benefits. If people take a variety of drugs to control or treat chronic illness, then the combined effects of several drugs can seriously disrupt sleep. It has been suggested that L-tryptophan, an amino acid found in foods such as milk, cheese, and meats, may help a person sleep, but research in this area has produced inconsistent and inconclusive results (McMahon, 1990b).

## Lifestyle

A person's daily routine may influence sleep patterns. An individual working a rotating shift (for example, 2 weeks of days followed by a week of nights) has difficulty adjusting to the altered sleep schedule. The body's internal clock might be set at 11 PM, but the work schedule forces sleep at 9 AM instead. The individual often can sleep only 3 or 4 hours because the body's clock perceives that it is time to be awake and active. Only after several weeks of working a night shift does a person's biological clock adjust. Brown (1988) documented the results of research in Australia into nurses' patterns of shift work which indicated that those who worked an evening shift followed by an early duty had an increased accident and error rate. Other alterations in routine that can disrupt sleep patterns include performing unaccustomed heavy work, engaging in late-night social activities, and changing evening mealtime.

### Sleep Patterns

The pattern and adequacy of sleep experienced each day affects an individual's functioning. Different times of day have been associated with an increased sleep tendency. These occur from about 2 to 7 AM and to a lesser degree from 2 to 5 PM. However, when sleep patterns are disrupted, the natural tendency to be sleeping at select times increases. An individual who experiences temporary sleep deprivation as a result of an active social evening or lengthened work schedule usually feels sleepy the next day; he or she may have difficulties in remaining attentive and in performing tasks, especially those that require speed or prolonged concentration, rather than physical effort (Hodgson, 1991). Occupational groups, such as pilots and long distance lorry drivers, have to comply with regulations that restrict continuous working hours (Roper *et al*, 1990).

Closs (1990) investigated sleep patterns in 200 patients/clients admitted to surgical wards and found that patients/clients retired to bed and rose almost an hour earlier than they did at home. Their normal period of sleeping was shortened by over an hour.

### Emotional Stress

Worry over personal problems or situations can disrupt sleep. Stress may also cause a person to try too hard to fall asleep, to awaken frequently during the sleep cycle, or to oversleep. Continued stress can cause poor sleep habits. For example, if older people experience losses that lead to emotional stress, such as retirement, death of a loved one or loss of economic security they may experience delays in falling asleep, earlier appearance of REM sleep, frequent awakening, increased total bed time, feelings of sleeping poorly, and early awakening (Colling, 1983).

### Environment

The environment has a significant influence on the ability to fall and remain asleep. Good ventilation is essential for restful sleep. The size, firmness, and position of the bed can affect the quality of sleep. Hospital beds are often harder than those at home, and Closs (1990) found that, for 35% of patients/clients in her study, hospital beds were a source of discomfort and dissatisfaction. If a person usually sleeps with another individual, sleeping alone can cause wakefulness.

Sound also influences sleep. The level of noise needed to awaken people depends on the stage of sleep (Webster and Thompson, 1986). Low noises are more likely to arouse a person from stage 1 sleep, whereas louder noises awaken people in stage 3 or 4 sleep. Some people require silence to fall asleep, whereas others prefer noise such as soft music.

In hospitals, noise creates a problem for patients/clients. Noise in hospitals is usually new or strange. Thus, patients/clients are prone to awaken. The level of noise in hospitals can be very loud. Normal conversation and bed changing measure about 60 decibels (Biley, 1993). People-induced noises (that is, nursing activities) are sources of increased sound levels. Intensive care units are sources of high noise levels. Close proximity of patients/clients, noise from confused and ill patients/clients, the ringing of alarm systems and telephones, and disturbances caused by emergencies make the environment unpleasant.

Light levels may affect the ability to fall asleep. Some individuals may prefer a dark room, whereas others, such as children, keep a soft light on at all times. Individuals may also have trouble sleeping depending on the temperature of a room. A room that is too warm or too cold can cause a person to become restless or to awaken. In one study, 46% of patients' reported being too hot in hospital, and waking up for this reason (Closs, 1990).

Constant environmental stimuli, such as noises from equipment, frequent monitoring by nurses, and ever-present lights can lead to the 'ICU' syndrome. In this situation the patient/client can become disorientated, and is unable to distinguish night from day. This can impair the individual's usual sleeping patterns.

### Exercise and Fatigue

A person who is moderately fatigued usually achieves restful sleep, especially if the fatigue is the result of enjoyable work or exercise. Exercising 2 hours before bedtime allows the body to cool down and maintains a state of fatigue that promotes relaxation. However, excess fatigue resulting from exhausting or stressful work can make falling asleep difficult. This can be a common problem for school-aged children and adolescents.

### Caloric Intake

Weight loss or gain influences sleep patterns. When a person gains weight, sleep periods become longer with fewer interruptions. Weight loss can cause short and fragmented sleep. Certain sleep disorders may be the result of the semi-starvation Ωdiets. In hospital, the last meal of the day, and evening drinks are often early. Some patients/clients may become hungry at night, which can interfere with sleep. Unless they or their visitors bring in suitable snacks they may find this a problem, as many wards now lack the facilities to provide these (McMahon, 1990b).

## SLEEP DISORDERS

**Sleep disorders** are conditions that repeatedly cause a disruption in sleep patterns. Sleep disorders may cause individuals to seek health care, or the effects of illness or hospitalization may create sleep disorders. The best way to diagnose sleep disorders is through the use of a night-time polysomnogram. This involves use of the EEG, EMG, and EOG to monitor stages of sleep and wakefulness. Patterns of inadequate sleep can cause numerous problems for individuals.

### Insomnia

**Insomnia** is a symptom of patients/clients who have chronic difficulty in falling asleep (initial insomnia), difficulty remaining asleep (intermittent insomnia), or an inability to go back to sleep after awakening (terminal insomnia). The insomniac complains of insufficient quantity and quality of sleep. Frequently, however, the person obtains more sleep than he or she realizes. Insomnia may signal an underlying physical or psychological disorder.

People may experience insomnia only temporarily, usually as a result of situational stresses such as family or work problems, jet lag, illness, or loss of a loved one. The condition can develop at any age. Insomnia may recur, but between episodes the person is able to sleep well. A temporary case of insomnia can lead to a chronic problem. Removal of a stressful situation may not cure the sleep problem. As a result a person loses confidence in the ability to fall asleep and develops anxiety about sleeping well.

Insomnia is most commonly associated with poor sleep habits. If the condition continues, the fear of not being able to sleep can be enough to cause wakefulness. During the day, a person with chronic insomnia may feel sleepy, fatigued, depressed, and anxious.

Because there are many causes of insomnia, management involves several approaches. First, it is important to treat underlying emotional or physical problems. Treatment is also symptomatic, including improved sleep preparation measures, biofeedback, cognitive techniques, and relaxation techniques such as hypnosis or aromatherapy. The exact cause of insomnia is unknown.

## Sleep Apnoea

The easiest description of **sleep apnoea** is the cessation of breathing for a time during sleep. Apnoea can be defined as the cessation of airflow through the nose and mouth for at least 10 seconds. There are three types: central, obstructive, and mixed.

The most common form, obstructive apnoea, occurs when muscles or structures of the oral cavity or throat relax during sleep. The upper airway becomes blocked, and nasal airflow stops for as long as 30 seconds. The person still attempts to breathe because chest and abdominal movement continue. During the apnoeic period, each successive diaphragmatic movement becomes stronger until the obstruction is relieved. Structural abnormalities such as a deviated septum, nasal polyps, or enlarged tonsils predispose a person to obstructive apnoea, although many patients/clients with sleep apnoea may have anatomically normal airways.

Obstructive apnoea causes a serious decline in arterial oxygen level (see Chapter 17). Patients/clients are at risk for cardiac dysrhythmias, right heart failure, pulmonary hypertension, anginal attacks, stroke, and hypertension. Middle-aged men tend to be more frequently affected, particularly when they have recently gained weight.

Central apnoea involves defects in the brain's respiratory-control centre. The impulse to breathe temporarily fails, and nasal airflow and chest wall movement cease. The oxygen saturation of the blood falls slightly. The condition is seen in patients/clients with brainstem injury, muscular dystrophy, and encephalitis. No treatment exists for central sleep apnoea.

A person with sleep apnoea typically snores at night. Cessation of breathing and then relief with marked snorting occurs. Near the end of each episode a brief arousal related to increased carbon dioxide levels occurs; the person rarely awakens. The individual is deprived of deep sleep periods. Complaints of excessive daytime sleepiness, sleep attacks, fatigue, morning headaches, and decreased sex drive are common. Treatment includes therapy for underlying cardiac or respiratory complications and emotional problems created by the disorder. A weight-loss programme and advice about sleeping habits can also help.

## Narcolepsy

**Narcolepsy** is a dysfunction of REM sleep processes and of mechanisms regulating alteration between sleep and awakened states. During the day a person may suddenly feel an overwhelming wave of sleepiness and fall asleep. REM sleep can occur within 15 minutes after sleep. Cataplexy, or sudden muscle weakness occurring during intense emotions such as anger, sadness, or laughter, may occur in the day. The person may lose muscle control and even fall to the floor. A person with narcolepsy may also have hallucinations that are like real dreams occurring just as he or she falls asleep. The person may not know the difference between a dream and reality. Sleep paralysis, or the feeling of being unable to move or talk just before waking or falling asleep, is another symptom.

The greatest problem with narcolepsy is that the individual falls asleep at inappropriate times. Unless a person understands the disorder, a sleep attack can easily be mistaken for laziness, lack of interest in activities, or drunkenness. A sufferer may be treated with stimulants that increase wakefulness and reduce sleep attacks and medications that suppress REM sleep. Brief daytime naps no longer than 20 minutes help reduce narcoleptic attacks. Factors that increase a narcoleptic person's drowsiness (for example, alcohol or exhausting activities) should be avoided.

## Sleep Deprivation

Although not a true sleep disorder, **sleep deprivation** is a problem that many individuals experience as a result of hospitalization, especially in intensive care units. Sleep deprivation involves decreases in the amount, quality, and consistency of sleep. When sleep becomes interrupted or fragmented, changes in the normal sequence of sleep stages occur, and cycles cannot be completed (McIntosh, 1989). Gradually a cumulative sleep deprivation develops.

A person's response to sleep deprivation is highly variable. Patients/clients may experience a variety of physiological and psychological symptoms (see box). The severity of symptoms is often related to the duration of sleep deprivation.

The most effective treatment for sleep deprivation is elimination or correction of factors that disrupt the sleep pattern. Nurses play an important role in treating sleep deprivation problems.

## Other Sleep Disorders

Sleep problems common in children include **somnambulism** (sleepwalking), night terrors, nightmares, **nocturnal enuresis** (bedwetting), and tooth grinding (bruxism). Specific treatment

## Sleep Deprivation Symptoms

### Physiological Symptoms
- Hand tremors
- Decreased reflexes
- Slowed response time
- Reduction in word memory
- Decreased reasoning, judgement, and association
- Cardiac dysrhythmias
- Decreased auditory and visual alertness

### Psychological Symptoms
- Moods
- Disorientation
- Irritability
- Decreased motivation
- Fatigue
- Sleepiness
- Hyperactivity
- Agitation

for these disorders varies. However, in all cases, it is important to support patients/clients and maintain their safety. For example, sleepwalkers are unaware of surroundings and are slow to react. Thus, the risk of falls is great. A nurse should not startle sleepwalkers but instead gently lead them back to bed.

## NURSING PROCESS AND SLEEP

 ASSESSMENT

To promote a normal restful sleep, the nurse assesses the person's sleep history, including factors that normally influence sleep. If sleep is adequate the nursing history can be brief.

Sleep is a subjective experience. Only the person can report whether it is restful. If the person is satisfied with the amount of sleep received, it may be considered normal (Closs, 1988). If a person admits to or the nurse suspects a sleep problem a more detailed history is required. However, Closs (1990) checked the reporting of sleep in nursing notes in relation to quantity, quality, use of medication and pre-sleep routine. Her findings indicated that recording of sleep was sparse and done on a random basis. She suggests that nurses should place more emphasis on comprehensive and reliable sleep assessment strategies for patients/clients.

### Sleep Assessment Tools
Most people can provide a reasonably accurate estimate of their sleep patterns, particularly if any changes have occurred. One of the most effective subjective methods for assessing sleep quality is use of a visual analogue scale (Closs, 1988). The nurse draws a straight horizontal line about 100 mm long. Opposing statements such as 'best night's sleep' and 'worst night's sleep' are at each end of the line. The middle represents an average night's sleep. Patients/clients are asked to place marks on the horizontal line at points corresponding to their perceptions of the previous night's

sleep. The distance of the mark along the line can be measured in millimetres and offers a numerical value for satisfaction with sleep. The scale can be re-used to show change over time.

Assessment is aimed at understanding the characteristics of any sleep problem and the person's usual sleep habits. Clapin-French (1986) strongly recommends the use of a sleep history, particularly in the care of older adults. Fig. 20-4 is one example of a framework through which to conduct a sleep history and assessment.

### Sources for Sleep Assessment
The individual is the best resource for describing a sleep problem. The person can also report the extent to which a sleep problem represents a change from normal. Often the person knows the cause for sleep problems, such as a noisy environment or worry over a relationship.

When caring for children, parents are often the best source of information. Parents are usually successful in learning why their children have trouble sleeping. Children often are able to relate fears or worries that inhibit their ability to fall asleep. If children frequently awaken in the middle of bad dreams, parents can identify the problem but perhaps do not understand the meanings of the dreams. Parents can also describe the typical behaviour patterns that foster or impair sleep. For example, excessive stimulation from active play or visiting friends may predictably impair sleep. With chronic sleep problems, parents can relate the duration of the problem, its progression, and the child's responses.

Information from patients'/clients' bed partners may reveal the nature of certain sleep disorders; for example, they can report on the patients'/clients' patterns. Partners of patients/clients with sleep apnoea often complain that their sleep is disturbed by clients' snoring and restless movements; as a result different beds or rooms are often required. The nurse should ask the partner whether the patient/client has pauses or interruptions of breathing or snoring during sleep. Some partners mention becoming fearful when patients/clients apparently stop breathing and then struggle before airflow returns. Partners may also be able to describe the frequency of clients' apnoeic attacks.

## DESCRIPTION OF SLEEPING PROBLEMS
When a person admits to, or the nurse suspects, a sleep problem, the nursing history must be detailed so that therapeutic care can be provided. Open-ended questions help a person to describe a problem more fully. A general description of a problem followed by more focused questions usually reveal specific characteristics that can be used in planning therapies. Assessment questions might include the following:
1. *Nature of the problem:* What type of problem do you have falling asleep? Why do you think your sleep is inadequate? Describe for me a typical night's sleep.
2. *Signs and symptoms:* Do you have difficulty in falling asleep or re-awakening? Do you snore loudly or have you been told that you snore loudly? Do you have headaches when awakening? Does your child awaken from nightmares?
3. *Onset and duration:* When did you first notice the problem?

How long has this problem lasted?

4. *Severity:* How long does it take to fall asleep? How often during the week you do have trouble falling asleep? Tell me how many hours of sleep you got this week; compare that to normal.

5. *Predisposing factors:* What you do just before going to bed? Have you recently had any changes at work or at home?

6. *Effect on patient/client:* How has the loss of sleep affected you? Ask a spouse or friend: have you noticed any changes in behaviour since the sleep problem started? Do you feel tired or irritable or have trouble concentrating?

Proper questioning helps the nurse determine the type of sleep disturbance and the nature of the problem.

## Normal Sleep Pattern

**Normal sleep** is difficult to define because individuals vary greatly. Knowing a person's normal sleep pattern allows a nurse to match sleeping conditions in a health care setting with those in the home. To determine the person's normal sleep pattern the nurse could ask the following questions:

1. What time do you usually go to sleep?
2. How quickly do you fall asleep?
3. What is the average number of hours you sleep during the night?
4. How many times do you awaken at night?
5. When do you typically awaken in the morning?
6. Do you rise once you awaken or do you stay in bed?

The nurse can then compare these data with the norm for the person's age and can begin to assess for patterns such as insomnia.

### Framework for Sleep Assessment

Name

Age

Normal pattern and quality of sleep during health

Current pattern and quality of sleep

Presence of dreams or nightmares

Present medication (including drugs which promote or inhibit sleep)

Current life events that may interfere with normal sleep

Emotional status, for example presence of anxiety/depression

Sleep related rituals, for example bedtime drinks, reading, television

Dietary factors

Sleeping environment preferred

Wake-time behaviour, for example daytime naps, mental efficiency

Adapted from Hodgson L: Why do we need sleep? Relating theory to practice. *J Adv Nurs*, 16: 1991.

**Fig. 20-4** Framework for assessing sleep.

Patients'/clients' sleep problems may show patterns drastically different from normal patterns, or they may be relatively minor.

## PHYSICAL ILLNESS

The nurse determines whether the person has any pre-existing health problems that might interfere with sleep.

If the person has recently undergone surgery he or she is at risk of a sleep disturbance. Pain is one of the most common causes of night time awakening in surgical patients/clients, and most patients/clients experience an increase in severity at night (Closs, 1992). Individuals often awaken frequently during the first night after surgery and receive little deep or REM sleep. Depending on the type of surgery, it may take several days for a normal sleep cycle to return. Effective pain assessment and control are vital if sleep disruption is to be minimized.

## PRESENT MEDICATION

The nurse also assesses the patient's/client's medication history, including a description of over-the-counter and prescribed drugs. If a patient/client takes medications to aid sleeping, the nurse determines the dosage.

## CURRENT LIFE EVENTS

The nurse establishes whether the person is experiencing any changes in lifestyle. A person's occupation may offer a clue to the nature of a sleep problem. Changes in job responsibilities, rotating shifts, or long hours can contribute to a sleep disturbance. Questions about social activities, recent travel, or mealtimes help clarify the sleep assessment.

## EMOTIONAL AND MENTAL STATUS

If a person is anxious, excitable, or angry, mental preoccupations can seriously disrupt sleep. The person may be experiencing emotional stress related to illness or situational crises such as loss of job or a loved one. Thus, the patient's/client's emotions may affect his or her ability to sleep.

## BEDTIME RITUALS

The nurse asks about the patient's/client's bedtime rituals, for example, he or she may drink a glass of milk, take a sleeping pill, eat a snack, watch television, or exercise. The nurse assesses habits that are beneficial compared with those that disturb sleep.

Hospitalization often interferes with bedtime rituals. Restrictions caused by illness may prevent the person from eating, drinking, or exercising. A nurse learns about the effects of the hospital environment and routines on the person's ability to fall asleep.

The nurse should pay special attention to a child's bedtime rituals. The parents can report whether it is necessary, for example, to read the child a bedtime story, rock the child to sleep, or engage in quiet play.

## DIETARY FACTORS

Assessment can reveal recent weight gain or weight loss. Crisp and Stonehill (1973) described how a reduction in total sleep, more broken sleep and earlier wakening were associated with weight loss, whereas weight gain has been linked to less broken sleep, later awakening and an increase in total sleep. Dietary habits, intake of calories and anorexia should all be assessed to determine if a problem exists.

## WAKE TIME BEHAVIOUR

The nurse should ask the patient/client about the number and duration of any daytime naps taken, which may increasingly account for periods of rest as a person becomes older (Clapin–French, 1986). If a person is taking sleeping medication, the nurse should ascertain whether 'hangover effects' are present during the day. It may be possible with careful questioning to establish a link between taking medication for other problems and the onset of sleeping disturbances.

## BEHAVIOURS OF SLEEP DEPRIVATION

Some individuals are unaware of their sleep problems. The nurse observes behaviours such as irritability, disorientation (similar to a drunken state), and slurred speech.

By carefully assessing the nature of a sleep disturbance, the nurse can design more effective interventions, for example, the nurse uses different therapies to help individuals who are unable to fall asleep versus patients/clients who have sleep attacks during the day.

Assessment should also identify the probable cause of the sleep disturbance. These causes become the focus of interventions for minimizing or eliminating the problem. For example, if a person is experiencing insomnia as a result of a noisy environment, the nurse could offer some basic recommendations such as controlling noise, reducing interruptions, or keeping doors closed. If the insomnia is related to worry, the nurse's actions could focus upon facilitating or supporting the patient's/client's coping strategies.

 PLANNING

An individualized care plan can be developed only after the nurse has gained an understanding of the patient's/client's current sleep pattern, the person's perception of a normal sleep pattern, and the factors disrupting sleep. Together the nurse and patient/client develop realistic interventions to promote rest and sleep in the home or health care setting (see care plan). The patient's/client's bed partner may have some useful suggestions.

In a hospital the nurse plans treatments or regimes so that the person will be able to rest; for example, in the intensive care unit, nurses check available electronic monitors to detect trends in vital signs without awakening the person each hour. Other staff members should be aware of the care plan so that they can cluster activities at certain times to reduce awakenings.

The nature of a sleep disturbance determines whether referrals to additional health care providers are necessary. It is also important to plan for continuity of care. For example, when a patient/client goes home following hospitalization, information about the sleep problem might be useful to the community nurse.

The success of sleep therapy depends on an approach that fits the person's lifestyle and the nature of the sleep disorder. The goals of any care plan for a patient/client needing sleep or rest might include the following:

1. Patient/client obtains a sense of restfulness and renewed energy following sleep.
2. Patient/client establishes a regular sleep pattern.
3. Patient/client understands factors that promote or disrupt sleep.
4. Patient/client assumes self-care behaviours to eliminate factors contributing to sleep disturbance.

 IMPLEMENTATION

Patient/clients need adequate sleep and rest to recover from physical illness. Nursing care in an acute-care setting differs from that provided in a patient's/client's home. The primary differences are in the environment and the nurse's ability to support normal sleep habits. The person's age also influences the type of therapies that are most effective. Interventions that promote normal sleep patterns include the general strategies listed below.

### Environmental Controls

All individuals require a suitable sleeping environment including a comfortable room temperature and proper ventilation, minimal sources of noise, a comfortable bed (see Procedures 20.1 and 20.2), and proper lighting. Infants sleep best when the room temperature is 18° to 21°C at night. Cots should be positioned away from open windows or drafts. The infant is covered with a light, warm blanket. Children and adults vary more with regard to what they consider to be a comfortable room temperature. Some prefer to sleep without covers. Older adults often require extra blankets or covers, while many sleep with their socks on.

It helps to eliminate sources of distracting noise so that the area is as quiet as possible. Noise and other environmental factors can cause chronic fatigue (World Health Organization, 1980). Hilton (1987) has discovered that sound levels of talking staff and noise from equipment are higher than the level of sound that raises pain perception.

In a hospital the nurse can control noise in several ways (see box). In addition, nurses should make equipment manufacturers aware of the need for quiet in future product designs. At home, it may require the cooperation of people living with the patient/client to reduce noise. For example, the volume of a television watched by family members in another room can be reduced.

A bed and mattress should provide support and comfortable firmness. Bed boards can be placed under mattresses to add support. The position of the bed in the room may make a difference for some people.

Some people experience disorientation or wandering at night. Bed side rails should not be used to stop these individuals getting out of bed, as they can cause injury. Placing the patient's/client's mattress on the floor can reduce the risk of injury if the person falls out of bed. A call bell should also be placed within the

## Control of Noise in Hospital

- Close door if patient/client is in a side room
- Reduce volume of nearby telephone
- Wear rubber-soled shoes
- Turn off bedside equipment that is not in use (e.g. oxygen, suction equipment)
- Avoid abrupt loud noises such as flushing a toilet or moving a bed
- Keep only necessary conversations at low levels, particularly at night
- Conduct discussions or nursing reports in a private, separate area away from patients/clients
- Turn off television or radio unless patient/client prefers soft music

patient's/client's reach so that he or she may ask for help as and when necessary.

Individuals vary in regard to the amount of light that they prefer at night. Older adults may sleep best with dimmed lights (see Chapter 26). This can help prevent falls if they get up during the night. If street lights shine through windows or if patients/clients sleep during the day, heavy curtains or blinds are helpful. Nurses can close curtains between patients/clients. Lights on a hospital ward or unit can be dimmed at night.

## Promoting Bedtime Rituals

Bedtime rituals relax patients/clients in preparation for sleep. It is easier for people to go to sleep when they feel fatigued or sleepy.

Newborns and infants sleep through so much of the day that a specific ritual is hardly necessary. However, quiet activities, such as holding them snugly in blankets, singing or talking softly, and gently rocking, helps infants to fall asleep.

A bedtime ritual (for example, same hour of sleep, snack, or quiet activity) used consistently helps young children avoid attempts to delay sleeping. Toddlers and preschool children may be too excited and full of energy to go to bed. Parents are advised to reinforce patterns of preparing for bedtime. Reading stories, allowing children to sit on the parent's or nurse's lap while listening to music, or listening to a prayer are routines that can be associated with preparing for bed. Quiet activities such as colouring and reading work well with school-aged children.

Working towards a consistent time for sleep helps most people gain a healthy sleep pattern and strengthens the rhythm of the sleep-wake cycle.

Relaxation exercises are a useful bedtime ritual. Slow, deep breathing for 1 or 2 minutes induces calm. Rhythmic contraction and relaxation of muscles (see Chapter 32) alleviates tension and prepares the body for rest (Hoch and Reynolds, 1986). Guided imagery, praying, meditation, and yoga may also promote sleep.

## Promoting Comfort

People fall asleep only after feeling comfortable and relaxed. The nurse can use several measures to promote comfort. Minor irritants can keep patients/clients awake. Nappies should be changed before placing infants in bed. Soft cotton nightclothes keep infants or small children warm and comfortable.

Hospital beds tend to be harder than ones at home and are often of a different height, length, or width. Keeping beds clean

and dry and in a comfortable position may help patients/clients relax (Procedures 20.1 and 20.2). Some individuals suffer painful illnesses requiring special comfort measures such as application of heat, use of supportive dressings or splints, and proper positioning.

A warm bath or shower before bedtime can be relaxing. Patients/clients restricted to bed should be offered the opportunity to wash the face and hands. Toothbrushing and care of dentures also help to prepare the person for sleep.

## Establishing Periods of Rest and Sleep

In a hospital or continuous care setting it is difficult to provide individuals with the time required to rest and sleep. However, the nurse plans care to avoid awakening patients/clients for nonessential tasks. The nurse can help by scheduling assessments, treatments and procedures for times when patients/clients are awake. For example, if a person's physical condition has been stable, the nurse should avoid awakening the person to check vital signs. Unless maintaining a drug's therapeutic blood level is essential, medications should be given during waking hours. The nurse should work with the radiology department and other support services to plan therapies at intervals that allow patients/clients time for rest.

When the person's condition demands more frequent monitoring, the nurse can plan activities to allow extended rest periods. For example, if a person needs frequent dressing changes, is receiving intravenous therapy, and has drainage tubes from several sites, the nurse should not make a separate trip to the bedside to check each problem. Instead, the nurse should use a single visit to change the dressing, regulate the intravenous system, and empty the drainage tubes. In the home, it may help to encourage individuals to stay physically active during the day so that they are more likely to sleep at night. Increasing daytime activity lessens problems with falling asleep.

Some people like to take a short nap during the day. Hayter (1985) suggests that older adults take afternoon naps to restore the body physically. Hoch and Reynolds (1986) recommend that naps be taken at the same time each day to maintain a consistent schedule.

## Controlling Physiological Disturbances

For patients/clients with physical illness, the nurse can help control symptoms that disrupt sleep. For example, a person with respiratory difficulties can sleep with two pillows or in a semi-sitting position to ease the effort to breathe. The person may benefit from taking prescribed bronchodilators before sleep to prevent airway obstruction. A patient/client with a hiatus hernia also needs special care. After meals the person may experience a burning sensation as a result of gastric reflux. To prevent sleep disturbances, the person should eat a small meal several hours before bedtime and sleep in a semi-sitting position. Patients/clients with pain, nausea, or other recurrent symptoms should receive any symptom-relieving medication at a time so that the drug's peak action takes effect at bedtime. Closs (1990) identified that giving analgesia was considered by postoperative patients/clients in her study to be one of the most helpful nursing

## Sample Care Plan for Sleep Pattern Disturbance

| Problem | Goal | Nursing Action | Evaluation | Rationale |
|---|---|---|---|---|
| Insufficient, poor quality sleep due to recent life changes and alteration in sleep scheduling | Elizabeth understands factors in present lifestyle that affect her ability to sleep and resumes normal sleep preparation habits | Outline process of normal sleep Assist patient/client to identify specific sleep preparation habits which are effective in promoting sleep Obtain verbal commitment to resume normal sleep preparation habits | Elizabeth will state that she resumed normal sleep preparation behaviour and discontinued activities which contributed to sleep disturbance at follow-up appointment in 2 weeks | Continuation of habits of normal bedtime intake promotes sleep (Fordham, 1988) Behavioural contracts between nurse and patient/client have demonstrated success for behavioural modification (Gilpatrick, 1989) |
| | Elizabeth will use relaxation therapies and retire to bed in state of relaxation | Discuss the importance of establishing relaxation time between study and retiring at night Promote resumption of usual relaxation activities Teach simple relaxation techniques | Elizabeth will incorporate one or more relaxation techniques into her sleep preparation routine within 1 week Elizabeth will state that she falls asleep regularly within 30 minutes of retiring at follow-up appointment in 2 weeks | Relaxation techniques have the potential to reduce psychological and physical tensions and promote sleep (Turton, 1986) |
| | Elizabeth will achieve a regular sleep pattern, feel rested, and have renewed energy following each night's sleep | Reinforce the importance of returning to previous established time of retiring | | |
| | | Outline measures that can be taken to promote a restful environment | Elizabeth will report a feeling of restfulness after waking each morning | Arousal threshold is dependent on the amount of prior sleep, and is higher following sleep deprivation (Downey and Bonnet, 1987) |
| | | Obtain commitment to complete a sleep diary for next 2 weeks | Elizabeth will report being able to complete work related responsibilities at follow-up appointment in 2 weeks | Provides a subjective view of success of strategies used and progress towards goals |

actions in assisting them to return to sleep when they woke in the night. Efforts to make them more comfortable, and taking time to talk were also appreciated as effective ways of promoting a return to sleep. As patient/client controlled analgesia and continuous administration of analgesia by infusion pump become more widely used, individuals' pain should be better controlled, and a positive effect on sleep can be expected as a result (see Chapter 27).

### Children's Nursing
### Promoting sleep in infants

Infants sleep best in softly lit rooms. Light should not shine directly on their eyes. Small table lamps in infants' rooms prevent total darkness. Infants' beds must be safe. To reduce the chance of suffocation, pillows or the ends of loose blankets should not be placed in cots. Loose-fitting plastic mattress covers should not be used, because infants might pull them over their faces and suffocate. Infants are usually placed on their backs or sides with the lower arm forward to stop them rolling over (DOH, 1993). This is because recent research suggests that cot death may be more common in infants who sleep prone. Some infants who require special care, or who have certain medical problems, need to be nursed prone. Infants should be kept warm, but they must not be allowed to get too warm, as overheating may also be a precipitating factor of cot death. Create a smoke free zone for the baby at all times.

### Stress Reduction

Sources of emotional stress can interfere with sleep. The inability to sleep can also make a person feel irritable and tense. When patients/clients feel emotionally upset, they should be encouraged not to force themselves to go to sleep. Otherwise, insomnia frequently develops, and soon bedtime is associated with the inability to relax. In the home, emotional calm and a sense of security can be promoted by attention to details such as checking doors are shut and locked, windows are open the right amount or wedged to prevent rattling, and pets are settled and confined to sleeping quarters (BUPA, 1985). A person who has difficulty falling asleep may find it helpful to get up and pursue a relaxing activity, such as reading or sewing, rather than stay in bed and think about sleep.

In a health care setting a nurse on the night shift should take time to sit and talk with patients/clients who are unable to sleep; thus helping him or her to ascertain what factors are keeping patients/clients awake. Explaining procedures or answering questions may give patients/clients the peace of mind needed to fall asleep. Massage can also be used to help patients/clients relax more thoroughly. If a sedative is indicated, the nurse confers with the doctor to ensure that the lowest dosage is used initially. Older adults can be particularly vulnerable to the side effects of sedatives, hypnotics, or analgesics because the medications are metabolized slowly.

Children often have bedtime fears, awaken during the night, or have nightmares. Fears (for example, fear of the dark, strange noises or intruders) are usually normal for this age. After nightmares, parents should enter children's rooms immediately and talk to them briefly about fears to provide a cooling-down period. Children are comforted but left in their own beds. Their fears should not be used as excuses to delay bedtime.

### Bedtime Snacks

Some people enjoy bedtime snacks, whereas others cannot sleep after eating. A full meal before bedtime can often cause gastrointestinal upset and interfere with the ability to fall asleep. Because of the association between weight loss and sleeping problems (Crisp and Stonehill, 1973) the nurse and dietitican have important roles to play in promoting sleep by devising ways of meeting the nutritional needs of patients/clients who have lost weight through disease, or who are anorexic.

Nurses should discourage patients/clients from drinking caffeine before bed. The stimulant can cause a person to stay awake or awaken throughout the night. Alcohol can interrupt sleep cycles and reduce the amount of deep sleep. Coffee, tea, colas, and alcohol act as diuretics and may cause a person to awaken in the night to void. However, as McMahon (1990b) points out, sudden withdrawal can lead to headaches and disturbed sleep patterns, so an established habit should be changed by the patient/client gradually reducing intake and substituting low caffeine equivalents.

### Adult Nursing
### Comfort measures for promoting sleep

- Administer any analgesics or sedatives about 30 minutes before bedtime
- Encourage patients/clients to wear loose-fitting nightwear
- Remove any irritants against the person's skin such as moist or wrinkled sheets or drainage tubing
- Position and support body parts to protect pressure areas and aid muscle relaxation
- Provide socks for people prone to cold
- Administer necessary hygiene measures
- Keep bed linen clean and dry
- Provide a comfortable mattress
- Encourage the person to void before going to sleep
- Provide a quiet environment

Infants require special measures to minimize night-time awakenings for feeding. It is common for children to have a need for middle-of-the-night bottle- or breast-feeding. Wong (1995) recommends offering the last feeding as late as possible. Eventually, it may help to gradually reduce the amount of formula or duration of breast-feeding. Infants should not be given bottles in bed.

## PROCEDURE 20-1 Making an Unoccupied Bed in Hospital

**SEQUENCE OF ACTIONS**

**RATIONALE**

1. Ensure patient is comfortable.
2. Assess clean linen required, according to patient's/client's needs (e.g. potential for incontinence).
3. Enlist assistance of a second nurse.

   To minimize time and energy of participating nurses.

4. Prepare needed equipment and take to bedside:
   a. linen bag
   b. appropriate clean linen
5. Wash hands and protect clothing if appropriate (e.g., plastic apron).

   Reduces transmission of microorganisms.

6. Pull out linen rest at foot of bed, or place two chairs to receive linen to be reused.

   Facilitates replacement.

7. Adjust bed to comfortable height for working.

   Provides easy access to bed. Minimizes strain on back and muscles.

8. With one nurse at each side of the bed, working together from top to bottom, loosen all bedclothes.
9. Remove pillowslips, discard into linen bag and place pillows on linen rest.
10. Remove each layer of bedlinen separately. If to be changed, place in linen bag. If to be reused, fold into 'Z' shape and place on linen rest in order of removal (*see illustration*)

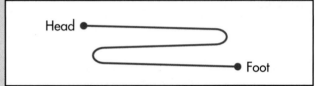

Reduces transmission of microorganisms. Promotes comfort.

11. Inspect mattress. Clean off any moisture/soiling with cleansing agent (and bacteriodial as appropriate), and dry thoroughly.
12. Replace bottom sheet, smoothing out all creases. Tuck in place with mitred corners, working from top to bottom (*see illustration*). Insert draw-sheet if required.

    Tucking excess under mattress anchors sheet in place to prevent sliding and wrinkling, which can contribute to pressure ulcers.

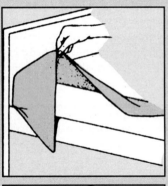
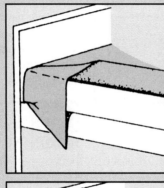
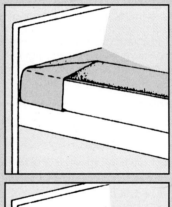
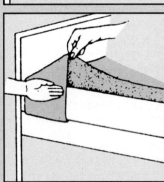
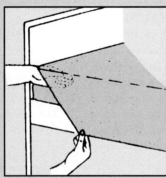
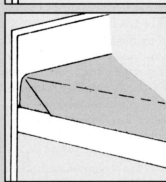

13. Replace top bedclothes separately, tucking in each at the foot of the bed with a modified mitred corner (*see illustration*), ensuring there is room for free movement of the patient's feet and adequate covering for the patient's shoulders.

    Modified mitred corner secures top linen, but keeps even edge of top sheet, blanket and spread draped over mattress. Avoids pressure on toes, ankles and heels. Provides adequate coverage for comfort.

14. Fold blanket down at top of the bed, then fold counterpane inwards to lie over blanket. Finally, fold sheet down over both.
15. Replace pillowslips and position pillows.
16. Replace linen rest or remove chairs. Remove soiled linen bag.
17. Wash hands and remove apron, if worn.

    Reduces transmission of microorganisms.

18. Evaluate patient's/client's condition and maximize opportunities for communication.

## PROCEDURE 20-2 Making an Occupied Bed in Hospital

| SEQUENCE OF ACTIONS | RATIONALE |
|---|---|
| 1. Assess clean linen required, according to patient's needs (e.g. potential for incontinence). Explain procedure to patient. Ensure comfort and maximize opportunities for communication and assessment. | |
| 2. Enlist assistance of a second nurse. | To minimize time and energy of participating nurses. |
| 3. Prepare needed equipment and take to bedside: a. linen bag b. appropriate clean linen | |
| 4. Wash hands and protect clothing if appropriate (e.g., plastic apron). | Reduces transmission of microorganisms. |
| 5. Pull out linen rest at foot of bed, or place two chairs to receive linen to be reused. | Facilitates replacement. |
| 6. Adjust bed to comfortable height for working. | Provides easy access to bed. Minimizes strain on back and muscles. |
| 7. Draw curtains around bedside. | |
| 8. Lie patient/client flat with one pillow, removing other pillows. Remove pillowslips, discard into linen bag and place pillows on linen rest. | |
| 9. With one nurse on each side, working together from top to bottom, remove each layer of bedlinen separately. Keep patient covered with a sheet or blanket. If linen is to be changed, place in linen bag. If to be reused, fold into 'Z' shape and place on linen rest in order of removal (see illustration). | Provides warmth and keeps body parts covered during linen removal. |
| 10. Roll patient/client to one side of bed, supported by second nurse, with pillow under head. Roll bottom sheet towards patient so that roll lies comfortably along length of body. | Ensures patient's/client's privacy. |
| 11. Inspect mattress. Clean off any moisture/soiling with appropriate cleansing agent and dry thoroughly. | Reduces transmission of microorganisms. Promotes comfort. |
| 12. Replace bottom sheet, smoothing out all creases. Tuck in place with mitred corners, working from top to bottom. Insert draw-sheet if required. | Tucking excess under mattress anchors sheet in place to prevent sliding and wrinkling, which could result in pressure ulcers. |
| 13. Carefully roll patient over the rolled sheets and remove the sheet to be changed. Roll the patient back to supine position and assist to a comfortable position with clean pillows. | |
| 14. Replace top bedclothes separately, tucking in each at the foot of the bed with a modified mitred corner. Ensure there is room for free movement of the patient's feet and sufficient bedclothes to cover the patient's shoulders. | |
| 15. Fold blanket down at top of the bed, then fold counterpane inwards to lie over blanket. Finally, fold sheet down over both. | |
| 16. Replace linen rest or remove chairs. Remove soiled linen bag. | |
| 17. Wash hands and remove apron, if worn. | Reduces transmission of microorganisms. |
| 18. Evaluate patient's/client's condition and ensure the patient is comfortable. | |

## Administering Sleep Medications

These drugs alleviate the specific symptoms of sleep problems, but do not alter the factors which cause them, so their use is non-curative (Schneider, 1991). They should be reserved for short courses of treatment after the cause of the sleeping difficulty has been established. Benzodiazepines such as nitrazepam, oxazepam, and lorazepam are the most commonly used hypnotics, as they have few side effects. However, the effects of hypnotics can last into the following day, and give rise to drowsiness, lethargy and headache (Henney *et al*, 1993).

It is now well established that the use of these drugs for more than short periods is associated with psychological and physical dependence, and leads to problems with their withdrawal (Kuhn, 1991) so reduction has to be a gradual process, and the decision to prescribe them should be a careful and considered one.

The use of nonprescription sleeping medications is not advisable. Patients/clients should be aware of the risks of such drugs, especially the long-term effects of sleep disruption. The nurse can help patients/clients use behavioural measures instead of drugs to cure sleep problems.

Regular use of any sleep medication can lead to tolerance, and withdrawal can then cause rebound insomnia. All patients/clients should understand the possible side effects of sleep medications. Routine monitoring of patient/client response to the medication is important.

 **EVALUATION**

Each patient/client has a different need for sleep and rest. For this reason the evaluation of therapies designed to promote sleep and rest must be individualized. Individuals in relatively good health may not need as much sleep or require as many adjustments to their sleep patterns as those whose physical conditions are poor.

The nurse ascertains whether expected outcomes have been met. Evaluative measures may be used shortly after a therapy has been tried (for example, observing whether a person falls asleep after reducing noise and darkening a room). Other evaluative measures may be used after a person awakens from sleep (for example, asking him or her to describe the number of awakenings during the previous night). The patient/client and partner can usually provide accurate evaluative information. Over longer periods, the nurse may use assessment tools such as a visual analogue scale to determine whether sleep has progressively improved or changed.

The nurse also assesses the level of understanding gained by the patient/client or family members after receiving instruction on sleep habits. Compliance with these practices may best be measured during a home visit, when the environment can be observed.

When expected outcomes are not met, the nurse revises nursing measures based on the patient's/client's needs or preferences. Finding an effective therapy depends on the person's sleep disturbance, age, and normal sleep pattern. The nurse documents the person's response to sleep therapies so that a continuum of care can be maintained. The nurse is effective in promoting rest and sleep if the goals of care are met.

## SUMMARY

Each day a person needs sleep to protect and restore body functions. Normally the sleep-wake cycle follows a 24-hour rhythm coordinated with other physiological functions such as body temperature and hormonal secretions. Sleep is a rhythm within a rhythm. After falling asleep, a person passes through stages that help the body rest and recover.

All age groups have different sleep requirements and sleep habits. Age affects the type of sleep therapies used by the nurse. The nurse's care may differ in the home compared with measures used to promote sleep in a hospital or extended-care setting.

Many factors can promote or disrupt sleep, and a number of sleep disorders can cause specific problems. The nurse assesses the nature of any sleep pattern. The patient's/client's participation in the care plan ensures an individualized approach to sleep therapy.

## CHAPTER 20 REVIEW

### Key Concepts

- Rest is not inactivity but a feeling of physical calm and freedom from worry.
- Sleep is believed to provide physiological and psychological restoration.
- The 24-hour sleep-wake cycle is a circadian rhythm that influences physiological function and behaviour.
- The control and regulation of sleep depends on a balance between central nervous system regulators.
- During a typical night's sleep a person passes through four to six complete sleep cycles. Each contains four NREM stages of sleep and a period of REM sleep.
- No specific number of hours of sleep is required by each person to rest and only a patient/client can report whether sleep is restful.
- Neonates, infants, and young children require more sleep than older children and adults.
- Symptoms of various diseases may disrupt sleep.
- Long-term use of sleeping pills may lead to difficulty in initiating and maintaining sleep.
- The hectic pace of a person's lifestyle, emotional and psychological stress, and alcohol ingestion disrupt the sleep pattern.
- An environment with a darkened room, reduced noise, comfortable bed, and good ventilation promotes sleep.
- The most common type of sleep disorder is insomnia, which is characterized by the inability to fall asleep, remain asleep during the night, or go back to sleep after awakening.
- If a person's sleep is adequate the nurse assesses the person's usual bedtime, normal bedtime ritual, and the preferred environment for sleeping.
- When a patient/client has a sleep problem, the nurse conducts a complete sleep history.
- Identifying sleep problems depends on identifying factors that impair sleep.
- When using environmental controls to promote sleep, the

nurse should consider the patient's/client's home and normal lifestyle.

- Noise can disrupt sleep and enhance pain perception.
- A bedtime ritual of relaxing activities prepares a person physically and mentally for sleep.
- Pain or other symptom control is essential to promote the ability to sleep.
- One of the most important nursing interventions for promoting sleep is establishing periods for sleep and rest.

## CRITICAL THINKING EXERCISES

1. Mrs Wills visits the community health centre for a routine visit. She is 78 years old. During a health history, she tells you that she normally gets only 5 hours of sleep and awakens as many as 3 times a night. Frequently, it may take her up to 30 minutes to fall asleep. Mrs Wills is concerned. What would you as the nurse tell her?

2. When conducting an assessment of a patient's/client's sleep pattern, what information can be gathered from a bed partner?

3. Mr John is a 55-year-old sheet-metal worker who works the evening shift. He typically drinks three to four pints of beer before going to bed. He normally sleeps about 6 hours a night after he goes to bed around 1 AM. It is common for him to arise during the night to urinate. His favourite way to relax is reportedly watching television in bed. As the nurse, what would you assess regarding Mr John's sleep history?

### Key Terms

Bed rest, p. 390
Biological clock, p. 391
Circadian rhythm, p. 391
Dreams, p. 393
Insomnia, p. 396
Narcolepsy, p. 397
Nocturnal enuresis, p. 397
Normal sleep, p. 399
NREM sleep, p. 392
Quality of sleep, p. 394
REM sleep, p. 392
Reticular activity system (RAS), p. 391
Sleep anpnoea, p. 397
Sleep deprivation, p. 397
Sleep disorders, p. 396
Sleep pattern, p. 392
Sleep, p. 390
Sleep-wake cycle, p. 391
Slow-wave sleep, p. 392
Somnambulism, p. 397

## REFERENCES

Biley F: Impact of noise in surgical wards, *Surg Nurs* :15, 1993.

Brown P: Shift work: punching the body clock, *Nurs Times* 84(44):26, 1988.

BUPA: *Facts about sleep and rest*, ed 3, London, 1985, BUPA

Medical Centre.

Canavan T: The psychobiology of sleep, *Nurs* 84(2):682, 1984.

Chase M, Weitzman ED, editors: *Sleep disorders: basic and clinical research*, New York, 1983, Spectrum.

Chuman MA: The neurological basis of sleep, *Heart Lung* 12:177, 1983.

Clapin-French E: Sleep patterns of aged persons in long-term care facilities, *J Adv Nurs* 11:57, 1986.

Closs SJ: Assessment of sleep in hospital patients: a review of methods, *J Adv Nurs* 13:501, 1988.

Closs SJ: Influences on patients' sleep on surgical wards, *Surg Nurs* 3(2):12, 1990.

Colling J: Sleep disturbances in aging: a theoretical and empiric analysis, *ANS* 6:36, 1983.

Crisp A, Stonehill E: Aspects of the relationship between sleep and nutrition, *Br J Psychiatry* 122:379, 1973.

Department of Health: *Sleeping position of infants and the risk of cot death (sudden infant death)*, London, 1993, DOH.

Downey R, Bonnet M: Performance during frequent sleep disruption, *Sleep* 10(4):354, 1987.

Fordham M: Sleep disturbance. In Wilson-Barnett J, Batchup L: *Patient problems: a research base for nursing care*, London, 1988, Scutari.

Gilpatrick D: Moving clients towards wellness, *Clin Nurs Specialist* 3(1):25, 1989.

Hayter J: Sleep behavior of older persons, *Nurs Res* 32:242, 1983.

Hayter J: To nap or not to nap? *Geriatr Nurs* 6:104, 1985.

Henney C *et al*: *A handbook of drugs in nursing practice*, ed 4, Edinburgh, 1993, Churchill Livingstone.

Hilton A: The hospital racket: how noisy is your unit? *Am J Nurs* 87:59, 1987.

Hoch C, Reynolds C: Sleep disturbances and what to do about them, *Geriatr Nurs* 7:24, 1986.

Hodgson L: Why do we need sleep? Relating theory to practice, *J Adv Nurs* 16:1503, 1991.

Kuhn M: Pharmacotherapies: a nursing process approach ed 2, Philadelphia, 1991.

McIntosh A: Sleep deprivation in critically ill patients, *Nurs* 3(35): 1989.

McKenna JJ: Rethinking 'healthy' infant sleep, *Breastfeeding Abstracts* 12(3):27, 1993.

McMahon R: Sleep management, *Surg Nurs* 3(4):25, 1990a.

McMahon R: Sleep therapies, *Surg Nurs* 3(5):17, 1990b.

McNeil BJ *et al*: Sleep questionnaire, *Am J Nurs* 86(1):261, 1986.

Roper N *et al*: *The elements of nursing*, ed 3, Edinburgh, 1990, Churchill Livingstone.

Schneider F. Sedatives and hypnotics. In Kuhn M, editor: *Pharmacotherapies: a nursing process approach*, ed 2, Philadelphia, 1991, FA Davis.

Torrance C: Sleep and wound healing, *Surg Nurs* 3(3):17, 1990.

Turton P: Relaxation techniques, *Nurs* 3(9):348, 1986.

Webster RA, Thompson DR: Sleep in hospital, *J Adv Nurs* 11:447, 1986.

Wong DL: *Nursing care of infants and children*, ed 5, St Louis, 1991, Mosby.

World Health Organization: *Noise*, Geneva, 1980, The Organization.

## FURTHER READING

### Adult Nursing

Gournay: Sleeping without drugs, *Nurs Times* 84(11):46, 1988.

Halfens R *et al*: Sleep medication in Dutch hospitals, *J Adv Nurs* 16:1422, 1991.

Jensen D, Herr K: Sleeplessness, *Adv Clin Nurs Res* 28(2):385, 1993.

Kearnes S: Insomnia in the elderly, *Nurs Times* 85(47):32, 1989.

Ogilvie A: Sources and levels of noise on the ward at night, *Nurs Times* 76:1363, 1980.

### Mental Health Nursing

Bhanji S: Treatment of depression by sleep deprivation, *Nurs Times* 73:540, 1977.

Bowden C: Current treatment of depression, *Hosp Community Psychiatry* 36(1):1192, 1985.

Brown RP, Mann JJ: A clinical perspective on the role of neurotransmitters in mental disorders, *Hosp Community Psychiatry* 36:489, 1985.

Field W: Physical causes of depression, *J Psychosoc Nurs* 23(10):7, 1985.

Wright J, Beck A: Cognitive therapy of depression theory and practice, *Hosp Community Psychiatry* 34(12):1119, 1983.

### Children's Nursing

Beal S, Finch C: An overview of retrospective case-control studies investigating the relationship between prone sleeping position and SIDS, *J Paed Child Health* 27:334, 1991.

Bernal J: Night waking in infants during the first 14 months, *Devel Med Child Neurol* 15:760, 1973.

Fardell J: Children who don't sleep, *Nurs Times* 85(17):39, 1989.

Gilbert R *et al*: Combined effect of infection and heavy wrapping in sudden infant death, *Arch Dis Child* 67:171, 1992.

McKenna JJ *et al*: Sleep and arousal patterns among co-sleeping mother-infant pairs: implications for SIDS, *Am J Phys Anthropol* 83:331, 1991.

hite M *et al*: Sleep onset latency and distress in hospitalised children, *Nurs Res* 39(3):134, 1990.

### Learning Disabilities Nursing

Quine L: Sleep problems with mental handicap, *J Mental Deficiency Research*, 35 (4): 269-90, 1991.

Quine L, Wade K: Sleep disturbance in children with severe learning difficulties: an examination and an intervention trial, Canterbury, 1991, University of Kent at Canterbury.

Stores G: Sleep studies in children with a mental handicap, *J Child Psychology & Psychiatry*, 33(8): 1303-17, 1992.

Wertheimer A: Stopping a long day's journey into night, *Search*, 9: 29-32, 1991.

# Nutrition

## CHAPTER OUTLINE

## LEARNING OUTCOMES

After studying this chapter, you should be able to:
- *Define the key terms listed.*
- *Explain the importance of maintaining a balance between energy intake and energy output from food metabolism.*
- *List the six categories of nutrients and explain why each is necessary for nutrition.*
- *List the end products of carbohydrate, protein, and lipid metabolism.*
- *Describe the digestive process and the role of enzymes in food breakdown.*
- *Describe the role of the intestines in the absorption, metabolism and elimination processes.*
- *Explain Nutritional Reference Values.*
- *Discuss dietary guidelines for health promotion.*
- *Identify factors that may influence the food intake of specific patient/client groups.*
- *Be aware of the alterations in nutritional needs throughout the life cycle.*
- *Discuss the major areas of nutritional assessment.*
- *Identify three major nutritional problems and describe patients/clients at risk for these problems.*
- *Identify environmental and other factors that may put the patient/client at risk for inadequate nutritional status in the health care setting.*
- *Discuss the role of the dietitian and the importance of diet counselling in evaluation and patient/client teaching in all settings.*
- *State what is meant by enteral and parenteral nutrition.*

The scientific approach to nutrition is relatively new. Previously, in the absence of other forms of treatments, early patient/client care relied heavily on the preparation and administration of food to maintain the body's strength and fight disease. Certainly, Florence Nightingale had no doubt as to its importance. In one of the first nursing text books, she wrote:

> What nursing ought to do .... It ought to signify the proper use of fresh air, light, warmth, cleanliness and the proper selection and administration of diet. (Nightingale, 1860)

The nurse's role in nutrition and **diet therapy** has changed over the years. Health professionals have become more aware of the direct links between good nutrition and good health. The link between good nutrition, wound healing and effective immunity is now well established, but it is possible that many other health problems are linked to nutrition. It is worth remembering that although good nutrition does not always lead to good health, good health is not achievable without adequate nutrition.

Today, there is also a greater awareness of the link between nutrition and the onset of acute and chronic illnesses. For instance, a possible link has been documented between food high in saturated fats, animal fats and cholesterol, and coronary artery disease. Foods high in starch are associated with a reduced risk of colorectal cancers.

This increased interest is not exclusive to health professionals: women's magazines frequently carry new pieces of dietary advice, and unwise or excessively vigorous dietary control that can cause more problems than solutions. Nurses must aquaint themselves with the facts about nutrition, and develop the ability to be discerning when reading research, so that this powerful tool for health promotion can be used effectively.

## PRINCIPLES OF NUTRITION

The body requires food to provide energy for organ function, body movement, and work; to maintain body temperature; and provide raw materials for enzyme function, growth, replacement of cells, and repair. **Metabolism** refers to all the chemical reactions within the body. It consists of **anabolic** reactions that build substances and body tissue from smaller substances, and **catabolic** reactions that break down substances. Food is eaten, digested, and absorbed to produce the energy needed for these reactions.

### Energy Balance
**Energy** is the ability to carry out work. It is measured in joules, which are symbolized by the letter J. A **joule** is defined as the energy released when one kilogram of weight falls one metre, under the influence of gravity. Energy is often measured in terms of kilojoules (kJ, one thousand joules) or megajoules (MJ, one million joules). One calorie (dietetic use) is equivalent to 4.2 kilojoules.

People's energy requirements vary and are influenced by many factors. The energy requirement of an awake person at rest is called the **basal metabolic rate (BMR).** The BMR is the energy needed at a person's lowest level of cellular function. The BMR varies with age, body size and temperature, environmental temperature, growth, gender and nutritional status. Activity increases energy requirements beyond those needed to fulfil BMR. With such variations, giving general rules for energy requirements can be misleading. However, it is useful to have an average: an adult man requires 10.6 MJ per day, and an adult woman 8.05 MJ per day, in order to fulfil his or her BMR. Each individual will require sufficient energy in order to fulfil his or her BMR, plus additional energy to meet energy requirements caused by all other activity.

The balance between energy intake and output directly affects changes in body weight:

$$\text{weight change} = \text{energy input} - \text{energy output}$$

When individuals consume more energy than they require, energy is stored within the body. The short-term energy reserve is glycogen, a complex carbohydrate that is osmotically inert. Glycogen is stored mainly in the liver and skeletal muscles. The liver stores approximately 500kJ of energy, or enough for 24 hours (Rich, 1982). The longer term energy stores are adipose, or fat tissue. The energy equivalent of a 1 kg change in body weight is 25 to 29 MJ. All body cells (except erythrocytes and central nervous system cells) can oxidize fatty acids for energy. In starvation, body protein, particularly skeletal muscle, is metabolized in order to obtain energy.

The catabolism of 1 g of pure carbohydrate produces 17 kJ of energy; 1 g of protein also yields 17 kJ and the catabolism of alcohol 29 kJ. Fats are a very concentrated source of energy, releasing 37 kJ per gram catabolized. In the West, many people eat too high a proportion of fat. In 1983 the National Advisory Council recommended that fat should provide only 20% of total energy intake.

**Nutrients** are substances that contain the elements necessary for body function. The six categories of nutrients are water, carbohydrates, proteins, lipids, vitamins and minerals. Water is required because nutrients must be in solution for absorption, transportation, and excretion. Vitamins and minerals act as co-enzymes in biochemical reactions.

### Water
Water is the most important nutrient, since the function of cells depends on a fluid environment. Water comprises 60 to 70% of total body weight (see Chapter 18). The bodies of lean people contain more water than bodies of obese people. Infants have the greatest percentage of total body weight as water, and older people have the least. Consequently, these groups are most vulnerable to water deprivation or loss. Yet no one, when deprived of water, can survive for more than a few hours in a desert or a few days in the most protective environment. The estimated daily fluid requirements for people of different ages are listed in Table 21-1.

**Children's Nursing**
**Diarrhoea and vomiting**

Nursing children with diarrhoea and vomiting requires close observation since the decreased intake of fluids, combined with an increased output of both fluid and electrolytes, can seriously threaten the body fluid economy of the infant. Such infants require fluid replacement with an oral electrolyte solution, such as oral rehydration solution or intravenous fluids. Infants who are breast-fed should continue to be breast-fed if possible and, if they are able to tolerate food, they should be given foods containing carbohydrates and potassium, such as cereals with mashed banana.

### Table 21-1 Ranges of Daily Fluid Requirements

| Age | Fluid Requirements *ml/kg/day* |
|-----|-------------------------------|
| 3 days | 80-100 |
| 10 days | 125-150 |
| 3 months | 140-160 |
| 6 months | 130-155 |
| 9 months | 125-145 |
| 1 yr | 120-135 |
| 2 yr | 115-125 |
| 4 yr | 100-110 |
| 6 yr | 100-110 |
| 10 yr | 90 -100 |
| 14 yr | 50 - 60 |
| 18 yr | 40 - 50 |
| 19-50 | 50 |

*Adapted from Behrman RE, Vaughan VC, editors: Nelson's textbook of pediatrics ed 3, Philadelphia, 1987, Saunders.*

Fluid needs are met by consumption of liquids and solid foods, such as fresh fruits and vegetables, and also by water produced when food is oxidized during metabolism. In a healthy individual the fluid intake from all sources equals the fluid output through elimination, respiration, and sweating (see Chapter 18). Disease, however can alter a person's fluid requirements.

## Carbohydrates

**Carbohydrates** are composed of carbon, hydrogen and oxygen. The hydrogen:oxygen ratio is the same as in water; two hydrogen ions for every oxygen ion. Carbohydrates are abundant in the diet, and also tend to be reasonably cheap to purchase. They are obtained primarily from plant foods. The only important source of animal carbohydrate is lactose (milk sugar).

Carbohydrates are classified according to the number of **saccharides** (sugar units) they contain. Monosaccharides cannot be broken down into more basic molecules. The most important monosaccharide is glucose. Glucose is the usual end-product of carbohydrate digestion. Disaccharides, such as sucrose (common table sugar), lactose, and maltose are formed by chemically combining two monosaccharides together, with water. Carbohydrates made of these small molecules taste sweet. Polysaccharides such as starch are composed of many sugar units. Polysaccharides are insoluble in water and do not taste sweet. They are digested into smaller molecules with varying degrees of completeness.

Plants store carbohydrates as **starch**. Starch is made up of granules enclosed by cell walls. When starch is cooked, the granules swell and burst their cellulose walls. Raw starch foods are more difficult to digest than the same foods after cooking because the freeing of the granules from the cellulose permits greater contact with digestive enzymes and more complete digestion. Starch digestion consists of several steps (Fig. 21-1).

Some polysaccharides cannot be digested because humans do not have enzymes capable of breaking them down. Nevertheless, these polysaccharides have a role in human nutrition because they

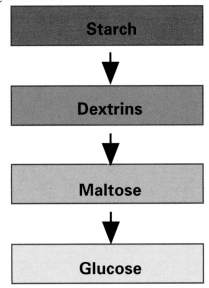

**Fig. 21-1** Digestion of starch.

add fibre to the diet. **Dietary fibre** consists of the fibrous substances in fruits and vegetables such as the structural polymers of cell walls. Fibre is receiving increasing attention as a dietary factor in disease prevention and treatment. The best sources are raw fruit, raw or lightly cooked vegetables and wholemeal (not brown) bread. However, some people find the rough texture of this diet difficult to chew. It is possible to add bran to the diet, which is easy to chew and swallow; however this should be accompanied by water, (since fibre is osmotically very active) as well as by plenty of minerals and vitamins, because high fibre diets increase faecal bulk.

## Proteins

**Proteins** are composed of hydrogen, oxygen, carbon and nitrogen. Most proteins also contain sulphur and phosphorus. The atoms are arranged into **amino acids** linked into a chain to form proteins. Proteins are large molecules, made up of many amino acids. They are essential for the synthesis of body tissue in growth, maintenance and repair. Protein intake is particularly important during periods of rapid growth, and after disease or injury.

Proteins are classified as simple, conjugated or derived. Simple proteins are hydrolysed (broken down) into amino acids or their derivatives. Albumin and globulin are simple proteins. The combination of a simple protein with a nonprotein substance produces a conjugated protein. Examples of conjugated proteins are mucoprotein, which is formed by the combination of a carbohydrate group and a simple protein, and lipoprotein, formed by a combination of a lipid and a simple protein. Derived proteins are formed during the hydrolysis of protein. Protein is metabolized to yield amino acids, nitrogen, and energy. Amino acids are anabolized into tissues, hormones, functional proteins (such as haemoglobin) and enzymes. Amino acids can also be converted into fat and stored as adipose tissue or catabolized into energy via **gluconeogenesis.**

There are 25 naturally occurring amino acids, and these can be classified as essential or nonessential. Since the body cannot manufacture essential amino acids, the diet must provide them. Nonessential amino acids do not have to be present in the diet because the body can form them from the metabolism of other amino acids (see box). Proteins that have an amino acid profile similar to dietary requirements are sometimes called foods of high biological value. Many traditional combinations of food, such as fish and chips, together provide a very healthy profile.

Protein is the body's only source of nitrogen, and 16% of protein is nitrogen. The body is in nitrogen balance when the intake and output of nitrogen are equal. When the intake of nitrogen exceeds the output, the body is in positive nitrogen balance: this is required for growth, normal pregnancy, and wound healing. The nitrogen retained by the body is used for building, repair, and replacement of body tissues.

Negative nitrogen balance occurs when the body loses more nitrogen than it gains. The increased nitrogen loss is the result of body tissue destruction. Negative nitrogen balance is associated with infection, fever, starvation, injury, and prolonged immobilization (see Chapter 24).

## Essential and Nonessential Amino Acids

### Essential
- Histidine
- Isoleucine*
- Leucine*
- Lysine*
- Methionine*
- Phenylalanine*
- Threonine*
- Tryptophan*
- Valine*

### Nonessential
- Alanine
- Arginine (essential for children)
- Asparagine
- Aspartic acid
- Citrulline
- Cysteine
- Cystine
- Glutamic acid
- Glutamine
- Glycine
- Hydroxyproline
- Norleucine
- Proline
- Serine
- Thyroxine
- Tyrosine

*Cannot be synthesized by man.*

**Protein sparing** is the provision of sufficient carbohydrate in the diet to meet the energy requirements of the body in order to spare protein for its role in nitrogen balance and tissue building.

The required daily allowance of protein ranges from 13 g for infants under 6 months to 55 g for men aged 15 years or older. Pregnant women require 60 g and lactating women 65 g.

### Lipids

**Lipid** is a comprehensive term applied to compounds that are insoluble in water but soluble in organic solvents (for example, ethanol, ether, benzene, and acetone). Lipids include fats that are solid at room temperature and oils that are liquid at room temperature. Lipids are composed of carbon, hydrogen, and oxygen, but the proportion of each element differs from that of carbohydrates.

Approximately 98% of dietary lipid and 90% of the lipid in the human body are in the form of triglycerides (Fig. 21-2). A triglyceride is a molecule composed of a glycerol backbone with three fatty acids attached to it.

There are approximately 50 commonly occurring **fatty acids**, these can be *saturated, unsaturated,* or *polyunsaturated*. A saturated fatty acid contains as much hydrogen as it can hold. An unsaturated fatty acid can take up another hydrogen atom, and a polyunsaturated fatty acid can take up many more hydrogen atoms. Unsaturated and polyunsaturated fatty acids are oils. They have a low melting point and are liquid at room temperature. Hydrogenation is a process by which these oils are made more solid by the addition of hydrogen. The addition of hydrogen also makes them more saturated. Fats are not usually composed of

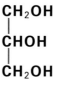

Glycerol (or Glycerine)

Triglyceride

**Fig. 21-2** Simplified structure of a triglyceride. Most dietary

fatty acids that are entirely saturated, unsaturated or polyunsaturated. Most animal fats have high proportions of saturated fatty acids. Most vegetable fats have higher amounts of unsaturated and polyunsaturated fatty acids.

Linoleic acid is the only *essential* fatty acid. Since the body is unable to synthesize linoleic acid, it is dependent on an adequate dietary intake. Linoleic acid is a polyunsaturated fatty acid found in sunflower, soybean, corn, cottonseed, and peanut oils.

### Micronutrients

**Micronutrients** are only required in small amounts, and are either vitamins or minerals.

### Vitamins

**Vitamins** are organic substances that are essential to normal metabolism. The body is unable to synthesize most vitamins in the required amounts, and therefore depends on dietary intake. Although they are contained in small amounts in many foods, vitamins are affected by processing, storage and preparation. Vitamin content is usually highest in fresh foods that are consumed quickly after minimal exposure to heat, air or water. Vitamins are classified as *water soluble* or *fat soluble*.

### WATER-SOLUBLE VITAMINS

The water-soluble vitamins (Table 21-2) are vitamin C and vitamin B complexes, (which consists of eight different vitamins). Water-soluble vitamins cannot be stored in the body and must be provided in the daily food intake. It was once assumed that, because water-soluble vitamins are not stored in the body, **hypervitaminosis** (a condition caused by excessive intake of a vitamin) of these vitamins would not occur. However, recent studies of people who have taken megadoses of vitamin C, riboflavin ($B_2$), and niacin indicate that toxicity can occur. When there is enough of any specific vitamin to meet the catalytic demands, the rest of the vitamin supply acts as a free chemical and may be toxic to the body.

## FAT-SOLUBLE VITAMINS

The fat-soluble vitamins — A, D, E, and K — (Table 21-3) can be stored in the body; therefore, daily intake is not needed. However, with the exception of vitamin D, these vitamins should be provided through dietary intake. Toxicity to some fat-soluble vitamins has been recognized for years. Toxicity is usually the result of large doses of synthetic vitamins, but it has also been reported in people whose diet includes a large intake of fish liver.

Processing, storage, and preparation of foods have less effect on fat-soluble vitamin content, and many foods, such as spreads, are fortified by the addition of vitamins A and D.

## Minerals

Minerals (Tables 21-4, 21-5) are inorganic elements essential to the body. Minerals are classified as *macrominerals* when the daily requirement is 100 mg or more, and as *microminerals* when less than 100 mg are needed daily. Since the required amount of microminerals is usually very small, they are also referred to as *trace elements.*

In addition to these minerals, arsenic, nickel, silicon, tin, vanadium, and possibly cadmium may play as yet unidentified roles in human nutrition. However, arsenic and cadmium have also been shown to be toxic.

## DIGESTION

### Ingestion

The only nutrients the body can utilize in their ingested form are monosaccharides, water, vitamins, some minerals, and alcohol. Digestion consists of the mechanical breakdown by chewing, churning, mixing with fluid, as well as by chemical reactions by which food is reduced to its simplest form.

Enzymes are an essential component in the chemistry of digestion. **Enzymes** are proteins that act as catalysts to speed up chemical reactions. As catalysts, enzymes are not part of the end product of the reaction. Most enzymes have one specific function, although some enzymes are involved in several closely related reactions. Each enzyme functions most effectively at a specific pH and is inactivated by major variations from that level. The secretions of the gastrointestinal tract have vastly different pH levels: saliva is relatively neutral, gastric juice is highly acidic, and the secretions of the small intestine are alkaline. Most enzymes are released as an inactive precursor, and they are converted to the active form once in the lumen of the gastrointestinal tract.

The mechanical, chemical, and hormonal activities of digestion are interdependent. Enzyme activity depends on the mechanical breakdown of food in order to increase its surface area for chemical action. Hormones regulate the flow of digestive secretions needed for enzyme supply, and digestion may also be slowed down or speeded up by strong emotional states. The secretion of digestive juice and motility of the gastrointestinal tract are regulated by physical, chemical, and hormonal factors, and they are intricately bound to psychological, emotional, and nervous system alterations.

Digestion begins in the mouth, where food is mechanically broken down by chewing. The food is mixed with saliva, which contains salivary amylase, an enzyme that acts on cooked starch to begin its conversion to maltose. The longer food is chewed, the more starch digestion occurs in the mouth. Proteins and fats are broken down physically but remain unchanged chemically because enzymes in the mouth do not react with these nutrients. Chewing reduces food particles to a size suitable for swallowing, and saliva provides lubrication to further ease swallowing of the **bolus** (food ready to be swallowed).

Swallowed food enters the oesophagus and is moved along by **peristalsis.** At the cardiac sphincter, the upper opening of the stomach, the presence of the food mass causes the sphincter to relax and allow food to enter the stomach. The stomach acts as a reservoir for food, and food remains in the stomach for varying periods, depending on the type of meal, gastric motility, and psychological influences. In the digestive sequence, carbohydrates are digested first, proteins second, and lipids last. Large meals and high fat intake decrease gastric motility and increase the length of time food remains in the stomach. Food remains in the stomach about 3 hours (range of 1 to 7 hours).

The activity of amylase continues in the stomach until hydrochloric acid decreases the pH enough to inactivate the amylase. The stomach churns the food mass, mixing it with gastric secretions and causing further breakdown in the size of the food particles. The acid environment favours the action of **pepsin,** an enzyme that splits proteins into smaller polypeptides.

Food leaves the stomach at the pyloric sphincter as an acidic, liquified mass known as **chyme.** Chyme flows into the duodenum and is quickly mixed with bile, intestinal juices, and pancreatic secretions. **Bile** is not an enzyme, but emulsifies fat to permit enzyme action and holds fatty acids in solution. Bile is manufactured in the liver and stored in the gall bladder.

Pancreatic and intestinal enzymes eventually hydrolyse polypeptides into amino acids. **Lipase,** an enzyme that functions best in an alkaline medium, is able to act on emulsified fats such as butter, egg yolk, milk, and cream at near-neutral pH levels. Lipase splits emulsified fats into fatty acids and glycerol.

Intestinal secretions contain seven enzymes: lipase for fat digestion, polypeptidase and dipeptidase for protein digestion, and amylase, sucrase, lactase, and maltase for carbohydrate digestion. **Pancreatic juice** contains five enzymes: amylase to digest starch, lipase to break down emulsified fats, and trypsin, chymotrypsin, and carboxypeptidases to break down proteins.

Peristalsis continues in the small intestine, mixing the secretions with the chyme. The mixture becomes increasingly alkaline, inhibiting the action of the gastric enzymes and promoting the action of the duodenal secretions. The major portion of digestion occurs in the small intestine, producing glucose, fructose, and galactose from carbohydrates; amino acids from proteins; and fatty acids and glycerol from lipids.

### Absorption

The small intestine is also the site of absorption of nutrients. It is lined with numerous villi that project into the lumen and greatly increase the surface area available for absorption.

When intestinal motility is increased, as in diarrhoea, the body loses nutrients and fluid that move through the small

## Table 21-2 Water-Soluble Vitamins

| Functions | Effects of Deficiency * | Effects of Excess | Sources |
|---|---|---|---|
| **Vitamin C (Asorbic Acid)** | | | |
| Production of collagen; integrity of capillary walls; formation of red blood cells; metabolism of amino acids; reduction of iron salts; protection of other vitamins from oxidation | Scurvy, poor wound healing, bleeding gums, loose teeth, bruising | Kidney stones, scurvy on withdrawal, urinary tract infection | Citrus fruits, potatoes, cabbage, tomatoes, broccoli, strawberries, cantaloupe, green peppers |
| **VITAMIN B COMPLEX** | | | |
| **Vitamin B₁ (Thiamine)** | | | |
| Component of enzymes; carbohydrate oxidation; oxidative conversion of pyruvic acid and hence citric acid cycle | Beriberi (rare), polyneuritis, mental confusion, muscular weakness, ataxia, cardiac rhythm disturbances, cardiac enlargement | Rapid pulse, headaches, weakness, irritability, insomnia | Pork, fish, eggs, poultry, dried beans, whole grains, wheat germ, oatmeal, bread, pasta |
| **Vitamin B₂ (Riboflavin)** | | | |
| Metabolism of nutrients; growth; oxidation and reduction of fat, carbohydrates, proteins | Ariboflavinosis: cracks at mouth corners, scaly desquamation of skin around mouth, eye irritation, glossitis (shiny tongue), photophobia (light sensitivity) | Ulcer, elevated blood glucose level, increased uric acid levels in blood | Milk, whole grains, green vegetables, liver |
| **Niacin** | | | |
| Protein utilization; glycolysis; fat synthesis; tissue repair | Pellagra: weakness, anorexia, indigestion; severe pellagra; dermatitis, diarrhoea, dementia | Ulcer, liver dysfunction, elevated blood glucose level, increased blood uric acid levels, diarrhoea, nausea, flushing | Meats, dairy products, whole grains, cereals, tuna |
| **Vitamin B₆ (Complex of Pyridoxine, Pyridoxal, Pyridosamine)** | | | |
| Metabolism of nutrients; synthesis of nonessential amino acids; conversion of tryptophan to niacin; proper function of blood and central nervous system cells | Anaemia, irritability, skin lesions, cracks at corners of mouth | Bloating, depression, fatigue, headache, nerve damage, irritability | Whole grains, liver, fish, poultry, green beans, nuts, meats, potatoes |
| **Folacin, Folic Acid, Folate** | | | |
| Metabolism of some amino acids; maturation of erythrocytes; synthesis of purines and pyrimidines, which are necessary for ribonucleic acid (RNA) and deoxyribonucleic acid (DNA) | Macrocytic anaemia, Neural tube defects in fetus of deficient pregnant women | Diarrhoea, insomnia, irritability, masking of vitamin B₁₂ deficiency | Liver, green leafy vegetables, meat, fish, poultry, whole grains. |
| **Vitamin B₁₂ (Cobalamin)** | | | |
| Manufacture of enzymes essential to metabolism of nutrients, nucleic acid, folic acid; proper function of cells of bone marrow, gastrointestinal tract, and nervous system; formation of purines and thus RNA and DNA | Pernicious anaemia and neurological disorders | None reported | Milk, eggs, cheese, meat, fish, poultry, foods of animal origin (Plant foods contain no vitamin B₁₂) |
| **Pantothenic Acid** | | | |
| Metabolism of nutrients; synthesis of cholesterol and steroid hormones; activity of adrenal cortex | None known | Increased need for thiamin, occasional diarrhoea, water retention | Meat, whole grain cereals, legumes |
| **Biotin** | | | |
| Synthesis of fatty acids; utilization of glucose; metabolism of protein; utilization of vitamin B₁₂ and folic acid | None known | None known | Liver, kidneys, dark green vegetables, egg yolk, green beans |

*Normal range for pantothenic acid is 4-7 mg/day, and for biotin, it is 30-100 µg/day. From Grant JA, Kennedy-Caldwll C: *Nutritional support in nursing*, New York, 1988, Grune & Stratton; and Whitney EN, Cataldo CB, Rolfes SR: *Understanding normal and clinical nutrition*, St Paul, Minn 1991, West.

intestine too rapidly for complete absorption.

The intestinal contents move into the large intestine by peristaltic action. Water is the only nutrient absorbed from the large intestine in large quantities. Other nutrients, on reaching the large intestine, are usually lost to the body and will be excreted as waste products. However, the large intestine also contains bacteria that produce useful nutrients, as by-products of metabolism. The most important of these is vitamin K.

## Metabolism

Nutrients absorbed in the intestines, including water, are transported through the circulatory system to body tissues, mostly via the liver. Through metabolism, the nutrients are converted into various substances which are then used by the body, or are stored. Carbohydrates, protein, and fat undergo metabolism to produce chemical energy and to maintain a balance between tissue build up and breakdown. The inter-relationships of protein, carbohydrate, and fat metabolism are shown in Fig. 21-3.

## Elimination

The intestinal contents move through the various segments of the large intestine by peristalsis. As the material moves towards the rectum, water is absorbed into the mucosa. The longer the material stays in the large intestine, the more water is absorbed and the firmer the remaining solid material becomes. The end products of digestion include cellulose and similar fibrous substances that the body is unable to digest, sloughed cells from the intestinal walls, mucus, digestive secretions, water, bile pigments and microorganisms.

## FOUNDATIONS OF AN ADEQUATE DIET

### Nutrition Reference Values (NRVs)

This concept was introduced in 1991 to replace recommended daily allowances. **Nutrition Reference Values (NRVs)** are an attempt to quantify nutritional requirements for people of different ages. They are average values, and therefore do not reflect demands of different lifestyles or states of health. They are based on a suggested number of servings of a variety of substances from the following four basic food groups: milk group (milk, yoghurt, cheese); vegetable/fruit group; bread/cereal group (bread, cereal, rice, pasta); meat group (poultry, fish, meat, dry beans, eggs, nuts) (DOH, 1991).

The labelling of food is now controlled by two pieces of legsislation: the Food Labelling Legislation of 1984 and the European Community Directive on Nutrition Labelling for Foodstuffs. Food labelling is not essential unless a claim is made regarding the nutritional value of a product. However, if nutrition information is provided, the label must supply the energy value of the food (in both kcal and kJ); the weight of protein, fat and carbohydrate in grams; plus the amount of nutrients about which specific claims are made — all this information must be provided per 100 g or 100 mls. Many manufacturers provide more information than the law requires. Some of this can be confusing

and more concerned with selling the product than with informing the purchaser; for example the use of emotive terms such as 'natural'.

### Other Dietary Guidelines

In 1992, the Department of Health, together with the Scottish, Welsh and Northern Ireland Offices, issued strategies for health in the various regions of the UK. These documents provided a picture of the current health status in the UK, and identified realistic targets for health improvement, including targets for nutrition (see box). As well as these targets, the strategies emphasized the importance of continuing research into diet and health, and in national surveillance of diet. The report also recognized the importance of disseminating nutrition information. One recommendation is the formation of a Nutrition Task Force, involving the government, statutory bodies, commercial organizations and charities. It is envisaged that such improvements will lead to better general health and, in particular, improvements in coronary artery disease.

### Alternative Food Patterns

Many people follow special patterns of food intake based on religion, cultural background, ethics, health beliefs, personal preference, or concern for the efficient use of land to produce food. A common dietary pattern is the vegetarian diet.

---

**Targets:
Diet and Nutrition**

- To reduce the average percentage of food energy derived by the population from saturated fatty acids by a least 35% by 2005 (to no more than 11% of food energy).
- To reduce the average percentage of food energy derived from total fat by the population by a least 12% by 2005 (to no more than about 35% of total food energy).
- To reduce the proportion of men and women aged 16-64 who are obese by at least 25% and 33% respectively by 2005 (to no more than 6% of men and 8% of women).
- To reduce the proportion of men drinking more than 21 units of alcohol per week and women drinking more than 14 units per week by 30% by 2005 (to 18% of men and 7% of women) (DoH, 1992).

Similar targets exist for other regions, but the problems may be differently emphasized. Scotland is deemed to have a more unhealthy diet than almost any other country in the Western world, which is one reason for the high numbers of death from coronary heart disease (Scottish Office, 1992). Wales is approximately mid-way in Europe for deaths from cardiovasular disease. The Welsh Office estimates that about 50% of Welsh hospitals have healthy eating policies. Their targets include healthy eating policies in all hospitals and a reduction of 35% in the numbers of overweight adults (NHS Cymru Wales, 1992). The Northern Ireland Office aims to reduce deaths from ischaemic heart disease among 35-64 year olds by 15% in the ten years to 1997 (Northern Ireland Office, 1991).

## Table 21-3 Fat-Soluble Vitamins

| Functions | Effects of Deficiency | Effects of Excess | Sources |
|---|---|---|---|
| **Vitamin A (Retinol, Retinal, Retonic Acid)** | | | |
| Growth and maintenance of epithelial tissue; maintenance of visual acuity in dim light; immune functions, especially antigen recognition | Night blindness, rough scaly skin, dry mucous membranes, decreased resistance to infection, faulty tooth and bone development | Nausea, vomiting, abdominal pain, and growth failure in children; weight loss in adults; mega-doses: hair loss, bone swelling and tenderness, joint pain, hepatomegaly, splenomegaly, headache | Whole milk products, eggs, green leafy vegetables, fish liver oil, liver |
| **Vitamin D (Cholecalciferol, Ergosterol)** | | | |
| Absorption and utilization of calcium in bone and tooth development | Rickets and delayed dentition in children, osteomalacia, (softening of bones) in adults | Megadoses : loss of appetite, vomiting, growth failure, weight loss, increased calcium deposits in soft tissue, blood vessels and kidneys | Sunlight, fortified milk, eggs, meats, cereals |
| **Vitamin E (Tocopherol )** | | | |
| Protection of vitamins A and C and polyunsaturated fatty acids from oxidation; synthesis of haeme | Increased haemolysis of erythrocytes and macrocytic anaemia in premature infants | Interference with utilization of vitamins A and K, prolonged prothrombin time, intestinal irritability, headache, fatigue, dizziness | Vegetable oils, green leafy vegetables, milk, eggs, meats, cereals |
| **Vitamin K** | | | |
| Prothrombin formation; blood clotting | Haemorrhagic disease of the newborn, prolonged clotting time in adults | Hyperbilirubinaemia in infants, vomiting in adults | Green leafy vegetables, liver, synthesis in gastrointentinal tract |

From Grant JA, Kennedy-Caldwell C : *Nutritional support in nursing* , New York, 1988, Grune & Stratton; and Whitney EN, Cataldo CB, Rolfes SR : *Understanding normal and clinical nutrition*, St Paul, Minn 1991, West.

Vegetarianism is the consumption of a diet free of meat. Lactovegetarians eat eggs, milk and butter, and some will also eat fish. Vegans consume only plant foods, avoiding dairy products and eggs. Vegans must be especially careful to eat a variety of foods, including legumes and nuts, because they can become deficient in micronutrients, particularly vitamin $B_{12}$ and calcium.

## Food, Culture and Religion

It is important to remember that culture may influence people's food intake in many different ways. For example, some feminist theorists argue that food and its intake may become a symbol of control and protest in some individuals (Orbach, 1978). On the other hand, meal times may have a special social and family meaning for some patients/clients. For some people, what is eaten, and how it is eaten and prepared, forms part of the expression of their religious and cultural identity. It is neither desirable nor possible to provide a list of laws, but some guidelines will be useful for the practising nurse (see also Chapter 8).

## JEWISH

Orthodox (or religious) Jews do not eat pork. Other meats must be rigorously cleansed of blood, and no dishes may be prepared or eaten involving both meat and milk together. Only fish with fins and scales may be eaten. There are also strict laws about the manner in which foods are prepared. Foods that are appropriate for strict Jews are called Kosher meaning 'fit' or 'proper'. The rules can sometimes be quite complex, and Jews who are guests in other cultures often choose vegetarian diets.

## CHRISTIAN

A revelation to one of the apostles (Acts, Chapter 10, verses 10-15) specifically encourages the eating of all animals and plants, as provided by God for humanity's sustenance. Some Christians choose to fast for short periods, either to mark a particular festival, or to assist in the individual's prayer life.

## Table 21-4 Macrominerals

| Functions | Effects of Deficiency | Effects of Excess | Sources |
|---|---|---|---|
| **Calcium** | | | |
| Formation of teeth and bones, contraction of muscle fibres; transmission of nerve impulses; activation of enzymes; permeability of cell membranes; coagulation of blood; cardiac function. | Tingling of fingers and area around mouth, muscle cramps, carpopedal (thumb or toe) spasm, tetany, convulsions, pathological fractures, stunted growth in children, bone loss in adults | Relaxed skeletal muscles, cardiac irregularities | Milk, milk products, leafy vegetables, fish and small edible bones |
| **Magnesium** | | | |
| Support of function of B vitamins; utilization of calcium, potassium, protein; maintenance of electrical activity in nerves and muscles | Neuromuscular irritability, confusion, hallucinations, growth failure | Lethargy, diarrhoea | Whole grains, nuts, legumes, green vegetables |
| **Phosphorus** | | | |
| Formation of bone and teeth; activation of B vitamins; transfer of energy in cells; promotion of muscle and nerve activity; metabolism of carbohydrates; regulation of acid-base balance; transmission of heredity traits | Haemolytic anaemia, defective white blood cell function, delayed clotting, bone pain, pathological fractures | Erosion of jaw, calcium loss | Pork, beef, dried peas and beans, milk and milk products |

From Grant JA, Kennedy-Caldwell C : *Nutritional support in nursing*, New York, 1988, Grune & Stratton; and Whitney EN, Cataldo CB, Rolfes SR : *Understanding normal and clinical nutrition*, St Paul, Minn 1991, West.

Some traditional Christian churches encourage the consumption of simple foods only on Fridays, the day of the Crucifixion. This has led to the tradition of eating meals without meat, often fish, on Fridays.

## MOSLEM

Moslem laws are derived from the Koran. Pork and alcohol are absolutely forbidden. Figs, olives, honey, milk and buttermilk are mentioned in the Koran as being of special value, and so are often considered of great benefit to people who are unwell. Ramadan, a period of 30 days in the ninth month of the Islamic lunar calendar, marks the time when Mohammed received the first of his revelations, and this is a very special time for Moslems. During this time, they abstain from all food and drink, even water, while the sun is up. Night times may be marked by feasting, but many Moslems choose to eat sparingly even then. The time at which it occurs varies, and the festival can be quite arduous if it falls during the summer.

## HINDU

Hindus believe in the reincarnation of the dead, possibly as animals, and so Hindus are usually strict vegetarians. Traditions with regard to fasting vary widely.

It must be stressed that individuals, and also different cultures, will vary as to how these practices are interpreted, in particular, how strictly they should be observed during sickness or pregnancy (see Chapter 8).

## DEVELOPMENTAL VARIABLES IN NUTRITION

### Infants

Infancy is marked by rapid growth and high energy requirements. The average birth weight of a baby in the West is 3.2 to 3.4 kg (7-7.5 lb). The infant usually doubles its birth weight at 4 to 5 months and triples it at 1 year. An energy intake of approximately 210 kJ per kilogram per day is required, just to fulfil BMR, (MAFF, 1985). A full-term newborn is able to digest and absorb simple carbohydrates, proteins, and a moderate amount of emulsified fat. Amylase, the starch-splitting enzyme, is not present until approximately 2.5 or 3.5 months. Infants require a high amount of fluid because a large portion of the total body weight is water.

### Breast-Fed Infants

Breast milk is the ideal food for infants, and it should be the major source of nutrients up to the age of 4 to 6 months. Breast milk is higher in protein than cow's milk and, in addition, it contains antibodies to protect against antigens in the environment which are not available in infant formulas and foods. As the infant grows, the gastrointestinal tract can fight against common bacteria and against proteins which cause allergies.

Breast-feeding promotes bonding between mother and child. The lipid content of breast milk is better absorbed than

## Table 21-5 Microminerals

| Functions | Effects of Deficiency | Effects of Excess | Sources |
|---|---|---|---|
| **Copper** | | | |
| Haemoglobin formation; synthesis of phospholipids; formation and activity of some enzymes; synthesis of prostaglandin | Abnormal blood cell development in infants, bone demineralization | Headache, dizziness, heart-burn, weakness, nausea, vomiting, diarrhoea, Wilson's disease | Liver, kidney, shellfish, nuts, raisins |
| **Fluoride** | | | |
| Formation of teeth; prevention of dental caries | Poor dental health | Mottling, pitting, and discolouration of tooth enamel | Fluorinated water, seafood, toothpaste, mouthwash |
| **Iodine** | | | |
| Basic component of thyroid hormones | Cretinism in infants, depressed thyroid activity | Toxic goitre | Iodized salt, seafood, food additives, dough oxidizers, dairy disinfectants, colouring agents |
| **Iron** | | | |
| Formation of haemoglobin; synthesis of vitamins, purines, and antibodies | Anaemia, fatigue, weakness, lethargy, lowered immunity | Haemosiderosis, poisoning from accidental ingestion in infants and children: cramps, abdominal pain, nausea, vomiting, black stools, cirrhosis | Liver, lean meats, whole grains, enriched breads and cereals, green leafy vegetables |
| **Zinc** | | | |
| Connective tissue integrity; immune response; formation of enzymes and insulin | Impaired wound healing, decreased sensations of taste and small, skin lesions, delayed growth | Anaemia, fever, nausea, vomiting, diarrhoea, muscle pain and weakness, decreased calcium absorption | Oysters, liver, meats, poultry, legumes, nuts |

From Grant JA, Kennedy-Caldwell C: *Nutritional support in nursing*, New York, 1988, Grune & Stratton; and Whitney EN, Cataldo CB, Rolfes SR: *Understanding normal and clinical nutrition*, St Paul, 1991, West.

that from other infant foods. Breast-feeding may prevent infant obesity and protect against **hypercholesterolaemia** (high blood cholesterol) later on in life. At the start of each feed, breast milk has a high water content which satisfies thirst, and at the end of a feed it has a higher fat content that provides satiety (satisfied feeling of being full), and stops the infant from suckling. The high cholesterol level of breast milk is thought to foster the development of a more efficient cholesterol metabolism.

Some authorities recommend supplementing breast-fed infants with vitamin C, fluoride, vitamin D and iron. After four months, when the fetal store of iron has become exhausted, the infant needs a dietary source of this nutrient.

There is some debate as to whether premature infants can obtain sufficient nutrients from breast milk alone.

### Formula-Fed Infants

Good quality formula milks are available for those who cannot, or do not wish to, breast feed. Great care must be taken in preparing these hygienically, and the temptation to give the baby the benefit of extra-strength feeds must be resisted, because they are unable to metabolize it.

Neither undiluted whole cow's milk nor skimmed milk should be used as a basis for infant formulas. Whole milk has excess protein and requires dilution, and skimmed milk does not contain linoleic acid and is too low in calories.

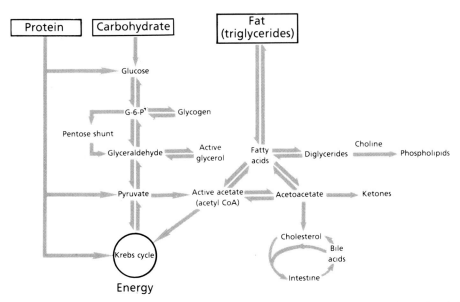

**Fig.21-3** Summary of metabolism of the nutrients. Note metabolic interrelationships of carbohydrate, protein, and fat (G-6-P is glucose-6-phosphate).From Williams SR, *Nutrition and diet therapy*, ed 6, St Louis, 1989, Mosby-Year Book.

## Introduction to Solid Food

The ability to swallow voluntarily is not fully developed until 10 to 12 weeks of age. Before that time, swallowing must be stimulated by suckling. The amount of saliva required to ease the swallowing of solid food is not secreted until about 3 months of age. The **extrusion reflex** (pushing food out of the mouth with the tongue) is the dominant reflex until the infant is 4 months old. Enzymes to digest complex carbohydrates (for example, cereals) and the ability to taste are not fully developed until 3 to 4 months of age.

Foods should be introduced gradually, one at a time, beginning initially between 4 and 6 months, depending on the infant's readiness. It is inadvisable to delay solids past this time. Most infants begin solids at 16 weeks of age. Foods should be pureed until smooth to begin with, then mashed, minced, and finally just cut up. To begin with bland starches such as potato or rice should be given, mixed with breast or formula milk.

The addition of foods to an infant's diet should be governed by his or her nutrient needs, physical readiness to handle different forms of foods, and the need to detect and control allergic reactions. Special baby foods are not required, and tend to be expensive, but can be used for convenience from time to time. Infants can and should be given samples of food that the family is eating, provided these are low in salt and sugar, and can be reduced to a suitable consistency.

## Toddlers and Preschool Children

Meal times should be an enjoyable experience for all concerned. Many parents worry about the diet of their young children, and may require reassurance that a healthy child will eat well, without the need for complex rules. The growth rate slows during toddler years (1 to 3 years). The toddler needs fewer calories but an increased amount of protein in relation to his or her body weight. Toddlers are more interested in their environment and in increasing motor skills than in food. For this reason finger food

is desirable as it allows children to participate in feeding themselves and sometimes to eat while on the move.

The toddler needs a minimum of two servings daily from the milk group to supply protein, calcium, riboflavin, and vitamins A and $B_{12}$. Whole milk should be used until the child reaches at least 5 years of age because of the linoleic acid in the milk fat, and the energy provided by the fat. Toddlers who consume excessive milk instead of other foods may develop **anaemia**. Lean red meats are a good source of iron. Whole grains, enriched cereals, and breads are also good sources, but are not well absorbed. When meat is given to a toddler, the portions should be cut into small pieces to avoid the possibility of choking. Foods the size of toddlers' tracheas (for example, hotdogs, peanuts and grapes) are dangerous for children at this age, unless they are cut in half. Peanuts are inadvisable for children under 6.

The toddler should receive four servings daily from the fruit and vegetable group. One serving should be a good source of vitamin C (for example, potatoes). Green leafy vegetables and deep yellow fruits and vegetables should be served frequently. Toddlers like bite-sized raw vegetables but should not be given these unsupervised because of the danger of choking.

A toddler also requires four servings from the bread and cereal group; and this should include whole grain or enriched

**Children's Nursing
Physiological anorexia**

The rate of growth slows between the ages of 12-18 months. This results in adjustment of calorific requirements. This reduction in need is termed *physiological anorexia* and toddlers usually respond by becoming fussy with food and developing food fads.

Parents should be advised not to worry about this apparent lack of interest in food and not to use meal times as punishment.

breads, cereals, and pastas. Sugar-coated cereals and sugar on cereals should be avoided. In addition to the **basic four food groups**, the toddler should have one to two teaspoons of margarine or butter both of which are sources for vitamin A. Vegetable oils, for example olive oil or sunflower oil, are preferable to butter, because they are lower in saturated fatty acids.

Growth slows down after 12 to 14 months, but energy and nutrient requirements are increased. Nutritious foods should be offered in small amounts. During the preschool years from the ages of 3 to 6, children gain an average of 2 kg (4.5 lb) of body weight and 5 to 8 cm (2 to 3 inches) in height a year. At the end of the preschool period, the child's weight is double that at 1 year, and his or her height is 1.5 times that at 1 year. The average 6-year-old weighs 19 kg (42 lb) and stands 105 cm (42 inches) high.

Daily protein needs are increased to 24 g. Calcium and iron are still important. The child should be encouraged to eat fruits and vegetables for vitamins A and C. Interest in food continues to be overshadowed by interest in the enlarging environment and motor skills. Several small meals may be preferable to the traditional three.

### School-Age Children

School-aged children, aged 5 to 12 years old, grow at a slower and steadier rate, with a gradual decline in energy requirements per unit of body weight. The school-aged child gains 3 to 5 kg (6.5 to 11 lb) in weight and 6 cm in height a year until puberty.

The appetites of school-aged children are greater than those of younger children, food intake is more varied, and parental control of food intake begins to lessen. Recommended intake includes two servings from the milk group, one serving of meat, four or more servings from the fruit and vegetable group (with a daily source of vitamin C and a source of vitamin A every other day), three to four servings from the bread and cereals group, and 1 to 2 teaspoons of margarine or butter.

Despite better appetites and more varied food intake, the diet of school-aged children should be carefully assessed for adequate protein and vitamin A and C. Milk intake usually exceeds recommendations, but failure to eat a proper breakfast and unsupervised intake at school may result in an improper or inadequate diet.

### Adolescents

During adolescence, physiological age is a better guide to nutritional needs than chronological age. Adolescence begins with the growth spurt of puberty at the end of childhood and ends with the completion of physical growth. Energy needs are greatly increased to meet increased metabolic demands. Protein needs increase to a daily requirement of 45 to 59 g. Calcium is essential for the rapid bone growth of the adolescent, and girls require a continuous source of iron to replace menstrual losses. Boys also need adequate iron for muscle development. Iodine supports increased thyroid activity, and B-complex vitamins support the heightened metabolic activity.

Adolescents' requirements from the basic groups include three or more servings from the milk group, two or more from

### Children's Nursing
### School meals

School meals have always been part of the school day and in some families the school meal has been a vital part of the child's diet.

In 1980, the government lifted price controls and removed the need for nutritional standards as part of its strategy of cutting local government subsidies and encouraged privatisation of its services including school meals. Councils began to move towards making school meals self-financing or stopping them altogether except for statutory provision for poorer families (Child Poverty Action Group, 1991).

Changes in benefit rules for families entitled to family credit have led to cash payments rather than free school meals. This has meant that low-income parents tend to spend this money on other things — equally important in their view.

Children's nurses need to be aware of government initiatives such as this, as potential problems may occur in the health of the children. Professionals can then put forward informed views on proposals and initiatives that may have a negative impact on the health and well-being of patients/clients.

the meat group, four or more from the vegetable fruit group (with a daily source of vitamin C and a source of vitamin A every other day), four to six or more from the bread and cereal group (with emphasis on whole grains), and 1 to 2 tablespoons of margarine or butter.

The adolescent's diet is influenced by several factors other than nutritional needs, including concern about body image and appearance, desire for independence, and fad diets. Many adolescents experience stressful times as their self identities begin to emerge, and food can become a symbol of this struggle. **Nutritional deficiencies** may occur as a result of dieting or using oral contraceptives. The nutrients involved are folic acid, vitamin $B_6$, vitamin C, thiamine, riboflavin, and iron. The adolescent boy's diet may be inadequate in total calories, protein, iron, folic acid, B vitamins and iodine. Teenagers, girls in particular, are sometimes at risk of anorexia or bulimia.

Snacks provide approximately 25% of the teenager's total dietary intake (Whitney *et al*, 1991). The irregular eating pattern of skipping meals or eating meals and the wrong choice of snacks, contribute to obesity and nutrient deficiencies. Snack foods from the milk and fruit–vegetable groups are good choices and contribute calcium, phosphorous, protein, zinc, vitamin A, vitamin C, and some of the B-complex vitamins.

'Fast food' eating is the norm but adds extra fat and energy and contributes to developing cardiovascular disease and weight-control problems.

Nutritional deficiencies can be a particular problem during pregnancy; counselling related to nutritional needs may prove difficult, and suggestions with regard to diet are probably better than rigid directions. The diet of a pregnant adolescent is often deficient in calcium, iron, and vitamins A and C.

### Mental Health Nursing
### Anorexia nervosa and bulimia nervosa

Anorexia nervosa is a biopsychosocial disorder in which self-imposed starvation is used to establish identity and control, marked by a belief of being grossly overweight and a denial of being underweight. It may be metabolic and in families there may be other relations who have also been anorexic. Often a problem in family dynamics is present. Early feeding patterns and attitudes towards food have also been implicated. The desirability of a slender figure in today's society may be a contributory factor but it is much more serious and dangerous than a case of 'dieting gone wrong'! Its increased incidences in the industrialized Western countries suggest that changing roles and expectations of young men and women may be contributory factors.

The patient/client with anorexia nervosa is usually a highly motivated adolescent girl. Extreme undernutrition leads to secondary endocrine disorders such as amenorrhoea, delayed sexual development, and depressed organ function such as cardiac dysrhythmias that can be life threatening. The treatment of anorexia nervosa is a long-term combination of psychotherapy, cognitive therapy, behaviour modification, and diet therapy.

**Bulimia nervosa**, or the binge-purge syndrome, occurs in half of the patients/clients with anorexia nervosa, but not all bulimic patients/clients have anorexia nervosa. The syndrome appears to develop with an abnormal craving for food accompanied by the desire to remain slender. The patient/client gorges on food to satisfy the craving and then induces vomiting to prevent the digestion of food. The patient/client may also use laxatives or enemas to increase gastrointestinal motility so that nutrients are not totally absorbed. The practice of secretly vomiting after eating usually starts with occasional binges and gradually becomes a daily activity and the preferred way of controlling weight. Frequent vomiting, laxative abuse, and overuse of enemas lead to electrolyte imbalances (hypokalaemia being the most serious), oesophageal lesions, dental caries, endocrine disturbances, and metabolic changes. Treatment includes dietary education, hospitalization, psychotherapy, drug therapy with phenytoin, group therapy, cognitive work and behavioural modification.

## Young and Middle-Aged Adults

The demands for most nutrients are reduced as the growth period ends. Mature adults require nutrients for energy, maintenance and repair. Energy requirements usually decline over the years. Obesity may become a problem due to decreased physical exercise, increased dining out, or the ability to afford more luxury foods. Obese individuals may also have a low proportion of brown adipose tissue (BAT), which metabolizes food more quickly than white adipose tissue.

Adult women who use oral contraceptives need extra folic acid, vitamin C, thiamin, riboflavin, vitamin $B_6$, and vitamin $B_{12}$. Iron and calcium intake are also necessary for all women.

Young and middle-aged adults are subject to the same recommendations from the basic food groups: two or more servings from the milk group, four or more from the vegetable-fruit group (with a daily source of vitamin C and three to four weekly servings of sources of vitamin A), four or more from the bread and cereal group, and 1 to 2 tablespoons of margarine or butter.

## Pregnancy

Poor nutrition during pregnancy may contribute to low birth weight in infants and decreased chances of survival. It can also cause birth defects, such as spina bifida, which is linked to a deficiency of folic acid in the mother. Generally, the fetus' needs are met at the expense of the mother's. However, if nutrient sources are not available, both suffer. The **nutritional status** of the mother at the time of conception is important in terms of nutritional reserves and basic eating habits. Significant aspects of fetal growth and development occur before pregnancy is even suspected. Women from low socioeconomic groups and some minority ethnic groups are at nutritional risk during pregnancy.

The energy requirements of pregnancy are related to body weight and activity. A total weight gain of 10 to 15 kg (22 to 35 lb) is recommended. Inadequate weight gain and weight gain above 15 kg (35 lb) are not desirable. In the event of undesirable gains or losses, food intake should be evaluated. Pregnant women should be cautioned against fasting as a method of weight control, because fasting leads to ketoacidosis, which can be dangerous to the fetus.

Food intake in the first trimester should include balanced portions of essential nutrients with emphasis on quality. Protein intake throughout pregnancy is increased by 6 g per day (DOH, 1991).

Calcium intake should be increased to 1200 mg per day. Calcium is necessary for fetal tooth and bone development, muscle contraction, and blood clotting. Calcium intake is especially critical in the third trimester, when fetal bones are mineralized.

### Adult Nursing
### People with physical disabilities

People with disabilities that interfere with independent food intake should be helped to do as much as possible for themselves. The nurse should discuss with the individual his or her thoughts and feelings and facilitate the person's choices. Special aids should be used if they will contribute to the person's independence. Some people with disabilities may become tired from their efforts to feed themselves. Patients/clients who stop eating may still be hungry and may need support or assistance. Small, frequent meals may be best in order to achieve adequate nutrition. The nurse who finds a way to help patients/clients in eating more independently should share this information by incorporating it into the care plan. It is important to include the patient's/client's family or carer in decision-making and care, where this is appropriate.

Pregnant women require more iron than can be supplied by most diets. Iron needs are increased to 30 mg per day, and a supplement is usually given. Iron is needed to correct pre-existing deficiencies and to provide for increased maternal blood volume, for fetal blood cell manufacture, and for blood loss during delivery.

Iodine needs are increased by 25 µg (15-17%) because of increased activity of the thyroid gland. Vitamin A is necessary for cell development, epithelial tissue maintenance, and tooth and bone development. Intake of this vitamin should be increased by 100 µg per day. However, there is evidence that excessive vitamin A (more than 3,300 µg/day) can cause birth defects. Pregnant women are therefore advised not to take supplements that contain vitamin A. Since liver can contain up to 40,000 µg/100g of vitamin A, it is advisable to avoid this food during pregnancy (DOH, 1991).

Pregnancy also increases requirements for B vitamins, which are needed for enzyme production necessitated by increased metabolic activity. Folic acid intake is particularly important for DNA synthesis and the increase in erythrocytes. Inadequate intake may lead to megaloblastic anaemia, a type of anaemia seen in women who have had many pregnancies. If there is a familial history of spinal problems in newborn babies, the woman may be advised to take high levels of Vitamin $B_6$, preferably from before she conceives.

Vitamin C requirements are increased by 10 mg to provide the intercellular cement in connective and vascular tissue and to enhance the absorption of iron. Vitamin D needs are increased by 5 µg (100%) because this vitamin promotes the absorption of calcium and phosphorus needed for tooth and bone development.

The pregnant woman should have four or more servings from the milk group; two or more from the meat group; five to seven from the vegetable-fruit group (including a citrus fruit and a potato daily and leafy green or dark yellow vegetables three to four times a week); four or more from the enriched or whole grain bread and cereal group; and at least 1 to 2 tablespoons of margarine or butter daily.

Pregnant women should increase their fluid intake by drinking at least eight glasses of water daily. They should avoid artificial sweeteners, alcohol, excessive caffeine, and all drugs not specifically prescribed. Adequate fluid intake can prevent constipation, commonly associated with pregnancy.

For many women, eating well in pregnancy is no problem, as there are no special rules, however, women who were poorly nourished before entering pregnancy need encouragement to take a healthy diet, and in particular to increase the amount of protein they eat.

## Lactation

The lactating woman needs 2 MJ more than her prepregnancy requirement. The production of breast milk increases energy requirements. Protein requirements are increased to 65 g per day. The need for calcium remains the same as during pregnancy. Although the lactating woman requires less protein, folic acid, and iron as compared to the pregnancy requirements, there is an increased need for vitamins A and C, niacin, riboflavin, iodine,

and zinc over pregnancy needs. The need for vitamins D, E, $B_6$, $B_{12}$, and thiamine and for the minerals calcium, phosphorus, and magnesium is the same for the pregnant and the lactating woman, but the lactating woman requires more fluid for optimal milk production.

The increased energy from the basic food groups should be provided by leafy green vegetables, citrus fruits, whole grains, milk, meat, and poultry to provide vitamins A and C, niacin, riboflavin, and zinc. Daily intakes of the water-soluble vitamins (B and C) are necessary to ensure adequate levels in breast milk. The lactating woman should try to drink 100 mls of milk daily or its equivalent from the milk group. Fluid intake should total at least 1500 mls per day. Caffeine, alcohol, and drugs are excreted in breast milk and intake should be minimized.

## Older Adults

This group is at particular risk of **malnutrition**. The reasons for this are multifactorial, and include social, psychological and physiological (see box). The older adult has lower energy requirements, due to a reduction of lean body mass, and they are more easily satiated. However, his or her requirements for protein, minerals and vitamins are at least as great. People often put on extra weight as they become older; indeed this can be quite desirable and associated with reduced morbidity, particularly osteoporosis in women. Income is probably the most important factor since a low income may reduce the amount of money available to buy food. People on lower incomes tend to have to spend a higher proportion of it on food, and economizing on food may appear to save money.

**Adult Nursing**
**Why are older adults at risk of becoming malnourished?**

- A reduction in the number of taste buds leads to less enjoyment of food.
- Reduced gastrointestinal motility can cause constipation, which leads to loss of appetite.
- Older people have lower energy requirements and reduced glucose tolerance.
- Many are lacking social stimulus, which could either increase or reduce appetite.
- Dental problems, absent or ill-fitting dentures, can make food difficult to chew, and also give an unpleasant taste.
- Many older people are poor and some are fearful of debt. This may lead to underspending on food.
- Older people with limited mobility often have difficulty in shopping for groceries, particularly fresh provisions. This is compounded by changing patterns of food shopping from small local shops to larger, centralized supermarkets.
- Joint problems are very common in older age, and can cause difficulties in preparing and eating food.
- Food fashions have changed much in recent years, and unfamiliar food can be unpalatable for older people.

Holmes S: Nutrition and older people: a matter of concern, *Nursing Times* 90 (42), 1994.

### Children's Nursing
### Nutrition while in hospital

North American studies have indicated a surprisingly high and worrying incidence of malnutrition among hospitalized children.

It is important to remember that these results may be transferrable to UK hospitals, particularly if children are in hospital for a long period of time have an acute/malignant illness or are undergoing chemotherapy. Dietary history and assessment should include information regarding preferred foodstuffs and utensils (toddlers may become very attached to a particular beaker), weight and height measurement, and appearance of the child on assessment.

Parents should be encouraged to continue to cook for a child and bring in the child's favourite dishes if hospital food is undesirable to the child.

### Mental Health Nursing
### Special considerations

People with mental distress and mental illness may refuse food and fluids because of their belief that the food may be tampered with and could harm them or that they are not worthy of the offer of food. Some people with long-term mental illness may have lost all skills, motivation and volition to budget, shop, cook and feed themselves. Those who abuse alcohol or other substances may place food as a very low priority.

People who have difficulty remaining in touch with 'here-and-now,' reality (e.g. those with Alzheimer's Disease) may become even more confused by ordering meals which do not arrive until the following day. Meal planning and menu systems should facilitate reality orientation.

nutrient requirements, because wound healing must take place. In addition the stress reaction following surgery, causes a rise in blood glucose, which is obtained by breaking down body tissues.

## PLANNING

Planning to maintain a proper nutritional status is better than having to correct deficits. Identifiying patients/clients at risk of nutritional problems should result in a care plan that will prevent or minimize nutritional problems. Nutrition education and counselling are important for individuals on regular diets, to prevent disease and promote health. Patients/clients on therapeutic diets who understand the rationale for the diet are more likely to accept responsibility for their own nutrition.

## IMPLEMENTATION

Ill or debilitated patients/clients usually have poor appetites despite the efforts of dietitians, nurses, families, friends, and other support people. Nurses can help by displaying interest in patient's/client's intakes, by understanding the influences that reduce appetite, and by being willing to do everything possible to improve intake.

One of the most disruptive influences on intake is diagnostic testing. Some blood and radiographic studies require the patient/client to fast. Therefore, the patient's/client's breakfast is usually withheld until the he or she returns from the test or the testing is completed.

Stress also influences intake. Individuals who are worried about their families, finances, employment, or illnesses are unable to eat or to eat enough to compensate for the effect of stress on their metabolism.

Drugs also affect intake and, in some cases, the utilization of nutrients. They can affect the sensations of taste or smell and, as a result, food is not as appetizing. In addition, drugs can cause nausea or vomiting. The patient/client is anorexic because of the nausea, or the nutrients are vomited before the person has

properly digested them. Drugs such as insulin and thyroid hormones can also affect metabolism.

Nurses design implementation measures around three general areas in order to promote nutrition. These areas include measures to stimulate the patient's/client's appetite, enteral nutritional therapies, and parenteral nutritional therapies.

### Stimulating Appetite

A nurse can help stimulate the patient's/client's appetite through environmental adaptations, consultation with a dietitian, special diets and food preferences, and patient/client and family counselling.

### ENVIRONMENT

Nurses are responsible for providing an environment that is conducive to eating. The ward or the patient's/client's room should be free of reminders of treatments and of odours. Mouth care should be provided when necessary to remove unpleasant tastes. The patient/client needs to be positioned comfortably so that the meal can be more enjoyable. If the patient/client has visitors or requires hygiene care before eating, sufficient time needs to be given to permit anticipation and preparation for the meal.

### DIETITIAN

After a meal, the patient's/client's intake may be evaluated and charted. The nurse shares responsibility with the dietitian for food intake. Sharing information about a person's concerns and response to **diet therapy** benefits the nurse, dietitian, and the individual. The patient's/client's education concerning the therapeutic diet should be a shared responsibility. The dietitian is the expert in diet therapy, but the nurse can relate the dietary modification to the patient's/client's condition and explain how the diet contributes to the care plan.

### SPECIAL DIETS

Nurses should be familiar with the special diets used so that they can select appropriate between-meal liquids and snacks, monitor food brought in by visitors, and offer acceptable food supplements. Numerous types of supplements are available, to be used with food or as the only nutrient source. Examples of formulas are milk based, lactose free, high protein feeds and formulas with extra fibre and calories, which range from 240 to 500 J/ml of formula.

## PSYCHOSOCIAL EFFECTS OF SPECIAL DIETS

Foods have symbolic meanings for people and are closely related to lifestyle, habits, cultural background, and other aspects of the individual. This causes many people to have difficulties in adjusting to special diets. Many would have considered mealtimes a pleasurable period distinct from routines or an interlude from work activities. A special diet, especially a **bland diet**, makes eating a dull affair. In addition, eating with others may have been a primary form of social interaction for the person, whereas now the patient/client may eat alone in a hospital room or at home and cannot eat the same foods as other family members. In such situations the nurse and other health care professionals should recognize the actual or potential psychosocial factors and make plans to counteract negative effects.

### Patient/Client and Family Counselling

Patients/clients discharged from a hospital with diet prescriptions often require dietary counselling in order to plan meals that meet specific dietary requirements or general nutrition needs. Similarly, in other health care settings, patients/clients with nutritional deficits or specific problems, such as obesity, may require assistance in menu planning and compliance with recommended diet therapies. The nurse's counselling role often includes families and information about community resources, and is central to the care offered by community nurses or health visitors.

Meal planning must take into account the family's budget and differences in the preferences of family members. Specific foods are chosen on the basis of the dietary prescriptions or standard dietary guidelines such as the four basic food groups. Meals should also provide a variety of foods and contrasting colours and consistencies. For families on limited budgets, substitutes can be used. For example, beans or cheese dishes can often replace meat in a meal, and evaporated or dry skimmed milk can be used for cooking. The method of preparation may also be modified when it is necessary to minimize certain substances. For example, baking rather than frying reduces fat intake, and lemon juice or spices can be used to replace salt in a low-sodium diet.

Planning menus a week in advance involves considerable self-discipline, but has several benefits. It helps ensure good nutrition or compliance with a specific diet and helps family members avoid impulse eating of less nutritional foods. Fruit and other nutritional items can be included in the plan for between-meal snacks. Careful advance planning can also help the family stay within the allotted budget because planned food buying is generally more economical. Last-minute shopping often includes more expensive processed and packaged foods. Often a simple tip can be of value in meal planning, such as advice to avoid grocery shopping when hungry, which can lead to spontaneous purchases

---

### General Guidelines for Assisting a Patient/Client to Eat and Drink

**Assessment**
- Determine why person needs assistance; for example, because of:
  - sensory-motor deficit in handling implements
  - lack of motivation/interest in food
  - sensory-motor deficit in coordination of swallowing/breathing
  - immaturity

**Planning**
- Involve patient/client in planning process as much as possible.
- Determine the person's nutritional requirements, how they should be distributed throughout the day, and which foods will fulfil these.
- Determine the person's food preferences.
- Determine if the person would benefit from adapted implements (seek assistance from occupational therapist).

**Implementation**
- As much as possible, ensure environment is pleasant and conducive to eating.
- Sit comfortably next to patient/client.
- Check person's preference for temperature of food, of eating, addition of salt and sugar (if permitted), and timing of sips of fluid.
- Let patient/client set the eating pace.

**Evaluation**
- Determine if the eating experience was pleasant for the patient/client.
- Determine if the patient/client has received adequate nutritional intake. Record if necessary.
- Determine if the menu should be changed.
- Determine if patient/client has progressed towards independence (if appropriate).

---

of more expensive or less nutritional foods not included in meal plans.

Finally, the nurse can assist the patient/client with referrals to community resources for assistance with dietary problems. This may involve using the services of the local authorities, such as meals-on-wheels or assistance with the cost of school meals.

### Oral Feedings
### ASSISTING PATIENTS/CLIENTS WITH FEEDING

Being fed by another person deprives patients/clients of the independence they gained over their food intake as toddlers. Nurses can improve patient/client feeding by carefully protecting his or her dignity and actively involving them in the process (see box above). Any material used to protect clothing should be referred to as a serviette or napkin, not a bib. The nurse should allow patients/clients time to empty their mouths after every spoonful, and ensure that they have sufficient fluids during the meal. They should carefully gauge the speed at which the person can manage the food. The nurse should also allow patients/clients to choose the order in which they wish to eat food items, and conversation about topics other than food should be an integral part of the process. The nurse who has several patients/clients to feed should use ingenuity to prevent an 'assembly line' approach, which is devastating to clients'/patients' self-esteem.

## Enteral Nutrition

**Enteral nutrition (EN)** refers to nutrients given via the intestinal tract. This includes ordinary meals, as well as blended foods and proprietary preparations. The oral route is the preferred method of meeting nutritional needs if the patient's/client's gastrointestinal tract is functioning by providing safe, economical, nutritional support. For individuals with eating difficulties, enteral nutrition may be supplied via nasogastric, jejunal, or **gastrostomy tube** (Robuck and Fleetwood, 1992). Patients/clients may be maintained indefinitely on tube feedings, which can provide all the essential nutrients except fibre. Although cramping and diarrhoea are commonly associated with tube feedings, these symptoms usually subside when the flow rate or concentration of the solution is reduced.

## Total Parenteral Nutrition

Parenteral nutrition is the use of an intravenous line to feed patients/clients, and **total parenteral nutrition (TPN)** is a nutritionally adequate hypertonic solution consisting of all the glucose, amino acids, lipids, minerals, and vitamins that he or she requires given through an indwelling peripheral or central intravenous catheter (see Chapter 18). It can be used when a patient/client is unable to meet his or her requirements orally, perhaps because of disease to the gastrointestinal tract, or because his or her needs have increased greatly. Total parenteral nutrition solutions are hyperosmolar (that is, highly concentrated), and as a result, they are infused through central lines. The solution itself is very precisely tailored to the individual's nutritional needs, with some common elements for all patients/clients.

## SUMMARY

Nurses must understand the functions of the basic nutrients and metabolism. An understanding of the guidelines for the selection of an adequate diet is essential so that nurses can teach patients/clients about nutrients and answer questions related to diet. Nurses should also be alert to current research findings and their impact on dietary recommendations. They should be familiar with alternative food patterns and know how age and health status influence dietary needs. They need to be observant and sensitive to people who, because of either mental illness or learning difficulties, are not always able to effectively communicate their needs.

Nurses must be able to assess the nutritional status of a patient/client. They must also recognize that many divergent factors influence food intake and consider these factors when attempting to modify food intake.

Nurses must be able to identify patients/clients at risk for nutritional problems and be aware of common nutritional conditions. They should be aware of the importance of their interactions with others in the area of food intake, be familiar with common hospital diets, and be able to assist patients/clients at mealtimes. Finally, nurses must evaluate their activities in the area of nutritional support, to revise those that prove ineffective and continue those that are beneficial.

## CHAPTER 21 REVIEW

### Key Concepts

- The principles of nutrition include energy balance, different nutrients, and their role in health.
- Food is mechanically prepared for digestion in the mouth and stomach, chemically digested, and then absorbed in the small intestine; water is absorbed in the large intestine. Finally, the undigested food residue and some cellular material is eliminated from the rectum.
- Dietary guidelines include the use of nutrition reference values, while recognizing that individuals will vary in their requirements.
- Individual differences in dietary intake may be due to consideration of religious or moral convictions, cultural background, or socioeconomic circumstance.
- Variations in diet occur throughout an individual's life span, for example between youngsters, older adults and pregnant women.
- It is a challenge to accurately assess nutritional status, include nursing and laboratory observations, and the patient/client history.
- Patients/clients who may be at particular risk of malnutrition include those who are ill, handicapped or obese, have anorexia nervosa, or are in hospital.
- When assisting patients to eat, it is important to maintain the patient's/client's dignity.
- A review is needed of the nursing skills required for patients/clients with special dietary needs.
- Enteral nutrition provides nutrients in an appropriate form and amount.
- Total parenteral nutrition is sometimes an appropriate means of providing adequate nourishment.

## CRITICAL THINKING EXCERSIES

1. Discuss the role of water- and fat-soluble vitamins with regard to function, needs, and patient/client teaching regarding food source and amounts needed.
2. Mrs McIntyre, aged 45 years, is concerned about weight gain. How would you assist her in reviewing her current dietary practices?
3. What concerns might the nurse have in relation to a 16-year-old girl whose parents have observed to be losing weight and refusing food consistently over a period of the previous two months?
4. The parents of Mina, a healthy 4-month-old baby girl are very worried about whether she is taking an adequate diet. How would you advise them?
5. Discuss the following statement:
   "Healthy eating is simply a matter of obtaining the correct nutrients"

## Key Terms

## REFERENCES

Child Poverty Action Group CPAG: *School meal fact sheet*, London, 1991, CPAG.

Department of Health: *Dietary reference values for the United Kingdom*, Report on health and social service no. 41. London, 1991, HMSO.

Department of Health: *The health of the nation: a strategy for health in England.* London, 1992, HMSO.

Grant JA, Kennedy-Caldwell C: *Nutritional support in nursing*, New York, 1988, Grune & Stratton.

Holmes S: Nutrition and older people: a matter of concern, *Nursing Times* 90(42), 1994.

Kennedy M: Solving the nutritional problem of people with a mental handicap, London, 1990, BDA Adviser.

Mills A, Tyler H, Infant Feeding Practice in Britain, Health Visitor, 63 (10) Oct, 1990

Ministry of Agriculture, fisheries and food: *Manual of nutrition*, London,1985, HMSO.

Nightingale F: *Notes on nursing: what it is and what it is not.* London, 1860, Harrison & Sons.

NHS Cymru Wales: *Caring for the future 1992*, Cardiff, 1992, Central Office of Information, The Welsh Office.

Northern Ireland Office: *A regional strategy for the Northern Ireland Health and Personal Social Services 1992-1997*, Belfast, 1991, Northern Ireland Office.

Orbach S, *Fat is a feminist issue*, London, 1978, Paddington Press

Rich AJ: The assessment of body composition in the clinical situation, Proc of Nutr Soc, 41: 389, 1982.

Robuck J, Fleetwood J: Nutrition support in the patient/client with cancer, *Focus Crit Care Nurs* 19(2):129, 1992.

Saul H, Fat is a pharmaceutical issue, New Scientist 1883:28, 1993.

Scottish Office: *Scotland's health: a challenge to you*, Edinburgh, 1992, Scottish Office.

US Department of Agriculture: *USDA's food guide pyramid*, USDA Human Nutrition Information Service Pub No 249, Washington, DC, 1992, US Government Printing Office.

Warnold I, Lunholm, K: Clinical significance of peropoerative nutritional status on 215 non cancer patients. *Ann Surg* 3:299, 1984.

Whitney EN, Catallo CB, Rolfes SR: *Understanding normal and clinical nutrition*, ed 3, St Paul, Minn, 1991, West.

## FURTHER READING

### Adult Nursing

Coates V: *Are they being served?* London, 1985, Royal College of Nursing.

Hamilton Smith S: *Nil by mouth?* London, 1972, Royal College of Nursing.

O'Brien M: Hospital food for ethnic minority patients, London, 1981, Haringey CHC.

Rifkind BM, Cholesterol lowering and reduced risk of coronary heart disease, *Pract Cardiol* 14:(suppl)3, 1988.

Stewart-Truswell A: *ABCs of nutrition.* (2nd ed) London, 1992, BMJ Press.

Williams SR: *Basic nutrition and diet therapy.* St Louis, 1992, Mosby.

Wardlaw GM, Insel PM, Seyler MF: *Contemporary nutrition: issues and insights*, St Louis, 1992, Mosby.

### Children's Nursing

Coles A *et al*, School Meals, Health Eating and Contract Specification, Health Education Journal, 52/1 10-12, 1993

Herschee P: *The joint breast feeding initiative.* London, 1987, HMSO

Duggan M: Cause and cure for iron deficiency in toddlers, *Health Visitor* 66 (7):750, 1993

Jackson C: No such thing as a free lunch, *Health Visitor*, 63 (8):261, 1990.

Mills A, Tyler H: Infant feeding practice in Britain, *Health Visitor* 63:10, 1990.

Mills A *et al*: Children's dietary habits in hospital, *Paed Nurs*, 5(8):17,1993

National Advisory Committee on Nutrition Education: *A discussion paper on proposals for nutrition guidelines for health education in Britain.* London, 1993, Health Education Council.

Palmer G: Any old iron, *Health Visitor*, 66,(7):248, 1993.

Wilkinson P, Davies D: When and why are babies weaned, *BMJ*, 1:1682, 1978.

Woolwridge M: Do changes in pattern of breast usage alter the baby's nutrient intake? *Lancet* 336(8712):395, 1990.

Young I: Health eating policies in schools; an evaluation of effects on pupils' knowledge, attitudes and behaviour, *Health Ed J* 52(1):5, 1993.

### Learning Disabilities Nursing

MacDonald NJ *et al:* Hypernaraemic dehydration in patients in a large hospital for the mentally handicapped, *BMJ* 299:1426, 1989.

Perry M: Learning disabilities: community nursing, Nursing Standard, 7 (11): 38-40, 1992.

Rotatori AF *et al:* Teaching nutrition, exercise and weight control to the moderate/mildly handicapped, London, 1985, Charles C Thomas.

Stewart L, Beango H: A surgey of dietary problems of adults with learning disabilities in the community, Mental Handicap Research, 7 (1): 41-50, 1994.

Wilson M, Parkingson K: Problems in promoting healthy eating, Mental Handicap, 21 (1): 25-8, 1993.

Mental Health Nursing:-

Chudley P: An unhealthy obsession, Nursing Times, March 26: 50, 1986.

Hofland SL, Dardis PO: Bulimia nervosa: associated physical problems, J Psychosoc Nurs Ment Health Serv, 30 (2): 23-7, 1992.

### Mental Health Nursing

Brownell KD, Foreyt JP: *The hardbook of eating disorders.* New York, 1986, Basic Books.

Orbach S: *Fat is a feminist issue.* London, 1978, Paddington Press.

# Urinary Elimination

## LEARNING OUTCOMES

After reading this chapter, you should be able to:
- *Define the key terms listed.*
- *Explain the function of each organ in the urinary system.*
- *Describe the process of micturition.*
- *Identify factors that may affect the characteristics of urine and describe normal and abnormal urine.*
- *Identify factors that influence urinary elimination.*
- *Compare and contrast common alterations in urinary elimination.*
- *Obtain a nursing history for a patient/client with urinary elimination problems.*
- *Obtain urine specimens.*
- *Describe the nursing implications of common diagnostic tests of the urinary system.*
- *Discuss nursing measures to promote normal micturition and reduce episodes of incontinence.*
- *Understand basic principles in selecting urinary catheters.*
- *Demonstrate insertion and irrigation of a urinary catheter.*
- *Discuss nursing measures to reduce urinary tract infection.*

Normal elimination of urinary wastes is a basic function most people take for granted. When the urinary system fails to function properly, virtually all organ systems can be affected. People with alterations in urinary elimination may also suffer emotionally from body image changes. The nurse can provide understanding and sensitivity to patients'/clients' needs. With older patients/clients in particular, the nurse must seek the reasons for problems and find acceptable solutions.

## PHYSIOLOGY OF URINE ELIMINATION

**Urinary elimination** depends upon the functioning of the kidneys, ureters, bladder, and urethra. The kidneys remove wastes from the blood to form urine. The ureters transport urine from the kidneys to the bladder. The bladder holds urine until the urge to urinate develops. Urine leaves the body through the urethra (Fig. 22-1).

### Kidneys
Kidneys are reddish-brown, bean-shaped organs that lie on either side of the vertebral column posterior to the peritoneum and against deep muscles of the back. The kidneys extend to the twelfth thoracic and third lumbar vertebrae. Normally the left kidney is 1.5 to 2 cm higher than the right because of the anatomical position of the liver. Each measures approximately 12 cm by 7 cm from the hilum to the cortex (in adults) and weighs 120 to 150 g. An adrenal gland lies on the superior pole of each kidney but is not directly related to urinary elimination. Each kidney is enclosed by several layers of supporting tissue: the medulla is surrounded by the outer cortex, which is covered by

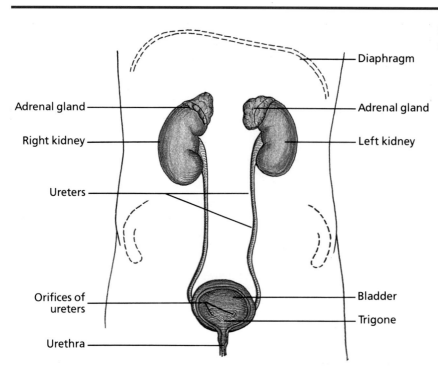

**Fig. 22-1** Organs of the urinary system.

Diaphragm

Adrenal gland

Right kidney

Left kidney

Adrenal gland

Ureters

Orifices of
ureters

Bladder

Trigone

Urethra

**Fig. 22-2** Section through a kidney. From Brooker C: *Human structure and function: nursing applications in clinical practice.* London, 1993, Mosby.

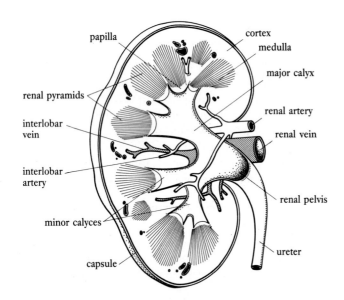

papilla

cortex

medulla

major calyx

renal pyramids

renal artery

interlobar
vein

renal vein

interlobar
artery

renal pelvis

minor calyces

capsule

ureter

the tough, fibrous renal capsule and is surrounded by a cushion of fat (Fig. 22-2). (For a detailed description of the structure and function of the kidney, refer to a detailed anatomy and physiology textbook).

Waste products of metabolism that collect in the blood are filtered in the kidneys. Blood reaches each kidney by the **renal artery** that branches from the abdominal aorta. The renal artery enters the kidney at the hilum. Approximately 20% to 25% of the cardiac output circulates daily through the kidneys. Each kidney contains 1 million nephrons. The **nephron**, the functional unit of the kidney, is capable of forming urine. The nephron is composed of the glomerulus, Bowman's capsule, proximal convoluted tubule, loop of Henle, distal tubule, and collecting duct (Fig. 22-3).

Blood reaches nephrons through the afferent arterioles. A cluster of these blood vessels forms the capillary network of the **glomerulus**, which is the initial site of urine formation. The glomerular capillaries are porous and permit filtration of water and substances such as glucose, amino acids, urea, creatinine, and major electrolytes into Bowman's capsule. This is the **filtrate**. Protein does not normally filter through the glomerulus, as the molecule is too large. Protein in the urine (**proteinuria**) is a sign of glomerular injury. The glomerulus filters approximately 125 ml of filtrate per minute.

Not all of the glomerular filtrate is excreted as urine. After the filtrate leaves the glomerulus, it passes through a system of tubules and collecting ducts, where water and substances such as

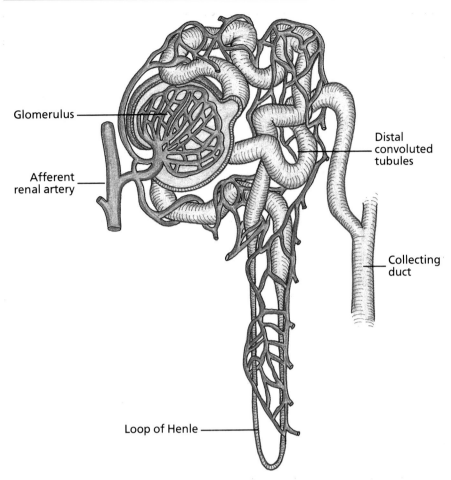

**Fig. 22-3** Renal nephron.

Glomerulus

Afferent renal artery

Distal convoluted tubules

Collecting duct

Loop of Henle

glucose, amino acids, uric acid, and sodium and potassium ions are selectively reabsorbed back into the plasma. Other substances such as hydrogen ions, potassium ions (in the presence of aldosterone), and ammonia are secreted back into the tubules. About 99% of the filtrate is reabsorbed into the plasma, with the remaining 1% excreted as urine. Thus the kidneys play a key role in fluid and electrolyte balance (see Chapter 18). The normal adult 24-hour output of urine is about 1500 to 1600 ml. An output of 60 ml of urine per hour is generally normal. An output of less than 30 ml per hour may indicate renal problems and should be reported. The kidneys also produce hormones vital to blood pressure regulation and production of erythrocytes (RBCs), and a substance concerned with bone mineralization.

The kidneys are responsible for maintaining a normal number of erythrocytes. They produce **erythropoietin**, a hormone released primarily from specialized glomerular cells that sense decreased erythrocytes oxygenation (local hypoxia). After it is released from the kidney, erythropoietin functions within the bone marrow to stimulate erythropoiesis (production and maturation of erythrocytes). **Renin** is another hormone produced by the kidneys. Its major role is the regulation of blood flow in times of renal ischaemia (decreased blood supply); this is frequently referred to as *autoregulation*. Renin is synthesized and released from juxtaglomerular cells, which are located on the juxtaglomerular apparatus of the nephron (Fig. 22-4).

Renin functions as an enzyme to convert angiotensinogen (a precursor substance synthesized by the liver) into angiotensin I. As angiotensin I circulates through the lungs, it is converted into angiotensin II. Angiotensin II exerts its effect on vascular smooth muscle to cause vasoconstriction and stimulates aldosterone release from the adrenal cortex. The effect of both of these mechanisms is an increase in arterial blood pressure.

The kidneys also play a role in calcium and phosphate regulation. They are responsible for producing a substance that converts vitamin D into its active form (see Chapter 18).

## Ureters

Urine leaves the tubules and enters collecting ducts that transport it to the renal pelvis. A ureter joins each renal pelvis at the initial exit route for urinary wastes (see Fig. 22-1). **Ureters** are tubular structures measuring 25 to 30 cm in length and 1.25 cm in diameter in the adult. They extend retroperitoneally to enter the urinary bladder in the pelvic cavity at the ureterovesical junction (the juncture of the ureters with the bladder). Urine draining from the ureters to the bladder is usually sterile.

Three layers of tissue form the wall of the ureter. The inner layer is a mucous membrane continuous with the lining of the renal tubules and urinary bladder. The middle layer consists of smooth muscle fibres that help transport urine through the ureters by peristaltic waves stimulated by distension with urine. An outer layer of fibrous connective tissue supports the ureters.

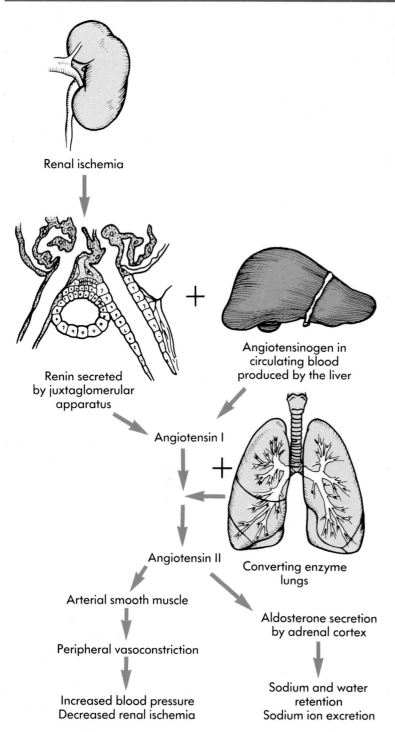

**Fig. 22-4** Juxtaglomerular apparatus of the nephron and the renin-angiotension system. From Ulric BT: *Nephrology nursing: concepts and practices*, Norwalk, Conn, 1989, Appleton and Lange.

Peristaltic waves cause the urine to enter the bladder in spurts rather than steadily. To prevent the reflux of urine from the bladder into the ureters, a small valve-like mechanism exists at the ureterovesical junction.

### Bladder

The urinary bladder is a hollow, distensible, muscular organ that is a reservoir for urine and the organ of excretion. When empty, the bladder lies in the pelvic cavity behind the symphysis pubis. In men the bladder lies against the rectum posteriorly, and in women it rests against the anterior wall of the uterus and vagina.

The bladder's shape changes as it becomes filled with urine. The walls of the bladder can expand. Normally it holds approximately 600 ml of urine. Pressure within the bladder is usually low, a factor that protects against infection. When the bladder is full, it expands and extends above the symphysis pubis. A greatly distended bladder may reach the umbilicus.

The **trigone** (a smooth triangular area on the inner surface of the bladder) is at the base of the bladder. An opening exists at each of the trigone's three angles. Two are at the base of the trigone for the ureters, and one is at the apex for the urethra.

The wall of the bladder has four layers: the inner mucous

coat, a submucous coat of connective tissue, a muscular coat, and an outer serous coat. The muscular layer has bundles of muscle fibres that form the detrusor muscle. Parasympathetic nerve fibres stimulate the detrusor muscle during micturition. The internal urethral sphincter, made of a ring-like band of muscle, is at the base of the bladder where it joins the urethra. The sphincter prevents escape of urine from the bladder and is under involuntary control.

### Urethra

Urine travels from the bladder through the urethra and passes outside of the body through the **urethral meatus**. Normally the turbulent flow of urine through the urethra washes it free of bacteria. Mucous membrane lines the urethra, and urethral glands secrete mucus into the urethral canal. The mucus is believed to be bacteriostatic and forms a mucus plug to prevent entrance of bacteria. Thick layers of smooth muscle surround the urethra.

In women the urethra is approximately 4 to 6.5 cm long. The external urethral sphincter, located about halfway down the urethra, permits voluntary flow of urine. The short length of the urethra in women provides an easy access for microorganisms. In men the urethra, which is a urinary canal and a passageway for cells and secretions from reproductive organs, is 20 cm long. It has three sections: the prostatic urethra, the membranous urethra, and the penile urethra.

In a woman the urinary meatus (opening) is located between the labia minora, above the vagina and below the clitoris. In a male the meatus is located at the distal end of the penis.

### Act of Micturition

**Micturition** and **voiding** are terms for the process by which urine is expelled from the urinary bladder. The bladder normally holds as much as 600 ml of urine. However, the desire to pass urine can be sensed when the bladder contains only a small amount of urine (150 to 200 ml in an adult and 50 to 200 ml in a child). As the volume increases, the bladder walls stretch, sending sensory

**Mother and Child Nursing**
**Effects of pregnancy on the bladder and urinary volume**

In a pregnant woman the enlarging uterus pushes against the bladder, causing a feeling of fullness and reducing the bladder's capacity. Hormones released during pregnancy result in a maternal net water gain of 7 litres. Most of this is due to increased plasma volume, resulting in haemodilution; 1 litre is due to amniotic fluid; and 1 litre is due to generalized oedema.

There is often increased urine production in pregnant women. At the beginning of pregnancy, before the uterus becomes an abdominal organ, and at the end of pregnancy as the fetal head engages, there is increased pressure on the bladder. These two factors result in increased frequency of micturition in the first and third trimesters.

Following delivery, there is a diuresis to remove the extra fluid, and women may void up to one litre on a single occasion. *(Bennett and Brown, 1989).*

impulses to the sacral spinal cord. Parasympathetic impulses from the sacral spinal cord stimulate the detrusor muscle to contract rhythmically. The internal urethral sphincter also relaxes so that urine may enter the urethra, although voiding does not yet occur. As the bladder contracts, nerve impulses travel up the spinal cord to the midbrain and cerebral cortex. A person is thus conscious of the need to urinate. If the person chooses not to void, the external urinary sphincter remains contracted, and the micturition reflex is inhibited. However, when a person is ready to void, the external sphincter relaxes, the micturition reflex stimulates the detrusor muscle to contract and the urethral sphincter to relax, and micturition occurs.

### Characteristics of Urine

The nurse inspects the patient's/client's urine for quantity, colour, clarity, and odour.

### Colour

Normal urine ranges from a pale, straw colour to amber, depending on its concentration. Urine is usually more concentrated in the morning or with dehydration. As the person drinks more fluids, urine becomes less concentrated.

Bleeding from the kidneys or ureters causes urine to become dark red; bleeding from the bladder or urethra causes a bright red urine. Various medications and foods also change urine colour. Beetroot, rhubarb, and blackberries may cause red urine. Special dyes used in intravenous diagnostic studies eventually discolour urine. Dark amber urine may be the result of high concentrations of bilirubin caused by liver dysfunction.

### Clarity

Normal urine appears transparent at voiding. Urine that stands several minutes in a container becomes cloudy. Freshly passed urine in patients/clients with renal disease may appear cloudy or foamy because of high protein concentrations. Urine also appears thick and cloudy as a result of bacteria.

### Odour

Urine has a characteristic odour, often described as 'newly mown hay'. The more concentrated the urine, the stronger the odour. Bacteria in the urine causes an ammonia odour, which is common in patients/clients who are repeatedly incontinent. A sweet or fruity odour occurs from ketones, by-products of incomplete fat metabolism, seen with diabetes mellitus or starvation.

## FACTORS INFLUENCING MICTURITION

Numerous factors influence the volume and quantity of urine and the patient's/client's ability to urinate. Disease processes can alter normal urinary elimination. For example, a decrease in renal perfusion leads to **oliguria** (diminished capacity to form urine) or, less commonly, **anuria** (inability to produce urine).

### Sociocultural Factors

Cultural norms can influence the design and acceptability of environments in which to void urine (for example, communal

**Children's Nursing**
**Micturition in children**

Infants and young children cannot concentrate urine and reabsorb water effectively. Their urine thus appears light yellow or watery. In relation to their small body size, infants and children excrete large volumes of urine. For example, a 6-month-old child who weighs 6–8 kg excretes 400–500 ml of urine daily. The child weights about 10% of an adult's weight but excretes 33% as much urine.

A child cannot control micturition voluntarily until the age 18–24 months. A child must be able to recognize the feeling of bladder fullness, to hold urine for 1 to 2 hours, and to communicate the sense of urgency to an adult. The young child needs parents' understanding, patience, and consistency. A child may not gain full control of micturition until the age of 4 or 5. Boys are generally slower than girls. Daytime control of micturition is easier to accomplish than night-time control and occurs earlier in the child's development, usually by 2 years of age.

**Adult Nursing**
**Influence of ageing on micturition**

Changes in the kidneys may begin as early as age 30. Common problems concerning micturition in older adults include:
- nocturia (the need to urinate at night), because the kidney's abilities to concentrate urine decline and the bladder is less elastic.
- urinary retention, particularly in older men with prostatic hypertrophy (enlargement of the prostate gland).
- urinary tract infections, because the bladder may not contract effectively and urine may remain after voiding (residual urine). This can increase the risk of bacterial growth.
- urgency (the need to void urgently). In young people, the sensation of bladder fullness and the urge to urinate is felt when the bladder is about half full. In older people, this urge may not be felt until the bladder is nearly full, and therefore requiring an immediate response.

Some older people experience continence problems, but incontinence is not an inevitable consequence of ageing. The condition may result from difficulties in walking to a lavatory, in retaining the urine for the necessary time, or in manipulating clothing.

Nurses can promote continence in older people by:
- recognizing underlying problems (for example, an infection)
- ensuring that the person can reach a lavatory quickly
- responding immediately to requests for assistance
- offering advice on clothing that can be removed easily
- offering health teaching (for example, pelvic floor exercises)
- referring for specialist advice or equipment

facilities) and preferred body positions for voiding. In addition, social expectations (for example, school breaks) influence the time of urination.

When the nurse is assessing a patient's/client's elimination needs, he or she must consider cultural and social habits. If a patient/client prefers privacy, the nurse tries to prevent interruptions as the patient/client voids. A patient/client who is less sensitive to the need for privacy should be treated with understanding and acceptance.

### Personal Habits

Privacy and adequate time to urinate are usually important to most people. Some people need distractions (for example, reading, or the sound of a running tap) to relax.

### Muscle Tone

Weak abdominal and pelvic floor muscles impair bladder contraction and control of the external urethral sphincter. Poor control of micturition can result from muscle wasting caused by prolonged immobility, stretching of muscles during childbirth, menopausal muscle atrophy (decrease in size of tissue), and damage to muscles from trauma.

Continuous drainage of urine through an indwelling catheter causes loss of bladder tone or damage to uretheral sphincters. The bladder remains relatively empty when a patient/client has an indwelling catheter in place, and thus it is never stretched to capacity. When a muscle is not stretched regularly, atrophy develops. When a catheter is removed, the patient/client may have difficulty regaining urinary control.

### Urinary Volume

The kidneys maintain a sensitive balance between retention and excretion of fluids (see Chapter 18). If fluids and the concentration of electrolytes and solutes are in equilibrium, an increase in fluid intake causes an increase in urine production. Ingested fluids increase the body's circulating plasma and thus increase the volume of glomerular filtrate and urine excreted. This amount varies with food and fluid intake. The volume of urine formed at night is about half that formed during the day because intake and metabolism decline. In a healthy person, the intake of water in food and fluids balances the output of water in urine, faeces, and insensible losses in perspiration and ventilation.

Ingestion of certain fluids directly affects urine production and excretion. Alcohol inhibits the release of antidiuretic

**Urinary Elimination**

Asian people may be uncomfortable using a lavatory with a high seat and toilet paper. Many prefer low-set toilets and washing with running water after using the lavatory. It is not uncommon for Asian women to position their feet on the lavatory seat in order to achieve the customary squatting position when passing urine or faeces.

People from some cultures, for example Hindus, may be very reluctant to discuss any problems with the genitourinary system. Sensitivity is needed when handling such discussions.

## Mental Health Nursing
## Psychological factors that influence micturition

Anxiety and emotional stress do not change the characteristics of urine but may cause a sense of urgency and increase frequency of urination. An anxious person may have the urge to void even after voiding only a few minutes earlier.

Anxiety may also prevent a person from being able to urinate completely. Emotional tension makes it difficult to relax abdominal and perineal muscles. If the external urethral sphincter is not completely relaxed, voiding may be incomplete, and urine is retained in the bladder.

In elderly patients/clients with organic brain dysfunction, micturition may become an area of concern. This may also become a source of embarrassment for the patient/client. Explanations for difficulties with micturition may be organic, psychological, social, or a combination of these.

hormone (ADH) and thus promotes urine formation. Coffee, tea, cocoa, and cola drinks that contain caffeine increase **diuresis** (increased formation and excretion of urine). Foods that contain a high fluid content, such as fruit and vegetables, may also increase urine production.

Febrile conditions influence urine production. The patient/client who becomes diaphoretic (sweaty) loses a large amount of fluids through insensible water loss, which decreases urine production. However, the increased body metabolism associated with fever increases accumulation of body wastes. Although urine volume may be reduced, it is highly concentrated because water is lost via sweat.

### Disease Conditions

Several diseases can affect the ability to micturate. Any lesion of peripheral nerves leading to the bladder causes loss of bladder tone, reduced sensation of bladder fullness, and difficulty in controlling urination. For example, diabetes mellitus and multiple sclerosis cause neuropathic conditions that alter bladder function.

Diseases that slow or hinder physical activity interfere with the ability to void. Rheumatoid arthritis, degenerative joint disease, and Parkinson's disease are examples of conditions that make it difficult to reach and use toilet facilities. A patient/client with rheumatoid arthritis often cannot sit on or rise from a toilet without an elevated seat.

### Surgical Procedures

The stress of surgery initially triggers what Selye (1946) described as the general adaptation syndrome (see Chapter 4). The posterior pituitary gland releases an increased amount of ADH, which increases water reabsorption and reduces urine output. The surgical patient is often in an altered state of fluid balance before surgery, which aggravates the reduction in urine output. The stress response also elevates the level of aldosterone, resulting in reduction in urine output in an effort to increase circulatory fluid volume.

Anaesthetic and opiate analgesics slow the glomerular filtration rate, reducing urine output. These pharmacological agents also impair sensory and motor impulses travelling between the bladder, spinal cord, and brain. Patients/clients recovering from anaesthesia and opiate analgesia are often unable to sense bladder fullness and are unable to initiate or inhibit micturition. Spinal anaesthetics, in particular, create the risk of urinary retention because of an inability to sense the need to void.

Surgery of lower abdominal and pelvic structures can impair micturition because of local trauma to surrounding tissues. The oedema and inflammation associated with healing may obstruct the flow of urine from the bladder or urethra, interfere with relaxation of pelvic and sphincter muscles, or cause discomfort during voiding. For this reason, after surgery involving the bladder and urethra, patients/clients may need urinary catheters.

### Medications

Diuretics (for example, frusemide) prevent reabsorption of water and certain electrolytes to increase urine output. Some medications and foods (for example warfarin, beetroot) change the colour of urine. Patients with impaired kidney function require dosage adjustments in medications excreted by the kidneys.

### Diagnostic Examination

Examination of the urinary system can influence micturition. Procedures such as an intravenous pyelogram or urogram require that the patient/client not take fluids orally before the test. A restriction in fluid intake commonly lowers urine output. Diagnostic examinations (for example, cystoscopy) that involve direct visualization of urinary structures may cause localized oedema of the urethral passageway and spasm of the bladder sphincter. The patient/client often has urinary retention after such a procedure and may pass red or pink urine because of bleeding resulting from trauma to the urethral or bladder mucosa.

## ALTERATIONS IN URINARY ELIMINATION

The most common urinary problems encountered by the nurse involve disturbances in the act of micturition. These disturbances result from impaired bladder function, obstruction to urine outflow, or inability to voluntarily control micturition. Some patients may have permanent or temporary changes in the normal pathway of urinary excretion.

### Urinary Retention

**Urinary retention** is accumulation of urine in the bladder with inability of the bladder to empty fully. Urine collects in the bladder, stretching its walls and causing feelings of pressure, discomfort, tenderness over the symphysis pubis, restlessness, and diaphoresis (sweating).

Urine production slowly fills the bladder and prevents activation of stretch receptors. After it distends beyond a certain point, the bladder becomes unable to contract.

A key sign is absence of urine output over several hours and formation of bladder distension. In severe urinary retention the bladder may hold as much as 2000 to 3000 ml of urine.

As retention progresses, retention with overflow may develop. Pressure in the bladder builds to a point where the external urethral sphincter is unable to hold back urine. The sphincter temporarily opens to allow a small volume of urine (25 to 60 ml) to escape. As urine escapes, the bladder pressure falls enough to allow the sphincter to regain control and close. With retention overflow the patient/client voids small amounts of urine 2 or 3 times an hour with no real relief of distension or discomfort. Bladder spasms may occur with voiding.

Retention occurs as a result of urethral obstruction (e.g., enlargement of the prostate gland), surgical trauma, alterations in motor and sensory innervation of the bladder, medication side effects, and anxiety.

### Lower Urinary Tract Infections

UTIs account for 40% of hospital-acquired (nosocomial) infections (Burgener, 1987). Bacteria in the urine (bacteriuria) may lead to the spread of organisms into the kidneys and bloodstream.

Microorganisms can enter the urinary tract through the urethral meatus, the bloodstream, or (less commonly) through a fistula between the bladder and the bowel. The ascending route through the urethra is more common. Bacteria inhabit the distal urethra, external genitalia, and vagina in women. Organisms enter the urethral meatus easily and travel up the inner mucosal lining to the bladder. Women are more susceptible to infection because of the proximity of the anus to the urethral meatus and because of the short urethra. In men, prostatic secretions contain an antibacterial substance that reduces UTIs. Older women, neonates and patients/clients with progressive underlying disease or decreased immunity are also at increased risk.

In a healthy person with good bladder function, organisms are flushed out during voiding. However, bladder distension reduces blood flow to the mucosal and submucosal layer, and tissues become more susceptible to bacteria. Residual urine in the bladder is an ideal medium for microorganism growth. The pH and chemical makeup of urine also affect the spread of organisms.

In hospital, the most common cause of infection is the introduction of instruments into the urinary tract. For example,

## TABLE 22-1 Types of Urinary Incontinence

| Description | Causes | Symptoms |
|---|---|---|
| **FUNCTIONAL** Involuntary, unpredictable passage of urine in patient/client with intact urinary and nervous system. | Change in environment; sensory, cognitive, or mobility deficits. | Strong urge to void that causes loss of urine before reaching appropriate receptacle. |
| **UNSTABLE BLADDER** Bladder muscle (detrusor) contractions are not under perfect voluntary control and contract unpredictably with relatively small volumes. | Often no obvious bladder or neurological pathology. However, does occur with neurological conditions such as multiple sclerosis and stroke. | Urgency, frequency and urge incontinence. Common precipitants include: standing, rain, cold, proximity to toilet, and bumpy journeys. Symptoms usually confined to certain times of the day. |
| **STRESS** Increased intra-abdominal pressure which causes leakage of a small amount of urine. | Coughing, laughing, vomiting, or lifting with a full bladder; obesity; full uterus in third trimester; incompetent bladder outlet; weak pelvic musculature. | Dribbling of urine with increased intra-abdominal pressure, urinary urgency and frequency. |
| **OUTFLOW OBSTRUCTION** Outflow of urine from the urethra is impeded, causing residual urine to accumulate in the bladder. | Most common cause in men is an enlarged prostate. Can be caused by faecal impaction in both sexes. | Dribbling overflow or stress incontinence. Frequency and double voiding, i.e. voiding twice in quick succession. Some may experience a feeling of incomplete emptying of the bladder. |
| **LOSS OF BLADDER TONE** A hypotonic bladder which will not contract effectively to empty — residual urine accumulates and overflows. | Common in diabetic patients/clients, and others with neurological problems. | Dribbling overflow or stress incontinence. Frequency and double voiding, i.e. voiding twice in quick succession. Some may experience a feeling of incomplete emptying of the bladder. |

the introduction of a catheter through the urethra provides a direct route for microorganisms. With an indwelling bladder catheter, bacteria ascend along the outside of the catheter on the urethral wall or travel up the catheter's lumen. The catheter interferes with the normal voiding mechanism that acts as a defence against organisms entering the urethra. Local irritation to the urethra or bladder further predisposes tissues to bacterial invasion. Infecting microorganisms tend to colonise catheter surfaces, forming a living 'biofilm', firmly attached to the catheter surface (Brown, 1988).

Poor perineal hygiene is a common cause of UTIs in women. Inadequate handwashing, failure to wipe from front to back after voiding or defaecating, and frequent sexual intercourse predispose women to infection. Passing urine after intercourse will reduce the incidence of UTIs. In some young girls, **cystitis** (inflammation of the bladder) develops from exposure to ingredients in bubble baths or shampoo used in the bath (Rogers, 1985). Any interference with the free flow of urine can cause infection. A kinked or obstructed catheter and any condition resulting in urinary retention increases the risk of a bladder infection.

Patients/clients with UTIs have pain or burning during micturition **(dysuria)** as urine flows past inflamed tissues. Fever, chills, nausea, malaise and confusion in older patients may develop as the infection worsens. An irritated bladder causes a frequent and urgent sensation of the need to void. Irritation to bladder and urethral mucosa results in blood-tinged urine **(haematuria)**. The urine appears concentrated and cloudy because of the presence of leucocytes or bacteria. If infection spreads to the kidneys **(pyelonephritis)**, loin pain, tenderness, low-grade fever, and chills are common.

## Urinary Incontinence

**Urinary incontinence** can be defined as an involuntary loss of urine resulting in a social or hygienic problem. Urinary incontinence may be differentiated into five different types: functional, bladder instability, stress, outflow obstruction, and loss of bladder tone (Norton, 1992) (see Table 22-1).

In the adult population, the prevalence of urinary incontinence is estimated to be 10 in 1000 known to the health and social services, and 71 in 1000 unknown to these services (Thomas *et al*, 1980). Incontinence can impair body image and

self-esteem, and some of its symptoms may cause severe disruption to an individual's life.

Physical limitations and environmental factors have to be taken into consideration. Restricted mobility can exacerbate incontinence because of an inability to reach toilet facilities in time, particularly if urgency of micturition is experienced. Older people often lack the energy to walk very far at one time when unwell. Low-set chairs and beds raised well above the floor may be obstacles for older adults, who must get up to reach a toilet. Some individuals may have difficulty undoing buttons or manipulating zips.

Continued episodes of incontinence create the potential for skin breakdown. The acidic character of urine is irritating to the skin. The immobilized patient/client who has frequent incontinence is especially at risk of developing pressure sores.

# NURSING PROCESS AND URINARY ELIMINATION

 **ASSESSMENT**

To assist in the identification of urinary elimination problems the nurse must obtain a detailed and comprehensive nursing history. This is an embarrassing subject for most people, hence time developing rapport is important; utmost privacy and maintenance of dignity is essential.

Patients/clients are asked about daily voiding patterns, including frequency and times of day, normal volume at each voiding, and recent changes. Keeping a chart which records the frequency and volume of urine output as well as fluid intake can assist in revealing the pattern of the underlying bladder disorder. This type of chart is easy to keep and in most cases the patients/clients or a relative can do it. During an assessment it is

---

 **Children's Nursing**
**Enuresis**

Enuresis is repeated involuntary urination in children who have reached the age when voluntary control is possible and where there is no indication or urological or neurological pathology. It is considered to be a problem at around the age of five years (Butler, 1987).

Episodes occur more commonly at night (nocturnal enuresis), usually during deep sleep (see Chapter 20). Enuresis may occur during the day (diurnal enuresis) when the child is engaged in play and unaware of a full bladder. Some children are enuretic during a temper tantrum or dispute with a sibling or playmate.

---

 **Learning Disabilities Nursing**
**Incontinence**

In addition to the various physiological causes of urinary incontinence among people with learning disabilities, there are some situations which are relatively simple to manage. One frequent cause of incontinence is the failure to recognize the need to micturate in time to get to the toilet. Nurses can overcome this by giving the patient/client regular, discreet reminders and opportunities to use the toilet. A second cause of incontinence, particularly in unfamiliar surroundings, is the inability to locate the toilet or to be able to ask where it is. A third 'simple' cause of incontinence is the inability of the person with a learning disability to appropriately adjust his or her clothing in order to use the toilet. These last two situations can cause considerable distress to individuals who are otherwise continent, yet can be wholly avoided if the nurse is alert to their abilities and needs; for example, by helping them to choose clothing which they can adjust themselves, or by helping them locate the toilets in an unfamiliar building.

## TABLE 22-2  Common Symptoms of Urinary Problems

| Symptoms | Description | Causes or Associated Factors |
| --- | --- | --- |
| Urgency | Feeling of needing to void immediately | Full bladder, inflammation or irritation of bladder mucosa from infection, incompetent urethral sphincter, psychological stress |
| Dysuria | Painful or difficult urination | Bladder inflammation, trauma or inflammation, increased pressure on bladder (e.g. pregnancy, psychological stress) |
| Frequency | Voiding at frequent intervals | Increased fluid intake, bladder inflammation, increased pressure on bladder (e.g. pregnancy, psychological stress) |
| Hesitancy | Difficulty initiating urination | Prostate enlargement, anxiety, urethral oedema |
| Polyuria | Voiding of large amount of urine | Excess fluid intake, diabetes mellitus or insipidus, use of diuretics, postobstructive diuresis |
| Oliguria | Diminished urinary output in relation to fluid intake (usually less than 400 ml in 24 hr) | Dehydration, renal failure, UTI, increased ADH secretion (SIADH), congestive heart failure |
| Nocturia | Urination, particularly excessive, at night | Excess intake of fluids (especially coffee or alcohol before bedtime), renal disease, ageing process |
| Dribbling | Leakage of urine despite voluntary control of micturition | Urine retention from incomplete bladder emptying, stress incontinence |
| Haematuria | Presence of blood in urine | Neoplasms of kidney, certain glomerular diseases, infections of kidneys or bladder, traumatic injury to urinary structure, calculi, blood dyscrasia |
| Retention | Accumulation of urine in bladder, with inability of bladder to empty | Urethral obstruction, bladder inflammation, decreased sensory activity, neurogenic bladder, prostate enlargement after anaesthesia, side effects of certain medications (e.g. anticholinergics, antispasmodics, antidepressants) |
| Residual urine | Volume of urine remaining in bladder after voiding (volumes of 100 ml or more) | Inflammation or irritation of bladder mucosa from infection, neurogenic bladder, prostatic enlargement, trauma or inflammation of urethra |

important to ask if the patient/client experiences any of the symptoms which are listed in Table 22-2. The nurse should also ask if the patient/client is aware of any conditions or factors which may precipitate or aggravate symptoms.

Urinary retention due to either obstructed outflow or the loss of bladder tone may only be excluded by measuring residual volume after a patient has emptied their bladder. This is achieved by the insertion of a plastic 'in and out' catheter in women, and a bladder ultrasound investigation in men. Patients with a residual volume of more than 100 ml have significant urinary retention.

### Factors Affecting Urination

Certain medications (for example, diuretics and sedatives) can affect patterns of voiding, or may cause or aggravate incontinence. The name, amount, and frequency of medications should be noted.

Enquiries need to be made into a patient's/client's social and environmental circumstances, as well as the presence of any functional disabilities and sensory impairments. For example, an older person living alone, with impaired mobility and poor eyesight, may have trouble reaching the toilet. Many older people may be coping with an underlying bladder disorder until one of a number of factors disturb their coping mechanism. This may be a urinary tract infection (causing frequency, urgency, and possible confusion), constipation (see Table 22-1), a reduction in mobility, a changed environment, or carers who are less sensitive to their needs.

Urinary incontinence is associated with a range of chronic neurological disorders which can include stroke, dementia, Parkinson's disease, multiple sclerosis, spina bifida, and diabetic autonomic neuropathy. Incontinence associated with these conditions may be difficult to correct. However, characterizing the type of underlying bladder disorder, irrespective of its cause, helps to plan effective treatment.

Personal habits also affect urination. If a patient is hospitalized the nurse needs to assess the extent to which personal habits are altered. Privacy is often difficult to accomplish in a health care setting, particularly if a patient must use a bedpan.

## Assessment of Urine

Assessment of urine involves measuring the patient's/client's fluid intake and urine output and observing characteristics of the patient's/client's urine.

### INTAKE AND OUTPUT

If a precise measurement of fluid intake is needed from the patient/client who is at home, the nurse may ask to see a commonly used glass or cup on which the intake estimate is based.

In a health care setting intake and output can be more accurately measured when necessary (see Chapter 18). The nurse includes all sources, including oral intake, intravenous fluid infusions, tube feedings, and fluid instilled into nasogastric tubes.

A change in urine volume is a significant indicator of reduced blood flow to the kidney or of kidney disease. For measuring urine output in a patient who is acutely ill, special urimeters can be attached between an indwelling catheter and the drainage bag. These are a convenient means of measuring urine volume on a regular basis (for example, hourly).

The nurse reports any extreme increase or decrease in volume. A repeated hourly output of less than 30 ml is cause for concern.

Similarly, high volumes of urine (**polyuria**), over 2000 ml daily, should be reported.

### URINALYSIS

A random routine urine specimen can be collected with a patient/client voiding naturally or through a Foley catheter. The specimen should be clean but need not be sterile. Dipped into the urine, most urine reagent strips used for urinalysis indicate measurements of specific gravity, pH, and levels of glucose, ketones, bilirubin, blood and protein in the urine (see Table 22-3).

It is easier to collect a specimen if the patient/client drinks a glass of fluid 30 minutes before the procedure. A patient/client should void before defaecating so that faeces do not contaminate the specimen. Women are also asked not to place toilet tissue in the bedpan.

**Midstream Specimen (MSU)** A midstream specimen is to test urine for culture and sensitivity (Procedure 22-1). After appropriate cleansing of the external genitalia, a patient/client begins the urinary stream allowing the initial portion to escape; then during the middle portion of voiding, the patient/client

### TABLE 22-3 Routine Urinalysis Values

| Measurement and Normal Value | Interpretation |
| --- | --- |
| pH (4.6-8.0) | pH helps indicate acid-base balance. Selected antibiotics (e.g. neomycin, streptomycin) are more effective against UTIs if pH is alkaline. Alkaline urine can result from bacteriuria. Urine which stands for several hours becomes alkaline due to subsequent bacterial colonization |
| Protein level (up to 10 mg/100 ml) | Normally protein is not present in urine. It is seen in renal disease because damage to glomerular membrane or tubules allows protein to enter urine. However, temporary presence of protein can occur after strenuous exercise, exposure to cold, psychological stress, or high dietary protein intake. Protein may also be present in urinary tract infection or haematuria. |
| Glucose level (not normally present) | Diabetic patients/clients have glucose in urine as result of inability of tubules to reabsorb high glucose concentration (over 8.0 mmol/l). Ingestion of high concentrations of glucose may cause some to appear in urine of healthy people. The renal threshold for glucose decreases in older people. |
| Ketone level (not normally present) | Patients/clients whose diabetes is poorly controlled experience breakdown of fatty acids. End products of fatty acid metabolism are ketones. Patients/clients with dehydration, starvation, or excessive aspirin ingestion also have ketonuria. |
| Blood level (up to two RBCs) | Damage of glomerulus or tubules may cause erythrocytes to enter urine. Trauma or disease of lower urinary tract also causes haematuria. In women, blood may be present in the urine if the specimen is collected during menstruation. |
| Urobilinogen (2-5 mg/24 hours) | The bile pigment, bilirubin, is altered in the intestine to urobilinogen. Increased urobilinogen in urine may indicate haemolytic jaundice. Decreased urobilinogen may indicated simple obstructive jaundice. |
| Specific gravity (1.010-1.030) | Specific gravity measures concentration of particles in urine. High specific gravity reflects concentrated urine, and low specific gravity reflects diluted urine. Dehydration, reduced renal blood flow, and increases in ADH secretion elevate specific gravity. Overhydration and inadequate ADH secretion reduce specific gravity. |

## PROCEDURE 22-1 Collecting Midstream Urine Specimen (MSU)

| SEQUENCE OF ACTIONS | RATIONALE |
|---|---|
| 1. Assess patient's/client's mobility and balance in being able to use toilet facilities independently. | Determines level of assistance required by patient/client. |
| 2. Assess patient's/client's understanding of purpose of test and method of collection. | Information allows you to clarify misunderstandings and promotes patient/client cooperation. |
| 3. Explain procedure to patient/client: <br> a. Reason MSU is needed | Helps patient/client provide specimen independently. |
| b. Way patient/client and family member can assist | |
| c. Way to obtain specimen free of faeces | Faeces change characteristics of urine and may cause abnormal values. |
| 4. If necessary, provide fluids to drink 0.5 hour before collecting the specimen, unless contra-indicated (i.e., fluid restriction). | Improves the likelihood of patient/client being able to void. |
| 5. Provide privacy for patient/client by closing bed curtain or door. | Maintenance of dignity. Allows patient/client to relax and, therefore, produce specimen more quickly. |
| 6. Wash hands and put on gloves. | Reduces risk of cross-infection. |
| 7. Assist or allow patient/client to independently cleanse perineum and collect specimen: | Cleansing the perineum helps prevent other organisms from contaminating the specimen. |
| a. Male: | |
| (i) Retract foreskin and clean the skin around the urethral meatus with soap and water, or sterile saline. Do not use a disinfectant solution. | Disinfectants may irritate or be painful to the urethral mucous membrane. They may also contaminate the specimen. |
| (ii) Ask the patient/client to direct the first and last part of the urine stream into the toilet or urinal. The middle portion is collected in a sterile container. | Helps prevent contamination of the specimen with microorganisms which normally accumulate at the urethral meatus and prevents their contamination of the specimen. |
| b. Female: | |
| (i) Cleanse urethral meatus with swabs soaked in soap and water or sterile saline. Do not use a disinfectant solution. | Disinfectants may irritate or be painful to the urethral mucous membrane. They may also contaminate the specimen. |
| (ii) Use separate gauze swab for each cleansing motion. | Prevents cross-infection. |
| (iii) Cleanse in one stroke, from front (above the urethral orifice) to back (towards the anus). | Prevents contamination of urethral meatus with faecal matter. |
| (iv) Ask the patient/client to micturate into a bed pan or toilet. Place a sterile receiver under the stream and remove before stream ceases. | Helps prevent contamination of the specimen with microorganisms which normally accumulate at the urethral meatus. |
| (v) Transfer the specimen into a sterile container. | |
| 8. Label the specimen container and attach laboratory requisition. | Prevents inaccurate identification that could lead to errors in diagnosis or therapy. |
| 9. Transport specimen to laboratory within 15 minutes or immediately refrigerate. | Bacteria grow quickly in urine. The specimen should be analyzed immediately to obtain correct results. |
| 10. Document the date and time the specimen was obtained in the nursing notes. | |

collects the specimen into a sterile container. The initial stream of urine cleans or flushes the urethral orifice and meatus of resident bacteria. It is easiest for a patient/client midstream specimens while using toilet facilities.

**Urine Culture** A urine culture requires a sterile or midstream sample of urine. It takes approximately 48 hours before the laboratory can report findings of bacterial growth. If bacteria are present, an additional test for sensitivity determines which

antibiotics are effective. If antibiotics are ordered pending the results (sensitivities) of a urine culture, the culture should be obtained before administering the medication.

**Sterile Specimen (CSU)** Another method for collecting a urine specimen for culture is by obtaining it from an indwelling catheter This method provides a **sterile specimen**. A urine specimen is not collected for culture from urine drainage bags unless it is the first urine drained into a new sterile bag. Bacteria grow rapidly in the drainage bags and would give a false measurement of bacteria.

For an indwelling catheter, a sterile syringe is used to withdraw urine. The nurse washes hands and applies nonsterile gloves to prevent transmission of microorganisms. Some catheter ports are of self-sealing rubber which requires the use of a needle. For some only a syringe is necessary. If a needle is used, a small-gauge is best to prevent creation of a permanent hole in the catheter port. Most urinary catheters have special ports to withdraw specimens. The tubing is clamped just below the site chosen for withdrawal, allowing fresh, uncontaminated urine to collect in the tube. While aspirating urine the nurse must be careful not to raise the tubing, which would cause urine to flow back into the bladder.

After obtaining the specimen transfer the urine into a sterile container carefully avoiding contamination (see Chapter 28).

## Timed Urine Specimens

Some tests of renal function and urine composition, such as measuring levels of adrenocortical steroids or hormones, creatinine clearance, or protein quantification tests, require collection of urine over 2-, 12-, or 24-hour intervals.

## Specific Gravity

The **specific gravity** is the weight or degree of concentration of a substance compared with an equal volume of water. Water will read as 1.000. To measure specific gravity the nurse uses a urinometer and cylinder (Fig. 22-5). The urinometer has a specific gravity scale at the top and a weighted mercury bulb at the bottom. The nurse pours a urine specimen into a clean, dry cylinder. Next the nurse suspends and lightly twirls the weighted urinometer into the cylinder of urine. The concentration of dissolved substances in the urine determines the depth at which the urinometer will float.

With the urinometer at eye level the nurse reads the measurement at the base of the meniscus at the level of the urine. The specific gravity of a morning urine specimen voided by a fasting patient/client reflects the kidney's maximum concentrating ability. A specific gravity below 1.010 reflects an inability of the kidneys to concentrate urine or an insufficient secretion of ADH. When the kidneys become diseased, they lose their ability to concentrate urine. Therefore the specific gravity becomes "fixed" at a low value (1.010). An elevated specific gravity can indicate dehydration.

## DIAGNOSTIC EXAMINATIONS

The urinary system is one of the few organ systems amenable to accurate diagnostic study by radiographic techniques. The two approaches for visualization of urinary structures, direct and indirect techniques, can be quite simple or very complex, requiring extensive nursing intervention. These procedures are further subdivided into invasive or noninvasive categories.

There will be established local/hospital procedures, in relation to nursing care, which deal specifically with all the following investigations. Prior to all investigations the preparation of a patient must include a thorough explanation of what is involved. There must also be ample opportunity thereafter for the patient to ask questions and express any anxiety they may have.

## Abdominal X-Ray

This is commonly used to assess the gross structures of the urinary tract for abnormalities. It can be used to determine size, symmetry, shape, and location of the kidneys, ureters, and bladder structures. It is also useful in visualizing calculi (if they are calcified) or tumours in these organs. In addition, the ribs or surrounding support structures can be assessed for fractures or abnormalities. This is important if the patient/client has suffered some type of traumatic injury. The lack of positive findings on the x-ray does not rule out the possibility

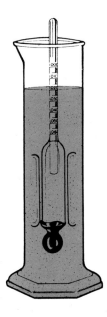

**Fig. 22-5** Measurement of urine specific gravity using a urinometer.

**Children's Nursing**
**Urine collection in children**

Specimen collection from infants and children is often difficult. Adolescents and school-aged children are usually able to cooperate, although they may be embarrassed. Preschool children and toddlers have difficulty voiding on request. Offering a young child fluids 30 minutes before requesting a specimen may help. The nurse must use terms for urination that the child can understand. A young child may be reluctant to void in unfamiliar receptacles. A potty chair or bedpan placed under the toilet is usually effective. The nurse must use special collection devices for infants or toddlers who are not toilet trained. Clear, plastic, single-use bags with self-adhering material can be attached over the child's urethral meatus.

  The nurse prepares an infant by first washing the genitalia, perineum, and surrounding skin with soap and water or an antiseptic. Thorough drying is necessary because the bag's adhesive does not stick to a moist, powdered, or oily surface. For a clean-voided specimen the nurse uses a sterile collection bag. Specimens should not be obtained by squeezing urine from the nappy material.

of abnormalities in the urinary tract. Additional diagnostic studies may be warranted.

## Intravenous Pyelogram (IVP)

An **intravenous pyleogram** (also called an *intravenous urogram*, IVU) visualizes the renal tissue and pelvis and outlines the ureters, bladder, and urethra. (The last two structures are better visualized by a cystourethrogram.) Although this procedure is non-invasive, it requires that the patient/client receive an intravenous injection of a radiopaque dye. Normally, the injected medium takes only a few minutes to circulate and be excreted. Because the kidneys and ureters lie behind the intestines, it is necessary that the patient/client receive a bowel preparation to empty the intestines before the procedure. Procedures using barium should not be performed 2 to 3 days before an IVP because residual barium in the intestines will obscure the view.

During the IVP, x-ray studies are taken at specific intervals over 30 to 60 minutes as the dye concentrates in the urinary tract. The patient/client may also be asked to void during the procedure to measure bladder emptying. Diseases or disorders of the urinary tract that should be investigated by this means include renal artery occlusion, tumours, cysts or calculi, vesicoureteral reflux, and traumatic injuries.

Nursing implications before the test include recognizing patients/clients at risk for alterations in renal function as a result of the intravenous injection of the contrast material. Any individual with renal insufficiency is at risk. Older people in particular are prone to the nephrotoxic effects of these substances because they can more easily become dehydrated during bowel preparation. Appropriate nursing assessment of fluid balance and its maintenance before and after this procedure is of utmost importance. Assess patients/clients for history of iodine allergy, which predicts allergies to the IVP dye, and warn them of possible transitory nausea as the dye is injected. Following the procedure, observe for signs of allergic reaction to dye (for example, respiratory distress, fall in blood pressure, and hives).

## Renal Scan

Radionuclide tests such as renal scans allow indirect visualization of urinary tract structures after an intravenous injection of radioactive isotopes. There are several different radiopharmaceutical agents used during this procedure. Their selection depends on the physiological process to be investigated. The emissions from the radionuclides can be photographed by special cameras. The isotope can be detected without the need of bowel preparation. A very low dosage of radioisotope is used. Its half-life is short. Therefore no precautions against radioactive exposure are needed.

After a radionuclide is injected, it circulates through the kidney and is excreted. The renal scan measures radioactive concentrations while the patient/client assumes a supine, prone, or sitting position. Except for the venepuncture, it is painless. The scanning procedure is completed in approximately 1 hour. Information pertaining to renal blood flow, anatomical structures, and their excretory function can be obtained from this procedure. The doctor can diagnose abnormalities such as renal artery occlusion, urinary obstruction, and many other diseases of the kidney. This procedure is indicated for patients/clients unable to receive IVP dyes.

## Computerized Tomography

**Computerized tomography** (CT) is a computerized x-ray procedure used to obtain detailed images of structures within a selected plane of the body. The tomographic scanner is a large machine that contains specialized computers and x-ray detector systems that function concomitantly to photograph internal structures in thin, transverse cross sections. The computer is able to 'reconstruct' the cross-sectional image as a recognizable photograph on the television monitor. With this procedure, it is possible to visualize abnormal pathological conditions such as tumours, obstructions, retroperitoneal masses, and lymph node enlargement. The CT scan can detect and characterize masses of less than 2 cm in size. Although this procedure is non-invasive, in some examinations, oral or intravenous contrast material is used to enhance the areas under study.

## Renal Ultrasound

**Ultrasonography** is another procedure gaining widespread acceptance as a valuable noninvasive diagnostic tool in the assessment of urinary disorders. It makes use of high-frequency, inaudible sound waves that reflect off tissue. A conductive gel is applied to the skin and functions as a transmitter for sound waves. A transducer passed over the conductive gel emits a beam as it is also passed over body tissues of varying density. Some of the sound waves are reflected to the transducer as echoes. The echoes are converted into electrical impulses that are displayed on an oscilloscope, presenting an image or photograph of the tissues being studied. The velocity of the sound waves varies with tissue density. The patient/client is usually prone during the procedure but can be positioned in a sitting position. No biological hazards have been identified with energy or sound wave emissions from this procedure. Ultrasound is frequently used to identify gross renal structures and structural abnormalities of the kidneys or lower urinary tract and to assist with percutaneous biopsy. Abnormalities such as tumours or cysts in the kidney are easily identified with this procedure. If a Doppler ultrasound is used with the transducer, examination of blood flow through the kidney can also be performed. This procedure is painless.

Nursing implications before the procedure include explaining the test and possibly encouraging the patient/client to ingest oral fluids to cause bladder distension. No specific patient care is indicated after the test.

## INVASIVE PROCEDURES

Invasive procedures include cystoscopy, biopsy, and arteriogram.

## Cystoscopy

To view the interior of the bladder and urethra a **cystoscopy** is performed. The cystoscope looks much like a urinary catheter, although it is not as flexible. It is inserted through the patient's/client's urethra. The instrument has an outer plastic or rubber sheath, an obturator that keeps the scope rigid during insertion, a telescope for viewing the bladder and urethra, and a channel for inserting catheters or special surgical instruments.

The procedure is painful during instrument insertion. Unless the patient/client lies still, there is risk of bladder perforation. Local, spinal, or general anaesthesia may be administered. Because the test requires insertion of a foreign object into a sterile cavity, the patient/client receives large amounts of fluids (intravenously or orally) before and during the procedure to maintain a continuous urine flow and to flush out any bacteria. Antibiotics may also be administered intravenously. During the test, urine and tissue specimens may be collected.

A patient who knows what to expect is likely to be more relaxed, which can lessen the spasms of the urethral sphincters and the associated discomfort.

When a lithotomy position is to be assumed, assure the patient that drapes will be applied to minimize exposure.

After the investigation has been performed it is important to observe characteristics of the urine (noting bloody or cloudy urine), encourage increased fluid intake, and monitor intake and output.

In addition to complete visual inspection of the bladder and urethra through the cystoscope, **retrograde pyelography** may also be performed. During this procedure, a small catheter is passed through the cystoscope into the bladder, which allows catheterization of the ureters and renal pelvis. Urine specimens are then collected separately from each ureter. Radio-opaque dye can be instilled into the renal pelvis while serial x-rays are taken to examine the filling of the renal collecting system. X-ray examinations to visualize the bladder and urethra are also considered invasive studies. These examinations include retrograde cystograms, voiding cystourethrograms (VCUGs), and cystourethrograms. All of these studies involve the instillation of a radiopaque fluid into the bladder via a catheter (urethral or suprapubic). Serial x-ray films taken during these procedures provide information regarding abnormalities in bladder mucosa, demonstrate **vesicoureteral reflux** (backflow of urine from bladder to ureter), provide information regarding bladder function, and provide an assessment of the size and shape of the ureters. Nursing implications for this procedure are the same as those for cystoscopy.

### Renal Biopsy

A renal biopsy is performed to determine the nature, extent, and prognosis of renal disease. This procedure involves obtaining a piece of renal cortical tissue for examination with sophisticated microscopic techniques. The procedure can be performed by percutaneous (closed) or surgical (open) methods. The use of ultrasound examinations to localize the kidney has revolutionized the percutaneous approach. Tissue diagnosis allows differentiation between disease processes causing alterations in renal function. Therefore more specific treatment interventions can be applied.

Nursing implications after the test include the following:

- Observe colour, amount, and character of urine, noting bloody urine.
- Monitor vital signs, noting changes consistent with haemorrhagic shock (see Chapter 4).
- Advise patient/client to remain in bed for prescribed time (usually 24 hours).

- Assess biopsy site for signs of bleeding and note complaints of pain.
- Maintain pressure dressings on biopsy site.

### Arteriogram (Angiogram)

A **renal arteriogram** is an invasive radiographic procedure that evaluates the renal arterial system. The arteriogram is most often used to examine the main renal artery or its segmental branches to detect any narrowing or occlusion. In addition, this procedure is useful in the evaluation of mass lesions (for example, neoplasms or cysts) to determine parity, collateral, or traumatic injury to blood vessels. The arteriogram is performed by placing a catheter into one of the femoral arteries and advancing it up the aorta to the level of the renal arteries. Radio-opaque contrast material is injected through the catheter while serial x-ray images are taken in rapid succession.

**Venograms** are most often performed to examine the excretory system and allow for sampling of renal vein blood to test for various renal hormonal levels (for example, renin and erythropoietin). During the venogram, a catheter is inserted into the femoral vein and advanced up the inferior vena cava to the level of the renal veins. Since there may be sensitivity to the radio-opaque iodide preparation, the precautions recommended for the IVP procedure should be followed. Following the investigation, vital signs should be monitored hourly until stable.

Nursing implications after the test include the following:

- Check pulse, assess the circulation in the cannulated extremity, and ensure that the extremity is kept in straight alignment.
- Observe for bleeding, increased tenderness, and haematoma formation at the catheter insertion site for 24 hours.
- Maintain a pressure dressing over the site for 24 hours.
- Observe patient/client for possible delayed reactions to the contrast material.
- Monitor the patient's/client's intake and output and report abnormalities in urine volume.

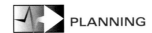 **PLANNING**

In collaboration with other members of the multi-disciplinary team, talk with the patient/client to plan interventions for urinary elimination problems. It is important to consider the patient's/client's home environment and normal elimination routines when planning care.

Alterations in urinary elimination can be embarrassing, uncomfortable, and often frustrating. Work with the patient/client to establish ways of maintaining his or her involvement in nursing care and to maintain normal elimination patterns when possible. Goals to promote normal urinary elimination may include the following:

- understanding normal urinary elimination
- promoting normal micturition
- enabling complete bladder emptying
- preventing infection
- maintaining skin integrity
- gaining a sense of comfort and dignity.

Planning should also include preparations for discharge. The patient's/client's educational needs, as well as any assistive devices he or she will require. It is important to teach the patient/client and, if necessary, relatives or carers, throughout the hospital stay. For example, a person being discharged with an indwelling catheter will need to perform catheter care, understand ways to empty the drainage bag and know signs and symptoms of urinary infection. The need for community services should be explored, and appropriate referrals should be made.

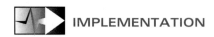 IMPLEMENTATION

## Promoting Normal Micturition

### STIMULATING MICTURITION REFLEX

The patient's/client's ability to void depends on feeling the urge to urinate, being able to control the urethral sphincter, and being able to relax during voiding. The nurse can foster relaxation and stimulate the reflex to void by helping the patient/client assume the normal position for voiding. A woman is better able to void in a squatting position. This position promotes contraction of the pelvic and abdominal muscles that assist in sphincter control and bladder contraction. If the patient/client is unable to use toilet facilities, the nurse positions the person in a squatting position on a bedpan (see Chapter 23) or bedside commode. A man voids more easily in the standing position. At times, it may be necessary for one or more nurses to assist a man in standing. If the man cannot reach toilet facilities, he may stand at the bedside and void into a urinal—a metal or plastic receptacle for urine.

Other measures that promote relaxation and the ability to void include sensory stimuli. Offering the patient/client a drink may also promote voiding. The sound of running water helps many patients/clients void through the power of suggestion. It is also easier for a person to relax and void when sitting on a bedpan that has been warmed.

### MAINTAINING ELIMINATION HABIT

Many people follow routines to promote normal voiding. In a hospital or long-term care facility the nurse's routines may conflict with those of patients/clients. Integrating patients'/clients' habits into the care plan fosters normal voiding.

Patients/clients usually require time to void. Asking patients/clients to void quickly so that they can be transported to x-ray testing or requesting a urine specimen as soon as possible does not contribute to normal voiding habits. Patients/clients should be given at least 30 minutes to provide a specimen. The nurse learns the times when patients/clients normally void, such as on awakening or before meals, and offers the opportunity to use toilet facilities then. Also important is the need to respond to patients'/clients' urges to urinate. Delay in assisting patients/clients to the toilet may interfere with normal micturition.

Privacy is essential for normal voiding. If the person cannot reach the toilet, the nurse makes sure that the bedside area is enclosed by a curtain. In the home the debilitated patient/client may prefer using a bedside commode enclosed behind a partition or room divider. Some patients are embarrassed by the sound of voiding. Running water or flushing the toilet masks the sound. Often young children are unable to void in the presence of people other than their parents.

If the patient/client typically uses special measures to void, the nurse should encourage their continued use at home and, when possible, in the institution. The patient may be able to relax and void more easily while reading or listening to music. Coffee or beer may also promote urination.

### MAINTAINING ADEQUATE FLUID INTAKE

A simple method of promoting normal micturition is maintaining good fluid intake. A patient/client with normal renal function who does not have heart disease or conditions requiring fluid restriction should drink 2000 to 2500 ml of fluid daily. However, an average daily intake of 1200 to 1500 ml of fluids is usually adequate.

When fluid intake is increased, the excreted urine flushes out solutes or particles that may collect in the urinary system. Because a patient/client is usually unwilling to drink 2500 ml of water daily, the nurse should offer fluid that the patient/client prefers. Vegetables and fruit also contain a high fluid content. At home it may help to set a schedule for drinking fluids (for example, with meals or medications). To prevent nocturia, fluids should be avoided 2 hours before bedtime.

## Enabling Complete Bladder Emptying

### FUNCTIONAL INCONTINENCE

A patient/client with functional incontinence may benefit from habit training, which helps improve voluntary control over urination. A flexible toileting schedule based on the patient's/client's pattern is established.

The patient/client is helped to the toilet before incontinent episodes occur, and fluids and medications are timed to prevent interference with the toileting schedule. Patients/clients with moderate or severe mental or physical disabilities can benefit providing successful voiding is rewarded with positive reinforcement. In an institutional setting, effective implementation of an individual toilet training programme is dependent upon staff who are aware of the aims and objectives of the exercise (Copperwheat, 1985). The difference between regular toileting of all patients/clients at intervals suited to the ward/home routine or staff availability, and regular toileting to suit an individual's need must be recognized. The former method is less likely to be successful because the enforced regimen may not coincide with individual bladder needs, and for this reason there is inappropriate reinforcement of behaviour (Rivers, 1986).

If it is necessary to contain symptoms, there are numerous aids and appliances available. Over 3,000 different items are listed in the Directory of Continence Aids and Appliances, published by the Association of Continence Advisors (ACA, 1990). Absorbent pads and pants remain the most common form of management (Norton, 1992). When choosing an aid or appliance to suit individual requirements expert knowledge and advice should be sought.

## UNSTABLE BLADDER

The primary mode of treatment is bladder retraining. This involves keeping a chart of voiding and incontinence from four to seven days, and identifying the times of day when incontinence is most likely to occur. The first objective is to achieve dryness, through more frequent trips to the toilet, or by a change in daily routine. Then the patient/client is asked to gradually extend the time between voiding to encourage the bladder to hold more. There will be more chance of success if the patient/client is motivated and cooperative. They will also need much ongoing support if they are to regain confidence and recover a feeling of self-control, which is often lacking as a result of the psychological and social consequences of this condition.

Drugs which diminish bladder contractions, such as anticholinergics, may also be used to help treat an unstable bladder. Imipramine hydrochloride and oxybutynin hydrochloride are commonly used. Both these drugs have unwanted side-effects (such as nausea and constipation) and it is necessary to be aware of these to ensure that they are closely monitored, especially with older patients.

## STRESS INCONTINENCE

If kept up conscientiously over a period of two to six months, pelvic floor (Kegel) exercises can greatly improve the symptoms of this condition. Once the patient is taught to exercise the correct groups of muscles, the exercises can be repeated conveniently and unobtrusively. The hospital or community physiotherapist can play a major role in treating/preventing stress incontinence (Castleden *et al*, 1984).

In cases of reduced hormone levels, particularly in post-menopausal women, either systemic or topical hormone replacement therapy may relieve symptoms of stress incontinence. In severe cases, surgery may be considered.

## OUTFLOW OBSTRUCTION

The commonest cause of obstruction in men is an enlarged prostate gland, which squeezes the urethra so that less urine can pass through. The prostate can now be routinely resected transurethrally under local anaesthetic. To relieve obstruction stents can also be inserted into the urethra. In both men and women faecal impaction is the cause of the obstruction; this obviously has to be dealt with immediately, perhaps with the aid of aperients, suppositories, and/or enemas. The patient/client will need advice relating to diet, fluid intake, and exercise to prevent further constipation.

If the cause of the outflow obstruction is neurological, specific drug therapy may be the solution. In some cases intermittent catheterization, once or twice a day to remove the residual urine, will restore continence.

## LOSS OF BLADDER TONE

A weak, insufficient detrusor which fails to empty the bladder can cause loss of bladder tone. If the patient is on drugs with anticholinergic side-effects (which dampen down bladder contractions), symptoms may be relieved if these are stopped. The choice of treatment is intermittent catheterization.

## CATHETERIZATION

**Catheterization** of the bladder involves introducing a rubber or plastic tube through the urethra and into the bladder. The catheter provides a continuous flow of urine in patients unable to control micturition or those with obstructions. It also provides a means of assessing hourly urine outputs in haemodynamically unstable patients/clients. Because bladder catheterization carries the risk of UTIs and trauma to the urethra, it is preferable to rely on other measures.

Types of Catheterization Intermittent and **indwelling retention** catheterization are the two forms of catheter insertion. With the intermittent technique a straight single-use catheter is introduced long enough to drain the bladder (5 to 10 minutes). When the bladder is empty, the nurse immediately withdraws the catheter. Intermittent catheterization can be repeated as necessary. An indwelling or Foley catheter remains in place for an extended period until a patient/client is able to void completely and voluntarily. It may be necessary to change indwelling catheters periodically, as per manufacturer's recommendations.

The straight single-use catheter has a single lumen with a small opening about 1.3 cm from the tip. Urine drains from the tip, through the lumen, and to a receptacle. An indwelling Foley catheter has a small inflatable balloon that encircles the catheter just below the tip. When inflated, the balloon rests against the bladder outlet to anchor the catheter in place. The indwelling retention catheter also has two or three lumens within the body of the catheter (Fig. 22-6). One lumen drains urine through the catheter to a collecting tube. A second lumen carries sterile water to and from the balloon when it is inflated or deflated. A third (optional) lumen may be used to instil fluids or medications into the bladder. It is easy to determine the number of lumens by the number of drainage and injection ports at the catheter's end.

Suggestions on how to make appropriate decisions regarding catheter selection are given in the box overleaf.

Indications for Catheterization Catheterization may be indicated for many reasons. When catheterization time will be short and minimizing infection is a priority, the intermittent method is best. Intermittent catheterization can be used for people with spinal cord injuries who have no bladder control; with neuromuscular degeneration; and with hypotonic bladders. People routinely using this method experience less incidence of the complications associated with indwelling catheters, such as infections, local abscesses, calculi, and urethral strictures (Smith and Clamp, 1991).

**Long-term catheterization has been shown to result in renal damage, hypertension (Carty *et al*, 1981; Warren *et al*, 1981) and increased mortality due to catheter-related UTIs (Platt *et al*, 1983).** Long-term indwelling catheterization, therefore, considered a last resort in treating urinary incontinence, after other methods have proved unsuccessful or are considered inappropriate. Whenever possible, the decision to catheterize should be a joint one between the patient/client, relative or carer, and health professionals. The psychological and social implications will have to be considered. The patient/client may need a great deal of ongoing education and support.

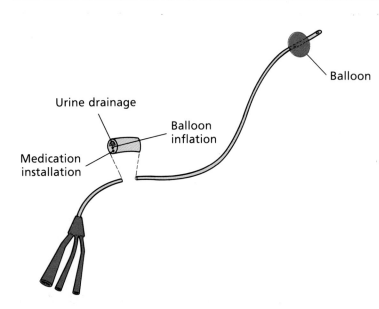

**Fig. 22-6** Triple-lumen Foley catheter with balloon inflated.

Balloon

Urine drainage

Balloon inflation

Medication installation

## Guidelines for Appropriate Catheter Selection

Catheter size is measured in the Charrier or French gauge (fg). The smallest size will provide good drainage and minimize trauma. In an adult this will normally be a 12, 14 or 16 fg. Unless haematuria is anticipated, sizes larger than a 16 fg should not be used. Paraurethral glands that bathe the urethra in its natural lubrication become blocked if a catheter lumen is too large. Large size catheters have been found to be associated with leakage, discomfort, and pain (Kennedy *et al*, 1983; Crow *et al*, 1986; Roe and Brocklehurst, 1987).

Women benefit from the use of shorter catheters. These are less prone to moving in and out of the urethra, and thus introducing bacteria into the urinary tract. When required, the shorter catheter also facilitates the attachment of a leg drainage bag above the dress line.

The length of the catheterization period should dictate the type of material selected:

| Plastic catheters | Intermittent catheterization |
| --- | --- |
| Teflon coated latex | Short term (up to 3 weeks) |
| Silicone elastomer coated latex | Medium (up to 6 weeks) |
| All silicone | Long term (up to 12 weeks) |
| Hydrogel coated Biocath | Long term (up to 12 weeks) |

Balloon sizes range from 3 ml (paediatric) to 30 ml. A 5-10 ml balloon is commonly used for standard adult catheterizations. The 30 ml should only be used if specifically requested, for example, for use after prostactectomies, as an aid in achieving postoperative haemostatis of the prostatic bed.

Only sterile water should be used to inflate the balloon. Normal saline crystallizes, thus causing incomplete deflation of the balloon on catheter removal.

**Catheter Insertion** Procedures for indwelling catheterization are well documented; every clinical area should have a copy of these procedures for reference. These may conform to a specific local/district criteria, but all will insist on the use of a strict aseptic technique (see Procedure 22-2 as an example). The steps for inserting a single-use catheter are similar, although a clean versus aseptic technique may be used in the home. While inserting an indwelling catheter, the opportunity can be used to obtain needed specimens.

**Self-Catheterization** A patient/client needs sufficient manual dexterity to put the catheter into the urethra, ability to understand the technique, a bladder capacity of over 100 ml, and a urethra free of stricture (Smith and Clamp, 1991). If necessary, an informed carer may be taught the technique, if willing. Teach the patient/client the structures of the external genitalia and the urinary tract, clean versus sterile technique, and the frequency of self-catheterization. Frequency may vary from four-hourly to daily, according to individual requirements (Rivers, 1986). Warn the patient/client about the early signs of bladder infections, such as bladder pain, frequency, and pyrexia.

**Closed Drainage Systems** After inserting an indwelling catheter, a **closed urinary drainage system** is maintained, to minimize the risk of infection (Burke *et al*, 1981). Urinary drainage bags are plastic and can hold up to 2000 ml of urine. The bag should hang on the bed frame without touching the floor when the bed is in its lowest position. A drainage bag should not be placed over or on the bed's side rails. The bag also fits on the frames of most wheelchairs. When the patient/client ambulates, the nurse or patient/client should carry the bag below the patient's/client's waist, or a leg drainage bag should be used. The nurse or other health care personnel should *never* raise a drainage bag and tubing above the level of the patient's/client's bladder. Urine in the bag and tubing can become a medium for bacteria, and infection is likely to develop if urine flows back into the bladder.

## PROCEDURE 22-2 Inserting a Urethral Catheter

| SEQUENCE OF ACTIONS | RATIONALE |
|---|---|
| 1. Ensure patient/client is comfortable. Maximize opportunities for communication. | |
| 2. Gather necessary equipment:<br>a. Catheterization pack containing receiver, cotton wool balls and/or swabs, disposable towels, forceps<br>b. Sterile gloves*<br>c. Sterile anaesthetic lubricating jelly<br>d. Two normal saline sachets<br>e. Sterile catheter of appropriate size<br>f. Incontinence pad<br>g. Disposable plastic apron<br>h. Appropriate size ampoule of sterile water<br>i. Sterile syringe and needle for drawing up the water<br>j. Urine drainage bag and holder<br>k. Sterile specimen container, if required | |
| 3. Explain procedure to patient/client. | Reduces anxiety and promotes cooperation. |
| 4. Arrange for extra nursing personnel to assist, if appropriate. | May be necessary to assist with positioning of patient/client and maintenance of correct position. To help in preparation of equipment trolley. |
| 5. Help patient/client to lie on his or her back, in the supine position. Cover patient/client with a blanket. | Supine position helps prevent tensing of abdominal and pelvic muscles. |
| 6. Ensure there is sufficient lighting by the bedside. | |
| 7. Place incontinence pad under the patient/client. | To keep bed clean and dry. |
| 8. Raise the bed to a comfortable working height. | Reduces strain on nurse's back |
| 9. Wash hands and put on disposable plastic apron. | Handwashing before catheterization helps prevent bacteria (Slade and Gillespie, 1985). |
| 10. Prepare the trolley, placing all the equipment on the bottom shelf. | |
| 11. Take the trolley to the patient's/client's bedside, taking care to disturb the bedside curtains as little as possible. | To minimize airborne contamination. |
| 12. Remove the blanket from the lower half of the patient/client. | |
| 13. Ask the FEMALE patient to relax her thighs so as to externally rotate them (legs may be supported by pillows) or position in side lying position with upper leg flexed at knee and hip , if unable to assume a supine position.<br>Ask the MALE patient/client to lie with legs extended. | Provides good view of perineal structures.<br><br><br><br><br>Assists access to penis |
| 14. Put on disposable gloves and wash perineal area with soap and water; dry. | Presence of microogranisms near urethral meatus is reduced. |
| 15. Remove and dispose of gloves. | Prevents cross-infection. |
| 16. Wash and dry hands. | |
| 17. Open the outer cover of the catheterization pack and slide the inner pack onto the top of the trolley. Open the inner pack. | |
| 18. Following principles of asepsis, open up the supplementary packs.* | The bladder is a sterile organ. |

* It is helpful, at this stage, to have assistance from another nurse to facilitate the maintenance of an aseptic technique. Once the first nurse has opened the inner pack, he or she can apply sterile gloves and arrange the contents onto the sterile field. The second nurse (having washed his or her hands) can open the supplementary packs without contaminating their contents. He or she can then pour the normal saline into the gallipot and hold the ampoule of sterile water while the first nurse withdraws its contents into a sterile syringe.

## Procedure 22-2 Inserting a Urethral Catheter (Cont'd)

**SEQUENCE OF ACTIONS**

19. Apply sterile gloves and organize the supplies on the sterile field. Apply the nozzle to the tube of anaesthetic lubricating jelly.

20. Apply some of the jelly to both sides of the catheter tip.

21. Drape the sterile towel across the patient's/client's thighs, allowing access for the female perineum; or make a slit in the towel through which the penis can protrude.

22. Cleanse the urethral meatus:

a. FEMALE
(i) Using the dominant hand, clean the vulva. Use a downward direction with a fresh swab soaked in saline each time. Take care not to contaminate the gloves. Forceps may be used to hold the swabs.

(ii) Using the non-dominant hand, separate the labia major and clean the labia minor and urethral meatus. Maintain separation of the labia.

b. MALE:
(i) Wrap a sterile swab around the penis. Retract the foreskin (if present) and clean the glans penis with normal saline. Forceps may be used to manipulate the swabs.

(ii) Squeeze the tube of anaesthetic lubricating jelly slightly, to prime the nozzle and nozzle tip.
(iii) Insert the nozzle of the anaesthetic lubricating jelly into the urethral meatus. Squeeze the jelly into the urethra. Remove the nozzle and discard the tube.

23. Place a kidney dish containing the catheter on the bed between the patient's thighs. Grasp the catheter with the dominant hand, approximately 5cm from the catheter tip.

24. Insert catheter:
a. FEMALE (see illustration):
(i) Slowly insert catheter (taking care not to contaminate the tip) through the meatus. (If no urine appears, catheter may be in vagina. If so, leave it in place; obtain and insert another catheter and remove first catheter.)
(ii) Advance catheter approximately 5-6 cm (in an adult) or until urine flows out of the catheter end. Either remove the catheter gently when urinary flow ceases or, if a retention catheter, advance another 5 cm after the urine appears. Do not force the catheter against resistance.

(iii) Release labia and hold catheter securely with non-dominant hand.

b. MALE (see illustration):
(i) Lift penis perpendicular to the patient's body and apply light traction upward.
(ii) Ask patient/client to bear down, as if voiding, and slowly insert catheter through meatus.
(iii) Advance catheter approximately 18-23 cm (in an adult) or until urine flows out of the catheter end.

**RATIONALE**

Lubrication reduces trauma in the urethra. The local anaesthetic properties of the jelly reduces discomfort.

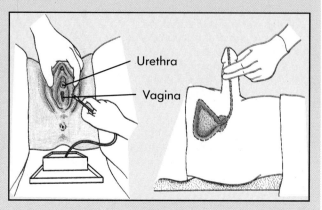

Step 24a                                      Step 24b

Insertion of nozzle into the urinary meatus will be more comfortable.

Collection of urine prevents soiling of bed linen and allows accurate measurement of urinary output.

Catheter in vagina is no longer sterile. Leaving first catheter in place helps prevent inserting second catheter in vagina.

The female urethra is short. Appearance of urine indicates that catheter tip is in bladder or lower urethra. Further advancement of catheter ensures bladder placement. Balloon of retention catheter must be advanced into bladder. Forceful insertion may traumatize urethra.

Bladder or sphincter contraction may cause accidental expulsion of catheter.

Straightens urethral canal to ease catheter insertion.
Relaxation of external sphincter aids in insertion of catheter.
The adult male urethra is long. Appearance of urine indicates that catheter tip is in bladder or urethra.

## Procedure 22-2 Inserting a Urethral Catheter (Cont'd)

| SEQUENCE OF ACTIONS | RATIONALE |
|---|---|
| (iv) If resistance is felt, apply steady 'gentle' pressure. If gentle pressure proves unsuccessful, withdraw the catheter; do not force it through the urethra. | Resistance may be due to spasm of the external sphincter, strictures of the urethra, or an enlarged prostate. Forceful insertion may traumatize the urethra. |
| (v) Either remove the catheter gently when urinary flow ceases, or if inserting a retention catheter, advance advance the catheter almost to its bifurcation. | Further advancement of catheter ensures that the catheter tip is well into the bladder before the balloon is inflated. |
| (vi) Release penis and hold catheter securely with dominant hand. | Bladder or sphincter contraction may cause accidental expulsion of catheter. |
| 25. Slowly inflate balloon of indwelling catheter. If the patient/client complains of sudden pain or if there is resistance against inflation, aspirate solution and advance catheter further. Inject no more fluid than is indicated by the manufacturers. | Inflation of the balloon anchors the catheter tip in place above the bladder outlet to prevent removal of catheter. Gentle withdrawal ensures proper placement and anchoring. Advancing the catheter slightly minimizes pressure on the bladder neck. |
| 26. Attach end of catheter to drainage bag. Place drainage bag in dependent position. Do not place bag on side rails of bed. | Closed system for urine drainage is established. The dependent position of the drainage bag promotes flow of urine away from bladder. Bags attached to side rails may be raised above the level of the bladder, if the rail is raised. |
| 27. Tape the catheter: | |
| a. FEMALE: tape catheter to inside of thigh. Allow for slack so that movement of thigh does not create tension on catheter. | Anchoring of catheter minimizes trauma to urethra and meatus during movement. |
| b. MALE: tape the catheter to the thigh or lower abdomen (with penis directed towards the abdomen). Allow some slack in catheter so that movement does not create tension on catheter. Reposition foreskin. | |
| 28. Make the patient/client comfortable. Ensure the area is dry. | |
| 29. Take a specimen of urine for laboratory examination, if required. | |
| 30. Dispose of gloves and equipment in a disposable plastic bag and seal the bag before moving the trolley. | Helps prevent cross-infection. |
| 31. Observe for colour, clarity, and volume of urine in the drainage system. | To determine whether urine is flowing adequately. |
| 32. Report and record type and size of catheter inserted, amount of fluid used to inflate balloon, and characteristics and amount of urine. | |

Most drainage bags contain an antireflux valve to prevent urine from re-entering the drainage tubing and contaminating the patient's/client's bladder. A tap at the base of the bag provides a means for emptying the bag. To keep the drainage system patent, check the tubing for kinks or bends. Avoid positioning the patient/client on the drainage tubing and observe for clots or sediment that may occlude the collecting tubing.

There are many types of drainage bags available and the choice of equipment is important in order to promote independence and self-care, particularly in people with long-term indwelling catheterization. It is the responsibility of the nurse to match choice with the individual. Where available, call upon the experienced advice of a continence advisor.

**Catheter Care** Patients/clients with indwelling catheters have a number of special care needs. Nursing measures are directed at preventing infection and maintaining unobstructed flow of urine through the catheter drainage system.

**Fluid Intake** All patients/clients with catheters should have a daily intake of 2000 to 2500 ml if permitted. This can be met through oral ingestion or intravenous infusion. A high fluid intake produces a large volume of urine that flushes the bladder and keeps catheter tubing free of sediment, although it does not prevent biofilm forming (Getliffe, 1993).

## Meteal Cleansing

Meatal cleansing or catheter toilet is often recommended with either soap and water or antiseptics. There is, however, no evidence to suggest that meatal cleansing actually inhibits or prevents catheter-associated infection (Burke *et al*, 1981; Stickler and Chawla, 1987). Personal hygiene, using mild soap and water, may be advisable for those with long-term indwelling catheters. It is most important to minimize cross-infection between catheterized patients/clients in institutional care, or patients/clients at home receiving help from health professionals or carers.

## Removal of Indwelling Catheter

When removing an indwelling catheter, it is important to promote normal bladder function and prevent trauma to the urethra. Loss of muscle tone in the bladder is a common problem after prolonged catheterization. **Bladder reconditioning**, which can reduce the loss of bladder tone, is begun at least 10 hours before catheter removal (Williamson, 1982). Clamp the indwelling catheter to allow urine to accumulate. The volume of urine stretches the bladder walls to stimulate muscle tone. Three hours later, unclamp the catheter and allow urine to drain for 5 minutes. The process is repeated twice more. After the conditioning procedure, remove the catheter. Patients/clients who receive bladder conditioning are believed to be able to feel the urge to void sooner than those who do not receive conditioning.

To remove a catheter the nurse requires a clean, disposable towel, and a sterile syringe the same size as (or larger than) the volume of solution within the catheter's inflated balloon. Disposable gloves are also recommended. The end of each catheter contains a label that denotes the volume of solution (5 to 30 ml) within a balloon.

Position the patient/client in the same position as during catheterization. Some institutions recommend collecting a sterile urine specimen at this time or sending the catheter tip for culture and sensitivity tests. After removing the tape, place the towel *between* the woman's thighs or *over* the man's thighs. Insert the syringe into the injection port. Most ports are self-sealing and require that only the tip of the syringe be inserted. Slowly withdraw all of the solution to deflate the balloon totally. The nurse must be aware of the possibility of an over-inflated ballon with a volume of solution above that recommended by the manufacturers. If a portion of the solution remains, the partially inflated balloon will traumatize the urethral canal as the catheter is removed. After deflation, explain that the patient/client may feel a burning sensation as the catheter is withdrawn. Then pull the catheter out smoothly and slowly.

It is normal for the patient/client to experience some dysuria, especially if the catheter has been in place several days or weeks. The catheter causes inflammation of the urethral canal. Until the bladder regains full tone, the patient/client may also experience frequency of urination.

Note when the patient/client first voids after catheter removal and assess for bladder distention. If over eight hours elapse, it may be necessary to reinsert the catheter. If the volume voided is small, residual urine may be in the bladder.

## ALTERNATIVES TO URETHRAL CATHETERIZATION

To avoid the risks associated with catheters inserted through the urethra, there are two alternatives for urinary drainage:

- **Suprapubic catheterization** involves surgical placement of a catheter through the abdominal wall above the symphysis pubis and into the urinary bladder. The procedure is performed under local or general anaesthesia. The catheter is anchored in place with sutures, a commercially prepared body seal, or both. Urine drains into a urinary drainage bag. The suprapubic catheter is relatively painless and reduces the incidence of infection commonly seen with self-retaining catheters. People who are wheelchair users, who are sexually active, or who experience problems with a urethral catheter (such as leakage, rejection) may benefit from a suprapubic catheter. Women who have undergone a vaginal hysterectomy may also benefit temporarily from the insertion of a suprapubic catheter after surgery.

The suprapubic catheter can become blocked by sediment, clots, or the abdominal wall itself. Nurses must monitor the patient's/client's intake and output carefully, observe for signs of kidney infection (for example, flank tenderness, chills, and fever), and monitor the appearance of urine. Spread of infection to the kidneys may indicate removal of the catheter. A suprapubic catheter must remain patent at all times. The nurse also administers skin care around the insertion site.

- The **urinary sheath** is the second alternative to catheterization. It is suitable for incontinent or comatose men who still have complete and spontaneous bladder emptying. The sheath is a soft, pliable, rubber and slips over the penis. It may be worn at night only or continuously, depending on the patient's/client's needs. It is held in place by either a strip of double-sided adhesive tape, or by adhesive already impregnated onto the inside of the sheath. Some types of sheath are applied with skin paste. Care must be taken not to contract the band tightly, or blood supply to the penis will be impaired. Never use standard adhesive tape to secure a urinary sheath, because it does not expand with change in penis size and blood supply to the penis is impaired.

The end of the sheath fits into a plastic drainage tubing. A drainage bag can be attached to the side of the bed or strapped to the patient's/client's leg. The urinary sheath poses little risk of infection. Infections with urinary sheaths usually result from buildup of secretions around the urethra, trauma to the urethral meatus, or buildup of pressure in the outflow tubing.

The nurse should change a urinary sheath daily to check for skin irritation, if the patient/client is unable to change it himself. With each catheter change, clean the urethral meatus and penis thoroughly. Twisting of the sheath at the drainage tube attachment irritates the skin and obstructs urine outflow. The drainage tubing must be checked often for patency.

For a man with a retracted penis, maintaining the intactness of a conventional urinary sheath may prove difficult. Special

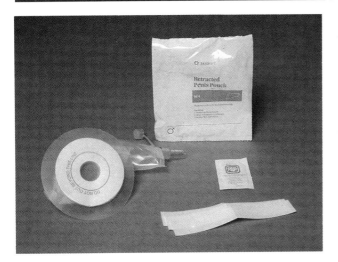

**Fig. 22-7** Retracted penis-pouch external urinary device.

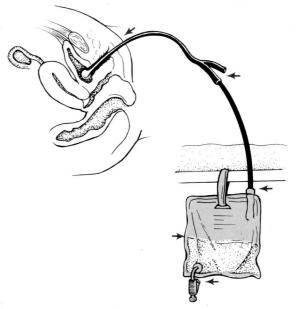

**Fig. 22-8** Potential sites for introduction of infectious organisms into a urinary drainage system.

devices are available to help alleviate this problem (Fig. 22-7). Manufacturers' guidelines for product application should be consulted.

The most frequently used incontinent devices for women are protective pads and protective clothing. There is a wide range of disposable and re-usable items available (ACA, 1990). Staff with sufficient skill and knowledge are required to help match appropriate devices with the requirements and needs of particular individuals.

### Preventing Infection

One of the most important considerations for a patient/client with urinary alterations is the need to prevent infection. Cleansing the genitalia and perineum, particularly after voiding, can help prevent infection. A daily fluid intake of 2000 to 2500 ml dilutes urine and promotes regular micturition.

Infection can develop in a catheterized patient/client in many ways. **Maintaining a closed urinary drainage system is important in infection control. A break in the system can lead to introduction of microorganisms** (Platt *et al*, 1983). Areas at risk are at the site of catheter insertion, drainage bag, tap, tube junction, and junction of tube and bag (Fig. 22-8). In addition, the nurse monitors the patency of the system to prevent pooling of urine within the tubing. Urine in the drainage bag is an excellent medium for microorganism growth. Bacteria can travel up the drainage tubing to grow in pools of urine. If this urine flows back into the patient's/client's bladder, an infection will likely develop. Effective handwashing techniques and the wearing of gloves should be employed whenever catheters and drainage bags are handled.

### CATHETER IRRIGATIONS AND INSTILLATION

To maintain the patency of indwelling urinary catheters, it sometimes becomes necessary to irrigate or flush a catheter. Blood, pus, or sediment can collect within tubing and result in bladder distention and the build-up of stagnant urine. Instillation of a sterile solution, usually normal saline, clears the tubing of accumulated material. For patients/clients with bladder

infections, bladder irrigations to include instillation of antiseptic or antibiotic solutions to wash out the bladder or treat local infection may be administered. In both irrigations, aseptic technique is followed.

There is evidence to suggest that the efficacy of using antiseptic bladder washouts to prevent or treat bladder infection is questionable (Brocklehurst, 1978; Davies et al, 1987). They may, moreover, lead to the development of resistant organisms (Stickla and Chawla, 1987). Infecting microorganisms tend to colonize catheter surfaces forming a 'biofilm' layer which is extremely difficult to remove and is very resistant to antiseptic or antibiotic agents (Brown *et al*, 1988).

The presence of these microorganisms precipitates the mineral encrustation of catheter surfaces which eventually leads to catheter blockage in up to 50% of catheterized patients (Roe and Brocklehurst, 1987). A study by Getliffe (1993) demonstrated that regular mini-washouts (20-30 ml) using an acidic reagent, can promote dissolution of encrustations within the catheter, suggesting catheter life may be extended, particularly in those who are prone to catheter blockage.

Burgener (1987) recommends that a closed system be maintained during intermittent irrigations or instillations. The nurse uses a sterile 30- to 50-ml syringe with a 19- to 22-gauge, 2.5cm needle to inject a prescribed solution into the catheter. This technique is effective for irrigating a partially blocked catheter or for bladder instillations.

A single intermittent irrigation is safer and less likely to introduce infections into the urinary tract. There are two additional methods for catheter irrigation. One is a closed bladder irrigation system. This system provides for frequent intermittent or continuous irrigation without disruption of the sterile catheter system. It is used most often in patients/clients who have had genitourinary surgery and are at risk for blood clots and mucus fragments occluding the catheter. The other system involves opening the closed drainage system to instil bladder irrigations. This technique poses greater risk for causing infection. However, it may be needed when catheters become blocked and it is undesirable to change the catheter.

## Maintaining Skin Integrity

The normal acidity of urine is irritating to skin. When urine becomes alkaline, encrustation or precipitate collects on the skin, fostering breakdown. Continuous exposure of the perineal area leads to gradual maceration and excoriation (see Chapter 25). Washing with mild soap and warm water is the best way to remove urine from skin. If frequent washes are required, use only warm water, as excessive washing with soaps can leave irritant deposits and remove the skin's protective barrier of surface lipids and sebum (Torrance, 1983). Patients/clients who wet their clothing should receive partial baths and clean sets of clothes after voiding.

## Promoting Comfort

Patients/clients with urinary alterations become uncomfortable as a result of the symptoms of urinary problems. Frequent or unpredictable voiding, dysuria, and painful distention are sources of discomfort.

The incontinent person gains comfort from having clean, dry clothing. When stress incontinence is the problem, a pad offers protection against soiling. Wet clothing adheres to the skin and can cause rubbing and irritation.

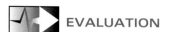 EVALUATION

To evaluate outcomes and responses to nursing care the nurse measures the effectiveness of all interventions. The optimal outcome is the patient's/client's ability to urinate voluntarily without symptoms (for example, urgency, dysuria, or frequency). The urine should be an amber colour, clear, without abnormal constituents, and within the normal range of pH and specific gravity. The patient/client should be able to identify factors that may influence normal voiding. The nurse also evaluates specific interventions designed to promote normal urinary function and prevent complications of urinary alterations.

Nursing interventions promote normal urination and provide support to patients/clients unable to maintain continence. Because of the urinary tract's vulnerability to infection, one of the nurse's primary concerns is infection control. The patient/client with urinary alterations may also suffer embarrassment, social isolation, and depression. Whether the alteration is temporary (for example, catheterization) or long term (for example, ureterostomy), the nurse must maintain the patient's/client's privacy and dignity. The nurse also evaluates the patient's/client's need for additional support services (for example, home care, physiotherapy, and counselling) and initiates the referral.

The provision of quality care delivery has become a paramount goal of the profession (Ulrich, 1989). To this end, nurses are actively involved in developing methods to systematically evaluate the nursing process. Nursing research is being conducted to validate nursing interventions. Quality improvement is evolving as a tool to evaluate nursing care delivery. The goal is to ensure the delivery of competent, state-of-the-art nursing care with positive outcomes for each patient/client.

## SUMMARY

Normal elimination of urinary waste requires maintenance of urinary function. Urinary elimination depends upon the functioning of the kidneys, ureters, bladder and urethra. The kidneys remove wastes from the blood to form urine, and the ureters transport urine from the kidneys to the bladder. Micturition is the process by which urine is expelled from the urinary bladder, and then leaves the body through the urethra.

Each patient/client has a different pattern of urinary elimination and the nurse must assess this pattern and aim to promote normal function. Factors which can influence micturition are sociocultural factors, personal habits, muscle tone, urinary volume, disease conditions, surgical procedures, and medications.

The most common urinary problems encountered by the nurse involve disturbances in micturition: urinary retention and urinary incontinence. Diagnostic investigations will help identify the underlying bladder disorder and enable effective treatment to be planned. In addition, a range of nursing interventions can be planned to enable the patient/client to return to his or her previous level of wellness. Whether the alteration is temporary or long term, the nurse can help the patient/client maintain his or her privacy and dignity, providing an understanding and sensitive approach to meeting patients'/clients' needs.

## CHAPTER 22 REVIEW

### Key Concepts

- Normal elimination of urinary wastes is a basic function most people take for granted and when it fails to function properly, this has physical and emotional effects on the person.
- The act of micturition or voiding is influenced by voluntary control from higher brain centres and involuntary control from the spinal cord.
- Symptoms common to urinary disturbances include urgency, frequency, dysuria, polyuria, oliguria, and difficulty in starting the urinary stream.
- A patient/client can appreciate the importance of perineal hygiene by knowing that the urinary tract is normally sterile.
- An increased fluid intake results in increased urine formation that flushes particles and solutes from the urinary system.
- Assessment of urine involves measuring the patient's/client's fluid intake and urine output and observing characteristics of the urine.
- Diagnostic examinations of the urinary system include abdominal X ray, intravenous pyelogram, renal scan, computerized tomography, and renal ultrasound.
- Invasive procedures include cytoscopy, biopsy and arteriogram.

- In collaboration with other members of the multidisciplinary team, plan with the patient/client interventions to reduce, minimize or control urinary elimination problems.
- Goals to promote normal urinary elimination may include: promoting normal micturition, enabling complete bladder emptying, preventing infection, maintaining skin integrity and promoting comfort.

## CRITICAL THINKING EXERCISES

1. A 64-year-old man returns from theatre after having undergone a trans-urethral prostatectomy. He has an indwelling Foley catheter. Identify potential complications resulting from the indwelling catheter.

2. You are asked to obtain a clean-voided midstream urine specimen for culture and sensitivity tests from a patient/client on your unit. What assessment data should be recorded in the nursing note regarding this specimen collection?

## Key Terms

Anuria, p. 433
Bacteriuria, p. 436
Bladder reconditioning, p. 450
Catheterization, p. 445
Closed urinary drainage system, p. 446
Cystitis, p. 437
Diuresis, p. 435
Dysuria, p. 437
Haematuria, p. 437
Intravenous pyelogram (IVP), p. 442
Micturition/voiding, p. 433
Mid-stream specimen (MSU), p. 439
Oliguria, p. 433
Polyuria, p. 439
Proteinuria, p. 430
Specific gravity, p. 441
Urinary elimination, p. 429
Urinary incontinence, p. 437
Urinary retention, p. 435
Urinary tract infections (UTIs), p. 436

## REFERENCES

Association of Continence Advisors: *Directory of continence aids,* London, 1990, ACA.

Bennett VR, Brown LK, editors: *Myles textbook for midwives,* Edinburgh, 1989, Churchill Livingstone.

Brocklehurst JC, Brocklehurst S: The management of indwelling catheters, *Br J Urol* 50:102, 1978.

Brown MRW *et al*: Resistance of bacterial biofilms to antibiotics: a growth related effect, *J Antimicrob Chemotherapy* 22:777,1988.

Burgener S: Justification of closed intermittent urinary catheter irrigation/installation: a review of current research and practice, *J Adv Nurs* 12:229, 1987.

Burke JP *et al*: Prevention of catheter associated urinary tract infections, *American Journal of Medicine,* 70: 665, 1981.

Butler RJ: *Nocturnal enuresis: psychological perspectives,* Bristol, 1987, Wright.

Carty M, Brocklehurst JC, Carty J: Bacteria and its correlates in old age, *Gerontology* 27:72, 1981.

Castleden CM *et al*: The effect of physiotherapy on stress incontinence, *Age Ageing* 13:235, 1984.

Copperwheat M: Putting continence into practice, *Geriatr Nurs* 5(3):4, 1985.

Crow R *et al*: *A study of patients with an indwelling catheter and related nursing practice,* Nurs Practice Research Unit, Guildford, 1986, University of Surrey.

Davies AJ *et al*: Does installation of chlorhexidine into the bladder of catheterized geriatric patients help reduce bacteriuria, *Journal of Hospital Infection,* 9: 72-75, 1987.

Getliffe K: Freeing the system, *Nurs Standard* 8:7, 1993.

Kennedy AP, Brocklehurst JC, Wye MDW: Factors related to the problems of long-term catheterization, *J Adv Nurs* 8:207, 1983.

Norton C: Incontinence in old age, *Nurs Elderly* 4:4, 1992.

Platt R *et al*: Reduction of mortality associated with nosomical urinary tract infection, *Lancet* 1:893, 1983.

Rivers PM: *Incontinence: a critical review of the literature and current initiatives,* Nursing Practice Research Unit, 1986, University of Surrey.

Roe BH, Brocklehurst JC: Study of patients with indwelling catheters, *J Adv Nurs* 12:713, 1987.

Rogers W: Shampoo urethritis (letter), *Am J Dis Child* 139:748, 1985.

Slade N, Gillespie WA: *The urinary tract and the catheter: infection and other problems.* Chichester, 1985, John Wiley and Sons.

Smith N, Clamp M: *Continence promotion in general practice,* Oxford, 1991, Oxford University Press.

Stickler DJ, Chawla JC: The role of antiseptics in the management of patients with long term indwelling bladder catheters, *Journal of Hospital Infections,* 10: 219-228, 1987.

Thomas TM *et al*: Prevalence of urinary incontinence, *BMJ* 281:1243, 1980.

Torrance C: *Pressure sores, aetiology, treatment and prevention,* London, 1983, Croom Helm.

Ulrich BT: *Nephrology nursing: concepts and strategies,* Norwalk, 1989, Appleton & Lange.

Warren JW *et al*: Sequalae and management of urinary tract infection in patients requiring chronic catheterization, *J Urol,* 125:1, 1981.

Williamson ML: Reducing post-catheterization bladder dysfunction by reconditioning, *Nurs Res* 31:28, 1982.

## FURTHER READING

### Adult Nursing

Association of Continence Advisors: *Directory of continence aids,* London, 1990, ACA.

Bates P: A troubleshooter's guide to indwelling catheters, *RN* 44:63, 1981.

Bello-Reuss E, Reuss L: Homeostatic and excretory functions of the kidney. In Klahr S, editor: *The kidney and body fluids in health and disease,* New York, 1983, Plenum.

Crummey V: Ignorance can hurt, *Nurs Times* 85(21):66, 1989.

Gibson LY: Bedwetting: a family recurrent nightmare, *MCN* 12(4), 1989.

Greengold BA, Ouslander JG: Bladder retraining, *J Gerontol Nurs* 12:31, 1986.

Kaltrieder DL *et al*: Can reminders curb incontinence? *Geriatr Nurs* 11(1):17, 1990.

Mandelstam D: Strengthening pelvic floor muscles, *Geriatr Nurs* 1:251, 1980.

Mares P: *In control: help with continence,* London, 1990, Age Concern.

Nurses' drug alert: Urinary tract irritation from shampoo, *Am J Nurs* 86:66, 1986.

Rees-Williams C *et al*: Making sense of urinary catheters, *Nurs Times* 84(40):46, 1988.

Robb SS: Urinary incontinence verification in elderly men, *Nurs Res* 34:278, 1985.

Roe B: *Catheter care:a guide for users and their carers,* Colchester, 1987, HG
    Wallace.
Smith N, Clamp M: *Continence promotion in general practice,* Oxford, 1991, Oxford
    University Press.


### Children's Nursing

Blackwell C: *A Guide to the Treatment of Enuresis for Professionals,* Bristol, 1989,
    Enuresis Resource and Information Centre.
Dean S: Caring for a child undergoing a circumcision using Roper's model. In While
    A (ed): *Caring for Children,* London, 1991, Edward Arnold.
Green C: *Toddler Taming,* Derby, 1985, Columbine.
Lybrand M, Medoff-Cooper B, Monro B: Periodic comparisons of specific gravity
    using urine from a diaper and collecting bag, *MCH* 15:238, 1990.


### Learning Disabilities Nursing

Bettison S: *Toilet training to independence: a manual for trainers,* London, 1982,
    Charles C Thomas.
Dalrymple NJ, Ruble LA: Toilet training and behaviours of people with autism:
    parent views, *J Autism & Dev Disorders,* 22 (2): 265-275.
Heilstrom PA *et al*: Bladder function in the mentally retarded, *B J of Urology,* 66 (5):
    475-8, 1990.


### Mental Health Nursing

Chambers K: Regained dignity... a regime that helped a woman with Alzheimer's
    disease achieve greater continence, *Continence,* 65, *Nursing Times,* 24-30,
    1993,
Jirovec MM, Wells TJ: Urinary incontinence in nursing home residents with
    dementia: the mobility-cognition paradigm, *Applied Nursing Research,* 3 (3):
    112-7, 1990.
McLean Hospital: Huntington's disease: helping the patient retain function,
    *American Journal of Nursing,* Belmont, MA, 93 (8): 62-4, 1993.
Palmer MH, German PS, Ouslander JG: Risk factors for urinary incontinence one
    year after nursing home admission, *Research in Nursing and Health,* 14 (6):
    405-12, 1991.
Watson R: Incontinence in perspective, *Nursing (London),* 4 (39): 7-10, 1991.

# Bowel Elimination

## CHAPTER OUTLINE

## LEARNING OUTCOMES

After reading this chapter, you should be able to:
- *Define the key terms listed.*
- *Discuss the role of gastrointestinal organs in digestion and elimination and describe the sequences involved.*
- *Describe the four interrelated functions of the large intestine.*
- *Discuss physiological and psychological factors that influence the elimination process.*
- *Describe common physiological alterations in elimination and suggest possible causes.*
- *Be aware of specific patient/client groups at risk for problems associated with bowel elimination.*
- *List common diagnostic examinations of the gastrointestinal tract and describe any instruments or equipment used.*
- *List nursing measures that promote normal elimination.*
- *Correctly administer an enema and a suppository.*
- *Provide support for the patient/client in the management of faecal incontinence.*
- *Describe the two basic types of stoma-forming surgery.*
- *Discuss the relationship between the structure and function of bowel stomas and nursing care required.*
- *Provide patients/clients with information on measures to promote optimum adjustment and comfort during postoperative rehabilitation for stoma formation.*

Regular elimination of bowel waste products is essential for normal body functioning. Alterations in elimination can cause problems with the gastrointestinal and other body systems. Because bowel function depends on the balance of several factors, elimination patterns and habits vary among individuals. However, there is increased evidence that frequent, high-volume, normal faeces is consistent with a lower incidence of colorectal cancer (Robinson and Weigley, 1989).

Patients/clients often need assistance from the nurse to maintain normal elimination habits which illness can prevent them from following. They might become physically unable to use normal toilet facilities. The home environment might present obstacles for people with altered mobility, requiring changes in bathroom fixtures.

To manage a patient's/client's elimination problems, the nurse must understand normal elimination and factors that promote or impede elimination. Supportive nursing care respects the person's privacy and emotional needs. Measures designed to promote normal elimination should also minimize discomfort.

## NORMAL DIGESTION AND ELIMINATION

The **gastrointestinal (GI) tract** is a series of hollow mucous membrane-lined muscular organs. The purposes of these organs are to absorb fluid and nutrients, prepare food for absorption and use by the body's cells, and provide for temporary storage of faeces (Fig. 23-1). The volume of fluids absorbed by the GI tract is high, making fluid balance a key function of the GI system. In addition to ingested fluids and foods, the GI tract also receives many secretions from organs such as the gallbladder and the pancreas (Table 23-1). A disorder that seriously impairs normal absorption or secretion of GI fluids causes fluid imbalance (see Chapters 18 and 21).

## Mouth

The GI tract mechanically and chemically breaks down nutrients into a suitable size and form. All digestive organs work together to ensure that the mass, or **bolus**, of food reaches the areas of nutrient absorption safely and effectively. Mechanical and

chemical digestion begin in the mouth. The teeth **masticate** (chew) food, breaking it down to a suitable size for swallowing. Saliva dilutes and softens the bolus of food in the mouth for easier swallowing.

## Oesophagus

As food enters the upper oesophagus, it passes through the upper oesophageal sphincter, which is a circular muscle that prevents air from entering the oesophagus and food from **refluxing** (moving backward) into the throat. The bolus of food travels approximately 25 cm down the oesophagus. Food is pushed along by slow peristaltic waves produced by alternating contractions of smooth muscle. As a portion of the oesophagus contracts behind the food bolus, the circular muscle in front of the bolus relaxes. A

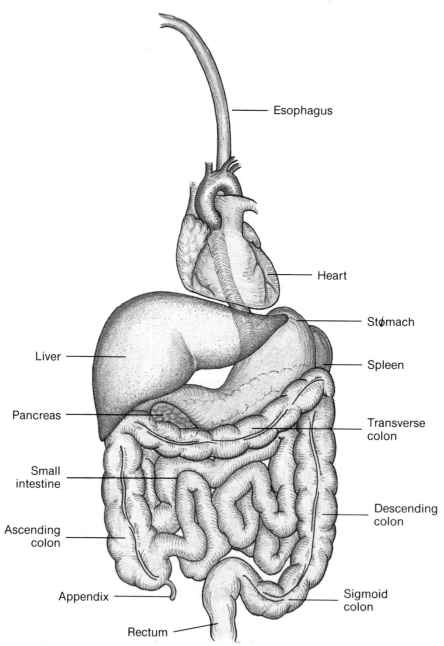

**Fig. 23-1** Organs of the GI tract (with the heart as a reference point).

Segmentation

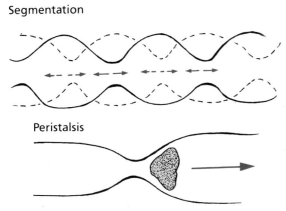

Peristalsis

**Fig. 23-2** Segmented and peristaltic waves.

peristaltic wave propels food towards the next wave (Fig. 23-2). **Peristalsis** moves food throughout the length of the GI tract.

In 15 seconds the bolus of food moves down the oesophagus and reaches the lower oesophageal sphincter. The lower oesophageal sphincter lies between the oesophagus and stomach, and a pressure difference exists at the lower end of the oesophagus (Tortora, 1989). The lower oesophageal pressure is 10 to 40 mmHg, whereas pressure within the stomach is 5 to 10 mmHg. The pressure gradient normally prevents reflux of stomach contents back into the oesophagus. Factors influencing lower sphincter pressure include antacids, which minimize reflux, and fatty foods and nicotine, which increase reflux.

## Stomach

In the stomach, food is temporarily stored and mechanically and chemically broken down for digestion and absorption. Before food leaves the stomach, it is changed into a semifluid material called **chyme**. Chyme is more easily digested and absorbed than solid food. People who have portions of their stomachs removed or who have rapid stomach emptying (as with gastritis) have serious digestive problems because food is not broken down into chyme. Food enters the small intestine before being adequately broken down to a semifluid form. Absorption is less efficient, and nutritional alterations can develop.

**TABLE 23-1**
**GI Tract Fluid Balance**

| Item | Ingested and secreted (ml) | Absorbed (ml) |
|---|---|---|
| Food and drink | 1500 | — |
| Saliva | 1500 | — |
| Gastric juice | 3000 | — |
| Pancreatic juice | 2000 | — |
| Bile | 500 | — |
| Small intestine fluid | | 5850 |
| Colon | | 2500 |
| Faeces | | 150 |
| **Total** | **8500** | **8500** |

## Small Intestine

During normal digestion, chyme leaves the stomach and enters the small intestine. The small intestine is a tube about 2.5 cm in diameter and 6 m in length. It contains three divisions: duodenum, jejunum, and ileum. Chyme mixes with digestive substances (such as bile and amylase) while travelling through the small intestine. **Segmentation** (alternating contraction and relaxation of smooth muscle) churns the chyme, further breaking down food for digestion (Fig. 23-2). As chyme mixes, forward peristaltic movement temporarily ceases to permit absorption. Chyme travels slowly down the small intestine to allow absorption.

## Large Intestine

The lower GI tract is the large intestine (**colon**) because its diameter is larger than the small intestine. However, its length of 1.5 to 1.8 m is much shorter. The large intestine is divided into the caecum, colon, and rectum (Fig. 23-3). It is the primary organ of bowel elimination.

## Caecum

Unabsorbed chyme enters the large intestine at the caecum through the ileocaecal valve, which is a circular muscle layer that prevents colon contents from **regurgitating** (returning to the small intestine).

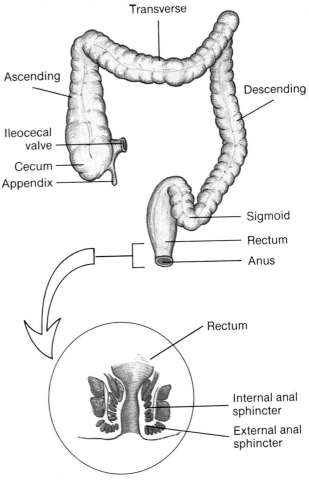

**Fig. 23-3** Divisions of the large intestine.

## Colon

Although watery chyme enters the colon, the volume of water lessens as chyme moves along it. The colon is divided into the ascending, transverse, descending, and sigmoid colons. The colon is made of muscular tissue, which allows it to accommodate and thus eliminate large quantities of waste.

The colon has four interrelated functions: absorption, protection, secretion, and elimination. A large volume of water and significant amounts of sodium and chloride are absorbed by the colon daily. As food passes through the colon, **haustral contractions** occur. These are similar to segmental contractions of the small intestine but last longer — up to 5 min. The contractions produce large sacs in the colon's wall, providing a large surface area for absorption.

As much as 2.5 L of water can be absorbed by the colon in 24 hours. On the average, 55 mmol of sodium and 23 mmol of chloride are absorbed daily. The amount of water absorbed from chyme depends on the speed at which colonic contents move. Chyme is normally a soft, formed mass. If the speed of peristaltic contractions is abnormally fast, there is less time for water to be absorbed and the stool will be watery. If peristaltic contractions slow down, water continues to be absorbed, and a hard mass of stool forms, resulting in **constipation**.

The colon protects itself by releasing a supply of mucus. Mucus is normally clear to opaque with a stringy consistency. Mucus lubricates the colon, preventing trauma to its inner walls. Lubrication is especially important near the distal end of the colon, where contents become drier and harder.

The secretory function of the colon aids in electrolyte balance. Bicarbonate is secreted in exchange for chloride. About 4 to 9 mmol of potassium is released each day by the large intestine. Serious alterations in colonic function can cause electrolyte imbalance.

Finally, the colon removes waste products and gas **(flatus)**. Flatus results from air swallowing, diffusion of gas from the bloodstream into the intestine, and bacterial action on non-absorbable carbohydrates. Fermentation of carbohydrates (such as in cabbage and onions) produces intestinal gas, which can stimulate peristalsis. An adult normally forms 400 to 700 ml of flatus daily.

Slow peristaltic contractions move contents through the colon. Intestinal content is the main stimulus for contraction. Waste products and gas exert pressure against the walls of the colon. The muscle layer stretches, stimulating the reflex that initiates contraction.

Mass peristaltic movements push undigested food towards the rectum. These movements are unlike the frequent peristaltic waves in the small intestine (which are usually heard during auscultation) in that they occur only three or four times daily.

When these mass peristaltic movements occur, large segments of the colon contract as a result of **gastrocolic** and **duodenocolic reflex responses**. These occur when the stomach or duodenum is filled with food. Filling initiates nerve impulses that stimulate the colon's muscular walls. Mass peristalsis is strongest during the hour after mealtime.

## Rectum

Waste products that reach the sigmoid portion of the colon are called **faeces**. The sigmoid colon stores faeces until just before defaecation.

The rectum is the final division of the GI tract. Its length varies according to age:
- infant 2.5 to 3.8 cm
- toddler 5 cm
- preschool child 7.5 cm
- school-aged child 10 cm
- adult 15 to 20 cm.

Normally the rectum is empty of faeces until defaecation. It contains vertical and transverse folds of tissue. Each vertical fold contains an artery and veins. If the veins become distended from pressure during the straining of defaecation, haemorrhoids form. Haemorrhoids can make defaecation painful.

When the faecal mass or gas moves into the rectum to distend its walls, **defaecation** begins. The process involves involuntary and voluntary control. The internal sphincter is a smooth muscle innervated by the autonomic nervous system. As the rectum distends, sensory nerves are stimulated and carry impulses that cause the internal sphincter to relax, allowing more faeces to enter the rectum. At the same time, impulses travel to the brain to create awareness of the need to defaecate.

As the internal sphincter relaxes, so does the external sphincter. A person who is toilet trained can voluntarily control the external sphincter. If the time for defaecation is not right, constriction of the levator ani muscles closes the anus and defaecation is delayed. At the time of defaecation, the external sphincter relaxes. Pressure can be exerted to expel faeces through an increase in intra-abdominal pressure or a Valsalva manoeuvre. A **Valsalva manoeuvre** is voluntary contraction of abdominal muscles during forced expiration with a closed glottis (holding one's breath while straining). Relaxation of the levator ani muscle allows faeces to be expelled. If the act of defaecation is voluntarily stopped, faeces remain in the rectum until the defaecation reflex is restimulated. Defaecation can be promoted by flexing the thigh muscles, which puts pressure on the abdomen, and sitting, which increases pressure down on the rectum.

## FACTORS AFFECTING ELIMINATION

Many factors influence the process of bowel elimination (Table 23-2). Knowledge of these factors allows the nurse to anticipate measures required to maintain a normal elimination pattern. Also, an understanding of the effects of these factors on normal elimination provides guidelines for reversing their effects.

### Age

Developmental changes that affect elimination occur throughout life. An infant has a small stomach capacity and less secretion of digestive enzymes. Some foods such as complex starches are tolerated poorly. Food passes quickly through an infant's intestinal tract because of rapid peristalsis. The infant is unable to

## TABLE 23-2 Factors Affecting Elimination

| Factors Promoting Elimination | Factors Impairing Elimination |
|---|---|
| Stress-free environment | Emotional stress (anxiety or depression) |
| Ability to follow personal bowel habits, privacy | Failure to heed defaecation reflex, lack of time or privacy |
| High-fibre diet | High-carbohydrate (refined), high-fat diet |
| Normal fluid intake (fruit juices, warm liquids) | Reduced fluid intake |
| Exercise (walking) | Immobility or inactivity |
| Ability to assume squatting position | Inability to squat because of immobility, advanced age, musculoskeletal deformities, pain, advanced pregnancy; pain during defaecation |
| Properly administered laxatives and cathartics | Use of narcotic analgesics, antibodies, and general anaesthetics and over use of laxatives |

control defaecation because of a lack of neuromuscular development. This development usually does not take place until 2 to 3 years of age.

During adolescence, there is rapid growth of the large intestine. The secretion of HCl (hydrochloric acid) increases, particularly in boys. Adolescents typically eat more.

Older adults often experience changes in the GI system that impair digestion and elimination. The amount of digestive enzyme in saliva and the volume of gastric acid decreases with ageing. The inability to digest fat-containing foods reflects a loss of the enzyme lipase. In addition, peristaltic action declines, and oesophageal emptying slows. Sluggish emptying of the oesophagus can cause discomfort in the epigastric region of the abdomen. Absorptive properties of the intestinal mucosa change, causing protein, vitamin, and mineral deficiencies. Older adults also lose muscle tone in the perineal floor and anal sphincter. Although the integrity of the external sphincter may remain intact, older adults may have difficulty controlling bowel evacuation. Because of slowing of nerve impulses, some are less aware of the need to defaecate and are likely to become constipated.

Hospitalized older adults are at particular risk of altered bowel function (Wright, 1974). One study indicated a 91% incidence of diarrhoea or constipation in a population of 33 hospitalized persons with a mean age of 76 years (Ross, 1990).

### Diet

Regular daily food intake helps maintain a regular pattern of peristalsis in the colon. The food that a person eats influences elimination. **Fibre**, the undigestible residue in the diet, provides the bulk in faecal material. Bulk-forming foods absorb fluids, thereby increasing stool mass. The bowel walls are stretched, creating peristalsis and initiating the defaecation reflex. An infant's immature bowel cannot usually tolerate fibre-containing foods until several years of age. By stimulating peristalsis, bulk foods pass quickly through the intestines, keeping the stool soft. The following foods contain a high amount of fibre:

- raw fruits (apples, oranges)
- cooked fruits (prunes, apricots)
- greens (spinach, kale, cabbage)
- raw vegetables (celery, carrots)
- whole grains (cereal, breads).

Convenience foods such as pizza, cooked pies, and sugar-coated cereals tend to be low in fibre. They are popular for people who have busy lifestyles or who live alone.

Ingestion of a high-fibre diet improves the likelihood of a normal elimination pattern if other factors are normal. Gas-producing foods such as onions, cauliflower, and beans also stimulate peristalsis. The gas formed distends intestinal walls, increasing colon motility. Some spicy foods can increase peristalsis but can also cause indigestion and watery stools.

Some foods, such as milk and milk products, are difficult or impossible for some people to digest. This is caused by a **lactose intolerance**. Lactose, a simple form of sugar found in milk, is normally broken down by the enzyme lactase. The incidence of primary lactose intolerance varies among different racial groups, from 5% in Caucasians to 70–80% among people of Asian and Afro-Caribbean origin. The inability to digest lactose results from a failure to produce lactase. Intolerance to specific foods may result in diarrhoea, gaseous distention, and cramping. Management involves simple avoidance of lactose-containing products.

### Fluid Intake

An inadequate intake of fluids or disturbances causing loss of fluid (such as vomiting) affect the character of faeces. Fluid liquifies intestinal contents, easing their passage through the colon. Reduced fluid intake slows passage of food through the intestine. An adult should drink 6 to 8 glasses (1400 to 2000 ml)

**Children's Nursing
Toddler diarrhoea**

Because food passes quickly through an infant's intestinal tract, infants often present with loose stools that contain undigested foodstuffs, such as carrots and peas. This is known as 'toddler diarrhoea' and is a normal phenomenon of early childhood.

of fluid daily. Hot beverages and fruit juices soften the stool and increase peristalsis. A large ingestion of milk may slow peristalsis in some people and cause constipation.

## Physical Activity

Physical activity promotes peristalsis, whereas immobilization depresses colonic motility. Early ambulation after illness is encouraged to promote maintenance of normal elimination.

Maintaining tone of skeletal muscles used during defaecation is important. Weakened abdominal and pelvic floor muscles impair the ability to increase intra-abdominal pressure and to control the external sphincter. Muscle tone may be weakened or lost as a result of long-term illness or neurological disease that impairs nerve transmission.

### Mental Health Nursing
### Constipation

When a person becomes severely depressed, many bodily functions slow down considerably. Bowel elimination may become a problem. In addition, many of the antidepressant medications prescribed cause varying degrees of constipation.

On the other hand, if a person is hyperactive, he or she may be too distracted, by a range of external stimuli, to pay attention to bowel elimination. When faecal content accumulates in the bowel and is not regularly eliminated, this will in turn cause bowel irritability. This makes the person uncomfortable and increases his or her restlessness.

These difficulties can be anticipated and prevented through careful nursing observation of the person's bowel habits and through ensuring that fluid intake does not become depleted.

## Psychological Factors

The function of almost all body systems can be impaired by prolonged emotional stress (see Chapter 10). If an individual becomes anxious, afraid, or angry, the stress response initiates impulses from the parasympathetic division of the autonomic nervous system. This response allows the body to restore defences. The digestive process is accelerated, and peristalsis is increased to provide nutrients needed for defence. Side effects of increased peristalsis are diarrhoea and gaseous distention. If a person becomes depressed, the autonomic nervous system slows impulses and peristalsis can decrease. A number of diseases of the GI tract may be associated with stress. These include ulcerative colitis, gastric ulcers, and Crohn's disease. Repeated research endeavours have failed to prove the myth that people with such diseases have underlying psychopathological conditions. Anxiety and depression may be a result of such chronic problems (Cooke, 1991).

A child's elimination pattern can be upset by the method of toilet training. Forcing a child to learn toilet training before cognitive, nervous and muscular systems are developed and coordinated is a waste of time. Punishing children for accidents makes toilet training stressful, and can lead to great difficulties.

## Personal Habits

Personal elimination habits influence bowel function. Most people benefit from being able to use their own toilet facilities at a time that is most effective and convenient for them. A busy work schedule may disrupt habits and result in alterations such as constipation. A person should learn the best time for elimination. The gastrocolic reflex is most easily stimulated to cause defaecation after breakfast.

Hospitalized individuals can rarely maintain privacy during defaecation. Wright (1974) found that 34% of people admitted to hospital had less frequent bowel action than when at home. Toilet facilities are often shared with other patients/clients whose hygienic habits might be quite different. The person's illness often limits physical activity and requires the use of a bedpan or bedside commode. Forty-four percent of the subjects in Wright's (1974) study who used bedpans or commodes reported constipation, compared with 26% who could walk to the lavatory. The sights, sounds, and odours associated with sharing toilet facilities or using bedpans are often embarrassing. Embarrassment prompts individuals to ignore the urge to defaecate, which can begin a vicious cycle of discomfort.

### Bowel Elimination

Some cultural or religious groups may have requirements for ritual cleansing of the anal area following defaecation. It is important to provide appropriate facilities for this whenever possible. If the person is bed-bound, and running water is not accessible, they may accept a wash with water poured from a jug.

Some Arabic or Asian people use one hand for food handling and the other for cleaning the anal area after defaecation. This can cause problems if one hand is paralysed. Nurses can also inadvertently cause offence by using the 'dirty' hand for 'clean' jobs, for example offering food.

The discussion of bowel problems may be difficult for people from some cultures. For example a Hindu women may be very reluctant to discuss her constipation with the doctor if her husband is present, although the Carak Samhita says that a husband or guardian must be present every time a doctor examines a Hindu woman. These situation require sensitive handling on the part of health care staff (Neuberger, 1994).

## Position During Defaecation

Squatting is the normal position during defaecation. Modern toilets are designed to facilitate this posture, allowing the person to lean forward, exert intra-abdominal pressure, and contract the thigh muscles. However, older or disabled people with joint disease, such as arthritis, may be unable to rise from a low toilet seat. Attachments that raise the seat enable the patient/client to get off the toilet without assistance. Individuals who use such attachments, as well as short people, might require a footstool for proper hip flexion. Adaptations and aids which may be required can be obtained for use in the person's home.

For the person immobilized in bed, defaecation is often

difficult. In a supine position, it is impossible to contract the muscles used during defaecation. Assisting the individual to a more normal sitting position on a bedpan enhances the ability to defaecate.

## Pain

Normally the act of defaecation is painless. However, a number of conditions, including haemorrhoids, rectal surgery, abdominal surgery, and childbirth can result in discomfort. In these instances the person often suppresses the urge to defaecate to avoid pain. Constipation is a common problem for people with pain during defaecation.

## Pregnancy

As pregnancy advances and the size of the fetus increases, pressure is exerted on the rectum. A temporary obstruction created by the fetus impairs the passage of faeces. Hence constipation is a common problem during the third trimester. A pregnant woman's frequent straining during defaecation can result in formation of permanent haemorrhoids.

## Surgery and Anaesthesia

General anaesthetic agents used during surgery cause temporary cessation of peristalsis (see Chapter 29). Inhaled anaesthetic agents block parasympathetic impulses to the intestinal musculature. The anaesthetic's action slows or stops peristaltic waves. The patient/client who receives local or regional anaesthesia is less at risk for elimination alterations because bowel activity is affected minimally or not at all.

Surgery that involves direct manipulation of the bowel temporarily stops peristalsis. This condition, called **paralytic ileus**, usually lasts about 24 to 48 hours. If the person remains inactive or is unable to eat after surgery, return of normal bowel function may be further delayed.

## Medications

Medications are available for promoting defaecation. **Laxatives** soften the stool and promote peristalsis. When used correctly, laxatives safely maintain normal elimination patterns. However, chronic use of laxatives causes the large intestine to lose muscle tone and become less responsive to stimulation by laxatives. Laxative overuse can also cause serious diarrhoea that can lead to dehydration and electrolyte depletion. Liquid paraffin, a common laxative in the past, decreases fat-soluble vitamin absorption. Laxatives can influence the efficacy of other medications by altering the **transit time** (that is, the time the medication remains in the GI tract for proper absorption).

Antispasmodic medications such as dicyclomine HCl suppress peristalsis and treat diarrhoea. Several medications have side effects that can impair elimination. Narcotic analgesics depress peristalsis in the GI tract. Opiates commonly cause constipation. Anticholinergic drugs, such as atropine or hyoscine, inhibit gastric acid secretion and depress GI motility. Although useful in treating hyperactive bowel disorders, anticholinergics can cause constipation. Many antibiotics produce diarrhoea by disrupting the normal bacterial flora in the GI tract. If the

diarrhoea and associated abdominal cramping become severe, the patient/client might need to change medications.

## Diagnostic Tests

Diagnostic examinations involving visualization of GI structures often require that portions of the bowel be empty of contents. A patient/client is not allowed to eat or drink after midnight of the day preceding examinations such as a barium enema, endoscopy of the lower GI tract, or an upper GI (UGI) series. In the case of a barium enema or endoscopy, the patient/client usually receives strong laxatives and an enema (for x-ray). Such emptying of the bowel can interfere with elimination until normal eating is resumed.

Barium examination procedures pose an additional problem. Barium hardens if allowed to stay in the GI tract. This can lead to constipation or bowel impaction. A patient/client should receive a laxative to promote elimination of barium. Failure to evacuate all the barium might require that the individual receive a cleansing enema.

## COMMON BOWEL ELIMINATION PROBLEMS

The nurse might care for patients/clients who have or are at risk of having elimination problems because of emotional stress (anxiety or depression), physiological changes in the GI tract, surgical alteration of intestinal structures, other prescribed therapy, disorders impairing defaecation, or physical disability such as paraplegia.

## Constipation

**Constipation** is a symptom, not a disease. It is a decrease in frequency of bowel movements, accompanied by the prolonged or difficult passage of hard, dry stools. Straining during defaecation is an associated sign. When intestinal motility slows, the faecal mass becomes exposed over time to the intestinal walls and most of the faecal water content is absorbed. Little water is left to soften and lubricate the stool. Passage of a dry stool may cause rectal pain.

Each person has an individual defaecation pattern that the nurse must assess. If daily records start to suggest a decrease in the frequency of defaecation there is cause for concern. The causes of constipation are summarized in the box.

Constipation is a significant hazard to health. Straining during defaecation causes problems to the person with recent abdominal or rectal surgery. The effort to pass a stool can cause sutures to separate, reopening the wound. In addition, people with histories of cardiovascular disease, diseases causing elevated intraocular pressure (glaucoma), and increased intracranial pressure should prevent constipation and avoid using the Valsalva manoeuvre. Exhaling through the mouth during straining avoids a Valsalva manoeuvre.

## Impaction

**Faecal impaction** results from unrelieved constipation. It is a collection of hardened faeces, wedged in the rectum, that cannot

## Common Causes of Constipation

- irregular bowel habits and ignoring the urge to defaecate can cause constipation
- a low-fibre diet that is high in animal fats (e.g. meats, dairy products, eggs) and refined sugars (rich desserts)
- a low fluid intake (slows peristalsis)
- lengthy bed rest or lack of regular exercise
- heavy use of laxatives (causes loss of normal defaecation reflex, and completely empties the lower colon which then requires time to refill with bulk)
- tranquillizers, opiates, anticholinergics, and iron
- slowed peristalsis, loss of abdominal muscle elasticity, and reduced intestinal mucous secretion in older adults
- GI abnormalities, such as bowel obstruction, paralytic ileus, and diverticulitis
- neurological conditions that block nerve impulses to the colon (e.g. spinal cord injury, tumour).

be expelled. In cases of severe impaction, the mass can extend up into the sigmoid colon. Patients/clients who are debilitated, confused, or unconscious are most at risk for impaction. They are too weak or unaware of the need to defaecate.

An obvious sign of impaction is the inability to pass a stool for several days, despite a repeated urge to defaecate. When a continuous oozing of diarrhoeal stool suddenly develops, impaction should be suspected. The liquid portion of faeces located higher in the colon seeps around the impacted mass. Loss of appetite (anorexia), abdominal distention and cramping, and rectal pain may accompany the condition. If you suspect, an impaction request the doctor to gently perform a digital examination of the rectum and palpate the impacted mass. There is a risk of causing vagal stimulation that slows heart rate during this procedure. Another danger with digital examination is bowel perforation, especially with older adults and people with neoplastic colon diseases.

### Diarrhoea

**Diarrhoea** is an increase in the number of stools and the passage of liquid, unformed faeces. It is a symptom of disorders affecting digestion, absorption, and secretion in the GI tract. Intestinal contents pass through the small intestine and colon too quickly to allow the usual absorption of fluid. Irritation within the colon can result in an increased mucus secretion. As a result, faeces become watery, so the individual may be unable to control the urge to defaecate.

It is often difficult to assess diarrhoea in infants. An infant who is bottle-fed may have one firm stool every second day, whereas a breast-fed baby may pass five to eight small, soft stools daily. The mother or nurse should note any sudden increase in number of stools, any reduction in faecal consistency with an increase in fluid content, and a tendency for faeces to be greenish.

Excess loss of colonic fluid can result in serious fluid and electrolyte imbalance. Infants and older adults are particularly susceptible to associated complications (see Chapter 18). Because repeated passage of diarrhoeal stools also exposes the skin of the perineum and buttocks to irritating intestinal contents,

meticulous skin care is needed to prevent skin breakdown (see Chapter 30). The person might experience abdominal cramping, nausea, and vomiting, depending on the cause of the diarrhoea.

Many conditions cause diarrhoea (Table 23-3). The aims of treatment are to remove precipitating conditions and to slow peristalsis. Any irritation to the intestinal mucosa must be eliminated.

### Incontinence

**Faecal incontinence** is the inability to control passage of faeces and flatus from the anus. Physical conditions that impair anal sphincter function or control may cause incontinence, such as obstetric trauma, perianal inflammatory bowel disease, rectal prolapse or severe haemorrhoids. The person who produces frequent, loose, large volume, watery stools may be unable to retain control and can experience minor soiling or major incontinence. Impaired pelvic or anorectal sensation, or motor function, can result from stroke, spinal cord injury, multiple sclerosis or brain tumours and these people may be unable to recognize or respond to normal rectal stimuli. Similarly, an individual with a mental disorder such as schizophrenia, severe depression or dementia may not respond to the stimulus to defaecate.

Incontinence can harm a person's body image. In many situations the person is mentally alert but physically unable to avoid defaecation. The embarrassment of soiling the clothes can lead to social isolation. The patient/client must depend on the nurse for a basic need. Individuals with mental or sensory alterations often are unaware that they have passed a stool. The nurse must understand and support the patient/client even though repeated cleaning of an incontinent individual can become frustrating.

Like diarrhoea, incontinence predisposes the skin to breakdown. The nurse must check often to be sure perianal and perineal regions are clean and dry.

### Flatulence

As gas accumulates in the lumen of the intestine, the bowel wall stretches and distends **(flatulence)**. It is a common cause of abdominal fullness, pain, and cramping. Normally, intestinal gas escapes through the mouth (belching) or the anus (passing of flatus). However, if there is a reduction in intestinal motility resulting from opiates, general anaesthetics, abdominal surgery, or immobilization, flatulence can become severe enough to cause abdominal distention. In addition, accumulation of gas forces the diaphragm up and reduces lung expansion, and shortness of breath can occur.

A person normally produces several hundred millilitres of gas. Swallowed air makes up over 75% of intestinal gas. Bacterial decomposition of food in the colon releases methane gas. Carbon dioxide is a product of fermentation in the bowel. Any factor that causes gas (for example, ingestion of onions, beans, and cauliflower) increases intestinal flatulence.

### Haemorrhoids

**Haemorrhoids** are dilated, engorged veins in the lining of the rectum. They are either external or internal. External

## TABLE 23-3
## Conditions That Cause Diarrhoea

| Condition | Physiological Effects |
|---|---|
| Emotional stress (anxiety) | Increased intestinal motility |
| Intestinal infection (streptococcal or staphylococcal enteritis) | Inflammation of intestinal mucosa, increased mucous secretion in colon |
| Food allergies | Reduced digestion of food elements |
| Food intolerance (greasy foods, coffee, alcohol, spicy foods) | Increased intestinal motility, increased mucous secretion in colon |
| Medications | |
| Iron | Irritation of intestinal mucosa |
| Antibiotics | Suprainfection allowing overgrowth of normal flora, inflammation and irritation of mucosa |
| Laxatives (short term) | Increased intestinal motility |
| Colon disease (colitis, Crohn's disease) | Inflammation and ulceration of intestinal walls, reduced absorption of fluids, increased intestinal motility |
| Surgical alterations Gastrectomy | Loss of reservoir function of stomach, improper absorption because food is moved into duodenum too quickly |
| Colon resection | Reduced size of colon, reduced amount of absorptive surface |

haemorrhoids are clearly visible as protrusions of skin. If the underlying vein is hardened, there can be a purplish discolouration. Internal haemorrhoids have an outer mucous membrane. Increased venous pressure from straining at defaecation, pregnancy, congestive heart failure, and chronic liver disease can cause haemorrhoids.

Haemorrhoids bleed easily when stretched. Passage of a hard stool commonly causes bleeding. The haemorrhoids become inflamed and tender, and sufferers might complain of itching and burning. Because pain worsens during defaecation, the urge to defaecate might be ignored, resulting in constipation. Untreated, bleeding haemorrhoids are a cause of anaemia. Rectal bleeding should always be investigated. The reason for this is that rectal bleeding is commonly associated with cancer of the rectum.

## STOMA-FORMING SURGERY

The normal passage of faeces through the intestine and their evacuation from the rectum can be disrupted in individuals with bowel disease. Some of these people may require a surgical operation to resolve the problem during which the bowel is opened and brought to the surface of the abdomen through an incision in the abdominal wall (a **stoma**, Fig. 23-4). Faecal material which passes through the stoma is collected in a plastic

pouch (ostomy appliance, stoma bag) which adheres to the skin and is emptied or changed as required. A stoma may be formed in the ileum (**ileostomy**) or the colon (**colostomy**) and may be temporary or permanent. It is estimated that there are more than 100,000 people in England and Wales with a permanent stoma and approximately 18,500 people will require stoma-forming surgery each year (Wade, 1989).

The patient's/client's general condition and medical problem will determine the location and type of stoma the surgeon creates. Two basic types of stoma are constructed:
1. *Loop* colostomy or ileostomy.
2. *End* colostomy or ileostomy.

Loop stomas are usually temporary and performed in emergency situations, often to relieve an obstruction. The surgeon pulls a loop of bowel to the surface of the abdomen, after which it is opened by diathermy. A communicating wall remains between the proximal and distal bowel. To prevent the loop of bowel from slipping back, a rod or bridge is placed under it and sutured to the skin. This is usually removed 7–10 days after surgery on the surgeon's instructions. A loop colostomy is a large stoma as it has two openings. The proximal side drains the stool. The distal side will discharge only mucus, which is normally produced by the bowel.

End stomas have one opening where the proximal end of the cut bowel is sutured to the skin. If the distal portion of the bowel is completely removed, the stoma will be permanent. Most end colostomies are done for carcinoma of the rectum. This is removed and the stoma is constructed from the descending or sigmoid colon. If the distal portion of bowel is not excised, the surgeon will either oversew the cut end and replace it in the abdominal cavity (Hartmann's pouch) or bring it to the surface of the abdomen as a separate distal nonfunctioning stoma (mucous fistula), which produces only mucus. It may later be possible to join together the proximal and distal ends of the bowel so that continuity is restored and the individual regains normal function of the bowel.

The volume and consistency of stomal output will vary according to its position along the intestine. For instance, an ileostomy will produce a liquid output at frequent intervals, whereas a sigmoid colostomy will usually produce a formed stool only once or twice daily. Successful management of the patient/client with a stoma begins with knowledge of the type of stoma, the expected nature and volume of the effluent and the ability to select an appropriate appliance to meet the person's individual needs.

All patients/clients who undergo stoma forming surgery have major adjustments to make if they are to become independent in the practical managment of the stoma and achieve the fullest quality of life of which they are capable physically, psychologically and socially (RCN, 1981). It is natural for them to grieve over the loss of a body part, alteration in physical appearance, loss of control over bowel action and to experience feelings of mutilation, disfigurement and negative body image. Nurses in hospital and the community have a major role within the multidisciplinary team in planning and implementing

## Fig. 23-4  FOUR TYPES OF STOMA AND IMPLICATIONS FOR MANAGEMENT

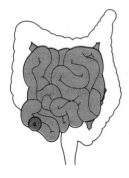 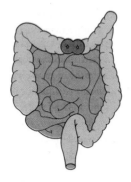 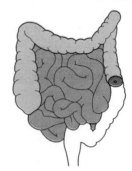 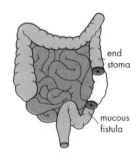

| A. End ileostomy | B. Transverse loop colostomy | C. End colostomy | D. End colostomy with mucous fistula |
|---|---|---|---|
| **STOMAL OUTPUT** | | | |
| Acts within 24 hours of surgery. Liquid/paste-like, fairly continuous. Contains digestive enzymes – highly corrosive in contact with skin. | Acts from 24–48 hours after surgery. Semi-formed to soft stool, with flatus, fairly continuous. Irritant to skin. | Acts from 48 hours after surgery, or later. Flatus produced first. Fairly firm to solid stool, once or twice daily. Fairly irritant to skin. | End stoma: see column 3. (N.B. A higher stoma may be formed - output will vary according to position) Mucous fistula: mucous discharge only. Varies in individuals from small to copious amounts. |
| **SUITABLE APPLIANCE** | | | |
| Drainable with clip/clamp at open end. Added skin protection, e.g. 'stomahesive' wafer. | Drainable with large enough opening to accommodate rod/bridge for first 7–10 days. Oval skin protective/adhesive backing provides larger area for attachment and greater security. | Closed appliance. Activated charcoal filter prevents appliance inflation by releasing flatus without odour – may be integral to pouch or applied separately. | End stoma: see column 3 and N.B. above. An activity pouch will accommodate a small output from mucous fistula. Copious amounts will require a drainable appliance with clip. |

**Fig. 23-4** Four types of stoma and implications for management. **A**, End ileostomy, **B**, transverse loop colostomy, **C**, end colostomy, **D**, end colostomy with mucous fistula.

individualized rehabilitation programmes to enable individuals to return to a normal life.

Advances in surgical knowledge and techniques now permit some patients/clients to avoid stoma formation. Stapling devices are used following large bowel resection to join the remaining bowel to the intact anal sphincter (ileoanal anastomosis). Surgeons can use sections of ileum to construct an internal reservoir for faeces (ileoanal pouch). These procedures avoid the stigma of a stoma and provide continence for suitable individuals.

## NURSING PROCESS AND BOWEL ELIMINATION

 ASSESSMENT

To assess bowel elimination patterns and determine abnormalities, the nurse takes a nursing history, inspects faecal characteristics, and reviews pertinent test results.

### Nursing History

It is essential that the nurse demonstrates sensitivity to the individual's feelings when obtaining information about elimination habits by conducting the interview in a private place where others cannot overhear (Roper *et al*, 1990). The nursing history (Fig. 23-5) provides a review of the patient's/client's usual bowel pattern and habits. What a person describes as 'normal' may be different from factors and conditions that tend to promote normal elimination. Identifying normal and abnormal patterns and habits allows the nurse to determine the patient's/client's problems. Much of the nursing history can be organized around the factors that affect elimination. The nurse then applies this knowledge through questions to determine the presence and extent of GI alterations. A typical nursing history of a person's elimination status includes the following:

1. Determination of the usual elimination pattern. Frequency and time of day are included.
2. Identification of routines followed to promote normal elimination. Examples are drinking hot liquids, using

laxatives, eating specific foods, or taking time to defaecate during a certain part of the day.

3. Description of any recent change in elimination pattern. This information is perhaps the most significant because elimination patterns are variable and the patient/client can best detect change. If there were changes in the person's last bowel movement, ask him or her to be very specific in describing the change and perhaps suggest a cause.

4. Patient's/client's description of usual characteristics of stool. Determine whether the stool is usually watery or formed, or soft or hard, as well as the typical colour. The patient/client also describes the stool's shape.

5. Diet history. Determine the patient's/client's dietary preferences for a day and note the intake of high and low fibre foods. Also determine whether mealtimes are regular or irregular, whether certain foods are eaten infrequently, and the reasons for this such as an inability to chew because of ill-fitting dentures.

6. Description of daily fluid intake. This includes the type and amount of fluid. The person might have to estimate the amount using common household measurements.

7. History of exercise. Ask the patient/client for a specific description of exercise patterns.

8. Assessment of the use of artificial aids at home. Assess whether the person uses enemas, laxatives, or special foods before having a bowel movement and the freqency with which he or she uses them. If the person is nursed at home, endeavour to follow his or her routine where possible. If aids are required the nurse should arrange these.

9. History of surgery or illnesses affecting the GI tract. This information can often help explain symptoms and provides an idea of the person's potential for maintaining or restoring a normal elimination pattern.

10. Presence and status of bowel diversions. If the person has a stoma, assess frequency of faecal drainage, character of faecal output, appearance and condition of the stoma (colour, swelling, and irritation), and type of appliance used.

11. Medication history. Ask whether the person takes medications (such as laxatives, antacids, iron supplements, and analgesics) that might alter defaecation or faecal characteristics.

12. Emotional state. The person's emotions can significantly alter frequency of defaecation. During assessment, observation of the patient's/client's emotions, tone of voice, and mannerisms can reveal significant behaviours that indicate stress.

13. Social history. If the patient/client is not independent in bowel management, determine who assists the individual and how.

14. Home environment. Establish the patient's/client's mobility and the location of the toilet. If the individual has difficulty reaching the toilet, ask if he or she has use of a commode or sanilav.

The objective of assessing a patient/client with faecal incontinence is to establish an effective plan to resolve or manage the incontinence. A careful history and assessment can establish

**Children's Nursing**
**Educating children about stomas**

Implementing individualized programmes is very important when caring for children and their families. The child's individual knowledge regarding his or her health problem needs to be assessed and coping strategies identified.

It is essential to know the child's developmental stage and how this relates to health related beliefs. For example, in early childhood some children view illness as a punishment. They may also imagine that their bodies are hollow containers for blood and fluid. When explaining stoma formation to these children, it is important to use dolls, teddies and diagrams of the body as teaching aids.

Children between 5–8 years rely less on what they see and more on what they know — that the body is made up of food, water, urine and faeces. They also recognize bones, brains and eyes. Body integrity is very important to children at this age and they are very sensitive if anything threatens it. The nurse must be aware of this, and must promote partnership and trust with the child.

Adolescents are more realistic about body parts and functions, but give greater importance to peer values and norms — anything that makes them look 'different' threatens their self concept and body image. In order to ensure an adaptive response, the children's nurse must understand the behaviour manifested during each developmental stage and should adapt his or her interventions to each individual child.

the cause of the problem, its severity and effect on the individual's normal lifestyle and ensure that realistic goals are set. An incontinence record or bowel function diary provides information about incontinent episodes, as well as any successful voluntary bowel movements, and can be used to assess the patient's/client's progress in bowel training programmes.

## Faecal Characteristics

Inspection of faecal characteristics (Table 23-4) reveals information about the nature of elimination alterations. Several factors can influence each characteristic. A key to assessment is knowing whether there have been any recent changes. The patient/client can best provide this information.

## Laboratory and Diagnostic Tests

Laboratory and diagnostic examinations yield useful information concerning elimination problems. Laboratory analysis of faecal contents can detect pathological conditions such as tumours, haemorrhage, and infection.

### FAECAL SPECIMENS

The nurse is directly responsible for ensuring that specimens are accurately obtained, properly labelled in appropriate containers, and transported to the laboratory on time. Institutions provide special containers for faecal specimens. Some tests require specimens to be placed in chemical preservatives.

Because about 25% of the solid portion of a stool is bacteria

Name _____ Sex   M ____   F ____   Age _____

**Duration of incontinence** _____

_____

**Degree of incontinence**

Discharge _____   Soiling _____   Urgency _____   Gas _____   Liquid _____   Solid _____

**Bowel habit**

Number of stool movements per day _____

**Stool consistency**

Watery _____   Loose _____   Formed _____   Hard _____

**Frequency of incontinence**

Number of episodes per day _____        Number of days of incontinence per week _____

Time of day _____   Time of night _____

**Relevant medical history**

Number of pregnancies/deliveries _____   Traumatic delivery? _____

History of anorectal surgery _____   Gastrointestinal surgery _____

Trauma to perineum _____   Trauma to spinal cord (level) _____

Neurological disease _____   Diabetes _____   Radiotherapy _____

Urinary incontinence _____   Impotence _____

Medication for diarrhoea _____   Other medications _____

Other illness _____

_____

**Fig.23-5  Form for assessment of patient history.** *From MacLeod JH: Endoscopy Rev **5**:45, 1988.*

from the colon, the nurse should wear disposable gloves when collecting and handling specimens.

Handwashing is necessary for anyone who might come in contact with the specimen. Often the patient/client can obtain the specimen if properly instructed. The nurse explains that faeces cannot be mixed with urine or water. For this reason the individual must defaecate into a clean, dry bedpan or special container placed under the toilet seat.

Tests performed by the laboratory for **occult blood** in the stool and **stool cultures** require only a small sample. The nurse collects about an inch of formed stool or 15 to 30 ml of liquid diarrhoeal stool. To avoid contact with faeces while transferring solid specimens to a container, the nurse should wear gloves and use the spoon attached to the lid of the container, or a wooden tongue depressor. The nurse must pour liquid specimens carefully into the proper container and ensure they do not contaminate the outer surface. Tests for measuring the output of faecal fat require a 3- to 5-day collection of stool. All faecal material must be saved throughout the test period.

After obtaining a specimen, removing the gloves and washing his or her hands, the nurse labels the sealed container and ensures the appropriate specimen request form has been completed. The nurse then records specimen collections in the patient's/client's nursing record. It is important to avoid delays in sending specimens to the laboratory. Some tests such as measurement for ova and parasites require the stool to be warm. When stool specimens are allowed to stand at room temperature, bacteriological changes that alter test results can occur.

## DIAGNOSTIC EXAMINATIONS

A person may have a diagnostic examination as an outpatient or inpatient. Visualization of GI structures may be by a direct or indirect approach.

**Direct Visualization**  Instruments introduced through the mouth (upper GI viewing) allow the doctor to inspect the integrity of mucosa, blood vessels, and organ parts. A **fibreoptic endoscope** is an optical instrument with a lens viewer, a long flexible tube, and a light source at the end. It allows viewing of structures at the tip of the tube and insertion of special

**TABLE 23-4 Faecal Characteristics**

| Characteristic | Normal | Abnormal | Cause |
|---|---|---|---|
| Colour | Infant: yellow; adult: brown | White or clay<br>Black or tarry (melaena) | Absence of bile<br>Iron ingestion or upper GI bleeding |
| | | Red | Lower GI bleeding, haemorrhoids |
| | | Pale with fat | Malabsorption of fat |
| Odour | Pungent; affected by food type | Noxious change | Blood in faeces or infection |
| Consistency | Soft, formed | Liquid | Diarrhoea, reduced absorption |
| | | Hard | Constipation |
| Frequency | Varies: infant 4 to 6 times daily (breast-fed) or 1 to 3 times daily (bottle fed); adult daily or 2 to 3 times a week | Infant more than 6 times daily or less than once every 1–2 days; adult more than 3 times a day or less than once a week | Hypomotility or hypermotility |
| Amount | 150 g per day (adult) | | |
| Shape | Resembles diameter of rectum | Narrow, pencil shaped | Obstruction, rapid peristalsis |
| Constituents | Undigested food, dead bacteria, fat, bile pigment, cells lining intestinal mucosa, water | Blood, pus, foreign bodies, mucus, worms | Internal bleeding, infection, swallowed objects, irritation, inflammation |

instruments for biopsy. The tube is flexible to minimize trauma and discomfort to the patient/client.

**Proctoscopes** and **sigmoidoscopes** are rigid, tube-shaped instruments with attached light sources. They are introduced through the rectum. These instruments are less flexible than fibreoptic scopes and more capable of causing discomfort.

UGI (upper gastrointestinal) **endoscopy** or **gastroscopy** allows visualization of the oesophagus, stomach, and duodenum. The doctor inspects for tumours, vascular changes, mucosal inflammation, ulcers, hernias, and obstructions. A gastroscope enables the doctor to remove tissue specimens **(biopsy)**, remove abnormal tissue growth **(polyps)**, and coagulate sources of bleeding. A flexible colonoscopy enables the doctor to examine the colon.

Sigmoidoscopy allows visualization of the anus, rectum, and sigmoid colon. Proctoscopy allows visualization of the anus and rectum. Both tests enable the doctor to collect tissue specimens and coagulate sources of bleeding.

**Indirect Visualization** When direct visualization is impossible (as with deeper GI structures), the doctor relies on indirect x-ray examination. The patient/client ingests a **contrast medium** or has the medium given as an enema. One of the most common media is barium, a white, chalky, radiopaque substance. It is used in UGI studies and barium enemas. Contrast media usually contain a flavouring agent for better taste.

UGI study is an x-ray study of an ingested contrast medium that allows the doctor to visualize the lower oesophagus, stomach, and duodenum. The doctor notes ulcerations, inflammation, tumours, and anatomical malposition of organs. The patency of organs and the pyloric valve are also observed.

Small bowel follow-through (continuation of UGI) allows the doctor to examine the small intestine. The flow of barium through the intestine may suggest motility problems. A barium enema allows indirect visualization of the lower colon to reveal location of tumours, polyps, and **diverticula**. The doctor can also detect positional abnormalities.

Specific instructions are given by the endoscopy and x-ray departments to prepare patients/clients for these investigations. On return to the ward, regular observation of the individual is often requested so that complications can be detected.

 **PLANNING**

Nursing assessment of the patient's/client's bowel function may indicate an actual or potential elimination problem. The care planning process includes measures to ensure maintenance of normal bowel function by incorporating the patient's/client's elimination habits or routines as much as possible. If the habits caused the elimination problem, the nurse helps the person learn new ones. Defecation patterns vary among individuals. For this reason, the nurse and patient/client must work together closely to plan effective interventions (see care plan).

When individuals are disabled or debilitated by illness, it is necessary to include the family in the care plan. Often family members have the same ineffective elimination habits as the patient/client. Thus patient/client and family teaching is an important part of the care plan. Other health team members such as dietitians and enterostomal therapists (stoma care nurse specialists) can be valuable resources.

The goals of care for individuals with elimination problems include:

- understanding normal elimination
- attaining regular defaecation habits
- understanding and maintaining proper fluid and food intake
- achieving a regular exercise programme
- achieving comfort
- maintaining skin integrity
- maintaining self-concept.

### Children's Nursing
### Constipation in children

Children who suffer from constipation may improve if nursing interventions include a 'stool chart': children who open their bowels successfully are praised and given a coloured star (usually gold); if they have their bowels open but soil, they receive a different coloured star. It is important to recognize that this method is based on praise and reward. Never punish a child for failing to meet the required goal.

'Retraining' usually means retraining the whole family. Research suggests that mothers tend to be tense, anxious and overprotective, and often use corrective methods during toilet training (Turner, 1991).

 ## IMPLEMENTATION

Success of the nurse's interventions depends on improving the patient's/client's and family members' understanding of bowel elimination. In the home, hospital, or long-term care facility, individuals capable of learning can be taught effective bowel habits.

The nurse should teach the patient/client and family about a healthy diet, adequate fluid intake, and factors that stimulate or slow peristalsis, such as emotional stress. The patient/client should also learn the importance of establishing regular bowel routines and regular exercise and taking appropriate measures when elimination problems develop. When complications develop from elimination problems, the nurse can teach the patient/client and family members to give proper skin care, administer enemas, and monitor drug effects.

The special needs of people with a stoma often require extensive education. Patients/clients learn the skills needed to apply stomal appliances and administer skin care.

### Promotion of Regular Bowel Habits

One of the most important habits a nurse can teach regarding bowel habits is to take time for defaecation. Ignoring the urge to defaecate and not taking time to defaecate completely are common causes of constipation. To establish regular bowel habits, a person must know when the urge to defaecate normally occurs.

The nurse advises the person to begin establishing a routine during a time when defaecation is most likely to occur, usually an hour after a meal. If attempts are made to defaecate during the time when mass colonic peristalsis occurs, the chances of success are great. If a person is restricted to bed or requires assistance in ambulating, the nurse should offer a bedpan or help the person reach the lavatory. The nurse must be prompt in assisting before the urge disappears or the individual becomes incontinent.

Many people have established rituals for defaecation. In a hospital or long-term care facility, the nurse should make certain that treatment routines do not interfere with these routines. This is important when the person is nursed at home. It is also important to provide privacy. When patients/clients are forced to

use a bedpan, pull the curtain around the area so the person can relax, knowing that interruptions will not occur. Always place the call bell within the person's reach. Close lavatory doors, but stand nearby in case the person needs assistance.

### Promotion of Normal Defaecation

To help people evacuate bowel contents normally and without discomfort, a number of interventions can stimulate the defaecation reflex, affect the character of faeces, or increase peristalsis.

### SQUATTING POSITION

Toilets may be too low for individuals unable to lower themselves to a squatting position because of joint or muscle diseases. Patients/clients can be provided with elevated toilet seats for the home. In orthopaedic and rehabilitation units in a health care centre, toilet seats are usually elevated.

### POSITIONING ON BEDPAN

Patients/clients restricted to bed must use bedpans for defaecation, but these can be extremely uncomfortable. The nurse should help position patients/clients comfortably.

Two types of bedpans are available (Fig. 23-6). The bedpan, made of metal or hard plastic, has a curved smooth upper end and a sharp-edged lower end and is about 5 cm deep. A **fracture pan**, designed for patients/clients with body or leg plasters, has a shallow upper end about 1.3 cm deep. The upper end of the pan fits under the buttocks towards the sacrum, with the lower end just under the upper thighs. The pan should be high enough so that faeces enter it. A metal bedpan should be warmed with water first, then dried.

When positioning a patient/client, it is important to prevent muscle strain and discomfort. A person should never be placed on a bedpan and then left lying flat unless activity restrictions demand it. If the person is flat, the hips remain hyperextended. It may be necessary to have the person flat when placing him or her on the bedpan. After the patient/client is on it, raise the head of the bed 30 degrees. Raising the person to a 90-degree angle makes positioning difficult. In a sitting position, the patient/client must rise straight up while using the strength of the arms as the nurse positions the pan. Most patients/clients are too

## SAMPLE NURSING CARE PLAN FOR A CLIENT WITH CONSTIPATION

Robert Fitzgerald is a student in his first term at University. He has moved from the family home to a flat and is responsible for buying, preparing and cooking his own food for the first time. Robert attended the Student Health Centre and, when seen by the doctor, described a change in bowel habit from a soft formed stool daily after breakfast to once every 3–4 days accompanied by straining. After a physical examination, he has been referred to the practice nurse.

### Assessment

Questioning and discussion enable the nurse to obtain a full nursing history and elicit the following information: stools passed are now brown, marblelike and hard. Typical daily food intake consists of white bread and butter, snacks of crisps and chocolate, a frozen convenience meal or 'fast food' takeaway. Fruit and vegetables are rarely eaten. Daily fluid intake is two cups of coffee, a glass of milk and one can of soft drink. Robert used to cycle and play squash but has not done so since he came to university.

| PROBLEM | GOALS | NURSING ACTION | EVALUATION | RATIONALE |
|---|---|---|---|---|
| Constipation due to low intake of dietary fibre, inadequate fluids and lack of exercise | Robert will describe and consume food and fluid required to promote soft formed stools within 48 hours | Outline process of normal elimination and factors which influence this Describe specific foods which are high in fibre and ascertain preferences Discuss the need for a fluid intake of 1.5–2 L a day and how this can be achieved | Robert will be able to list a range of high fibre foods for inclusion in his diet Robert's written meal plans will include foods and fluid suited to his elimination needs which promote normal defaecation | High fibre foods increase peristalsis and help propel intestinal contents through GI tract by increasing stool mass and fluid content (Brown and Everett, 1990) Adequate fluid intake helps keep faecal material soft (Ewing, 1989) |
| | | Assist Robert to develop 2 daily meal plans Obtain commitment to follow meal plans, to plan and eat appropriate meals for a further 5 days, and to keep a written record of intake during this time | Robert will state that his diet and fluid intake matched his meal plans over the previous 7 days | Behavioural contracts between nurse and Robert have demonstrated success for behavioural modification (Gilpatrick, 1989) |
| | | Give Robert educational booklet, about healthy eating to read at home | | Written material provides reinforcement of verbal instruction and facilitates retention of information (Castledine, 1988) |
| | Robert will resume regular exercise within 1 week | Discuss benefits of walking and cycling in relation to normal elimination | Robert will be able to describe one form of exercise in which he has participated daily during the previous 7 days | Physical activity increases muscle tone (Wright, 1974), facilitating voluntary contraction during defaecation |
| | | Provide verbal and written information on location of sports facilities and opportunities for use | | |
| | | Obtain verbal commitment from Robert to participate in at least one form of exercise daily over the next 7 days | | (Cont'd) |

## SAMPLE NURSING CARE PLAN FOR A CLIENT WITH CONSTIPATION (Cont'd)

| PROBLEM | GOALS | NURSING ACTION | EVALUATION | RATIONALE |
|---------|-------|----------------|------------|-----------|
| Constipation due to low intake of dietary fibre, inadequate fluids and lack of exercise. | Robert will return to usual defaecation pattern within 3 days | Discuss the importance of responding to urge to defaecate when it occurs for resumption of normal pattern of elimination | Robert will describe appropriate actions undertaken to resume normal bowel elimination routine | |
| | | Inform Robert of the optimum time for defaecation in relation to previous habits i.e. half to 1 hour after breakfast | Robert will demonstrate an understanding of actions which promote normal defaecation by listing those he has incorporated into his routine during the previous 7 days | Gastrocolic reflex is most sensitive in the morning and after meals (Goldfinger, 1991) |
| | | Discuss Robert's present daily morning routine and suitable strategies for making time available for defaecation to occur | Robert will state that he is now able to pass soft stools without straining | |
| | | Obtain verbal commitment from Robert to implement appropriate actions to promote normal defaecation during the next 7 days | Robert will state that his regular pattern of daily defaecation after breakfast has returned | |

weak to accomplish this. Those who have had abdominal surgery are hesitant to exert strain on suture lines. The nurse should not risk injury by trying to lift a weak person onto the bedpan alone, but should ask a colleague for help.

Fig. 23-7 shows proper and improper positions on bedpans. The best method is to be sure the patient/client is positioned high in bed. Raise the individual's head about 30 degrees, to prevent hyperextension of the back, and provide support to the upper torso as the person raises his or her hips, by bending the knees and lifting the hips upward. The nurse places a hand palm under the patient's/client's sacrum, resting the elbow on the mattress and using it as a lever to help in lifting, while slipping the pan under the patient/client.

If the patient/client is immobile or it is unsafe to allow him or her to exert such effort, he or she can roll onto the bedpan by using the following steps:

1. Flatten the backrest, remove excess pillows and assist the patient/client to roll onto one side, backside towards you.
2. Apply powder lightly to back and buttocks to prevent skin from sticking to the pan.
3. Place the bedpan firmly against the buttocks, down into the mattress with the open rim towards the patient's/client's feet (Fig. 23-8).
4. Keeping your hand against the bedpan, place the other around the patient's/client's far hip. Ask him or her to roll back onto the pan, flat in bed.
5. With the patient/client positioned comfortably, raise the head of the bed 30 degrees.
6. Place a rolled towel or small pillow under the lumbar curve of the patient's/client's back for added comfort.
7. Ask the patient/client to bend his or her knees to assume a squatting position, unless this is contraindicated.

Always maintain the privacy of a patient/client using a bedpan. Place the call bell and a supply of toilet paper within easy reach. When the person finishes, respond to the call signal *immediately* and remove the pan. The patient/client might require assistance with wiping. To remove the pan, ask the person to roll off to the

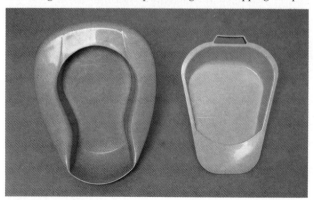

**Fig. 23-6** Types of bedpans. From left, usual bedpan and fracture bedpan.

side or to raise his or her hips. Hold the pan steady to avoid spilling. Avoid pulling or pushing the pan from under the patient's/client's hips, because this can pull the patient's/client's skin and cause tissue injury. Wear gloves to clean the anal and perineal areas. Provide a bowl of water, soap and a towel for the patient/client to handwash after bedpan use.

After assessing the stool, immediately empty the bedpan's contents into the toilet or in a special receptacle in the utility room. Rinse the bedpan thoroughly before placing it in the bedpan washer. In the client's home wash and dry the bedpan thoroughly. Dispose of disposable bedpans according to manufacturer's instructions. Chart the characteristics of the faeces.

Offer the bedpan often. Patients/clients may accidentally soil bedclothes if forced to wait. Many individuals try to avoid using a bedpan because it is embarrassing and uncomfortable. They may try to get to the lavatory even though their conditions prohibit ambulation. The nurse must warn patients/clients about the risk of falls or accidents. If the patient's/client's condition permits, defaecation is easier if assisted onto a bedside commode, or the person can be wheeled on a sanichair to the lavatory where privacy is assured.

## TABLE 23-5 Common Types of Oral Laxatives

| Agent/Brand Name | Action | Indications | Risks |
|---|---|---|---|
| **BULK FORMING**<br>Methylcellulose | High-fibre content absorbs water and increases faecal mass. | Agents are least irritating, most natural, and safest laxatives | Agents can cause obstruction if not mixed with at least 240 ml of water or juice and swallowed quickly. |
| Sterculia<br>Ispaghula husk<br>Unprocessed wheat bran | Agents stretch intestinal wall to stimulate peristalsis | Agents are drugs of choice for chronic constipation (e.g. pregnancy, low-residue diet).<br>Agents may also be used to relieve mild, watery diarrhoea. | Caution is used with bulk-forming laxatives that also contain stimulants. Agents are not used in clients for whom large fluid intake is contraindicated.<br>Full effect may take some days to develop. |
| **FAECAL SOFTENERS**<br>Docusate sodium<br><br>Liquid paraffin | Stool softeners are detergents that lower surface tension of faeces, allowing water and fat to penetrate. They may increase secretion of water by intestine. | Agents are used for short-term therapy to relieve straining on defaecation (e.g. haemorrhoids, perianal surgery, pregnancy, recovery from myocardial infarction). | Agents are of little value for treatment of chronic constipation.<br>Liquid paraffin can lead to anal seepage and irritation with prolonged use. |
| **OSMOTIC LAXATIVES**<br>Magnesium hydroxide<br><br>Magnesium sulphate<br><br>Lactulose | Agents contain salt preparation not absorbed by intestines.<br>Osmotic effect increases pressure in bowel to act as stimulant for peristalsis.<br>Agents may also lubricate faeces. | Agents are normally used only for acute emptying of bowel (e.g. endoscopic examination, suspected poisoning, acute constipation). | Agents are not used in long-term management of constipation.<br>Agents are not used in patients/clients with kidney dysfunction (toxic build-up of magnesium). |
| **STIMULANT LAXATIVES**<br>Bisacodyl<br>Castor oil<br>Senna | Agents irritate intestinal mucosa to increase motility.<br>Agents decrease absorption in small bowel and colon. | Agents may be used to prepare bowel for diagnostic procedures. | Agents may cause severe cramping.<br>Agents are not for long-term use.<br>Chronic use may cause fluid and electrolyte imbalances.<br>Agents are avoided during pregnancy and lactation. |

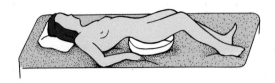

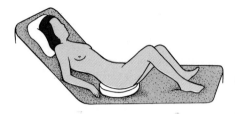

Fig. 23-7 Positions on a bedpan. *Top*, Improper positioning of patient/client. *Bottom*, Proper position reduces patient's/client's back strain.

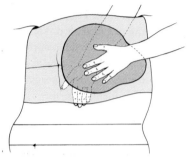

Fig. 23-8 Positioning an immobilized patient/client on a bedpan.

## LAXATIVES

Often a patient/client is unable to defaecate normally because of pain, constipation, or impaction. Laxatives have the short-term action of emptying the bowel. They are also used in bowel evacuation for people undergoing GI tests and abdominal surgery. Laxatives which have a very strong action on the intestines are sometimes referred to as *cathartics* or *purgatives* (Table 23-5).

Laxatives are available in oral, enema and suppository dosage forms. Although the oral route is more commonly used, laxatives that come prepared as suppositories are more effective because of their stimulant effect on the rectal mucosa.

Teach patients/clients about the potential harmful effects of repeated use of laxatives and that they are not meant for long-term maintenance of bowel function.

## ANTIDIARRHOEAL AGENTS

For individuals with diarrhoea, frequent passage of liquid stools can severely restrict their normal lifestyle. Opiates, such as codeine phosphate and diphenoxylate (lomotil), are effective antidiarrhoel agents. Antidiarrhoeal opiate agents decrease intestinal muscle tone to slow passage of faeces. Opiates inhibit peristaltic waves that move faeces forward, but they also increase segmental contractions that mix intestinal contents. As a result, more water is absorbed by the intestinal walls. Antidiarrhoeal agents should be used with caution because opiates are habit forming.

Loperamide HCl (Imodium) controls diarrhoea by reducing the motility of the GI tract. Adsorbent mixtures of chalk and kaolin may be effective in controlling diarrhoea. Bulk forming drugs such as methylcellulose increase faecal mass and can be used effectively in treating diarrhoea as well as constipation. Methylcellulose is especially useful for increasing faecal consistency when used with individuals who have ileostomy and colostomy and experience troublesome fluid output. Antidiarrhoeal drugs relieve symptoms but do not treat the cause of diarrhoea, which should always be investigated if it persists.

## ENEMAS AND SUPPOSITORIES

An **enema** is instillation of a fluid into the rectum and sigmoid colon. An evacuant enema promotes defaecation by stimulating peristalsis. The volume of fluid instilled into the bowel breaks up the faecal mass, stretches the rectal wall and initiates the defaecation reflex. Evacuant enemas can be used to provide temporary relief from constipation, remove impacted faeces, empty the bowel before diagnostic tests or surgery and before commencing a programme of bowel training.

The basic principles in administering an enema are shown in Procedure 23-1.

Soap and water enemas of a large volume have fallen into disrepute, because they have been associated with shock following bowel distension and irritation of the bowel lining (Clarke, 1988). Fletcher's phosphate enema is commercially prepared and consists of a plastic sachet containing 128 ml of solution with a rectal tube for administration. Once in the bowel, the hypertonic solution pulls fluid out of the interstitial spaces. The colon fills with fluid and the resulting distension promotes defaecation. Microenemas contain a wetting agent or faecal softener in only 5 ml of solution. This low volume is especially suitable for the frail and elderly who often have less competent anal sphincters and cannot retain large amounts of fluid, and may be at more risk of dehydration from fluid depletion if stronger hypertonic solutions are used.

Retention enemas are intended to remain in the bowel for a specified period of time. This is achieved by enabling the patient/client to remain in bed in a comfortable position after the enema is given and elevating the foot of the bed by 35–45 degrees. A commercially prepared 120 ml arachis oil retention enema should be warmed to 37–40°C in a small bowl of water before it is given and will soften faeces and make them easier to pass. The patient/client may defaecate in the normal way or the enema may be followed by an evacuant enema.

Medicated enemas contain drugs which either act locally or are effectively absorbed through the bowel mucosa. Corticosteroid retention enemas contain hydrocortisone or prednisolone and are used to relieve the inflammation of ulcerative colitis or proctitis. The patient/client is taught how to administer the enema at bedtime, which should be retained for a least an hour. It is helpful if a parent is present to comfort and calm a child who requires an enema. Explain each step of the procedure to them both and allow the child to see and touch the equipment beforehand.

## PROCEDURE 23-1   GIVING AN ENEMA

| SEQUENCE OF ACTIONS | RATIONALE |
|---|---|
| 1. Inform the patient/client of the intended activity and explain the procedure. | To obtain consent and cooperation and reduce anxiety of the patient/client during the prodedure (Wilson-Barnett, 1978). |
| 2. Allow the patient/client to empty his/her bladder. | A full bladder can cause discomfort during the procedure. |
| 3. Collect appropriate equipment: | |
| • disposable, prepackaged enema warmed in a bowl/jug of water to 37 - 40°C, measured with a bath thermometer | • a cold solution can cause abdominal cramping and is difficult to retain. A hot solution can scald and damage rectal mucosa |
| • lubricating jelly | • eases introduction of rectal tube by reducing friction and mucosal irritation |
| • waterproof incontinence pad | • to protect bedclothes and prevent soiling |
| • toilet tissues and gauze squares | • to maintain patient's/client's personal hygiene |
| • disposable gloves | • prevents transmission of microorganisms from faeces and reduces risk of cross infection |
| 4. Pull curtains around the patient's/client's bed or close the door to the room. | To provide privacy and reduce embarrassment. |
| 5. With the patient/client on the bed, arrange clothing so that hips and buttocks are exposed. Place an incontinence pad under the person, then cover with a blanket so that only the anal area is exposed. | Prevents faecal soiling of clothing and bedlinen if enema is not completely retained. Provides warmth, minimizes embarrassment, demonstrates concern for dignity and helps reduce anxiety. |
| 6. Position the patient/client on the left side with buttocks near the edge of the bed and the right knee well flexed. | Facilitates downward flow of enema solution by gravity into the rectum and sigmoid colon. Flexing the knee permits easier insertion of the administration tubing. |
| 7. Wash hands thoroughly, dry, and put on disposable gloves. | Reduces risk of cross infection through faecal contamination. |
| 8. Use gauze to apply lubricant jelly to tubing, then remove cap from the tip of tubing. | Facilitates insertion and reduces the  risk of trauma to the rectal mucosa. |
| 9. Instruct the patient/client to breathe slowly and deeply through the mouth while tube and fluid are inserted. | Promotes relaxation of external anal sphincter and facilitates introduction of administration tube. |
| 10. Administer the enema by separating the buttocks and inserting enema tube to about 10 cm. Slowly roll the tubing from the bottom upwards until all solution has been given. | Ensures fluid is delivered into the rectum. Slow administration prevents irritation and distension of the bowel wall, and avoids the risk of premature evacuation due to increased peristalsis. |
| 11. Gently withdraw the tube and wipe dry the patient's/client's perianal area with gauze or toilet tissue. | Reduces risk of immediate bowel evacuation. Prevents irritation/excoriation of the perianal area and promotes patient/client comfort and cleanliness. |
| 12a. Ask patient/client to remain in bed and retain evacuant solution for 10–15 minutes. | Longer retention promotes more effective stimulation of peristalsis and defaecation. |
| 12b. If a retention enema is given, raise the foot of the bed about 45° and ask patient/client to remain in bed and retain enema as long as prescribed. | Position aids retention of the enema by the patient/client for the desired period. |
| 13. Discard used items and gloves into yellow disposable bag. | To prevent accidental crossinfection through faecal contamination. |
| 14. Provide call bell for patient/client. Check that toilet is available or bring a bedpan/commode to bedside. If necessary, assist patient/client to use toilet facilities. | Access to appropriate facilities prevents accidental soiling and decreases anxiety. |
| 15. Note and record in nursing notes character of stool and fluid passed. | Communicates relevant information to other health team members and provides a record of bowel function. |
| 16. Assist patient/client to meet personal hygiene needs and rearrange clothing if required. | Faeces are irritant to the skin. Promotes feelings of cleanliness and maintainance of dignity. |

A **suppository** is a solid or semisolid pellet introduced into the anal canal which acts by dissolving at body temperature to release medication, to sooth and treat haemorrhoids or itching or to empty a constipated bowel. Less uncomfortable to the patient/client and easier to administer, they are often preferred to an enema. Glycerine or Bisacodyl suppositories promote peristalsis by increasing intestinal motility. The basic principles in administering a suppository (see Procedure 31-2) are to:

- collect the appropriate items of equipment
- prepare the patient/client for the procedure
- perform the procedure safely and effectively
- maintain the dignity, comfort and personal cleanliness of the patient/client
- record relevant information accurately in the patient's/client's nursing records.

## MANAGEMENT OF FAECAL INCONTINENCE

The individual with faecal incontinence is unable to maintain bowel control. Environmental measures can promote continence. These include easy access to toilet facilities, ensuring aids to walking are at hand, and rails fitted to toilet walls. Clothing with velcro fastenings or elasticated waistbands prevent delay when the patient/client feels the urge to defaecate. Stools of normal consistency and volume can be produced by manipulation of the diet and the use of appropriate medication can enable some individuals to regain control. If faecal continence cannot be achieved, it will need to be contained. Pads and pants with a variety of fastenings are available. Protective garments need to be tried and their effectiveness evaluated and it may take some time before the product which best meets the person's individual needs is found. External collection devices consist of a drainable plastic pouch with an adhesive skin barrier placed over the perianal area. The use of such a device ensures that **excoriation** is prevented, comfort maintained and odour avoided if the person with acute diarrhoea is faecally incontinent.

Biofeedback therapy, muscle toning exercises, bowel training programmes or a combination of these methods help some individuals, including those with sensory and motor deficits and the elderly, to achieve normal control of defaecation. In a bowel training programme, a daily routine is set up which is normal and acceptable for the individual and his or her lifestyle.

By attempting to defaecate at the same time each day and using measures that promote defaecation, the patient/client gains control of bowel reflexes. The programme requires time, patience, and consistency. The doctor determines the person's physical readiness and ability to benefit from bowel training. A successful programme includes:

1. Assessing the normal elimination pattern and recording times when the patient/client is incontinent.
2. Choosing a time in the individual's pattern to initiate defaecation-control measures and establishing a regular time for bowel movement which is appropriate for the individual.
3. Giving stool softeners orally every day or an evacuant suppository at least half an hour before the selected defaecation time. Rectal emptying can be stimulated if necessary by using suppositories or microenemas.

4. Offering a hot drink or fruit juice (or whatever fluids normally stimulate peristalsis for the patient/client) 0.5–1 hour before the defaecation time.
5. Assisting the person to the toilet within 15 minutes of the designated time, and also whenever rectal distension or the urge to defaecate are felt.
6. Providing privacy and setting a time limit for defaecation (15–20 minutes).
7. Instructing the person to lean forward at the hips while sitting on the toilet, to apply manual pressure with the hands over the abdomen, and to bear down but not strain to stimulate colon emptying.
8. Not criticizing or conveying frustration if the person is unable to defaecate.
9. Providing regular meals with adequate fluids and fibre to normalize stool consistency.
10. Maintaining normal exercise within the patient's/client's physical ability.

The patient/client will require positive reinforcement and encouragement. It often takes several days to weeks before training is successful.

**Caring for the person with a stoma** In hospital, individuals with a newly formed temporary or permanent stoma face uncertainty about their future lives and need to acquire knowledge and information about practical issues and the basic skills to deal with the stoma (Kelly and Henry, 1992). It is essential to assess each individual's needs, concerns and unique circumstances and then implement a planned programme of teaching in which realistic, specific, short-term goals are set (Curry, 1991; Donaldson, 1989). The box on p.475 lists specific areas for inclusion.

Teaching should proceed at the individual's own pace and not be attempted with a person who is in pain or tired. Motivation to learn can be increased by encouraging the patient/client to evaluate his or her progress towards goal achievement, and through providing genuine praise and positive feedback.

### Promoting self-care

The patient's/client's ability to change the appliance successfully is usually the criteria for discharge (Donaldson, 1989). A transparent, drainable appliance is fitted in the operating theatre and remains in place for several days. This allows frequent observation of the stoma. A healthy stoma with a good blood supply is dark pink (similar to the inside of the mouth) and shiny. Dullness and a change of colour to blue-black indicates a reduced blood supply and should be reported immediately, as should a stoma that either becomes much longer or seems to disappear

---

**Children's Nursing**
**Retention enemas in children**

Never give a retention enema to a child younger than six years of age. The child won't be able to retain it. For older children the amount of solution is important; smaller children require smaller amounts.

below the skin surface. The stoma will be swollen and oedematous at first, gradually decreasing in size over 6–8 weeks. Some stomas will act and produce faecal material very soon after surgery. The postoperative appliance can be emptied without disturbing the patient/client. Emptying is done when the bag is a quarter to a third full, before the weight of faecal fluid becomes enough to pull the appliance away from the skin and cause leakage. The postoperative appliance is changed for a suitable ostomy pouch after considering the type, site and size of the stoma, volume of output, patient's/client's body contours and skin condition, manual dexterity and eyesight, normal activity levels and lifestyle.

At first, the patient/client will not usually want to look at the stoma, but will closely observe the nurse's facial expression and reactions as he or she deals with the appliance for signs of distaste or revulsion. A positive and accepting attitude is essential as negative responses can have a devastating effect on self image and subsequent adjustment. Despite preparation, many patients/clients are shocked at the first sight of the stoma. They should never be forced to look until they are ready. Once this has

been achieved, the individual can be encouraged to participate in stoma care, and gradually assume full responsibility for stoma management.

As soon as the patient/client is able, stoma care activities are done away from the bedside and in the bathroom, so that privacy can be provided and dignity and self esteem regained.

Psychologically and emotionally, patients/clients are extremely vulnerable as they begin to come to terms with their stoma management and thoughtful care is important. For instance, providing the person with a deodorant spray for his or her own use is an appropriate and supportive act, whereas the liberal use of this spray by the nurse adjacent to the bedside after the person has performed an appliance change is not.

Ewing (1989) investigated self-care preparation in appliance management provided for patients/clients by ward nursing staff. She identified nine aspects of physical care of the stoma which have to be mastered by the individual in order to be able to manage the appliance successfully:

* preparation of the equipment
* preparation of the patient/client
* removal of old appliance
* skin care
* skin protection
* selection of new appliance
* preparation of new appliance
* application
* disposal.

A total of 53 appliance changes were carried out by nurses on 12 subjects under observation. Data analysis revealed that none of the subjects had been observed to perform all nine aspects of care independently before nurses discontinued teaching or the patient/client was discharged home. An uncoordinated approach to providing this care existed. Subjects were observed to develop self-care skills in some aspects of appliance management, then revert to nonparticipation and dependency on subsequent occasions so that practice opportunities were insufficient Although it is not appropriate to generalize the study findings, they can be used by nurses in similar units as a basis for reflecting on and questioning the quality and effectiveness of their own nursing practice. To ensure continuity and coordination of the patient's/client's preparation for self care, good verbal communication and written documentation of progress is essential. This may be in the care plan or as a separate record.

## APPLIANCE SELECTION

There are many different disposable appliances available for the patient/client with a stoma which are manufactured from several layers of plastic with different physical characteristics. This enables the production of pouches which are leakproof, odourproof, noiseless, comfortable, and inconspicuous. Pouches are transparent or coloured white or beige.

The nature of stomal output determines the choice of a drainable or nondrainable pouch. The patient/client with a sigmoid colostomy may have a fluid output in the early postoperative period. A drainable pouch can later be changed

## TOPICS TO INCLUDE IN PATIENT/CLIENT EDUCATION ABOUT STOMAS

| The Stoma | Resuming A Normal Lifestyle |
|---|---|
| Construction of the stoma | Diet |
| | Clothing |
| Position of the stoma | Work — returning, coping with the stoma |
| How the stoma will function | |
| What the stoma will look like | Social activities — sport, holidays, travel, going out |
| Specific cultural issues | Personal relationships — partner/spouse, family members, disclosure to others |
| Caring for the stoma and peristomal skin | |
| Type of appliance required | Sexual relationships, pregnancy |
| Obtaining supplies | Sources of help — support groups, contact with a fellow ostomist, health care professionals, appliance manufacturers' helplines, information booklets |
| Storage of supplies | |
| Disposal of used appliances | |
| Exemption from prescription charges | |
| Recognizing complications | |
| Dealing with problems — leakage, soreness, odour, flatus | |

## Steps in Appliance Selection

1. Drainable or closed pouch?
2. One- or two-piece appliance?
3. Starter hole or precut and sized?
4. What skin protection is required?
5. Select one pouch from the suitable appliances which meet individual needs

for a closed one when the faeces become more formed. Drainable appliances can be changed every 2–3 days, whereas a closed appliance is changed after the bowel has acted.

One-piece appliances are easy to apply by peeling off the protective backing paper, inconspicuous and flexible so they conform well to body contours. They can be useful for individuals with limited manual dexterity or difficultly remembering steps in the pouching procedure. A two-piece appliance has an adhesive baseplate and flange. A plastic ring around the aperture of the pouch is placed over the flange and pushed down so that it is secure. The flange remains undisturbed for two to five days. Some are attached to skin protective wafers which promote healing of sore or excoriated skin as they do not have to be removed each time an appliance is changed. A flange with a microporous backing is more flexible. Two-piece systems enable the patient/client to use different pouches when required, such as an activity pouch for swimming or other sports. Reasonable dexterity is required to use a two-piece appliance.

A choice is also made between an appliance with a starter hole which is cut to an appropriate size and shape and one which has a precut aperture. A starter hole is suitable in the early weeks after surgery and for stomas which are irregular in shape. A template cutting service is offered by appliance manufacturers for patients/clients with poor eyesight or limited dexterity who require an individually cut aperture. An appliance with a previously cut aperture of an approximate diameter enables the patient/client to carry out his or her stoma care more quickly as the appliance requires no preparation.

The patient/client is assisted to select a suitable appliance from a range of appropriate alternatives before discharge home as this helps to promote responsibility for stoma care management (Ewing, 1989). Some people try several appliances before making a final choice.

## CONTINUITY OF CARE IN THE COMMUNITY

Individuals may take about a year to adapt to life with a stoma (Wade, 1989) and to resume their previous lifestyle. The stoma care nurse usually works in the hospital and the community, developing a close relationship with the client. Liaison with the primary health care team is important. The nurse marks the proposed site of the patient's/client's stoma and provides essential information and teaching on practical aspects of care and appliance selection. The nurse's overall responsibility is to coordinate the rehabilitation programme from admission to hospital until the individual resumes a normal lifestyle. The nurse liaises with other multidisciplinary team members in hospital and in the community to ensure that care and management is directed

## The main goals in changing an appliance are to:

- collect the appropriate items of equipment
- prepare the patient/client for the procedure and ensure he or she is comfortable during the procedure
- clean the stoma and protect the peristomal skin to maintain its integrity
- prepare the correct appliance and fit it correctly so that leakage does not occur
- dispose of the used appliance and equipment safely and correctly

towards this goal. The nurse uses his or her knowledge and expertise to enable the patient/client to adapt physically, psychologically and socially to life with a stoma.

Stoma nurses give a specialist service. As the NHS reforms continue and fundholders increasingly influence purchasing of nursing in the community, the role of such specialists could alter. This would influence patient care.

## Maintaining Proper Fluid and Food Intake

In choosing a diet for promoting normal elimination, consider the frequency of defaecation, characteristics of faeces, and types of foods that impair or promote defaecation. The person with frequent constipation or impaction requires an increased intake of high-fibre foods and more fluids. However, he or she should realize that diet therapy provides only long-term relief of elimination problems and may not give immediate relief from problems such as constipation.

When diarrhoea is a problem, recommend foods with a low fibre content and discourage foods that typically cause gastric upset or abdominal cramping. The person with diarrhoea is susceptible to potassium loss from heavy loss of GI contents. Fruits and vegetables contain potassium but are not ideal because they have a high fibre content. Baked chicken, seafood, pork, veal, and evaporated and dry nonfat instant milk are better choices.

Diarrhoea caused by illness can be debilitating. If the person cannot tolerate foods or liquids orally, intravenous therapy (with potassium supplements) is necessary. The patient/client returns to a normal diet slowly, often beginning with fluids. Excessively hot or cold fluids stimulate peristalsis, causing abdominal cramps and further diarrhoea. As the tolerance to liquids improves, solid foods are ordered.

People with a stoma are able to eat a varied and nutritional diet. It is not appropriate to introduce strict dietary guidelines as there is considerable variation in the extent to which different foods affect stomal action or give rise to problems such as gas and odour (Elcoat, 1986). In the early postoperative period, high fibre foods may cause very liquid ileostomy output and so should gradually be reintroduced into the diet over a period of several weeks. A food which has once caused problems can be tried in small amounts later and may then be tolerated (Bosantco, 1988). Incompletely digested high fibre foods such as mushrooms, celery, potato skins, peanuts and unpeeled apples can obstruct the ileostomy (bolus obstruction). The patient/client has colicky pain until, in most cases, the mass of food is passed through the stoma by peristaltic movement. To avoid this problem, advise the individual to chew these foods throughly, not to eat them on an empty stomach, to take in low fibre foods at the same time and to avoid large quantities. Fluids should be taken freely, because the person with an ileostomy loses more salt and water than other people. A fluid intake of about two litres per day from drinks and food is usually sufficient. Discuss with the patient/client how to incorporate this requirement into his or her normal eating and drinking routine. The passage of noisy flatus, odour, and fluid effluent are problems that can be linked to dietary intake. A dietary history helps to identify foods responsible. Liquid stool may follow ingestion of greens, fruit or fish. Greens, beans, onions, some fruit and fizzy drinks can cause wind (Elcoat, 1986). There may not always be a direct link between the types of food eaten and stomal problems. Other relevant factors include emotional stress or irregular eating habits.

A person with a stoma is encouraged to resume a normal lifestyle and the activity of eating and drinking is an essential part of this. The nurse's role is to provide sufficient accurate information and practical advice to enable patients/clients to make their own decisions. For example, alcoholic drinks such as beer are enjoyed by many people as part of social activities and events. For the person with a stoma, this can cause liquidity, increased output and flatulence. If the individual understands and is prepared to deal with the consequences, the nurse can offer practical suggestions, such as using a drainable appliance and the need for more frequent emptying, so that participation can be continued.

### Promoting Regular Exercise

A daily exercise programme helps prevent elimination problems. Walking, riding a stationary bicycle, swimming, or other sports stimulate peristalsis. People who are sedentary at work are most in need of regular exercise.

For a patient/client temporarily immobilized, the nurse should attempt ambulation as soon as possible. If the condition permits, assist postoperative patients/clients in walking to a chair on the evening of the day of surgery. The patient/client should walk farther each day.

Some individuals have difficulty passing stool because of weak abdominal and pelvic floor muscles. Exercises help bedridden people using a bedpan. The person can practise the exercises as follows:

1. Lie supine; tighten the abdominal muscles as though pushing them to the floor. Hold them tight to three; relax. Repeat 5–10 times, as tolerated.
2. Flex and contract the thigh muscles by raising one knee slowly towards the chest. Repeat for each leg at least five times and increase frequency, as tolerated.

### Promoting Comfort

Many people have discomfort from alterations in elimination. Pain results when haemorrhoidal tissues are directly irritated. Flatulence can also create discomfort, particularly if distention develops.

### Mother and Child Nursing
### Stomas and pregnancy

An ileostomy or colostomy for urinary or alimentary diversion should not affect the course of pregnancy. Approximately 75% of women with stomas have a normal vaginal delivery. Problems that may occur include:

- changes in shape and position of the stoma as the uterus enlarges
- leakage from the stoma as the opening changes shape
- hormonal changes that alter the skin secretion, leading to reduced adhesiveness of the appliance
- reduced absorption of nutrients (e.g. vitamin $B_{12}$, folic acid), thus requiring supplementation
- increased risk of intestinal obstruction from gynaecological laparoscopy; the consequent abdominal pain is difficult to distinguish from appendicitis or labour (Kammerer, 1979).

Most of these problems are manageable if the caregivers and patient/client are observant and appropriately informed.

The primary goal for the person with haemorrhoids is to have soft-formed, painless stools. Proper diet, fluids, and regular exercise improve the likelihood of stools being soft. If the person becomes constipated, passage of hard stools may cause bleeding and irritation.

Often, haemorrhoids become so enlarged that they cover the rectum. To prevent trauma to tissues, the nurse must use caution when inserting suppositories, or if a rectal thermometer has to be used. A generous amount of lubricating jelly reduces friction when inserting an object past a haemorrhoid. Fear of pain may cause extreme tension and often the patient/client is better able to insert an object safely into the rectum. Never attempt to force an object into the rectum without full view of the anus. Soothing agents, often containing local anaesthetics, can be prescribed as creams or suppositories. They may cause sensitization of the skin, so should only be used for short periods. When haemorrhoids cause chronic pain, surgical removal is the best treatment.

To relieve the discomfort of flatulence, use measures that reduce flatus or promote its escape. Swallowing air increases flatus. The patient/client can reduce the amount of air swallowed by not drinking carbonated beverages, not using straws for drinking, and not chewing gum or hard-boiled sweets. When flatulence becomes severe as a result of reduced peristalsis, a nasogastric tube is often used.

When flatulence results in abdominal cramping, ambulation promotes passage of flatus. Assisting the individual to walk about may be enough to stimulate peristalsis and relieve gas. If conservative measures fail, flatulence can be relieved by insertion of a rectal tube. The patient/client assumes a side-lying position while the nurse inserts the tube in the same manner as for an enema.

Continual use of rectal tubes can cause irritation and eventual **excoriation** of the anus and rectal mucosa. A rectal tube should

## Adult Nursing
## Older adults with stomas

Living with a stoma can be difficult at any age, but there may be special issues to consider for older people. For example, older people may have:

- generational and cultural preconceptions about bodily elimination and the handling of body wastes
- already had to cope with alterations in body image (due to ageing); a stoma may be an additional, unacceptable change
- no immediate family who could help with changing an appliance or obtaining supplies, and may find it difficult to ask their children for assistance
- decreased mobility and difficulty travelling to shops for appliances
- reduced dexterity (e.g. due to arthritis), thus difficulty changing the appliance
- sensitive skin due to ageing, which may lead to skin breakdown or tissue trauma around the stoma site
- financial difficulties which may reduce their ability to follow a special diet in order to control the consistency of the stools, or to buy new clothing to conceal the stoma site and bag.

not remain in place longer than 30 minutes. The doctor determines the frequency with which the tube can be inserted. If flatulence persists, the nurse should notify the doctor.

The rectal lavage enema is another means used to expel flatus. The alternating instillation and drainage of fluid into and out of the colon and rectum stimulates passage of flatus.

### Maintaining Skin Integrity

The person with diarrhoea or faecal incontinence is at risk for skin breakdown when faecal contents remain on the skin. The same problem exists for the patient/client with a stoma that drains liquid stool. Liquid stool is usually acidic and contains digestive enzymes. Irritation from repeated wiping with toilet tissue aggravates skin breakdown. Bathing the skin after soiling helps but may result in more breakdown unless the skin is thoroughly dried.

Teach the patient/client to cleanse the perianal area with mild soap and water after each passage of stool. When a person with a stoma removes the pouch covering the stoma, the surrounding skin should be gently and thoroughly cleaned, and then dried carefully to promote good adhesion of the appliance and prevent leakage.

When caring for a debilitated, incontinent person who is unable to ask for assistance, check often for defaecation. The perianal area can be protected with a barrier cream such as zinc oxide, which will also prevent drying and cracking. Yeast infections of the skin can develop easily. Several powdered antifungal agents are effective against yeast. Baby or talcum powder should not be used because they frequently cake on the skin and become difficult to remove.

### Promoting Self-Concept

When a person has a bowel elimination problem, a threat to self-concept may be experienced. Frequent incontinence, foul, odourous stools, and a stomal appliance are just a few factors that may cause a person to perceive a change in body image. The result could be that the person avoids socializing with others or is unwilling to assume responsibility for self-care. The person with a stoma often sees this as a form of mutilation. This person may have difficulty maintaining or initiating sexual relations with a partner. The nurse can play an important role in restoring a person's self-concept through the following interventions:

- give the patient/client an opportunity to discuss concerns or fears about elimination problems.
- provide the individual and his or her family with information to understand and manage the elimination problem.
- give positive feedback when he or she attempts self-care measures.
- help the person manage the condition but do not expect him or her to like it.
- provide privacy during care.
- show acceptance and understanding.

Often, a person with an elimination problem goes through a process similar to grieving (see Chapter 11). The nurse's support is essential to help him or her return to a more normal lifestyle.

 EVALUATION

The effectiveness of care depends on success in meeting realistic, patient/client-centred goals. Optimally, the individual will be able to:

- regularly defaecate soft-formed, painless stools
- gain information needed to establish a normal elimination pattern
- demonstrate ongoing success measured at specific intervals over an extended period of time
- accomplish normal defaecation by manipulating natural components of daily living such as diet, fluid intake, and exercise
- have minimal reliance on artificial means of defaecation such as enemas and laxative use
- be comfortable and competent in the daily management of stoma care
- have appropriate information and support to resume a normal lifestyle.

## SUMMARY

The normal elimination of faecal wastes requires maintenance of GI function. Bowel elimination depends upon the functioning of the GI tract ; a series of organs comprising the mouth, oesophagus, stomach, and the small and large intestines. Fluid and nutrients from food are gradually broken down for absorption by mechanical and chemical processes as they progress along the GI tract through the mechanism of peristalsis. Food breakdown and digestion begins during mastication in the mouth and continue during the subsequent conversion into chyme in the stomach and small intestine. Chyme progresses into the large intestine where further fluid and nutrients are absorbed. Unabsorbed waste products that reach the rectum are called faeces. Elimination is the process through which faeces are expelled from the rectum and then leave the body through the anus.

Each patient/client has a different pattern of bowel elimination and the nurse must assess this pattern and aim to promote normal function. Factors which can influence bowel elimination are developmental age, dietary intake of food and fluids, physical activity, psychological and sociocultural factors, personal habits, pain, pregnancy, surgical procedures/anaesthesia, and medications. The most common bowel elimination problems encountered by the nurse include disturbances in the frequency and control of excretion: constipation (sometimes leading to impaction), diarrhoea, and faecal incontinence. Associated problems include flatulence and haemorrhoid development. Diagnostic investigations will help identify the underlying bowel disorder and enable effective treatment to be planned. A range of nursing interventions can also be implemented to enable the patient/client to return to his or her previous level of wellness. Where the alteration is long term (e.g. following stoma-forming surgery), the nurse can help the patients/clients by demonstrating sensitivity to and understanding of the physical and emotional needs of patients/client during readjustment.

## CHAPTER 23 REVIEW
### Key Concepts

- A primary function of the elimination process is fluid balance.
- Mechanical breakdown of food elements, gastrointestinal motility, and selective absorption and secretion of substances by the large intestine influence the character of faeces.
- Mass peristalsis in the large intestine is strongest an hour after a meal.
- Food high in fibre content and an increased fluid intake keep faeces soft.
- Regular use of laxatives can lead to constipation.
- Vagal stimulation, which slows the heart rate, may occur during straining while defaecating, taking rectal temperatures, and enemas.
- The greatest danger from diarrhoea is the development of fluid and electrolyte imbalance.
- The location of a stoma influences consistency of the stool.
- Assessment of elimination patterns should focus on bowel habits, factors that normally influence defaecation and recent changes in elimination.
- Indirect and direct visualization of the lower gastrointestinal tract requires cleansing of the bowel before the procedure.
- The nurse should consider frequency of defaecation, faecal characteristics, and effect of foods on gastrointestinal function when selecting a diet promoting normal elimination.
- Proper positioning on a bedpan allows the patient/client to assume a position similar to squatting without experiencing muscle strain.

- Laxatives should be administered shortly before the usual time of defaecation.
- Proper administration of an enema is the slow instillation of a warm solution.
- The site, size and shape of the stoma, volume and nature of faecal output, body contours, skin condition, manual dexterity, eyesight and normal lifestyle should be considered when selecting an appliance for a patient/client.
- A correctly fitting ostomy appliance should prevent leakage, odours and be comfortable to wear.
- Skin breakdown can occur after repeated exposure to liquid stool.

### Key Terms

Colon, p. 457
Colostomy, p. 463
Constipation, p. 458, 462
Defaecation, p. 458
Diarrhoea, p. 462
Endoscopy, p. 466
Enema, p. 472
Faecal incontinence, p. 462
Faecal impaction, p. 461
Faeces, p. 458
Gastrointestinal (GI) tract, p. 455
Gastroscopy, p. 467
Ileostomy, p. 463
Laxatives, p. 461
Peristalsis, p. 457
Protoscope, p. 467
Sigmoidoscope, p. 467
Stoma, p. 463
Stool culture(s), p. 466
Suppository, p. 474

## CRITICAL THINKING EXERCISES

1. A 24-year-old man with a history of good health is admitted to your unit after a motor vehicle accident. He will rest in bed for the next 2 weeks. What type of plan would you design to prevent him from becoming constipated during this period of immobility?

2. An older woman with a new, permanent colostomy is about to be discharged from your unit to her daughter's home. The skin around her stoma has no breakdown. She and her daughter realize the importance of maintaining this skin integrity. How would you go about advising them?

## REFERENCES

Bosantco S, editor: *The Ileostomy Book, Mansfield*, 1988, Ileostomy Association of Great Britain and Ireland.

Brown M, Everett I: Gentler bowel fitness with fibre, *Geriatr Nurs* 11(1):26, 1990.

Castledine G: Preoperative information, *Surg Nurs* 1(1):11, 1988.

Clarke B: Making sense of enemas, *Nurs Times* 84(30):40, 1988.

Cooke D: Inflammatory bowel disease: primary health care management of ulcerative colitis and Crohn's disease, *Nurs Pract* 16(8):27, 1991.

Curry A: Returning home with confidence, *Prof Nurs* 4(5):242, 1991.

Donaldson I: Communication can help ostomists accept their stoma, *Prof Nurs* 4(5):242, 1989.

Elcoat C: *Stoma care nursing,* London, 1986, Baillière Tindall.

Ewing G: The nursing preparation of patients for self care, *J Adv Nurs* 14:411, 1989.

Gilpatrick D: Moving clients towards wellness, *Clin Nurs Spec* 3(1):25, 1989.

Goldfinger S: Constipation: the hard facts, *Harvard Health Letter* 16(4):1, 1991.

Kammerer WS: Non-obstetric surgery during pregnancy, *Med Clin NA* 63: 1157, 1979.

Kelly M, Henry T: A thirst for practical knowledge, *Prof Nurs* 7(6):350, 1992.

Neuberger J: *Caring for dying people of different faiths,* ed 2, London, 1994, Mosby.

Robinson C, Weigley E: *Basic nutrition and diet therapy,* ed 6, New York, 1989, Macmillan.

Roper N, Logan W and Tierney A: *The elements of nursing,* ed 3, Edinburgh, 1990, Churchill Livingstone.

Ross D: Constipation among hospitalized elders, *Orthopaedic Nurs* 9(3):73, 1990.

Royal College of Nursing: *Stoma care: a team approach*, London, 1981, RCN.

Tortora G: *Basic principles of human anatomy,* ed 5, New York, 1989, Harper & Row.

Turner AF: Encorporesis: family support must accompany treatment. In Glasper A, editor: *Child care: some nursing perspectives,* London, 1991, Wolfe.

Wade B: *A stoma is for life,* London, 1989, Scutari.

Wilson-Barnett J: Patients' emotional responses to barium x-rays *J Adv Nurs* 3(1):37, 1978.

Wright L: *Bowel function in hospital patients,* London, 1974, RCN.

## FURTHER READING

### Adult Nursing

Burns S: Assessing bowel function *Surg Nurs* 4(1):23, 1991.

Curry A: Returning home with confidence, *Prof Nurs* 6(9):536, 1991.

Davis K: Impotence after surgery, *Nurs* 4(18):23, 1990.

Doughty D, editor: *Urinary and faecal incontinence: nursing management,* St Louis, 1991, Mosby.

Hogstel M, Nelson M: Anticipation and early detection can reduce bowel elimination complications, *Geriatr Nurs* 13(1):28, 1992.

Hughes A: Life with a stoma, *Nurs Times* 87(25):67, 1991.

Jeffries E: At home with stoma care, *Nurs Times* 89(14):59, 1993.

Martinsson E, Josefsson M, Ek A: Working capacity and quality of life after undergoing an ileostomy, *J Adv Nurs* 16(9):1035, 1991.

Poulton L: Preoperative bowel preparation, *Surg Nurs* 4:12, 1991.

Price B: *Body image: nursing concepts and care,* New York, 1990, Prentice Hall.

Roe B: *Clinical nursing practice: the promotion and management of incontinence,* New York, 1992, Prentice Hall.

Salter M: *Altered body image: the nurse's role,* Chichester, 1988, John Wiley & Sons.

### Children's Nursing

Candy L: Recent advances in the care of children with acute diarrhoea: giving responsibility to the nurse and parents, *J Adv Nurs* 12:95, 1987.

Donaldson M : *Children's minds,* London, 1978, Fontana.

Gelbert E: What do I have inside me? How children view their bodies. In *Psychosocial aspects of pediatric care,* New York, 1978, Grune & Stratton.

Glen S: Altered body image in children. Salter M, editor: *Altered body image,* Chichester, 1988, John Wiley & Sons.

Johnson H: Stoma care for infants, children and young people, *Paediatr Nurs* :8-11, 1992.

Johnson H: Growing up with a stoma, *Nurs Times Commun Outlook* 84:15, 1988.

Lister J, Webster P, Mirza S: Colostomy complications in children, *Practitioner* 227:229, 1983.

Lyall J: A simple solution, *Nurs Times* 86(19):16, 1990.

Webster P: Forging a role, *Paediatr Nurs* 1(6):8, 1989.

Webster P: Special babies, *Community Outlook* **vol:**19, 1985.

### Learning Disabilities Nursing

Bettison S: *Toilet training to independence: a manual for trainers,* 1982, Charles C Thomas.

Capra SM, Hannan-Jones M: A controlled dietary trial for improving bowel function in a group of training centre residents with severe or  profound intellectual disability, *Australia & New Zealand Journal of  Developmental Disabilities,* 18(2): 111-121, 1992.

Dalrymple NJ, Ruble LA: Toilet training and behaviours of people with  autism: parent views, *Journal of Autism & Developmental Disorders,* 22(2): 265-275.

Jansson LM: Encopresis in a multihandicapped child: rapid multidisciplinary treatment, *Journal of Developmental and Physical Disabilities,* 4(1): 83-90, 1992.

# Mobility and Immobility

## LEARNING OUTCOMES

After reading this chapter you should be able to:
- *Define the key terms.*
- *Describe the roles of the skeleton, skeletal muscle and nervous system in regulation of movement.*
- *Discuss physiological and pathological influences on body alignment and joint mobility.*
- *Identify changes in physiological function during immobilization and suggest possible psychosocial effects on the patient/client.*
- *Assess body alignment and mobility.*
- *Describe common lifting, transferring, and positioning techniques, and suggest appropriate use of equipment where applicable.*
- *List the devices available to assist patient/client ambulation, and describe their correct usage.*
- *Suggest nursing interventions to minimize the hazards of immobility in all the main areas of concern.*
- *Evaluate care plans for maintaining body alignment and mobility.*

Clinical nursing requires nurses to incorporate knowledge and skills into practice. One component of this knowledge and skill is body mechanics, a broad term used to describe the coordinated efforts of the musculoskeletal and nervous systems.

Body mechanics includes knowing how and why certain muscle groups are used. To use proper body mechanics nurses need to understand the regulation of movement, including how coordinated body motion involves integrated functioning of the skeletal system, skeletal muscle, and the nervous system.

Mobility serves many purposes, such as expression of emotions, self-defence, satisfaction of basic needs, activities of daily living, and recreational activities. To maintain optimal physical mobility, the nervous, muscular, and skeletal systems of the body must be intact and functioning properly.

## OVERVIEW OF BODY MECHANICS

**Body mechanics** is the coordinated effort of the musculoskeletal and nervous systems to maintain balance, posture, and body alignment during lifting, bending, and moving. Use of proper body mechanics reduces the risk of injury and allows movement without muscle strain and excessive use of muscle energy.

### Body Alignment
**Body alignment** refers to the positioning of the joints, tendons, ligaments, and muscles while standing, sitting and lying. Correct body alignment reduces strain on musculoskeletal structures, maintains adequate muscle tone and contributes to balance.

## Body Balance

Body balance is achieved when the **centre of gravity** is balanced over a wide, stable base of support. When the body is improperly balanced, the centre of gravity is displaced, increasing the force of gravity and the possibility of falling.

Body balance is enhanced by **posture**. Proper body alignment and posture are enhanced by two simple techniques. The base of support can be widened by separating the feet and balance is increased when the centre of gravity is moved closer to the base of support. This is achieved by bending the knees, flexing the hips and maintaining proper back alignment by keeping the trunk erect (Stamps, 1989).

## Coordinated Body Movement

**Weight** is the force exerted on something by gravity. When an object is lifted, the lifter must overcome the object's weight and know its centre of gravity. In symmetrical objects the centre of gravity is exactly in the centre.

The human body is not geometrically perfect; therefore, the centre of gravity is usually at 55% to 57% of standing height and is located in the midline of the body. The force of weight is always directed downward, which is why an unbalanced object falls. People who are unsteady fall because their centres of gravity become unbalanced (for example, when leaning backwards while walking with a frame), and the gravitational force of their weight eventually causes them to fall.

**Friction** is a force that opposes movement. As a nurse turns, transfers, or lifts a patient/client, friction must be overcome. The greater the surface area of the object to be moved, the greater the friction. For example, if a patient/client is unable to assist you in moving up in bed you place the person's arms across his or her chest to decrease surface area and reduce friction.

A passive or immobilized person produces greater friction to movement. Thus, whenever possible, use some of the person's strength and mobility when lifting, transferring, or positioning. This can be done by explaining the procedure and telling him or her when to move. The individual can then participate, thus decreasing friction.

Friction can also be reduced by *lifting*, rather than *pushing*, a patient/client. Lifting decreases the pressure between the individual and the bed or chair. The use of lifting slings reduces friction, because the person is more easily moved along the bed's surface. Similarly, hoists should be used wherever possible.

## REGULATION OF MOVEMENT

## Skeletal System

The skeleton is the body's supporting framework and comprises four types of bones: long, short, flat, and irregular. **Long bones** contribute to height (for example, the femur, fibula, and tibia in the leg) and length (for example, the phalanges of the fingers and toes). **Short bones** occur in clusters and, when combined with ligaments and cartilage, permit movement of the extremities. Examples of short bones are the tarsal bones in the foot. **Flat bones** provide structural contour, such as the bones of the ribs. **Irregular bones** make up the vertebral column and some bones of

the skull, such as the mandible.

The skeleton provides attachments for muscles and ligaments. These attachments allow movement of parts of the skeleton, such as in opening and closing the mouth or extending an arm or a leg. The skeleton also protects vital organs. For example, the skull protects the brain, and the ribs protect the heart and lungs. Bones assist in regulation of calcium balance. Bones store calcium and release it into the circulation as needed. People with altered calcium regulation and metabolism are at risk of developing osteoporosis and **pathological fractures** (fractures caused by diseased bone tissue), which can occur in all bones, but are most common in the ribs and weight-bearing bones. Bones contain bone marrow which participates in erythrocyte production, and acts as a reservoir for blood. Patients/clients with altered bone marrow function or diminished erythrocyte production are usually weakened and fatigue easily, which decreases mobility and places them at risk of falling.

## Characteristics of Bone

The characteristics of bone include **firmness, rigidity,** and **elasticity**. Firmness results from inorganic salts, such as calcium phosphate, which are laid down in the bone matrix. Firmness is related to the bone's rigidity, which is necessary to keep long bones straight, and enables bones to withstand weight bearing. Elasticity and skeletal flexibility change with age. For example, the newborn has a large amount of cartilage and is highly flexible; toddler's bones are more pliable than those of older people and are better able to withstand falls.

## Joints

**Joints** are the connections between bones and are classified according to structure and degree of mobility. There are four classifications of joints: **synostotic, cartilaginous, fibrous,** and **synovial**.

The **synostotic joint** occurs when bones are jointed by bones. No movement is associated with this type of joint, and the bony tissue that forms between the bones provides strength and stability. The classic example of this type of joint is the sacrum.

The cartilaginous joint, has little movement but is elastic and uses cartilage to unite body surfaces. Cartilaginous joints are found where bones are exposed to constant pressure, such as the costosternal joints between the sternum and ribs.

The fibrous joint, has a tough layer of fibrous **connective tissue** that binds bones firmly together. Because of the flexibility of connective tissue, some movement of the joint is permitted. For example, the connective tissue between the tibia and fibula joins the bones in a fibrous joint at their distal ends, where they provide a socket for the upper part of the tarsal bones of the foot. Together, these bones and connective tissues form the ankle joint, which permits plantar and dorsal flexion of the foot.

The synovial joint, or true joint, is a freely movable joint in which contiguous bony surfaces are covered by articular cartilage and connected by ligaments lined with a synovial membrane. Joining of the humeral radius and ulna by cartilage and ligaments forms a pivotal joint. Other types of synovial joints are ball-and-socket joints, such as the hip joint, and hinge joints, such as the interphalangeal joints of fingers.

## Ligaments

**Ligaments** are flexible bands of fibrous tissue that bind joints together and connect bones and cartilages. Ligaments aid joint flexibility and support. Some ligaments also have a protective function. For example, ligaments between the vertebral bodies, nonelastic ligaments, and the ligamentum flavum prevent damage to the spinal cord during movement of the back.

## Tendons

**Tendons** are fibrous bands of tissue that connect muscle to bone. They are strong, flexible and inelastic, and occur in various lengths and thicknesses. The Achilles tendon (tendo calcaneus) is the thickest and strongest tendon in the body. It begins near the middle of the back of the leg and attaches the gastrocnemius and soleus muscles in the calf to the calcaneal bone in the back of the foot.

## Cartilage

**Cartilage** is nonvascular, supporting connective tissue located chiefly in the joints and thorax, trachea, larynx, nose, and ear. The fetus has a large amount of temporary cartilage, which is replaced by bone during infancy. Permanent cartilage is unossified, except in advanced age and diseases such as osteoarthritis.

## Skeletal Muscle

**Skeletal muscles**, with their ability to contract and relax, are the working elements of movement. Muscle contraction is stimulated by an electrochemical impulse which travels from the nerve to the muscle across the neuromuscular junction. The electrochemical impulse causes the thin, actin-containing filaments to shorten, thus contracting the muscle. Removal of the stimulus results in muscle relaxation.

There are two types of muscle contractions: isotonic and isometric. In **isotonic contraction**, increased muscle tension results in muscle shortening. **Isometric contraction** causes an increase in muscle tension or muscle work but no shortening or active movement of the muscle. Voluntary movement is a combination of isotonic and isometric contractions. For example, when the nurse lifts a patient/client up in bed, the person's weight causes increased tension in the muscles of the nurse's arms, until the tension (isometric) is equal to the weight to be lifted and the weight of the lower arm. When this equilibrium is reached, continued stimulation results in muscle shortening (isotonic) and bending of the elbow (active movement), until the patient/client is lifted.

Although isometric contractions do not result in muscle shortening, energy expenditure is increased. This type of muscle work is comparable to having a car in neutral, continually depressing the accelerator and racing the engine. The car is not going anywhere, but expends a large amount of energy.

Some skeletal muscles are concerned primarily with movement, whereas others are concerned with posture.

## Muscles Concerned with Movement

Muscles concerned mainly with movement are located near the skeletal region where the movement is caused by leverage. Leverage occurs when specific bones, such as the humerus, ulna, and radius, and the associated joints, such as the elbow joint, act together as a lever. Thus, the force applied to one end of the bone to lift a weight at another point tends to rotate the bone in the direction opposite that of the applied force. The muscles attached to such bones provide the necessary strength to move the object.

## Muscles Concerned with Posture

Muscles of the trunk, neck, and back are concerned primarily with posture. These muscles are short and featherlike in appearance, and converge obliquely at a common tendon. They work together to stabilize and support body weight, allowing sitting or standing posture to be maintained.

## MUSCLE REGULATION OF POSTURE AND MOVEMENT

Posture and movement can be reflections of personality and mood. For example, a person with a dramatic personality may make expansive hand gestures and a person who is fatigued or depressed may slouch.

Posture and movement also depend on the skeleton and the shape and development of skeletal muscles. Coordination and regulation of different muscle groups depend on muscle tone and the activity of antagonistic, synergistic, and antigravity muscles.

### Muscle Tone
Muscle tone, or tonus, is the normal state of balanced muscle tension. Tension is achieved by alternate contraction and relaxation, without active movement. Muscle tone enables a body part to be maintained in a functioning position without muscle fatigue. Muscle tone also promotes venous return to the heart, as in the case of leg muscles.

Muscle tone is maintained through continual use of muscles. As a result of immobility or prolonged bed rest, activity level and muscle tone decrease.

### Muscle Groups
The antagonistic, synergistic, and antigravity muscle groups are coordinated by the nervous system and work together to maintain posture and initiate movement.

**Antagonistic muscles** work together to bring about movement. During movement, the active muscle contracts, and its antagonist relaxes. For example, when flexing the arm, the active biceps brachii contracts, and its antagonist, the triceps brachii, relaxes. During extension of the arm, the active triceps brachii contracts, and the new antagonist, the biceps brachii, relaxes.

**Synergistic muscles** contract together to accomplish the same movement. When the arm is flexed, the strength of contraction of the biceps brachii is increased by contraction of the synergistic muscle, the brachialis. Thus, with synergistic muscle activity, there are two active movers, the biceps brachii and the brachialis, that contract while the antagonistic muscle, the triceps brachii, relaxes.

**Antigravity muscles** are specifically involved with stabilization of joints. These muscles continuously oppose the effect of gravity on the body, and permit maintenance of an upright or sitting posture. The antigravity muscles are the extensors of the leg, gluteus maximus, quadriceps femoris, soleus muscles, and muscles of the back.

### Nervous System

Movement and posture are regulated by the nervous system. The major voluntary motor area, located in the cerebral cortex, is the precentral gyrus or motor strip. Most motor fibres descend from the motor strip and cross at the level of the medulla. Thus the motor fibres from the right motor strip initiate voluntary movement for the left side of the body, and motor fibres from the left motor strip initiate voluntary movement for the right side of the body.

During voluntary movement, impulses descend from the motor strip to the spinal cord. An impulse exits from the spinal cord through efferent motor nerves and travels through the nerves to the muscles, where movement occurs. Synapses control the impulse and keep it travelling in one direction.

Transmission of the impulse from the nervous system to the musculoskeletal system is an electrochemical event and requires a neurotransmitter. **Neurotransmitters** are chemicals, such as acetylcholine, that transfer the electric impulse from the nerve across the neuromuscular junction to the muscle. When the neurotransmitter reaches a muscle and stimulates it, movement occurs.

Movement can be impaired by disorders that alter neurotransmitter production, transfer from the nerve to the muscle, or activation of muscle activity. Posture is also regulated by the nervous system and requires coordination of proprioception and balance.

### Proprioception

**Proprioception** is the sensation achieved through interpretation of stimuli regarding spatial position and muscular activity. It is monitored by **proprioceptors**, which are nerve endings located in muscles, tendons, and joints that continuously monitor muscle activity and body position. For example, the proprioceptors on the soles of the feet contribute to correct posture while walking. As a person walks, the proprioceptors on the bottom of the feet monitor pressure changes. Thus, when the bottom of the moving foot comes into contact with the walking surface, the individual automatically moves the stationary foot forward. Proprioceptors allow people to walk without having to watch their feet.

### Balance

Standing, running, lifting, or performing activities of living require balance. Balance is assisted by the nervous system, the cerebellum and the inner ear. The cerebellum coordinates voluntary movement, particularly highly skilled movements such as those required in golf and skiing (Strand, 1978). The cerebellum also assists in balance, by permitting a person to stand on one foot with his or her eyes closed (Romberg test of cerebellar function).

Balance is also facilitated by the **semicircular canals**, three fluid-filled structures in the inner ear. When the head is suddenly rotated in one direction, the fluid remains stationary for a moment while the canals turn with the head, allowing sudden position changes without loss of balance.

## PRINCIPLES OF BODY MECHANICS

Proper body mechanics is equally important to the nurse and the patient/client. It affects well-being and is necessary for promoting health and preventing disability.

The nurse uses a variety of muscle groups during nursing activities. Weight and friction influence body movement. Used correctly, these forces increase the nurse's efficiency. Incorrect use can affect safety and cause injury. The main principles of body mechanics in all settings are:

- stability is increased by a wide base of support and a low centre of gravity
- the stronger the muscle group, the more work it can safely perform
- facing the direction of movement prevents abnormal twisting of the spine
- levering, rolling, turning or pivoting requires less work than lifting
- reducing friction reduces the force required to move any object (Corlett, 1992)

## PATHOLOGICAL INFLUENCES ON BODY ALIGNMENT AND MOBILITY

Many pathological conditions affect body alignment and mobility. Although a complete description of each is beyond the scope of this chapter, four main types are presented here: postural abnormalities, impaired muscle development, damage to the central nervous system, and direct trauma to the musculoskeletal system.

### Postural Abnormalities

Congenital or acquired postural abnormalities affect the efficiency of the musculoskeletal system, as well as body alignment, balance, and appearance. During any physical assessment, the nurse should observe body alignment and range of motion (ROM). Postural abnormalities can impair alignment, mobility, or both.

Knowledge about the characteristics, causes, and treatment of common postural abnormalities can be used to improve the patient's/client's body alignment during lifting, transferring, and positioning. Nursing interventions should be planned to strengthen affected muscle and joint groups, improve the individual's posture, and use affected and unaffected muscle groups.

### Impaired Muscle Development

Inadequate development of skeletal muscles affects body alignment, balance, and mobility. **Muscular dystrophies** are the most common developmental impairments of skeletal muscles. These are a group of genetically transmitted diseases characterized by progressive pathological changes in the skeletal muscles, resulting in muscle wasting and weakness (Gröer and Shekleton, 1989).

### Adult Nursing
### Posture, mobility and ageing

An adult who has correct posture and body alignment feels good, looks good, and generally appears self-confident. The healthy adult also has the necessary musculoskeletal development and coordination to carry out all activities of living.

The ageing process can result in musculoskeletal changes. Degenerative joint changes may decrease range of motion. Skeletal muscle mass and strength may be reduced. Changes in the structure of the bone matrix may result in fragile, brittle bones (Pinel, 1989).

Older people may walk more slowly and appear less coordinated. They may also take smaller steps, keeping the feet closer together, which decreases the base of support. Thus, body balance is unstable, and they have a greater risk of falls and injuries.

## Damage to the Central Nervous System

Damage to any component of the central nervous system that regulates voluntary movement results in impaired body alignment and mobility. The motor strip in the cerebrum can be damaged by trauma from a head injury, ischaemia from a cerebrovascular accident (stroke), or bacterial infection from meningitis. **Motor impairment** is directly related to the amount of destruction of the motor strip. For example, an extensive right-sided cerebral haemorrhage which destroys the motor strip will result in a left-sided hemiplegia. However, a person with a right-sided head injury may have cerebral oedema and damage (but not destruction) of the motor strip, and should regain voluntary movement with intensive physiotherapy.

The voluntary motor fibres descend from the motor strip in the cerebrum down the spinal cord; therefore, trauma to the spinal cord also impairs mobility. If the motor fibres are cut, complete bilateral loss of voluntary motor control below the level of the trauma is caused. Spinal cord trauma frequently results from diving, industrial, sports and car accidents, or gunshot and knife wounds to the neck and back.

## Direct Trauma to the Musculoskeletal System

Direct trauma to the musculoskeletal system can result in bruises, contusions, sprains, and fractures. A **fracture** is a disruption of bone tissue continuity. Fractures most commonly result from external trauma, but they can also occur as a consequence of some deformity of the bone (for example, the pathological fractures of osteoporosis, Paget's disease, and osteogenesis imperfecta).

The fractured bone initiates a cellular process that results in bone formation. Young children are able to form new bone more easily than adults and therefore have fewer complications. Treatment includes positioning the fractured bone in proper alignment and immobilizing it to promote healing. Immobilization causes some muscle atrophy, loss of tone, and joint stiffness.

## IMPAIRED MOBILITY

**Mobility** is a person's ability to move about freely. Mobility is often essential to the patient's/client's perception of health

(Rubin, 1988a, 1988b; Tompkins, 1980). Complete unrestricted mobility requires voluntary motor and sensory control of all body regions.

A partial loss of mobility may be temporary (for example, the result of a fracture) or permanent (for example, the result of paralysis). In some cases, restriction of mobility is beneficial for the person's recovery (for example, after application of a plaster cast).

The hazards associated with partial mobility depend on the degree and duration of immobilization (Rubin, 1988b; Greenleaf, 1984). The resulting hazards are usually temporary and resolve shortly after complete mobility is restored (Greenleaf, 1984). Nursing care should be directed towards minimizing such hazards because it is easier to prevent complications than to treat or cure them (Reddy, 1986).

Four main conditions (either in isolation or combined) may result in immobility:

- physical inactivity, such as bed rest
- physical restriction or limitation of movement (for example, by cast or traction) forces reduced movement
- restriction of changes in position and posture result in a loss of the body's ability to adapt to such changes
- sensory deprivation causes reduction in stimuli that cause movement and may result in even greater physical inactivity

The degree of immobility depends on the extent that these conditions are present (Gröer and Shekleton, 1989).

## Bed Rest

**Bed rest** involves restricting the patient/client to bed for therapeutic reasons. The general objectives of bed rest include the following:

- reducing physical activity and oxygen needs
- reducing pain and the need for large doses of analgesics
- enabling ill, debilitated or exhausted patients/clients to rest and regain strength.

Bed rest has physiological and psychological benefits only if the patient/client finds it restful and if the client can freely move and change positions. People who are resistant to bed rest may actually expend more energy fighting bed rest than they would if they were allowed to move more freely (Hinchliff and Montague, 1992).

## Immobility

**Immobility** occurs when an individual is unable to move or change positions independently. The effects of immobility are systemic and functional. No body system is immune. Healthy people who are exposed to periods of immobility or prolonged bed rest also suffer physiological and psychological effects (Deitrick, 1948; Bliss, 1990). Such effects can be gradual or immediate. The greater the extent and the longer the duration of immobility, the more pronounced the consequences.

## Physiological Effects

The severity of the impairment depends on the person's age, overall health and the degree of immobility. Older individuals

**Children's Nursing
How does physiological development affect posture and mobility?**

**Infants:** The newborn infant's spine is flexed and lacks the anteroposterior curves of the adult. The first spinal curve occurs when the infant extends the neck from the prone position. As growth and stability increase, the thoracic spine straightens, and the lumbar spinal curve appears, allows sitting and standing. The infant's musculoskeletal system is flexible. The extremities are flexed and joints have complete ROM. As the newborn matures, the musculoskeletal system becomes stronger, and the infant is able to resist movement and reach out and grasp objects. As the baby grows, musculoskeletal development permits support of weight for standing and walking. Posture is awkward because the head and upper trunk are carried forward. Because body weight is not evenly distributed along a line of gravity, posture is off balance and frequent falls occur.

**Toddlers:** The toddler's posture — slightly swaybacked with a protruding abdomen — is awkward. As the child walks, the legs and feet are usually far apart and the feet are slightly everted. Towards the end of toddlerhood, posture appears less awkward, curves in the cervical and lumbar vertebrae are accentuated, and foot eversion disappears.

**Preschool and School-aged Children:** By the third year the body is slimmer, taller, and better balanced. Abdominal protrusion is decreased, the feet are not as far apart, and arms and legs have increased in length. The child also appears more coordinated. From the third year to the beginning of adolescence the musculoskeletal system continues to develop. Long bones in the arms and legs grow. Muscles, ligaments, and tendons become stronger, resulting in improved posture and increased muscle strength. Greater coordination enables the child to perform tasks that require fine motor skills.

**Adolescents:** Adolescence is usually initiated by a tremendous growth spurt. Growth is frequently uneven and the adolescent may appear awkward and uncoordinated. Adolescent girls usually grow and develop earlier than boys. Hips widen, and fat is deposited in the upper arms, thighs, and buttocks. Boys experience long-bone growth and develop increased muscle mass. Legs become longer and hips narrower. Muscular development increases in the chest, arms, shoulders, and upper legs.

**Mother and Child Nursing
The effects of pregnancy on posture**

Normal changes in posture and body alignment occur in pregnant women. These changes result from the body's adaptive response to the growing fetus. The centre of gravity shifts towards the anterior, and the pregnant woman leans back and becomes slightly swaybacked.

with chronic illnesses develop complications more quickly (Bliss, 1990).

## METABOLIC CHANGES

Reduced mobility results in:

- **decrease in basal metabolic rate (BMR)**. BMR falls in response to the decreased energy requirement of the cells, which is directly related to cellular oxygen demands (Hinchliff and Montague, 1992). However, if infection is present, immobilized clients may have an increased BMR as a result of fever. Fever and wound healing also increase cellular oxygen requirements (McCance and Huether, 1990).

- **decreased pancreatic activity**, which thus decreases the body's ability to tolerate glucose. These effects can be seen within 3 days but can reverse 7 days after resuming activity (Rubin, 1988b).

- **negative nitrogen balance** that results when the excretion of nitrogen from the breakdown of protein exceeds protein intake (Hinchliff and Montague, 1992). Since protein metabolization produces nitrogen as an end product, nitrogen balance therefore provides a reliable indicator of protein use by the body. During periods of immobility, urinary excretion of nitrogen increases, increasing the risk of a negative nitrogen balance. The urinary excretion of nitrogen increases on about the fifth or sixth day of immobilization (Exton-Smith, 1985; Hinchliff and Montague, 1992). Decreased mobility also increases the percentage of body fat, which results from the loss of lean body mass as a result of protein breakdown (Hinchliff and Montague, 1992).

- **major shifts in blood volume** — there is an immediate diuretic response during the first day of bed rest. The person loses an average of 600 ml of fluid (Rubin, 1988b). In addition, there is an increase in urinary excretion of calcium, chloride, and sodium (Hinchliff and Montague, 1992).

- **increased urinary excretion of calcium** is due to **bone reabsorption**. Immobility causes the release of calcium into the circulation. Normally the kidneys can excrete the excess calcium. However, if the kidneys are unable to respond appropriately, hypercalcaemia results (Rubin, 1988b; Brocklehurst, 1990).

- **impairments in gastrointestinal functioning** vary, but result from decreased gastrointestinal motility. Constipation is a common symptom. Diarrhoea can occur as the result of faecal impaction, (when liquid stool passes around an area of impaction). Left untreated, faecal impaction can result in a mechanical bowel obstruction that may partially or completely occlude the intestinal lumen, blocking normal propulsion of liquid and gas. The resulting fluid in the intestine produces distention and increases intraluminal pressure. Over time, intestinal function becomes depressed, dehydration occurs, absorption ceases, and fluid and electrolyte disturbances worsen.

## RESPIRATORY CHANGES

In the recumbent position, the lungs shift position 90 degrees and the abdominal contents push against the diaphragm causing a decrease in lung volume (Rubin, 1988b).

The majority of respiratory problems associated with immobility are caused by:
- **decreased haemoglobin**, which can result from the disease process causing reduced mobility or from restricted mobility itself. Haemoglobin is the carrier that transports oxygenated blood to tissues. When the oxygen-carrying capacity is reduced, there is a reduction in oxygen delivery to the tissues. Initially the body tries to adapt by increasing pulse and respiratory rates, but this is a short-term adaptive response and ultimately increases cardiac workload.
- **decreased lung expansion** — any changes in the individual's position changes the distribution of ventilation and blood flow through the lung. Consequently, the dependent lung is better oxygenated (Olsen and Thompson, 1990). The exception to this principle occurs when the patient/client has a pathological condition of the lung. All lung volumes, except tidal volumes, are reduced during immobilization (Olsen and Thompson, 1990).
- **weakened respiratory muscles and stasis of secretions** which increase the work of breathing (Bliss, 1990). There is a proportional decline in the patient's/client's ability to cough productively. Ultimately, the distribution of mucus in the bronchi increases, particularly when the individual is in the supine, prone, or lateral position. Mucus accumulates in the dependent regions of the airways. Because mucus is an excellent medium for bacterial growth, hypostatic bronchopneumonia may result.

## CARDIOVASCULAR CHANGES

Three major cardiovascular changes associated with immobility are:
- **postural hypotension** which affects people on bed rest and those experiencing prolonged immobility in the sitting position (Hinchliff and Montague, 1992). Postural hypotension is a drop of 15 mmHg or more in blood pressure when the client rises from a lying or sitting position to a standing position. Immobility causes decreased circulating fluid volume, pooling of blood in the lower extremities and decreased autonomic response. These factors result in decreased venous return, followed by a decrease in cardiac output, which is reflected by a decline in blood pressure (Winslow, 1985; McCance and Huether, 1990).
- **increased cardiac workload** — which is demonstrated by rate changes. Prolonged bed rest increases resting heart rate by 4 to 15 beats/min. When the immobilized person is asked to undertake physical activity the increase in rate is more pronounced (Winslow, 1985). As the workload of the heart increases, its oxygen consumption does too. The heart therefore works harder and less efficiently during periods of prolonged rest. As immobilization increases, cardiac output falls, further decreasing cardiac efficiency and increasing workload.
- **thrombus formation** an accumulation of platelets, fibrin, clotting factors, and the cellular elements of blood. The thrombus attaches to the interior wall of a vein or artery,

sometimes occluding the lumen of the vessel (Fig. 24-1, overleaf). Causes of thrombi formation include:
(i) hypovolaemia (lowered blood volume), which increases the haematocrit (blood cell concentration), and the circulating blood is more viscous (Hinchliff and Montague, 1992);
(ii) more procoagulants in the blood and shortened thrombastin (clotting factor) time after 8 days of bed rest (Rubin, 1988b)
(iii) compressed blood vessels of the calves from the weight of the patient/client causing vessel wall injury and stasis of blood (Rubin, 1988b; THRIFT, 1992)
(iv) increased fibrinolytic activity (Rubin, 1988b).

## MUSCULOSKELETAL CHANGES

The effects of immobility on the musculoskeletal system include:
- permanent impairment of mobility
- restricted mobility, which affects endurance, muscle mass and stability
- impaired calcium metabolism
- impaired joint mobility.

**Muscle** Reduced muscle endurance for physical activity results from changes in the muscles and altered cardiovascular functioning. As cardiac workload increases, muscle endurance decreases due to the reduced ability of the cardiopulmonary system to meet the tissue's oxygen needs (Winslow, 1985).

Because of protein breakdown, the patient/client loses lean body mass, which is composed partially of muscle. The reduced muscle mass is unable to sustain activity without increased fatigue. Metabolic causes and disuse (including lack of exercise) lead to further reduction in mass.

The muscle atrophy caused by immobility is observable and measurable. As muscle atrophies, the size of the muscle decreases (Bliss, 1990). The antigravity muscles in the legs appear to be the most affected, suggesting that the normal stresses of gravity are important in maintaining function, development, and therefore mobility (Gröer and Shekleton, 1989).

Decreased stability results from loss of endurance, decreased muscle mass, atrophy, and actual joint abnormalities. Patients/clients are unable to move steadily, and their risk of falling increases.

**Skeletal Effects** Immobilization causes two skeletal changes: impaired calcium metabolism and joint abnormalities. Immobilization results in bone reabsorption, decreased density of bone tissue, and osteoporosis (Brocklehurst, 1990). When osteoporosis occurs, the patient/client is at risk of pathological fractures. Bone reabsorption also causes calcium to be released into the blood, which can lead to hypercalcaemia.

Immobility also causes **joint contractures**. A joint contracture is an abnormal and usually permanent condition characterized by flexion and fixation of the joint. It is caused by disuse, atrophy, and shortening of the muscle fibres. When a contracture occurs, the joint cannot maintain full ROM and the joint is often left in a nonfunctional position (Hinchliff and Montague, 1992). One common and debilitating contracture is footdrop (Fig. 24-2). When footdrop occurs, the foot becomes permanently fixed in plantar flexion, and walking becomes extremely difficult.

Joint mobility can also be altered by joint inflammation, degeneration, or articular disruption.

**Arthritis** is an inflammation of the joints characterized by swelling and pain. It can result from a direct inflammatory reaction in the joint tissue such as gouty arthritis, an infectious process such as septic arthritis, or an immune-mediated inflammatory process such as rheumatoid arthritis.

Joint degeneration is demonstrated by changes in articular cartilage combined with changes at the articular bone ends (Gröer and Shekleton, 1989). Synovial and cartilaginous joints are equally affected, and degenerative changes commonly affect weight-bearing joints. Although degenerative joint disease is not caused by inflammation, it is frequently termed osteoarthritis.

## SKIN CHANGES

The skin is affected by immobility and by the resulting impaired metabolism, the loss of lean body mass, and negative nitrogen balance (Gröer and Shekleton, 1989). Thus any break in the skin's integrity is difficult to heal.

A **pressure sore**, or decubitus ulcer, is a localized area of tissue necrosis that develops when soft tissue is compressed between a bony prominence and an external surface for a prolonged period. Usually, sores form over bony prominences. Ischaemia develops when pressure on the skin is greater than the pressure inside the small peripheral blood vessels supplying blood to the skin (Clarke and Kadhom, 1988). Older individuals have a greater risk of developing pressure sores (Waterlow, 1991). Impairments in skin integrity have significant impact on well-being, nursing care, and length of hospital stay (see Chapter 30).

## URINARY ELIMINATION CHANGES

Changes in urinary elimination include:

- **urinary stasis** — in the upright position, urine flows out of the renal pelvis and into the ureter and bladder because of gravitational forces. When the patient/client is recumbent or flat, the kidneys and the ureters move towards a more level plane. Urine formed by the kidney must enter the bladder against gravity. Because the peristaltic contractions of the ureters are insufficient to overcome gravity, the renal pelvis may fill before urine enters the ureters. This condition increases the risk of urinary tract infection and renal calculi (see Chapter 22).

- **renal calculi** — calcium stones that lodge in the renal pelvis and pass through the ureters. Immobilized patients/clients are at risk because of altered calcium metabolism leading to hypercalcaemia (Brocklehurst, 1990). During the initial period of immobility urine volume is increased secondary to fluid shifts and a natural diuresis (Dietrick *et al*, 1948; Bliss, 1990). As the period of immobility continues, fluid intake often diminishes, and other factors, such as fever, increase the risk of dehydration. Urinary output therefore declines on or about the fifth or sixth day and becomes highly concentrated. This concentrated urine increases the risk of calculi formation and infection. Poor perineal care after bowel movements, particularly in women, increases the risk of urinary tract

contamination by bowel organisms, such as *Escherichia coli* bacteria. Catheterization increases the risk of infection.

## Psychosocial Effects

Immobilization has emotional, intellectual, sensory, and sociocultural implications. Changes in emotional status usually occur gradually, but older people are particularly vulnerable. The most common emotional changes are depression, behavioural changes, changes in the sleep-wake cycle, and impaired coping.

## NURSING PROCESS FOR IMPAIRED BODY ALIGNMENT AND MOBILITY

 ASSESSMENT

Both mobility and immobility should be assessed regularly.

### Mobility

Assessment of mobility focuses on range of motion, gait, exercise and activity tolerance, and body alignment.

### RANGE OF MOTION

**Range of motion** is the maximum amount of movement possible at a joint in one of the three planes of the body: sagittal, frontal, and transverse (Fig. 24-3, overleaf). The sagittal plane is a line that passes through the body from front to back, dividing the body into a left and a right side. The frontal plane passes through the body from side to side and divides the body into front and back. The transverse plane is a horizontal line that divides the body into upper and lower portions.

Joint mobility in each of the planes is limited by ligaments, muscles, and construction of the joint. However, some joint movements are specific to each plane. In the sagittal plane,

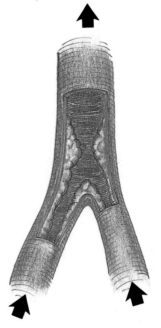

**Fig. 24-1** Thrombus formation in a vessel.

Some religious or cultural practices include physical movement or body positioning as part of their ritual practice. Some Hindu people, for example, may combine physical exercise with meditation and prayer into Hatha Yoga. In some eastern cultures T'ai Chi (a ritual sequence of smooth body movements and postures) is practised every morning, or morning and evening.

movements are flexion and extension (fingers and elbows) and hyperextension (hip). In the frontal plane, movements are abduction and adduction (arms and legs), and eversion and inversion (feet). In the transverse plane, movements are pronation and supination (hands), internal and external rotation (knees), and dorsiflexion and plantar flexion (feet).

When assessing ROM, the nurse collects data about joint stiffness, swelling, pain, limited movement, and unequal movement. Patients/clients whose joint mobility is restricted because of illness, disability, or trauma require passive movement of joints to reduce the hazards of immobility. These exercises are called passive ROM exercises.

## GAIT

**Gait** is the manner or style of walking, including rhythm, cadence, and speed. Observing a patient's/client's gait allows the nurse to assess balance, posture, safety, and ability to walk without assistance.

Normally, during walking, the adult posture is well aligned. The actual activity of walking takes place in a four-phase sequence: heel strike, stance, push-off, and swing. During heel strike, the foot is almost at right angles to the leg. The knee is extended but not locked and ready for slight flexion as the body weight is shifted forward into the stance phase. During stance, the trunk is maintained in a vertical position with the head and neck properly aligned. At push-off, there is plantar flexion of the foot and hyperextension of the metatarsophalangeal joints of the toes. During swing, the foot easily clears the floor with good alignment. Walking is rhythmic and coordinated.

## EXERCISE AND ACTIVITY TOLERANCE

Exercise conditions the body, improves health, and maintains fitness. It can also be used as therapy for correcting a deformity or restoring the patient/client to maximum health. There is an overall improvement of physiological functioning as a result of exercise. All systems become stronger and function more efficiently. When a person exercises, physiological changes occur.

Assessment of the patient's/client's energy level includes the physiological effects of exercise and activity tolerance. **Activity tolerance** is the kind and amount of exercise or work that a person is able to perform. Assessment of activity tolerance is necessary when planning activity such as walking, ROM exercises, activities of living and nursing interventions.

The person who experiences changes in physiological function during exercise, such as dyspnoea or chest pain, will not tolerate activity as well as the person who does not. Similarly, a weak or debilitated person will be unable to sustain activity.

People who are depressed, worried, or anxious are frequently

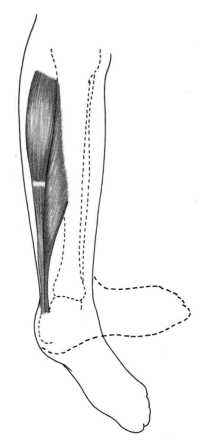

**Fig. 24-2** Footdrop. Ankle is fixed in plantar flexion. Normally the ankle is able to flex (dotted line), which eases walking.

unable to tolerate exercise. Depressed people may be difficult to motivate. Similarly, drugs, including alcohol and nicotine, can impair performance. Patients/clients who are worried or anxious fatigue easily because they expend a great deal of energy in worry and anxiety. Thus, they may experience physical and emotional exhaustion.

Developmental changes also affect activity tolerance. As the infant becomes a toddler, activity increases and the need for sleep declines. The child entering school expends mental energy in learning and may require more rest. During puberty more rest may be required because much of the body's energy is expended for growth and hormone changes.

As the person grows older, activity tolerance changes. Muscle mass is reduced, posture changes, and the composition of bones is altered. The individual may still exercise but will do it at a reduced intensity.

## BODY ALIGNMENT

Body alignment can be assessed with the patient/client standing, sitting, or lying down. Assessment has the following objectives:
- determining normal physiological changes in body alignment resulting from growth and development
- identifying deviations in body alignment caused by poor posture
- identifying learning needs of patients/clients for maintaining correct body alignment

- identifying trauma, muscle damage, or nerve dysfunction
- obtaining information concerning other contributing factors such as fatigue, malnutrition, and psychological problems.

The first step in assessing body alignment is to put patients/clients at ease so that unnatural or rigid positions are not assumed.

**Standing** The nurse should focus assessment on the following points:
1. The head is erect and midline.
2. When observed posteriorly, the shoulders and hips are straight and parallel.
3. When observed posteriorly, the vertebral column is straight.
4. When observed laterally, the head is erect and the spinal curves are aligned in a reversed S pattern. The cervical vertebrae are anteriorly convex, the thoracic vertebrae are posteriorly convex, and the lumbar vertebrae are anteriorly convex.
5. When observed laterally, the abdomen is comfortably tucked in and the knees and ankles are slightly flexed. The person appears comfortable.
6. The patient's/client's arms are comfortably at the sides.
7. Feet are placed slightly apart to achieve a base of support, and the toes are pointed forward.
8. When the patient/client is viewed anteriorly, the centre of gravity is in the midline, and the line of gravity is from the middle of the forehead to a midpoint between the feet. Laterally, the line of gravity runs vertically from the middle of the skull to the posterior third of the foot (Fig. 24-4).

**Sitting** The nurse assesses using the following observations:
1. The head is erect, and the neck and vertebral column are in alignment.
2. Weight is evenly distributed over the buttocks and thighs.
3. Thighs are parallel and in a horizontal plane.
4. Both feet are supported on the floor and the ankles are comfortably flexed (Fig. 24-5, overleaf).
5. A 2- to 4-cm space is maintained between the edge of the seat and the popliteal space at the back of the knee. This space ensures that there is no pressure on the popliteal artery or nerve to decrease circulation or impair nerve function.
6. The patient's/client's forearms are supported on the armrest, in the lap, or on a table in front of the chair.

It is particularly important to assess alignment when sitting if the individual has muscle weakness, muscle paralysis, or nerve damage. Because of these alterations, the patient/client will have diminished sensation and may be unable to perceive pressure or decreased circulation. Proper alignment reduces the risk of damage to the musculoskeletal system.

**Lying** Healthy people have voluntary muscle control and normal perception of pressure. As a result, they usually assume a position of comfort when lying down. Because their range of motion, sensation, and circulation are within normal limits, they change positions when they perceive muscle strain and decreased circulation.

Assessment of body alignment while lying requires that the patient/client be placed in the lateral position with all but one pillow and all positioning supports removed from the bed (Fig. 24-6, overleaf). The body should be supported by an adequate mattress. The vertebrae should be in straight alignment without observable curves.

The following people will be at risk of damage to the musculoskeletal system when lying down:
- those in traction or with arthritis

**Mental Health Nursing
Emotional adjustment to immobility**

Temporary or permanent immobility can impair a person's ability to carry out activities of living (ALs). Inability to perform ALs can contribute to low self-concept in some patients/clients. Impaired self-concept, in turn, can lead to self-defeating and self-destructive behaviours that may impede the patient's/client's rehabilitation and recovery.

Nursing care for these patients/clients should include interventions that contribute to increasing the individual's sense of worth, in addition to competency in managing daily activities.

From Haber J *et al: Comprehensive psychiatric nursing*, ed 4, St Louis, 1992, Mosby-Year Book.

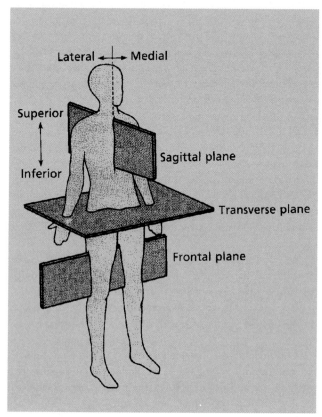

**Fig. 24-3** Planes of the body.

- those with decreased sensation, such as people with hemiparesis resulting from a stroke
- those with impaired circulation, such as people with diabetes
- those with lack of voluntary muscle control, such as people with spinal cord injuries.

If a patient/client is at risk, interventions are directed at maintaining proper body alignment through positioning (see later section).

## Immobility

The nurse assesses an immobilized patient/client for complications of immobility by performing a head-to-toe physical, psychological and developmental assessment.

### PHYSIOLOGICAL FACTORS

The physiological complications of immobility that may be identified during a nursing assessment are summarized in Table 24-1.

**Metabolic System** When assessing metabolic functioning the nurse uses intake and output charts to evaluate fluid and electrolyte status, assesses wound healing to evaluate alterations in the exchange of nutrients, and assesses the client's food intake, elimination patterns and weight to determine gastrointestinal functioning.

Intake and output measurements assist the nurse in determining whether a fluid imbalance exists. Dehydration and oedema increase the risk of skin breakdown.

If an immobilized patient has a wound, the rate of healing indicates how well nutrients are being delivered to tissues (see Chapter 30). Normal progression of healing indicates that the metabolic needs of injured tissues are being met.

Anorexia occurs commonly in immobilized patients/clients. The person's food intake should be assessed at each mealtime. Dietary patterns and food preferences should be assessed early in immobilization (see Chapter 21).

**Respiratory System** A respiratory assessment should be performed at least every 4 hours for individuals with restricted activity. The patient's/client's colour should be noted and the rate and quality of respirations recorded.

**Mother and Child Nursing**
**How does pregnancy affect energy tolerance?**

Pregnancy causes fluctuations in energy tolerance. During the first trimester tiredness is common, because hormonal changes and fetal development use energy. The second trimester usually results in a return of activity tolerance to the prepregnancy state. In fact, some women feel their activity tolerance is greater during this period. During the last trimester, fetal development consumes a great deal of the mother's energy. In addition, because of the size and location of the fetus, the pregnant woman's ability to take a deep breath is decreased and less oxygen is available for physical activities.

**Cardiovascular System** Cardiovascular assessment of the immobilized patient/client includes:

- **blood pressure monitoring** — because of the risk of postural hypotension, the individual's blood pressure should be measured, particularly when changing from a lying to a sitting or standing position. In this way, the ability to tolerate postural changes can be assessed before the person leaves the safety of bed.
- **evaluation of apical and peripheral pulses** — recumbency increases cardiac workload and results in an increased pulse rate. In some individuals, particularly older people, the heart may not tolerate the increased workload, and a form of cardiac failure may develop. A third heart sound, heard at the apex, can be an early indication of congestive heart failure. Monitoring peripheral pulses allows the nurse to evaluate the heart's ability to pump blood. The absence of a peripheral pulse, particularly one that was previously present, should be documented and reported to the medical team.
- **observation of signs of venous stasis** (oedema, poor wound healing) — oedema may indicate the heart's inability to handle increased workload. Because oedema moves to dependent body regions, assessment should include the sacrum, legs, and feet. If the heart is unable to tolerate the workload, peripheral body regions, such as the hands, feet, nose, and earlobes, will be colder than central body regions. In addition, **deep vein thrombosis** is a common hazard of restricted mobility. A dislodged thrombus, called an **embolus,** may travel through the circulatory system to the lungs or brain, impairing circulation and posing a threat to life.

Observe the calves for redness, warmth, and tenderness at least once each shift. In addition, measure calf circumference daily. To do this, mark a point on each calf and use this mark each day for

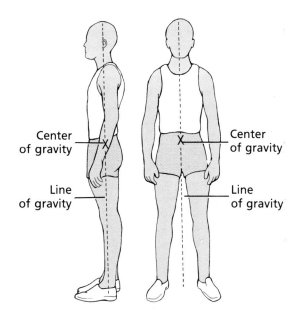

Fig. 24-4 Correct body alignment when standing.

placement of the tape measure. One-sided increases in calf diameter can be an early indication of thrombosis. Because deep vein thrombosis can also occur in the thigh, take thigh measurements daily if the patient/client is prone to thrombosis. In many people, deep vein thrombosis can be prevented by active exercise and elastic stockings.

### Musculoskeletal System

Musculoskeletal abnormalities that may be identified during nursing assessment include decreased muscle tone, loss of muscle mass, and contractures.

Assessment of ROM is important as a baseline against which later measurements can be compared to evaluate whether a loss in joint mobility has occurred.

Disuse osteoporosis cannot be identified by physical assessment. However, postmenopausal women and people with increased serum and urine calcium levels probably have a greater risk of bone demineralization and this should be considered when planning nursing interventions.

### Skin

The nurse must continually assess the patient's/client's skin for signs of breakdown. The skin should be observed each time that the individual is turned or when hygiene measures are performed (see Chapter 30).

### Elimination

The patient's/client's input (orally and/or parenterally) and output status should be evaluated on each shift.

Inadequate intake and output or fluid and electrolyte imbalances can increase the risk of renal system impairment, ranging from recurrent infections to kidney failure. Dehydration can also increase the risk of skin breakdown, thrombi formation, respiratory infections, and constipation. Such physical complications can decrease the overall level of mobility and can increase duration and cost of care.

Assessment of elimination status should also include the frequency and consistency of bowel movements (see Chapter 24). Accurate assessment enables the nurse to intervene before constipation and faecal impaction occur.

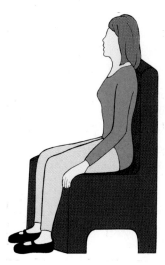

**Fig. 24-5** Correct body alignment when sitting.

## PSYCHOSOCIAL FACTORS

Changes in the patient's/client's psychosocial status are often overlooked by health care personnel. The nurse should therefore:

- **be alert to changes in emotional status** — if the individual appears to be becoming depressed due to boredom or isolation, such depression can often be alleviated by increasing bedside activities and occupational therapy.
- **observe for behavioural changes** — such as the cooperative patient/client who becomes argumentative — try to determine the reasons for such alterations to identify specific nursing interventions.
- **identify and correct unexplained changes in the sleep-wake cycle** — most can be prevented or minimized, such as those occurring because of nursing activities, a noisy environment, or discomfort. They may also occur because of medications such as analgesics, sedatives, or cardiovascular drugs.
- **observe for changes in the patient's/client's use of normal coping mechanisms** to adapt to immobilization. Decreased coping ability may cause the patient/client to become disoriented, confused, or depressed, or to experience other behavioural changes.

### Developmental Factors

Assessing the immobilized person should include developmental considerations.

**Children**: Determine whether the young child is achieving developmental milestones and is progressing normally. The child's development may regress or be slowed because of immobilization, and nursing interventions should be designed to maintain normal development. Parents may also need reassurance that developmental delays are usually temporary.

**Older people**: Determine the older patient's/client's ability to meet his or her needs independently and to adapt to developmental changes, such as declining physical functioning and altered family and peer relationships. A decline in developmental functioning needs prompt investigation to determine why the change occurred and what can be done to return to optimal levels of function as soon as possible.

 **PLANNING**

Body alignment and mobility are interrelated. Alterations in body alignment can result from developmental changes, postural abnormalities, abnormalities in bone formation, impaired muscle development, damage to the central nervous

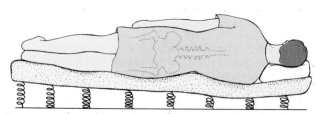

**Fig. 24-6** Correct body alignment when lying down.

## Table 24-1 Physiological Hazards of Immobility

| System | Abnormal Findings |
| --- | --- |
| Metabolic | Slowed wound healing, abnormal<br>Abnormal laboratory data<br>Muscle atrophy<br>Decreased amount of subcutaneous fat<br>Generalised oedema resulting from<br>hypoalbuminaemia |
| Respiratory | Asymmetrical chest wall movement,<br>dyspnea<br>Crackles, wheezes, increased<br>respiratory rate |
| Cardiovascular | Orthostatic hypotension<br>Incrased heart rate, third heart sound,<br>weak peripheral pulses, peripheral<br>oedema |
| Musculoskeletal | Erythema, increased diameter in calf or<br>thigh<br>Decreased ROM, joint contracture<br>activity intolerance, muscle atrophy,<br>joint contracture |
| Skin | Break in skin integrity |
| Elimination | Decreased urine output, cloudy or<br>concentrated urine<br>Decreased frequency of bowel<br>movements<br>Distended bladder and abdomen<br>Decreased bowel sounds |

system, and direct trauma to the musculoskeletal system.

**Too often, nurses focus purely on the physiological dimension of care, neglecting the psychosocial and developmental dimensions which are vitally important to health.**

For example, during immobilization, social interaction and stimulation are decreased. Ultimately, the patient/client may become isolated, withdrawn, and bored. Such individuals may frequently use the call bell to request minor physical attention, when their real need is greater socialization.

Care plans should be individualized and should consider the patient's/client's developmental stage, level of health, lifestyle and home environment. Planning care also involves an understanding of the individual's need to maintain motor function and independence. The nurse and patient/client should work together to establish ways to keep him or her involved in nursing care and to maintain optimal body alignment and mobility, whether the individual is in hospital or at home.

The care plan may contain one or more of the following long-term goals:

• maintaining proper body alignment

• regaining proper body alignment or optimal level of body alignment
• reducing injuries to the skin and musculoskeletal system
• achieving full or optimal ROM
• preventing contractures
• maintaining a patent airway
• achieving optimal lung expansion and gas exchange
• mobilizing airway secretions
• maintaining cardiovascular function
• increasing activity tolerance
• achieving normal elimination patterns
• maintaining normal sleep-wake patterns
• achieving socialization
• achieving independent completion of self-care activities
• achieving physical and mental stimulation.

These should be individualized and broken down into short-term achievable, and realistic steps.

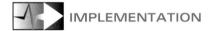 IMPLEMENTATION

### Body Alignment

To maintain proper body alignment lift, move and position the person correctly using hoists, as appropriate.

### LIFTING TECHNIQUES

Most occupational injuries are back injuries that are the direct result of improper lifting and bending techniques (Newman and Callaghan, 1993). The most common back injury is strain to the lumbar spine. Injury to this area affects the ability to bend forward, backward, and side to side. In addition, the ability to rotate the hips and lower back is decreased.

Before lifting, the nurse should consider:

1. Is lifting necessary or can the patient/client move him or herself under supervision and guidance?
2. Can a hoist be used?
3. Position of weight. The weight to be lifted should be as close to the lifter as possible.
4. Height of the patient/client or object.
5. Body position; the body should normally be positioned with the trunk erect so that multiple muscle groups work together in a synchronized manner.
6. Maximum weight. European Community directives 1992 (cited Corlett, 1992) have tightened up both employer and employee requirements regarding the safe manual handling of loads. Each nurse should know the maximum weight that is safe to carry — safe for the nurse and for the patient/client. An object is too heavy if its weight is 35% or more of a person's body weight. Therefore a nurse who weighs 59 kg should not try to lift an immobilized 45.5 kg person. Although the nurse may be able to do it, there is a risk of dropping the patient/client or injuring the nurse's back.

When lifting, the nurse should follow a procedure designed to maintain safety.

## Positioning Techniques

Patients/clients with impaired mobility often require help to attain proper body alignment while in bed or sitting. The nurse can use the following items for this purpose:

- a **good supply of pillows**. Before using a pillow, determine whether it is the proper size. A thick pillow under the patient's/client's head increases cervical flexion. A thin pillow under bony prominences may be inadequate to protect skin and tissue from damage caused by pressure.
- a **footboard** prevents footdrop by maintaining the feet in dorsiflexion. It must be placed perpendicular to the mattress, parallel to and touching the plantar surfaces of the patient's/client's feet .
- a **trochanter roll or pillow** prevents external rotation of the legs when the patient/client is in a supine position. When correct alignment of the hip is achieved, the patella faces directly upward.
- **sandbags** are sand-filled, material bags that can be shaped to body contours. They can be used in place of, or in addition to, pillows to immobilize an extremity or maintain body alignment.
- **hand rolls** maintain the hand, thumb, and fingers in a functional position (thumb in slight adduction and in opposition to the fingers).
- **hand-wrist splints** are individually moulded for the patient/client to maintain proper alignment of the thumb (slight adduction) and the wrist (slight dorsiflexion).
- a **trapeze** is a triangular device attached to the bed frame. It allows the pateint/client to raise the trunk off the bed or to perform upper arm exercises (Fig. 24-7).
- **side rails**, bars positioned along the sides of the bed, can help ensure patient/client safety and are also useful for increasing mobility. They allow the weak person to roll from side to side or sit up in bed. However, side rails should be used cautiously with people who are confused or disorientated: they may be injured if they try to get out of bed over the top of the rails (RCN, 1992).

The nurse should follow these universal steps for patients/clients who require positioning assistance:

1. Keep joints supported to prevent impaired alignment.
2. Position joints in a slightly flexed position, to prevent decreased mobility.
3. Assess pressure areas during positioning. When actual or potential pressure areas exist, nursing interventions involve reducing pressure, thus decreasing the risk of pressure sore development (see Chapter 30) and further trauma to the musculoskeletal system.

## Supported Fowler's Position

In the supported Fowler's position (Fig. 24-8, overleaf), the head of the bed is elevated 45 to 60 degrees and the patient's/client's knees are slightly elevated. The angle of head and knee elevation and the length of time that the individual should remain in the Fowler's position are influenced by his or her illness and overall condition. Supports must permit flexion of the hips and knees and proper alignment of the normal curves in the cervical, thoracic, and lumbar vertebrae.

The following problems may occur for the individual in the Fowler's position:

- increased cervical flexion because the pillow behind the head is too thick and pushes the head forward
- knees fully extended, allow the patient/client to slide to the foot of the bed
- pressure on the back of the knees, decreasing circulation to the feet
- hips externally rotated
- arms hanging unsupported at the patient's/client's sides
- unsupported feet
- unprotected pressure areas at the sacrum and heels.

## Supine Position

The supine position (Fig. 24-9, overleaf), where the client rests on his or her back, is also called the dorsal recumbent position, and the relationship of body parts is essentially the same as in standing. Pillows, trochanter rolls and arm splints are used to increase comfort and reduce injury.

The mattress should be firm enough to support the cervical, thoracic, and lumbar vertebrae (if the bed is very soft, place plywood under the mattress to give extra support). Shoulders must be supported and elbows slightly flexed to control shoulder rotation. A foot support should be used to prevent footdrop. The following problems may occur for the patient/client in the supine position:

- pillow at the head too thick, increasing cervical flexion
- head flat on the mattress
- shoulders unsupported and internally rotated
- elbows extended
- thumb not in opposition to the fingers
- hips externally rotated
- unsupported feet
- unprotected pressure areas at the back of the head, lumbar vertebrae, elbows, and heels.

## Prone Position

The patient/client in the prone position (Fig. 24-10, overleaf), lies face down, ensuring a safe airway. The head pillow should be thin enough to prevent cervical flexion or extension and maintain alignment of the lumbar spine. Placing a pillow under the lower leg permits dorsiflexion of the ankles and some knee flexion, which promotes relaxation. If a pillow is unavailable, the ankles should be in dorsiflexion over the end of the mattress. The nurse should assess for and correct any of the following potential trouble points:

- neck hyperextension
- hyperextension of the lumbar spine
- plantar flexion of the ankles
- unprotected pressure areas at the chin, elbows, hips, knees, and toes.

## Side-Lying Position

In the side-lying (or lateral) position (Fig. 24-11, overleaf) the patient's/client's major portion of body weight rests on the dependent hip and shoulder. Trunk alignment should be the same as in standing. For example, the structural curves of the spine should be maintained, the head should be supported in line with the midline of the trunk, and rotation of the spine should be avoided. The following trouble points are common:

- lateral flexion of the neck
- spinal curves out of normal alignment
- shoulder and hip joints internally rotated, adducted, or unsupported
- lack of support for the feet
- lack of protection for pressure points at the ear, ilium, knees, and ankles.

### Sims' Position

The Sims' position (Fig. 24-12, overleaf) differs from the side-lying position in the distribution of the patient's/client's weight. In the Sims' position the weight is placed on the anterior ilium, humerus, and clavicle. Trouble points include:

- lateral flexion of the neck
- internal rotation, adduction, or lack of support to the shoulders and hips
- lack of support for the feet
- lack of protection for pressure areas at the ilium, humerus, clavicle, knees, and ankles.

## TRANSFER TECHNIQUES

The following guidelines should be used in any transfer procedure:

1. Assess the patient's/client's mobility and strength to determine if he or she can assist during the transfer.
2. Determine the need for assistance or a hoist.
3. Explain the procedure and describe what is expected of the patient/client.
4. Elevate the level of the bed to a comfortable height.
5. Raise the side rail on the side of the bed opposite the nurse to prevent the patient/client from falling out of bed. Apply the brake on hospital beds to prevent the bed from falling.
6. Assess body alignment and pressure areas after each transfer.

The nurse who is attempting transfer or moving techniques for the first time should request help to reduce the risk of injury to the patient/client and nurse. Moving a completely immobile patient/client alone is dangerous.

### Moving Patients/Clients

Patients/clients will require various levels of assistance to move in bed, change to a side-lying position, or sit up at the side of the bed. For example, a young, healthy woman may need only a little support as she sits at the side of the bed for the first time after childbirth, whereas an older man may need help from one or more nurses to do the same task one day after an appendicectomy.

To determine what the individual is able to do alone, whether a hoist should be used and how many people are needed to help, the nurse should:

1. Assess the patient/client to determine whether the illness contradicts exertion (for example, cardiovascular disease).
2. Determine whether the patient/client understands what is expected (for example, a person who has recently received medication for postoperative pain may be too lethargic to

understand instructions). To ensure safety, two nurses are needed to move the person in bed.

3. Determine the comfort level of the patient/client and whether he or she is too heavy or immobile for the nurse to complete the procedure alone. **In doubtful cases, always request assistance from another person and/or use a hoist**.

### Transferring a Patient/Client from Bed to Chair

Transferring a patient/client from bed to chair by one nurse (Fig. 24-13, A-D on p. 498-9) requires assistance from the person and should not be attempted with a patient/client who cannot help.

1. Explain the procedure to the patient/client before the transfer and prepare the environment by removing obstacles.
2. Place the chair next to the bed with the chair back in the same plane as the head of the bed. This enables the nurse to pivot with the individual and to transfer the person's weight efficiently and safely.
3. Request assistance, if there is any doubt. A safe transfer is the first priority. The patient/client should sit on the side of the bed for at least a minute before standing, and provision should be made so that he or she can quickly be lowered back into bed in case of dizziness or fainting.

### Transferring a Patient/Client From Bed to Trolley

An immobilized patient/client who must be transferred from bed to trolley, or bed to bed (Fig. 24-14 on p. 499), requires a three (or more) person lift. This technique is best implemented when personnel who are doing the lifting are similar in height. If the individual has spinal cord trauma, spinal alignment must be maintained during the transfer.

1. Prepare patient/client for the transfer and ask him or her to help if possible by, for example, crossing his or her arms.

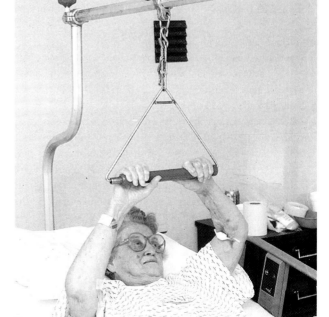

Fig. 24-7 Patient/client using a trapeze bar.

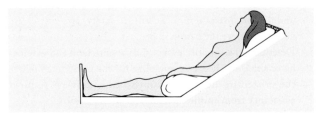

**Fig 24-8** Supported Fowler's position.

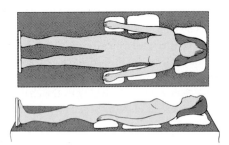

**Fig 24-9** Supine position.

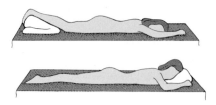

**Fig 24-10** Prone position.

do not cause pain
- never force a joint beyond its capacity; repeat each movement five times during the session
- when performing passive ROM exercises, stand at the side of the bed closest to the joint being exercised
- if an extremity is to be moved or lifted, place a cupped hand under the joint to support it (Fig. 24-15 A on p. 500), support the joint by holding the adjacent distal and proximal areas (Fig. 24-15 B on p. 500), or support the joint with one hand and cradle the distal portion of the extremity with the remaining arm (Fig. 24-15 C on p. 500).

## Walking

In the normal walking posture the head is erect; the cervical, thoracic, and lumbar vertebrae are aligned; the hips and knees have appropriate flexion; and the arms swing freely with the legs.

## ASSISTING A PATIENT/CLIENT TO WALK

As with any other procedure, assisting the patient/client to walk requires preparation:

1. First assess the individual's activity tolerance, strength, presence of pain, coordination, and balance to determine the amount of assistance needed.
2. Explain why walking is important, how far the patient/client should try to walk, who is going to help and when the walk will take place.
3. Determine with the patient/client how much independence he or she can assume.
4. Remove obstacles so that the individual has ample room to walk safely.
5. Establish rest points before starting, in case activity tolerance is less than estimated or the person becomes dizzy. For example, place a chair in the corridor for the patient/client to sit on if needed.
6. Minimize the effects of postural hypotension, by helping the patient/client to sit on the side of the bed for 1 to 2 minutes before standing.
7. After standing, allow the patient/client to remain stationary for 1 to 2 minutes before moving, to allow his or her balance to stabilize. The longer the period of immobility, the greater the risk of hypotension when the individual stands.
8. Provide support at the waist so that the patient's/client's centre of gravity remains midline. While walking, the individual should not lean to one side because this alters the centre of gravity, distorts balance, and increases the risk of falling.
9. Return the individual who appears unsteady or complains of dizziness to a nearby bed or chair. If the person faints or begins to fall, assume a wide base of support with one foot in

2. Clear the environment of obstacles and remove unnecessary equipment from the bedside.
3. Place the trolley at right angles to the bed, so the lifters can pivot towards the trolley and transfer the patient/client efficiently.
4. Work together, as with all procedures, safety is the priority. Safety is increased in all lifts if the lifters work together. Therefore, one person should assume the leadership role.

### Joint Mobility

Nursing interventions should be designed to maintain maximum joint mobility. The nurse and physiotherapist can teach the patient/client ROM exercises but if the individual does not have voluntary motor control, the nurse should carry out passive range of motion exercises.

## RANGE OF MOTION EXERCISES

To ensure that patients/clients receive these exercises (see Table 24-1) regularly, the nurse should schedule them at specific times, perhaps alongside another nursing activity, such as during the individual's bath.

ROM exercises may be active (the person is able to move all joints through their ROM unassisted), passive (the person is unable to move independently and the nurse moves each joint through its ROM), or somewhere in between. With a weak patient/client, for example, the nurse may merely provide support while the individual performs most of the movement, or the individual may be able to move some joints actively while the nurse passively moves others.

Key points for ROM exercises include:
- exercises should be as active as the patient's/client's health and mobility allow
- contractures may develop in joints if they are not moved periodically through their full ROM
- unless contraindicated, begin passive ROM exercises as soon as the person's ability to move the extremity or joint is lost
- ensure movements are carried out slowly and smoothly and

front of the other and gently lower the patient/client to the floor, protecting the head.

For individuals with **hemiplegia** (one-sided paralysis) or **hemiparesis** (one-sided weakness), always stand on the person's affected side and support him or her by holding one arm around the waist and the other arm around the inferior aspect of the upper arm so that the nurse's hand is under the patient's/client's axilla. Holding only the individual's arm is incorrect because the nurse cannot easily lower the person to the floor if that person faints or falls. Also, if the patient/client falls with the nurse holding an arm, a shoulder joint may be dislocated.

Many patients/clients will need to be assisted by two nurses. The two-nurse method helps distribute the person's weight evenly:

1. Stand on either side of the patient/client.
2. Each nurse places his or her near arm around the patient's/client's waist, and the other arm around the inferior aspect of the patient's/client's arm so that both nurses' hands are supporting the patient's/client's axillae.

## USING ASSISTIVE DEVICES FOR WALKING

Walking frames are extremely light, movable devices, about waist height, made of metal tubing. They have four widely placed, sturdy legs (sometimes with wheels attached). The patient/client holds the handgrips on the upper bars, takes a step, moves the walker forward, and takes another step (Fig. 24-17 on p. 501).

Walking sticks are used to support and balance a client with decreased leg strength. The walking stick should be kept on the stronger side of the body. For maximum support when walking, the person places the walking stick forward, keeping body weight on both legs. The weaker leg is moved forward 15–25 cm to the walking stick so that the body weight is divided between the walking stick and the stronger leg. The stronger leg is advanced past the walking stick so that the weaker leg and the body weight are supported by the walking stick and weaker leg. To walk, the person continually repeats these steps.

Crutches are also used to increase mobility. Their use may be temporary, such as after ligament damage to the knee or permanent (for example, by the client with spina bifida and leg calipers). There are three types of crutches:

- **axillary crutch** (Fig. 24-17 A on p.501), which has a padded curved surface at the top, which fits under the axilla. A handgrip in the form of a crossbar is held at the level of the palms to support the body.
- **gutter crutch** (Fig. 24-17 B on p. 501), which has a trough to contain the forearm and is suitable for individuals with weakened hands and wrists.
- **elbow crutch** (Fig. 24-17 C on p.501), which has a handgrip and a metal band that fits around the forearm. Both the metal band and the handgrip are adjusted to fit the person's height.

Crutches must be selected and measured by the physiotherapist. Patient/clients must be taught to use their crutches safely.

### Reducing the Hazards of Immobility

Nursing interventions should focus on preventing or minimizing the hazards of immobility. Interventions should therefore be directed at maintaining optimal function of all body systems.

## METABOLIC SYSTEM

The immobilized patient/client requires a high-protein, high-calorie diet with vitamin B and C supplements. Protein is needed to repair injured tissue and rebuild depleted protein stores. A high-calorie intake provides sufficient fuel to meet metabolic needs and to replace subcutaneous tissue.

Vitamin C supplements are necessary to replace protein stores. Vitamin B complex is needed for skin integrity and wound healing.

If the individual is unable to eat, nutrition must be provided parenterally or enterally. Enteral feedings include delivery through a nasogastric, gastrostomy, or jejunostomy tube (see Chapter 21). Total parenteral nutrition involves delivery of nutritional supplements through a central or peripheral intravenous catheter.

## RESPIRATORY SYSTEM

Nursing interventions for the respiratory system are aimed at promoting expansion of the chest and lungs, preventing stasis of pulmonary secretions, maintaining a patent airway, and promoting adequate exchange of respiratory gases.

### Promoting Expansion of Chest and Lungs

Changing the position of the patient/client at least every 2 hours allows the dependent lung regions to re-expand. Re-expansion maintains the elastic recoil property of the lungs and clears the dependent lung regions of pulmonary secretions.

The nurse should encourage the patient/client to deep breathe and cough or huff every 1 to 2 hours. Alert individuals can be taught to deep breathe every hour. This action expands all lobes of the lungs and prevents atelectasis. Coughing reduces the stasis of pulmonary secretions. For unconscious individuals with an artificial airway, the nurse can expand the chest and lungs by using an Ambu bag (see Chapter 17).

The nurse must use caution when administering post operative pain medication. These medications can depress the respiratory centre, so the rate of respiration or expansion of the lungs is decreased.

If abdominal binders and rib supports are required, with permission from the medical staff, they should be removed every

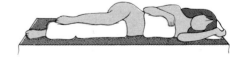

**Fig 24-11** Side-lying position.

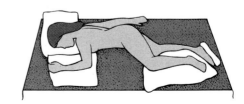

**Fig 24-12** Sims' position.

2 hours to allow the patient/client to breathe deeply. Removal may be contraindicated, however, for the person who has just had surgery or has just suffered trauma.

### Preventing Stasis of Pulmonary Secretions

Stagnant secretions accumulating in the bronchi and lungs can lead to growth of bacteria and subsequent development of pneumonia. However, pulmonary infections may still develop despite interventions to prevent them.

Stagnation of secretions can be reduced by frequent changes of position which repositions the dependent lung and mobilizes secretions.

Chest physiotherapy is an effective method of preventing pulmonary secretions. Physiotherapists use positioning techniques to drain secretions from specific segments of the bronchi and lungs into the trachea. The patient/client then expels secretions by coughing.

### Maintaining a Patent Airway

Immobilized patients/clients and those on bed rest are generally weakened. If weakness progresses, the cough reflex gradually becomes inefficient. If the person is too weak or unable to cough up

secretions, the nurse must maintain a patent airway using suctioning techniques (see Chapter 17). The stasis of secretions in the lungs may be life threatening for an immobilized person, because hypostatic bronchopneumonia can easily develop. Symptoms of this condition include productive cough with greenish-yellow sputum, fever, pain on breathing, crackles, wheezes, and dyspnoea. Dislodging and mobilizing stagnant secretions reduces the risk of pneumonia.

An obstructed airway is usually the result of a mucus plug. Several therapies can help reduce the risk of mucus plugs and to maintain a patent airway (see Chapter 17 for more details):

- Patients/clients can be asked to deep breathe and cough or huff every 1 to 2 hours. The nurse instructs the individual to take in three deep breaths and cough or huff with the third exhalation. This technique produces a more forceful, productive cough without excessive fatigue.
- Tracheal suction can be used to remove secretions in the upper airways of someone who is retaining secretions, is distressed and unable to cough productively. This procedure must be performed aseptically. The nurse inserts a catheter via the patient's/client's nose or mouth and applies suction.
- The nurse can suction secretions from an artificial airway,

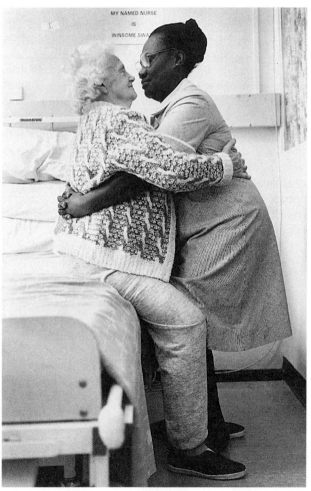
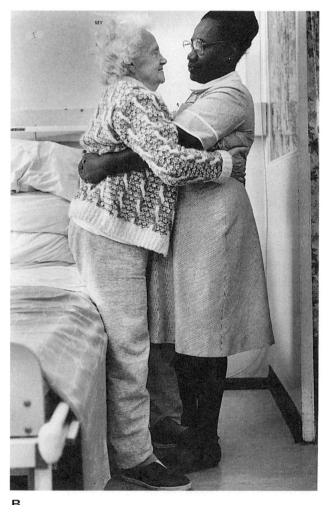

A              B

**Fig 24-13** Transferring a patient/client from bed to chair by one nurse. A. Place hands firmly around patient's/client's back, B. rock patient/client up to standing while straightening your hips and legs, keeping knees slightly flexed.

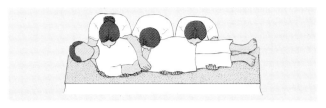

**Fig 24-14** Transferring a patient/client from bed to trolley. Lifters' arms are placed under patient's/client's head and shoulders, hips, and thighs and lower legs, with their fingers securely around the other side of patient's/client's body.

such as an endotracheal or tracheal tube. Using aseptic technique, the nurse inserts a catheter into the artificial airway and removes pulmonary secretions from the upper and lower airways (see Chapter 17).

## CARDIOVASCULAR SYSTEM

**Reducing Postural Hypotension** After a period of bed rest, patients/clients usually have an increased pulse rate, a decreased pulse pressure, and increased fainting when standing (Winslow, 1985). The following interventions can reduce or eliminate the effects of **postural hypotension**:

- attempt to get the patient/client out of bed as soon as

possible, even if the move is only to a chair, because activity maintains muscle tone and increases venous return
- when being moved from bed to chair, the individual should change positions gradually and any changes in vital signs should be documented
- obtain baseline vital signs with the individual in the supine position; then raise him or her to a high Fowler's position and measure the vital signs again to evaluate decreases in blood pressure or elevations in pulse
- remain with the patient/client for a few moments to allow the body to adapt to any changes
- monitor the person for any dizziness and light-headedness and ask the person to sit on the side of the bed with feet on the floor for a few minutes before attempting the transfer.

Frequent sitting or standing minimize the hypotensive effects of bed rest. These interventions counteract the headward fluid shift that occurs with bed rest and redistributes venous volume (Winslow, 1985).

**Preventing Thrombus Formation** Immobilized patients/clients are frequently prescribed low-dose heparin

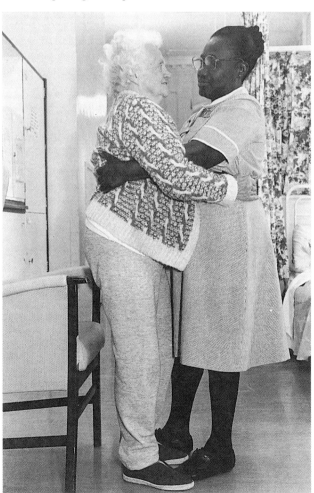

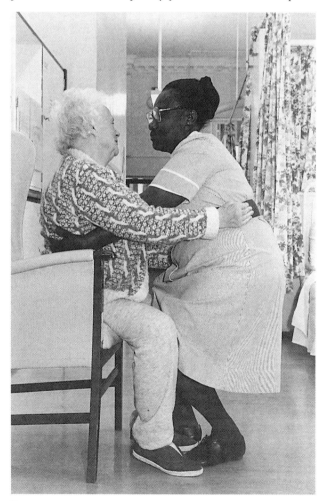

**C**       **D**

C. pivot on foot that is farther from chair, D. flex your hips and knees while lowering patient/client into chair.

therapy to minimize the risk of venous thromboembolism. Heparin is an anticoagulant which suppresses clot formation. Heparin therapy requires a medical prescription. The usual route of administration is subcutaneous injection. Because of the action of this medication, the nurse must continually assess the patient/client for signs of bleeding, such as increased bruising, guaiac positive stools, haematuria and bleeding gums. Although most people receiving low-dose heparin do not experience side effects, the risk remains present. Other interventions to prevent thrombus formation include:

- Intermittent pneumatic compression (IPC) devices that are designed to provide rhythmic external extremity compression through inflatable 'stockings'. IPC has proven effective in reducing deep vein thrombosis in general surgical, high-risk oncology, orthopaedic, and neurological patients/clients (THRIFT, 1992).

- therapeutic elastic stockings with graded compressions reduce the risk of thrombus formation (THRIFT, 1992). Elastic stockings help maintain external pressure on the leg muscles and thus may promote venous return. The stockings must be applied properly and removed and reapplied at least daily.

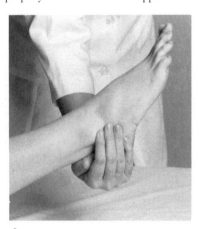

**A**

- Proper positioning. When positioning patients/clients, care should be taken to prevent pressure behind the knee and on the deep veins in the lower extremities.
- ROM exercises also have beneficial effects in preventing thrombi. Exercise causes contraction of the skeletal muscles, which in turn exerts pressure on the veins and promotes venous return, reducing venous stasis.

If deep vein thrombosis is suspected, the nurse should report it to the medical staff immediately. The leg should be elevated with no pressure on the thrombus. The family, patient/client, and all health care personnel should be instructed not to massage the area because of the danger of dislodging the thrombus.

## MUSCULOSKELETAL SYSTEM

Some orthopaedic procedures, such as joint replacement, require more frequent passive ROM exercises to restore function after surgery. Patients/clients with such conditions may use automatic equipment for passive ROM exercises. The equipment extends an extremity to a particular angle for a prescribed period. This is beneficial when the patient/client must gradually increase the degree and duration of extension.

Individuals on bed rest should have active ROM exercises incorporated into their daily schedules. They can perform these exercises during activities of living. The box describes joint movements that occur with daily activities.

Active ROM exercises maintain functioning of the musculoskeletal system and progressive exercise programmes are vital in helping the transition back to normal (or optimal) functioning.

Exercise programmes should be individualized to the patient's/client's health, age, weight, illness, and motivation, gradually increasing activity to reverse the deconditioning associated with bed rest (Winslow and Weber, 1980). Before beginning the programme, warm-up exercises should be performed, unless they are contraindicated.

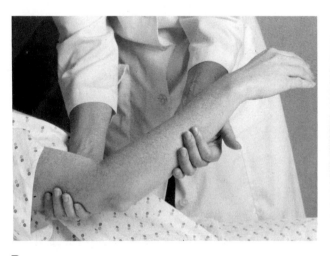

**B**

**Fig. 24-15** Methods for supporting a joint: A. Cupped hand, B. holding adjacent, distal and proximal areas, C. cradling distal portion.

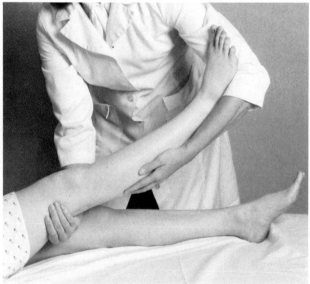

**C**

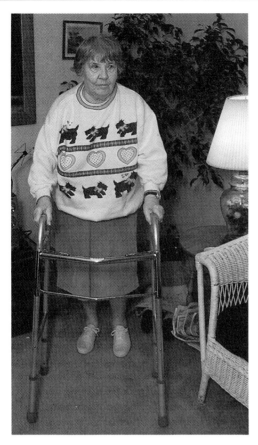

**Fig 24-16** Patient/client using a walking frame.

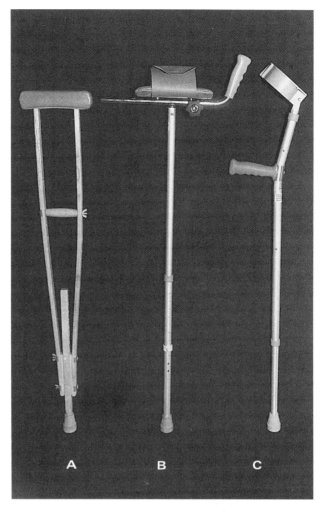

**Fig 24-17** Types of crutches. A. axiliary crutch B. gutter crutch, C. elbow crutch. © Bruce Bailey/ Select Photos, London.

## SKIN

The major risk to skin from restricted mobility is **pressure sores**. Nursing interventions should therefore focus on prevention and treatment (see Chapter 30).

## ELIMINATION

Nursing interventions for maintaining optimal urinary functioning are directed at keeping the patient/client well hydrated (without causing bladder distention) and preventing urinary stasis, calculi, and infections.

Adequate hydration (for example, 2000 to 3000 ml daily) helps prevent renal calculi and urinary tract infections. The well hydrated individual will void large amounts of dilute urine. To prevent bladder distention, assess the frequency and amount of urinary output. A patient/client who continually dribbles urine and whose bladder is distended often has overflow incontinence. If the immobilized person does not have voluntary control of urinary elimination, an indwelling catheter (as a last resort) may be necessary to prevent distention, promote comfort, preserve skin integrity and enable accurate monitoring of output (see Chapter 22).

The nurse must also record the frequency and consistency of bowel movements. A diet rich in fruits, vegetables, and bulk can facilitate normal peristalsis. If a patient/client is unable to maintain a regular bowel pattern, the doctor may prescribe stool softeners, laxatives, or enemas (see Chapter 23).

## PSYCHOSOCIAL CHANGES

The nurse should anticipate changes in the patient's/client's psychosocial status and provide regular and informal socialization:

- Plan nursing activities so that the individual can talk and interact with staff.
- If possible the person should be placed in a room with others who are mobile and interactive. If a private room is required, staff and family members should visit frequently.
- Provide stimuli to maintain orientation. A daily newspaper helps people keep track of events and time. Conversation should engage the patient's/client's nursing activities, meals, and visiting hours. Books help occupy the person when alone. The individual can participate in craft activities. Radio and television provide stimulation and help pass the time.
- Encourage patients/clients to maintain their body image by wearing their glasses or dentures, shaving or applying make-up. Maintenance of body image can help alleviate depression resulting from immobilization.
- Patients/clients should be involved in their care and enabled to be as independent as possible.
- Schedule nursing care to minimize interruptions of sleep. For

## Learning Disabilities Nursing
## Working with mobility problems

Many people with learning disabilities have associated mobility problems, ranging from mild, but significant, ataxia to profound handicaps that render them incapable of unaided movement. The key to minimizing these disabilities lies in a thorough, realistic and carefully planned multidisciplinary assessment. This should be followed by a carefully planned physiotherapy and rehabilitation programme that is consistently implemented. Ensuring that such a programme is carried out every day requires meticulous coordination and the ability to motivate team members to what often seems a hopeless task. Close and continued work with the physiotherapist and other health professionals, combined with the imaginative incorporation of physiotherapy programmes and exercises into everyday activities, are key elements in the success of such programmes.

Some people with learning disabilities have developed gait and posture disorders that label them as 'handicapped'. In many cases, tactful but firm guidance on normal ways of walking and correct posture can be beneficial. The use of music and dance can help patients/clients with uncoordinated movement to develop confidence and poise.

example, administer medications and assess vital signs when the client is turned or receives special skin care.

- Assess and promote the individual's coping strategies. If selected strategies are ineffective, a counsellor, social worker or spiritual advisor may be needed. Their recommendations should be incorporated into the care plan.

## DEVELOPMENTAL CHANGES

Ideally, immobilized patients/clients continue normal development. This is sometimes unrealistic for the very young or very old; however, the following nursing interventions can help.

- Involve mental and physical stimulation. Incorporate play activities into the care plan. Completing puzzles or playing computer games, for example, helps a child to develop fine motor skills, and reading helps the child develop cognitively.
- Place an immobilized child with children of the same age who are not immobilized, unless a contagious disease is present.
- Design nursing activities, such as dressing changes, cast care, and care of traction, to require participation of the child.
- Recognize significant changes from normal behavioural patterns.

Restricted mobility in older patients/clients presents unique nursing challenges. (Chapter 6 describes measures to assist older people in meeting developmental needs). Chronic illnesses often place them at increased risk from the complications of immobility. Inactive older patients/clients are at greater risk of confusion, depression, and disorientation which may result from immobilization, chronic illness and medications. For example, frail older clients may need position changes every hour instead of

every 2 hours, and may need more frequent ROM exercises. An individualized care plan should be designed to prevent or minimize these hazards. To assist in maintaining orientation to time, keep a calendar and a clock with a large face in view (see Chapter 26). The calendar should be marked so that the patient/client can immediately identify the correct day and date. In addition, encourage independence through nursing care.

 ## EVALUATION

To evaluate outcomes and response to nursing care, the nurse must measure the effectiveness of all interventions, including patient/client and family teaching. The nurse also investigates the patient's/client's and family's need for additional support services (for example, home care, community nurse, meals-on-wheels) and initiates the referral process.

Evaluation of nursing care for patients/clients with altered body alignment and mobility should be based on objective criteria for each nursing goal.

Maintaining good body alignment and mobility, and preventing the hazards of immobility increases independence and overall mobility. The best approach to problems with body alignment and joint mobility is prevention, which begins early in the care plan.

## Incorporating Active Exercises into Activities of Living

- Nodding head 'yes' exercises neck (flexion and extension).
- Shaking head 'no' exercises neck (rotation).
- Moving right ear to right shoulder exercises neck (lateral flexion).
- Moving left ear to left shoulder exercises neck (lateral flexion).
- Reaching to turn on overhead light exercises shoulder (flexion).
- Reaching to bedside stand for book exercises shoulder (abduction).
- Scratching back exercises shoulder (hyperextension and inward rotation).
- Rotating shoulders toward chest exercises shoulder.
- Rotating shoulders toward back exercises shoulder.
- Eating, bathing, shaving, and grooming exercise elbow (flexion, extension).
- All activities requiring fine motor coordination, such as writing and eating, exercise fingers and thumb (flexion, extension, abduction, adduction, opposition).
- Walking exercises hip (flexion, extension, hyperextension).
- Rolling toes outward exercises hip (external rotation).
- Walking exercises knee (flexion, extension).
- Walking exercises ankle (dorsiflexion, plantar flexion).
- Pointing toe toward head of bed exercises ankle (dorsiflexion).
- Pointing toe toward foot of bed exercises ankle (plantar flexion).
- Walking exercises toes (extension, hyperextension).
- Wiggling toes exercises toes (abduction, adduction).

## SUMMARY

The nurse uses an understanding of the physiological principles of movement and body mechanics to transfer and position patients/clients safely, and to assist patients/clients in the correct use of walking frames, crutches and other mobility-promoting devices. A knowledge of the pathological influences of body alignment and of the risk factors associated with immobility enables the nurse to develop an effective care plan for patients/clients with potential or actual alterations in these areas.

Planning is vital in the prevention of the numerous secondary physical complications associated with immobility. The psychosocial effects of immobilization affect every aspect of the patient's/client's life, and continuous assessment by the nurse can ensure optimum levels of both physical and mental patient/client health. A range of nursing interventions can also be implemented to promote optimum comfort, mobility, and joint range-of-motion flexibility for each individual.

An understanding of body mechanics can be used to protect both the nurse and patient/client from injuries to the musculoskeletal system. Correct use of lifting, positioning, and transfer techniques are fundamental to all aspects of nursing care, ensuring maximum comfort for the patient/client and nurse during every procedure.

## CHAPTER 24 REVIEW

### Key Concepts

- Body mechanics refers to the coordinated efforts of the musculoskeletal and nervous systems as the person moves, lifts, bends, stands, sits, lies down, and completes daily activities.
- Coordinated body movement requires integrated functioning of the skeletal system, skeletal muscles, and nervous system.
- The skeleton provides a bony support structure for movement, attachment of ligaments and muscles, protection of vital organs, and contributes to the regulation of calcium and blood cell production.
- The nervous system initiates and provides voluntary control of movement.
- Coordination and regulation of muscle groups depend on muscle tone and activity of antagonistic, synergistic, and antigravity muscles.
- Balance is assisted by the cerebellum and inner ear.
- Body alignment is the relationship of joints, tendons, ligaments, and muscles in various body positions.
- Body balance is achieved when there is a wide base of support, the centre of gravity falls within the base of support, and a vertical line falls from the centre of gravity through the base of support.
- Developmental stages influence body alignment and mobility; the greatest impact of physiological changes on the musculoskeletal system is observed in children and older people.
- Normal physical mobility depends on intact and functioning nervous and musculoskeletal systems.

- The risk of disabilities related to immobilization depends on the extent and duration of immobilization.
- Immobility may result from illness or trauma or may be prescribed for therapeutic reasons. Immobility presents physiological, psychological and developmental hazards.
- The nursing process is used to provide care for patients/clients experiencing, or at risk for, the adverse effects of impaired body alignment and immobility.
- After a comprehensive assessment, the nurse plans and implements interventions to prevent or minimize the hazards and complications of impaired body alignment and immobilization.
- Range of motion exercises include one or all of the body joints.
- Mechanical devices to promote walking include walking sticks, walking frames, and crutches.

## CRITICAL THINKING EXERCISES

1. You are caring for a patient/client who is in bilateral leg traction. How do you determine what type of mobility this person can safely perform and how this can be incorporated into the care plan?
2. When caring for a patient/client with a spinal cord injury, you note that his or her legs 'stiffen' and resist motion occasionally during ROM exercises. What do you do so that further injury does not occur to the musculoskeletal system?
3. Mrs Miller's mobility is limited after a stroke that left her with hemiplegia. She has a history of chronic constipation. What measures can the nurse independently implement to reduce potential complications? What criteria could be used to determine effectiveness?
4. You're caring for a 27-year-old mother who is immobilized after spinal cord trauma. You note that she is becoming increasingly depressed and withdrawn. What actions would you take?

### KEY TERMS

Bed rest, p. 485
Body alignment/posture, p. 481, 482
Body mechanics, p. 481
Cartilage, p. 483
Centre of gravity, p. 482
Connective tissue, p. 482
Embolus, p. 491
Fracture, p. 485
Gait, p. 490
Joint contracture(s), p. 487
Joints, p. 482
Ligaments, p. 483
Mobility/immobility, p. 485
Pathological fractures, p. 482
Range of motion (ROM), p. 488
Skeletal muscles, p. 483
Tendons, p. 483
Thrombus (formation)/deep vein thrombosis, p. 487, 491
Weight, p. 482

## REFERENCES

Bliss M: Medical implications of the sedentary posture: *Care Science Practice* 8(3):104, 1990.

Brocklehurst JC: Bone disease in the elderly, *Nurs Elderly* 2(1):16, 1990.

Clarke M, Kadhom HM: The nursing prevention of pressure sores in hospital and community patients, *JAN* 13(3):365, 1988.

Corlett EN: *The guide to the handling of patients*, Teddington, 1992, National Back Pain Association.

Deitrick JE *et al*: Effects of immobilization upon various metabolic and physiologic functions of normal men, *Am J Med* 4:3, 1948.

Exton-Smith AN: *Practical geriatric medicine*, Edinburgh, 1985, Churchill Livingstone.

Greenleaf JE: Physiological responses to prolonged bedrest and fluid immersion in humans, *J Appl Physiol* 57(3):619,1984.

Gröer MW, Shekleton ME: Basic pathophysiology: a conceptual approach, ed 3, St Louis, 1989, Mosby.

Hinchliff S, Montague S: *Physiology for nursing practice*, London, 1992, Baillière Tindall.

McCance KL, Huether SE: *Pathophysiology: the biologic basis for disease in adults and children*, St Louis, 1990, Mosby.

Newman S, Callaghan C: Work related back pain, *Occupational Health* 45(6):201, 1993.

Olson EV, Thompson LF: The hazards of immobility: effects on respiratory function, *Am J Nurs* 90(3):47, 1990.

Pinel C: Metabolic bone disease, *Nurs* 3(37):22, 1989.

Reddy MP: A guide to early mobilization of bedridden elderly, *Geriatrics* 41(9):59, 1986.

RCN: *Focus on restraint: guidelines on the use of restraint in the care of older people*, London, 1992, Royal College of Nursing.

Rubin M: How bedrest changes perception, *Am J Nurs* 88:55, 1988a.

Rubin M: The physiology of bedrest, *Am J Nurs* 88:50, 1988b.

Stamps JL: "Back" to basics, *Emerg Med Services* 18(2):38, 1989.

Strand FL: *Physiology: a regulatory systems approach*, New York, 1978, Macmillan.

THRIFT (Thromboembolic Risk Factors) Consensus Group: risk of and prophylaxis for venous thromboembolism in hospital patients, *BMJ* 305: 567, 1992.

Tompkins ES: Effect of restricted mobility and dominance on perceived duration, *Nurs Res* 29:333, 1980.

Waterlow J: A policy that protects: the Waterlow pressure sore prevention/treatment policy, *Prof Nurs* 6(5): 258, 1991.

Winslow EH: Cardiovascular consequences of bedrest, *Heart Lung* 14(3):236, 1985.

## FURTHER READING
### Adult Nursing

Bliss MR: Is bed really bad for older people? *Geriatric Med* 22(1):41, 1992.

Braggins S: *The Back — functions, malfunctions and care*, London, 1993, Mosby.

Corlett EN: *The guide to the handling of patients*, ed 2, Teddington, 1992, National Back Pain Association.

Hall J, Clarke AK: An evaluation of crutches, *Physiotherapy* 77(3):156, 1991.

Lane PL, LeBlanc R: Crutch walking, *Orthop Nurs* 9(5):31, 1990.

Pitson D *et al*: Effectiveness of knee replacement surgery in arthritis, *International Journal of Nursing Studies*, 31 (1): 49-56, 1994.

RCN: *Comprehensive guide to lifting and handling*, London, 1991, Royal College of Nursing.

Turnbull N: Prevalence of spinal pain among the staff of a DHA, *Occupational Medicine* 42(3): 143, 1992.

### Children's Nursing

Bee H: *The developing child*, ed 6, New York, 1992, Harper Collins.

McCormack A: *Coping with your handicapped child*, Edinburgh, 1985, W & R Chambers.

STEPS: *Tulipes — a handbook for parents*, Cheshire, 1981, Lymm.

STEPS: *Lower limb deficiency — a booklet for parents*, Cheshire, 1992, Lymm.

### Learning Disabilities Nursing

Hari M, Akos K: *Conductive education*, London, 1988, Tavistock/Routledge.

Leonard CT *et al*: The development of independent walking in children with cerebral palsy, *Developmental Medicine & Child Neurology*, 33 (7): 567-77, 1991.

Pointer B: *Movement activities for children with learning difficulties*, London, 1993, Jessica Kingsley.

Presland JL: *Paths to mobility in 'special care': a guide to teaching gross motor skills to very handicapped children*, London, 1982, BIMH.

Swindle M: Encouraging independent movement, *Focus*, 7: 11-13, 1992.

# Hygiene

## CHAPTER OUTLINE

## LEARNING OUTCOMES

After studying this chapter, you should be able to:
- *Define the key terms listed.*
- *Describe the structure and functions of healthy skin.*
- *Describe factors that influence personal hygiene practices and that should be recognized during assessment.*
- *Perform a complete bed bath, maintaining the dignity and comfort of the patient/client.*
- *Discuss factors that influence the condition of the nails and feet.*
- *Explain the importance of foot care for the diabetic patient/client.*
- *Develop a care plan based on patient/client preferences and hygiene practices.*
- *Discuss conditions that may put a patient/client at risk for impaired oral hygiene.*
- *Assist with or provide oral hygiene to meet specific patient/client needs.*
- *Care for patients'/clients' hair.*
- *Offer hygiene skills to meet the needs of patients/clients requiring eye, ear, and nose care.*

Maintenance of personal hygiene is necessary for comfort, safety, and well-being. Healthy individuals are capable of meeting their own hygiene needs. However, ill or *physically challenged* people may require the nurse's assistance to carry out routine hygiene practices. The nurse assesses a person's ability to perform self-care, plans necessary interventions with the patient/client in order to meet any deficit, carries out these interventions, and evaluates the effectiveness of the care.

## CARE OF THE SKIN

One of the principal purposes of good hygiene is to maintain healthy skin. The skin is an active organ with the functions of protection, secretion, excretion, temperature regulation, and sensation. Throughout our lifespan our skin changes to meet our developmental needs. The skin has three primary layers: epidermis, dermis, and subcutaneous. The **epidermis** (outer layer) is composed of several thin layers of cells undergoing different stages of maturation. It shields underlying tissue against water loss and mechanical and chemical injury and prevents the entry of disease-producing microorganisms. The innermost layer of the epidermis generates new cells that migrate slowly towards the epidermal surface or top layer (called the **stratum corneum**). These cells replace the dead cells that are continuously shed from the skin's outer surface. The epidermis also contains **melanocytes**, special cells that produce the melanin or dark pigment of the skin. Exposure to sunlight causes melanocytes to produce **melanin**, which gives some people a tan. Darker-skinned races have more active melanocytes, which produce more melanin. The distribution of pigmentation in dark-skinned people varies widely.

Bacteria commonly reside on the skin's outer surface. These resident bacteria (for example, *Corynebacterium* species) are normal flora that do not cause disease but instead inhibit the multiplication of disease-causing microorganisms.

The **dermis** is a thicker skin layer containing bundles of collagen and elastic fibres to support the epidermis. Nerve fibres, blood vessels, sweat glands, sebaceous glands, and hair follicles course through the dermal layer. Sebaceous glands secrete **sebum**,

### Mental Health Nursing
### Teaching hygiene skills
People who have received care in large mental institutions may have a reduced ability in recognizing and attending to their hygiene needs. In addition to this, their mental health may be such that they do not appreciate their hygiene needs. Nurses involved with such individuals need to work closely with them, carefully assessing their hygiene needs
and their ability to meet these needs. An individualized programme should be established, in which the nurse teaches and demonstrates how the client may meet his or her hygiene needs. The nurse/client relationship provides the context within which the nurse can demonstrate genuine interest in and concern for the client's well-being, thus creating a safe environment for the client to relearn some of

an oily, odourless fluid, into the hair follicles. Sebum lubricates the skin and hair to keep them supple and pliant. There are two types of sweat glands: eccrine and apocrine. The **eccrine glands** are distributed throughout the skin but are more abundant in the forehead, palms, and soles. Sweat excreted from the eccrine glands assists in temperature control through evaporation. The **apocrine glands** can be found in the axillary and genital areas. The bacterial decomposition of sweat from these glands is responsible for body odour. In the ears, ceruminous glands secrete **cerumen** into the external ear canal. This heavy, oily substance (ear wax) traps any foreign material entering the ear.

The **subcutaneous** tissue layer contains blood vessels, nerves, lymph vessels, and loose connective tissue filled with fat cells. The fatty tissue serves as a heat insulator for the body. Subcutaneous tissue also provides support for upper skin layers, enabling it to withstand stresses and pressure without injury. Very little subcutaneous tissue can be found underlying the oral mucosa.

The skin exchanges oxygen, nutrients, and fluid with underlying blood vessels; synthesizes new cells; and eliminates dead, nonfunctioning cells. The cells of the integument require adequate nutrition and hydration to resist injury and disease. Adequate circulation is essential to maintain cell life (see Chapter 30). The skin often reflects a change in physical condition by alterations in colour, thickness, texture, turgor, temperature, and hydration. As long as the skin remains intact and healthy, its physiological function remains optimal.

 **ASSESSMENT**

When individuals are unable to meet their personal hygiene needs, the nurse must assist them or assume full responsibility for providing this aspect of care. In order to do this the nurse must first carry out a thorough assessment. Roper *et al* (1990) suggest that all activities of living are influenced by physical, psychological, sociocultural, environmental and politico-economic factors and that these should be considered when assessing a patient/client.

### Physical Influences
Assess the patient's/client's physical condition and ability to tolerate possible nursing interventions, many of which can be exhausting. Other physical factors to consider may be the degree of mobility the patient/client has, either as a result of illness or pain. Finally, any equipment which is connected to the patient/client, including intravenous lines and drainage bags, may restrict his or her ability to participate in care and may limit the nursing interventions possible.

### Psychological Influences
Personal hygiene is often affected by an individual's psychological state. This may be as a result of lack of interest, low self-esteem or a changing body image. Work with the person to motivate and educate him or her while remaining nonjudgemental.

### Sociocultural Influences
The social and cultural groups to which a patient/client belongs may influence his or her personal hygiene. For some cultural groups, cleanliness has deep religious significance and is a priority of their care. Others may attach less importance to hygiene. It is important to respect the individual's wishes without becoming judgemental.

### Environmental Influences
These include availability of hot or running water, a bathroom and indoor toilet.

Special consideration is important for the hygiene practices of patients/clients from some ethnic or religious groups. Many people from European, Asian and Arab countries prefer to shower under running water than to sit in a bath. For example, Sikh people may wish to wash under running water before prayer. Hindu people believe that purification of the body helps to purify the mind. Many Hindus like to wash early in the day before prayer. Muslims may also wish to perform Al-Whudu (ritual ablutions) before their Salah (prayers). They may pray to Allah at least five times a day.

Even if people from these groups are unable to get out of bed, they may still appreciate the offer of washing facilities.

Some cultures, for example Muslims, find nakedness offensive. If possible Muslim women should be offered the opportunity to be helped to wash by female nurses, and Muslim men by male nurses.

## Politicoeconomic Influences

Finally, a person's economic resources may control his or her normal practices and use of toiletries. Not all individuals will be able to afford to buy toiletries such as soap, deodorant, toothpaste and shampoo.

## Continuing Assessment of the Patient/Client

While helping meet the patient's/client's personal hygiene needs, continue the physical assessment. Using the skills of looking and touching, determine the condition of the skin by observing its colour, texture, thickness, turgor, temperature, and hydration. Chapter 4 describes in detail the techniques for assessing each of these characteristics.

Also assess for skin problems, noting areas of dry skin, **maceration** (softening), possibly as a result of improper drying or sweating, and calloused areas on the feet or hands that might benefit from soaking and the application of lotion. A lanolin hand cream can be used to moisturize dry areas.

### Learning Disabilities Nursing Hygiene considerations

Personal hygiene and self-care are particularly important for people with learning disabilities. Good self-hygiene is required not only to maintain physical health, but also to promote positive social development. Since many self-care tasks are complex, a highly systematic and individualized approach is required to help the person achieve these tasks independently. If a person is profoundly handicapped and unable to perform self-hygiene independently, these needs must be given careful attention by that person's carers. Poor oral hygiene, for example, may lead to tooth decay and gum disease. This can be a particular risk for people who are taking liquid medication on a long-term basis.

Anti-convulsant drugs can cause gum hyperplasia, which can lead to pain, halitosis and poor appearance. This, in turn, can lead to tooth loss, which will cause eating problems, and can lead to physical distancing in social situations.

 PLANNING

Once the individual's needs have been fully assessed, a care plan can be developed. Planning should focus on the methods of skin care that the nurse will deliver and on the variety of nursing care measures the nurse can perform. Educate the patient/client, and provide emotional support and values clarification while assisting with hygiene needs.

The individual's condition influences the plan for meeting his or her hygiene needs. A seriously ill patient/client usually needs a daily bath, because body secretions accumulate and the person is unable to maintain cleanliness. If an individual is normally inactive during the day and his or her skin tends to be dry, the nurse may need to bathe the person only twice a week. Plan for necessary assistance for patients/clients who are weakened or possess poor muscle strength and coordination. For example, an elderly client at home, who has had difficulty getting out of the bath, may need a bath hoist and assistance from a nurse.

Timing is also important in planning hygiene care. Being interrupted in the middle of a bath to go to an x-ray examination can frustrate and embarrass a patient/client. Try to plan care around tests and procedures the patient/client must undergo. This can be difficult in a hospital, because tests may not be scheduled for specific times.

Finally, each patient/client has individual desires and preferences on when and how to bathe, shave and care for his or her hair. These preferences should be accommodated where possible to provide individualized care. For example, one person may prefer to bathe in the evening, another to shave following a shower.

Goals for patients/clients requiring assistance with personal hygiene include the following:

* Skin will remain free from body odours.
* The patient/client states that he or she feels clean and fresh.

 IMPLEMENTATION

### Bathing

Bathing a patient/client is a part of total hygiene care. Baths can be categorized as **cleansing** or **therapeutic**. A doctor's order is necessary for baths designed for therapeutic purposes. The order prescribes bath temperature, the body part being treated (in the case of soaks), and any medicated solution used (for example potassium permanganate, used to treat some skin conditions).

The underlying principles for bathing a patient/client or assisting a patient/client with a wash are to:

* **ensure thorough preparation:** assemble all the required equipment prior to the procedure to ensure you do not have to leave the patient/client during the procedure

### Children's Nursing Bathing infants

Infants do not need a daily bath, although it is common practice to do this. 'Topping and tailing' is satisfactory and preferred if the infant is sick and requires minimal handling. Bathing the baby provides an opportunity to examine his or her skin for signs of infection, e.g. sticky eyes or septic spots (Adamson, 1987). The two principles of care that must be adhered to are:
a. the infant must be safe throughout the bathing routine
b. the infant must not lose body temperature

Toddlers are often frightened at being bathed by strangers in a strange environment. Every attempt must be made to ensure that they are bathed by their parents, or other significant adult and, if this is not possible, by their named nurse.

- **provide privacy:** close the door, and pull curtains around the bed and at the window; ensure that only the area being washed is exposed at any one time
- **maintain safety:** ensure side rails are replaced, if in use, when leaving the patient/client; position the nurse call bell within patient's/client's reach
- **maintain warmth:** reduce all draughts and expose only the minimum body area to keep the patient/client warm
- **promote independence:** allow patients/clients to do as much for themselves as they feel able to do
- **communicate:** explain fully the entire procedure to the patient/client.

The extent of the patient's/client's bath and the methods used for bathing depend on the person's physical capabilities and the degree of hygiene required. A **complete bed bath** is needed for patients/clients who are totally dependent (see Procedure 25-1).

A **partial bed bath** consists of bathing only body parts that would cause discomfort or odour if left unbathed (for example, hands, face, perineal area, and axillae). Some patients/clients are able to carry out most of their wash themselves, but require assistance in washing those parts that they cannot reach (see Procedure 25-2).

The bath or shower can be used to give a more thorough bath than a bed bath. Washing and rinsing all body parts are easier. Safety is of primary concern because the surface of a bath or shower is often slippery. Patients/clients vary in how much help they will need. Some baths are specially designed for dependent patients/clients and there are a variety of aids to help a person in and out of a bath, whether in hospital or in their own home.

### Perineal Care

Usually **perineal care** is part of the complete bed bath. Patients/clients most in need of meticulous perineal care are those at greatest risk for acquiring an infection, for example, patients/clients who have indwelling urinary catheters, those who are recovering from rectal or genital surgery, or those who have undergone childbirth. A patient/client able to perform self-care should be facilitated in doing so. Many nurses are embarrassed about providing perineal care, particularly to patients/clients of the opposite sex. Male nurses often seek a female team member to provide hygiene to female patients/clients, and vice versa. Embarrassment should not cause the nurse to overlook the patient's/client's hygiene needs. A professional, dignified attitude can reduce embarrassment and put the person at ease. However, the patient's/client's wishes must be respected — for example a Muslim woman cannot be cared for by a male nurse.

If a patient/client performs self-care, various problems, such as vaginal or urethral discharge, skin irritation, and unpleasant odours may go unnoticed. Be alert for complaints of burning during urination, or localized soreness, excoriation or pain in the perineum and inspect the patient's/client's bed linen for signs of discharge.

## EVALUATION

During and at the completion of the patient's/client's bathing and skin care, evaluate the success of the interventions. For each goal established in the care plan, evaluate the accomplishment of expected outcomes. Evaluation involves physical assessment measures, as well as questions directed towards the patient/client.

## CARE OF THE FEET AND NAILS

The feet and nails often require special attention to prevent infection, odours, and injury to tissues. Often, people are unaware of foot or nail problems until pain or discomfort occurs. Problems result from abuse or poor care of the feet and hands, such as biting nails or trimming them improperly, exposure to harsh chemicals, and wearing poorly fitted shoes.

The feet are important to physical and emotional health. Foot pain can cause a person to walk differently, causing strain on different muscle groups. Many people must walk or stand comfortably to perform their jobs effectively.

## ASSESSMENT

### Physical Factors

Assessment of the feet involves a thorough examination of all skin surfaces; the shape, size, and number of toes; the shape of the foot; and the condition of the toenails. Inspect for lesions and note whether areas of dryness, inflammation, or cracking are present. The areas between the toes should be carefully checked. The heels, soles, and sides of the feet are prone to irritation from poorly fitted shoes. The toes are normally straight and flat. The feet should be in straight alignment with the ankle and tibia.

Patients/clients with peripheral vascular disease, including those with diabetes, are particularly at risk for foot lesions. They should be carefully assessed for the adequacy of circulation to the feet. Palpation of the dorsalis pedis and posterior tibial pulses indicates whether adequate blood flow is reaching peripheral tissues. Oedema and changes in skin colour, texture, and temperature can indicate that the patient/client is in need of special care. Any lesions detected should be carefully monitored and referred to the person's doctor if necessary.

### Developmental Factors

The nurse's assessment also considers the special needs of older adults, who are often unable to maintain proper foot and nail care. Note the presence of poor vision, hand tremors, obesity, or the inability to bend over to establish the level of assistance required by the older patient/client. If foot or nail problems stay unresolved, an older adult can easily become disabled. Also assess common problems of old age, such as hardening of skin, callous formation, and thickened nails. A thorough nursing assessment should integrate these changes with the symptoms of chronic diseases and treatable conditions.

## PROCEDURE 25-1 Bedbathing a Patient/Client

| SEQUENCE OF ACTIONS | RATIONALE |
|---|---|
| 1. Assess the patient's/client's needs. | Prerequisite for planning care. |
| 2. Plan the required care with the patient/client taking into account his or her personal preferences. Ensure comfort throughout and utilize opportunities for communication. | Promotes participation and independence. |
| 3. Assemble all equipment required.<br><br>(i) towel(s)<br>(ii) flannel(s)<br><br>(iii) washbasin reserved for patient/client and warm water<br>(iv) soap and toiletries as preferred by patient/client<br>(v) drawsheet<br>(vi) clean night clothes<br>(vii) clean bedlinen if required<br>(viii) laundry skip<br>(ix) bedpan or commode | Nurse will not have to leave during procedure. While it is preferable to use a separate flannel/towel for the face and body, many patients/clients are not used to this. The nurse must avoid being judgemental.<br><br>Minimizes risk of cross-infection (Greaves, 1985).<br><br>Increases independence.<br><br>To cover patient/client during procedure.<br><br><br><br><br>For patient/client to use prior to procedure. |
| 4. Prepare bed area, ensuring it is free from draughts, with sufficient privacy and room to carry out the procedure. | Patient/client comfort/privacy. Ease of manoeuvre for nurse. |
| 5. Offer patient/client a bedpan, urinal or commode. | Patient/client comfort. Avoids disruption of procedure. |
| 6. Loosen top covers at foot of bed. Cover patient/client with drawsheet and fold back bedclothes. | Avoids bedclothes becoming damp during procedure. Ensures patient/client remains warm and covered. |
| 7. Ask patients/clients if they use soap on their face. Wash, rinse and dry face, neck and ears. | Many people find soap drying on their face and prefer plain water. |
| 8. Remove top half of nightclothes. If an extremity is injured or if an intravenous infusion is present, remove nightclothes on unaffected side first. | Minimum exposed at one time. Removal of nightclothes on unaffected limb is easier and less uncomfortable for the patient/client. |
| 9. Wash, rinse and dry top half of body. Apply toiletries as requested by patient/client. Replace nightclothes as each area of wash completed. | Enhances patient/client well-being. Avoids large areas being exposed at one time. Provides privacy, warmth. |
| 10. Repeat with lower half of body/back. Change the water when it becomes cold or scummy. If the patient/client is to remain in bed, change the bottom sheet while the person is being turned. | Enhances patient's/client's well-being. Avoids large areas being exposed at one time. Provides privacy, warmth. |
| 11. When all areas have been washed and dried ensure that patient/client is dressed in clean nightclothes. | Warmth and privacy of patient/client. |
| 12. Comb patient's/client's hair as desired. | Promotes positive body image. |
| 13. Remake bed, removing and replacing dirty linen. | Provides clean, fresh environment. Protects against pressure ulcers. |
| 14. Tidy bed area, replace personal possessions within reach. | Promotes patient well-being. |
| 15. Wash hands. | Prevents cross-infection. |
| 16. Evaluate the effectiveness of the procedure against the pre-set goal, and effects on patient/client. Check patient's/client's condition and ensure comfort. | Completes the nursing process cycle. Assesses patient/client tolerance prior to planning the next day's care. |

## PROCEDURE 25-2 Assisting a Patient/Client with a Wash

| SEQUENCE OF ACTIONS | RATIONALE |
|---|---|
| 1. Assess patient's/client's needs, including his or her need to wash, and most suitable area for carrying out the procedure. | Prerequisite for planning care. |
| 2. Plan the care with the patient/client, taking into account his or her personal preferences. Utilize opportunities for communication. | Promotes participation and independence. |
| 3. Assemble all equipment required in the designated area — this may be in the bathroom or at the patient's/client's bedside. | Avoids interruption of procedure. |
| 4. Assist the patient/client to assume a suitable and comfortable position. | Patient/client comfort and safety. |
| 5. Allow the patient/client to perform as much of the procedure as possible. It may not be necessary to remain with the patient/client throughout, but care must be taken to ensure patient's/client's safety. | Encourages independence. Ensures safety. |
| 6. Assist the patient/client by washing any areas that he or she is unable to wash. | Enhances patient/client well-being. |
| 7. Help the patient/client to dress in clean nightclothes if he or she is able to do so. | Provides warmth, privacy and positive self-esteem. |
| 8. Help the patient/client back to the bedside. Tidy away equipment as necessary. | Enhances patient/client well-being and safety. |
| 9. Evaluate the effectiveness of the procedure against the pre-set goal and the effect on the patient/client. Check patient's/client's condition and ensure comfort. | Completes nursing process cycle and helps with future planning. |

## Knowledge of Foot and Nail Care Practices

Determine the person's knowledge about foot and nail care to assess their educational needs. Observe whether patients/clients know how to cut nails or use over-the-counter products for nail care and grooming. It is especially important to assess the knowledge of diabetic patients/clients and those with peripheral vascular disease because they must inspect their feet daily. Due to vascular insufficiency and neuropathy they are at risk of injury to their feet which can easily lead to infection (Thurston and Beattie, 1984).

 **PLANNING**

The nurse may provide foot and nail care during the bed bath or at a separate time in the day, according to the patient's/client's preference. Many community nurses visit patients/clients at home solely to provide foot and nail care. Individuals requiring specialist care will be referred to a chiropodist.

Goals for patients/clients receiving nail and foot care include the following:

- skin and nail surfaces will remain intact and smooth
- patient/client can state that his or her feet feel clean and comfortable
- patient/client will walk and bear weight normally
- patient/client will care for his or her own feet and nails correctly.

 **IMPLEMENTATION**

Foot and nail care involves soaking to soften cuticles and layers of horny cells, thorough cleansing, drying, and proper trimming of nails.

For patients/clients assessed at particular risk of foot injury due to peripheral vascular disease, restrict care to careful washing and drying of the feet. All other aspects of foot care will be referred to a chiropodist.

 **EVALUATION**

A patient's/client's response to nail and foot care is best evaluated over several days. If the person has any existing problems, it may take time for the alterations to improve. Also teach the patient/client on ways to evaluate personal nail and foot care practices.

### ORAL HYGIENE

**Oral hygiene** helps maintain the healthy state of the mouth, teeth, gums, and lips. Brushing cleanses the teeth of food particles, plaque, and bacteria; massages the gums; and relieves discomfort resulting from unpleasant odours and tastes. Flossing or using interdental brushes/sticks further helps remove plaque and tartar between teeth to reduce gum inflammation and infection. Complete oral hygiene gives a sense of well-being and thus can stimulate appetite.

The nurse's responsibilities in oral hygiene are maintenance and prevention. The nurse can help patients/clients maintain good oral hygiene by teaching them correct techniques or by actually performing hygiene for weakened or disabled patients/clients. Often the nurse must make referrals to a dentist or hygienist for problems requiring special care. Education about common gum and tooth disorders and methods of prevention can motivate patients/clients to follow good oral hygienic practices (Griffiths and Boyle, 1993).

 ASSESSMENT

### Physical Factors
Assess the patient's/client's lips, teeth, buccal mucosa, gums, palate, and tongue for colour, hydration, texture, and lesions. Patients/clients who do not follow regular oral-hygiene practices may have receding gum tissue, inflamed gums, discoloured teeth (particularly along gum margins), dental caries, missing teeth, and halitosis. Localized pain is a common symptom of a gum disease and certain tooth disorders. An infection of the mouth may involve organisms such as *Herpesvirus hominis*.

### Developmental Factors
Throughout a person's life span, physiological changes affect the condition and appearance of structures in the oral cavity. As a person grows older, oral-hygiene practices change to further influence the teeth and mucosa. Age-related changes in the mouth, combined with chronic disease, physical disabilities, and prescribed medications that have side effects in the mouth, can result in poor oral care. Effects of inadequate care include dental caries and loss; periodontal disease; onset of systemic infections; and long-term effects on self-esteem, ability to eat, and the maintenance of relationships (Danielson, 1988). Assessment of a patient's/client's developmental level helps in determining the types of hygienic problems to expect.

### Common Oral Problems
A nurse should be familiar with common oral problems. Each problem presents recognizable signs and symptoms and influences the type of hygiene teaching provided.

The two major types of problems are dental caries (tooth decay) and periodontal disease. **Dental caries** is the most common oral problem of younger people. The development of cavities is a pathological process that involves the eventual destruction of the tooth enamel through decalcification. Decalcification is a result of an accumulation of mucin, carbohydrates, and lactic acid bacilli in the saliva normally found in the mouth, which forms a coating on the teeth called **plaque**. Plaque is transparent and adheres to the teeth, particularly near the base of the crown at the gum margins. The plaque prevents normal acid dilution and neutralization, impeding the dissolution of bacteria in the oral cavity. The acid eventually destroys the

tooth enamel and in severe cases the pulp or inner spongy tissue of the tooth. A cavity first begins as a chalky white discolouration of the tooth. As the cavity advances, the tooth takes on a brown or black discolouration.

For people aged over 35 years, the most common problem is **periodontal disease**. This is a long-term process involving infection and destruction of the supporting teeth structures: the gingiva (gums), cementum, ligaments, and alveolar bone. Periodontal disease progresses in four stages (Levine, 1973):
1. Gingivitis or inflammation of the gums.
2. Periodontitis.
3. Acute necrotizing ulcerative gingivitis.
4. Destruction of the tooth-supporting structures.

Symptoms of periodontal disease include bleeding gums, swollen inflamed tissues, receding gumlines with the formation of gaps or pockets between the teeth and gums, and the eventual loss of teeth. If proper oral care is not maintained, dead bacteria, called *tartar*, can collect at the gumline. The tartar attacks the gums and fibres attached to the teeth, resulting in the loss of teeth. The best preventive measures are regular flossing using interdental brushes/sticks and brushing.

Other oral problems include **stomatitis**, an inflammatory condition of the mouth resulting from contact with irritants such as tobacco or from vitamin deficiency, infection by bacteria, viruses, or fungi or use of chemotherapeutic drugs; **glossitis**, an inflammation of the tongue resulting from infectious disease or injury from a burn, bite, or other injury; and **gingivitis**, an inflammation of the gums usually resulting from poor oral hygiene or occurring as a sign of leukaemia, vitamin deficiency, or diabetes mellitus.

**Halitosis** (bad breath) is a common problem of the oral cavity. It may be the result of poor oral hygiene, the ingestion of certain foods, or an infection or disease process. Proper oral hygiene can eliminate the odours unless the cause is a systemic condition such as liver disease or diabetes.

The nurse frequently encounters **cheilosis** in patients/clients. The disorder involves cracking of the lips, especially at the angle of the mouth. Vitamin B deficiency, mouth breathing, and excess salivation may cause cheilosis. Lubrication of the lips with petroleum jelly helps retain moisture, and antifungal or antibacterial ointments discourage microorganism growth.

**Oral malignancies** appear as lumps or ulcers in or around the mouth. They are commonly found in patients/clients with a history of pipe smoking or use of chewing tobacco. The most common site is at the base of the tongue. Early detection is vital to the success of treatment. Any sore in the mouth that does not heal should be brought to the attention of a dentist or doctor.

 PLANNING

Developing a care plan for patients/clients in need of oral hygiene involves considering the person's personal preferences, emotional status, and physical capabilities. It is necessary to establish a good relationship with the patient/client, in order to assist with oral hygiene practices. Some individuals are very sensitive about the condition of their mouth and are reluctant to let someone else care for them. In many cases, patients/clients are also unaware that they are at risk for serious dental and periodontal disease and thus require extensive education. Goals for patients/clients in need of oral hygiene include the following:

- oral mucosa will be intact and well hydrated
- patient/client will be able to care for his or her own teeth and gums
- patient/client will state that his or her mouth is fresh and comfortable.

 **IMPLEMENTATION**

### Oral Hygiene

Good oral hygiene requires preventive and therapeutic measures. Proper care prevents oral disease and tooth destruction. Oral care must be provided on a regular daily basis. The frequency of hygienic measures depends on the condition of the patient's/client's oral cavity.

Brushing, flossing or using interdental brushes/sticks, and irrigation are necessary for proper cleansing. Patients/clients also benefit from a well-balanced diet, which excludes foods promoting plaque formation and tooth decay and promotes healthy periodontal structures. Patients/clients of all ages should have a dental check-up at least every six months.

### Diet

To prevent tooth decay, patients/clients may have to change their eating habits, reducing the intake of carbohydrates, especially

**Children's Nursing**
**Mouthcare for children**
Most hospitalized children do not require special mouthcare unless the child is immunocompromised or receiving chemotherapy, as this reduces the normal flora in the mouth and infections are common. Mouth care or oral toilet is similar to that for adults, except that since the use of forceps would be dangerous a disposable glove is worn and the mouth is cleaned with a swab wrapped around the little finger.

sweet snacks between meals. Sweet or starchy food adheres to tooth surfaces. After eating sweets, a person should brush within 30 minutes to reduce the action of plaque. Eating acid-containing fruits (for example, apples and fibrous foods such as fresh vegetables) also reduces plaque. The acidic quality of fruits eliminates bacteria that form on teeth. A well-balanced diet ensures the integrity of oral tissues.

For pregnant women, appropriate nutrients are essential for development of primary teeth in the fetus.

### Methods of Cleaning the Mouth
#### BRUSHING

Research has shown brushing to be the most effective way of cleaning the teeth and removing plaque (Howarth, 1988).

Thorough brushing of the teeth at least four times a day with a fluoride toothpaste (after meals and at bedtime) is basic to an effective oral-hygiene programme. A toothbrush should have a straight handle and a brush small enough to reach all areas of the mouth. Individuals with reduced dexterity and grip may require an enlarged toothbrush handle that provides an easier grip. This can be accomplished by piercing a soft rubber ball and pushing the brush handle through, or by gluing a short piece of plastic tubing around the handle. An even, rounded brushing surface with soft, multi-tufted, nylon bristles is best. Rounded soft bristles stimulate the gums without causing abrasion and bleeding. All tooth surfaces — inner, outer, and chewing — should be brushed thoroughly. Following brushing, careful rinsing with water is needed to remove dislodged food particles and excess toothpaste.

#### FOAM STICKS AND GAUZE SWABS

For patients/clients unable to tolerate brushing because of oral trauma or bleeding tendencies, a foam stick or finger wrapped in gauze may be used to clean the mouth. The use of plain swabs is preferable to flavoured varieties, as some of these can have a harmful effect on the teeth and mucosa. Glycerin has an astringent effect, drying and shrinking gums and mucous membranes. It also provides nourishment for bacteria within the mouth. Lemon, if used extensively, changes the natural pH of the oral cavity, exhausts the salivary reflex through overstimulation, and can erode tooth enamel (Pettigrew, 1989). As swabbing fails to cleanse teeth adequately, plaque accumulates around the base of the teeth.

Other preparations often used for cleaning the mouth include sodium bicarbonate and hydrogen peroxide.

**Sodium Bicarbonate:** This is used to dissolve mucin and loosen debris when crusting has occurred. It is prepared by dissolving one teaspoon (8 g) of sodium bicarbonate in 500 ml of warm water. Stronger solutions are unpleasant and are harmful to the mucosa.

**Hydrogen Peroxide:** Prepare immediately prior to use according to the pharmacist's instructions, as concentrations vary. Although useful in loosening debris and dissolving crusts, it is irritant to the mucosa and should be rinsed away with warm water following use.

The amount of assistance needed by the person in brushing the teeth may vary; many can perform their own oral care and should be encouraged to do so. Observe the patient/client to ensure proper techniques are used. Some patients/clients require total assistance with hygiene.

### Special Oral Hygiene

Some patients/clients require special oral-hygiene methods because of their level of dependence on the nurse or the presence of oral mucosa problems. The principles underlying procedures for mouthcare are to:

- **ensure thorough preparation:** assemble all required equipment prior to the procedure to ensure you do not have to leave the patient/client during the procedure
- **communicate:** explain fully the procedure to the patient/client; patients/clients who are unconscious can still hear.

## PROCEDURE 25-3 Performing Mouthcare for an Unconscious Patient/Client

| SEQUENCE OF ACTIONS | RATIONALE |
|---|---|
| 1. Assess the patient's/client's needs, including presence of gag reflex. | Prerequisite for planning care. |
| 2. Plan the required care for the patient/client and explain it to him or her. | Hearing is the last sense to go. Careful explanations are needed even though the patient/client is unconscious. |
| 3. Prepare all the necessary equipment:<br><br>(i) toothbrush<br>(ii) toothpaste and petroleum jelly<br>(iii) towel<br>(iv) kidney dish and beaker of water<br>(v) gauze swabs<br>(vi) suction machine | Toothbrush is most effective way of cleaning teeth. |
| 4. Place towel under patient's/client's head, with kidney dish positioned against chin. | Protects bed.<br>To catch any discharge from the mouth. |
| 5. Carefully clean the teeth with toothbrush and small pea-sized piece of toothpaste. | Toothbrush is most effective way of cleaning teeth. |
| Rinse by wiping with damp gauze. | Necessary to restore normal pH balance of mouth. |
| Suction away any remaining secretions. | Removes secretions from back of mouth and reduces risk of aspiration. |
| 6. Apply petroleum jelly to patient's/client's lips. | Prevents drying and cracking of lips. |
| 7. Clear away equipment and wash hands. | Prevents cross-infection. |
| 8. Evaluate effectiveness of care. Check patient's/client's condition and ensure comfort. | Completes the nursing process cycle and guides future care. |

## UNCONSCIOUS PATIENTS/CLIENTS

These patients/clients are susceptible to drying of mucosa-thickened salivary secretions because they are unable to eat or drink and frequently breathe through the mouth. They also often receive oxygen therapy and oropharyngeal suction, all of which have been shown to cause stress to the oral mucosa (De Walt and Haines, 1969). In addition, the unconscious patient/client cannot swallow salivary secretions that accumulate in the mouth. These secretions often contain gram-negative bacteria that can cause pneumonia if aspirated into the lungs. Consequently, the nurse must protect the patient/client from choking and aspirating. Good oral hygiene is an important aspect of the care of an unconscious patient (see Procedure 25-3).

## PATIENTS/CLIENTS WITH DIABETES

Visits to the dentist are needed every three or four months. All tissues should be handled gently with a minimum of trauma. Patients/clients should be taught to follow rigid cleansing routines.

## PATIENTS/CLIENTS WITH ORAL INFECTIONS

Notify a doctor when signs of an infection, such as coated ulcerations or a red, dry, swollen tongue, are seen. Yoghurt (containing active cultures) with every meal is effective against yeast infections (Wilson, 1986). In some cases, topical liquid antibiotics may be prescribed.

### Flossing

Dental flossing is necessary for effective removal of plaque and tartar between teeth, and should be carried out once a day if possible. **Flossing** involves insertion of waxed or unwaxed dental floss between all tooth surfaces, one at a time. The seesaw motion used to pull floss between teeth removes plaque and tartar from tooth enamel. To prevent bleeding, patients/clients receiving chemotherapy or radiation should use unwaxed floss and avoid vigorous flossing near the gumline.

### Denture Care

Patients/clients should be encouraged to clean their own dentures as frequently as natural teeth, to prevent gingival infection and irritation. The nurse may be required to assist with denture care if patients/clients are unable to do so. To do this, ask the patient/client to remove dentures and place them in an emesis basin. If necessary, assist the person to remove the dentures, by wrapping your thumb and index finger in gauze, grasping the upper plate at the front with your thumb and index finger, and gently pulling downward. Remove lower dentures by gently lifting the denture from the jaw and rotating one side downward to remove it from the mouth. Place the dentures in a basin.

When cleaning the surface of the outer tooth, apply dentrifice to the dentures and brush the surface horizontally, using short strokes. When cleaning the undersurface of the dentures, hold the brush horizontally and use a back-and-forth movement.

When the dentures are clean, assist the patient/client to gently brush his or her gums, palate and tongue, and to rinse his or her mouth thoroughly.

 **EVALUATION**

The beneficial outcomes of oral hygiene may not be seen for several days. Repeated cleansing is often needed to remove thick encrustations of the tongue and to restore the mucosa hydration to normal.

## HAIR CARE

A person's appearance and feeling of well-being often depend on the way the hair looks and feels. Illness or disability may prevent patient's/client's from caring for their hair. An immobilized patient's/client's hair soon becomes tangled. Dressings may leave sticky blood or antiseptic solutions on the hair. Brushing, combing, and shampooing are basic hygienic measures for all patients/clients. Individuals should be permitted to shave when their conditions allow.

Hair growth, distribution, and pattern can be indicators of general health status (see Chapter 4). Hormonal changes, emotional and physical stress, ageing, infection, and certain diseases or drugs can affect characteristics of the hair. The hair shaft is an inert structure. Changes in its colour or condition occur as a result of hormonal activity and nutrient supply to the follicle.

 **ASSESSMENT**

### Physical Assessment
Before performing hair care, assess the condition of the hair and scalp (see Chapter 4). Normally the hair is clean, shiny, and untangled, and the scalp is clear. The hair of black-skinned patients/clients is usually thicker, drier, and curlier than lighter-skinned patients/clients. The loss of hair (**alopecia**) can result from improper hair-care practices or the use of chemotherapy medications.

### Self-Care Ability
Assess a patient's/client's physical ability to care for hair. Painful conditions of the upper extremities such as arthritis, a weakened hand grip, fatigue, and physical encumbrances (for example, an intravenous infusion or dressing) are just some of the conditions that impair a patient's/client's ability to perform hair care.

### Hair-Care Practices
One way to assess a person's hair-care practices is by observing the appearance of the hair. Dull, tangled, dirty hair indicates improper care. Unkempt hair may be the result of lack of interest, depression, or physical inability to care for the hair.

By assessing a patient's/client's preferred hairstyle and hair type, the nurse can attempt to arrange the patient's/client's hair in the same manner. Asking the patient/client to assist or teach the nurse how to style the hair correctly gives the patient/client a greater sense of independence and helps the nurse avoid making a mistake that can damage hair.

Also assess the type of hair-care products a patient/client prefers to use, as well as the time of day when hair care is usually performed. Assessment of shaving products is necessary with male patients/clients.

 **PLANNING**

Good hair care practices must be done routinely to meet patients'/clients' hygiene needs. Goals for patients/clients in need of hair and scalp care include the following:
*   the hair and scalp will be clean and healthy
*   the patient/client can state that his or her hair feels clean and comfortable
*   the patient's/client's hair is styled to his or her preference.

 **IMPLEMENTATION**

### Brushing and Combing
Frequent brushing helps keep hair clean and distributes oil evenly along hair shafts. Combing merely styles the hair and prevents it from becoming tangled. Short-tooth combs are adequate for short hair, but large-tooth wide spaced combs are preferred for curly hair.

Black-skinned patients/clients have thick, coarse, curly hair that often becomes very dry and brittle. It is therefore important that the nurse should seek the patient's/client's advice and follow the individuals normal hair care practices to avoid damage to the hair.

### Shampooing
Frequency of shampooing depends on a person's daily routine. Remind hospitalized patients/clients that staying in bed, excess perspiration, or treatments that leave blood or solutions in the hair may require more frequent shampooing. For patients/clients at home, the nurse's greatest challenge may be to find ways the patients/clients can shampoo their hair without injury.

If patients/clients are able to take showers or baths, their hair can usually be shampooed without difficulty. If the patient/client can sit in a chair, the hair can usually be shampooed in front of a sink or over a washbasin. However, bending is limited or contraindicated in certain conditions (for example, after certain eye surgery or total hip replacement surgery). In these situations, teach the patient/client the degree of bending allowed.

If the patient/client is unable to sit in a chair, it may be necessary to shampoo his or her hair in bed. This is done by removing any pillows and positioning the patient's/client's shoulders level with the top of the mattress. Ensure the patient/client can breathe properly while lying flat. Place a washbasin on a table below the patient's/client's head and pour clean water from a jug to wash the hair. Check the water temperature. Take care to protect the patient/client with towels and to support the head at all times. After shampooing, patients/clients may want their hair rolled on curlers or styled. Most hospital wards and day centres have portable hair dryers (Wells and Trostle, 1984).

**Adult Nursing
Hair care: multicultural considerations**

Afro-Caribbean patients/clients usually apply various types of oil preparations to their hair before or after shampooing. The hair and scalp have a natural tendency to be dry and require daily combing and gentle brushing. Oil prevents drying and subsequent breaking of hair at the follicles or ends. Grier (1976) recommends a solution of alcohol and mineral oil to remove old oil that adheres to the hair shaft. The alcohol is an antiseptic and cleansing agent. The mineral oil cleanses and lubricates the hair. Discuss with patients/clients the preferred type of oil preparation. Olive oil, baby oil, or Vaseline® hair oil are commonly used. Applying an oil generally makes combing easier.

## Shaving

Shaving of facial hair can be done after the bath or shampoo. When assisting a patient/client, take care to avoid cutting the person with razor blades. Suicidal patients/clients are not allowed to use razor blades. Patients/clients prone to bleeding, such as those receiving anticoagulant medications (heparin or warfarin) or high doses of aspirin, and those with bleeding disorders (haemophilia or leukaemia) are instructed to use an electric razor.

When a razor blade is used for shaving, the skin must be softened to prevent pulling, scraping, or cuts. For example, placing a warm flannel over the male patient's/client's face for a few seconds, followed by the application of shaving cream or a lathering of mild soap, effectively softens the skin. If the male patient/client is unable to shave his own face, the nurse may perform the shave. To avoid causing discomfort or razor cuts, hold the razor at a 45-degree angle to the skin and gently pull the skin taut while using short, firm razor strokes in the direction that the hair grows. Short downward strokes work best to remove hair over the upper lip. Often, a patient/client can explain the best way to move the razor. After the shave is completed, wash the patient's/client's face thoroughly to remove soap and hair. After drying the face, assist in applying powder or an after-shave lotion to the patient's/client's face.

## Moustache and Beard Care

Male patients/clients with moustaches or beards require daily grooming. Keeping these clean is important, because food particles can easily collect in the hair. If patients/clients are unable to care for themselves, the nurse should trim, comb, or wash beards or moustaches when needed or on request. Never shave off a moustache or beard without the patient's/client's consent. Facial hair has important significances in certain religions.

 **EVALUATION**

Evaluation of nursing care measures for the patient's/client's hair care are based on the expected outcomes and goals of care. Use evaluative measures, such as asking the patient/client to demonstrate hair-care practices or re-inspecting the condition of the hair and scalp, to determine the success of nursing interventions.

## CARE OF THE EYES, EARS, AND NOSE

Special attention is given to the cleansing of the patient's/client's eyes, ears, and nose during the patient's/client's bath. However, individuals may also have special problems that require cleansing of these organs throughout the day. Nursing care centres on preventing infection and maintaining the patient's/client's normal organ function.

### Eyes

Normally, no special care is required for the eyes because they are continually cleansed by tears, and the eyelids and lashes prevent the entrance of foreign particles. A person needs only to remove any dried secretions that have collected on the inner canthus or on the eyelashes. Patients/clients who are unconscious are at risk for eye injury because the blink reflex may be absent. In these patients/clients, excessive drainage frequently collects along eyelid margins. Special attention is also required for patients/clients who have had eye surgery or an eye infection that can result in increased discharge or drainage. The nurse often assists patients/clients in the care of eyeglasses, contact lenses, or artificial eyes.

### Ears

Hygiene of the ears has implications for hearing acuity when wax or foreign substances collect in the external ear canal and interfere with sound conduction. The nurse should be sensitive to any behavioural cues that might indicate a hearing impairment (see Chapter 4). When caring for a patient/client with a hearing aid, teach the patient/client about proper cleansing and maintenance, and on communication techniques that promote hearing the spoken word.

### Nose

The nose provides for the sense of smell but also controls the temperature and humidity of inhaled air, and prevents the entrance of foreign particles into the respiratory system. Accumulation of encrusted secretions within the nares can impair olfactory sensation and breathing. Irritation of nasal mucosa can cause swelling, leading to obstruction of the nares. Typically, hygienic care of the nose is simple, but patients/clients with nasogastric, enteral feeding, or endotracheal tubes that enter the nose may require special attention.

**ASSESSMENT**

### Physical Factors

Chapter 4 describes the techniques used to assess the condition and function of the eyes, ears, and nose. Normally the eyes are free of infection. The conjunctivae are clear, pink, and without inflammation. The eyelid margins are in close approximation with the eyeball, and the lashes are turned outward. The lid margins are without inflammation, drainage, or lesions. The eyebrows should be symmetrical.

Assessment of the external ear structures includes inspection of the auricle and external ear canal. While performing hygiene care, the nurse is most concerned with noting the presence of accumulated cerumen or drainage in the ear canal, local inflammation, or pain.

Inspect the nares for signs of inflammation, discharge, lesions, oedema, and deformity. The nasal mucosa is normally pink and clear and has no discharge. If patients/clients have any form of tubing exiting the nose, look at the nares surfaces that come in contact with the tubing for tissue sloughing, localized tenderness, inflammation, and even bleeding.

### Use of Sensory Aids

If patients/clients wear eyeglasses, contact lenses, artificial eyes, or hearing aids, assess the patient's/client's knowledge, the methods used to care for the aids, and the presence of any problems caused by the aids. The following factors should be assessed for patients/clients using sensory aids. The nurse's findings have implications for patient/client education.

### EYEGLASSES

- purpose for wearing glasses (for example, reading, distance or both)
- methods used to clean glasses
- presence of symptoms (for example, blurred vision, photophobia, headaches).

### CONTACT LENSES

- type of lens worn
- frequency and duration of time that lenses are worn
- presence of signs and symptoms (for example, burning, excessive tear formation, redness, irritation, swelling)
- techniques used to insert, clean and store lenses
- use of eye drops or ointments
- use of an emergency identification bracelet to warn others that contact lenses are in place (optional).

### ARTIFICIAL EYES

- method used to insert and remove the eye
- method of cleaning the eye
- presence of symptoms (for example, pain in the orbit).

### HEARING AID

- type of aid worn
- methods used to clean aid
- patient's/client's ability to change the battery and adjust the volume of the hearing aid (see Chapter 26).

### Self-Care Ability

Assess the patient's/client's physical ability to perform eye, ear, and nose care, as well as care of any sensory aids. Patients/clients who are unable to grasp small objects, who have limited mobility in the upper extremities, who have reduced vision, or who are very tired may require assistance from the nurse.

Assessment may reveal an actual alteration in the function of sensory organs, a problem in the patient's/client's ability to perform personal hygiene, or a deficit in the patient's/client's understanding of hygiene.

 **PLANNING**

The patient's/client's personal preferences and habits are considered when planning hygiene care. The eyes, ears, and nose are sensitive to irritating or painful stimuli. Extra care must be taken to avoid injury to tissues. The goals of care for the patient/client include:

- absence of infection
- optimal sensory organ function
- the patient/client understands how to care for his or her eyes, ears, and nose.

 **IMPLEMENTATION**

### Basic Eye Care

Cleansing the eyes is usually performed during the bath and involves washing with a clean flannel moistened in water. Soap is usually omitted, because it may cause burning and irritation. Wipe from the inner to the outer canthus of the eye, to prevent secretions from draining into the lacrimal sac. Use a separate section of the flannel each time to prevent the spread of infection. If a patient/client has dried secretions that are not removed easily with wiping, place a damp cloth or cotton ball on the lid margins to loosen the secretions. Never apply direct pressure over the eyeball because it may cause serious injury.

The unconscious patient/client may require more frequent eye care. Secretions may collect along the lid margins and inner canthus when the blink reflex is absent or when the eye does not close totally. If necessary to prevent corneal drying, administer lubricating eyedrops according to the doctor's orders. The principles underlying eye care for these individuals are to:

- **ensure thorough preparation:** assemble all required equipment prior to the procedure to ensure you do not have to leave the patient/client during the procedure
- **communicate:** explain fully the entire procedure to the patient/client; patients/clients who are unconscious can still hear.

### CLEANSING GLASSES

Glasses are made of hardened glass or plastic that is impact resistant to prevent shattering. Nevertheless, because of the cost of glasses, use care when cleaning glasses, and protect them from breakage or other damage when the patient/client is not wearing them. Glasses should be put in their case and in a drawer of the bedside locker when not in use. Label with patient's/client's name if there is any possibility of loss.

Warm water is sufficient for cleansing glass lenses. A soft tissue is best for drying to prevent scratching. Plastic lenses may scratch easily, and may require special cleaning solutions and drying tissues.

## CONTACT LENS CARE

A contact lens is a thin, transparent, oval disk that fits directly over the cornea of the eye. The lens floats on the tear layer that lubricates the eye. There are different types of contact lenses including hard, soft and gas permeable. These all differ in the care they require.

Individuals who wear contact lenses generally care for their contact lenses themselves. However, the nurse may need to remove a patient's/client's contact lenses in an emergency, as prolonged wearing of contact lenses can cause serious corneal damage. Patients/clients who are confused, unconscious or who are restricted from moving their hands should have their lenses removed immediately by a person familiar with the procedure.

## ARTIFICIAL EYES

Patients/clients with artificial eyes have had an enucleation of an entire eyeball as a result of tumour growth, severe infection, or eye trauma. Some artificial eyes are permanently implanted. Others should be removed for routine cleaning. Patients/clients with artificial eyes usually prefer to care for their own eyes. The nurse should respect the patient's/client's wishes and help by providing him or her with the necessary equipment. If it is necessary to remove an artificial eye from an unconscious patient/client, obtain advice from someone familiar with the procedure.

### Cleaning the Ears

The nurse cleanses the patient's/client's ears as a routine part of a bed bath. The clean end of a moistened flannel, rotated gently into the ear canal, works best for cleaning. When cerumen is visible, gentle downward retraction at the entrance of the ear canal may cause the wax to loosen and slip out. Instruct patients/clients never to use sharp objects to remove ear wax. The use of such objects can cause trauma to the ear canal and rupture of the tympanic membrane. Use of cotton-tipped applicators should also be avoided because they can cause wax to become impacted within the canal. Excessive or impacted cerumen can be removed by irrigation on the orders of a doctor and by someone qualified to do so.

### Nose Care

The patient/client can usually remove secretions from the nose by gently blowing into a soft tissue. This is done by closing one nostril by pressing on the side of the nostril, and blowing gently to clear the other side. The procedure is then reversed. This may be all the daily hygiene needed. Caution the patient/client against harsh blowing that creates pressure capable of injuring the eardrum, nasal mucosa, and even sensitive eye structures. Bleeding from the nares is a key sign of harsh blowing, mucosal irritation, or dryness.

If the patient/client cannot remove nasal secretions, assist by using a wet flannel or a cotton-tipped applicator moistened in water or saline. The applicator should never be inserted beyond the length of the cotton tip. Excessive nasal secretions can also be removed by suctioning. Nasal suctioning is contraindicated in nasal or brain surgery.

When patients/clients have feeding or suction tubes inserted through the nose, change the tape anchoring the tube at least once a day (see Chapter 29). When the tape becomes moist from nasal secretions, the skin and mucosa can easily become macerated. The up-and-down movement of tubing causes tissue injury. The nurse should know how to tape tubing correctly to minimize tension or friction on the nares (see Chapter 29). When tissue injury occurs, it may be necessary to remove the tube and insert one through the other naris. Always cleanse the nares thoroughly around the tubing because secretions accumulate.

 EVALUATION

Evaluation of eye, ear, and nose care must be individualized on the basis of the patient's/client's existing sensory function. Hygiene care alone will not improve sensory function beyond a patient's/client's baseline level.

## SUMMARY

Hygiene measures cover a variety of basic physical needs that individuals are often unable to meet themselves. A fundamental principal of good hygiene is the maintenance of healthy skin. Skin care provision has important physical and psychological implications for the patient/client. Cleanliness helps the skin to remain healthy, and washing stimulates circulation to the skin, stimulates the rate and depth of respirations, and provides range of motion exercise. On a psychological level, a bath or shower helps the individual to relax, promotes feelings of well-being, and improves self-image. These therapeutic benefits can be as great as the physical benefits of hygiene maintenance. Promoting independence and participating in personal hygiene is a vital part of the nurse's role.

The nurse should take time for therapeutic communication, teaching, and provision of emotional support when delivering hygiene measures. The implementation of suitable nursing interventions can ensure that no aspect of patient/client hygiene is omitted. Thorough assessment enables the specific, actual or potential problems of each individual to be identified, and helps prevent neglect in general areas of concern, such as oral hygiene. It is important that the nurse recognizes the special hygiene needs of every patient/client throughout their period of dependency and responds accordingly, while respecting the personal practices and dignity of the individual.

## CHAPTER 25 REVIEW
### Key Concepts
- Hygiene is a personal matter, and all factors influencing personal hygiene routine must be considered.

- The nurse assumes responsibility for meeting patients'/clients' daily hygiene needs if they are unable to care for themselves adequately.
- Meeting hygiene needs provides an opportunity to assess all external body surfaces and the patient's/client's emotional state.
- Meeting hygiene needs also allows use of teaching and communication skills to develop a meaningful relationship with the patient/client.
- The patient's/client's personal preferences must always be considered when planning daily hygiene care.
- Maintain the person's privacy and comfort when providing daily care.
- Helping patients/clients with personal hygiene involves care of the skin, feet, nails, mouth, hair, eyes, ears and nose.
- The evaluation of hygiene care is based on the patient's/client's expression of a sense of comfort, relaxation, well-being, and an understanding of personal hygiene techniques.

## CRITICAL THINKING EXERCISES

1. You are working with a community nurse caring for a 77-year-old woman suffering from severe arthritis. Identify the factors you need to consider when helping her with her personal hygiene.
2. Mr Johannson is a 43-year-old, insulin-dependent diabetic who has been admitted with an infected ulcer on his right foot. What special care would he require in relation to his hygiene needs?
3. Jamie Taylor is a 6-year-old boy who was admitted following an accident on his bike. He is unconscious and requires total nursing care. Plan the nursing interventions that he will require to meet his hygiene needs. Which aspects of this care can his mother perform?

### Key Terms

Apocrine glands, p. 506
Bath (cleansing/therapeutic), p. 507
Cerumen, p. 506
Complete bed bath, p. 508
Dental caries, p. 511
Dermis, p. 506
Eccrine glands, p. 506
Epidermis, p. 505
Flossing, p. 513
Gingivitis, p. 511
Glossitis, p. 511
Halitosis, p. 511
Maceration, p. 507
Oral hygiene, p. 510
Partial bed bath, p. 508
Perineal care, p. 508
Periodontal disease, p. 511
Plaque, p. 511
Sebum, p. 506
Stomatitis, p. 511

## REFERENCES

Adamson F: *Essential paediatric nursing*, Edinburgh, 1987, Churchill Livingstone.
Danielson KH: Oral care and older adults, *J Gerontol Nurs* 14:6, 1988.
De Walt EM, Haines AK: The effects of specific stressors on healthy oral mucosa, *Nurs Res* 18(1):22, 1969.
Greaves A: We'll just freshen you up ear, *Nurs Times* 81(36):3, 1985.
Grier ME: Hair care for the black patient, *Am J Nurs* 76:1781, 1976.
Griffiths JE, Boyle SJ: A colour guide to holistic oral care, London, 1993, Mosby.
Howarth H: Mouthcare procedures for the very ill, *Nurs Times* 73:354, 1988.
Levine P: Safeguarding your patients against periodontal disease, *RN* 36:38, 1973.
Pettigrew D: Investing in mouth care, *Geriatr Nurs* 10:22, 1989.
Roper N, Logan WW and Tierney AJ: *The elements of nursing*, ed 3, Edinburgh, 1990, Churchill Livingstone.
Thurston R, Beattie C: Foot lesions in diabetics, predisposing factors, *Nurs Times* 80(34):44, 1984.
Wells R, Trostle K: Creative hairwashing techniques for immobilised patients, s*Nursing* 14(1):47, 1984.
Wilson D: Make mouth care a must for your patients, *RN* 49:39, 1986.

## FURTHER READING
### Adult Nursing

Allbright A: Oral care for the cancer chemotherapy patient, *Nurs Times* 80(21):40, 1984.
England PM *et al*: An experiment in health education, *Nurs Times* 75(35):1491, 1979.Greaves A: We'll just freshen you up dear, *Nurs Times* 81(36):3, 1985.
Hallett N: Mouthcare, *Nurs Mirror* 159(21):31, 1984.
ohnson A: Dental care during pregnancy, *Nurs Times* 81(50):28, 1985.
Neeson JD, May KA: *Comprehensive maternity nursing: nursing process and the childbearing family*, New York, 1986, Lippincott.
Roberts S: Getting to know you..., *Nurs Times* 83(14):36, 1987.
Wagnild G, Manning RW: Convey respect during bathing procedures, *J Geront Nurse* 11(12):6, 1985.
Wong DL: *Nursing care of infants and children*, ed 4, St Louis, 1995, Mosby.
Wilson M: Personal cleanliness, *Nurs* 3(2):80, 1986.

### Children's Nursing

Griffiths JE, Boyle SJ: *A colour guide to holistic oral care*, London, 1993, Mosby.
Henningson A *et al*: Bathing or washing babies after birth? *Lancet* 2:1401, 1981.
Jolly H: *Book of childcare*, London, 1975, Unwin Paperbacks.
Leach P: *Baby and child*, London, 1979, Penguin Books.
Powell C: Privacy in the paediatric unit, *Paediatr Nurs*, 1991.
Robertson N: *A manual of normal neonatal care*, London, 1988, Edward Arnold.
Spocke B: *Baby and child care*, London, 1979, Allen and Co.

### Learning Disabilities Nursing

Anderson RC: The need to modify health education programes for the mentally retarded and developmentally disabled, *Journal of Developmental & Physical Disabilities*, 5 (2): 95-108, 1993.
Hindle J: Dental care courses for adults with disabilities, *Dental Health London*, 31 (2): 3-5, 1992.
Richardson N: Fit for the future, *Nursing Times*, 89 (44): 36-38, 1993.
Roth S, Brown N: Advocates for health, *Nursing Times*, 87 (21): 62-64, 1991.
Rose V: Health education for parents with special needs, *Health Visitor*, 67 (3): 95-96, 1994.

# unit 5

# Nursing Practice and Nursing Skills

# Sensory Alterations

## LEARNING OUTCOMES

After studying this chapter, you should be able to:
- *Define the key terms listed.*
- *List and describe seven senses of the human body.*
- *Differentiate between the processes of reception, perception, and reaction to sensory stimuli.*
- *Discuss common causes and effects of sensory alterations.*
- *Discuss common sensory changes that normally occur with ageing.*
- *Identify factors to assess in determining sensory status.*
- *Perform a nursing assessment relevant to individuals with sensory alterations.*
- *Develop a plan of care for individuals with visual, auditory, tactile, speech, and olfactory deficits.*
- *Identify key factors that need to be considered when interacting with infants and children who have sensory deficits.*
- *Describe how an individual's sensory alteration influences the nursing care approaches selected to improve sensory function.*
- *List interventions for preventing sensory deprivation and helping to control sensory overload.*

Part of the uniqueness of human beings is their ability to sense a variety of stimuli within the environment, perceive and organize those stimuli, and respond appropriately. Stimulation comes from many sources inside and outside the body, particularly through the senses of sight **(visual)**, hearing **(auditory)**, touch **(tactile)**, smell **(olfactory)**, and taste **(gustatory)**. The body also has a **kinaesthetic** sense that enables a person to be aware of the position and movement of body parts without seeing them. **Stereognosis** is a sense that allows a person to recognize an object's size, shape, and texture. The ability to speak is not considered a sense, but it is similar in that the patient/client may lose the ability to interact in a meaningful way with other human beings. Meaningful stimuli enable a person to learn about the environment and are necessary for healthy functioning and the normal development of the sensory organs. From birth, infants have a highly defined repertoire of senses; for example, they can focus both eyes on the same point, with 20 cm being the best focal point. Within a few weeks, babies can follow a moving object with their eyes and from 8–12 weeks, they can discriminate between their mother's face and those of strangers. Babies can hear sounds from birth and can discriminate their mother's voice. They can also discriminate between the four basic tastes (sweet, sour, bitter and salt).

When sensory function is altered, the patient's/client's ability to relate to, and function within, the environment changes. The extent of this change is dependent upon the type and extent of the sensory alteration.

Many people enter the health care system with pre-existing sensory alterations or may develop sensory alterations as a result of treatment (for example, cataract removal). Individuals who have partial or complete loss of a major sensory function must find alternative ways to function safely within the environment. If sensory deficits, or alterations, occur early in life, individuals may experience developmental and socialization problems because of the difficulty in responding to people and the environment.

Others may enter health care settings with normal sensory function. However, a health care setting, particularly a hospital, is often a place of unfamiliar sights, sounds, and smells. Hospitalization may also result in a reduction of contact with family and friends. If individuals feel isolated and alienated, they may be less receptive to meaningful stimuli. Thus, there is the potential for sensory alterations to develop which may become serious and may interfere with the progress of such an individual towards wellness.

The nurse must understand and help meet the needs of individuals with sensory alterations, and must recognize those individuals most at risk for developing sensory problems. The nurse helps individuals who have sensory alterations learn how to interact, and react, safely and effectively.

## NORMAL SENSATION

The nervous system continually receives thousands of pieces of information from sensory nerve organs, relays the information through appropriate channels, and integrates the information into a meaningful response. **Sensory stimuli** reach the sensory organs and can elicit an immediate reaction or present information to the brain to be stored for future use. The nervous system must be intact for sensory stimuli to reach appropriate brain centres and for the individual to perceive the sensation. After interpreting the significance of a sensation, the person can then react to the stimulus.

The three components of any sensory experience are reception, perception and reaction. **Reception** begins with stimulation of a nerve cell called a *receptor,* which is usually designed for only one type of stimulus, such as light or sound. Nerve impulses then travel along pathways from the receptor to the spinal cord or directly to the brain. For example, the retina of the eye receives light, with impulses travelling along the optic nerve to the occipital lobe of the brain.

Only pain receptors receive several forms of stimuli, such as pressure, chemicals, and heat. The movement of a body part stimulates **proprioceptors** to send impulses along peripheral spinal nerves to the spinal cord. From the spinal cord a second set of nerve fibres conducts the sensation of position, travels up the cord, crosses over at the medulla, and travels to the thalamus. At the thalamus, impulses synapse with a third pathway and are sent to the cerebral cortex. **Sensory nerve pathways** usually cross over to send stimuli to opposite sides of the brain. For example, if a person touches an object with the right hand, it is the left side of the brain which receives the stimulus.

The actual **perception** or awareness of individual sensations depends on the receiving region of the cerebral cortex, where specialized brain cells interpret the quality and nature of the sensory stimuli. A person's level of consciousness influences how well stimuli are perceived and interpreted. Factors that lower consciousness can impair sensory perception. Perception includes an integration and interpretation of the stimuli based on the person's experiences. If sensation is incomplete, or if past experience is inadequate for understanding the stimuli, the person may react inappropriately.

It is impossible to **react** to each of the multiple stimuli constantly entering the nervous system. The brain is normally capable of discarding and storing sensory information to prevent sensory bombardment. A person usually reacts to stimuli that are most meaningful or significant at the time. After continued reception of the same stimulus, however, a person stops responding and the sensory experience goes unnoticed. For example, a person reading a good book is not aware of the pressure of resting the body against the back of a chair. This phenomenon of **adaptability** occurs with most sensory stimuli, except for those of pain (see Chapter 27).

The balance between sensory stimuli entering the brain and those actually reaching the conscious awareness maintains a person's well-being. If an individual attempts to react to every stimulus within the environment, or if a variety and quality of stimuli are lacking, sensory alterations will occur.

## TYPES OF SENSORY ALTERATIONS

Many factors alter the capacity to receive or perceive sensations (see box). The types of **sensory alterations** commonly seen by the nurse are sensory deficits, sensory deprivation, and sensory overload. When an individual suffers from more than one sensory alteration, the ability to function and relate effectively within the environment is seriously impaired.

### Sensory Deficits
A defect in the normal function of sensory reception and perception is a **sensory deficit**. An individual may not be able to receive certain stimuli (for example, the individual may be blind or deaf), or stimuli may become distorted (for example, the individual may have cataracts or be confused). A sudden onset of a sensory loss can cause feelings of fear, anger, or of helplessness. Initially, a person may withdraw by avoiding communication or socialization with others in an attempt to cope with the sensory loss. It becomes difficult for the person to interact safely with the environment until new skills relying on existing functions are learned. When a deficit develops gradually or when considerable time has passed since the onset of an acute sensory loss, the person learns to rely on unaffected senses. Some senses may even become more acute to compensate for an alteration. For example, an individual who is visually impaired often learns to utilize his or her sense of hearing more effectively.

People with sensory deficits may respond to their situation in positive or negative ways. For example, someone with a hearing impairment may turn the unaffected ear towards a speaker to hear better, whereas someone else may shun other people to avoid the embarrassment of their speech not being understood.

Young children suffer from frustration at not being able to make themselves understood. In addition, adults may react differently to deaf children, for example, by not fully explaining why they should not do something, but simply saying 'no'. Deaf children may find this hard to understand — not only do they not know why they cannot do something, but also they do not know why they may have been punished (Lansdown, 1980). Gregson

(1976) found more tantrums among deaf children than among four-year-old children with normal hearing (Freeland, 1989).

## Sensory Deprivation

Sensory stimulation must be of sufficient quality and quantity to maintain a person's awareness. When someone experiences an inadequate quality or quantity of stimulation, such as monotonous or meaningless stimuli, **sensory deprivation** may occur. There are three types of sensory deprivation:

- a reduction in sensory input (sensory deficit from visual or hearing loss)
- the elimination of order or meaning from input (for example, individuals exposed to strange environments)
- restriction of patient's/client's environment (for example, bed rest) that predisposes to monotony and boredom (Ebersole and Hess, 1990).

Sensory deprivation may affect individuals in a variety of ways (see box). The symptoms can easily cause nurses and medical staff to believe someone is psychologically ill, unbalanced or confused, or is suffering from severe electrolyte imbalance, or perhaps is under the influence of psychotropic drugs. Therefore, the nurse must always be aware of the individual's existing sensory function and the quality, and quantity, of stimuli within the surrounding environment.

## Sensory Overload

When a person receives multiple sensory stimuli and cannot perceptually disregard or selectively ignore some stimuli, **sensory overload** occurs. Excessive sensory stimulation prevents the brain from appropriately responding to, or ignoring, certain stimuli. Due to the multitude of stimuli leading to overload, the person may no longer perceive the surrounding environment in a way that makes sense. Overload interferes with, and may prevent, appropriate response by the brain; for example, the person's thoughts race, attention moves in many directions, and therefore, restlessness occurs. As a result, overload causes a state similar to that produced by sensory deprivation.

An acutely ill individual may fall victim to sensory overload. The constant pain from the disease process, the nurse's frequent monitoring of vital signs, and the irritation from drainage tubes protruding from the body combine to cause overload. Even if the

---

### Factors that Influence Sensory Function

#### AGE
- Infants are unable to differentiate easily between sensory stimuli. Nerve pathways are immature.
- Visual changes during adulthood include presbyopia and the need for glasses for reading (usually occurring from ages 40 to 50).
- Hearing changes, which begin at 30, include decreased hearing acuity, speech intelligibility, pitch discrimination, and hearing threshold. Tinnitus often accompanies a hearing loss. Older adults hear low-pitched sounds the best but have difficulty hearing conversation over background noise.
- Older adults have reduced visual fields, increased glare sensitivity, impaired night vision, reduced accommodation and depth perception, and reduced colour discrimination.
- Older adults may have difficulty discriminating some consonants (f, s, th, ch). Speech sounds are garbled, and there is often a delayed reception and reaction to speech.
- Gustatory and olfactory changes include a decrease in the number of taste buds in later years and reduction of olfactory nerve fibres by age 50. Reduced taste discrimination and sensitivity to odours are common.
- Proprioceptive changes after age 60 include increased difficulty with balance, spatial orientation, and coordination.
- Older adults often experience tactile changes, including declining sensitivity to pain, pressure, and temperature.

#### MEDICATIONS
- Some antibiotics (e.g. streptomycin, gentamicin, aspirin) are ototoxic and can permanently damage the auditory nerve; chloramphenicol can irritate the optic nerve. Narcotic analgesics, sedatives, and antidepressant medications can alter the perception of stimuli.

#### ENVIRONMENT
- Excessive environmental stimuli (for example, equipment noise and staff conversation in an intensive care unit) can result in sensory overload, marked by confusion, disorientation, and the inability to make decisions. Restricted environmental stimuli (e.g. with isolation) can lead to sensory deprivation. Poor quality of environment (e.g. reduced lighting, narrow walkways, background noise) can heighten sensory impairment.

#### COMFORT LEVEL
- Pain and fatigue often alters the way a person perceives and reacts to stimuli.

#### PRE-EXISTING ILLNESSES
- Peripheral vascular disease can cause reduced sensation in the extremities and impaired cognition. Chronic diabetes can lead to reduced vision, blindness, or peripheral neuropathy. Strokes often produce loss of speech. Some neurological disorders impair motor function and sensory reception.

#### SMOKING
- Chronic tobacco use can atrophy the taste buds, lessening the perception of flavours.

#### NOISE LEVELS
- Constant exposure to high noise levels (e.g. on a construction site) can cause hearing loss.

#### ENDOTRACHEAL INTUBATION
- Temporary loss of speech results from insertion of an endotracheal tube through the mouth or nose into the trachea.

nurse offers a comforting word or provides a gentle massaging touch, patients/clients may not benefit because their attention and energy are focused on more stressful stimuli (see Chapter 27 for discussion of Gate Control Theory).

Sensory overload differs from sensory deprivation in that the level of stimuli that can cause the condition depends more on individual factors. The point at which stimuli become sufficient to tax endurance changes according to a person's level of fatigue, temperament, and emotional and physical well-being. Continued overload may cause a person to (eventually) develop many of the same symptoms as are found with sensory deprivation.

## NURSING PROCESS AND SENSORY ALTERATIONS

 **ASSESSMENT**

When assessing individuals with, or at risk of developing, sensory alterations, it is important to consider all the factors influencing sensory function (see box on previous page), particularly age. When obtaining a history also assess the degree to which a sensory deficit affects the individual's lifestyle, psychosocial adjustment, and ability to relate to the environment. The assessment must also focus on the quality and quantity of the surrounding environmental stimuli.

### People at Risk

You can quickly assess sensory function for those most at risk. Older adults are a high risk group because of normal

---

### Effects of Sensory Deprivation

COGNITIVE
Reduced capacity to learn, inability to solve problems, poor task performance, disorientation, bizarre thinking.

AFFECTIVE
Boredom, restlessness, increased anxiety, emotional lability, increased need for physical stimulation and socialization.

PERCEPTUAL
Reduced attention span, disorganized visual and motor coordination, temporary loss of colour perception, disorientation, confusion of sleeping and waking states.

---

physiological changes involving sensory organs. Patients/clients who are immobilized due to bed rest or physical encumbrances (for example, limbs encased in plaster-casts or on traction) are unable to experience all the normal sensory sensations of free movement. Other groups at risk include people with altered consciousness and individuals who are isolated in a health care setting or at home. For example, a person who is isolated because of an infection (see Chapter 28) is often alone in a room and may be restricted with regard to visitors.

An individual with a known sensory deficit is obviously at risk

for sensory alterations. The length of time a person has had a sensory deficit may, or may not, affect that individual's response to the environment. Magilvy (1985) found that women with a later onset of hearing loss considered themselves to have a lowered quality of life compared with women who experienced hearing loss at a younger age. Walsh and Eldredge (1989) suggest that an individual who loses his or her hearing at an early age experiences cumulative developmental effects and socialization problems that are compounded with ageing.

A hospital environment is full of sensory stimuli, including conversation between staff members, the sounds of electrical monitors and equipment, bright lighting, and the odours of body fluids. A hearing-impaired individual accustomed to living alone may find it difficult to cope with the cacophony often found in a hospital environment. The individual may find it difficult to distinguish between the different sounds: telephones ringing, equipment bleeping, footsteps tapping, crockery and cutlery clinking and rattling, as well as to understand the unfamiliar speech patterns and words (Tolson and McIntosh, 1992). Remember, however, that noise can mean different things to different people (Gough, 1986).

### Physical Assessment

To identify sensory deficits, an individual is assessed for sight, hearing, olfaction (smell), taste, and the ability to discriminate

---

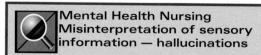 **Mental Health Nursing**
**Misinterpretation of sensory information — hallucinations**

In some instances people with a mental illness may experience altered perceptions in the absence of any impinging stimuli — hallucinations. Altered perceptions can arise in any of the five senses. The experience is not pleasant; it leaves the person distracted, anxious, frightened and embarrassed. It is essential to remember that while the nurse may not be able to experience those sensations described by the patient/client, the sensations nevertheless feel very real and are very pertinent to the individual. The nurse's task is to develop appropriate communication skills in order to support patients/clients through these experiences and to help them focus increasingly on reality-based communication. Where these sensations become troublesome and are unmanageable, psychotropic medications may be given.

The safety of the patient/client is of paramount importance in any situation where he or she is experiencing sensory alterations, since this can affect his or her judgement of situations and people.

---

experiences such as light, touch, temperature, pain, and position (see Table 26-1). The nurse should note whether an individual uses sensory aids (for example, glasses or hearing aids) and whether that person is functioning properly. While giving care, the nurse may observe an individual exhibiting behaviours that indicate specific sensory alterations.

A neurological assessment of an individual's level of consciousness, orientation, and cognitive thought processes should reveal any symptoms of sensory deprivation or overload. This procedure also assesses levels of perception. It should be remembered that factors other than sensory deprivation or overload may cause impaired perception (for example, medication, pain, hypoxia).

## Ability to Perform Self-Care

Individuals with sensory or perceptual alterations are often unable to perform, or have difficulties with, the activities of living. An individual's **functional abilities** are assessed in his or her home or in the hospital setting, including feeding, dressing, grooming, and toileting activities. For example, whether or not someone with altered vision can find items on a meal tray and can read directions on a prescribed medicine. An assessment should be undertaken to ascertain a visually impaired individual's ability to perform daily tasks such as reading bills and writing cheques, discriminating between coins and notes of differing monetary values, and driving a vehicle at night. This assessment is usually carried out by an occupational therapist. If the person's ability to perform self-care alters, it is necessary to assess the resources within the home prior to discharge from the acute care setting. Arrangements should be made to organize any modifications necessary for the person to function as safely and as independently as possible.

## Environment

The environment can either minimize or heighten sensory alterations. In some cases the environment may be the cause of the problem. It is necessary to assess the quality and quantity of stimuli within the health care environment and the individual's home environment.

Effective lighting within the home environment is important for people with visual impairments. Often, lighting is too dim and/or is poorly positioned within the main living and working areas of the home such as the kitchen and living room. In addition, there is often a low level of light in the hallway and stairwell. Lighting levels can be remedied by increasing the wattage of lightbulbs, or by the judicious positioning of ceiling-based fittings. Lowering the central light may be all that is required: halving the distance from the light source increases illumination four-fold (Cullinan, 1991). A lamp fitted with a red bulb can be left on at night, as this colour gives less brightness and is easier for the eyes to adjust to, initially, upon waking during the night; for instance, to use the bathroom.

## HAZARDS

An individual with sensory alterations may be at risk of injury if the environment is unsafe. Cluttered furniture, dimly lit corridors and stairways, and torn carpets are dangerous for people with visual impairments (see Chapter 19). In addition, because an older adult may experience more glare in very bright light, shiny objects such as metal furniture, highly waxed floors, and bright, direct lighting can pose problems. Consideration of potential hazards is also particularly important for children. A child with normal vision may be prone to accidents, for example if toys are placed carelessly; but for blind children these hazards are accentuated. Children who have hearing impairments rely upon

---

 **Children's Nursing**
**Key points for those working with blind babies and young children**

### MOVEMENT

Blind babies often go still when their mother approaches. This is not a sign of rejection; it is an indication that the baby is concentrating. Sighted babies lift their head and later try to walk because they can see that this is of value. The blind baby needs encouragement.

Blind babies' hands are often 'dead'. The baby needs help to guide them, perhaps with a bell on one wrist at a time.

### SOUND AND LANGUAGE

Blind people do not develop superhuman hearing, but they do learn to use their hearing more efficiently than most sighted people. Background noise is bad; radios, televisions, and stereos should be turned off unless they are being listened to.

Blind babies need conversation to help them learn to talk and to enable them to keep track of where the other person is. It is helpful to keep up a running commentary, reinforced with frequent touching, to provide babies with a sense of security.

No blind child should be touched without a prior warning word or sound.

As a sighted child builds up a vocabulary of words, so a blind child must develop a vocabulary of sounds. These include footsteps, differences in the sound of water from a tap and from a teapot, and other everyday sounds the sighted take for granted.

Cause and effect can be taught via sound, for example, by having a toy which makes a noise when shaken (Landsdown, 1980).

### Key points for those working with hearing-impaired children

Most children have some residual hearing; it should be used to the full.

Children with intermittent deafness often seem to be naughty when in fact they cannot hear.

The speaker's face should be well illuminated.

A moustache or a beard are barriers to lip reading.

If an object is being shown it should be held as near the speaker's mouth as possible.

Speech should be clear and natural, using phrases and sentences which would be used with a hearing child of the same age.

The same word should be used consistently for the same object.

Children should not have their attention caught with a pull or a poke; they may come to imagine that this is normal behaviour (Lansdown, 1980).

---

visual input to help make sense of their environment. When walking, for example, these children often look around rather than watching where they are going. Thus, they may appear to be clumsy, poorly coordinated and accident prone.

The person with a hearing impairment should be assessed to ascertain whether sounds such as a doorbell, the telephone, a

## TABLE 26-1 Assessment of Sensory Function

| Assessment | Behaviour Indicating Deficit (Children) | Behaviour Indicating Deficit (Adult) |
|---|---|---|
| **VISION — WITH GLASSES, IF WORN**<br>Assess whether patient/client can read newspaper, magazine, or lettering on menu. | Self-stimulation, including eye-rubbing, repeated blinking, squinting, body rocking, sniffing or smelling, arm twirling. Reluctance to crawl in infancy, clumsiness. | Poor coordination, squinting, underreaching or overreaching for objects, persistent repositioning of objects, impaired night vision, accidental falls. Clumsiness. |
| **HEARING —**<br>**WITH HEARING AID, IF WORN**<br>Observe patient/client conversing with others.<br>Compare patient's/client's ability to recognize consonants with ability to distinguish vowels.<br>Assess patient's/client's perception of hearing ability and history of tinnitus.<br>Inspect ear canal for hardened cerumen. | Frightened when unfamiliar people approach, no reflex or purposeful response to sounds, failure to be awakened by loud noise, slow or absent development of speech, greater response to movement than to sound, avoidance of social interaction with other children, self-absorption, clumsiness, behavioural difficulties. | Blank looks, decreased attention span, lack of reaction to loud noises, increased volume of speech, positioning of head towards sound, inappropriate smiling and nodding of head in approval when someone speaks, use of other means of communication such as lip reading or writing, complaints of ringing in ears. |
| **TOUCH**<br>Assess patient/client for sensitivity to light, touch and temperature.<br>Check patient's/client's ability to discriminate between sharp and full stimuli.<br>Assess whether patient/client can distinguish objects (coin or safety pin) in the hand with eyes closed.<br>Ask whether patient/client feels unusual sensations. | Inability to perform developmental tasks related to grasping objects or drawing, repeated injury from handling of harmful objects (e.g. hot stove, sharp knife). | Clumsiness, overreaction or underreaction to painful stimulus, failure to respond when touched, avoidance of touch, sensation of pins and needles, numbness. |
| **SMELL**<br>Have patient/client close eyes and identify several nonirritating odours (e.g. coffee, vanilla). | Difficult to assess until child is 6 or 7 years old, difficulty discriminating noxious odours. | Failure to react to noxious or strong odour. |
| **TASTE**<br>Ask patient/client to sample and distinguish different tastes (e.g. lemon, sugar, salt). (Have patient/client sip water and wait 1 min between each taste.)<br>Ask patient/client if recent weight change has occurred. | Inability to tell whether food is salty or sweet, possible ingestion of strange-tasting things. | Change in appetite, excessive use of seasoning and sugar, complaints about taste of food, weight change. |
| **POSITION SENSE**<br>Perform conventional tests for balance and position sense. | Clumsiness, extraneous movement, excessive arm swinging in those with hyperactivity or learning difficulty. | Poor balance and spatial orientation, shuffling gait, reduced response to brace self when falling, more precise and deliberate movements. |

smoke alarm, and an alarm clock can be heard, and also whether he or she can discriminate between them. It is possible to alter auditory alarms to visual ones, for example, with flashing lights.

## MEANINGFUL STIMULI

Meaningful stimuli reduce the incidence of sensory deprivation. The home environment is assessed for stimuli such as pets, a record player or television, pictures of family members, and a calendar and clock. In a health care setting the nurse notes whether patients/clients have visitors or are able to socialize with others in the ward, as the presence of others can offer positive stimulation. However, sharing a ward area with someone who constantly watches television, persistently tries to talk, or continuously keeps lights on can also contribute to sensory overload.

It is possible to become disorientated in a barren environment that gives few signals for normal sensory perception. The presence or absence of meaningful stimuli can enhance or inhibit alertness and the ability to participate in care. It is important to check the environment for bright colours, comfortable furnishings, adequate lighting, good ventilation, and clean surroundings.

## AMOUNT OF STIMULI

Excessive stimuli in an environment can cause sensory overload. In an acute care setting, the nurse assesses the level of care required. The frequency of observations and procedures performed may be stressful. If the individual is in pain, has many tubes and dressings, or is restricted by plaster casts or traction, overstimulation can be a problem. If the patient's/client's bed is near the nurses' station, the kitchen, the sluice or the door leading to the stairs, the noise may be excessive and inhibit the patient/client in his or her efforts to rest and recuperate.

## Social Development and Support

The degree of contact with supportive family members and significant others can influence the degree of isolation an individual feels. It should be established whether an individual lives alone and whether family and friends visit frequently. A pattern of social isolation can contribute to sensory changes. The ability to discuss fears or concerns with loved ones is an important coping mechanism for most people. A lack of effective communication can cause sensory deprivation which may not become apparent until behavioural changes occur.

Sensory losses can often impair a person's ability to socialize with others. For example, a hearing-impaired child will often find it difficult to successfully initiate interactions with others and thus may not be able to relate to, and socialize with, those in his or her environment. Another example is older adults who are frequently aware of developing sensory problems with their hearing or vision. When older adults suspect that sensory functions are deteriorating, they may avoid social interactions to avoid embarrassment. Burton (1986) suggests that older adults who are hard of hearing have a tendency to withdraw from social interaction with others when it becomes not only embarrassing, but also too tiring. Thus, the difficulties experienced may cancel out the advantages that are normally associated with communication.

When individuals have socialization problems resulting from sensory deficits, it can become difficult for care givers to adequately plan care. In the case of the severely hearing impaired, nursing staff may have difficulty planning routine care, negotiating and providing instructions for self-care, and involving the patient/client directly in nursing interventions. It is important to provide ample cues and clues as to the context of the conversation for a hearing impaired individual so that he or she can participate effectively (Rye, 1990; Verney, 1989; Levene, 1983).

## Communication Methods

Individuals with existing sensory deficits often develop alternative ways of communicating; it is important to be aware of these and to be able to respond appropriately and also promote interaction with others. Someone who is deaf or hearing-impaired may lip-read, use a form of sign language (there are several), listen with

### Children's Nursing
### Providing a stimulating environment

Wards catering for infants and young children should have plenty of toys available. Play is more than purely a way of passing the time; it is how children learn about their environment. Children's play influences their physical, emotional and social development (Cohen, 1993). The play area should have toys and play materials that are appropriate for children of various developmental levels, including items of different sizes, shapes, textures and colours. The play area should be clean, bright, and decorated attractively with continual access allowed to the play materials for the children and their families.

the help of a hearing aid, read and write notes, or may prefer to use speech. Visual input is constantly used in communication as an accompaniment to hearing.

Individuals who are visually impaired are unable to observe facial expressions and other nonverbal behaviours that help clarify the content of spoken communication. Instead, they rely on voice tones and inflections to detect and determine the emotional tone of communication. Younger people with visual deficits often learn to read Braille (based upon a system of raised dots) or use the Moon System (based upon the Roman alphabet), but older individuals who have lost their sight or who have become partially sighted, often find it difficult to master either (Brocklehurst and Allen, 1987).

People with **aphasia** may be unable to produce or understand language. Aphasia can be caused by trauma or by degenerative disorders. **Expressive aphasia,** a motor type of aphasia, is the inability to name common objects or to express simple ideas in words or writing. For example, a person may understand a question but be unable to express an answer. **Sensory** or **receptive aphasia** is difficulty in understanding written or spoken language. The individual may be able to express words but is unable to understand inquiries or comments of others. **Global aphasia** is the inability to understand language or communicate orally.

The temporary or permanent loss of the ability to speak is extremely traumatic to an individual. It is important to be aware of, and assist with an individual's alternative method of communication to minimize unease and anxiety. Patients/clients who have undergone laryngectomies often write notes, use communication boards, speak with mechanical vibrators, or use oesophageal speech. With individuals who have endotracheal or tracheostomy tubes the loss of speech is usually temporary. Most use a notepad to write their questions and requests on. However, they may become incapacitated and unable to write messages. The nurse ascertains whether the patient/client has developed a sign language, or system of symbols, to communicate needs, and if not organizes a system of communication for him or her. Some individuals require permanent assistance with speech via tracheal cannulation and speaking-valves, which allow the passage of exhaled air through the vocal cords. This is an important consideration in infants and small children who have yet to learn language.

To understand the nature of a communication problem, it is necessary to know whether an individual has trouble speaking, understanding, naming objects, reading, or writing. The most appropriate method of communication is dependent on the nature of the difficulty. Although the patient/client should remain the nurse's primary source of information, you may also have to seek information from the person's relatives or friends if he or she cannot communicate effectively.

## Mental Status

Mental status assessment is an important component of any evaluation of sensory function. Observation of the individual during history taking, the physical examination, and care giving provides valuable data that can serve as the basis for an evaluation of mental status.

## Self-Perception of Sensory Loss

It is important to understand the way sensory losses are perceived by affected individuals. Many people believe that the quality of their lives has been altered because of sensory alterations (Salter, 1988). Of all the disadvantages of ageing, sensory deficits are the

### Learning Disabilities Nursing
### Sensory alterations

There are approximately 200,000 people with learning disabilities in the United Kingdom who have additional physical and sensory handicaps. Sometimes these additional disabilities remain undiagnosed and can result in the patient/client functioning at a level below their real potential.

When patients/clients with learning disabilities have impaired vision or hearing capable of being improved by the use of appropriate aids (e.g. glasses or hearing aids), the introduction of such aids will need to be carefully planned, and a structured approach taken in order to ensure that the aid is tolerated and used as intended.

The nurse will also need to ensure that the regular cleaning and maintenance of equipment such as hearing aids takes place in order that these remain in working condition and are useful to the patient/client, as he or she may not indicate that the appliance is no longer working.

In addition to the most commonly recognized sensory handicaps of vision and hearing, many people with learning disabilities appear to have altered or impaired sensitivity to pain and extremes of temperature, resulting in an increased risk of accidental injury. This may remain undisclosed for some time, as the patient/client does not appear to be in any discomfort.

For example, an able patient/client with impaired sensitivity to heat and pain may habitually sit on or next to an extremely hot radiator or get into a scalding bath, resulting in extensive burns which may not be discovered unless the nurse happens to observe the patient/client undressing and notes the condition of his or her skin. A patient/client such as this will need to be regularly supervised and taught strategies to help keep safe from injury.

most likely to cause social isolation (Bernardini, 1985). Simply observing an individual interact with others may reveal the person's sense of confidence. It may be necessary to ask questions about the individual's feelings towards his or her loss of hearing (or sight, or speech). Subsequently, strategies can be identified that can help the individual to adjust his or her perceptions with regard to sensory loss. Goffman (1963) suggests that: "When a person's differentness is not immediately apparent, he then has to decide whether to tell or not to tell, to let on or not to, to lie or not to lie." Denial of difficulties, particularly with the hard of hearing, is common (Burton, 1986; Lindsay, 1988).

Loss of independence is often the most difficult aspect of adjustment. Today, many assistive devices and technological advances enable people with sensory impairments to participate in mainstream society and thus reduce their isolation. Many cinemas and theatres, for example, have induction/infrared loop systems to assist people with hearing impairments. Some television programmes and videotapes are subtitled. New advances include the development of a commentary on the soundtrack of cinema films and television programmes to assist people with visual impairments to understand actions that are not obvious from the programme's dialogue.

After gathering data about the individual's sensory status, the nurse and patient/client agree upon a plan of care.

 **PLANNING**

The plan of care depends on the nurse's assessment of the individual's perception and acceptance of the sensory alteration. It also depends on the extent to which the individual has adjusted to the sensory loss. Every effort should be made to provide care that will enable the individual to adapt to the health care setting and to the home. The individual should be encouraged to actively participate in selecting interventions and strategies for the plan of care. Individuals who have sensory alterations at the time of entering a health care setting are usually most informed about how to adapt interventions to their routines and lifestyles, and partnership in their care can be negotiated. It is particularly important for children to have a voice in the planning of their care, to enable true partnership between children, families and health professionals to evolve.

Some sensory alterations are short term, for example, a patient suffering sensory/perceptual alterations as a result of sensory overload in an intensive care unit. Appropriate interventions are thus likely to be only temporary. Sensory alterations such as permanent loss of vision require long-term goals of care. Occasionally, it becomes necessary for the individual to make major changes in the way activities relating to self-care, communication, and socialization are performed.

It is important to consider all resources available to patients/clients. The family can play a key role in providing effective and meaningful stimulation and in learning ways to help their relative adjust to any limitations. Referrals may need to be made to other health care professionals. Early referrals to occupational or speech therapists, for example, can speed recovery.

RNIB produces the following information for ethnic minority visually impaired people:

1. 'Introducing RNIB' : this is a leaflet which is produced in Bengali, Chinese, English, Greek, Gujarati, Hindi, Punjabi, Turkish, Urdu and Welsh.

2. 'Your Benefit' booklet: this is produced in a taped version only in Bengali, Chinese, Greek, Gujarati, Hindi, Punjabi, Turkish Urdu.

3. RNIB Talking Books: about 100 talking books are available in Hindi, as well as a very small number in Bengali, Gujarati, Urdu and Punjabi. These are being added to continuously.

There are various organizations that can provide information and support in the form of advice, equipment and aids, such as the Royal National Institute for the Deaf, The British Deaf Association and the Royal National Institute for the Blind (see box). Most organizations have local groups that provide social contact and/or practical help. The nurse may be able to arrange for a volunteer to visit a patient/client or have printed materials made available that describe ways to cope with sensory problems.

Goals for the care of a patient/client with actual, or potential, sensory alterations include:

- ensuring the optimal functioning of existing senses
- controlling the environment to provide effective sensory stimuli
- establishing and maintaining a safe environment
- preventing additional sensory loss
- communicating effectively with regard to existing sensory alterations
- understanding the nature and the implications of sensory loss
- achieving self-care.

Priorities must be established between the goals of care. For example, an individual who temporarily loses vision following eye surgery will require more assistance in establishing a safe environment than receiving interventions that prevent additional sensory loss. Many individuals receive treatment for sensory problems either on an outpatient basis or only after a short stay in a hospital. For this reason, strategies and treatments should be planned that can be continued in the home.

 IMPLEMENTATION

Nursing interventions involve the individual and family so that a safe, pleasant, and stimulating sensory environment can be maintained. The most effective interventions enable the individual with sensory alterations to function safely with existing deficits. The individual is generally able to continue a normal lifestyle. Nursing interventions are chosen depending on the nursing assessment formulated and any related factors which may contribute to the difficulties encountered.

## Promoting Function of Existing Senses

Nursing assessment reveals the functional level of an individual's senses. Nursing measures are then implemented that enhance the remaining sensory functions or enhance other senses. Sensory testing detects sensory problems early so that corrective devices can be made available.

## VISION

The most common visual problem during childhood is a **refractive error** such as shortsightedness. Vision screening of school-aged children and adolescents can achieve early detection of visual impairment. Children are screened at various stages during their early years by health visitors, school nurses and by clinical medical officers: any problems identified are referred for further testing by an ophthalmologist who will prescribe corrective lenses. Visual problems that may require more invasive methods, such as a pronounced strabismus (squint), are referred to an ophthalmic surgeon (Chandna, 1989; Watkinson, 1989).

Since an adult develops visual changes with age (most commonly presbyopia), several strategies may be employed to help individuals adapt to these changes. An individual who wears corrective contact lenses or spectacles should make sure they are kept clean, accessible, and functional, in that they fit properly and that the lenses are not badly scratched. Regular ophthalmic examinations ensure that the proper lenses are worn. There are

### USEFUL ADDRESSES

**Royal National Institute for the Blind,** 224 Great Portland Street, London W1N 6AA

**RNIB Customer Services,** Production and Distribution Centre, Bakewell Road, Orton, Southgate, Peterborough PE2 0XU

**RNIB Talking Book Service,** Mount Pleasant, Alperton, Wembley, Middlesex HA0 1RR

**The Guide Dogs for the Blind Association,** Head Office, Alexandra House, Park Street, Windsor, Berkshire SL4 1JR

**Partially Sighted Society,** Queens Road, Doncaster DN1 2NX

**Disabled Living Foundation,** 380/384 Harrow Road, London W9 2HU

**\*Royal National Institute for the Deaf,** 105 Gower Street, London WC1E 6AH

**\*British Association for the Hard of Hearing,** 7-11 Armstrong Road, London W3 7JL

**\*British Deaf Association,** 38 Victoria Place, Carlisle CA1 1HU

**\*National Deaf Children Society (NDCS),** 45 Hereford Road, London W2 5AH

**\*NDCS Technology Information Centre,** 4 Church Road, Birmingham B15 3TD

**NDCS Family Services Centre,** 24 Wakefield Road, Rothwell Haigh, Leeds LS26 0SF

**British Telecom's Action for Disabled Customers,** Room B4036, BT Centre, 81 Newgate Street, London EC1A 7AJ

\*Telephones at these offices can be operated using voice or minicom.

## Strategies to Enhance Sensory Functioning: Vision

### UTILIZING RESIDUAL VISION

- Spectacles or contact lenses to be kept clean, functional, and protected from damage.
- Aids for visual impairment should be utilized: hand-held magnifiers, talking alarm clocks, writing guides, wristwatches with large faces, raised numerals or Braille, adapted telephones, large print books.
- Additional wing mirrors should be added to vehicles to enhance visual field perception.
- Large print used for labelling items such as medicines.
- Large print and contrasting colours used for any teaching materials.

### UTILIZING SHARP CONTRAST

- Colours that provide sharp contrast can be used to highlight: electrical fittings and switches, the edges of worktops, furniture, steps and stairs.
- Lighting should be adequate.
- Tactile cues can be added to the controls and dials on household and kitchen appliances, promoting safety and enhancing independence.

### REDUCE GLARE

- Lightbulbs can be changed to 'soft-tone' type which will cut down on glare and reflection.
- Non-carpeted areas of flooring should have a matt finish.

### UTILIZING OTHER SENSES

- Tape-recorded books (check if eligible for Talking Book Service).
- Having a purse, or wallet, with separate compartments for various types of notes and change.
- Having a system for positioning food on plates and items on trays that is easily memorized.
- Pouring salt/pepper into palm of hand so that their addition to food is easier for the individual to control.
- Provision of tactile cues in various parts of the surrounding environment to assist with orientation and promote independence.
- Spectacles can have tinted lenses or clip-on sunglasses. Sunvisors or wide-brimmed hats should be worn in bright sunlight.
- Night driving, and driving in poor light, should be avoided.

### EVALUATION

- Observation of visually impaired individual's ability to perform activities of living.
- Discussion with visually impaired individual and family/carers.

### Adult Nursing
### Home aids for people with hearing impairment

In the home, light-signalling devices for burglar alarms, doorbells, alarm clocks, smoke detectors, special baby-alarms and telephones are available. The hearing impaired patient/client is entitled to these technical aids under the 1970 Chronically Sick and Disabled Persons Act. The individual can apply for them through local Social Services Departments or the assigned Social Worker for the Deaf (Burton, 1984). Advice on technical aids is also available from the Royal National Institute for the Deaf (RNID). Signalling devices allow the deaf person to enjoy greater independence. The patient/client may also be eligible for a Hearing Dog for the Deaf which acts as the 'ears' of a person with a hearing impairment (Rye, 1990).

Anyone who calls on a regular basis should be asked to let the telephone, or doorbell, ring for a longer period of time. A telecommunications device is available for the deaf (a Minicom). It comprises a computer and printer that transfer written words via the telephone. Both the sender and receiver, however, must have a Minicom to complete a communication. Individuals who are registered as deaf or speech impaired are eligible for rebates of up to 60% on their telephone bills from British Telecom, through the RNID. The proposed advent of the video-telephone will also prove beneficial to hearing impaired and deaf individuals who lip-read, and/or use manual means of communication, such as signing (Winstanley, 1993).

Older adults may be unable to hear with background noise. The nurse can suggest that radios, televisions, and other appliances are turned off during conversations. It is also helpful to have conversations in settings where floor coverings and soft furnishings muffle extraneous background noises (Bernardini, 1985). If a hearing aid is worn, it should be properly cleaned and adjusted and checked for battery function. The hearing impaired individual should wear it at all times, except for when swimming, bathing, when washing hair or when asleep. Ensure the individual knows how and when to change the batteries (Fountain, 1987; Levene, 1983).

Deaf patients/clients who require care in the community can apply for assessment of their needs to the local social services department under the terms of the NHS Community Care Act, 1990.

various methods that can assist in the maintenance of existing visual function (see box). The individual can be taught to strengthen visual stimuli, use other senses, use sharp visual contrasts, and minimize the effects from glare.

## HEARING

Children with chronic middle ear infections — a common cause of impaired hearing — should undergo auditory testing. Repeated ear infections can lead to the condition known as 'glue ear' which is the build-up of sticky, viscous secretions in the middle ear that impair the conduction of sound: **conductive hearing loss**. Parents must be warned of the risks and should seek medical care when the child has symptoms of earache or upper respiratory infection. Even a mild hearing loss can create developmental problems in a child (Tate, 1989). As soon as they are able to cooperate, children should be taught how to blow their noses in order to help clear secretions from the middle ear. Children should also be immunized against childhood diseases (for example, measles, rubella, and mumps) that can cause hearing loss and should not be treated with ototoxic medications, if at all possible.

Older adults frequently experience hearing impairment as a result of impacted cerumen. With ageing, cerumen has a

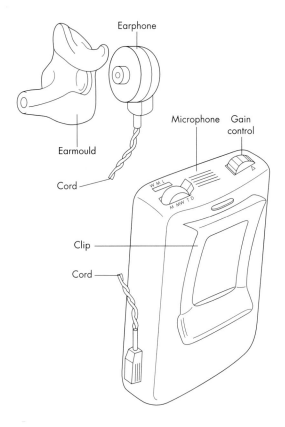

**Fig 26-1** National Health Service hearing aids: a typical body-worn aid.

tendency to thicken and build up in the ear canal, often becoming impacted on the tympanic membrane. This excess of cerumen occluding the ear canal often causes a conductive hearing loss. Removal of cerumen can improve hearing ability (Lewis-Cullinan, 1990) and improve the quality of sound experienced by those who use hearing aids (Rye, 1990). When appropriate, hearing aids should be recommended (Fig. 26-1).

## TASTE

The sense of taste can be promoted by using measures to enhance remaining taste perception. Good oral hygiene keeps the taste buds well hydrated. Taste perception will be heightened if foods are well seasoned, differently textured, and eaten separately. The use of vinegar or lemon juice can add tartness to food. The nurse should determine which foods taste the most appealing to the patient/client. If taste perception is improved, food intake and appetite should also improve.

Stimulation of the sense of smell with aromas such as brewed coffee and baked bread can heighten taste sensation. The individual should try to avoid blending or mixing foods because the effect is to make it difficult to identify tastes. Older people have far fewer taste buds and should, therefore, try to chew food thoroughly to allow more contact with those remaining, though this may prove difficult for individuals with dentures (Bee and Mitchell, 1980).

## TOUCH

Individuals with reduced tactile sensation usually have the impairment over a limited portion of their bodies. Existing function can be stimulated by utilizing therapeutic touch. If the individual is willing to be touched, hair brushing and combing, a gentle massage, and touching of the arms or shoulders are ways of increasing tactile contact. When sensation is reduced, a firm pressure may be necessary for the individual to feel the nurse's hand. Turning and repositioning can also improve the quality of tactile sensation.

If an individual is overly sensitive to tactile stimuli (hyperaesthesia), then endeavours must be made to keep irritating stimuli to a minimum. Keeping bed linen loose to reduce direct contact with the individual (perhaps with a bed cradle) and protecting the skin from exposure to irritants are other helpful measures.

## SMELL

An individual's sense of smell can be improved by strengthening pleasant olfactory stimulation. The immediate environment can be made more pleasant with smells such as cologne, mild room deodorizers, fragrant flowers, and perfumed sachets. Individuals can also be encouraged to sniff food before eating as this may enhance the ability to taste. Alternatively, when preparing a meal tray, or when assisting with eating, naming the foods on the tray may help individuals imagine the aromas. However, it is important to ascertain which aromas are considered pleasant or appetizing as some smells may actually decrease an individual's appetite.

Removal of unpleasant odours can improve the quality of a person's environment. It is important to ensure an individual's room is kept clean, and that items such as bedpans, or urinals, are dealt with promptly.

### Maintaining Meaningful Stimulation

When an individual's environment presents the risk of understimulation or overstimulation of the senses, endeavours should be made to eliminate confusing or irritating stimuli and replace them with others which are more pleasing or meaningful for that person. He or she may wish to have something with them from a familiar environment, for example, a photograph or a cushion. **To avoid sensory deprivation:**

- arrange for alterations in the immediate environment that stimulate all the senses, but do not force these changes if the individual is more concerned with basic functions such as comfort and nutrition.

A bedridden individual may have a limited view of his or her environment. Long intervals of staring at ceilings and walls can heighten sensory problems. **To reduce sensory problems:**

- provide comfort measures, such as frequent positioning, washing the face and hands, and gentle massage
- plan time to talk with the individual
- provide access to reading materials, a radio or cassette tapes, or television for those who are not well enough to stimulate themselves.

**Control excessive stimuli for individuals at risk for sensory overload:**

- ensure patient/client has the time needed for rest and

freedom from stresses caused by frequent monitoring and repeated tests

- sit quietly with the person or involve him or her in a simple activity, such as combing hair or brushing teeth
- offer to read aloud to provide a peaceful form of stimulation
- ask the patient/client at home to participate in tasks such as meal planning and household chores, as these are simple activities which often do not require too much thought
- provide re-orientation to the environment by wearing name tags on uniforms, addressing the individual by name, and using conversational cues as to time or location
- reduce the tendency for individuals to become disorientated by offering short and simple repeated explanations and reassurance
- help individuals to become as mobile and independent as possible, within their prescribed limits
- advise the family not to argue with, or contradict, the confused individual, but to calmly explain location, identity, and time of day and to repeat these as often as is necessary.

**Organize the care plan to coordinate care:**
- combine activities, such as dressing changes, bathing, and observation of vital signs to prevent the individual from becoming overly tired
- schedule time for rest and quiet, and engender cooperation from family and visitors
- coordinate with laboratory and radiology departments to reduce the amount of time required for tests and examinations
- anticipate needs, such as elimination, to reduce uncomfortable stimuli.

**Control extraneous noise in and around the ward area:**
- ask for the volume on a nearby television to be lowered or perhaps move the patient/client to a quieter area
- monitor equipment noise and keep it to a minimum, where possible
- turn off bedside equipment, such as suction and oxygen apparatus, when not in use
- avoid abrupt loud noises such as the clattering or rinsing of bed pans
- control laughter or conversation at the nurses' station
- allow the doors of individual rooms or cubicles to be closed, where appropriate.

## Providing a Safe Environment

The nurse has a responsibility to protect individuals with existing sensory loss from injury, whereas those at risk for sensory loss must learn to avoid injury. The nature of the actual or potential sensory loss determines the safety precautions that need to be taken (see Chapter 19).

### VISION LOSS

The patient/client with recent visual impairment often requires assistance with mobility. The nurse should stand at the individual's nondominant side approximately one step in front.

The nondominant hand can be used to grasp the nurse's arm while reaching forward with the dominant hand to feel for any obstacles or familiar landmarks. Describe the course to be taken and ensure that obstacles have been removed. Never leave a visually impaired individual standing alone in an unfamiliar area. For individuals undergoing eye surgery, it is important to teach family members how to assist their relative.

### HEARING LOSS

Nurses sometimes rely on patients/clients in health care settings to report unusual sounds, such as suction apparatus running improperly or an intravenous pump alarm. However, the individual with a hearing loss may not hear such sounds and thus requires more frequent visits by the nurse. A person with a hearing impairment can also benefit from learning to use his or her vision to discover sources of risk and danger .

### REDUCED OLFACTION

A reduced sensitivity to odours may result in the inability to smell leaking gas, a smouldering cigarette or fire, and tainted food. The installation of smoke detectors is recommended plus other alternative precautions such as checking ashtrays or placing cigarette butts in water. It is essential to check the dates on food packaging and also the colour and texture of food. Pilot flames on any gas appliances must be checked visually.

### REDUCED TACTILE SENSATION

Individuals with reduced tactile sensation risk injury when their illnesses, or conditions, confine them to bed as they are unable to sense pressure on bony prominences or the need to change position. These patients/clients rely on nurses, or relatives, for repositioning, moving tubes or devices that the patient/client may lie on, and regular turning to preserve skin integrity.

If the ability to sense temperature variation is reduced, extra caution is required when using treatments that include the application of heat and cold (see Chapter 27) and when preparing bath water, for example, running cold water in prior to the addition of the hot. The condition of the individual's skin should be checked frequently.

### SPEECH ALTERATIONS

An individual lacking the ability to speak cannot call out for assistance. Those who have aphasia, a laryngectomy, or an artificial airway (see Chapter 17) need alternative methods of communication, such as message boards and note pads. In the hospital a call bell should always be near. For someone at home, a small bell or alarm at the bedside is helpful. Alarms are available which can be worn on the person's wrist and can be used to alert a close neighbour.

## Understanding Sensory Loss

It is necessary to understand all the implications of sensory loss. The individual with impaired hearing must learn that excessive background noise interferes with the ability to hear conversation, as must those who are participating in the communication. Similarly, an older person with visual loss must be aware of the need to install proper lighting in hazardous areas to reduce the risk of injury. Individuals can learn to adapt to sensory alterations so that living and working environments can be safe as well as appropriately stimulating. All family members should understand the ways in which an individual's sensory loss may affect normal daily activities. Family and friends will be more supportive when they understand sensory deficits and the types of elements that worsen or lessen sensory problems. If an individual feels socially unaccepted, he or she is more likely to perceive sensory losses as seriously impairing his or her quality of life.

## Preventing Sensory Loss

Occupation or lifestyle may place a person at risk for sensory loss. Persons working with, or in the vicinity of, loud noise need to be aware of the potential dangers to hearing function. The use of protective ear covers, or ear plugs, is essential if exposure to loud noise is frequent or continuous. Ringing of the ears, a form of **tinnitus**, may be an early sign of hearing impairment. Data from the Institute of Hearing Research, using figures based upon the 1981 Population Census for Great Britain and Northern Ireland, show that 13.6 million people (approximately 24% of the population) have degrees of hearing loss in excess of 25 decibels. It is further suggested that an incidence of 10–15% hearing impairment will be apparent in people in their fourth decade, attributable to increased levels of environmental and leisure noise (Sympathetic Hearing Scheme, 1988).

People exposed to dangerous chemicals or airborne debris in their working environment should wear safety glasses for protection. A chemical burn to the cornea or a penetrating eye injury can cause permanent blindness. Children should be discouraged from playing with any kind of sharp object, because they can be accidentally blinded by a playmate. Care must also be taken to prevent children from placing sharp objects in their ears.

## Promoting Communication

A sensory deficit can cause a person to feel isolated, because of an inability to communicate with others. This problem can complicate a nurse's effectiveness in teaching information and skills. The nature of the sensory loss influences the methods and styles of communication that nurses can use. The methods described in the following box can also be taught to family members and significant others.

The patient/client with a hearing impairment may be able to speak normally. However, the deaf patient's/client's inability to hear self-spoken words may cause serious speech alterations. A child born deaf, or who has been deafened pre-lingually, cannot reproduce speech that does not sound distorted. Some individuals may use sign language or lip reading, write with a pad and pencil, rely on a hearing aid, or learn to use a computer for communication. Special communication boards contain common terms used in nursing care and help individuals express their needs. If an individual has a hearing aid, there are guidelines that can help to ensure the aid works properly (Procedure 26-1).

Depending on the type of aphasia, the inability to communicate can be frustrating and frightening. The nurse should initially establish very basic communication and recognize

### Communication Methods

PATIENTS/CLIENTS WITH APHASIA
- Listen to the patient/client and wait for the patient/client to communicate.
- Do not shout or speak loudly (hearing loss is not the problem).
- If the patient/client has problems with comprehension, use simple, short questions and facial gestures to give additional clues.
- If the patient/client has problems speaking, ask questions that require simple yes or no answers or blinking of the eyes. Offer pictures or a communication board so that the patient/client can point.
- Give the patient/client time to understand.
- Do not pressure or tire the patient/client.

PATIENTS/CLIENTS WITH AN ARTIFICIAL AIRWAY
- Use pictures, objects, or word cards so that the patient/client can point.
- Offer a pad and pencil or magic slate for the patient/client to write messages.
- Do not shout or speak loudly.
- Provide an artificial voice box (vibrator) for the patient/client with a laryngectomy to use to speak words and phrases.

PATIENTS/CLIENTS WITH HEARING IMPAIRMENT
- Get the patient's/client's attention. Do not startle the patient/client when entering the room. Do not approach a patient/client from behind. Ensure the patient/client knows you wish to speak.
- Face the patient/client. Ensure your face and lips are illuminated to promote lip reading.
- If the patient/client wears glasses, ensure they are clean so that your gestures and face can be seen. If the patient/client wears a hearing aid, ensure it is in place and working.
- Speak slowly and articulate clearly. Older adults may take longer to process verbal messages. Use a normal tone of voice and inflections of speech. Refrain from speaking with something in your mouth.
- When you are not understood, rephrase rather than repeat the conversation.
- Use visible aids. Speak with your hands, face and eyes.
- Do not shout. Loud sounds are usually higher pitched and may impede hearing by accentuating vowel sounds and concealing consonants.* If it is necessary to raise your voice, speak in lower tones.
- Talk towards the patient's/client's best or normal ear.
- Use gestures or written information to enhance the spoken word.
- Do not restrict a deaf patient's/client's hands. Never have intravenous lines in both of the patient's/client's hands if the preferred method of communication is sign language.†

*Data from Bernardini L: *Top Clin Nurs,* Jan 1985, p 72.
†Data from Chovaz C: *Can Nurs* 85(3):34, 1989.

that these difficulties do not indicate intellectual impairment or the degeneration of personality.

## Promoting Self-Care

The ability to perform self-care is essential for self-esteem. Frequently, family members and nurses believe sensory impaired persons require assistance, when in fact they can help themselves.

## PROCEDURE 26-1 Care of a Behind-the-Ear (Postaural) Hearing Aid

| SEQUENCE OF ACTIONS | RATIONALE |
|---|---|
| 1. Assess patient's/client's knowledge of and routines for cleansing and caring for hearing aid. | Determines patient's/client's understanding and need for health education. Adapts method of care to patient's/client's procedure. |
| 2. Determine whether patient/client can hear clearly with use of the aid by talking slowly and clearly in normal voice tone. | Inability to hear may indicate faulty function of hearing aid. |
| 3. Have patient/client suggest any additional tips for care; explain that you are going to clean and replace hearing aid. | Patient/client becomes uncomfortable when unable to hear clearly. Minimizes confusion and anxiety. |
| 4. Turn aid off, then assess whether hearing aid is working by removing from patient's/client's ear. Close battery case and turn volume slowly to high. Cup hand over earmould. If aid emits no sound, replace batteries and assess again. | Determines need for new battery. Feedback squeal will cause harsh whistling sound. |
| 5. Check to ensure plastic connecting tube is not twisted or cracked. | Cracked or twisted tube prevents transmission of sound. |
| 6. Check to see if earmould is cracked or has rough edges. | Can cause irritation to external ear canal. |
| 7. Check for accumulation of cerumen around earmould and plugging of opening in mould. | Prevents clear sound reception and transmission. |
| 8. Prepare necessary equipment and supplies: | |
|    a. Basin | Used to soak earmould. |
|    b. Mild soap and warm water | |
|    c. Nail brush (optional) | Used to clean plastic connecting tube. |
|    d. Soft towel | |
|    e. Dry cloth | |
|    f. Storage case | |
| 9. Clean ear mould: | |
|    a. Wash hands. | Reduces transmission of microorganisms. |
|    b. Assemble supplies at bedside table or sink area. | Procedure can be performed without delays. |
|    c. Detach earmould from battery device. Pull tubing away from the elbow of the aid. **Do not pull the tubing out of the mould** (see illustration). | Moisture entering battery and transmitter will cause permanent damage to aid. |
|    d. Add warm water and soap to emesis basin. Soak ear mould for several minutes. | Soaking removes cerumen that can accumulate on mould. |
|    e. Wash ear mould with cloth moistened in soap and water. Rinse and dry. | Removes cerumen and debris. |
|    f. If cerumen has built up in hole of earmould, carefully cleanse hole with a nail brush. | Wax will prevent normal sound transmission. |
|    g. Rinse earmould thoroughly with clear water. | Soap may form residue that blocks opening in mould. |
|    h. Allow mould to dry thoroughly after wiping with soft towel. | Water droplets left in connecting tube could enter hearing aid and damage parts. |
|    i. Cleanse connecting tube with nail brush (optional). | Removes moisture and debris that can interfere with sound transmission and hearing aid function. |
|    j. Reconnect earmould to hearing aid device before inserting or storing hearing aid. | Reassembly allows check of functioning. |
|    k. Store hearing aid in case if patient/client is about to bathe, use hair dryer, sit under sun lamp or heat, go to surgery or major procedure, or go to sleep. | Protects hearing aid against damage and breakage. |
| 10. Insert hearing aid: | |
|    a. Check batteries (see Step 4); replace batteries as needed. | Necessary for proper sound amplification. Always change batteries over soft surface (e.g. towel or bed) to avoid breakage. |

## PROCEDURE 26-1 Care of a Behind-the-Ear (Postaural) Hearing Aid (Cont'd)

| SEQUENCE OF ACTIONS | RATIONALE |
|---|---|
| b. Turn aid off and turn volume control down. | Protects patient/client from sudden exposure to sound. |
| c. Place earmould in external ear canal. Ensure that ear bore (hole) in mould is placed into canal first. Shape of mould indicates correct ear. Gently press and twist until mould feels snug. | Proper fit ensures optimal sound transmission. |
| d. Gently bring connecting tube up and over towards back of ear, avoiding kinking. Battery device fits around upper ear. | Ensures correct function of hearing aid device and maintains patient's/client's comfort. |
| e. Adjust volume gradually to comfortable level for talking to patient/client in normal voice at 1–1.25 m distance. | Gradual adjustment prevents exposing patient/client to harsh squeal or feedback. Patient/client should hear nurse comfortably. |
| 11. Return to patient/client to assess whether hearing is clear or hearing aid is producing inappropriate feedback sound. | If earmould is not securely in place, it will squeal or not function. |
| 12. Document that aid is worn if patient/client is to undergo surgery or special procedure and inform theatre staff. | Protects from liability of loss of hearing aid. |
| 13. Report difficulties patient/client has in communicating to nursing staff. | Improves continuity of care in communication techniques for patient/client. |
| 14. Note on nursing notes that patient/client uses hearing aid. | Alerts personnel to hearing impairment. |

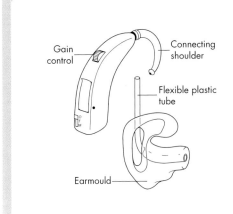

Labels: Gain control, Connecting shoulder, Flexible plastic tube, Earmould

**What the letters mean**

**O**  hearing aid is off

**T**  hearing aid can pick up signals from a telephone or television — listener will hear only the signal (e.g. the voice on the telephone) and will not be bothered by background noise

**M**  listener can hear through hearing aid microphone

**N**  normal listening

**H**  low tones are filtered out — helps reduce background noise

The following useful guidelines can assist those with visual or tactile impairment when help is required with activities of living:

- Arrange meal trays so the food and drink on the tray are numbers on the face of a clock. Orientate the visually impaired patient/client to see positions and explain each item's location.
- Facilitate easier dressing for people with diminished sense of touch by encouraging them to use zips or velcro fastenings, pullover-type sweaters or blouses, and elasticated waists. If an individual has partial paralysis and reduced sensation, the affected side should be dressed first.
- Encourage family members responsible for selecting clothing for the visually impaired to follow the individual's own preferences. Any sensory impairment has a significant influence on body image, and it is important for the individual to feel well groomed and attractive. Offer assistance, if needed, in brushing, combing, and shampooing hair.

- Assist individuals with visual problems in reaching toilet facilities safely. Safety bars should be installed near the toilet, and toilet paper and the call bell cord should be within easy reach. Patients/clients with proprioceptive problems may lose their balance when attempting to use the toilet. Supervise these individuals while walking and sitting, to help prevent falls, and caution against leaning too far forward.

 **EVALUATION**

When caring for someone with a sensory alteration, it is necessary to evaluate whether the nursing interventions being implemented improve, or at least maintain, that individual's ability to interact and function within the environment. The nature of an individual's sensory alteration influences the way the nurse evaluates the care given. The evaluation of care needs to be adapted to the individual's sensory deficit to determine whether actual outcomes are the same as expected outcomes. For example, use appropriate communication techniques to evaluate whether someone with a hearing deficit has gained the ability to hear more effectively. Similarly, use large printed materials to test a visually impaired individual's ability to read a prescription. When expected outcomes have not been achieved, there may be a need to change the nursing interventions planned to alter the individual's environment. Family members may need to become more involved in the support that is necessary for that person.

If nursing care has been directed at improving sensory acuity, the integrity of the sensory organs and the individual's ability to perceive stimuli should be evaluated. Any interventions designed to relieve problems associated with sensory alterations are evaluated on the basis of the individual's ability to function normally without injury. When the nurse attempts to directly, or indirectly (through education), alter the individual's environment, evaluation is directed at observing whether the changes have been made. When teaching is designed to improve an individual's sensory function, it is important to determine whether the recommendations are being followed. Asking the individual to explain or demonstrate self-care skills is an important strategy in evaluating the level of learning that has occurred. It may be necessary to reinforce previous instruction if learning has not taken place.

When an individual is discharged from an acute care setting to the home environment, hospital-based nurses should communicate with colleagues in the community about the types of intervention that helped the process of adaptation to sensory problems. Similarly, it is essential that information describing that individual's existing sensory deficits should be communicated. Continuity of care is achieved when an individual is required to make only minimal changes to his or her care to adapt it for the home setting.

## SUMMARY

The individual with sensory alterations often faces a lonely and frightening world. The inability to interact effectively with the environment may result in a loss of security and self-esteem. A healthy balance between incoming sensory stimuli, and stimuli to which the person is able to respond, is necessary for the person's well-being.

Nurses work with a variety of people who have actual or potential sensory alterations. Specific physiological changes can create sensory deficits. Exposure to excessive environmental stimulation causes sensory overload. Isolation in an environment without meaningful stimulation causes sensory deprivation. Individuals most at risk for sensory problems include older adults, immobilized individuals, and those who are socially isolated.

The nature of any sensory alteration influences the choice of nursing interventions. The nurse promotes the ability of the sensory impaired individual to maintain normal functioning with the existing sensory deficits. Similarly, the nurse attempts to make changes within the individual's environment to provide safe and appropriate stimulation. Sensory changes can affect various aspects of an individual's lifestyle. The nurse uses creative interventions to assist individuals to interact effectively with their environments.

## CHAPTER 26 REVIEW

### Key Concepts

- Sensory reception involves the stimulation of sensory nerve fibres and the transmission of impulses to higher centres within the brain.
- Sensory perception involves the organization and integration of sensory information into meaningful and conscious awareness.
- Because a person learns to develop and rely on unaffected senses after experiencing a sensory loss, the nurse designs interventions to preserve function of these senses.
- Sensory deprivation results from an inadequate quality or quantity of sensory stimuli.
- Ageing results in a gradual decline of acuity in all senses but there are no specific changes.
- Environmental stimuli within an intensive care unit can place an individual at risk from sensory overload.
- Individuals who are older, immobilized, or confined in isolated environments may develop sensory alterations.
- Even when physical senses are intact perceptions of, processing of, and reaction to stimuli may be altered.
- The extent of support from family members and significant others can influence the quality of sensory input experienced.
- Assessment of sensory function includes a physical examination and measurement of functional abilities.
- Sensory losses can impair a person's ability or desire to socialize.
- An assessment of environment includes identifying potential dangers or health hazards, sources of stimuli, risk of over-stimulation, and presence of meaningful stimuli.
- The plan of care for individuals with sensory alterations should include participation by family members.
- Nursing care for individuals with sensory alterations includes using stronger sensory stimuli, compensating with other senses, and modifying the environment to promote remaining sensory function.
- Individuals with existing sensory deficits can learn alternative methods of communication.
- Care of individuals at risk for sensory deprivation includes the introduction of appropriate and pleasant stimuli for all senses.
- To prevent sensory overload, the nurse controls stimuli, orientates the individual to the environment, and promotes rest by minimizing interruptions.
- To improve communication with the hearing impaired, the nurse speaks clearly, avoids shouting, and ensures that facial and lip movements can be seen clearly.
- Individuals with artificial airways can communicate effectively with communication boards and written messages.
- Technical aids and practical support enable individuals with various sensory impairments to function as independently as possible

## CRITICAL THINKING EXERCISES

1. Describe features that should be incorporated into the design of a nursing home for older adults with visual deficits.

2. On entering Mrs James' room, you discover that she is disorientated to time and place. She appears restless and has a reduced attention span. How would you determine whether Mrs James is suffering from sensory deprivation or from electrolyte imbalance?

3. Describe ways of communicating with a visually impaired individual who has an artificial airway.

4. Mr Peters has recently been transferred to a medical ward after spending 6 days in intensive care. As the nurse caring for Mr Peters, what interventions would you use to create an appropriate and effective sensory environment?

### Key Terms

## REFERENCES

Bee HL, Mitchell SK: *The developing person: a life-span approach,* San Francisco, 1980, Harper & Row.

Bernardini L: Effective communication as an intervention for sensory deprivation in the elderly client, *Top Clin Nurs* 6(4):72, 1985.

Burton D: Communication, behaviour and relationships. In Royal National Institute for the Deaf: *Breaking the sound barrier,* London, 1986, RNID.

Burton D: Social and communication needs of the deaf, *Midwife Health Visitor Commun Nurs* 20:54, 1984.

Chandna A, Chandna A: Assessment of visual function in infants and children, *Matern Child Health* 14(11):358, 1989.

Cohen D: *The development of play,* ed 2, London, 1993, Routledge.

Cullinan TR: Sight. In SJ Redfern: *Nursing elderly people,* Edinburgh, 1991, Churchill Livingstone.

Ebersole P, Hess P: *Toward healthy aging,* ed 3, St Louis, 1990, Mosby.

Fountain D: Hearing: aids and their care, *Geriatr Nurs Home Care* 7(2):12, 1987.

Freeland A: *Deafness: the facts,* Oxford, 1989, Oxford University Press.

Goffman E: *Notes on the management of spoiled identity,* New Jersey, 1963, Prentice Hall.

Gregson S: *The deaf chld and his family,* London, 1976, Allen & Urwin.

Lansdown R: *More than sympathy,* New York, 1980, Tavistock Publications.

Lewis-Cullinan C, Janken JK: Effect of cerumen removal on the hearing ability of geriatric patients, *J Adv Nurs* 15:594, 1990.

Lindsay M: Sensory impairment and body image. In M Salter, editor: *Altered body image: the nurse's role,* Chichester, 1988, John Wiley & Sons.

Magilvy JK: Quality of life of hearing-impaired older women, *Nurs Res* 34:140, 1985.

Rye S: A confusion of sound, *Nurs Times* 86(37):42, 1990.

Salter M: *Altered body image: the nurse's role,* Chichester, 1988, John Wiley & Sons.

Sympathetic Hearing Scheme: *The hearing impaired population of the United Kingdom,* London, 1988, BAHOH.

Tate M: Deafness in children, *Midwife, Health Visitor & Community Nurse,* 25(10):438, 1989.

Tolson D, McIntosh J, Swan IRC: Hearing impairment in elderly residents, *Br J Nurs,* 1(14):705, 1992.

Verney A: The patient with hearing impairment, *Nurs* 3(35):17, 1989.

Walsh C, Eldredge N: When deaf people become elderly, *J Gerontol Nurs* 15(12):27, 1989.

Watkinson S: Visual handicap in childhood, *Nurs* 3(45):13, 1989.

Weibley TT: Inside the incubator, *MCN,* 14: 96, 1989.

Winstanley T: Lifting the wraps on technology, *Talk* 148:10, 1993.

## FURTHER READING

### Adult Nursing

Corrado OJ: Everyday aids and appliances: hearing aids, *BMJ* 296:33, 1988.

Coni N, Davidson W, Webster S: *Ageing: the facts,* ed 2, Oxford, 1992, Oxford University Press.

Dudley NJ: Everyday aids and appliances: aids for visual impairment, *BMJ* 301:1151, 1990.

Ford M, Heshel T: *The in touch handbook: BBC Radio 4's guide to services for people with a visual handicap,* ed 7, London, 1990, Broadcasting Support Services.

French S: Understanding partial sight, *Nurs Times* 84(3):32, 1988.

Illingworth M: *Visual handicap for community nurses: a handbook,* London, 1986, Disabled Living Foundation.

Kelly JS: Visual impairment among older people, *Br J Nurs,* 2(2):110, 1993.

Latham J: *Pain control,* ed 2, London, 1995, Mosby.

Martin M, Glover B: *Hearing loss: causes, treatment and advice,* Edinburgh, 1986, Churchill Livingstone.

Nelligan B: Ophthalmic nursing: eye investigations, *Nurs* 3(45):10, 1989.

Royal National Institute for the Blind: *Information for people who are losing their sight,* London, RNIB.

Royal National Institute for the Deaf: *Breaking the sound barrier,* London, 1986, RNID

### Children's Nursing

Hayhow R: Who should see a speech therapist? *Matern Child Health* 11(1):98, 1986.

Kittel R: Choices for the deaf child, *Matern Child Health* 15(7): 214, 1990a.

Kittel R: Making the right choices for your deaf child II, *Matern Child Health* 15(12): 374, 1990 b.

Powell CA: Choices for the deaf child, *Matern Child Health* 16(4): 106, 1991.

### Mental Health Nursing

Hume A: Let me whisper in your ear, *Nurs Times* 84(16):39, 1988.

Hume A: Sound remedies, *Nurs Times* 84(18):42, 1988.

Williams CA: Perspectives on hallucinatory process, *Issues Mental Health Nurs* 10:99, 1989.

# Controlling Pain

## LEARNING OUTCOMES

After studying this chapter, you should be able to:
- *Define the key terms listed.*
- *Discuss common misconceptions about pain.*
- *Identify the three main physiological components of the pain experience and describe the sequences involved in pain transmission.*
- *Explain the relationship of the gate-control theory to selected nursing interventions for pain relief.*
- *Discuss the three phases of behavioural response to pain.*
- *Be aware of patterns of patient/client behaviour that may indicate pain.*
- *Anticipate possible causes of pain in commonly occurring medical conditions.*
- *Differentiate between acute and chronic pain and respective patient/client care needs.*
- *Identify factors which may affect an individual's response to pain.*
- *Perform an assessment of a patient/client experiencing pain.*
- *Discuss the guidelines for implementing individualized pain control measures.*
- *Identify the techniques and rationales for selecting pain control measures.*
- *Describe three nonpharmacological methods which can help the patient/client to reduce or to avoid pain.*
- *Describe the use of analgesics in the provision of effective pain relief.*
- *Provide ongoing nursing interventions that prevent or reduce a patient's/client's pain.*

Everyone has experienced some type or degree of pain. Yet the concept of pain is difficult to communicate. It is the most common reason to seek health care. A person in pain feels distress or suffering and seeks relief. The nurse uses a variety of interventions to bring relief. However, the nurse cannot see or feel the patient's/client's pain. No two people experience pain in the same way, and no two painful events create identical responses or feelings in a person. Pain is one of the most common problems faced by nurses, yet it is a source of frustration and is often one of the most misunderstood problems that the nurse confronts. The International Association for the Study of Pain (IASP) defined pain as "an unpleasant, subjective sensory and emotional experience associated with actual or potential tissue damage, or described in terms of such damage" (IASP, 1979). Pain can be a major factor inhibiting the ability and motivation to recover from illness.

Nurses care for people in many settings and situations in which interventions are provided to promote comfort (for example, the community nurse caring for a dying patient/client with cancer, the school nurse delivering first aid to an injured child, and a rheumatology nurse suggesting pain relief measures for chronic arthritic pain). The nurse has a responsibility to understand the experience of pain and to initiate measures that provide relief or help the patient/client learn to cope.

## NATURE OF PAIN

Pain is much more than a single sensation caused by a specific stimulus. Pain is subjective and highly individualized, and the interpretation and meaning of pain involve psychosocial and cultural factors. The person experiencing pain is the only authority on it. According to McCaffery (1980), "Pain is whatever the experiencing person says it is, existing whenever he says it does". Pain cannot be objectively measured, such as with an x-ray examination or blood test. Although certain types of pain create predictable signs and symptoms, often the nurse can only assess pain by relying on the patient's/client's words and behaviour. Only the patient/client knows whether pain is present and what the experience is like. To help that person gain relief, the nurse must first believe that the pain exists.

Pain is a protective physiological mechanism. A person with a sprained ankle, for example, avoids bearing full weight on the foot to prevent further injury. Pain is a warning that tissue damage has occurred. The patient/client who is unable to feel sensations, such as one with a spinal cord injury may be unaware of pain-inducing tissue damage.

Pain is a leading cause of disability. As the average life span increases, more people have chronic disease, in which pain is a common symptom. In addition, medical advances have resulted in diagnostic and therapeutic measures that are often uncomfortable. Nurses care daily for individuals in pain. One of the earliest fears of any patient/client with a diagnosed illness is the concern about the pain that might be experienced.

## Prejudices and Misconceptions

Health care personnel often hold prejudices against patients/clients in pain. Unless a patient/client has objective signs of pain, a nurse may not believe that the person is uncomfortable. The attitudes many nurses have concerning pain are caused in part by the traditional medical model of illness. This model suggests that physical problems result from physical causes. Thus, pain is viewed as a physical response to organic dysfunction. When no obvious source of pain can be found, nurses may stereotype pain sufferers as complainers or difficult patients/clients. This is particularly so for patients/clients who suffer from chronic pain (Taylor *et al*, 1984).

The extent to which nurses make assumptions about patients/clients in pain may seriously limit their ability to offer effective pain relief. Unfortunately, all people are influenced by prejudices based on their culture, education, and experience. Too often, nurses allow misconceptions about pain (see box below) to affect their willingness to intervene. Some nurses may even avoid acknowledging a patient's/client's pain because of their own fear and denial.

### Common Biases and Misconceptions about Pain

- Drug abusers and alcoholics overreact to discomfort.
- Patients/clients with minor illnesses have less pain than those with severe physical illness.
- Administering analgesics regularly will lead to drug dependence.
- The amount of tissue damage in an injury can accurately indicate pain intensity.
- Health care personnel are the best authorities on the nature of the patient's/client's pain.
- Psychogenic pain is not real.

To help a patient/client gain comfort or relief, the nurse must view the experience through that person's eyes. Acknowledging personal prejudices or misconceptions also helps the nurse address the patient's/client's problem more professionally. Often a nurse who has personally experienced pain is more able to provide support (Holm, 1989). The nurse who becomes an active, knowledgeable observer of a patient/client in pain will make a more objective analysis of the total pain experience. The patient/client alerts the nurse that pain is present, and the nurse works to apply knowledge and skills that ultimately provide effective pain relief.

## PHYSIOLOGY OF PAIN

Pain is a complex mixture of physical, emotional, and behavioural reactions. To best understand the pain experience, it helps to describe its three physiological components: **reception**, **perception**, and **reaction**. A patient/client in pain cannot discriminate among the components. However, understanding each component helps the nurse recognize factors that can cause pain, symptoms that accompany pain, and the rationale and actions of selected interventions.

### Reception

Nerve receptors in the skin and tissues respond to stimuli resulting from actual or potential tissue damage. **Noxious** (pain) stimuli may be thermal, mechanical, chemical, or electrical. **Thermal** stimuli result from skin contact with hot or cold substances. Pressure, friction, tension, and stretching are **mechanical** stimuli. **Chemical stimuli** originate from substances within the body, such as gastric enzymes, or from substances outside the body, such as caustic chemicals. An electrical current causes an **electrical stimulus.** Table 27-1 summarizes the physical alterations that elicit pain-producing stimuli.

Not all tissues contain receptors that transmit pain signals. The brain and alveoli of the lung are examples of tissues insensitive to pain. Some receptors respond to only one type of pain stimulus, whereas others are also sensitive to temperature and pressure. The **pain threshold** is reached when a stimulus is sufficiently intense to create a nerve impulse. Normally the physiological pain threshold does not differ among individuals, even those of different racial or cultural backgrounds (Melzack and Wall, 1988).

Nerve impulses resulting from the pain stimulus travel along afferent peripheral nerve fibres. Two types of peripheral nerve fibres conduct painful stimuli: the fast, myelinated A-delta fibres and the very small, slow, unmyelinated C-fibres. The A-delta fibres send pricking sensations that localize the source of pain and detect pain intensity. C-fibres relay impulses of a deeper and more diffuse nature. For example, after stepping on a nail, a person initially feels a sharp, localized pain, which is the result of A-delta fibre transmission. Within a few seconds pain becomes more diffuse and widespread until the whole foot aches because of C-fibre innervation (Fig. 27-1).

A-delta and C-fibres transmit impulses from peripheral

projections to the end of the fibre in the dorsal horn of the spinal cord. Within the dorsal horn, **neurotransmitters** such as substance P are released, causing a synaptic transmission from the afferent (sensory) peripheral nerve to spinothalamic tract nerves (Paice, 1991). This allows the pain impulse to be transmitted further within the central nervous system (Fig. 27-2). Pain stimuli travel through nerve fibres in the spinothalamic tracts that cross to the opposite side of the spinal cord. Pain impulses then travel up the spinal cord. Fig. 27-3 shows the normal pain reception pathway. After the pain impulse ascends the spinal cord, information is transmitted quickly to higher centres in the brain, including the reticular formation, limbic system, thalamus, and sensory cortex.

A **protective reflex response** also occurs with pain reception (Fig. 27-4). A-delta fibres send sensory impulses to the spinal cord, where they synapse with spinal motor neurones. The motor impulses travel via a reflex arc along efferent (motor) nerve fibres back to a peripheral muscle near the site of stimulation. Contraction of the muscle leads to a protective withdrawal from the source of pain. For example, when a person accidentally touches a hot iron, a burning sensation is felt, but the hand also reflexively withdraws from the iron's surface. When superficial fibres in the skin are stimulated, a person moves away from the pain source. If internal tissues such as muscle or mucous membranes become stimulated, tightening and guarding of muscles occur.

Pain reception requires an intact peripheral nervous system and spinal cord. Common factors that disrupt pain reception include trauma, drugs, tumour growth, and metabolic disorders.

## Neuroregulators

**Neuroregulators**, or substances that affect the transmission of nerve stimuli, are divided into two groups: neurotransmitters and neuromodulators (see box overleaf). **Neurotransmitters** such as substance P send electrical impulses across the synaptic cleft between two nerve fibres. They are excitatory or inhibitory. **Neuromodulators** modify neurone activity without directly transferring a nerve signal through a synapse. They are believed to act indirectly by increasing and decreasing the effects of particular neurotransmitters (Melzack and Wall, 1988). Endorphins are an example of a neuromodulator.

## Gate Control Theory of Pain

There have been several attempts to explain the complexity of pain in terms of the relationship of physiological, psychological, and cognitive variables. The **gate control theory**, proposed by Melzack and Wall (1965), is the most comprehensive. The theory suggests that pain impulses can be regulated or even blocked by gating mechanisms along the central nervous system. The proposed location of the gates is in the dorsal horn of the spinal cord. Further findings have suggested that other gates exist (Melzack and Dennis, 1978). When gates are open, pain impulses flow freely, when gates are closed, pain impulses become blocked. Partial opening of the gates may also occur.

Excitation of A-delta and C-fibres inhibits gating mechanisms so that pain stimuli flow easily to cortical centres of the brain. Larger A-beta fibres pass through the same gating mechanisms (see Fig. 27-1). Whether the gates remain open or closed depends on whether competing passages from larger A-beta nerve fibres stimulate the gating mechanism. A bombardment of A-beta fibre sensory impulses, such as those from the pressure of a backrub or the heat of a warm compress, closes the gates to pain stimuli. Transmission of pain impulses from the spinal cord to the cerebral cortex can be inhibited or facilitated, thus altering pain perception.

It is also believed that the reticular formation in the brainstem can send inhibitory signals to gating mechanisms. When there is excess sensory input (for example, with pain), the reticular

## TABLE 27-1 Examples of Physical Sources of Pain

| Type of Stimulus | Source | Pathophysiological Process |
|---|---|---|
| Mechanical | Alteration in body fluids<br>Duct distension | Oedema distending body tissues<br>Overstretching of duct's narrow lumen (e.g. passage of kidney stone through ureter) |
| | Space-occupying lesion (tumour) | Irritation of peripheral nerves by growth of lesion within confined space |
| Chemical | Perforated visceral organ | Chemical irritation by secretions on sensitive nerve endings (e.g. ruptured appendix, duodenal ulcer) |
| Thermal | Burn (heat or extreme cold) | Inflammation or loss of superficial layers of epidermis, causing increased sensitivity of nerve endings |
| Electrical | Burn | Skin layers burned with muscle and subcutaneous tissue injury, causing injury to nerve endings |

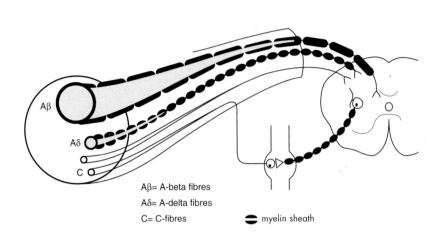

**Fig. 27-1** Components of a cutaneous nerve.

Aβ= A-beta fibres
Aδ= A-delta fibres
C= C-fibres   ⬤ myelin sheath

**Fig. 27-2** Substance P and other neurotransmitters are released from primary afferent fibres that terminate in the dorsal horn of the spinal cord.
From Paice JA: *Oncol Nurs Forum* 18(5):843, 1991.

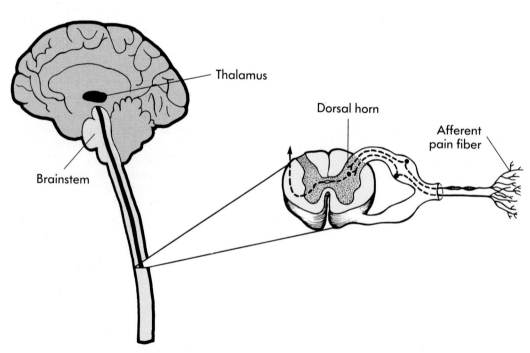

**Fig. 27-3** Pain reception pathway. Pain is transmitted from primary afferent fibres to the dorsal horn of the spinal cord. The fibres synapse with spinothalamic tract neurons, which cross over and then ascend the spinal cord to the thalamus.

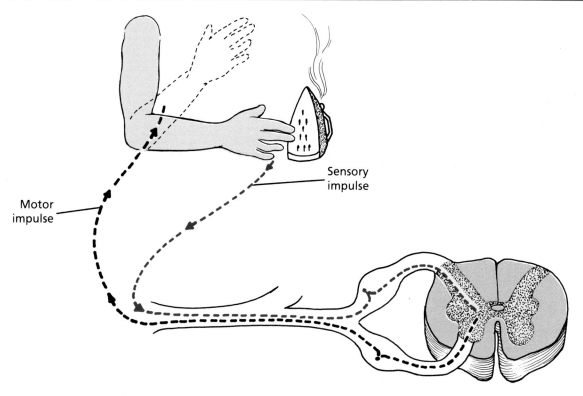

**Fig. 27-4** Protective reflex to pain stimulus.

Motor impulse

Sensory impulse

## Neurophysiology of Pain: Neuroregulators

### NEUROTRANSMITTERS
Substance P
- Is found in the pain neurones of the dorsal horn (excitatory peptide)
- Is needed to transmit pain impulses from the periphery to higher brain centres
- Causes vasodilatation and oedema

Serotonin
- Is released from the brainstem and dorsal horn to inhibit pain transmission

Prostaglandins
- Are generated from the breakdown of phospholipids in cell membranes
- Are believed to increase sensitivity to pain

### NEUROMODULATORS
Endorphins
- Are the body's natural supply of morphine-like substances
- Are activated by stress and pain
- Are located within the brain, spinal cord, and gastrointestinal tract
- Cause analgesia when they attach to opioid receptors in the brain
- May be present in higher levels in people who have less pain than others, with a similar injury

Bradykinin
- Is released from plasma that leaks from surrounding blood vessels at the site of tissue injury
- Binds to receptors on peripheral nerves, increasing pain stimuli
- Binds to cells that cause the chain reaction producing prostaglandins

formation can close gates. Some patients/clients can be distracted from pain by removing the sensation of pain from their centre of attention. Auditory or visual stimuli can distract patients/clients and help make pain more tolerable.

The gate-control theory provides a conceptual basis for pain-relief measures. However, some studies have failed to support the theory.

## Perception
**Perception** is the point at which a person experiences pain. Pain stimuli are transmitted up the spinal cord to the thalamus and midbrain. From the thalamus, fibres transmit the pain message to various areas of the brain, including the sensory cortex and association cortex (both in the parietal lobe), the frontal lobe, and the limbic system (Fields, 1987). After nerve transmission ends within the higher brain centres, a person actually perceives the sensation of pain.

There is an interaction of psychological and cognitive factors with neurophysiological ones in the perception of pain. Meinhart and McCaffery (1983) describe three interactional systems of pain perception as sensory-discriminative, motivational-affective, and cognitive-evaluative (see box).

The gate control theory suggests that gating mechanisms can also be altered by thoughts, feelings, and memories. The cerebral cortex and thalamus can influence whether pain impulses reach a person's consciousness. The realization that, in a sense, there is conscious control over pain perception helps explain the different ways people react and adjust to pain.

## Reaction

The **reaction** to pain comprises the physiological and behavioural responses that occur after pain is perceived.

## Physiological Responses

As pain impulses ascend the spinal cord towards the brainstem and thalamus, the autonomic nervous system becomes stimulated as part of the stress response. Acute pain, of low to moderate intensity, and superficial pain elicit the 'flight-or-fight' reaction of the general adaptation syndrome (see Chapter 10). Stimulation of the sympathetic branch of the autonomic nervous system results in physiological responses (Table 27-2). If the pain is unrelenting, severe, or deep, typically originating from involvement of the visceral organs (such as with a myocardial infarction and colic from gallbladder or renal stones), the parasympathetic nervous system goes into action. Sustained physiological responses to pain could cause serious harm to an individual. Except in cases of severe acute pain, which may send a person into shock, most people reach a level of adaptation in which physical signs return to normal. Thus, a patient/client in pain will not always exhibit physical signs.

## Behavioural Responses

Meinhart and McCaffery (1983) describe three phases of a pain experience: anticipation, sensation, and aftermath. The anticipation phase occurs before pain is perceived. A person knows that pain will occur. The **anticipation** phase is perhaps most important, because it can affect the other two. In situations

### Learning Disabilities Nursing Assessment of pain

If a person has a relatively mild learning disability then recognizing and treating pain is no different from treatment for any other individual. However, the patient/client is likely to have difficulty describing the nature, intensity and location of the pain, due to his or her limited vocabulary and comprehension (particularly with descriptive nouns and metaphors).

A person with a profound handicap presents other problems that need to be addressed:

- recognizing they are in pain — to determine this, the nurse must have a comprehensive knowledge of the individual and how he or she behaves in order to detect and assess variations from their normal behaviour. For example, is the patient/client more physically agitated than usual? Unusually still and tense? Unusual posture or repetitive activity can also provide clues to discomfort; for example, head banging can indicate a headache, and face-slapping can indicate an earache or toothache.
- understanding how pain affects the autonomic nervous system — this will enable the nurse to evaluate alteration in heart rate, respiration rate, and skin colour, and use such information to assess the pain.
- evaluating changes in behaviour (both subjective and objective) — this will help the nurse manage the patient's/client's pain.

When working with profoundly handicapped patients/clients, particularly those with gross physical disabilities such as limb contractures and muscle spasm, pain management may be best achieved by using many different strategies. Massage, gentle heat, changes of position, and passive movements have all been shown to be of value. Providing a calm, relaxing environment, with gentle music, subdued lighting and soft furnishings can also help induce a calm and relaxed state, which helps reduce the experience of pain in these individuals.

### Interactional Systems of Pain Perception

#### SENSORY-DISCRIMINATIVE
- Nerve transmission occurs between the thalamus and sensory cortex.
- A person perceives the location, severity, and character of pain.
- Factors that lower consciousness (e.g. analgesics, anaesthetics, cerebral disease) decrease pain perception.
- Factors that increase the awareness of stimuli (e.g. anxiety, sleep deprivation) increase pain perception.

#### MOTIVATIONAL-AFFECTIVE
- Interaction between the reticular formation and limbic system results in pain perception.
- The reticular formation creates a defensive response, causing a person to interrupt or avoid pain stimuli.
- The limbic system controls emotional response and the ability to cope with pain.

#### COGNITIVE-EVALUATIVE
- Higher cortical centres in the brain influence perception.
- Culture, experience of pain, and emotions influence evaluation of the pain experience.
- This system helps a person to interpret the intensity and quality of pain so that action can be taken.

of traumatic injury or unforeseen painful procedures a person will not anticipate pain.

Anticipation of pain often allows a person to learn about pain and its relief. With adequate teaching and support, patients/clients learn to understand pain and control anxiety before it occurs. Nurses play an important role in helping patients/clients during the anticipatory phase. With proper guidance, patients/clients become aware of the unknown and thus cope with their discomfort. In situations in which a person is too fearful or anxious, anticipation of pain can heighten the perception of pain severity (Walding, 1991).

**Sensation** of pain occurs when pain is felt. The ways that people choose to react to discomfort vary widely. A person's **tolerance** of pain is the point at which there is an unwillingness to accept pain of greater severity or duration. The extent to which a person tolerates pain depends on attitudes, motivation, and values.

Pain threatens physical and psychological well-being. Patients/clients may choose not to express pain, considering it a

## TABLE 27-2 Physiological Reactions to Acute Pain

| Response | Cause or Effect |
|---|---|
| SYMPATHETIC STIMULATION* | |
| Dilation of bronchial tubes and increased respiratory rate | Provides greater oxygen intake |
| Increased heart rate | Provides greater oxygen transport |
| Peripheral vasoconstriction (pallor, elevation in blood pressure) | Elevates blood pressure with shift of blood supply from periphery and viscera to skeletal muscles and brain |
| Increased blood glucose level | Provides additional energy |
| Diaphoresis | Controls body temperature during stress |
| Increased muscle tension | Prepares muscles for action |
| Dilation of pupils | Affords better vision |
| Decreased gastrointestinal motility | Frees energy for more immediate activity |
| PARASYMPATHETIC STIMULATION† | |
| Pallor | Causes blood supply to shift away from periphery |
| Muscle tension | Results from fatigue |
| Decreased heart rate and blood pressure | Results from vagal stimulation |
| Rapid, irregular breathing | Causes body defences to fail under prolonged stress of pain |
| Nausea and vomiting | Causes return of gastrointestinal function |
| Weakness or exhaustion | Results from expenditure of physical energy |

\* Pain of low to moderate intensity and superficial pain
† Severe or deep pain

sign of weakness. Often patients/clients believe that being a 'good patient' means not expressing pain to avoid bothering people around them. In addition, patients/clients may not express pain because maintaining self-control is important in their culture. The patient/client with high pain tolerance may endure periods of severe pain without assistance. Often a nurse must encourage such an individual to accept pain-relieving measures so that mobility or sleep are not adversely affected.

In contrast, a patient/client with low pain tolerance may seek relief in anticipation of pain. The patient's/client's ability to tolerate pain significantly influences the nurse's perceptions of the degree of the discomfort. The nurse may be more willing to attend to the patient/client whose pain tolerance is higher. Yet it is unfair to ignore the needs of a person who has difficulty in coping with pain.

Typical body movements and facial expressions that indicate pain include holding the painful part, bent posture, and grimaces. A patient/client may cry or moan. Often a patient/client expresses discomfort through restlessness and frequent requests to the nurse. The nurse soon learns to recognize patterns of behaviour that reflect pain. However, lack of pain expression does not necessarily mean that the patient/client is not experiencing pain. Unless a patient/client openly reacts to pain, it is difficult to determine the nature and extent of the discomfort. The nurse can help patients/clients communicate their pain response effectively. Knowledge of the disease or illness may help the nurse to anticipate the patient's/client's pain. For example, a ruptured

intravertebral disk in a lower lumbar vertebra typically causes severe low-back pain and pain that radiates or extends down the leg. Table 27-3 summarizes common disorders that cause pain.

The **aftermath** phase of pain occurs when pain is reduced or stopped. Even though the source of discomfort is controlled, a patient/client may still require the nurse's attention. Pain is a crisis, and after a painful experience, patients/clients may experience physical symptoms such as chills, nausea, vomiting, anger, or depression. If there are repeated episodes of pain, aftermath responses can become serious health problems. The nurse can help patients/clients gain control and self-esteem to minimize fear over potential pain experiences.

### Matching Physiological Conditions with Pain Relief Interventions

It helps for the nurse to understand the effect of interventions on the human body. In the case of pain relief, several treatment

**Mental Health Nursing
Masochistic behaviours**

In mental health care a nurse may encounter referrals for counselling for individuals with particular variations in sexual expression. Sexual sado-masochism, for example, involves deriving intense sexual arousal through acts and fantasies where physical pain and humiliation have a major focus.

## TABLE 27-3 Common Disorders That Cause Pain

| Disorder | Pain Characteristics |
| --- | --- |
| Kidney disease | Abdominal aching |
| Angina pectoris | Tenderness and pain in back area of costovertebral angle <br> Crushing sensation in chest, often radiating down left shoulder and arm |
| Ruptured intravertebral disk | Low-back pain accompanied by pain radiating down leg |
| Gastric ulcer | Burning pain around umbilicus, referred pain in shoulder |
| Trigeminal neuralgia | Lightening-like or stabbing pain along distribution of trigeminal nerve, involving gums, lips, mouth, nose, and chin |

options are available. Use of a combination of interventions may bring relief of pain, especially if several different physiological actions are used:

- Nonsteroidal anti-inflammatory drugs (NSAIDs) act by inhibiting the action of the enzyme that forms prostaglandins (Paice, 1991). With less prostaglandin released peripherally, the generation of pain stimuli is blocked. A reduction in pain sensitivity also occurs.
- Neurotransmitters and opioid receptors are located in the dorsal horn of the spinal cord. Administration of opioids such as morphine results in the opioids binding to receptors and inhibiting the release of substance P. As a result, transmission of painful stimuli to the spinal cord is blocked. Opioids may be given orally, intramuscularly, subcutaneously, intravenously or epidurally.
- The administration of tricyclic antidepressants such as amitriptyline creates an analgesic effect, as well as an antidepressant effect. The tricyclics inhibit the normal re-uptake of serotonin at nerve terminals (Paice, 1991). With more serotonin present in nerve terminals, pain transmission is inhibited.
- Spinothalamic nerve tracts are localized in a region of the spinal cord. As a result of the nerve tract location, surgeons can ablate, or remove, the nerves and reduce pain isolated to one side of the body. The procedure is called a *cordotomy* and is generally used only in patients/clients with a limited life expectancy.
- Nonpharmacological methods of pain management (see Implementation section).

## ACUTE AND CHRONIC PAIN

Everyone experiences some level of pain throughout the day. Common examples include the ache of over-exercised muscles, the burning discomfort from eye strain, and pressure from sitting in one position for too long. These minor discomforts rarely cause a person to seek health care.

The pain that nurses most often observe in patients/clients includes three types: acute, chronic malignant, and chronic nonmalignant (Engber, 1986). **Acute pain** follows acute injury,

disease, or types of surgery and has a rapid onset, varying in intensity (mild to severe) and lasting for a brief time (Meinhart and McCaffery, 1983). The function of acute pain is to warn individuals of impending injury or disease. Acute pain eventually resolves with or without treatment after a damaged area heals.

Patients/clients in acute pain are frightened and anxious, and expect relief quickly. The time sequence of acute pain usually results in a willingness by health care team members to treat acute pain rapidly. However, conflict between the nurse and patient/client may arise if the nurse does not provide quick relief. Acute pain is self-limiting and the patient/client can anticipate that pain will cease in a relatively short period of time. However, this does not necessarily make the pain easier to cope with while it is experienced.

Acute pain seriously threatens a patient's/client's recovery and should be one of the nurse's priorities of care. For example, acute postoperative pain hampers the patient's/client's ability to become mobile and increases the risk of complications from immobility (see Chapter 24). Rehabilitation may be delayed and hospitalization may be prolonged if acute pain is not controlled. There cannot be physical or psychological progress as long as it persists because the patient/client focuses all interests on pain relief. The nurse's efforts at teaching and motivating the patient/client towards self-care will also prove less effective. After pain is relieved, the mobile patient/client and health care team can direct full attention towards recovery.

**Chronic pain** is prolonged, varies in intensity, and usually lasts more than 6 months (Anderson *et al*, 1987). Chronic pain caused by uncontrolled cancer or other progressive disorders is called **intractable pain**. In some cases it can be prolonged until death, but techniques of pain control are being developed.

Chronic pain can arise in people whose tissue injury is nonprogressive or healed but whose pain is ongoing and often does not respond to treatment. Frequently the cause for this pain is unknown. An injured area may have healed long ago, yet pain persists. In chronic pain, endorphins often cease to function (Meinhart and McCaffery, 1983). An example of this type of chronic pain is low-back pain.

Health care workers are usually willing to treat chronic malignant pain as energetically as acute pain. In contrast, treatment for nonmalignant pain may not be as rigorous. If the

## USEFUL ADDRESSES

PANG (Pain and Nociception Group)
c/o Ms D Wood
Department of Anaesthesia
Charing Cross Hospital
London W6 8RF

IASP (International Association for the Study of Pain)
c/o Louisa E Jones
Executive Officer
909 NE 43rd Street, Suite 306
Seattle, WA 98105
USA.

RCN Pain Forum
Royal College of Nursing
20 Cavendish Square
London W1M 0AB

The Pain Society
(The British and Irish Chapter of the International
    Association for the Study of Pain)
9 Bedford Square
London WC1B 3RA

National Back Pain Association
31–33 Park Road
Teddington
Middlesex TW11 0AB

cause of pain is unclear, care givers may question the severity of a patient's/client's discomfort. For patients/clients with cancer, family members may be unwilling to administer strong opioids for fear of causing side effects such as lethargy and drug dependence.

The patient/client with chronic pain often has periods of **remission** (partial or complete disappearance of symptoms) and **exacerbations** (increase in severity). The unpredictability of chronic pain frustrates the patient/client, frequently leading to psychological depression. The pain becomes part of every aspect of life. Chronic pain is a major cause of psychological and physical disability, leading to problems such as loss of job, inability to perform simple daily activities, sexual dysfunction, and social isolation from family and friends.

The person with chronic pain often does not show overt physiological symptoms. The individual does not adapt to the pain but seems to suffer more with time as physical and mental exhaustion occur. Chronic pain creates an insecurity of never knowing how one will feel from day to day. Symptoms of chronic pain include fatigue, insomnia, anorexia, weight loss, depression, hopelessness, and anger.

The quality of life of a person with chronic pain can be severely diminished. Typically, the person consults many doctors and therefore accumulates various medications and therapies. However, taking several medications may result in undesirable side effects. Patients/clients desperate for pain relief may also fall prey to quackery (for example, unproven liniments, diets, or pain-relief devices). Fortunately, pain clinics are available throughout the United Kingdom to help individuals find more acceptable methods of pain control. Doctors and other health care professionals at the clinics understand pain better and offer measures other than pharmacological interventions such as complementary therapies (acupuncture, relaxation techniques, massage) and psychological support.

Caring for the patient/client with chronic pain is a challenge. The nurse should not become frustrated when relief measures fail to fully control pain. Similarly, the nurse should not offer false hope for a cure. The nurse's primary goal may be to reduce the person's perception of pain, and to promote patient/client and family adaptation through identification and enhancement of coping strategies.

## FACTORS INFLUENCING PAIN

Since pain is complex, numerous factors influence an individual's pain experience (Fig. 27-5). The nurse must consider all factors that affect the patient/client in pain, as this is necessary to obtain an accurate assessment of the person's pain and to select appropriate pain relief interventions.

### Age

Age is an important variable that influences pain, particularly in children and older adults. Developmental differences among these age groups can influence how children and older adults react to the pain experience. Young children have difficulty understanding pain and the procedures administered by nurses that may cause pain. Young children who have not developed full vocabularies also have difficulty in describing and expressing pain to parents or care givers. Cognitively, toddlers or pre-schoolers are unable to recall explanations about pain or associate pain as experiences that can occur in various situations.

The ability of older people to interpret pain can be complicated by the presence of multiple diseases with vague symptoms that may affect similar parts of the body. When older adults have more than one source of pain, a nurse should gather detailed assessments. The manifestations of different diseases can cause an atypical presentation of painful conditions. In other words, different diseases can cause similar symptoms; for example, chest pain does not always indicate a myocardial infarction or heart attack. Instead, chest pain can be a symptom of arthritis of the spine, herpes zoster infection or an abdominal disorder (Zoob, 1978).

Herr and Mobily (1991) note that older adults may not report pain because:

- They may believe that pain is something they must live with. Care givers and older patients/clients may believe that pain is a natural result of ageing and so complaints are often ignored.
- They may deny pain because of fear of unknown consequences. Older adults may have considerable fear of the loss of independence.
- They may choose not to admit having pain for fear of serious illness or death.
- They may believe that it is not acceptable to show pain. Older individuals may use a variety of mechanisms to distract attention from pain (McCaffery and Beebe, 1994a).

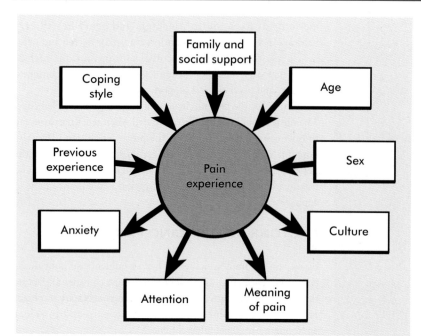

**Fig. 27-5** Factors that influence the pain experience.
*From Gil K: Anesthesiol Report 2(2):246, 1990.*

**Children's Nursing**
**Helping children understand pain**

It has been suggested that children possess a pain vocabulary and a nurse must use simple but appropriate communication techniques to help children understand and describe pain. For example, asking children, "Tell me where you hurt" or "What helps take away the hurt?" can help accurately assess pain. The nurse may also show a series of pictures depicting different facial expressions, such as smiling, frowning, or crying. Children may point to the picture that best describes how they feel (Wong and Baker, 1988).

**Adult Nursing**
**The experience of pain in older adults**

During the ageing process, changes occur in both the sensory and peripheral nervous systems. In older adults, these changes may manifest as a slower reaction time to pain, or a generally reduced ability to respond to any stress (Schultz, 1982).

In older adults pain impulses may be less clearly defined, so their experience of pain may be very different from that of younger people. For example, when older people experience myocardial infarction (heart attack), they may not experience the acute pain that younger people characteristically feel. For this reason, myocardial infarction in older people is often described as 'silent'.

The emotional component of the pain response is important at any age. Schultz suggests that older people's responses consist of different emotions occurring simultaneously, due to their accumulation of life experiences. Research demonstrates that chronic pain in older people is associated with low self-esteem and depression.

It is important, therefore, for nurses to consider the older person's psychological and emotional needs, as well as the relief of their physical pain.

## Gender

Generally, men and women do not differ significantly in their responses to pain (Gil, 1990). It is doubtful whether gender by itself is a factor in the expression of pain. There are cultural influences on gender (for example, making it appropriate for a little boy to be brave and not cry, whereas a little girl in the same situation is allowed to cry). Pain tolerance has been the subject of research involving men and women. Burns *et al* (1989) studied postoperative opioid requirements in patients undergoing abdominal surgery. Male patients required significantly more morphine than female patients to achieve similar levels of pain relief.

## Culture

Culture influences how people learn to react to and express pain (Zborowski, 1969). People respond to pain in different ways, and the nurse must never assume to know how patients/clients will respond. However, an understanding of cultural background,

socioeconomic status, and personal attributes helps the nurse more accurately assess pain and its meaning for patients/clients (Lipton and Marbach, 1984).

Several studies have demonstrated that more educated and affluent patients/clients respond more quickly to symptoms and seek medical care for conditions that people in lower social classes ignore (Townsend *et al*, 1992). Expression of pain by children in different cultures also varies; for example, Eskimo children learn to laugh in response to pain, and Chinese children learn to respond favourably to surgery, whereas American children view hospitalization as traumatic (Ross and Ross, 1988). Nurses must learn that there are ways to respond to pain other than their own. Assessment of cultural influences on the way patients/clients respond to or react to pain assists in determining the significance of pain to patients/clients and measures that will be effective in providing relief.

## Meaning of Pain

The meaning that a person attributes to pain affects the experience of pain. A person will perceive and cope with pain differently if it suggests a threat, loss, punishment, or challenge; for example, the degree and quality of pain experienced by a woman in labour will be perceived quite differently from a woman experiencing pain from a recent back injury.

### Controlling Pain

People from different cultures may express pain differently. The traditional British 'stiff-upper-lip' discourages the expression of feelings. In other cultures, the expression feelings is more encouraged.

Certain religious groups, for example Muslims, may believe that it is God's will for them to experience pain. They may also be unwilling to take drugs, although those for medical treatment are usually accepted. They may try to avoid taking analgesics and may benefit from a visit from a religious leader or a member of the local religious group (for example from the local Islamic centre).

Patients who are fasting may be unwilling to take anything into the body by mouth, injection or suppository. This can make pain control difficult to achieve and alternative methods, for example massage, can be tried if these are acceptable. If patients do refuse medication on religious grounds, they may gain considerable spiritual comfort from this, despite their physical pain.

Some people may be unwilling to accept medication in case it clouds or impairs their senses. Buddhists, for example, may prefer to use meditation techniques to help to relieve their pain.

## Attention

The degree to which a patient/client focuses on pain can influence pain perception. Increased attention has been associated with increased pain, whereas distraction has been associated with a diminished pain response (Gil, 1990). This concept is one that nurses can apply in various pain-relief interventions such as relaxation, guided imagery, and massage. By focusing a patient's/client's attention and concentration on other stimuli, the nurse places pain on the periphery of awareness. Usually, this results in an increased tolerance for pain that lasts only during the time of distraction (McCaffery and Beebe, 1994b).

## Anxiety

The relationship between pain and anxiety is complex. Anxiety often increases the perception of pain, but pain may also cause feelings of anxiety. Autonomic arousal patterns are similar in pain and anxiety (Gil, 1990), and it is therefore difficult to separate

aspects of the two concepts. Emotionally healthy people are usually able to tolerate moderate or even severe pain better than those whose emotions are less stable. Research suggests that anxiety may be a major influence on how pain is perceived by people with cancer (Spiegel and Bloom, 1983; Twycross and Lack, 1983). Endorphins may cause differences in sensitivity to pain, and in some people, anxiety over pain may release endorphins.

## Fatigue

Fatigue heightens perception of pain. This intensifies pain and decreases coping abilities. Pain is often experienced less after a restful sleep than at the end of a long day.

## Previous Experience

Each person learns from painful experiences. Previous experience does not necessarily mean that a person will accept pain more easily in the future. If a person has had frequent episodes of pain without relief or bouts of severe pain, anxiety or even fear may recur. In contrast, if a person has had repeated experiences with the same type of pain but the pain has successfully been relieved, it becomes easier to interpret the pain sensation. As a result, the patient/client is better prepared to take necessary actions in relieving the pain.

When a person has had no experience of pain, the first perception of it can impair the ability to cope with it; for example, after abdominal surgery, it is common for a patient to experience severe incisional pain for several days. Unless the patient is aware of this, the onset of pain may be viewed as a serious complication. Rather than participate actively in postoperative breathing exercises (see Chapter 29), the patient may lie immobile in bed and maintain shallow breathing because of the fear that something has gone wrong. The nurse should prepare the patient with a clear explanation of the type of pain that will be experienced and methods to reduce it (Hayward, 1975).

## Coping Style

The experience of pain can be lonely. When individuals experience pain in health care settings such as hospitals, the loneliness can be unbearable. Frequently, patients feel a loss of control and an inability to control their environment or the outcome of events. Coping style thus influences the ability to deal with pain.

People with **internal loci of control** perceive themselves as having personal control over their environment and the outcome of events, such as pain (Gil, 1990). In contrast, people with **external loci of control** perceive other factors in their environment, such as nurses, as being responsible for the outcome of events. Individuals with internal loci of control report less severe pain than those with external loci (Schultheis et al, 1987). This concept is applied in the use of **patient-controlled analgesia** (PCA). Patients/clients who are able to self-administer small doses of intravenous pain medication during an acute episode successfully achieve pain control more quickly than those who rely on nurses to administer intermittent doses of analgesics.

Research by Copp (1985) suggests that although people cope

with the psychological and physical effects of acute pain in a variety of ways, there are a number of common strategies which could be beneficial to both nurses and patients/clients. These coping strategies have been broadly classified into those which involve internal mental processes, and those where patients/clients use external stimuli/objects to reduce pain perception. They can include rubbing an area adjacent to the pain, rocking movements, the presence of other people, focusing on environmental objects/stimuli, visualization, dreams, and separation of the mind from the physical sensation of pain. It is important to understand a patient's/client's coping strategies during a painful experience. These strategies, such as communicating with a supportive family, exercise, or singing, can be used in the nurse's care plan to support the person and offer a degree of pain relief.

Coping strategies are more than just methods or techniques. A patient/client may depend on the emotional support of a spouse, children, other family members, or friends. Although pain still exists, the presence of a loved one can minimize loneliness and fear. A patient's/client's religious beliefs can also provide comfort. Reading scriptures or saying a prayer gives many individuals an inner strength to cope more effectively with discomfort. Being actively involved in housework or other tasks can be another mechanism for coping.

### Family and Social Support

Another factor that can significantly affect the pain response is the presence and attitudes of significant others. People of different sociocultural groups have different expectations of people to whom they complain about pain (Meinhart and McCaffery, 1983). People in pain often depend on family members for support, assistance, or protection. An absence of family or friends can often make the pain experience more stressful. The presence of parents is especially important for children experiencing pain.

## NURSING PROCESS AND PAIN

In order to understand a patient's/client's pain and provide appropriate interventions, there is a need for a systematic approach to pain management. The nursing process is a structured approach which can ensure accurate assessment and management of pain.

### Possible Sources of Error in Pain Assessment

- Bias, which causes nurses to consistently overestimate or underestimate the pain that patients/clients experience
- Vague or unclear assessment questions, which lead to unreliable assessment data
- Use of pain assessment tools that have not been proven reliable and valid with identical patients/clients (a reliable assessment tool focuses only on pain cues that provide a reliable measure of relevant clinical changes)
- Patients/clients who may not be able to provide complete, pertinent, and accurate pain details

 ## ASSESSMENT

Accurate pain assessment is critical for evaluating a patient's/client's progress, arriving at proper nursing goals, and selecting appropriate interventions. Although pain assessment is one of the most common activities a nurse performs, it is one of the most complex. The key to assessing pain is in maximum involvement of the patient/client. The nurse must explore the pain experience through the eyes of the patient/client. Nurses should not allow personal biases to prejudice assessment of pain (Taylor *et al*, 1984). Viewing the pain from the patient's/client's perspective enables the nurse to make a more accurate assessment. It is important also to carefully interpret pain expression and remember that psychological and physical components of pain, among others, influence the reaction to it.

When assessing pain, the nurse must be sensitive to the patient's/client's level of discomfort. If pain is acute or severe, it is unlikely that the patient/client can provide a detailed description of the entire experience. During an episode of acute pain the nurse primarily assesses how the person feels, determining physiological responses to pain and the location, severity, and quality of the pain. A more thorough pain assessment takes time and should be conducted when the person is more comfortable.

For patients/clients with chronic pain, assessment may best be focused on affective and evaluative aspects of the pain experience and on its history and context (Reuler *et al*, 1980). In the case of chronic nonmalignant pain, assessment should include the level of function because it may not be possible to achieve complete pain relief. Numerous factors can cause errors in assessment (see box). The nurse should be aware of these factors and adapt assessment strategies to minimize error (Harrison, 1991). Some factors deal with the nature of the pain experience, and others deal with the types of assessment cues available for nurses and doctors.

### Patient's/Client's Expression of Pain

Some patients/clients may be reluctant to discuss pain, remaining silent and trying to appear calm (Cartwright, 1964). A complication in pain assessment is that many nurses believe that patients/clients will report pain if they have it. This is not always true.

Patients/clients must trust a nurse and perceive the nurse's willingness to help if they are to discuss their pain experience openly. If patients/clients sense that the nurse doubts that pain exists, they will share little information. The nurse must develop supportive relationships and give patients/clients time to discuss pain. Attempting to find comfortable positions for patients/clients before asking questions may help patients/clients sense the nurse's interest. The nurse should avoid aggravating pain with a lengthy assessment.

The nurse should ascertain the patient's/client's method of communicating discomfort; for example whether the person can communicate verbally or whether nonverbal behaviours will be the best source of information. If the patient/client speaks a different language, pain assessment can be difficult. A family member or interpreter may be necessary to describe the patient's/client's feelings and sensations.

## Classification of the Pain Experience

It is helpful to know the phase of pain patients/clients are experiencing. The phase – anticipatory, sensation, or aftermath – influences not only patients'/clients' symptoms but also the types of interventions most likely to relieve pain. Individuals likely to be in the anticipatory phase include those scheduled to undergo invasive diagnostic or therapeutic procedures or surgery and those with histories of recurring pain such as the pain of myocardial ischaemia. These patients/clients may be anxious or fearful, or they may ask questions about anticipated pain.

Individuals in the sensation phase generally demonstrate signs and symptoms of discomfort. Individuals with traumatic injuries and those who have had surgery are uncomfortable, so the nurse should not ask detailed questions. Patients/clients who are experiencing pain, especially severe pain, need rapid relief. After the pain has been relieved, the nurse must assess carefully for physical and psychological effects. Patients/clients may later express apologies to the nurse for acting 'improperly' during the pain experience.

## Characteristics of Pain

The nature of the pain experience provides more detailed information for the nurse. Assessment data help establish medical and nursing goals and determine pain relief interventions.

## ONSET AND DURATION

The nurse asks questions to determine the onset, duration, and time sequence of pain. Ask when the pain began, how long it lasted, whether it occurs at the same time each day, and how frequently it recurs.

It may be easier to diagnose the nature of pain by identifying time factors. For example, certain types of headaches can be characterized by the time of day when they occur. The onset of sudden and severe pain is easier to assess than gradual, mild discomfort. An understanding of the time cycle of pain helps you to know when to intervene before the pain occurs or worsens (Table 27-4).

## LOCATION

To assess pain location ask the person to point to all areas of discomfort. To localize the pain more specifically, ask the patient/client to trace the area from the most severe point outward. This is difficult to do if pain is diffuse, involves several sites, or involves large segments of the body. Some assessment tools have figures of the body (Fig. 27-6) on which you can draw the location of the pain. This can be useful as a baseline if the pain should change.

When recording pain location, use anatomical landmarks and descriptive terminology. The statement "The pain is localized in the upper right abdominal quadrant" is more specific than "The patient/client states that the pain is in the abdomen". Knowing a patient's/client's disease or illness can help you locate pain more easily. Pain, classified by location, may be superficial or cutaneous, deep or visceral, or referred or radiating (Table 27-5).

## SEVERITY

The most subjective characteristic of pain may be its severity, or intensity. Patients/clients are often asked to describe pain as mild, moderate, or severe. However, the meaning of these terms differs for the nurse and patient/client. This type of information is also difficult to verify over time.

Descriptive **pain scales** are a more objective means of measuring pain severity (Fig. 27-7). A **verbal descriptor scale (VDS)** consists of a line with three- to five-word descriptors equally spaced along the line. The descriptors are ranked from 'no pain' to 'unbearable pain'. The word chosen by a patient/client determines the intensity of the sensation. Numbers may also be used on scales instead of word descriptors. The VDS enables a patient/client to choose a category for describing pain. The scale works best when assessing the intensity of pain before and after interventions (McGuire, 1984).

A **visual analogue scale** does not have labelled subdivisions. It consists of a straight line (usually 10 cm in length), representing a continuum of intensity, and has verbal descriptors at each end. This scale gives the patient/client total freedom in identifying the severity of pain. The visual analogue scale may be a more sensitive measure of pain severity because patients/clients

## TABLE 27-4 Implications of Pain Assessment for Nursing Interventions

| Assessment Criteria | Nursing Interventions |
| --- | --- |
| Onset and duration | Administer analgesics so that peak action occurs when pain is most acute (e.g. during dressing change or physiotherapy). |
| Location | Position patient/client off affected area. Apply local treatments (e.g. elastic bandage and splinting) directly over painful site. |
| Severity | Change or revise interventions, depending on success of selected intervention. |
| Precipitating or aggravating factors | Avoid activities that cause or aggravate pain. Teach patient/client or family to avoid the same activities. |
| Relief measures | Use measures that the patient/client uses to relieve pain, as long as they are safe and appropriate. |

mark at any point on the continuum rather than being forced to choose one word (McGuire, 1984).

A pain scale should be designed so that it is easy for the nurse to administer and is not time consuming for the individual to complete. If the patient/client can easily understand the scale, the description of pain severity should be more accurate. Descriptive scales are useful not only in assessing the severity of pain but also in evaluating changes in intensity. You can use the scales after interventions or when symptoms become aggravated to evaluate whether the pain has decreased or increased.

Do not use pain scales to compare one patient/client with another. Although the scales lend relative objectivity to measurement, the severity of pain is too subjective to permit comparisons between individuals.

## QUALITY

Another subjective characteristic of pain is its quality. Since there is no common or specific pain vocabulary in general use, the words a patient/client may choose to describe pain can apply to any number of things. Often, a patient/client describes pain as crushing, throbbing, sharp, or dull. A patient's/client's pain can often be indescribable.

The nurse should not provide descriptive words for a patient/client. Assessment is more accurate if a patient/client can describe the sensation after open-ended questions. For example, the nurse might say, "Tell me what your pain feels like". The only time that the nurse offers to list descriptive terms is when the patient/client cannot describe pain. Meinhart and McCaffery (1983) report that the qualities of pricking, burning, and aching

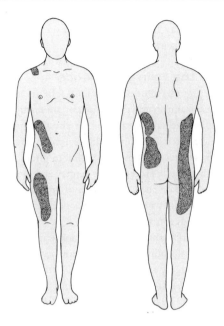

**Fig. 27-6**
Diagrammatic figures used to locate a patient's/client's pain.

are useful to describe pain initially. Later the patient/client may choose more descriptive terms.

There is some consistency in the way people describe certain types of pain. The pain associated with a myocardial infarction is often described as *crushing* or *vice-like*, whereas the pain of a surgical incision is often described as *sharp* and *stabbing*. When the patient's/client's descriptions fit the pattern forming in the nurse's assessment, a clearer analysis can be made of the nature and type of pain.

## TABLE 27-5 Classification of Pain by Location

| Definition | Characteristics | Examples |
|---|---|---|
| **SUPERFICIAL OR CUTANEOUS** | | |
| Pain resulting from stimulation of skin | Pain is of short duration and is localized. It is usually a sharp sensation | Venepuncture; small cut or laceration |
| **DEEP VISCERAL** | | |
| Pain resulting from stimulation of internal organs | Pain is diffuse and may radiate in several directions. Duration varies but it usually lasts longer then superficial pain. Pain may be sharp, dull, or unique to organ involved | Crushing sensation (e.g. angina pectoris); burning sensation (e.g. gastric ulcer) |
| **REFERRED** | | |
| Common phenomenon in visceral pain because many organs themselves have no pain receptors; entrance of sensory neurones from affected organ into same spinal cord segment as neurones from areas where pain is felt; perception of pain in unaffected areas | Pain is felt in part of body separate from source of pain and may assume any characteristic | Myocardial infarction, which may cause referred pain to jaw, left arm, and left shoulder; kidney stones, which may refer pain to groin |
| **RADIATING** | | |
| Sensation of pain extending from initial site of injury to another body part | Pain feels as though it travels down or along body part. It may be intermittent or constant | Low-back pain from ruptured intravertebral disk accompanied by pain radiating down leg from sciatic nerve irritation |

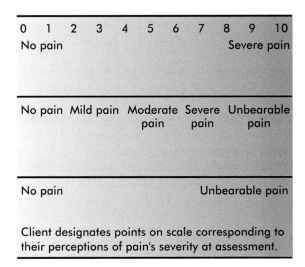

0  1  2  3  4  5  6  7  8  9  10
No pain                          Severe pain

No pain  Mild pain  Moderate  Severe  Unbearable
                      pain      pain      pain

No pain                          Unbearable pain

Client designates points on scale corresponding to their perceptions of pain's severity at assessment.

Fig. 27-7 Sample pain scales. A, Numerical. B, Verbal descriptive. C, Visual analogue.

## PAIN PATTERN

Various factors can affect the character of pain. It helps to assess specific events or conditions that induce or exacerbate pain. You may ask the person to demonstrate actions that elicit a painful response such as coughing or movement. After you have identified precipitating or exacerbating factors, it is easier to plan interventions that avoid making the pain worse.

**Relief Measures** It is useful to know whether a patient/client has an effective way for relieving pain such as changing position, eating, or applying heat to the painful site. Patients/clients gain comfort from knowing that the nurse is willing to try their relief measures. In the home, the nurse must be sure that relief measures are being used safely. Assessment of relieving factors should also include identification of practitioners (for example, masseur, acupuncturist, chiropractor, or osteopath) whose services the patient/client has sought. Patients/clients with chronic pain are more likely to try complementary health care therapies (see Chapter 32).

## CONCOMITANT SYMPTOMS

Symptoms that often occur with pain include nausea, headache, breathlessness, constipation, and restlessness. Certain types of pain have predictable accompanying symptoms, for example, severe rectal pain often results in constipation. The pain of an inflamed gallbladder or kidney

---

**Children's Nursing**
**Pain relief for children**

There are two main categories of pain relief methods; pharmacological and nonpharmacological. Non-pharmacological utilizes interventions such as distraction, relaxation, guided imagery and massage with the use of hot or cold compresses. Analgesia may be used very successfully — but must be given regularly and at an effective dosage to relieve pain. The dosage must be carefully calculated to achieve its desired effect and must not be harmful to the child.

---

stone frequently causes nausea and vomiting. **Concomitant symptoms** may be as much a treatment priority as the pain itself.

### Effects of Pain on the Patient/Client

By recognizing the effects of pain on a patient/client, the nurse can identify the nature and existence of the pain.

### PHYSICAL SIGNS AND SYMPTOMS

The physiological response to pain can reveal the existence and nature of pain and the potential threat to the patient's/client's welfare. When a patient/client experiences discomfort, the nurse should assess vital signs and observe for autonomic nervous system involvement (see Table 27-2). Physiological signs can reveal pain in a patient/client who tries not to complain or admit discomfort. There is no predictable level or extent of change in a patient's/client's vital signs that indicates pain severity.

Do not confuse signs and symptoms of pain with other behavioural or pathological changes. For example, a patient/client who is highly anxious also exhibits elevated heart and respiratory rates. A patient/client who is seriously dehydrated has an increased pulse because of volume depletion. The nurse must consider all signs and symptoms before determining that pain is the cause.

It helps to determine patients/clients at greater risk for having pain; the patient/client who has had surgery and the victim of serious trauma are just two examples of individuals who probably experience acute pain.

If pain is unrelieved, look for signs of physical exhaustion. Decreasing vital sign values indicate parasympathetic nerve response. The patient/client becomes less responsive to stimuli within the environment. Vital signs should be measured more often if the patient's/client's condition deteriorates.

### BEHAVIOURAL EFFECTS

When a patient/client has pain, the nurse assesses vocal response, facial and body movements, and social interaction (see box). A verbal report of pain is a vital part of the total assessment. The person's verbalization of pain may depend on the nurse's willingness to listen or understand. A number of patients/clients cannot verbalize discomfort owing to an inability to communicate; for example an infant, someone who is unconscious, a disoriented or confused person (Marzinski, 1991), an aphasic person, or someone who speaks a foreign language. In these cases, it is especially important to be aware of behaviours that indicate pain.

Groaning, grunting, and crying are examples of vocalizations used to express pain. Certain vocalizations may be involuntary and may occur without warning when acute pain occurs. For some patients/clients, vocalizations are culturally acceptable ways to communicate.

Subtle facial expressions or body movements often reveal more about the character of pain than precise questioning. For example, the person may grimace or begin to toss and turn at regular intervals. The amount of restlessness or protective movement may increase as the assessment progresses. The individual may also react more uncomfortably while assuming different positions.

Some nonverbal expressions characterize sources of pain. The person with chest pain often grabs or holds the chest. A child or adult with severe abdominal pain often assumes a fetal position. An adult with a severe headache may squint or rub the temples. The nonverbal expression of pain may support or contradict other information about pain. If a woman in labour reports that her labour pains are occurring more frequently and if she begins to massage her abdomen more frequently, her report is confirmed. If a person complains of severe abdominal pain but continues to grasp the chest, a more detailed assessment may be necessary.

The nature of pain causes a person to attend to the discomfort and fight it or give in to the discomfort and withdraw socially. The extent to which a patient/client interacts with the environment can provide a clue about the intensity or nature of pain.

## INFLUENCE ON ACTIVITIES OF LIVING

Patients/clients who live with daily pain experience changes in their ability to participate in routine activities. Assessment of these changes reveals the extent of the person's disability and adjustments necessary to help individuals to participate in self-care.

The nurse asks whether pain interferes with sleep. There may be difficulty falling asleep. Sleeping pills or other medications

### Behavioural Indicators of Effects of Acute Pain

VOCALIZATIONS
- Moaning
- Crying
- Screaming
- Gasping
- Grunting

FACIAL EXPRESSIONS
- Grimace
- Clenched teeth
- Wrinkled forehead
- Tightly closed or widely opened eyes or mouth
- Lip biting
- Tightened jaw

BODY MOVEMENT
- Restlessness
- Immobilization
- Muscle tension
- Increased hand and finger movements
- Pacing activities
- Rhythmic or rubbing motions
- Protective movement of body parts

SOCIAL INTERACTION
- Avoidance of conversation
- Focus only on activities for pain relief
- Avoidance of social contacts
- Reduced attention span

may be needed to induce sleep. The pain may awaken the person during the night, or he or she may have insomnia as a result of the pain (see Chapter 20).

Depending on the location of pain, the person may have difficulty performing normal hygiene measures. It is important to determine whether the patient/client can dress independently or shampoo hair. The pain may restrict mobility to the point where the individual is no longer able to bathe normally. The person may have problems performing other activities of daily living, for example, a patient/client with severe arthritis may find it painful to grasp eating utensils. It is important to determine the individual's need for assistance with self-care activities, and to consider the need for family members or friends to assist the person with basic hygiene.

Pain can impair the ability to maintain normal sexual relations. Conditions such as arthritis, degenerative diseases of the hip, and chronic back pain make it difficult for a person to assume usual positions during intercourse. When assessing the extent to which pain has affected sexual activity, it is important to distinguish whether a patient/client is physically unable to participate or if the desire for sexual intercourse has been reduced by the pain.

The ability of people to work can be seriously threatened by pain. The more physical activity required in a job, the greater the risk of discomfort when the pain is associated with musculoskeletal and certain visceral disorders. Pain related to emotional stress is probably increased in individuals whose jobs involve tension-laden decision making. The nurse can assess the work that patients/clients do and their abilities to function in certain types of employment. The daily activities of those working within the home are assessed in the same manner as the duties involved in other employment. Assess whether it is necessary for patients/clients to stop the activity occasionally because of pain. In conjunction with an occupational therapist, the nurse can help patients/clients select ways of minimizing or controlling the pain so that they can remain productive.

It is also important to include an assessment of the effect of pain on social activities. The pain may be so debilitating that the patient/client becomes too exhausted to socialize. The nurse identifies the patient's/client's normal social activities, the extent to which they have been disrupted, and the person's wish to participate.

## NEUROLOGICAL STATUS

A patient's/client's neurological function can easily influence the pain experience. Any factor that interrupts or influences normal pain reception or perception affects the patient's/client's awareness and response to pain. For example, a person who has a spinal cord injury, peripheral neuropathy, or a neurological disease such as multiple sclerosis or intracerebral lesions, may experience pain differently to a patient/client who has normal neurological function. Some interventions influence pain perception and response. Analgesics, sedatives, and anaesthetics depress functions of the central nervous system. It is important to be aware of situations or conditions which may lead to a patient/client being at risk due to altered pain perception. An individual could suffer injury easily and thus require preventive nursing care; for example, an overly sedated patient/client would not be able to sense the discomfort of a tight plaster cast or dressing.

## Determining Patient/Client Needs

The nurse should focus on the specific nature of the pain to help identify the most useful types of interventions for alleviating pain and minimizing its effect on the patient's/client's lifestyle and function.

The extent to which pain affects a person's lifestyle and general state of health determines whether additional patient/client needs are relevant. For example, the nurse's assessment may reveal that a patient/client suffers from pain in the hands and shoulders, due to arthritis. As a result, the individual is unable to remove or fasten necessary items of clothing. The person's needs are therefore twofold: that of relief of chronic musculoskeletal pain, and that of assistance with dressing and personal grooming.

 PLANNING

For each patient/client need or nursing problem identified, the nurse develops a care plan (see care plan). Together the nurse and patient/client discuss realistic expectations for pain-relief measures and the degree of pain relief to expect. Expected outcomes and goals are selected on the basis of the type of pain present and the person's underlying medical condition. Appropriate interventions are chosen on the basis of the related factors contributing to the patient's/client's pain or health problem. For example, pain related to acute incisional pain responds to appropriate analgesics, whereas pain related to early

labour contractions can be reduced with relaxation exercises.

An intervention that works for one individual will not necessarily work for all. It is often necessary for the person to understand that complete pain relief cannot be guaranteed but that it will be attempted by combining appropriate strategies from both the patient/client and health care professionals.

When compiling the care plan, develop priorities based on the patient's/client's level of pain and its effect on the person's condition. For acute severe pain it is important to provide relief as soon as possible. Analgesics can provide relatively rapid relief and lessen the chance of pain worsening. After a patient/client gains some relief from pain, the nurse may plan other interventions such as relaxation or thermal applications to enhance the effect of analgesics.

A comprehensive plan includes a variety of resources for pain control. It is important to include the family in the care plan. The family may need to administer care in the home. In an acute care setting the family must understand the nature and extent of the patient's/client's pain and the types of interventions to be used. Additional resources available include clinical nurse specialists, physiotherapists, and occupational therapists. An oncology nurse specialist is very familiar with measures most effective for chronic, malignant pain. Physiotherapists can plan exercises that strengthen muscle groups and lessen pain in affected areas. Occupational therapists may devise splints to support painful body parts. When the nurse is caring for a person experiencing pain, patient/client-centred goals might include the following:

- Stating a sense of well-being and comfort
- Maintaining the ability to perform self-care
- Maintaining existing physical and psychosocial function
- Explaining factors contributing to the pain experience.

## SAMPLE NURSING CARE PLAN FOR ACUTE PAIN RELIEF

### Patient/client problem: Pain related to abdominal incision movement

| GOALS | EXTENDED OUTCOMES | INTERVENTIONS | RATIONALE |
|---|---|---|---|
| Patient/client will achieve control of pain within 24 hr of surgery. | Patient/client will express relief during PCA infusion. | Explain to patient/client purpose of patient-controlled analgesia device, method for initiating device, and expected response. | Patient/client who has control over own pain achieves greater pain relief. |
| | | Demonstrate and teach patient/client through relaxation exercise. | Use of comfort measures aimed at distracting patient/client may potentiate effect of analgesia. |
| | Patient/client will initiate movement in bed without painful behavioural cues. | Position patient/client anatomically on side with knees flexed and small pillow between legs. | Flexion of knees minimizes strain on abdominal muscles. |
| | | Have colleague available to lift patient/client in bed for repositioning; encourage patient/client to ask for assistance. | Lifting of patient/client prevents patient/client from pulling self up in bed, aggravating abdominal pain. |

To establish an effective care plan, the nurse develops a therapeutic relationship with the patient/client and together they explore the nature of the pain and decide upon the appropriate pain relief measures to be employed.

## Therapeutic Relationship

Patients/clients in pain are highly vulnerable, and may not always be convinced that someone is concerned about their welfare. They therefore need someone to trust. If the nurse is unable to establish a therapeutic relationship with patients/clients, any resultant mistrust can heighten the awareness of pain. Unless patients/clients have the means to express concerns or fears about pain, their reactions to the pain may become inappropriate. Individuals may become angry or complain about the nurse's care when needs for pain relief are ignored.

The nurse can best help by viewing the patient/client as a total person and conveying a sense of caring. Paying careful attention to the patient's/client's concerns during assessment is one way of building confidence in the nurse. Promptness in attending to the patient's/client's needs further establishes a strong therapeutic relationship. Making judgements about the validity of pain, bargaining pain relief in return for 'good' patient/client behaviour, and controlling sources of pain relief destroy the patient's/client's trust in the nurse.

A successful relationship with the patient/client depends in part on your ability to respect the patient's/client's response to pain. Many nurses value firm self-control; however, a patient/client may need to cry or moan or even become angry. The person should never feel ashamed or fearful that you will not accept his or her unique response to pain.

## Education

People are better prepared to handle almost any situation when they understand it, and the experience of pain is no exception. Teaching patients/clients about their pain experience reduces anxiety and helps them to achieve a sense of control. For example, a person entering a clinic or hospital for the first time may know that tests will be performed but may not understand them. As a result, they might fantasize about the experience. Fears are enhanced if friends have had unpleasant experiences in similar circumstances, and fear increases the perception of painful stimuli.

During the anticipatory phase of the pain experience, teach patients/clients about the procedures and associated discomfort. Price *et al* (1980) found that when patients/clients received instruction about a forthcoming painful experience, they perceived the actual experience as less unpleasant. Patients/clients changed the way they evaluated the pain sensation and thus tolerated pain more effectively.

For some individuals, early warning of pain can be a problem. The highly anxious or fearful patient/client may be less rational and unable to learn from the nurse's explanations. Such people tend to fantasize horrible events if they receive information too early about painful procedures. If an individual seems unlikely to benefit from advance preparation, it is best to explain invasive procedures a short time before they occur. It is not always easy to know whether patients/clients can accept impending unpleasant experiences. If an individual is overtly anxious or if previous teaching has not relieved anxiety, you use your judgement as to when to tell the individual about procedures.

Relevant play is a type of teaching that works well with children. Play reduces anxiety that might otherwise be created if the nurse tries to explain complicated procedures. For example, if a child is to have a laceration of the arm sutured, it helps to let the child put sutures into a doll's arm. Almost any procedure or situation can be acted out with dolls or other appropriate toys (McCaffery and Beebe, 1994b).

 **IMPLEMENTATION**

The nature of pain and the extent to which it affects physical and psychosocial well-being should determine the choice of pain relief interventions. However, nurses can independently use pain-relief measures that complement those prescribed by a doctor. Witt (1984) describes the following characteristics of ideal nursing interventions for chronic pain management:

1. Interventions should be within the scope of the nurse's education and training to use them effectively.
2. They use equipment which is really available.
3. Nursing interventions should not interact adversely with the patient's/client's medical treatments.
4. Nursing interventions should not be subject to a doctor's approval or supervision.

The nurse can play an important role in helping patients/clients use techniques for acute and chronic pain relief. If there is doubt about a nursing intervention, the nurse should consult a clinical nurse specialist or the patient's/client's doctor.

## Guidelines for Individualizing Pain Relief Measures

When providing pain-relief measures, choose interventions suited to the patient's/client's unique pain experience. McCaffery (1979) suggests nine useful guidelines for individualizing pain therapy (see box).

## Nonpharmacological Management of Pain

A basic nursing responsibility is protecting the patient/client from harm. One simple way to promote comfort is by removing or preventing painful stimuli (see box). This is especially important for people who are immobilized or unable to sense discomfort.

Often, pain can be avoided by maintaining normal body function. For example, a person who is allowed to become constipated may suffer from abdominal distention and cramps. The nurse actively intervenes to ensure that the normal elimination process continues.

Pain can also be prevented by anticipating painful procedures or activities. Before performing procedures, consider the patient's/client's condition, aspects of the procedure that may be

## Guidelines for Individualizing Pain Relief

• *Establish a relationship of mutual trust.* Always believe the patient/client and convey concern. An adversarial relationship between nurse and patient/client lessens the effectiveness of pain relief measures.

• *Use different types of pain-relief measures.* Using more than one intervention has an additive effect in reducing pain. In addition, the character of pain may change throughout the day, requiring several different approaches.

• *Provide pain-relief measures before pain becomes severe.* It is easier to prevent severe pain than to relieve it once it exists. Giving an analgesic 0.5 hr before a patient/client must walk or perform an activity is an example of controlling pain early.

• *Consider the patient's/client's ability or willingness to participate in pain-relief measures.* Some patients/clients cannot actively assist with pain-relief interventions because of fatigue, fear, or altered levels of consciousness. However, there are some pain-relief measures that require limited activity such as relaxation exercises in bed or listening to music as a distraction.

• *Choose pain-relief measures on the basis of the patient's/client's behaviour reflecting the severity of pain.* It would be poor judgement to administer a strong opioid if a patient/client has only mild pain. The nurse carefully assesses the patient's/client's comments and behaviour before choosing an intervention. Some patients/clients acquire relief from severe pain after using only mild analgesics. Only the patient/client can determine the efficacy of a specific intervention.

• *Use measures that the patient/client believes are effective.* The patient/client may have ideas about measures to use (e.g. rubbing lotion on a swollen finger) and particular times to use them that will make pain relief measures successful

• *If an intervention is ineffective at first, encourage the patient/client to try it again before abandoning it.* Often anxiety or doubt prevents an intervention from relieving pain, or the measure may require adjustment or practice to become effective. The nurse should be patient and understanding in helping the patient/client learn to use measures that do not afford immediate relief.

• *Keep an open mind about what may relieve pain.* New ways are often found to control pain. There is still much to be learned about the pain experience. Rejecting unconventional therapies leads to mistrust. The nurse should be sure all therapies are safe.

• *Keep trying.* The nurse can easily become frustrated when efforts at pain relief fail. The nurse should *not* abandon the patient/client when pain persists but reassess the situation and consider alternative interventions.

• *Protect the patient/client.* A pain relief measure should not cause more distress then the pain itself. The nurse always observes the patient's/client's response to interventions. The nurse's aim is to relieve pain without disabling the patient/client mentally, emotionally, or physically.

• *Educate the patient/client about pain.* When possible, the nurse should explain the cause of the pain, times of occurrence, duration and quality, and ways to gain relief. Education promotes the prevention of pain.

uncomfortable, and techniques to avoid causing pain. For example, for a person with knee pain caused by arthritis, the nurse knows that any extreme flexion of the knee causes much pain. Before walking the patient/client to the bathroom make sure that an elevated toilet seat is available. The patient/client can then be seated and stand up with minimal discomfort.

It takes only simple consideration of the patient's/client's comfort and a little extra time to avoid pain-producing situations. Knowledge of factors that precipitate or aggravate pain helps you prevent or minimize the patient's/client's discomfort. Learning proper lifting techniques and avoiding sudden turning movements can help a person with a history of back pain to avoid discomfort.

## CUTANEOUS STIMULATION

One way to prevent or reduce pain perception is through **cutaneous stimulation,** the stimulation of a person's skin to relieve pain. A massage, warm bath, application of liniment, hot or cold pads, and transcutaneous electrical nerve stimulation (TENS) are simple ways to reduce pain perception. The specific way in which cutaneous stimulation works is unclear. One suggestion is that it causes the release of endorphins, thus

blocking the transmission of painful stimuli. Based on the gate control theory, it is suggested that cutaneous stimulation activates large-diameter A-beta sensory nerve fibres, decreasing the transmission of painful stimuli through small-diameter A-delta and C fibres. Synaptic gates close to the transmission of pain impulses.

Cutaneous stimulation requires the nurse to touch the patient/client. Work by Krieger (1975) suggests that therapeutic touch alone may result in a patient's/client's improved sense of well-being. Touch can communicate caring and thus help patients/clients relax.

Cutaneous stimulation can provide effective, temporary pain relief. To enhance its effects, help the patient/client assume a comfortable position, eliminates environmental distractions such as noise and bright lights, and explain the purpose of the intervention. Cutaneous stimulation should not be used directly on sensitive skin areas (for example burns, rashes, or bruises), incisions, inflamed areas, or underlying fractures.

Massage and aromatherapy (see Chapter 32) are low-cost, safe ways to use cutaneous stimulation. Massage by a trained practitioner may lessen pain by promoting muscular relaxation.

## Controlling Potentially Painful Stimuli in the Patient's/Client's Environment

- Tighten and smooth wrinkled bed linen.
- Remove tubing on which patient/client is lying.
- Loosen constricting bandages (unless specifically applied as a pressure dressing).
- Position patient/client in anatomical alignment unless contraindicated.
- Check temperature of hot or cold applications, including bath tub water.
- Lift patient/client in bed — do not pull or drag.
- Position patient/client correctly on bed pan.
- Avoid exposing skin or mucous membranes to irritants (e.g. diarrhoea, wound drainage).
- Prevent urinary retention.
- Prevent constipation with fluids, diet, and exercise.

Cold and heat applications are routine measures that can be used in the hospital or home; the advantage of these is that they give patients/clients and families some control over pain symptoms and treatment. Ice bags, warm and cold sitz baths, heating pads, and hot or cold compresses can relieve pain and promote healing of injured tissues. The selection of heat versus cold therapies varies according to the person's condition; for example, moist heat relieves the early morning stiffness of arthritis, but cold applications reduce the acute pain and inflamed joints of the disease (Ceccio, 1990). When using any

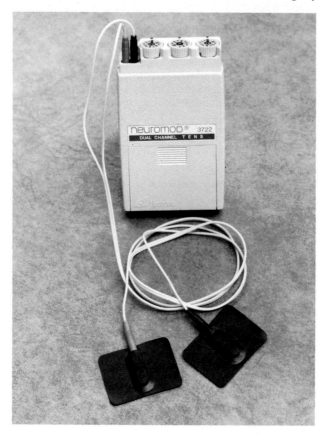

**Fig. 27-8** TENS.

form of cold or heat application, teach the patient/client to avoid injury to the skin. People can easily be burned by the incorrect use of heat applications; especially at risk are individuals with spinal cord or other neurological injuries, older adults, and confused individuals.

Application of cold packs is a type of cold therapy that is particularly effective for pain relief. It takes about 5 to 10 minutes to use a cold application, and placement near the actual site of pain tends to work best. The patient/client feels cold, burning, and aching sensations and numbness. When numbness occurs, the ice should be removed. Cold applications are also effective before invasive needle punctures such as intramuscular injections, bone marrow punctures, and lumbar punctures.

**Transcutaneous electric nerve stimulation** involves stimulation of nerves beneath the skin with a mild electrical current passed through external electrodes. The therapy may require a doctor's agreement before use. The TENS unit consists of a battery-powered transmitter, lead wires, and electrodes (Fig. 27-8). The electrodes are placed directly over or near the site of pain. Hair or skin preparations should be removed before attaching the electrodes. When a patient/client feels pain, the transmitter is turned on. The TENS unit creates a buzzing or tingling sensation. The patient/client may adjust the intensity and quality of skin stimulation. The tingling sensation can be applied as long as pain relief lasts. In a study conducted by Taylor *et al* (1983), people who received TENS reported greater pain relief than people who received opioid analgesics. TENS may be effective for postsurgical pain control and, in some cases, reduction of pain caused by postoperative procedures (for example, removing drains and cleaning and repacking surgical wounds) (Hargreaves and Lander, 1989).

## DISTRACTION

The reticular activating system inhibits painful stimuli if a person receives sufficient or excessive sensory input. With meaningful

### Effects of Relaxation

- Decreased pulse, blood pressure, and respirations
- Decreased oxygen consumption
- Decreased muscle tension
- Decreased metabolic rate
- Heightened concentration
- Lack of attention to environmental stimuli

### Body Positions for Relaxation

SITTING
- Sit with entire back resting against back of chair.
- Place feet flat on floor.
- Keep legs separated.
- Hang arms at the side or rest on chair arms.
- Keep head aligned with spine.

LYING
- Keep legs separated with toes pointed slightly outward.
- Rest arms at sides without touching sides of body.
- Keep head aligned with spine.
- Use thin, small pillow under head.

sensory stimuli, a person can try to ignore or become less aware of pain. Pleasurable stimuli also cause the release of endorphins to relieve pain. People who are bored or in isolation have only their pain to think about and thus perceive it more acutely. **Distraction** may work best for short, intense pain lasting a few minutes such as pain experienced by a patient/client during a procedure or while waiting for an analgesic to work (Mayer, 1985).

The nurse should ask the patient/client which distractions he or she uses; these might include singing, praying, describing photos or pictures aloud, listening to music, and playing games.

One effective distraction is music. Some institutions have music therapists. However, the nurse can use music creatively in many clinical situations, particularly as a means to promote relaxation in an individual with chronic pain.

## RELAXATION AND GUIDED IMAGERY

Patients/clients can alter affective-motivational and cognitive pain perception through relaxation and guided imagery. The ability to relax physically also promotes mental relaxation. **Relaxation techniques** provide patients/clients with self-control when pain occurs, reversing the physical and emotional stress of pain. People who use relaxation techniques successfully may experience several physiological and behavioural changes (see lower boxes opposite). Relaxation techniques can include meditation, yoga, Zen, guided imagery, and progressive muscle relaxation exercises.

Relaxation with or without guided imagery can relieve tension headaches, labour pain, and chronic pain disorders. It may take five to ten training sessions before patients/clients can effectively minimize pain. Relaxation training can be practised indefinitely and usually has no side effects (Anderson et al, 1987).

In **guided imagery** the patient/client creates an image in the mind, concentrates on that image, and gradually becomes less aware of pain. The nurse assists the patient/client to form an image and to concentrate on the sensory experience. Initially, ask the patient/client to think of a pleasant scene or experience that promotes use of all senses. The patient/client describes the image and the nurse records it so that it can be used during later exercises. Use specific information given by the patient/client and do not make changes to the patient's/client's image. The use of any formal relaxation technique or guided imagery exercise should only be undertaken by a nurse who is trained in the appropriate use of these complementary therapies (see Chapter 32).

## ANTICIPATORY GUIDANCE

Modifying anxiety directly associated with pain relieves pain and enhances the effects of other pain-relief measures. Moderate anxiety may be useful when a patient/client anticipates a painful experience, because patients/clients can learn what is to be expected during a painful procedure or event. Knowledge about pain helps an individual control anxiety and cognitively gain a level of pain relief (Walding, 1991).

It is important to give patients/clients information that prevents misinterpretation of the painful event and promotes understanding of what to expect. Information given to patients/clients includes explanation of the following:

- Occurrence, onset, and expected duration of pain
- Quality, severity, and location of pain
- Information on how the patient's/client's safety is ensured
- Cause of the pain
- Methods nurse and patient/client use for pain relief
- Expectations of the patient/client during a procedure.

An example of **anticipatory guidance** is preoperative teaching (see Chapter 29). Explanation of the incisional pain the patient/client will feel and methods used to control it helps the person adapt postoperatively.

The nurse cannot say that the patient/client will experience no pain. Anticipatory guidance provides an honest explanation of the pain experience. The nurse also gives instruction on pain-relief techniques so that the person will be prepared to cope with discomfort.

## BIOFEEDBACK

**Biofeedback** is a behavioural therapy that involves giving individuals information about physiological responses (such as blood pressure or tension) and ways to exercise voluntary control over those responses (Flor et al, 1983). Electrodes are attached externally and measure skin tension in microvolts. A polygraph machine visibly records the tension level for the patient/client to see. The individual learns to achieve optimal relaxation using feedback from the polygraph while lowering the actual level of tension experienced. The therapy takes several weeks to learn. This technique, however, is not readily available within the National Health Service.

## Pharmacological Management of Pain

Several pharmacological agents provide pain relief, and all require a doctor's prescription. The nurse's judgement in the use of medications and assessment of patients/clients receiving pharmacological management helps ensure the best pain relief possible.

## ADMINISTERING ANALGESICS

**Analgesics** are the most common method of pain relief. However, nurses and doctors often have misconceptions about the dangers and effects of analgesics. Frequently, nurses and doctors undertreat patients/clients because of incorrect pharmacological knowledge, concerns about addiction, anxiety over errors in judgement while using a strong opioid analgesic, and administration of less analgesia than was prescribed (Marks and Sachar, 1973). Rankin and Snider (1984) studied nurses' perceptions of pain suffered by cancer patients/clients. The study showed that 89% of nurses believed that patients/clients had adequate pain control. However, 67% assessed that the patients/clients suffered moderate pain. Often nurses' uncertainty over the correct administration of analgesics leads only to a reduction in pain, not significant relief. However, recent research suggests that, at least in the domain of cancer care, the majority of doctors understand the basic principles of pain control, and fears of addiction and respiratory depression are no longer major determinants in the use of strong opioid analgesics (White et al, 1991).

There are four types of analgesics: nonopioid analgesics, weak opioid analgesics, strong opioids, and adjuvants or co-analgesics (see following box). Nonopioid analgesics (non-narcotic analgesics or nonsteroidal anti-inflammatory drugs — NSAIDs) and weak opioids provide relief for mild to moderate pain, such as the pain associated with rheumatoid arthritis, minor surgical and dental procedures, episiotomy, and low back pain problems. Strong opioids are generally prescribed for severe pain such as the pain caused by major surgical procedures or malignant pain, whereas co-analgesics may enhance **analgesia** (lack of pain) or relieve other signs and symptoms associated with pain such as depression and nausea.

Nurses must understand the drugs available for pain relief and their pharmacological effects. Pharmacological agents act at different levels of the nervous system to create pain relief. A drug may act at the peripheral receptor level or at the central nervous system level. The most common peripheral analgesics and NSAIDs act primarily on peripheral receptors to diminish transmission and reception of pain stimuli. All except paracetamol inhibit the synthesis of prostaglandins at the site of injury.

**Strong opioid analgesics**, when given orally or by injection, act on higher centres of the brain and spinal cord by binding with opioid receptors to modify perception of and reaction to pain. Morphine sulphate and diamorphine hydrochloride have the two following characteristic analgesic effects:

1. Raising the pain threshold, thereby reducing pain perception.
2. Reducing anxiety and fear, which are components of the affective reaction to pain.

A consideration in the use of morphine sulphate and other strong opioid analgesics is the potential for depression of vital nervous system functions. Strong opioids can cause respiratory depression by depressing the respiratory centre within the brainstem. This effect can usually be avoided by careful titration of the dose of the drug against the severity of the pain being experienced (Hanks and Hoskin, 1987). Some patients/clients may also experience side effects such as nausea, vomiting, constipation, and altered mental processes. The following are characteristics of an ideal analgesic:

1. Rapid onset.
2. Effective action over a prolonged time.
3. Availability for all ages.
4. Oral and parenteral use.
5. Lack of severe side effects.
6. Low addiction potential .
7. Inexpensive.

Anticonvulsants, antidepressants, and muscle relaxants are **co-analgesics** often prescribed for those patients/clients whose pain is less responsive to analgesics alone, usually due to specific co-existing pathophysiology such as neuropathic pain due to nerve compression or muscle spasm associated with severe musculoskeletal pain (Hanks, 1988).

Analgesics require careful assessment, application of pharmacological principles (see Chapter 31), and common sense.

## Examples of Analgesics

### NONOPIOID ANALGESICS
- Paracetamol
- Acetylsalicylic acid (aspirin)

### WEAK OPIOID ANALGESICS
- Dihydrocodeine
- Co-proxamol (paracetamol and dextropropoxyphene)
- Codeine phosphate

### STRONG OPIOIDS
- Diamorphine hydrochloride
- Morphine sulphate
- Pethidine
- Papaveretum
- Buprenorphine

### NSAIDs
- Flurbiprofen
- Naproxen
- Indomethacin
- Piroxicam

### CO-ANALGESICS
- NSAIDs, e.g. flurbiprofen
- Anticonvulsants, e.g. carbemazepine
- Antidepressants, e.g. amitryptyline
- Anxiolytics, e.g. diazepam
- Antispasmodics, e.g. baclofen

A person's response to an analgesic is highly individualized, whereby a weak opioid may prove as effective as a more potent analgesic for some patients/clients, or an orally administered analgesic may bring the same relief as an injectable form of analgesic. It is the nurse's responsibility to follow a few basic principles (see following box).

The nurse should always know the equianalgesic dosages of analgesics in oral and injectable form. **Equianalgesic** means approximately equal analgesia, i.e. doses of medication that provide about the same pain relief when switching from one route of administration to another or when switching from one drug to another. For example, a doctor may order pethidine 50 to 100 mg intramuscularly or orally every 2 to 3 hours as necessary. This order leaves much to the judgement of the nurse and requires clarification. Such an order would create confusion where several nurses must select the best dose, route, and time interval of administration. The maximum dose of pethidine (100 mg) by mouth has about the same analgesic strength as 13 mg morphine intramuscularly (Heidrich and Perry, 1982). The lowest dose, 50 mg, by mouth is equal to the strength of two aspirin. If nurses on subsequent shifts choose different routes for the same doses, the patient/client will not receive the same level of analgesia, and pain control will be poor. Nurses must provide controlled, sustained pain relief.

## PATIENT-CONTROLLED ANALGESIA (PCA)

Patients/clients benefit from having control over pain therapy. When patients/clients depend on nurses for analgesia, an erratic cycle of alternating pain relief and breakthrough pain can occur, particularly when the prescription is for 'prn' or 'as required' administration. The individual feels pain and asks for an analgesic, but the nurse may be unable to administer the drug promptly. Within an hour of drug administration, analgesia finally occurs. Pain relief may last only 1–2 hours then, gradually, the patient/client again feels discomfort, and the cycle begins again.

A drug delivery system called **patient-controlled analgesia (PCA)** allows patients/clients to safely administer pain medications when they want them. The PCA is a portable pump (usually computerized) containing a chamber for a syringe. The pump delivers a small preset dose of medication either intravenously or subcutaneously. The analgesic of choice is diamorphine hydrochloride because of its high solubility and stability in solution (Jones and Hanks, 1986). To receive a dose the person pushes a button attached to the pump. The system is designed to deliver no more than a specified number of doses every hour to avoid the potential for overdosage. For example, a PCA device can deliver a dose as small as 1 ml or 1 mg of diamorphine hydrochloride every 6 minutes. Most pumps have locked safety systems that prevent tampering by patients/clients or their family members, and a dose can be released only at a preset time interval. Benefits of PCA include the following:

1. Patients/clients have increased control over their pain.
2. Pain relief does not depend on nurse availability.
3. Patients/clients tend to take less medication, achieving a balance between the pain-relieving properties and the sedative effects.
4. Small doses of analgesics delivered at short intervals stabilize serum drug concentrations for sustained pain relief.

PCA has been found to be effective in controlling postoperative, traumatic, obstetric, and cancer pain. The nurse and doctor assess the appropriateness of PCA for patients/clients. Often, individuals receive test doses of the drug before PCA is started to establish an appropriate regimen in terms of dose and frequency to be set on the pump. Patients/clients should be capable of handling the pump and understanding correct use. The nurse explains the purpose of PCA therapy, operating instructions for the pump, expected pain relief, precautions, and potential side effects; patients/clients should be informed that it is a safe method of drug delivery as well as its ability to prevent the risk of an overdose. Family members or friends should never operate the PCA device for patients/clients. The patient/client should be alert while an explanation is being given; a demonstration of its operation often increases the person's confidence in its use. The nurse should not wait until immediately after surgery to instruct patients/clients because at this stage they are likely to be sedated. Even though patients/clients control administration of analgesics, the nurse must routinely check that the PCA pump operates correctly. The nurse also documents drug dosages administered by the pump and records any wastage of controlled drugs in the appropriate ward drug register.

## LOCAL ANAESTHETICS
**Local anaesthesia** is the loss of sensation to a localized body part. Doctors use local anaesthesia while suturing a wound,

moving a body part in which the patient/client is experiencing pain, delivering an infant, and performing some surgery. Local anaesthesia has fewer risks than **general anaesthesia**, which causes loss of consciousness and depression of vital functions.

Local anaesthetics can be applied topically on skin and mucous membranes or injected to anaesthetize a part of the body. Local anaesthetics block the function of sensory, motor, and autonomic neurons supplying the affected area. Thus, when the person temporarily loses sensation in a body part, motor and autonomic function is also lost. Smaller sensory nerve fibres are more sensitive to local anaesthetics than the larger motor fibres. As a result, the person loses sensation before losing motor function, and conversely, motor activity returns before sensation.

Local anaesthetics can cause side effects, depending on their absorption into the systemic circulation. Itching or burning of the skin or a localized rash is common after topical applications. Application to vascular mucous membranes increases the chance of systemic effects such as a change in heart rate. Injection of anaesthetics increases the risk of systemic side effects, depending on the amount of drug used and the area injected.

Table 27-6 summarizes the types of local anaesthesia by injection. Each produces a different level of anaesthesia as a result of the amount of anaesthetic used and location of the spinal nerve affected.

The nurse assists the doctor during use of local anaesthesia by providing emotional support to patients/clients, watching for systemic side effects, and protecting patients/clients from injury. Many individuals are apprehensive about whether an anaesthetic will prevent pain. The nurse explains the application of the anaesthetic and the sensations experienced. Injection of anaesthetics can be painful if the doctor does not first numb the injection site. The nurse can prepare patients/clients for such discomfort.

Before the person receives an anaesthetic, the nurse determines any history of allergies, monitors systemic effects of local anaesthetics, assesses blood pressure and pulse.

After administration of a local anaesthetic the nurse protects the patient/client from injury until full sensory and motor function returns. Pain is a normal protective mechanism, therefore until the local anaesthetic is absorbed and metabolized, the patient/client must be careful in using an anaesthetized body part. For example, after an injection into a joint, warn the patient/client to avoid using the joint until function returns. For individuals with topical anaesthesia avoid applying heat or cold to numb areas. After spinal anaesthesia the person stays in bed until sensory and motor function returns; thereafter the nurse assists the patient/client during the first attempt to get out of bed.

## EPIDURAL ANALGESIA
The administration of medication into the spinal epidural space for acute and chronic pain management is becoming a more common intervention. Initially used for the management of acute

## Nursing Principles for Administering Analgesics

| | |
|---|---|
| **Know the Patient's/Client's Previous Response to Analgesics** | • Determine whether relief was obtained.<br>• Ask whether a weak analgesic was as effective as a more potent analgesic.<br>• Identify previous doses and routes of administration to avoid undermedication. |
| **Select Appropriate Medication When More Than One is Prescribed** | • Use nonopioid analgesics or weak opioids for mild to moderate pain.<br>• Remember that morphine sulphate and diamorphine hydrochloride are the strong opioids of choice for long-term management of severe pain.<br>• Know that injectable medications act quicker and can relieve severe, acute pain within 1 hour and that oral medication may take as long as 2 hours to relieve pain.<br>• Use a weak opioid with a nonopioid analgesic for moderate pain because such combinations treat pain peripherally and centrally (e.g. co-proxamol).<br>• For chronic pain, give an oral drug for sustained relief. |
| **Know the Accurate Dosage** | • Remember that doses at the upper end of normal are generally needed for severe pain.<br>• Adjust doses, as appropriate, for children and older patients/clients.<br>• Titrate the dosage to control the pain without inducing excessive side effects. |
| **Assess the Right Time and Interval for Administration** | • Administer analgesics as soon as pain occurs and before it increases in severity.<br>• Do not give analgesics only as required. Remember that a regular administration schedule is usually best, especially in chronic pain.<br>• Give analgesics before pain-producing procedures or activities.<br>• Know the average duration of action for a drug and the time of administration so that the peak effect occurs when pain is most intense, and breakthrough pain is avoided. |

pain during childbirth or following surgery, epidural infusions are now used to successfully treat selected patients/clients with chronic cancer pain (Turnage *et al*, 1990). The use of epidural analgesia permits control or reduction of severe pain without the central sedative effects normally associated with the administration of strong opioids. Epidurals can be short or long term, depending on the person's condition and life expectancy. Short-term therapy is used for pain after surgery or caesarean section, whereas long-term therapy may be appropriate for pain caused by cancer.

Epidural analgesia is administered into the spinal epidural space and the ventricles of the brain (Wilkie, 1990). Analgesics can also be introduced the intrathecal route, the spinal subarachnoid space, creating the same effects as epidural analgesia. Each route requires a slightly different approach for placement of a small plastic catheter. A doctor (usually an anaesthetist) enters the epidural and subarachnoid spaces by inserting the catheter into the lumbar region (level L3 and L4). If the catheter is only temporary, it is connected to tubing positioned along the spine and over the patient's/client's shoulder. The entire catheter and tubing length is taped for stability and protection, and the end of the catheter can then be placed on the patient's/client's chest for the nurse's ready access (Lonsway, 1988). Permanent catheters may be tunnelled subcutaneously through the skin and exit at the patient's/client's side.

Due to the location of the catheter, strict surgical aseptic technique (see Chapter 28) is required to prevent serious and potentially fatal infection. Doctors should be notified immediately of any signs or symptoms of infection or pain at the insertion site. Thorough nursing care is needed during hygiene procedures to keep the catheter system clean and dry.

Nurses receive special training for the administration of epidural analgesia. Opioid analgesics such as preservative-free morphine sulphate is one of the more common medications given. The opioids act like large doses of endorphins, blocking pain transmission. A local anaesthetic such as bupivacaine may also be administered. The anaesthetic blocks pain conduction through local peripheral nerve fibres around the site of insertion. Bupivacaine also blocks the sympathetic nervous system, causing side effects such as hypotension, reduced intestinal peristalsis, and bladder dysfunction. Infusions may be given by intermittent injection or continuously through established epidural catheters (see Chapter 31). Continuous infusions must be administered through electronic infusion devices for proper control.

The nursing implications for managing epidural analgesia are considerable. Monitoring of the medication's effects differs, depending on whether infusions are intermittent or continuous, with respiratory depression as the most serious side effect. When patients/clients are started on epidural anaesthesia, monitoring can occur as often as every 15 minutes. The patient/client must receive thorough education about epidural analgesia in terms of the action of the medication and its advantages and disadvantages. A patient/client on long-term therapy can be taught to safely administer infusions in the home with minimal ongoing intervention by the nurse.

## Promoting Wellness

Pain can seriously disable and immobilize an individual, resulting in impaired self-care ability. Pain can also change self-esteem and desire to socialize with others. The nurse can help the individual and family members to find ways to cope with pain and maintain a normal lifestyle.

The nurse acts to minimize potential effects of immobilization (see Chapter 24) by practising effective positioning techniques. Regular turning, range-of-motion exercise, and anatomical alignment of body parts can prevent painful contractures from developing. When a patient/client is mobile, the nurse ensures that painful body parts are protected. Elastic bandages, braces, splints, or even pillows can support injured parts during movement. If crutches or other aids are required, the nurse ensures that they are used properly, in conjunction with the physiotherapist or occupational therapist. This reduces the patient's/client's risk of further injury or pain.

Painful disorders of the upper extremities can create difficulty in eating, bathing, grooming, and dressing. The nurse may refer a patient/client to an occupational therapist who can devise ways to maintain function, even when finger movement or grasp is impaired. Eating utensils, a comb and brush, and a toothbrush can be attached to extension devices. These devices have enlarged handles or splints that allow patients/clients to pick up the items. Clothing fasteners made from Velcro tape® make it easier for patients/clients to remove or apply clothing, and shirts or blouses can be sewn so that garments can simply be pulled on or off over the head.

A warm bath can be relaxing and personal cleanliness can also promote comfort. If chronic pain exists, encourage family members to help patients/clients maintain their personal hygiene in the home.

With fatigue, pain perception can increase. Therefore, wherever possible, procedures within a health care setting should be planned around rest periods. Patients/clients with chronic discomfort should be encouraged to rest before social activities in the home.

A person with pain may avoid sexual activity for fear that it will cause or aggravate discomfort. However, the need for sexual warmth is not negated by pain (Cash, 1984). Patients/clients can learn to express themselves sexually regardless of pain. A person whose movement is restricted by pain may not be able to assume the positions for intercourse. Alternative positions may be less uncomfortable and strenuous. Nurses should also advise patients/clients that tranquilizers, muscle relaxants, and strong analgesics can all decrease libido and potency.

## Surgical Measures for Pain Relief

When a patient's/client's pain persists despite medical treatment and it is clear that the pain is physical and not psychological, surgical interventions may give relief. A **posterior rhizotomy** involves surgically cutting the dorsal (posterior) roots of a spinal nerve. The resection involves the posterior root of the spinal cord. It is effective for relieving localized acute pain in the area supplied by the nerve root and deep visceral pain. The patient/client loses sensation of pain but retains full motor function.

A **chordotomy** is more extensive and involves resection of the thoracic or cervical spinal cord at various levels. The procedure is used to treat intractable or unrelieved pain. The higher the focus of pain, the higher the site selected for a chordotomy. For example, pain in the thorax, upper extremities, and shoulders requires a high cervical chordotomy. The risks of the procedure are great because permanent paralysis may result from oedema of the spinal cord or accidental resection of motor nerves. After the procedure the patient/client has a permanent loss of pain and temperature sensation in the affected areas. If the surgery is uncomplicated, the senses of touch and position are retained.

## TABLE 27-6 Types of Local Anaesthesia by Injection

| Type | Area of Injection | Area Anaesthetized | Indications for Use |
|---|---|---|---|
| Infiltration | In superficial area under skin or mucous membranes | Small peripheral nerves to area infiltrated | Small incisions of skin, insertion of sutures to close cuts or wounds, minor dental repairs |
| Peripheral nerve block | In area surrounding large peripheral nerve at point above bifurcation of nerve | Wider area than with infiltration, numbing entire body part (e.g. hand, upper gums, foot) | Major dental repairs, manipulation or reduction of extremity fractures, minor hand and foot surgery |
| Epidural or peridural nerve block | In lumbosacral region of spinal cord, around major nerve roots exiting base of spinal cord at site outside dura mater | Lower trunk and extremities | Delivery of newborn, major surgery to lower trunk and extremities (e.g. haemorrhoidectomy, vascular repair) |
| Spinal nerve block | Around major nerve root within subarachnoid space of spinal cord | Lower trunk and extremities | Major surgery to lower trunk and extremities, patients/clients at risk with general anaesthesia |

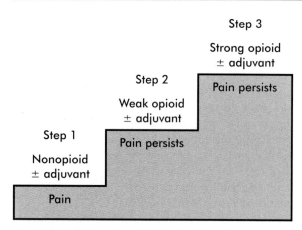

Step 3
Strong opioid
± adjuvant

Pain persists

Step 2
Weak opioid
± adjuvant

Pain persists

Step 1
Nonopioid
± adjuvant

Pain

**Fig. 27-9** WHO's analgesic ladder is a three-step approach to using drugs in cancer pain management. ± *adjuvant*, With or without adjuvant medications.
From World Health Organization: *Cancer pain relief and palliative care: report of a WHO Expert Committee*, WHO Tech Rep Series NO 804, Geneva, 1990, The Organization.

## Patients/Clients with Chronic Cancer Pain

**Intractable pain** cannot be permanently relieved, and the pain can become so debilitating that it encompasses a patient's/client's total existence. Cleeland (1984) notes that one in three people with metastatic cancer report pain that interferes with their quality of life. One of the greatest nursing challenges is to care for the patient/client with intractable pain.

When treatment to control the spread of cancer fails, analgesic medication may be one of the only ways to alleviate suffering. Administration of analgesics in treatment of cancer-related pain requires application of principles different from those used to treat acute pain. The World Health Organization (1986) recommends a three-step approach to managing cancer pain (Fig. 27-9). Basically, therapy begins with nonopioids and then progresses to strong opioids if pain persists. When a person with cancer first experiences pain, it is important to begin with a dosage that is adequate for relief. In addition, there is rigorous treatment of the side effects of analgesia, such as nausea and constipation, so that analgesia can be continued.

Studies show that drug dependence is low among people with cancer-related pain (Porter and Jick, 1980). Administering the right drug and the required dose at the proper interval alleviates the fear of pain, protects the person from drug-seeking behaviour, and reduces the incidence of dependence. It has also been shown that some dying patients/clients with prolonged pain develop a physiological tolerance to analgesics. As a result, these people may require higher doses of analgesics to attain the same level of pain relief. Higher analgesic doses in individuals who have become tolerant to strong opioids are not usually dangerous because patients/clients also develop tolerance to central nervous system depression (Hanks and Hoskin, 1987).

The aim of drug therapy for patients/clients with cancer is to anticipate and minimize pain, as well as to provide complete relief. It is therefore necessary to give required doses on a regular basis. Prescribing analgesics on an as-required basis for people who have cancer is ineffective and causes more suffering. The cancer patient/client must take an analgesic regularly, even when the pain subsides.

### Adult Nursing
### Patient-controlled analgesia in the home

In the home, patients/clients may use ambulatory infusion pumps. The pumps are lightweight and compact (about the size of a transistor radio) and allow free movement. The pump is battery powered and worn in a pouch attached to a belt or harness. The bag or syringe fits inside the pump. A dosage of diamorphine, delivered continuously over 24 hours, is usually slowly infused via a subcutaneous infusion device, or if one is already *in situ* following cancer therapy, a central venous catheter. These large catheters, inserted into the patient's/client's subclavian vein in the hospital, are relatively easy to maintain and can be left in place for an extended period. The patient/client and family learn to manage the pump, observe for side effects, and maintain function of the administration set. Because the individual is established on a stable dose of analgesic in the hospital prior to going home, the risk of side effects is not as great unless a significant increase in the dose of the drug is required. A community or Macmillan nurse makes routine visits to ensure that the individual and his or her family are supported and are managing the pump correctly. The fluid reservoir and tubing are usually changed at least once a week by the nurse, to maintain the sterility of the drug delivery system.

## Pain Clinics and Hospices

During the last decade, health professionals from the United Kingdom and America have recognized pain as a significant health problem. With an increased awareness of the multiple problems that pain can cause for patients/clients, specialist centres have been established for pain management. Pain clinics offer several options. A comprehensive pain clinic can treat individuals on an inpatient and outpatient basis. Staff members representing all health care disciplines such as nursing, medicine, physiotherapy, and dietetics work with patients/clients to find the most effective pain-relief measures. This may include the use of a range of recognized complementary therapies (see Chapter 32). A comprehensive clinic provides not only diverse therapy but also research into new treatments and training for professionals.

**Hospices** care for those who are dying and for their families. Hospice comes from the Latin word *hospes*, which means 'a place to rest'. These services help dying people continue to live at home in comfort and privacy with the help of home care teams. Individuals can receive the proper dosage and forms of analgesics that provide pain relief, and under the guidance of specialist nurses, families learn to monitor clients' symptom control and become the primary care givers.

 **EVALUATION**

The patient/client is the best resource for evaluating the effectiveness of pain-relief measures. The nurse must continually determine whether the character of the patient's/client's pain changes and whether individual interventions are effective. The

## Sample Evaluation of Interventions for Pain

| Goals | Expected Outcomes | Evaluative Measures |
|---|---|---|
| Patient/client will achieve control of pain within 24 hr of surgery. | Patient/client will express relief during PCA infusion. | Have patient/client report severity of pain on scale of 1 to 10, 2 hr after initiating PCA and at least every 4 hr thereafter. |
| | Patient/client will initiate movement in bed without painful behaviour cues. | Observe patient's/client's posture in bed, ease of position change, and facial expression. |
| Patient/client will perform self-care by discharge. | Patient/client will independently perform self-care activities. | Observe patient/client while dressing, eating, bathing, and grooming. |
| Patient/client will use pain-relief measures in the home. | Patient/client will state he/she understands the prescribed analgesic regime. | Ask patient/client to demonstrate relaxation techniques. Patient/client will perform relaxation exercise. Have patient/client explain analgesic use. |

family is often another valuable resource, particularly in the case of the person with cancer who may not be able to express discomfort during the latter stages of advanced illness. The nurse is successful in relieving pain when the mutually determined goals of care are met. The nurse uses evaluative criteria in determining the outcome of pain-relief interventions (see evaluation box).

While the majority of pain assessment/evaluation is obtained and communicated verbally, it is of paramount importance that this information is accurately documented in writing in order to enhance continuity of patient/client care (Albrecht *et al*, 1992). This can be achieved through the use of formal pain assessment tools/charts or through succinct written documentation in the patient's/client's nursing notes.

If the nurse determines that a patient/client continues to have discomfort after interventions, it may be necessary to try different or additional measures. For example, if an analgesic provides only partial relief, the nurse may add relaxation or guided-imagery exercises. The nurse may also consult with the doctor about trying different analgesics.

The nurse also evaluates the patient's/client's perceptions of the effectiveness of pain management. The patient/client may help decide the best times to attempt an intervention. For example, the patient/client is the best judge of whether a nursing intervention works better when anxiety and irritability are absent or when the pain is most severe.

The nurse and patient/client jointly determine the response to interventions and the overall relief obtained. For example, if a nurse administers an analgesic, side effects from the medication and the patient's/client's reported pain relief must be assessed. Similarly, after turning a patient/client, the nurse should return to determine whether the patient/client is tolerating the new position and whether pain has subsided. If an intervention aggravates discomfort, the nurse must stop it immediately and seek an alternative.

The nurse and patient/client should not become frustrated if

an intervention does not work quickly. Time and patience may be necessary to observe the maximum effect of a pain relief measure. The nurse considers factors that may be influencing the patient's/client's perceptions or reactions to pain. For example, a massage may prove ineffective if the patient/client has just learned the results of diagnostic tests and has had no opportunity to express concerns. The nurse should evaluate the entire pain experience to determine which are the most effective interventions and the times at which they should be administered.

## SUMMARY

Pain is a common problem faced in all health care settings. Although a subjective and highly individualized experience, the meaning that pain conveys, the threat it poses to comfort, and its potential as an indicator of serious illness, means it can cause very real feelings of fear and distress.

Pain comprises the three components of reception, perception, and reaction. It can result from either mechanical, chemical, thermal or electrical sources, each of which are associated with particular types of conditions. A basic understanding of the relationship between the physiological, psychological, and cognitive variables, as described in the gate control theory of pain, provides the nurse with a conceptual basis for pain-relief measures.

It is also important that the nurse is aware of the common behavioural responses to pain, in order to meet patient/client needs. The nurse should be alert for patterns of behaviour that may indicate pain and should encourage patients/clients to communicate their pain response effectively. This enables the nurse to understand the experience as fully as possible and to match the patient's/client's physiological condition with suitable pain-relief interventions. The different methods of pain relief required by individuals with acute or chronic types of pain is another important consideration.

The experience of pain is unique to each individual, and the nurse should always be aware of the developmental or environmental factors that may influence the pain response. The measures of pain control implemented for each patient/client should also be individualized. An understanding of the role of pain as a protective physiological mechanism, and an awareness of any personal prejudices and misconceptions, enables the nurse to work closely with the patient/client to provide effective relief.

## CHAPTER 27 REVIEW

### Key Concepts
- Pain is frequently a protective mechanism that warns of tissue injury.
- A nurse's misconceptions about pain may result in doubt about the extent of the patient's/client's suffering and in an unwillingness to provide relief.
- Knowledge of the three components of the pain experience – reception, perception, and reaction – provides the nurse with guidelines for determining pain-relief measures.
- An interaction of affective and cognitive factors affects pain perception.
- The pain experience is influenced by a variety of variables, including age, gender, culture, anxiety, meaning of pain, and previous experience.
- The difference between acute and chronic pain involves duration of discomfort, physical signs and symptoms, and the patient's/client's perceptions regarding their pain and pain relief.
- Chronic pain can affect every aspect of life and lead to psychosocial problems.
- The nurse does not conduct a pain assessment when the patient/client is experiencing severe discomfort.
- Pain assessment scales are used to objectively evaluate the effectiveness of pain relief interventions.
- Pain can cause physical signs and symptoms similar to the signs and symptoms of certain disease processes.
- To provide maximum pain relief the nurse develops a therapeutic relationship with the patient/client and provides patient/client education about pain.
- The nurse individualizes pain relief measures by collaborating closely with the patient/client, using assessment findings, and trying a variety of interventions.
- Eliminating sources of painful stimuli is a basic nursing measure for promoting comfort.
- Proper administration of analgesics requires the nurse to know the patient's/client's response to the drugs, select the correct medication, and administer an appropriate dose in a timely manner.
- Using a regular schedule for analgesic administration is more effective than an as-required schedule in controlling pain.
- A patient-controlled analgesic device gives patients/clients control of their pain relief.

- While caring for a patient/client who receives local anaesthesia, the nurse protects the patient/client from injury.
- Nursing implications for administering epidural analgesia include preventing infection and monitoring closely for signs of respiratory depression.
- The aim of pain management for patients/clients with cancer is to anticipate and prevent pain rather than treat it once it has recurred.
- Evaluation of the patient's/client's pain management requires consideration of the changing character of pain, response to interventions, and the patient's/client's perceptions of their effectiveness.

## CRITICAL THINKING EXERCISES

1. What factors influence the way in which a person communicates his or her experience of pain?
2. Outline the gate theory of pain transmission.
3. Describe formal and informal methods of pain assessment.
4. Mrs Duncan has chronic pain associated with metastatic cancer in her pelvis and both femurs. The pain makes it difficult for her to attend to her own personal hygiene needs, or to mobilize freely. Morphine sulphate elixir 30 mg every 4 hours has been prescribed for Mrs Duncan.

   What principles of analgesic use should the nurse follow in administering morphine sulphate? If morphine sulphate proves ineffective, what other measures could be employed?
5. Mr McKeown returned from theatre 6 hours ago, following a laparotomy, he has yet to require analgesia from ward staff. The nurse notices Mr McKeown having difficulty turning onto his side and grimacing when he moves. His blood pressure and pulse rate are moderately elevated.

   What pain relief measures would be appropriate for the nurse to use with Mr McKeown?

### Key Terms

Acute pain, p. 544
Aftermath (of pain), p. 543
Analgesia, p. 557
Analgesics, p. 557
Anticipation phase, p. 542
Biofeedback, p. 557
Chemical stimuli, p. 538
Chordotomy, p. 561
Chronic malignant pain, p. 544
Chronic nonmalignant pain, p. 544
Co-analgesics, p. 558
Concomitant symptoms, p. 551
Cutaneous stimulation, p. 555
Descriptive pain scales, p. 549
Electrical stimuli, p. 538
Equianalgesic dosage, p. 558

# REFERENCES

Albrecht MN *et al*: Factors influencing staff nurse's decisions for non-documentation of patient response to analgesia administration *J Clin Nurs* 1: 243, 1992.

Anderson S et al, editors: *Chronic non-cancer pain*, London, 1987, MTP Press Ltd.

Burns JW et al: The influence of patient characteristics on the requirements for postoperative analgesia, *Anaesthesia* 44:2, 1989.

Cartwright A: *Human relations and hospital care*, London, 1964, Routledge & Kegan Paul.

Cash JT: Sexuality and chronic pain, *Am j Nurs*, 84:1417, 1984

Ceccio CM: Heat vs cold as treatment for arthritic pain, *RN* 53:83, 1990.

Cleeland CS: The impact of pain on the patient with cancer, *Cancer* 54(suppl):2635, 1984.

Copp LA: Pain coping. In Copp LA, editor: *Perspectives on pain: recent advances in nursing*. London, 1985, Churchill Livingstone.

Engber E: Report on the NIH consensus development conference on pain, *J Pain Symptom Manage* 1:165, 1986.

Fields HL: *Pain,* New York, 1987, McGraw-Hill.

Flor H et al: Efficacy of EMG biofeedback, pseudotherapy and conventional medical treatment for chronic rheumatic back pain, *Pain* 17:21, 1983.

Gil K: Psychologic aspects of acute pain, *Anesthesiol Report* 2(2):246, 1990.

Hanks GW, editor: Pain and cancer, *Cancer Surveys* 7:1, 1988.

Hanks GW, Hoskin PJ: Opioid analgesics in the management of pain in patients with cancer: a review, *Palliative Medicine* 1:1, 1987.

Hargreaves A, Lander J: Use of transcutaneous electrical nerve stimulation for postoperative pain, *Nurs Res* 38(3):159, 1989.

Harrison A: Assessing patients' pain: identifying reasons for error, *J Adv Nurs* 16:1018, 1991.

Hayward J: *Information - A Prescription against pain*, London, 1975, Royal College of Nursing.

Heidrich G, Perry S: Helping the patient in pain, *Am J Nurs* 82:1828, 1982.

Herr KA, Mobily PR: Complexities of pain assessment in the elderly, *J Gerontol Nurs* 17(4):12, 1991.

Holm K et al: Effect of personal pain experience on pain assessment, *Image J Nurs Scho* 21(2):72, 1989.

International Association for the Study of Pain, Subcommittee on Taxonomy: Pain terms: a list with definitions and notes on usage, *Pain* 6:249, 1979.

Jones VA, Hanks GW: New portable infusion pump for prolonged administration of opioid analgesics in patients with advanced cancer, *BMJ* 292:1496, 1986.

Krieger D: Therapeutic touch: the imprimatur of nursing, *Am J Nurs* 75:784, 1975.

Lipton JA, Marbach JJ: Ethnicity and pain experience, *Soc Sci Med* 19(12):1279, 1984.

Lonsway RA: Care of the patient with an epidural: an infection-control challenge, *JIV Nurs*, 11

Marks RM, Sachar EJ: Undertreatment of medical inpatients with narcotic analgesics, *Ann Intern Med* 78:173, 1973.

Marzinski LR: The tragedy of dementia: clinically assessing pain in the confused, nonverbal elderly, *J Gerontol Nurs* 17(6):25, 1991.

Mayer DK: Non-pharmacologic management of pain in the person with cancer, *Adv Nurs* 10:325, 1985.

McCaffery M: *Nursing management of the patient with pain*, ed 2, Philadelphia, 1979, Lippincott.

McCaffery M: Understanding your client's pain, *Nurs* 80(10):26, 1980.

McCaffery M, Beebe A: Pain in the elderly: special considerations. In McCaffery M, Beebe A, Latham J (editor): *Pain: clinical manual for nursing practice,* London, 1994a, Mosby.

McCaffrey M, Beebe A: Pain in children: special considerations. In McCaffery M, Beebe A, Latham J, editors: *Pain: clinical manual for nursing practice,* London, 1994b, Mosby.

McGuire DB: The measurement of clinical pain, *Nurs Res* 33(3): 152, 1984.

Meinhart NT, McCaffery M: *Pain: a nursing approach to assessment and analysis*, Norwalk, Conn, 1983, Appleton-Century-Crofts.

Melzack R, Dennis FG: Neurophysiological foundations of pain. In Sternbach RA, editor: *The psychology of pain*, New York, 1978, Raven.

Melzack R, Wall PD: *The challange of pain*, ed 2, UK, 1988, Penguin Books.

Paice JA: Unraveling the mystery of pain, *Oncol Nurs Forum* 18(5):843, 1991.

Porter J, Jick H: Addiction rare in patients treated with narcotics, *N Eng J Med* 302:123, 1980.

Price DD et al: Psychophysical analysis of experimental factors that selectively influence the affective dimension of pain, *Pain* 8(2):137, 1980.

Rankin MA, Snider B: Nurses' perceptions of cancer patients' pain, *Cancer Nurs* 7:149, 1984.

Reuler JB et al: The chronic pain syndrome: misconceptions and management, *Ann Intern Med* 93:5588, 1980.

Ross DM, Ross SA: *Childhood pain: current issues, research, and management,* Baltimore, 1988, Urban & Schwarzenberg.

Schultheis K et al: Preparation for stressful medical procedures and person-treatment interactions, *Clin Psych Rev* 7:329, 1987.

Schultz R: Emotionality and ageing: a theoretical and empirical analysis, *J Gerontol* 37(1), 1982.

Spiegel D, Bloom J: Pain in metastatic breast cancer, *Cancer* 52(2):341, 1983.

Taylor AG et al: How effective is TENS for acute pain? *Am J Nurs* 83:1171, 1983.

Taylor AG et al: Duration of pain, condition, and physical pathology as determinants of nurses' assessment of patients in pain, *Nurs Res* 33:4, 1984.

Townsend P et al: *Inequalities in health: the Black Report; the health divide,* Harmondsworth, 1992, Penguin Books.

Turnage G et al: Spinal opioids: a nursing perspective, *J Pain Symptom Manag* 5(3):154, 1990.

Twycross RG, Lack SA: *Symptom control in far advanced cancer: pain relief,* London, 1983, Pitman.

Walding MF: Pain, anxiety and powerlessness, *J Advs Nurs* 16:388, 1991.

White ID et al: Analgesics in cancer pain: current practices and beliefs, *Br J Cancer* 63:271, 1991.

Wilkie DJ: Cancer pain management: state-of-the-art nursing care, *Nurs Clin North Am* 25(2):331, 1990.

Witt J: Relieving chronic pain, *Nurs Pract* 9:36, 1984.

Wong DL, Baker CM: Pain in children: comparison of assessment scales, *Ped Nurs* 14(1):9, 1988.

World Health Organization: *Cancer pain relief,* Geneva, 1986, The Organization.

Zborowski M: *People in pain,* San Francisco, 1969, Jossey-Bass.

Zoob M: Differentiating the causes of chest pain, *Geriatrics* 33:95, 1978.

# FURTHER READING

## Adult Nursing

Bast C, Hayes P: Patient-controlled analgesia, *Nurs 86* 16(1):25, 1986.

Bast C, Hayes P: PCA: a new way to spell pain relief, *RN* 49(8):18, 1986.

Churchill W: The point of health. *Nursing Times* 84(44): 38, 1988.

Craig KD: Social modelling influences in pain. In Sternbach RA, editor: *The psychology of pain*, ed 2, New York, 1986, Raven.

Dimotto JW: Relaxation, *Am J Nurs* 84:754, 1984.

Hannon D et al: Pain: portable relief for terminal patients, *RN* 48:37, 1985.

Holm K et al: Effect of personal pain experience on pain assessment, *Image J Nurs Sch* 21(2):72, 1989.

Kanner RM, Portenoy RK: Are the people who need analgesics getting them? *Am J Nurs* 86:589, 1986.

Keller E, Bzdek VM: Effects of therapeutic touch on tension headache pain, *Nurs Res* 35:101, 1986.

LaFoy J, Geden EA: Postepisiotomy pain: warm versus cold sitz bath, *JOGNN* 18:399, 1989.

Melzack R: The McGill pain questionnaire: major properties and scoring methods, *Pain* 1:277, 1975.

Proctor MR, Warfield CA: Biofeedback pain control, *Hosp Pract* 12:104, 1984.

Wells N: The effect of relaxation on postoperative muscle tension and pain, *Nurs Res* 31:236, 1982.

Williams DJ: Pushbutton pain relief puts the patient in control, *Am J Nurs* 85:1458, 1985.

Zahourek RP: Hypnosis in nursing practice: emphasis on the 'problem patient' who has pain, *J Psychosoc Nurs* 20:13, 1982.

## Children's Nursing

Côté JJ, Morse JM, James SG: The pain response of the postoperative newborn. *J Adv Nurs* 16: 378, 1991.

Levitt G: Pain relief in babies – a not so simple problem, *Matern Child Health* 121, 1989.

Mc Grath PA: Issues in pediatric symptom control: Part 1 - Evaluating a child's pain. *J Pain Symptom Manag* 4(4): 1989.

Mercer G: A child's magic world where pain melts away, *The Independent* 17.2.87:13, 1987.

Price S: Pain: its experience, assessment and management in children, *Nurs Times* (occasional paper) 86(9):42, 1990.

Reape D: Children and pain, *Nurs Stand* 4(16):33, 1990.

Ross D, Ross S: *Childhood pain: current issues, research and management,* Baltimore, Maryland, 1988, Urban & Schwartzenberg.

Schultz N: How children perceive pain, *Nurs Outlook* 19:760, 1971.

# Controlling Infection

## CHAPTER OUTLINE

**Nature of Infection**
*Chain of infection*
*Course of infection*
*Defences against infection*

**Nosocomial Infections**
*Concept of asepsis*

**The Nursing Process in Infection Control**
*Assessment*
*Planning*
*Implementation*
*Evaluation*

## OBJECTIVES

After studying this chapter, you should be able to:
- *Define the key terms listed.*
- *Explain the cyclical nature of the chain of infection and factors involved at each stage.*
- *Give an example for preventing infection for each element of the infection chain.*
- *Describe the development of inflammation during the inflammatory response, differentiating between vascular and cellular responses.*
- *Explain the difference between cell-mediated and humoral immunity.*
- *Discuss the causes of nosocomial infection transmission in the health care setting and differentiate between medical and surgical aseptic techniques.*
- *Perform an assessment of a patient/client at risk of infection and describe symptoms of localized and systemic infection.*
- *Identify the techniques and rationales of infection control.*
- *Compare body substance isolation with universal blood and body fluid precautions.*
- *Discuss the psychosocial needs of the isolated patient/client.*
- *Correctly perform protective isolation and thorough handwashing techniques.*
- *Correctly apply a surgical mask, sterile gown, sterile gloves, and other protective equipment.*

Good health depends in part on a safe environment. Infection control practices control or eliminate sources of infection and help protect patients/clients and health care staff from disease and infection. A person entering a health care setting (for example a hospital, a health centre or a residential home) could be at risk for acquiring infections because of lowered resistance to infectious microorganisms, increased exposure to numbers and types of disease-causing organisms, and invasive procedures. Nurses come into contact with a variety of microorganisms and thus must practise infection-control techniques to avoid spreading them to patients/clients.

In the home an individual must recognize sources of infection and be able to institute protective measures. The nurse is responsible for teaching patients/clients about infection, mode of transmission, reasons for susceptibility, and infection control.

The nurse's knowledge of infection, application of infection control principles, and use of common sense help protect patients/clients from infection. **Control of infection is an important part of every action the nurse performs.**

## NATURE OF INFECTION

An **infection** is an invasion of the body by **pathogens**, that is any microorganism capable of producing disease. If the microorganisms fail to cause serious injury to cells or tissues, the infection is **asymptomatic**. Disease and disorders result if the pathogens multiply and cause an alteration in normal tissue function. If the infection can be transmitted directly from one person to another, it is an **infectious** or **contagious disease**, which may be communicable.

## Chain of Infection

The presence of a pathogen does not mean that an infection will begin. Development of an infection occurs in a cyclical process that depends on the following elements:

- an infectious agent or pathogen
- a reservoir or source for pathogen growth
- a portal of exit from the reservoir
- a mode of transmission
- a portal of entry to host
- a susceptible host.

An infection will develop if this chain remains intact (Fig. 28-1). Nurses use aseptic practices to break an element of the chain so that infection will not develop.

## Infectious Agent

Pathogenic organisms include bacteria, viruses, fungi, and protozoa (Table 28-1). Pathogens on the skin are resident or transient. **Resident** pathogens are normally present and stable in number. They survive and multiply on the skin. Most are found in superficial skin layers, but some inhabit deep epidermal layers. Resident pathogens are not easily removed by handwashing with plain soaps and detergents unless considerable friction is used. Resident microorganisms in deep skin layers are usually killed only by handwashing with products containing antimicrobial agents.

**Transient** pathogens attach to the skin when a person has contact with another object during normal activities of living. For example, if you touch a bedpan or a contaminated dressing, transient bacteria adhere to the skin. The organisms attach loosely to the skin in dirt and grease or under fingernails. Frequent, thorough handwashing removes transient pathogens easily.

The potential for microorganisms or parasites to cause disease depends on the following factors:

- number of organisms
- **virulence**, or ability to produce infection
- ability to enter and survive in the host
- susceptibility of host.

Many resident skin microorganisms are not highly virulent and cause only minor skin infections. However, they can cause serious infection when surgery or other invasive procedures allow them to enter deep tissues or when a patient/client is severely **immunocompromised** (impaired immune system).

## Reservoir

Microorganisms have many sources or reservoirs for growth. One of the most common is the body itself. A variety of organisms live on the surface of the skin and within body cavities, fluids, and discharges. The presence of microorganisms does not always cause a person to be ill. **Carriers** are people or animals who show no symptoms of illness but who have pathogens on or in their bodies that can be transferred to others. For example, a person can be a carrier of hepatitis B virus or *Staphylococcus* organisms without having manifestations of infection.

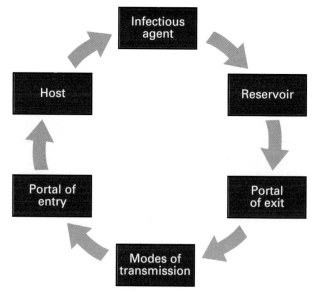

**Fig. 28-1** Chain of infection.

Some areas of the body contain larger populations of resident flora than others; these include the skin, respiratory tract, mouth, vagina, colon, and lower urethra. Areas of the body normally considered sterile, without organism growth, are the bloodstream, spinal fluid, peritoneal cavity, urinary tract, muscles, bones, and chambers of the eye. The entrance of a foreign object into a sterile site increases the risk for infection.

Animals, plants, insects, and inanimate objects (such as hospital sinks and baths) are also reservoirs for infectious organisms, for example, shellfish can become contaminated with *Vibrio cholerae*, the bacterium that causes cholera. Suction drainage bottles collect fluids that become a reservoir for microorganisms such as *Pseudomonas* organisms.

Food, water, and milk are additional reservoirs for pathogens. *Clostridium botulinum* toxin survives in improperly stored food, such as unrefrigerated milk products, to cause botulism. The bacterium, *Legionella pneumophila*, which causes legionnaires' disease, lives in contaminated, pooled water.

To thrive, organisms require food and a conducive environment to survive. Characteristics of an environment that supports organism growth include food, oxygen, water, temperature, pH, and light.

### FOOD

Microorganisms require nourishment. Some, such as *Clostridium perfringens*, the microbe that causes gas gangrene, thrive on organic matter. Others, such as *E. coli*, consume undigested foodstuffs in the bowel. Carbon dioxide and inorganic material such as soil provide nourishment for other organisms. In a health care environment, bed linens and work surfaces soiled with body secretions can become food sources for microorganisms.

### OXYGEN

**Aerobic bacteria** require free oxygen for survival and for multiplication sufficient to cause disease. Aerobic organisms tend to cause more infections in humans. Examples of aerobic

## TABLE 28-1 Common Pathogens and Some Infections or Diseases They Produce

| Organism | Reservoir | Infection or Disease |
| --- | --- | --- |
| **Bacteria** | | |
| *Escherichia coli* | Colon | Enteritis |
| *Staphylococcus aureus* | Skin, hair, anterior nares | Wound infection, pneumonia, food poisoning, cellulitis |
| *Streptococcus* (beta-haemolytic group A) organisms | Oropharynx, skin, perianal area | 'Strep throat', rheumatic fever, scarlet fever, impetigo |
| *Streptococcus* (beta-haemolytic group B) organisms | Adult genitalia | Urinary tract infection, wound infection, endometritis |
| *Mychobacterium tuberculosis* | Lungs | Tuberculosis |
| *Neisseria gonorrhoeae* | Genitourinary tract, rectum, mouth, eye | Gonorrhoea, pelvic inflammatory disease, infectious arthritis, conjunctivitis |
| *Staphylococcus epidermidis* | Skin | Wound infection, bacteraemia |
| **Viruses** | | |
| Hepatitis A virus | Faeces, blood, urine | Infectious hepatitis |
| Hepatitis B virus | Faeces, blood, all body fluids and excretions | Serum hepatitis |
| Herpes simplex virus (type 1) | Lesions of mouth, skin, blood, excretions | Cold sores, aseptic meningitis, sexually transmitted disease |
| Human immunodeficiency virus (HIV) | Blood, semen, vaginal secretions (also isolated in saliva, tears, urine, breast milk but not proven to be sources of transmission) | Acquired immunodeficiency syndrome (AIDS) |
| **Fungi** | | |
| *Aspergillus* organisms | Mouth, skin, colon, genital tract | Thrush, dermatitis |
| Candida albicans | Soil, dust | Aspergillosis |
| **Protozoa** | | |
| *Plasmodium falciparum* | Mosquito | Malaria |

organisms are *S. aureus* and strains of *Streptococcus* organisms.

**Anaerobic bacteria** thrive where little or no free oxygen is available. Infections deep within the pleural cavity, in a joint, or in a deep sinus tract are typically caused by anaerobes. Bacteria that cause tetanus, gas gangrene, and botulism are anaerobes.

## WATER
Most organisms require water for survival. The spirochete that causes syphilis, *Treponema pallidum*, lives only in a moist environment. Some bacteria assume a form resistant to drying. These spore-forming bacteria, such as those that cause anthrax, botulism, and tetanus, can live without water.

## TEMPERATURE
Microorganisms can live only in certain temperature ranges. However, some can survive temperature extremes that would be

fatal to humans. Some viruses are resistant to boiling water. Cold temperatures tend to prevent growth and reproduction of bacteria (**bacteriostasis**). A temperature that destroys bacteria is **bacteriocidal**.

## pH
The acidity of an environment determines the viability of microorganisms. Most microorganisms prefer an alkaline environment within a pH range of 5 to 8. Bacteria in particular thrive in urine with a high pH. Organisms cannot survive the acid environment of the stomach.

## LIGHT
Microorganisms thrive in dark environments such as those under dressings and within body cavities. Ultraviolet light is effective in killing certain forms of bacteria.

## TABLE 28-2 Modes of Transmission

| Routes and Means | Examples of Organisms |
|---|---|
| **CONTACT** | |
| Direct contact, or direct physical transfer between infected person and susceptible host (e.g. turning patients/clients, giving baths, having sexual contact with infected person) | *Staphylococcus* organisms, *T. pallidum* (syphilis), herpes simplex virus |
| Indirect contact, personal contact of susceptible host with contaminated inanimate object (e.g. needles, bedpan, intravenous tubing, instruments and dressings, linen, dishes, cutlery) | Measles virus, hepatitis B virus, *Enterococcus* and *Pseudomonas* organisms |
| Droplet contact or infectious agent coming in contact with conjunctivae, nose, mouth of susceptible host (droplets travel less than 1 metre and therefore contact is not airborne) (e.g. coughing, sneezing) | Influenza virus, *Mycobacterium tuberculosis* (tuberculosis) |
| **AIR** | |
| Droplet nuclei, or residue of evaporated droplets remaining suspended in air (e.g. coughing, sneezing, talking) | Influenza virus, pneumococcus (pneumonia, meningitis, other infections), varicella-zoster virus (chickenpox) |
| Dust (contains infectious agent) | *Aspergillus* organisms (aspergillosis) |
| **VEHICLES** | |
| Contaminated items | *M. tuberculosis* (tuberculosis) |
| Liquids | |
| Water | *Bivrio cholerae* (cholera) |
| Drugs, solutions | *Pseudomonas* organisms |
| Blood | Hepatitis B virus |
| Food (improperly handled or stored, fresh fruits and vegetables) | *Salmonella, Staphylococcus, Enterobacter,* and *Klebsiella* organisms |
| **VECTORS** | |
| Insects | |
| Mosquitoes | *Plasmodium falciparum* (malaria) |
| Fleas, ticks, lice | *Rickettsia typhi* and *R. prowazekii* (typhus) |
| Animals (cows, pigs) | *Brucella* organisms (brucellosis) |

### Portal of Exit

After microorganisms find a site to grow and multiply, they must find a portal of exit if they are to enter another host and cause disease. When the human is the reservoir, microorganisms can exit through a variety of sites, for example:

* skin and mucous membranes
* respiratory tract
* urinary tract
* gastrointestinal tract
* reproductive tract
* blood.

### Modes of Transmission

There are many vehicles for transmission of microorganisms from the reservoir to the host. Table 28-2 summarizes common modes of transmission. Certain infectious diseases tend to be transmitted more commonly by specific modes. However, the same microorganisms may be transmitted by more than one route. For example, herpes zoster may be spread by the airborne route in droplet nuclei or by direct contact.

Almost any object within the environment (for example, a stethoscope or thermometer) can become a means of transmitting infection. All hospital personnel providing direct care and performing diagnostic and support services must follow practices to minimize the spread of infection. Each group follows procedures for handling equipment and supplies used by a patient/client. Certain devices and diagnostic procedures provide avenues for growth and spread of pathogens. Invasive procedures such as cystoscopy (visualization of the bladder) facilitate diagnosis of problems but also increase the risk of transmitting infection. Since so many factors can promote the spread of infection to a patient/client, all health care workers must be conscientious in using infection-control practices.

### Portal of Entry

Organisms can enter the body through the same routes they use for exiting. For example, when a contaminated needle pierces a person's skin, organisms enter the body. Any obstruction to the flow of urine from a urinary catheter allows organisms to travel up the urethra. Mishandling of sterile bandages over an open wound permits pathogens to enter exposed tissues. Factors that reduce the body's defences enhance the chances of pathogens entering the body.

## Susceptible Host

Whether a person acquires an infection depends on susceptibility to an infectious agent. **Susceptibility** is the degree of resistance an individual has to pathogens. Although everyone is constantly in contact with large numbers of microorganisms, an infection will not develop until an individual becomes susceptible to the strength and numbers of those microorganisms. The more virulent an organism, the greater the likelihood of a person's susceptibility. A person's natural defences against infection, as well as a number of other factors, influence susceptibility.

## Course of Infection

By understanding the chain of infection, the nurse can intervene to prevent infections from developing. When the patient/client acquires an infection, the nurse is able to observe signs and symptoms of infection and take appropriate actions to prevent its spread. Infections follow a progressive course (see box overleaf). The severity of the patient's/client's illness depends on the extent of the infection, the **pathogenicity** of the microorganisms, and susceptibility of the host.

If infection is **localized** (limited to a particular area such as a wound infection), proper care will control the spread and minimize the illness. Only localized symptoms such as pain and tenderness at the wound site will develop. An infection that affects the entire body instead of just a single organ or part is **systemic.** A systemic infection can progress and become fatal.

The course of an infection influences the level of nursing care provided. The nurse is responsible for properly administering prescribed antibiotics and monitoring the response to drug treatment.

Regardless of whether infection is localized or systemic, the nurse plays a dominant role in minimizing its spread. The organism causing a simple wound infection can spread to involve a recent surgical incision if the nurse uses poor technique during a dressing change. Nurses who have breaks in their own skin can also acquire infections from patients/clients if their techniques for controlling infection transmission are inadequate.

### Adult Nursing
### Infection in older adults

An infection in older adults may not present with typical signs and symptoms. Often older adults have advanced infection before it is identified because of their reduced inflammatory and immune responses. A reduced or absent fever response may occur from chronic use of aspirin or nonsteroidal anti-inflammatory drugs. Atypical symptoms such as confusion, incontinence, or agitation may be the only symptoms of an infectious illness (Tideiksaar, 1987).

## Defences Against Infection

The body has normal defences against infection. Normal body flora that reside inside and outside of the body protect a person from several pathogens. Each organ system has defence mechanisms that minimize exposure to infectious microorganisms. The **inflammatory response** is a protective vascular and cellular reaction that neutralizes pathogens and repairs body cells. Normal flora, body system defences, and inflammation are all nonspecific defences that protect against microorganisms regardless of prior exposure. The immune system is composed of separate cells and molecules resistant to disease. Certain responses of the immune system are nonspecific, whereas others are specific defences against specific pathogens. If any of the body's defences fail, an infection can quickly progress to a serious health problem.

## Normal Flora

The body normally contains microorganisms that reside on the surface and deep layers of skin, in the saliva and oral mucosa, and in the gastrointestinal tract. A person normally excretes millions of microbes daily through the intestines. The skin also has a large population of resident flora. Normal flora do not cause disease but instead participate in maintaining health.

Flora of the large intestine exist in large numbers without causing injury. These bacterial flora compete with disease-producing microorganisms for food. Flora also secrete antibacterial substances within the intestine's walls. The skin's flora exert a decontaminative action by inhibiting multiplication of organisms landing on the skin. The mouth and pharynx are also protected by flora that impair growth of invading microbes. The mass of normal flora maintains a sensitive balance with other microorganisms to prevent infection. Any factor that disrupts this balance places a person at serious risk for acquiring an infectious disease.

## Body System Defences

A number of the body's organ systems have unique defences against infection (Table 28-3). The skin, respiratory tract, and gastrointestinal tract are easily accessible to microorganisms. Pathogenic organisms easily adhere to the skin's surface, are inhaled into the lungs, or are ingested with food. Each organ system has defence mechanisms physiologically suited to its structure and function; for example, the lungs cannot completely control the entrance of microorganisms. However, the airways are lined with hair-like projections, or cilia, that

People from different ethnic groups may be susceptible to particular infections. Qureshi (1994) suggests that ethnic Asian people are genetically predisposed to bovine tuberculosis, which arises in the skin and upper cervical region. Qureshi claims that this arises in part because cow's milk is not pasteurized and because the cow, being a sacred animal in India, escapes the rigourous control of antitubercular vaccination.

Qureshi B T: *Transcultural medicine: dealing with patients from different cultures*, London, 1994, Kluwer Academic Publishers.

## Course of Infection by Stage

**INCUBATION PERIOD**
- Interval between entrance of pathogen into body and appearance of first symptoms (e.g. chickenpox, 2-3 weeks; common cold, 1-2 days; influenza, 1-3 days; mumps, 18 days).

**PRODROMAL STAGE**
- Interval from onset of nonspecific signs and symptoms (malaise, low-grade fever, fatigue) to more specific symptoms. (During this time, micro-organisms grow and multiply, and the patient/client is more capable of spreading disease to others.)

**ILLNESS STAGE**
- Interval when patient/client manifests signs and symptoms specific to type of infection (e.g. common cold manifested by sore throat, sinus congestion, rhinitis; mumps by earache, high fever, parotid and salivary gland swelling).

**CONVALESCENCE**
- Interval when acute symptoms of infection disappear. (Length of recovery depends on severity of infection and patient's/client's general state of health; recovery may take several days to months.)

rhythmically beat to move a blanket of mucus and adherent organisms up to the pharynx to be swallowed. Conditions that impair an organ's specialized defences increase susceptibility to infection.

## Inflammation

The body's cellular response to injury or infection is **inflammation**. Inflammation is a protective vascular reaction that delivers fluid, blood products, and nutrients to interstitial tissues in an area of injury. The process neutralizes and eliminates pathogens or dead **(necrotic)** tissues and establishes a means of repairing body cells and tissues. **Signs of inflammation include swelling, redness, heat, pain or tenderness, and loss of function in the affected body part.** When inflammation becomes systemic, other signs and symptoms develop, including fever, leucocytosis, malaise, anorexia, nausea, vomiting, and lymph node enlargement.

The inflammatory response may be triggered by physical agents, chemical agents, and microorganisms. Mechanical trauma, exposure to temperature extremes, and radiation are physical agents. Chemical agents include external and internal irritants such as harsh poisons or gastric acid. Microorganisms were previously discussed.

After tissues are injured, a series of well-coordinated events occurs. The inflammatory response includes the following:
1. vascular and cellular responses
2. formation of inflammatory exudate
3. tissue repair.

### VASCULAR AND CELLULAR RESPONSES

Acute inflammation is an immediate response to cellular injury. Arterioles supplying the infected or injured area dilate, allowing more blood into local circulation. The increase in local blood flow causes the characteristic redness of inflammation. The symptom of localized warmth results from a greater volume of blood at the inflammatory site. If the inflamed area is deep within the body, local warmth does not occur because the maximum body temperature is at the body's core. Local vasodilation delivers blood and leucocytes to injured tissues.

Injury causes tissue necrosis, and as a result the body releases histamine, bradykinin, prostaglandin, and serotonin. These chemical mediators increase the permeability of small blood vessels. Fluid, protein, and cells enter interstitial spaces. Accumulated fluid appears as localized swelling **(oedema)**.

Another sign of inflammation is pain. The swelling of inflamed tissues increases pressure on nerve endings, causing pain. Chemical substances such as histamine stimulate nerve endings. As a result of physiological changes occurring with inflammation, the involved body part usually undergoes a temporary loss of function. For example, a localized infection of the hand causes the fingers to become swollen, painful, and discoloured. Joints may become stiff as a result of swelling, but function of the fingers returns when inflammation subsides.

The cellular response of inflammation involves leucocytes arriving at the site. These pass through blood vessels and into the tissues. Through the process of **phagocytosis**, specialized leucocytes, neutrophils and monocytes, ingest and destroy microorganisms or other small particles. As inflammation becomes systemic, other signs and symptoms develop. **Leucocytosis**, or an increase in the number of circulating leucocytes, is the body's response to leucocytes leaving blood vessels. A serum leucocyte count is normally 5000 to 10,000/mm$^3$ but may rise to 15,000 to 20,000/mm$^3$ during inflammation. Fever is caused by phagocytic release of pyrogens from bacterial cells that cause a rise in the hypothalamic set point. Other systemic signs and symptoms include malaise, anorexia, and lymph node enlargement.

### INFLAMMATORY EXUDATE

Accumulation of fluid and dead tissue cells and leucocytes forms an **exudate** at the site of inflammation. Exudate may be **serous** (clear like plasma) or **sanguineous** (containing red blood cells). Eventually the exudate is cleared away through lymphatic drainage. Platelets and plasma proteins such as fibrinogen form a meshlike matrix at the inflammation to prevent its spread.

 **Children's Nursing
Immunity in infants and children**

Throughout the life span, susceptibility to infection changes. An infant has reduced defences against infection. Born with only the antibodies provided by the mother, the infant's immature immune system is incapable of producing the necessary immunoglobulins and leucocytes. As the child grows, the immune system matures, but the child is still susceptible to organisms that cause the common cold, intestinal infections, and infectious diseases, such as mumps and measles.

## TABLE 28-3 Normal Defence Mechanisms against Infection

| Defence Mechanisms | Action | Factors That May Alter Defence |
| --- | --- | --- |
| **SKIN** | | |
| Intact multilayered surface (body's first line of defence against infection) | Provides barrier to microorganisms | Cuts, abrasions, puncture wounds, areas of maceration |
| Shedding of outer layer of skin cells | Removes organisms that adhere to skin's outer layers | Failure to bathe regularly |
| Sebum | Contains fatty acid that kills some bacteria | Excessive bathing |
| **MOUTH** | | |
| Intact multilayered mucosa | Provides mechanical barrier to micro-organisms | Lacerations, trauma, extracted teeth |
| Saliva | Washes away particles containing microorganisms | Poor oral hygiene, dehydration Contains microbial inhibitors (e.g. lysozyme) |
| **RESPIRATORY TRACT** | | |
| Cilia lining upper airway, coated by mucus | Trap inhaled microbes and sweep them outward in mucus to be expectorated or swallowed | Smoking, high concentration of oxygen and carbon dioxide, decreased humidity, cold air |
| Macrophages | Engulf and destroy microorganisms that reach lung's alveoli | Smoking |
| **URINARY TRACT** | | |
| Flushing action of urine flow | Washes away microorganisms incapable of surviving low pH | Administration of antacids |
| Intact multilayered epithelium | Provides barrier to microorganisms | Introduction of urinary catheter, continual movement of catheter in urethra |
| **GASTROINTESTINAL TRACT** | | |
| Acidity of gastric secretions | Chemically destroys microorganisms incapable or surviving low pH | Administration of antacids |
| Rapid peristalsis in small intestine | Prevents retention of bacterial contents | Delayed motility resulting from impaction of faecal contents in large bowel or mechanical obstruction by masses |
| **VAGINA** | | |
| At puberty, normal flora causing vaginal secretions to achieve low pH | Inhibit growth of many microorganisms | Antibiotics and oral contraceptives disrupting normal flora |

## TISSUE REPAIR

When there is injury to tissue cells, healing involves the defensive, reconstructive, and maturative stages. Damaged cells are eventually replaced with healthy new cells. The new cells undergo a gradual maturation until they take on the same structural characteristics and appearance as the previous cells. If inflammation is chronic, tissue defects may fill with fragile **granulation tissue**. Granulation tissue is not as strong as tissue collagen and assumes the form of scar tissue.

## Immune Response

When an invading microorganism enters the body, it is first attacked by monocytes. Remnants of the microorganism then trigger the immune response. The remaining foreign material **(antigen)** causes a series of responses that changes the body's biological makeup so that reactions to future exposures are different from the first reaction. These altered responses are known as **immune responses**. In a normal immune response, the antigen is neutralized, destroyed, or eliminated.

Antigens are usually composed of proteins that are not normally found in a person's body. Often, antigens exist as part of the structure of a bacterium or virus. After an antigen enters the body, it travels in the blood or lymph and initiates cell-mediated or humoral immunity.

**Adult Nursing
Immunity in older people**

Defences against infection change with ageing. The immune response, particularly cell-mediated immunity, declines. Older adults also undergo alterations in the structure and function of the skin, urinary tract, and lungs. For example, the skin loses its turgor and the epithelium thins. As a result, the skin is more easily abraded or torn. This increases exposure to pathogens.

Alterations in the immune system may even trigger the ageing process. Cells of the immune system such as lymphocytes become more diversified with age, and the body undergoes a progressive loss of cellular regulation. When viruses or other antigens and corresponding antibodies lodge in sites such as the kidney and arteries, factors injurious to the tissues are released, and deterioration begins. With ageing and autoimmune diseases (alterations of the immune system), cellular changes such as depletion of lymphoid tissues occur. The basic mechanism for the ageing process is not understood. However, it is known that immunity to infection decreases with advancing age.

## CELL-MEDIATED IMMUNITY

There are two classes of lymphocytes. These are T lymphocytes (T cells) and B lymphocytes (B cells). T cells play a major role in **cell-mediated immunity**. There are antigen receptors on the surface membranes of T cells. When an antigen meets a T cell whose surface receptors fit the antigen, a binding occurs. This binding activates the T cell to divide rapidly to form sensitized T cells. Sensitized T cells travel to the area of inflammation or injury, bind with antigens, and release chemical compounds called *lymphokines*. The lymphokines attract macrophages and stimulate them to attack antigens. Eventually the antigens are killed.

## HUMORAL IMMUNITY

Stimulation of B cells triggers the **humoral immune response**, causing synthesis of immunoglobulins **(antibodies)** that destroy antigens. After a B cell binds with an antigen, it causes formation of plasma and memory B cells. Plasma cells synthesize and secrete large amounts of antibodies, which are proteins normally found in the body that provide general immunity. Memory B cells prepare the body against future antigen invasion. Thus, when an antigen enters the body again, antibodies form more rapidly than during the first exposure, and immunoglobulin levels remain high to attack the antigen.

Antibodies are large protein molecules; there are five classes of antibody immunoglobulins, which are identified by the letters M, G, A, E, and D. Immunoglobulin M (IgM) is the predominant antibody formed after initial contact with an antigen. This initial contact is the primary immune response. The most abundant circulating antibody is IgG, which is formed after subsequent contacts with antigens or during the secondary immune response. The IgG antibody is important in providing resistance to infection and can cross the placenta from mother to child, giving the infant **passive immunity**.

Formation of antibodies is the basis of immunization against disease. **Natural immunity** is an inherited resistance to infection. **Acquired immunity**, which occurs after an exposure to a foreign antigen, is the result of antibody production. For example, when children are vaccinated against diseases such as diphtheria or whooping cough, the vaccine produces an acquired immunity.

## NOSOCOMIAL INFECTIONS

Patients/clients in health care environments can easily acquire infection because they are in high-risk groups. **Nosocomial infections** result from delivery of health services in a health care facility. A hospital is one of the most likely places for acquiring an infection because it harbours a high population of virulent strains of microorganisms that are usually resistant to antibiotics. The intensive care unit (ICU) is one area in the

**Sites and Causes
for Nosocomial Infections**

URINARY TRACT
• Insertion of urinary catheter
• Closed drainage system becoming open
• Catheter and tube becoming disconnected
• Drainage bag port touching dirty surface
• Poor specimen collection technique
• Obstruction or interference with urinary drainage
• Urine in catheter or drainage tube being allowed to re-enter bladder (reflux)
• Poor handwashing technique
• Repeated catheter irrigations with solutions

SURGICAL OR TRAUMATIC WOUNDS
• Improper skin preparation (shaving and bathing) before surgery
• Poor handwashing before and after dressing changes
• Failure to cleanse skin surface properly
• Failure to use aseptic technique during dressing changes
• Use of contaminated antiseptic solutions

RESPIRATORY TRACT
• Contaminated respiratory therapy equipment
• Failure to use aseptic technique while suctioning airway
• Improper disposal of mucous secretions

BLOODSTREAM
• Contamination of intravenous fluids by tubing or needle changes
• Insertion of drug additives to intravenous fluid
• Addition of connecting tube or stopcocks to intravenous system
• Improper care of needle insertion site
• Contaminated needles or catheters
• Failure to change intravenous access site when inflammation first appears
• Poor technique during administration of multiple blood products
• Improper care of peritoneal or haemodialysis shunts

hospital where the risk of acquiring a nosocomial infection is especially high (see box).

**Iatrogenic infections** are a type of nosocomial infection resulting from a diagnostic or therapeutic procedure. A urinary infection that develops after catheter insertion is an example of an iatrogenic nosocomial infection. Health care workers may also acquire nosocomial infection as a result of contacting infectious organisms. The acquisition of hepatitis B from contact with a contaminated needle is an example of nosocomial infection. Illich (1988) defines clinical iatrogenesis, such as hospital acquired infections, as 'all clinical conditions for which remedies, physicians or hospitals are the pathogens or "sickening" agents'.

The number of health care personnel having direct contact with patients/clients, type and number of invasive procedures, treatment received, and length of hospitalization influence the risk of infection. Major sites for nosocomial infection include the urinary tract, surgical or traumatic wounds, respiratory tract, and bloodstream.

### Concept of Asepsis

The nurse's efforts to minimize the onset and spread of infection are based on the principles of aseptic technique. **Asepsis** is the absence of infectious microorganisms on living tissues; thus, an aseptic technique is a procedure performed to eliminate and exclude all infectious microbes (Burton, 1992). Effective handwashing is a major contributor to a state of asepsis.

### Surgical Asepsis

Surgical asepsis or sterile technique requires a nurse to use different precautions from those of medical asepsis. Surgical asepsis requires the absence of all microorganisms, including pathogens and spores, from an object. **The nurse working with a sterile field or with sterile equipment must understand that the slightest break in technique results in contamination.** The nurse also practises surgical asepsis (for example, filling a syringe or changing a dressing on a wound) to keep microorganisms away from an area.

Although surgical asepsis is commonly practised in the operating theatre, labour and delivery area, and major diagnostic areas, the nurse may also use surgical aseptic techniques at the patient's/client's bedside. This would include, for example, inserting intravenous or urinary catheters, and reapplying sterile dressings.

### ASEPTIC PROCEDURES

**Patient/Client Preparation** Explain how the procedure is to be performed and what the patient/client can do to avoid contaminating sterile items, including:
- refraining from touching sterile supplies or drapes
- avoiding coughing and sneezing, or talking over a sterile area.

Also:
- administer prescribed analgesics no more than half an hour before a sterile procedure begins (if necessary)
- allow the patient/client to have elimination needs met
- help the patient/client assume the most comfortable position possible.

### PRINCIPLES OF SURGICAL ASEPSIS

1. A sterile object remains sterile only when touched by another sterile object. This principle guides you in placement of sterile objects and how to handle them.

   a. Sterile object touching sterile object remains sterile; for example, sterile gloves are worn, or sterile forceps are used to handle objects on a sterile field.

   b. Sterile object touching clean object becomes contaminated; for example, if the tip of a syringe or other sterile object touches the surface of a clean disposable glove, the syringe or object is contaminated.

   c. Sterile object touching contaminated object becomes contaminated; for example, when the nurse touches a sterile object with an ungloved hand, the object is contaminated.

   d. Sterile object touching questionable object is contaminated; for example, when a tear or break in the covering of a sterile object is found, it is discarded regardless of whether the object itself appears untouched.

2. Only sterile objects may be placed on a sterile field. All items are correctly sterilized before use. Sterile objects are kept in clean, dry storage areas for only a prescribed time; thereafter they are considered unsterile. Before use, all sterile packages are checked for sterilization dates or expiry dates on labels. The package or container holding a sterile object must be intact and dry. A package that is torn, punctured, wet, or open is unsterile, and must not be used.

3. A sterile object or field out of the range of vision or an object held below a person's waist is contaminated. Never turn your back on a sterile tray or leave it unattended. Contamination can occur accidentally by a dangling piece of clothing, falling hair, or an unknowing patient/client touching a sterile object. Any object held below waist level is considered contaminated because it cannot be viewed at all times. Sterile objects should be kept in front with hands as close together as possible.

4. A sterile object or field becomes contaminated by prolonged exposure to air. Avoid activities that may create air currents, such as excessive movements or rearranging linen after a sterile object or field becomes exposed. When sterile packages are being opened, it is important to minimize the number of people walking into the area. Microorganisms also travel by droplet through the air. No one should talk, laugh, sneeze, or cough over a sterile field or when gathering and using sterile equipment. A nurse with a cold or other respiratory ailment should not perform aseptic procedures. Microorganisms travelling through the air can fall on sterile items or fields if the nurse reaches over the work area. When opening sterile packages, hold the item or piece of equipment as close as possible to the sterile field without touching the sterile surface. Minimal movement or rearranging of sterile items also reduces contamination by air transmission.

5. When a sterile surface comes in contact with a wet, contaminated surface, the sterile object or field becomes

contaminated. If moisture seeps through a sterile package's protective covering, microorganisms travel to the sterile object. When stored, sterile packages become wet, the nurse discards the objects immediately or sends the equipment for resterilization. When working with a sterile field, the nurse may have to pour sterile solutions. Any spill can be a source of contamination unless the object or field rests on a sterile surface that cannot be penetrated by moisture. For example, if a nurse places a piece of sterile gauze in its wrapper on a patient's/client's bedside table and the table surface is wet, the gauze is considered contaminated.

6. Fluid flows in the direction of gravity. A sterile object becomes contaminated if gravity causes a contaminated liquid to flow over the object's surface. To avoid contamination during a surgical hand wash, the nurse holds the hands above the elbows. This allows water to flow downward without contaminating your hands and fingers. The principle of water flow by gravity is also the reason for drying from fingers to elbows with hands held up, after the wash.

7. The edges of a sterile field or container are considered to be contaminated. Frequently, nurses place sterile objects on a sterile towel or drape. Since the edge of the drape touches an unsterile surface, such as a table or bed linen, a 2.5 cm border around the drape is considered contaminated. The edges of sterile containers become exposed to air after they are opened and are thus contaminated. After a sterile needle is removed from its protective cap or after forceps are removed from a container, the objects must not touch the container's edge. The lip of an opened bottle of solution also becomes contaminated after it is exposed to air. When pouring a sterile liquid, first pour a small amount of solution and discard it. The solution washes away microorganisms on the bottle lip. Then pour out the sterile liquid for a second time (on the same side) in order to fill a container with the desired amount of solution.

## THE NURSING PROCESS IN INFECTION CONTROL

 **ASSESSMENT**

To prevent or manage an infection appropriately, assess the patient's/client's defences against infection and susceptibility to infection. A review of the person's clinical condition may detect signs and symptoms of infection. An analysis of laboratory findings provides information about a patient's/client's defence against infection. By knowing the factors that increase susceptibility or risk for infection, you are more able to plan preventive therapy that includes aseptic technique. By recognizing early signs and symptoms of infection, you can alert the doctor to the potential need for treatment and initiate appropriate nursing measures.

### Status of Defence Mechanisms

A review of assessment findings and the patient's/client's health reveals the status of normal defence mechanisms against infection. For example, any break in the skin or mucosa is a potential site for infection. Similarly, a chronic smoker is at greater risk for acquiring a respiratory tract infection after general surgery because the cilia of the respiratory tract are less likely to be active and able to propel retained mucus from the lung's airways. Any reduction in the body's primary or secondary defences against infection places a patient/client at risk (see box below).

### Patient/Client Susceptibility

Many factors influence susceptibility to infection. The nurse gathers information about each factor through the nursing history.

### NUTRITIONAL STATUS

When protein intake is inadequate as a result of poor diet or debilitating disease, the rate of protein breakdown can exceed that of tissue synthesis. As a result, the body is in a negative nitrogen balance; in other words, the output of nitrogen sources such as protein exceeds nitrogen intake. A reduction in the intake of protein and other nutrients such as carbohydrates and fats reduces the body's defences against infection and impairs wound healing (see Chapter 30).

Patients/clients with illnesses or problems that increase protein requirements are at further risk. These problems include traumatic injury, extensive burns, and conditions causing fever. Individuals who have had surgery also have this problem.

Assess patients'/clients' dietary intakes and abilities to tolerate solid foods. People who have difficulty with swallowing, who experience alterations in digestion, or who are too confused or weak to feed themselves are at risk from inadequate dietary intake. A dietitian may be called to assist in calculating the patient's/client's calorific requirements.

### STRESS

The body responds to emotional or physical stress by the general adaptation syndrome (see Chapter 10). During the alarm stage, the basal metabolic rate increases as the body uses energy stores. Adrenocorticotropic hormone (ACTH) acts to increase serum

> **Risk Factors for Infection**
>
> **INADEQUATE PRIMARY DEFENCES**
> - Broken skin or mucosa
> - Traumatized tissue
> - Decreased ciliary action
> - Obstructed urine outflow
> - Altered peristalsis
> - Change in pH of secretions
>
> **INADEQUATE SECONDARY DEFENCES**
> - Reduced haemoglobin level
> - Suppression of leucocytes (drug or disease related)
> - Suppressed inflammatory response (drug or disease related)
> - Low leucocyte count (leucopenia)

### Adult Nursing
### Assessing the risk of infection in older adults

| Component | Possible Changes With Age | Outcome |
| --- | --- | --- |
| Skin | Thinner dermal and epidermal layers, decreased collagen strength, decreased skin elasticity, decreased sweat | Pressure ulcers |
| Peripheral nerves | Reduced sensitivity, particularly in patients/clients with history of alcohol abuse, vitamin $B_{12}$ deficiency, and diabetes mellitus | Pressure ulcers, ignored trauma leading to infection |
| Circulation | Congestive heart failure, calcified mitral and aortic valves | Pneumonia, bacterial endocarditis |
| Peripheral circulation | More elastic veins, less effective venous valves, blood pooling in lower extremities | Venous stasis ulcers |
| Mouth | Dehydration, loss of saliva production, functional inability to maintain oral hygiene | Parotid gland infection, periodontal disease, localized abscess, bacteraemia |
| Gastrointestinal tract | Loss of ability to secrete stomach acid in 30% of persons over 70 | Salmonellal diarrhoea |
| Pulmonary system | Increased colonization of oropharynx, impaired mucociliary clearance, decreased macrophage function, decreased cough reflex | Viral and bacterial pneumonia |
| Urinary tract | Prostatic hyperplasia, urethral strictures, age-related hormonal changes in vaginal wall, pelvic floor relaxation, ureterocele or cystocele, degeneration of nerves leading to neurogenic bladder, use of tricyclic antidepressants, dehydration | Asymptomatic bacteriuria, cystitis, pyelonephritis |
| Nutrition | Malnutrition, vitamin deficiency (vitamin A, pyridoxine, and riboflavin), protein and caloric malnutrition | Impaired immune response to infection |
| Drug therapy | Corticosteroid and cytotoxic drugs | Impaired immune response to infection |
| Nursing home residency | Exposure to nosocomial infections, including influenza, *Proteus* and *Providencia* organisms with an indwelling catheter, tuberculosis, and wound infections (incidence of bacteraemia after admission is 50%) | Frequent serious infection, increased risk of pneumonia |

Adapted from Tideiksaar R: Infections in the elderly: diagnosis and treatment, *Physician Assist* 11(2):17, 1987.

glucose levels and decrease unnecessary anti-inflammatory responses through the release of cortisone. If stress continues or becomes intense, elevated cortisone levels result in decreased resistance to infection. Continued stress leads to exhaustion, wherein energy stores are depleted and the body has no resistance to invading organisms. The same conditions that increase nutritional requirements such as surgery or trauma also increase physiological stress.

## DISEASE PROCESS

Patients/clients with diseases of the immune system are at particular risk for infection. Leukaemia, acquired immunodeficiency syndrome (AIDS), lymphoma, and aplastic anaemia are examples of conditions that compromise a host by weakening defences against infectious organisms. Patients/clients with leukaemia are unable to produce enough leucocytes to ward off infection.

People affected by chronic disease such as diabetes mellitus and multiple sclerosis are also more susceptible to infection because of general debilitation and nutritional impairment. Diseases that impair body system defences, such as pulmonary emphysema and bronchitis (which impair ciliary action and thicken mucus), cancer (which alters the immune response), and peripheral vascular disease (which reduces blood flow to injured tissues), increase susceptibility to infection.

## MEDICAL TREATMENT

Some drugs and medical treatments compromise immunity to infection. Assess the patient's/client's history to ascertain whether he or she takes medications at home that increase infection susceptibility. A review of treatments received within the health care setting may reveal further risks. For example, adrenal corticosteroids, prescribed for several conditions, are anti-inflammatory drugs that cause protein breakdown and impair the inflammatory response against bacteria and other pathogens. Cytotoxic or antineoplastic drugs attack cancer cells but cause side effects of bone marrow depression and normal cell toxicity. With bone marrow depression the body is unable to produce lymphocytes and sufficient leucocytes. When normal cells become altered by antineoplastic agents, cellular defences against infection fail. Cyclosporine and other immunosuppressant drugs, which decrease the body's immune response, are commonly taken by people who receive organ transplants. The immunosuppressants prevent organ and tissue rejection; yet they increase susceptibility to infection.

### Clinical Appearance

The signs and symptoms of infection are **local** or **systemic**. Localized infections are most common in areas of skin or mucous membrane breakdown such as surgical and traumatic wounds, pressure ulcers, and mouth lesions (see Chapter 30). Infections also develop locally in cavities beneath the skin; for example, an abscess.

To assess an area for localized infection, first inspect the area for redness and swelling caused by inflammation. There may be drainage from open lesions or wounds. Infected drainage may be yellow, green, or brown, depending on the site of infection. Ask the person about pain or tenderness around the site. The person may complain of tightness caused by oedema. If the infected area is large enough, movement of a body part may be restricted. Gentle palpation of an infected area usually results in some degree of tenderness.

Systemic infections cause more generalized symptoms than local infection. They usually result in fever, fatigue, and malaise. Lymph nodes that drain the area of infection often become enlarged, swollen, and tender during palpation. For example, an abscess in the peritoneal cavity may cause enlargement of lymph nodes in the groin. Systemic infections commonly cause a loss of appetite, nausea, and vomiting.

Systemic infections often develop after treatment for localized infection has failed. Be alert for changes in the person's level of activity and responsiveness. As systemic infections develop, the patient/client may become lethargic and complain of a loss of energy. An elevation in body temperature may lead to episodes of increased heart and respiratory rates. Involvement of major body systems produces specific signs. For example, a pulmonary infection results in a productive cough with purulent sputum. A urinary tract infection may result in cloudy, foul-smelling urine.

## Patients/Clients with Infection

A person with infection may have a variety of health problems. It is important to assess the influences of the infection on the patient's/client's needs, which may be physical, psychological, social, or economic. For example, a person with AIDS may experience serious psychological problems as a result of decreased self-esteem or rejection by family and friends.

During assessment, gather *objective findings*, such as an open incision or a reduced calorific intake, and subjective data, such as a patient's/client's complaint of tenderness over a surgical wound site. Interpret the data carefully, looking for clusters of defining characteristics or risk factors that create a pattern suggesting a specific nursing problem. It may be necessary to validate data (for example, by inspecting the integrity of a wound more carefully and more regularly). Similarly, additional data such as laboratory findings may help.

**Mental Health Nursing**
**Special needs of people with mental illness**

In the mental health environment, some patients/clients may be too distracted by their mental distress or mental illness to acknowledge the discomfort that may arise from a local or systemic infection. Some patients/clients may be so distrusting of others, that they are afraid to, or feel unable to, register any discomfort caused by infections. Many patients/clients may lack the appropriate social skills to communicate their symptoms to others, or may do so in a bizarre way, which requires careful deciphering by the nurses.

Many patients/clients in large psychiatric institutions may have acquired habits, such as hoarding 'rubbish', or may collect items from bins or refuse sites. This increases their risk of infection, unless nurses pay particular attention to their hygiene and address their behaviour.

When working with individuals who are mentally ill or who have mental distress, nurses must be particularly careful in assessing the patient's/client's physical health as well as mental health needs. Physical care and psychological care must go hand-in-hand.

## PLANNING

The nursing problems identified for a patient/client direct the nurse's selection of interventions for a care plan. As always, involve the patient/client and any family in establishing goals of care and the specific nursing measures required. When there is a high risk for infection or the person has a known infection, common goals of care may include the following:

- preventing exposure to infectious organisms
- controlling or reducing the extent of infection
- maintaining a resistance to infection

- understanding infection-control self-care practices.

Prioritize the goals of care; for example, a patient/client has developed an open wound, suffers from a debilitating disease such as cancer, and has been unable to tolerate solid foods. The priority of administering therapies that promote wound healing exceeds the goal of educating the person to assume self-care therapies at home. When the person's condition improves, the priorities will change, and patient/client education becomes an essential intervention. The development of a care plan (see care plan) includes measures involving use of aseptic technique.

### Nursing Care Plan for Urinary Tract Infection in Person with Urinary Catheter

**Problem: Urinary tract infection. Patient/client has a urinary catheter.**

| Goals | Nursing Interventions | Rationale |
|---|---|---|
| Eradicate infection (Wright, 1988a). Prevent cross-infection by direct and indirect contact, maintaining a safe environment (Wright, 1988b). Prevent backflow of urine (Crow *et al*, 1988). Remove catheter when appropriate to do so, or on instructions from medical staff. | 1. Explain problem of urinary tract infection to the patient/client and the need for precautions. Give an overall view of the nursing care required to allow the patient/client to gain an understanding. | 1. To inform the patient/client of what is happening. To provide an explanation of what actions will be undertaken, when they will be undertaken and why. To assist in developing interpersonal skills. To provide an opportunity for the person to ask questions. |
| | 2. Review the continued need for the catheter and remove if possible. | 2. To keep a urinary catheter *in situ* for longer than is necessary is disadvantageous to the patient/client in several ways. For example, promotion of infection, promotion of further discomfort and weakening of urethral sphincter muscles. |
| | 3. Institute precautions as detailed below: <br> a) wear gloves and apron when emptying urine drainage bag or handling the catheter <br> b) discard the urine collected in a sterile measuring jug <br> c) remove gloves and apron, then wash and dry hands thoroughly. <br> d) use gloves to perform catheter care as required. | 3. To lessen the risk of infection caused through poor hygiene. To apply a safe standard of nursing care with the use of appropriate hospital/clinic policies. |
| | 4. Check catheter is strapped securely to the inner aspect of the thigh and ensure patient/client comfort. | 4. To prevent 'dragging' and, therefore, greater discomfort. To promote patency of the catheter. |
| | 5. Ensure the drainage bag is always below the level of the bladder. | 5. To allow for gravitational drainage and prevent back flow and stasis of urine. |
| | 6. Ensure patient/client drinks at least 1.5–2 litres of fluid per day (if not on fluid restriction). | 6. To prevent urine infection and to maintain adequate hydration. |
| | 7. Administer prescribed antibiotics and monitor the effect. | 7. To enable the urinary tract infection to be monitored. A change in prescribed antibiotic therapy may be required. |
| | 8. If possible, do not nurse next to another patient/client. | 8. To prevent cross infection with other patients/clients. |

**IMPLEMENTATION**

The nurse's primary goals in controlling infection are preventing the onset and spread of infection and administering measures for treatment of infection. By recognizing and assessing a patient's/client's risk factors for infection and implementing appropriate measures, you can reduce the risk of infection.

Through the application of knowledge about the chain of infection, try to prevent an infection from developing or spreading by minimizing the numbers and kinds of organisms transmitted to potential infection sites. Eliminating reservoirs of infection, controlling portals of exit and entry, and avoiding actions that transmit microorganisms prevent bacteria from finding a site to grow. Proper use of sterile supplies and protective garments and effective handwashing are examples of aseptic methods that the nurse uses to control the spread of microorganisms. A final preventive measure is to strengthen a potential host's defences against infection, for example, nutritional support and rest.

Treatment of an infectious process includes eliminating the infectious organisms and supporting the patient's/client's defences. Collect specimens of body fluids or drainage from infected body sites for cultures. When the disease process or causative organism has been identified, the doctor prescribes an anti-infective or antibiotic drug — whichever is most effective for the situation. The nurse correctly administers the antibiotics in accordance with hospital policy, observing for allergic reactions and assessing the progress of the infection.

Systemic infections require measures to prevent complications of fever. Maintaining intake of fluids prevents dehydration. The patient's/client's increased metabolic rate requires an adequate nutritional intake. Rest preserves energy for the healing process.

During the course of infection the nurse supports the patient's/client's body defence mechanisms. For example, if a person has infectious diarrhoea, the nurse must maintain skin integrity to prevent breakdown and the entrance of microorganisms. Routine hygiene measures such as cleansing the oral cavity and bathing protect the skin and mucous membranes from organism spread.

A patient/client with an infection has many needs. By monitoring the infection's course carefully, you can choose the most appropriate measures to maintain or restore health, and keep the patient/client comfortable.

## CONTROLLING OR ELIMINATING INFECTIOUS AGENTS

Proper cleansing, disinfection, and sterilization of contaminated objects significantly reduce and often eliminate microorganisms. In hospitals a central department disinfects and sterilizes reusable supplies. However, you may encounter situations that require use of these techniques. Many principles of cleansing and disinfection also apply to the home.

When cleaning equipment that is soiled by organic material such as blood, faecal matter, mucus, or pus, the nurse must ensure that hospital or community infection control policies and standards are adhered to at all times.

**Disinfection and Sterilization** **Disinfection** is the destruction or removal of infectious or harmful microorganisms from non-living objects by physical or chemical methods (Burton, 1992). **Sterilization** is defined as the complete destruction or removal of all microbes, including spores. It can be achieved by heat, chemicals, irradiation and filtration (Brunner and Suddarth, 1992).

The two primary methods for disinfection and sterilization

## TABLE 28-4 Examples of Disinfection and Sterilization Processes

| Characteristics | Examples of Use |
|---|---|
| **MOIST HEAT** Moist heat includes steam (moist heat under pressure). When exposed to high temperature, water vapour can attain temperatures above boiling point to kill all pathogens and spores. | Autoclave is used to sterilize surgical instruments, parenteral solutions, and surgical dressings. |
| **RADIATION** Ionizing radiation penetrates deeply into objects for effective sterilization and disinfection. | Radiation is used in sterilizing drugs, foods, and other heat-sensitive items. |
| **CHEMICALS** Chemicals are effective disinfectants because they attack all types of microorganisms, act rapidly, work with water, retain no odour, are stable in light and heat, are inexpensive, are not harmful to body tissues, do not destroy article being disinfected, and are not inactivated by inorganic material. | Chemicals are used for disinfection of instruments and equipment. |
| **BOILING WATER** Boiling is the least expensive for use in home. Bacterial spores and some viruses resist boiling. It is not used in hospitals. | The items should be boiled for at least 15 minutes. |

(Table 28-4) are physical processes, which involve the use of heat or radiation, and chemical processes, which use various solutions or gases. Both disrupt the internal function of microorganisms by destroying cell proteins. Sterilization and disinfection occur when heat reaches a level sufficient to destroy organisms or when a concentration of chemicals has adequate exposure to microorganisms.

A **disinfectant** is a chemical solution that is used when cleaning only inanimate objects. Examples of disinfectants are alcohol, chlorine, glutaraldehyde, and phenol. The solutions can be caustic and toxic to tissues. A **germicide** is a chemical preparation that can be applied on skin and tissues, as well as inanimate objects.

## CONTROLLING OR ELIMINATING RESERVOIRS

To control or eliminate reservoir sites for infection, eliminate sources of body fluids, drainage, or solutions that might harbour microorganisms. Also carefully discard articles that become contaminated with infectious material (see box). All health care institutions must have guidelines for the disposal of infectious waste material — these must be adhered to (RCN, 1994).

## CONTROLLING PORTALS OF EXIT

Follow aseptic practices to minimize or prevent infectious organisms from exiting the body. To control organisms exiting via the respiratory tract, avoid talking directly into patients'/clients' faces or talking, sneezing, or coughing directly over surgical wounds or sterile dressing fields. Cover your mouth or nose when sneezing or coughing. Teach patients/clients to protect others when they sneeze or cough and provide them with tissues to control the spread of microorganisms.

A nurse who has a mild cold and continues to work with

---

patients/clients can wear a mask, especially when changing a dressing or performing a sterile procedure. The same nurse should refrain from working with patients/clients who are highly susceptible to infection.

Another way to control the exit of microorganisms is the careful handling of body substances (such as urine, faeces, emesis, and blood). Contaminated fluids can easily splash while being discarded. Wear disposable gloves, gowns, and eye wear if there is a chance of contact with any fluids. Bag and dispose of soiled items appropriately. Laboratory specimens from all patients/clients are handled as if they were infectious.

## CONTROLLING TRANSMISSION

Effective control of infection requires a nurse to remain aware of the modes of transmission and ways to control them. In the hospital, home, or extended care facility a patient/client should

---

**Adult Nursing**
**Working with clients in the home**

At home, a client's risk of infection is reduced because the client is not exposed to alien pathogens. However, high standards of asepsis should be maintained. Nurses working with clients at home should follow these tips to control infection:
- recognize that the environment in the home is planned as a living area, not as a treatment area as in a hospital or clinic; therefore, be adaptable and make the best and safest use of circumstances in the home
- use aseptic technique for client care when appropriate (it is neither necessary nor acceptable to offer a lower standard of asepsis in the home than in the hospital)
- carry paper towels for drying your hands and small bottles of hand wash lotions, in case the soap and towels in the client's home are not clean
- dispose of dressings and sharps appropriately (never put dirty dressings, sharps or other clinical waste in the client's waste disposal system)
- follow local infection control policy
- improvise and adapt, but never compromise standards of care

---

**Infection Control to Reduce Reservoirs of Infection**

BATHING
- Use soap and water to remove drainage, dried secretions, excess perspiration, or sediment from disinfectants.

DRESSING CHANGES
- Change dressings that become wet and soiled (see Chapter 30).

CONTAMINATED ARTICLES
- Place tissues, soiled dressings, or soiled linen in moisture-resistant bags for proper disposal.

CONTAMINATED NEEDLES
- Place syringes and uncapped hypodermic needles and intravenous needles in moisture-resistant, puncture-proof containers, which should be located in patient/client rooms or treatment areas so that exposed, contaminated equipment need not be carried more than a small distance.
- Do not recap needles or attempt to break them.

BEDSIDE UNIT
- Keep table surfaces clean and dry.

BOTTLED SOLUTIONS
- Do not leave bottled solutions open for prolonged periods.
- Keep solutions tightly capped.
- Date bottles when opened.

SURGICAL WOUNDS
- Keep drainage tubes and collection bags patent to prevent accumulation of serous fluid under the skin surface.

DRAINAGE BOTTLES AND BAGS
- Empty and dispose of drainage suction bottles according to local policy.
- Empty all drainage systems at appropriate intervals.
- Never raise a drainage system (e.g. urinary drainage bag) above the level of the site being drained unless it is clamped off.

have a personal set of care items. Sharing bedpans, urinals, bath basins, and eating utensils can easily lead to transmission of infection. Glass thermometers, even when individually used, warrant special care.

Because certain microorganisms travel easily through the air, linens or bedclothes should not be shaken. Dusting with a treated or dampened cloth prevents dust particles from entering the air.

To prevent transmission of microorganisms through indirect contact, soiled items and equipment must be kept from touching the nurse's clothing. A common error is to carry dirty linen in the arms against the uniform. Special linen bags should be used, or soiled linen carried with hands held out from the body. Laundry bags should not be allowed to overflow.

Anything that touches the floor is contaminated. If you accidentally drop a piece of equipment, dispose of it appropriately. When you stoop or bend, your uniform should not touch the floor. Never place clean or soiled linen on the floor.

Handwashing  The most important and most basic technique in preventing and controlling transmission of pathogens is **handwashing** (Sedjwick, 1984). A thorough and effective handwashing technique involves soaping all of the hand surfaces  paying attention to detail, particularly the areas around the nails, nail beds and the interdigital clefts. The hands should be rinsed thoroughly and dried carefully on paper towels.

An alternative method of hand hygiene is the application of an alcohol-based solution to physically clean hands and rubbing them dry. The solution must be applied to all hand surfaces, because the alcohol can kill only the organisms it touches (Taylor, 1978a). Studies have shown that up to 89% of staff miss some part of the hand surface during handwashing (Taylor, 1978b).

Contaminated hands are a prime cause of cross-infection. For example, a nurse caring for a patient/client who has excessive pulmonary excretions assists the patient/client in expectorating mucus and disposes of the tissues in a bedside container. The patient's/client's neighbour asks the nurse for assistance with his meal. The nurse then leaves the patient's/client's bedside to pour a dose of medication due in 5 minutes. If the nurse fails to wash his or her hands before each of these actions, organisms from the first person's mucus could easily be transmitted to the neighbour's food and to the medication container. Chauduri (1993) found that the cost of all hospital acquired infections (HAI) was estimated at £111 million in 1986, with a total of 950,000 bed days lost. Some HAIs result from poor handwashing techniques. A 20% reduction in the incidence if HAIs would save the NHS £15.6 million.

The need for handwashing depends on the type, intensity, duration, and sequence of activity. It is recommended that nurses wash their hands between different patients/clients and activities and especially before:

1. Contact with patients/clients who are susceptible to infection (for example, newborn infants or immunosuppressed clients [patients/clients with leukaemia, organ transplant recipients, and patients/clients who are HIV-positive]).
2. After caring for an infected patient/client.
3. After touching organic material.
4. Before performing invasive procedures such as administration of injections, catheterization, and suctioning.
5. Before and after handling dressings or touching open wounds.
6. After handling contaminated equipment.
7. Between contact with different patients/clients in high-risk units (for example, nursery and critical care units).

---

**Fieldman's Criteria for Handwashing Evaluation**

**SCORES**

**Used soap**
2 Visible lather
0 No contact with soap

**Used continuously running water**
2 Did
0 Did not

**Positioned hands to avoid contaminating arms**
2 Held hands down so that water drained from fingertips into sink
1 Held hands parallel with arms so that water drained from hands into sink
0 Held hands so that water drained onto arm

**Avoided splashing clothing or floor**
2 No splashing
1 Minimal splashing
0 Vigorous splashing

**Rubbed hands together vigorously**
2 Vigorous rubbing
1 Minimal rubbing
0 No rubbing

**Used friction on all surfaces**
2 Dorsal, ventral, interdigital
1 One or two of the above
0 Did not use friction

**Rinsed hands thoroughly**
2 All surfaces: dorsal, ventral, interdigital
1 One or two of the above
0 Did not rinse

**Held hands down to rinse**
2 Did
0 Did not

**Dried hands thoroughly**
2 Dried all surfaces
1 Dried one or two surfaces
0 Did not dry

**Turned tap off with paper towel**
2 Did
0 Did not

From Hinchliff SM, Norman SE, Schober JE: Nursing practice and health care, London, 1993, Edward Arnold.

The ideal duration of handwashing is unknown. Nurses' compliance with handwashing is important. Failure to follow effective handwashing techniques may be due to concern over the effects repeated handwashing has on the condition of skin. Feldman's Criteria for Handwashing Evaluation may be used as a guideline for effectiveness (Phillips, 1989).

Teach patients/clients and visitors about the proper technique and times for handwashing. Teaching handwashing is particularly important if health care is to continue at home. Patients/clients should wash their hands before eating or handling food; after handling contaminated equipment, linen, or organic material; and before and after elimination. Visitors are encouraged to wash their hands before eating or handling food, after coming in contact with infected patients/clients, and after handling contaminated equipment or organic material.

## CONTROLLING PORTALS OF ENTRY

A number of measures that control the exit of microorganisms similarly control the entrance of pathogens. Maintaining the integrity of skin and mucous membranes reduces the chances of microorganisms reaching a host. The patient's/client's skin should be kept clear and supple. Immobilized and debilitated patients/clients are particularly susceptible to skin breakdown. Individuals should not be positioned on tubes or objects that might cause breaks in the skin. Dry, wrinkle-free linen also reduces the chances of skin breakdown. Turning and positioning should be undertaken as soon as a patient's/client's skin becomes reddened. Frequent oral hygiene prevents drying of mucous membranes. A water-soluble ointment keeps the person's lips well lubricated (see Chapters 25, 30).

Patients/clients, health care personnel, and others are at risk from acquiring infections from accidental needlesticks. After administering an injection, carefully dispose of contaminated needles without resheathing them. A stray needle lying in bed linen or carelessly thrown into a wastebasket is a prime source for pathogens. Hepatitis B, or serum hepatitis, is the infection most commonly transmitted by contaminated needles. A needle stick injury should be reported immediately and the appropriate incident form should be completed.

Another cause for entrance of microorganisms into a host is improper handling and management of urinary catheters and drainage sets. The point of connection between a catheter and drainage tube should remain closed and intact. As long as such systems are closed, their contents are considered sterile. Outflow of spigots on drainage bags should also remain closed to prevent entrance of bacteria. Movement of the catheter at the urethra should be minimized to reduce chances of microorganisms ascending the urethra into the bladder.

The nurse may care for patients/clients with closed drainage systems that collect wound drainage, bile, or other body fluids. In each example, the site from which a drainage tube exits should remain clear of excess moisture or accumulated drainage. All tubing should remain connected and kink free throughout use. Drainage receptacles should only be opened when it is necessary to discard or measure volume of drainage.

At times the nurse obtains specimens from drainage tubes.

Disinfect tubes and ports by wiping outward with an alcohol or an iodine solution before entering the system. Temporarily place squares of sterile gauze around the ends of an opened drainage tube to provide further protection against bacteria.

A final method for reducing the entrance of microorganisms is the technique for cleansing wounds (see Chapter 30). The wound itself is considered to be sterile. To prevent entrance of microorganisms, into the wound, clean outward from a wound site. When applying a disinfectant or cleansing solution, wipe around the wound edge first and then clean outward. For example, use clean gauze for each revolution around the wound's circumference.

Isolation Practices  The risk of transmitting nosocomial infection or infectious disease among patients/clients is high. When a patient/client has a known source of infection, health care workers become alerted and follow infection-control practices. However, health care workers may not be aware that patients/clients have infections. Most organisms causing nosocomial infections are found in the **colonized** body substances of individuals regardless of whether a culture has confirmed infection and a diagnosis has been made (Lynch and Jackson, 1988). Body substances such as faeces, urine, mucus, and wound drainage always contain potentially infectious organisms.

**Isolation** precautions can control the transmission of pathogens. Barriers such as protective gowns and gloves, masks, eyewear and single rooms keep pathogens in a confined area. Follow proper procedures to prevent organisms from leaving the room of patients/clients or to prohibit organisms from entering the rooms of susceptible patients/clients. Always wear gloves

---

### Universal Precautions

#### If an accident occurs, follow these guidelines:

**Needle Stick Injury**
In the event of a sharps or needle stick injury:
1. Encourage bleeding from the puncture wound. Do not suck.
2. Wash the area thoroughly with soap and water.
3. Cover with a waterproof dressing.
4. If known, note the name of the patient.
5. Report to occupational health department.
6. Notify line manager and document incident.

**Conjunctiva/Mucous Membrane**
- If splashed with blood/body fluids, irrigate with copious amounts of saline. Follow steps 4-6.

**Spillages**
- Wear household gloves and plastic apron. Spills should be covered with disposable towels which are then treated with sodium hypochlorite solution 10,000 ppm. These should be left for two minutes before being disposed of as infected waste.

From: DOH: Guidance for clinical health care workers, protection against infection with HIV and hepatitis viruses: recommendations of the expert advisory group on AIDS, London, Smith and Nephew Medical, on behalf of the Royal College of Nursing AIDS Forum, 1990. Reprinted with permission.

when dealing with blood and other body fluids. Note, however, that while gloves are protective, they can become damaged and allow the passage of bacteria (Lascelles, 1982).

## Universal precautions for infection control

The following general guidelines on **universal precautions** should be practised by health care personnel at all times. For additional details on universal precautions, consult the Department of Health's *Guidelines for clinical health care workers, protection against infection with HIV and hepatitis viruses*, 1990.

- Universal precautions apply to blood and to other body fluids.
- Wear gloves when handling blood, body fluids such as urine, pleural fluid, peritoneal fluid, cerebrospinal fluid, and vaginal and seminal secretions.
- Wear gloves when handling items or surfaces soiled with blood or body fluids (for example, vaginal secretions, pleural fluid, and peritoneal fluid) and when performing venepuncture and other vascular access procedures.
- Change gloves after contact with each patient/client.
- Wear a mask, disposable apron, and sometimes protective eyewear during procedures (for example, irrigations) that are likely to generate droplets of blood or other body fluids containing blood, to prevent exposure of mucous membranes of the mouth, nose, and eyes.
- Wear gowns during procedures that are likely to generate splashes of blood or other body fluids containing blood.
- Wash hands and other skin surfaces immediately and thoroughly if contaminated with blood or other body fluids.
- To prevent needlestick injuries, do not resheath needles; purposely bend, break, or remove needles from disposable syringes. Place used needles in puncture-resistant containers in the work area. Do not allow the containers to get overfull.
- To reduce the need for mouth-to-mouth resuscitation use mouthpieces, resuscitator bags, or other ventilation devices.
- Refrain from all direct patient/client care and from handling patient/client care equipment if you have any exudative lesions.
- Place all contaminated waste into yellow clinical sacks and leave for incineration, according to local unit policy.

Regardless of the type of isolation system, always follow the following basic principles:

- Wash hands thoroughly before entering and leaving the room of the patient/client receiving isolation.
- Dispose of contaminated supplies and equipment in a manner that prevents spread of microorganisms to other persons and in accordance with local policy.
- When using protective barriers be sure to know the disease process and the means of infection transmission.
- All persons who might be exposed during transport of a patient/client outside the isolation room must be protected.

## Psychological Implications of Isolation

An individual who requires isolation in a single room will often feel slightly lonely because normal social relationships become disrupted. This situation can be psychologically harmful, particularly for children.

As a result of the infectious process, patients'/clients' body images are altered. They may feel unclean, rejected, lonely, or guilty. Aseptic practices further intensify these beliefs of difference or undesirability. Isolation in a single room limits sensory contact. Unless the nurse acts to minimize feelings of psychological and physical isolation, patients'/clients' emotional states can interfere with recovery.

- Before isolation measures are instituted explain the nature of the disease or condition, the purposes of isolation, and steps for carrying out specific precautions to the patient/client and family.
- Improve the patient's/client's sensory stimulation during isolation. Reading materials, a radio or television set, a clock, and hobby materials should be available. However, if a book or other inanimate object comes in contact with infected material, it must be disinfected or discarded.
- Ensure the room environment is clean and pleasant. Curtains or shades should be opened, and excess supplies and equipment removed.
- Listen intently to the patient's/client's concerns or interests. If the nurse rushes through care or shows a lack of interest, the person will feel rejected and even more isolated. Mealtime is a particularly good opportunity for conversation.
- Provide comfort measures, such as repositioning, or a gentle massage. If the person's condition permits, encourage him or her to walk and sit up in a chair.
- Ensure the isolation room or an adjoining anteroom contains handwashing, bathing, and toilet facilities and that soap and antiseptic solutions are made available. Ensure personnel and visitors wash their hands before coming to the patient's/client's bedside and again before leaving the room.
- Ensure that the isolation room contains a special impervious bag for soiled or contaminated linen, as well as a rubbish container with plastic liners. Impervious receptacles prevent transmission of microorganisms by preventing seepage to and soiling of the outside surface. A disposable impervious container should be available in the room to discard used needles, syringes, and sharp objects.
- Avoid taking any article or piece of equipment into a patient's/client's room that is to be reused outside the isolation area. If such an article becomes contaminated, it must be discarded or disinfected and sterilized. Keep the patient's/client's chart outside the room. Equipment such as a sphygmomanometer, stethoscope, or other examination devices should be left in the patient's/client's room until isolation precautions are no longer required. Afterwards, all reusable equipment must be disinfected.

### PROTECTION FOR PERSONNEL

Sufficient isolation supplies should be readily available for personnel to wear before entering an isolation room. A special area outside the room holds supplies of gowns, masks, gloves, handwashing equipment and supplies of clean materials, for example, linen.

**Gowns** The primary reason for gowning is to prevent soiling clothes during contact with the patient/client. Gowns protect health care personnel and visitors from coming in contact with infected material and also protect patients/clients from organisms on other people's clothing.

Isolation gowns open at the back and have ties at the neck and waist to keep them closed and secure. Gowns should be long enough to cover all outer garments. Long sleeves with tight-fitting cuffs provide added protection. There is no special technique required for applying clean gowns as long as they are fastened securely. However, the nurse must remove gowns carefully to minimize contamination of the hands and uniform and then discard them after removal.

**Masks** A mask can protect you from inhaling microorganisms from a patient's/client's respiratory tract and can prevent transmission of pathogens from your respiratory tract to the patient/client. Different types of masks vary in the degree of protection they offer.

A properly applied mask fits snugly over the mouth and nose so that pathogens and body fluids cannot enter or escape through the sides. If a person wears glasses, the top edge of the mask fits below the glasses so that they will not cloud over as the person exhales. Talking should be kept to a minimum while wearing a mask to reduce respiratory air flow. A mask that has become moist does not provide a barrier to microorganisms and thus is ineffective. It should be discarded. A mask should never be reused. Patients/clients and family members should be warned that a mask can cause a sensation of smothering. If family members become uncomfortable, they should leave the room and discard the mask.

Before removing a mask, remove gloves (if worn) or wash hands if they have been in contact with infectious material. The mask is disposed of by holding it at the tie, avoiding contact with the soiled surface. It is placed in a waste receptacle.

**Gloves** Gloves prevent the transmission of pathogens by direct and indirect contact. Reasons for wearing gloves include:

* reducing the possibility of personnel coming in contact with infectious organisms that infect patients/clients (for example, handling contaminated dressings or cleaning an incontinent person with hepatitis B)
* reducing the likelihood that personnel will transmit their own endogenous flora to patients/clients
* reducing the possibility that personnel will become transiently colonized with microorganisms that can be transmitted to other patients/clients (transient colonization can usually be prevented with handwashing).

Nurses should use gloves when there is risk of exposure to infected material, when performing venepuncture or finger or heel sticks, when they expect to spill blood or other body fluids on the hands, and when they are inexperienced. In most cases, disposable, single-use gloves are worn. When full protective clothing is needed, first apply a mask, wash and dry hands, apply a gown and then apply gloves. Disposable gloves are easily applied and designed to fit either hand. The glove's thin rubber, however, can be easily torn. The glove cuffs should be pulled up over the wrists or cuffs of a gown.

After coming in contact with any infected material, gloves should be changed. Researchers have determined that repeated manipulations of gloved hands can allow bacteria to pass through the rubber. Korniewicz et al (1989) suggest that gloves should be changed frequently after high-stress use in high-risk situations.

Family members often believe that they can touch any object after they have applied gloves. The nurse should explain that gloves can also become contaminated after touching infected material or another contaminated object. It is very important to wash hands after removing gloves. Bacteria can cross through rubber gloves, especially if the rubber is thin or if the gloves have been worn for a prolonged period of time under stress (Korniewicz et al, 1989).

Reverse barrier nursing is used to prevent transmitting an infection to a patient/client; for example, a person who is immunosuppressed.

**Protective Eyewear** When participating in an invasive procedure that creates droplets or splashing of blood or other body fluids, a nurse may be required to wear protective eyewear. This will help prevent infectious agents entering the bloodstream through the eye. Examples of invasive procedures include irrigation of a large abdominal wound and insertion of an arterial catheter in which the nurse assists a doctor. Eyewear may be available in the form of plastic glasses or goggles. The eyewear should fit snugly around the face so that fluids cannot enter between the face and glasses.

**Delivering Care When Barrier Nursing** Remain aware of the aseptic technique while working with patients/clients in protected environments. You should feel comfortable in performing all procedures and yet remain conscious of infection-control principles. If you bring any article into the room or expose an article to infected material and then touch or remove the article, the risk of transmitting infection to other patients/clients or personnel is increased.

Regardless of the form of barrier nursing, the nurse follows certain precautions when handling equipment and supplies. The following guidelines limit transmission of microorganisms:

* keep medication trolleys or trays outside of the patient's/client's room
* discard unsheathed needles, sharp objects, and syringes in puncture-proof receptacles in the patient's/client's room
* keep equipment for assessing vital signs in the patient's/client's room for the duration of isolation. Use disposable thermometers. Avoid bringing electronic thermometers into isolation rooms
* when plastic, rubber, or glass reusable items become soiled, place them in separate bags because methods of sterilization differ.

**Specimen Collection** Many laboratory studies may be required when a patient/client is suspected of having an infectious disease. Body fluids and secretions suspected of containing infectious organisms are collected for culture and sensitivity investigations. The specimen is placed in a medium that

**TABLE 28-5 Specimen Collection Techniques**

| Amount Needed* | Collection Device* | Specimen Collection and Transfer |
|---|---|---|
| **WOUND CULTURE** | | |
| As much as possible (after cleaning skin to remove flora) | Cotton-tipped swab or syringe | Place clean test tube or culturette tube on clean paper towel. After swabbing centre of wound site, grasp collection tube by holding it with a paper towel. Carefully insert swab without touching outside of tube. After washing hands and securing tube's top, transfer labelled tube into bag for transport to laboratory. |
| **BLOOD CULTURE** | | |
| 10 ml per culture bottle, from two different venepuncture sites (volume may differ based on collection containers) | Syringes and culture media bottles | Perform venepuncture at two different sites to decrease likelihood of both specimens being contaminated by skin flora. Inject 10 ml of blood into each bottle. Wash hands. Secure tops of bottles, label specimens, and send to laboratory. |
| **STOOL CULTURE** | | |
| Small amount, approximately size of a walnut | Clean cup with seal top (not necessary to be sterile) and tongue blade | Place cup on clean paper towel in patient's/client's bathroom. Using tongue blade, collect needed amount of faeces from bedpan. Transfer faeces to cup without touching cup's outside surface. Wash hands and place seal on cup. Transfer specimen cup into clean bag for transport to laboratory. |
| **URINE CULTURE** | | |
| 1-5 ml | Syringe and sterile cup | Place cup or clean towel in patient's/client's bathroom. Use syringe to collect specimen if patient/client has Foley catheter. Have patient/client follow procedure to obtain clean-voided specimen if not catheterized. Transfer urine into sterile container by injecting urine from syringe or pouring it from used container. Wash hands and secure top of labelled container. Transfer labelled container to laboratory. |

*Local policies may differ on type of containers, amount of specimen material required, and bagging.

promotes growth of organisms. A laboratory technician then identifies the microorganisms growing in the culture. Additional test results indicate the antibiotics to which the organisms are resistant or sensitive. Sensitivity reports determine the antibiotics to be used in treatment.

Obtain all culture specimens using disposable gloves and sterile equipment. Collecting fresh material from the site of infection, such as in the case of wound drainage, ensures that the specimen will not be contaminated by neighbouring microbes. Each specimen container should be sealed tightly to prevent spillage and contamination of the outside of the container. Table 28-5 describes techniques for collecting specimens from the patient/client with a suspected infection.

## Bagging Articles

Use special bagging procedures for removing contaminated items from the patient's/client's environment. Bagging articles prevents accidental exposure of personnel to contaminated articles and prevents contamination of the surrounding environment.

Suggested guidelines for handling soiled linen (Weinstein *et al*, 1989) include:

1. Placing it in the appropriate laundry bag in the patient's/client's room.
2. Labelling the bag or having a specific colour (for example, red) designated for such linen so that it is easily recognized.
3. Using bags that are soluble in hot water as they require less handling. However, these may need to be double bagged as they puncture or tear easily.

If double bagging is followed, the procedure requires the nurse in the patient's/client's room to place all soiled linen into a bag and close it tightly. The nurse then places the first bag into a second bag held by a 'clean nurse' or into a self-supporting linen holder outside the patient's/client's room. The outer bag is specially labelled or coloured. The clean nurse secures the outer bag and sends it to the laundry. Nurses should familiarize themselves with infection control policies and the regulations employed for discarding soiled and/or infected linen, equipment and other materials.

## ROLE OF THE INFECTION CONTROL NURSE

Many hospitals employ nurses who are specially trained in infection control. These nurses are responsible for advising hospital personnel on safe aseptic practices and for monitoring infection outbreaks within the hospital. Duties of an infection control nurse include the following:

1. Providing staff education on infection control.
2. Reviewing infection-control policies and procedures.
3. Reviewing patient's/client's records and laboratory reports to recommend appropriate isolation procedures.
4. Screening patient/client records for community-acquired infections.
5. Consulting with occupational health departments concerning recommendations to prevent and control the spread of infection among personnel such as tuberculosis testing.
6. Gathering statistics regarding the epidemiology of nosocomial infections.
7. Notifying public health department of incidences of communicable diseases.
8. Conferring with all hospital departments to investigate unusual events or clusters of infection.
9. Educating patients/clients and families.
10. Identifying infection-control problems with equipment.
11. Checking microorganism sensitivity to antibiotics in use and reminding medical staff of resistance.
12. Liaising with hospital and community health care personnel.

## INFECTION CONTROL FOR HOSPITAL PERSONNEL

Health care workers are continually at risk for exposure to infectious microorganisms. Suggested guidelines to protect employees from infectious hazards in the workplace include:

1. Compliance with universal precautions. Employees should follow universal precautions to prevent contact with blood or other infectious materials during the routine care of patients/clients.
2. Domestic staff. Workplaces are to be maintained in a clean and sanitary condition. Routine cleaning and decontamination procedures are established, depending on surfaces to clean and the procedures performed in the work area. For example, containers of contaminated needles must be replaced regularly and not allowed to overfill.
3. High-risk exposure. If health care workers have needle stick injury or mucous membrane exposure to blood or other infectious body fluids, the incident should be reported immediately. Evaluation and preventive treatment for hepatitis B and HIV is critical. The staff member may be screened, and appropriate treatments provided. Immunization programmes should also be made available to protect employees from becoming infected. Hepatitis B vaccinations are now widely available for student nurses. Other vaccinations may be made available by employers.

## PATIENT/CLIENT EDUCATION

Apart from the need to administer self-injections, it is more practical for patients/clients to learn clean rather than strict sterile techniques that can be practised at home. Family members who may care for such a patient/client, however, must be involved in the nurse's teaching plan. Teach patients/clients and family members a commonsense approach to controlling and preventing infection.

## PERFORMING STERILE PROCEDURES

All the necessary equipment should be assembled before a procedure is undertaken. Thus, the nurse avoids having to leave a sterile area unattended because equipment is missing. A few extra supplies should be available in case objects accidentally become contaminated. Prior to the procedure, each step should be explained so that the patient/client can cooperate fully. If an object becomes contaminated during the procedure, the nurse should not hesitate to discard it immediately.

**Opening Sterile Packages** Sterile items such as syringes, gauze dressings, or catheters are packaged in paper or plastic containers impervious to microorganisms as long as they are dry and intact. Some institutions wrap reusable supplies in a double thickness of linen or muslin.

Sterile supplies have dated labels or chemical tapes that indicate the date when the sterilization period expires. The tapes change colour during the sterilization process. Failure of the tapes to change colour means the item is not sterile. A sterile supply or piece of equipment should never be used after the expiration date. The item is either discarded or returned to the institution's supply area for resterilization.

Before opening a sterile item wash your hands thoroughly. Assemble the supplies in the work area such as the trolley or table top before opening packages. The work area should be above waist level. Sterile supplies should not be opened in a confined space where a dirty object might fall on or strike them.

**Preparing a Sterile Field** When performing sterile procedures, the nurse needs a sterile work area that provides room for handling and placing of sterile items. A **sterile field** is an area

## PROCEDURE 28-1 Preparing a Sterile Field

| SEQUENCE OF ACTIONS | RATIONALE |
|---|---|
| 1. Prepare sterile field just before planned procedure. Supplies are to be used immediately. | Prevents exposure of sterile field and supplies to air and contamination. |
| 2. Select clean work surface above waist level. | Sterile object held below waist is contaminated. |
| 3. Assemble necessary equipment:<br>  a. Sterile drape<br>  b. Assorted sterile supplies | Preparation of equipment in advance prevents break in technique. |
| 4. Check dates or labels on supplies for sterility of equipment. | Equipment stored beyond expiration date is considered unsterile. |
| 5. Wash hands thoroughly. | Prevents transmission of infection. |
| 6. Place pack containing sterile drape on work surface and open as described. | Ensures sterility of packaged tape. |
| 7. With fingertips of one hand, pick up folded top edge of sterile drape (see illustration). | 2.5 cm border around drape is unsterile and may be touched. |

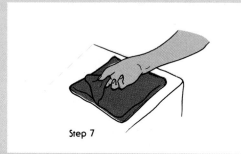

Step 7

| | |
|---|---|
| 8. Gently lift drape up from its outer cover and let it unfold by itself without touching any object. Discard outer cover with your other hand. | If sterile object touches any other nonsterile object, it becomes contaminated. |
| 9. With other hand, grasp adjacent corner of drape and hold it straight up and away from your body. | Drape can now be properly placed while using two hands. Drape must be held away from unsterile surfaces. |
| 10. Holding drape, first position the bottom half over intended work surface (see illustration). | Prevents nurse from reaching over sterile field. |

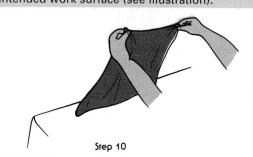

Step 10

| | |
|---|---|
| 11. Allow top half of drape to be placed over work surface last (see illustration). | Creates flat, sterile work surface. |

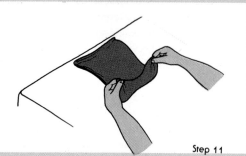

Step 11

### ADDING STERILE ITEMS

| | |
|---|---|
| 12. Open sterile item (following package directions) while holding outside wrapper in nondominant hand. | Frees dominant hand for unwrapping outer wrapper. |
| 13. Carefully peel wrapper onto nondominant hand. | Item remains sterile. Inner surface of wrapper covers hand, making it sterile. |

## PROCEDURE 28-1 Preparing a Sterile Field (Cont'd)

| SEQUENCE OF ACTIONS | RATIONALE |
|---|---|
| 14. Making sure wrapper does not fall down on sterile field, place item onto field at angle. Do not hold arm over sterile field | Prevents reaching over field and contaminating its surface. |
| 15. Dispose of outer wrapper. | Prevents accidental contamination of sterile field. |
| 16. Perform procedure using sterile technique. | Prevents transmission of infection to patient/client. |

free of microorganisms and prepared to receive sterile items. The field may be prepared by using the inner surface of a sterile wrapper as the work surface or by using a sterile drape. Procedure 28-1 describes the preparation of a sterile field. After the surface for the field is created, add sterile items by placing them directly on the field or by transferring them with sterile forceps. When transferring sterile items, carefully place objects onto the sterile field. An object that comes in contact with the 2.5 cm border should be discarded.

You may choose to wear sterile gloves while preparing items on the field. If this is the case, you can touch the entire drape, but sterile items must be handed over by an assistant. Your gloves must not touch the wrappers of sterile items.

 ## EVALUATION

The success of the nurse who practises infection-control techniques is measured by determining whether the goals for reducing or preventing infection are achieved. A comparison of the patient's/client's response, such as absence of fever or development of wound drainage, with expected outcomes determines the success of nursing interventions. Similarly, a determination is made about whether interventions should be revised or eliminated. To correctly assess wounds for healing and to conduct a physical assessment of body systems are important skills in evaluation. Closely monitor patients/clients, especially those at risk, for signs and symptoms of infection.

The patient/client at risk for infection must understand the measures needed to reduce or prevent microorganism growth and spread. Providing patients/clients or family members with the opportunity to discuss infection-control measures or to demonstrate procedures will reveal their ability to comply with therapy. You may determine that patients/clients require new information or that previously instructed information requires reinforcement.

Accurately document the patient's/client's response to treatments for infection control. A clear description of any signs and symptoms of systemic or local infection is necessary to give all nurses a baseline for comparative evaluation. The efficacy of any intervention in reducing infection must also be reported.

## SUMMARY

In every aspect of practice the nurse encounters situations that present a risk of an infection developing or being transmitted. Pathogens, or microorganisms capable of causing disease, are widespread in the environment and can cause infection to develop. Aseptic practice helps break the chain of infection in a susceptible host. An awareness of the conditions that cause pathogens to thrive, and the modes of their transmission, is therefore essential in the identification of nursing interventions for infection control.

Knowledge of the role of normal body flora, the healthy immune response, and other body mechanisms that defend against infection helps the nurse identify those patients/clients most at risk. An ability to recognize the signs of inflammation that indicate the body's cellular response to injury or infection enables the nurse to be alert to changes in any body part and to act accordingly.

It is also vital that the nurse recognizes all those procedures that can cause nosocomial infections in the health care setting and factors that increase the risks of inter-patient/client transmission. The principles of asepsis need careful implementation during all routine nursing actions, and the universal precautions guidelines should be followed at all times by all health care personnel. Where surgical asepsis is required, the nurse should be especially alert to the strict guidelines that must be adhered to.

It should be remembered that failure to follow the required aseptic procedure for any nursing action, using the relevant protective equipment, may seriously hamper the recovery of the individual or the maintenance of good health in either the nurse or patient/client involved.

## CHAPTER 28 REVIEW

### Key Concepts

- Handwashing is the most important technique in preventing and controlling transmission of infection.
- The potential for microorganisms to cause disease depends on the number of organisms, virulence, ability to enter and survive in a host, and susceptibility of the host.
- Normal body flora resist infection by releasing antibacterial substances and inhibiting multiplication of pathogenic microorganisms.
- The signs of local inflammation and infection are identical.
- Immunity to infection is a biological response that changes the body's response to future exposure to antigens.
- An infection can develop as long as the six elements composing the infection chain are uninterrupted.
- Microorganisms are transmitted by direct and indirect contact, by airborne spread, and by vectors and contaminated vehicles.
- Increasing age, poor nutrition, stress, inherited conditions,

chronic disease, and treatments or conditions that compromise the immune response increase susceptibility to infection.

- The major sites for nosocomial infections include the urinary and respiratory tracts, bloodstream, and surgical or traumatic wounds.
- Invasive procedures, medical treatments/investigations, long hospitalization, and contact with health care personnel increase a hospitalized patient's/client's risk for acquiring a nosocomial infection.
- Patients/clients within an intensive care unit have a higher risk for infection than patients/clients who are not in this area.
- Isolation practices prevent personnel and patients/clients from acquiring infections and prevent transmission of microorganisms to other persons.
- Proper cleansing requires mechanical removal of all foreign material from an object or area.
- Universal blood and body fluid precautions serve to prevent the spread of the HIV virus and other blood-borne pathogens.
- A patient/client in isolation is subject to sensory deprivation because of the restricted environment.
- A clinical nurse specialist (infection control) monitors the incidence of infections within an institution and provides educational and consultative services to maintain infection control practices.
- If the skin is broken or if the nurse performs an invasive procedure into a body cavity normally free of microorganisms, surgical aseptic practices are followed.

## CRITICAL THINKING EXERCISES

1. Maintain a reflective record of how often, in what situations, and for what reasons you should have washed your hands and/or worn gloves to undertake nursing procedures on the patients/clients you have been caring for over a period of two days. Highlight why you did or did not follow the correct procedures.
2. The infection chain consists of six elements. Identify the elements of the infection chain created by the introduction of an urinary catheter into a patient/client. Explain the risks to the individual and nurse.
3. What are the cardinal signs of a wound infection?
4. Discuss with a senior colleague or tutor why stringent cross-infection measures and barrier nursing techniques have to be undertaken in some instances.
5. The cleansing of patient/client care equipment breaks which element of the infection chain?

## Key Terms

Antibodies, p. 574
Antigen, p. 573
Asepsis, p. 575
Bacteria, p. 568, 569
Bacteriocidal, p. 569
Bacteriostasis, p. 569
Colonization, p. 583
Disinfection, p. 580
Iatrogenic infections, p. 575
Immune response, p. 574
Immunocompromised, p. 568
Inflammatory response, p. 571
Isolation, p. 583
Nosocomial infections, p. 574
Pathogens, p. 567
Sterile field, p. 587
Sterilization, p. 580
Universal precautions, p. 584
Virulence, p. 568

## REFERENCES

Burton GRW: *Microbiology for the health sciences*, ed 4, Philadelphia, 1992, JB Lippincott.

Brunner LS, Suddarth DS: *The textbook of adult nursing*, London, 1992, Chapman & Hall.

Chauduri AK: Infection control in hospitals: has its quality - enhancing and cost-effective role been appreciated? *J Hosp Infect*, 25: 1, 1993.

Crow R *et al*: Indwelling catheterisation and related nursing practice. *J Adv Nurs* 13(4): 489, 1988.

Department of Health: *Guidance for clinical health care workers, protection against infection with HIV and hepatitis viruses*, London, 1990, Smith & Nephew Medical

Illich I: *Limits to medecine—medical nemesis: the expropriation of health*, London, 1988, Penguin Books.

Korniewicz DM *et al*: Integrity of vinyl and latex procedure gloves, *Nurs Res* 38(3):144, 1989.

Lascelles I: Wound dressing technique, *Nurs* 2(8):217, 1982.

Lynch P, Jackson MM: Isolation practices: how much is too much or not enough? *Asepsis* 10(3):12, 1988.

Royal College of Nursing: *Universal precautions against Hepititis B and AIDs*. London, 1994, Royal College of Nursing.

Sedjwick J: Handwashing in hospital wards, *Nurs Times*, 80(20): 64, 1984.

Taylor LJ: An evaluation of handwashing techniques, *Nurs Times* 74(**Jan**):12, 1978a.

Taylor LJ: An evaluation of handwashing techniques, *Nurs Times* 74(2):54, 1978b.

Tideiksaar R: Infections in the elderly: diagnosis and treatment, *Physician Assist* 11(2):17, 1987.

Weinstein SA *et al*: Bacterial surface contamination of patient's linen: isolation precautions versus standard care, *Am J Infection Control*, 17(5):264, 1989.

Williams WW: CDC guidelines for infection control in hospital personnel, *Infect Control* 4(4):325, 1983.

Wright E: Catheter care: The risk of infection, *Prof Nurs*, 4(12):63, 1988a.

Wright E: Minimising the risk of a urinary tract infection, *Prof Nurs*, 4(2):63, 1988b.

## FURTHER READING
### Adult Nursing
Burton GRW: *Microbiology for the health sciences*, Philadelphia, 1992, JB Lippincott.

Centers for Disease Control: Update: universal precautions for prevention of transmission of human immunodeficiency virus, hepatitis B virus, and other bloodborne pathogens in health care settings, *MMWR* 37(24):377, 1988.

### Children's Nursing
Ayliff G AJ *et al* eds: *Control of Hospital infection: apractical handbook* 3/e, London, 1992, Chapman & Hall

Brown G, Evans S: Immunization — uptake study, *Paed Nurs* 1(4), 1989.

Rudd P, Nicoll A: *British paediatric association manual on infections and immunizations in children*, Oxford, 1991, Oxford University Press.

# Perioperative Nursing

## LEARNING OUTCOMES

After studying this chapter, you should be able to:
- *Define the key terms listed.*
- *Explain the concept of perioperative nursing care.*
- *List and discuss the many factors to include in the preoperative assessment of a surgical patient/client.*
- *List the common preoperative screening tests undertaken and describe their purposes.*
- *Recognize the importance of a preoperative teaching programme.*
- *Demonstrate postoperative exercises.*
- *Prepare a patient/client for surgery on the morning of a scheduled operation.*
- *Describe correct preoperative documentation procedures.*
- *Explain the role of the nurse during transport to theatre, theatre admission, and in the operating theatre.*
- *Describe the nurse's role in the recovery unit.*
- *Identify factors to include in the postoperative assessment of a patient/client in recovery.*
- *Describe the rationale for nursing interventions designed to prevent postoperative complications.*

A patient/client faces a variety of stressors when confronting surgery. Anticipating surgery can lead to fear and anxiety for people who associate surgery with pain, possible disfigurement, dependence, and perhaps even loss of life. Family members often fear a disruption in lifestyle and experience a sense of powerlessness as the surgery approaches. The trauma sustained during surgery creates physical and psychological needs, requiring close supervision and skilled intervention by the nurse and doctor. The individual is more able to participate in the planned care if the nurse has provided information about events occurring before and after surgery.

Modern surgical techniques, for example key hole surgery, laser procedures, and contemporary surgical nursing practice, have helped reduce the length of inpatient stay. Many patients/clients now attend day surgery or five-day wards. Early discharge is advocated to reduce the risk of hospital-acquired infection and to promote earlier recovery, enhancing physical and psychological independence. Surgical nurses, therefore, often work under increased pressure to maintain a high quality of care in an area with a fast throughput of patients/clients.

To promote effective and appropriate care within all surgical settings, surgical nurses are encouraged to practise a shared philosophy of care, identify or create a nursing model that demonstrates the application of the philosophy in practice, write standards of care, and undertake an audit of their area which includes their patients'/clients' perspectives of the care received. A prerequisite for these strategies is reflection on practice, which enables the surgical nurse to assess the efficacy of his or her actions, question current practices and create innovative changes based on assessment and evaluation. Surgical nurses require specialist knowledge and skills to ensure their patients/clients receive a high standard of care.

The surgical patient/client is in a vulnerable position. His or her surgery may be medically classified as a minor operation and considered routine, but to the individual it is of major significance. The role of the surgical nurse is to ensure each person receives individualized perioperative care within a nursing framework that meets the person's physical, psychological, sociocultural and spiritual needs in a safe and effective manner. It is important, also, to ensure there is good communication between the hospital and community nursing service so that clients receive appropriate and timely follow-up after discharge.

## PERIOPERATIVE NURSING CARE

**Perioperative nursing** refers to the role of the nurse during the preoperative, intraoperative, and postoperative phases of a patient's/client's surgical experience. The concept of perioperative nursing stresses the importance of providing **continuity of care**. The system of ward organization complements this aim. Primary nursing or team nursing should ensure that the same nurses provide care for the same patients/clients and should also promote a supportive environment. In some hospitals preoperative visiting is undertaken by the theatre nurse, and patients/clients and their relatives may be invited to view the theatre suite to reduce their fear of the unknown. The theatre nurse assesses the individual's health status, identifies specific needs, reinforces preoperative teaching, attends to the patient's/client's needs in the operating department, and cares for the person in the recovery area. **The nurse's main responsibility is to provide safe, effective and consistent nursing care during each phase of surgery.**

## PREOPERATIVE PHASE

Surgical patients/clients enter the health care setting in different stages of health. A person may enter the hospital on a predetermined day feeling relatively healthy and prepared to face elective surgery. In contrast, a victim of a road traffic accident may face emergency surgery with no time to prepare.

Surgical patients/clients undergo tests and procedures to determine their physical status in preparation for surgery. Tests may be performed in a pre-admissions clinic or as an outpatient. Pre-admission clinics also provide preoperative patient information and education (Pape, 1990). This negates the need for earlier hospitalization prior to surgery. Pellett (1990) provides a succinct account of the preparation for day surgery in children.

 **ASSESSMENT**

Assessment of the surgical patient/client involves collecting a nursing history, reviewing the patient's/client's and family members' emotional health, and analysing risk factors and diagnostic data. Day surgery patients/clients may receive a less detailed assessment. The assessment establishes normal values for

the patient/client and alerts the nurse to possible postoperative complications.

The nurse conducts an initial interview to collect information that will enable him or her to plan individualized care. In the day ward setting, the history may be shorter than that collected when the person is hospitalized before surgery. If a patient/client is unable to relate all necessary information, the nurse may ask family members, partners or close friends.

On admission, most individuals should be encouraged to remain in their everyday clothes for as long as possible. This enables them to retain their personal identity and to feel 'normal'. Biographical details and information is recorded on the admission form.

The assessment provides the nurse with specific information to devise an individualized care plan for each person. The documentation provides information regarding actual or potential patient/client problems. Figure 29-1 illustrates part of a pre-printed preoperative care plan with room to add individual patient/client needs. In this care plan the actual and potential problems are identified using the Roper *et al* (1990) model for nursing which provides a theoretical framework for clinical practice. The numbering system relates to the appropriate activity of living.

Surgical assessment also enables the nurse to identify the patient's/client's gaps in knowledge and the need for health education. While specific patient information materials may be helpful, the nurse should ensure that the patient/client understands them (Taylor *et al*, 1982).

### Documenting the Nursing Assessment

The assessment part of the nursing care plan, based on the model of care, will guide the area of questioning. If, for example, the Roper *et al* (1990) model is utilized as a framework for care, the nurse will determine the patient's/client's level of independence in each of the activities of living (ALs).

One of the original ALs, *dying*, has been replaced by *personal worries*. It could be considered inappropriate to discuss the concept of dying with most surgical patients/clients. Thompson (1992) addresses the needs of terminally ill patients/clients on an acute surgical ward. McRobb (1993) provides a poignant account of her experience for the benefit of all nurses. Although nursing as a profession strives to care for the whole person, spiritual care is often delegated to the hospital chaplain or other spiritual leaders. Burnard (1985) asserts that the spiritual aspect of the person remains largely unexplored in both the nursing literature and nursing practice. Sims (1987), however, provides guidelines for nurses to assess patients'/clients' spiritual needs.

The physical, psychological, sociocultural, politicoeconomic factors that enhance or inhibit independence should be identified within each of the ALs as appropriate. The patient's/client's perception of independence, however, needs to be elicited as it may not be congruent with that of the nurse. Fulbrook (1992) supports the view that the Roper *et al* model could be considered appropriate for nursing surgical patients. Fraser (1990) notes, however, that although it has become one of the best known and widest used models of nursing in the United Kingdom, there are no research findings that demonstrate the validity of the model in practice.

| ACTIVITIES OF LIVING: (A) ACTUAL (P) POTENTIAL PROBLEMS | PATIENT'S PROBLEMS | AIM/EVENTUAL OUTCOME | PREOPERATIVE NURSING CARE PLAN | SIGNED |
|---|---|---|---|---|
| 2(A) | Anxiety due to impending surgery | Patient/client is able to express anxieties and fears | • Discuss preoperative and anticipated postoperative care, including methods of pain relief | |
| | | | • Allow patients and relatives time to talk and ask questions, reinforcing previous explanations | |
| | | | • Arrange visit by outside agency if appropriate (specify) | |
| | | | • Offer night sedation as prescribed | |
| | | | • Prescribed premedication to be given at (TIME)          (DATE) | |
| | | | • After which patient to remain in bed with a call bell | |
| | | | | |
| 3(P) | Respiratory problems due to (a) inhalation of gastric contents while unconscious | Minimize risk of chest infection/inhalation of gastric contents | • Report any breathing difficulties | |
| | (b) underlying respiratory disorder | Identify any respiratory problems | • Discourage smoking | |
| | | | • Reinforce physiotherapist's teaching of deep breathing exercises | |
| | | | • NO FOOD FROM | |
| | | | • NIL BY MOUTH FROM | |
| | | | | |
| 8(P) | Decreased mobility leading to circulatory problems | Patient will remain mobile/perform leg exercises as appropriate | • Encourage mobility during postoperative period | |
| | Pressure sore risk assessment score | | • Reinforce physiotherapist's teaching of leg exercises | |
| | | | • Apply TED stockings YES/NO | |
| | | | | |
| 1 (P) | Wound infection from skin flora | Patient's skin to be clean prior to surgery | • Patient to have bath/shower – no talcum powder to be used | |
| | | | • Shave only if specifically requested by surgeon | |
| | | | • Check nails and umbilicus—remove make-up as appropriate | |
| | | | • Patient to have clean theatre gown and cap | |
| | | | • Remake bed with clean linen when patient is in theatre | |
| | | | | |
| 5(P) | Full bowel causing problems during surgery | Ensure patient has bowel action before surgery | • Bowel preparation required YES/NO | |
| | | Bowel clearance prior to major bowel surgery | (SPECIFY) | |

**Fig. 29-1** Pre-printed, preoperative care plan that can be individualized. Note: Activities of living are numbered here according to the originally proposed order. Courtesy of Joyce Green Hospital, Dartford, Kent.

Whenever posssible, the nursing care plan should be written *with* the patient/client. Many clinical areas now place the care plan at the bedside for the patient/client to read. This should facilitate communication, understanding and participation by the individual.

## PATIENTS'/CLIENTS' AND FAMILY MEMBERS' PERCEPTIONS OF SURGERY

Each person brings his or her fears and expectations to the surgical setting. Some fears are due to past hospital experiences, warnings from friends and family, or lack of knowledge. If someone has had surgery previously, the nurse assesses what the experience was like. The course of recovery, occurrence of complications, or perception of the quality of care given by nurses can influence a person's feelings about anticipated surgery. Incongruent perceptions of environmental stressors between nurses and surgical patients/clients may lead to inappropriate care (Biley, 1989; see Table 29-1).

The nurse faces an ethical dilemma when a person is misinformed or unaware of the reason for surgery. Manley (1990) discusses ethical principles in relation to surgical patients/clients. The nurse asks for a description of the patient's/client's understanding of the surgery and its implications. The nurse might ask questions such as, "Tell me what you think will happen before and after surgery", or "Explain to me what you know about surgery". The nurse usually confers with the doctor before

### TABLE 29-1 Nurses' and Patients' Perceptions of Surgical Stressors*

| Staff | (Patients) | Surgical Stressors |
|---|---|---|
| 1 | (6.5) | Right number of visitors |
| 2 | (1) | Getting to know patients |
| 3 | (2) | Adapting to a new routine |
| 4 | (12) | Amount of noise |
| 5 | (5) | Sleeping in a different bed |
| 6 | (3) | Asking staff questions |
| 7 | (6.5) | Meeting different staff |
| 8 | (15) | Unsuitable/unsatisfactory food |
| 9 | (4) | Sleeping in a strange environment |
| 10 | (16) | Nurses having too little time |
| 11 | (11) | Using a bedpan/bottle |
| 14 | (18) | Being a nuisance to nursing staff |
| 14 | (20) | Away from relatives |
| 14 | (13) | Lack of privacy |
| 14 | (23) | Being away from home/work |
| 14 | (8) | Staff discussing you |
| 17.5 | (9) | Having tests |
| 17.5 | (19) | Questions not answered |
| 19 | (17) | Doing something embarrassing |
| 20.5 | (10) | Having drips/injections |
| 20.5 | (25) | Not understanding instructions |
| 22 | (22) | Not enough information |
| 23 | (26) | Being in pain |
| 24.5 | (21) | Having an operation |
| 24.5 | (14) | Overall feeling since admission |
| 26 | (24) | Not knowing test results |

*ranked from 1 (least stressful) to 26 (most stressful)

From Biley F: Nurses' perceptions of stress in preoperative surgical patients, *J Advanced Nurs* 14:575, 1989.

revealing specific information related to the medical diagnosis. The nurse should also determine the person's knowledge of routine preoperative and postoperative procedures, although these will not appear routine to the patient/client. Hayward (1975) identified the need to provide information preoperatively to reduce anxiety in the postoperative phase.

It is important for the nurse to determine the extent of support from family members, partners and friends. Surgery may result in temporary or permanent disability that requires added assistance during recovery. The patient/client cannot always immediately assume the same level of physical activity enjoyed before an illness. Often an individual returns home with dressings to change or exercises to perform.

The family will also provide the emotional support needed to motivate the person to return to a previous state of health and his or her optimum level of independence. The family may need considerable support themselves. Social support is exceptionally important if the person, or family, has recently experienced a major life event or crisis. Life events, as identified by Holmes and Rahe (1967), can influence the person's attitude to surgery and the rehabilitation process.

## MEDICATION HISTORY

If a person regularly uses prescription or over-the-counter medications, the doctor may temporarily discontinue them before surgery or adjust the dosages. However, many patients/clients will continue to take their medication, unless contraindicated, until the immediate preoperative period.

### Safe Environment
### LEVEL OF ORIENTATION

During the assessment, the nurse observes the patient's/client's level of orientation, alertness, and mood, noting whether the person answers questions appropriately and can recall recent and past events. A person who is going to have surgery for neurological disease (for example, brain tumour or aneurysm) is likely to demonstrate an impaired level of consciousness or altered behaviour.

Undergoing surgery may also be particularly difficult for women from cultures which require them to keep their bodies totally covered.

In some cultures a woman belongs to her husband and difficulties can arise if she wants an operation and her husband does not wish her to have surgery.

Preoperative shaving may not be willingly accepted in some cultures, for example Rastarfarian.

In some cultures, the wearing of specific articles of jewellery is significant. For example, an adult initiated Sikh wears a Kara, a steel bangle around the wrist of their dominant hand. This bangle is a symbol of the unity of God, and should not be removed without permission from the individual person. Before surgery, the kara can be covered with tape. If removal is essential, for example in order to operate on that wrist, the nurse could sensitively suggest that the bangle could be placed on the other wrist, or kept it close to hand in a pocket or under a pillow.

## Children's Nursing
## Special considerations for children undergoing surgery

Children who undergo surgery have very different psychological and physiological needs than do adults undergoing surgery.

**Psychological care** is very important. Visitainer and Wolfer (1975) have identified various stress points before and after surgery, and it is useful for the nurse to be aware of these and to plan care accordingly. These stress points include: admission, blood tests, afternoon of the day before surgery, injections, and transport to and from the theatre and recovery room.

Children also have very different fears; for example, children under 5 years old worry about where they will wake up and who will be there. Nurses must also use appropriate terminology with this age group; for example, never describe anaesthesia as 'putting to sleep' as this may evoke memories of pets being 'put to sleep' and not waking up. Children aged 5-8 years are more concerned about how the anaesthetic works; adolescents are concerned with the operation, and potential physical deformities and death.

It is now common procedure to allow parents to accompany their child to the anaesthetic room. While this is helpful, the parents must be fully supported, informed and prepared for the event. If they are not prepared, their anxiety may rise, which may adversely affect the child.

**Physiological care** also differs for children, although the principles for care remain the same. For example, fasting time must be calculated carefully; infants must receive a carbohydrate mixture 3 hours preoperatively, and children must receive some fluid 4 hours preoperatively. Theatre delays must not result in longer periods of fasting.

Premedication in children under 7 years is usually oral and should be administered 2 hours prior to theatre. At the same time, EMLA (eutetic mixture of local anaesthetic) cream may be applied to the back of each hand to provide local anaesthesia prior to the intravenous induction of anaesthesia.

For the majority of children under 16 years, informed consent is obtained from the next of kin who take parental responsibility. However, the Children's Act (1989) re-emphasizes that minors below the age of 16 years have the right to consent to treatment if deemed competent. Whatever the child's age, it is important to ensure that the child is fully informed about the nature of his or her health problem and the intervention required.

## ALLERGIES

The nurse is particularly alert for allergies to drugs, for example penicillin, or to iodine, which may be applied to the skin prior to surgery. Hypoallergic tape should be used whenever possible to avoid an allergic skin reaction. The nurse informs the doctor of any allergies and should also highlight the information in the nursing care plan and in the relevent documentation sent with the patient/client to the operating theatre.

## Safe Psychological Environment
### FEELINGS

The nurse may be able to detect the patient's/client's feelings about surgery from **verbal** and **nonverbal behaviours**. A fearful person may ask many questions or alternatively become rather quiet and withdrawn, may seem uneasy with strangers or may actively seek the company of friends and relatives.

It is often difficult to assess feelings thoroughly when day surgery is scheduled. The nurse usually has limited time to establish a relationship with the patient/client. Fears may be allayed if the person attends a pre-admission clinic. Some surgical wards and theatre departments have produced patient information leaflets and videos providing general and specific details of the operation and care. The aim is to reduce anxiety by providing information. The nurse, however, should choose a time for discussion to explain that it is normal to have fears and concerns. The patient's/client's ability to share feelings depends on the nurse's willingness to listen, to be supportive, and to clarify misconceptions.

If the person feels powerless, the nurse ascertains why. The medical diagnosis may generate apprehension of increased dependence and loss of physical or mental function. The thought of being 'put to sleep' under anaesthesia creates concern about loss of control. Many people feel the need to retain the power to make decisions about treatment. The nurse must assure patients/clients of their right to ask questions and to seek information.

Patients/clients of ethnic and religious minorities may feel powerless and fearful that their cultural and spiritual needs may not be met. There may be language difficulties. Lack of insight by the nurse may cause anxiety and even offence to the person. The nurse must strive to ensure that he or she provides high quality, individualized care to all patients/clients. Marr (1993) and McCall (1991) provide insight into meeting the needs of patients/clients from various ethnic groups.

### PERSONAL IDENTITY

**Self-concept** People with a positive **self-concept** are more likely to approach surgical experiences appropriately. The nurse assesses self-concept by asking the person to identify his or her personal strengths and weaknesses. Those who are quick to criticize or scorn personal characteristics may have little self-regard or may be testing the nurse's opinion of their characters. Poor self-concept hinders the ability to adapt to the stress of surgery and aggravates feelings of guilt or inadequacy.

**Coping resources** Assessment of feelings and self-concept helps reveal whether the patient/client can cope with the stress of surgery. The nurse also asks the person about past stress management. If the patient/client has had previous surgery, the nurse determines behaviours that helped resolve any tension or nervousness. The nurse may instruct the person on relaxation exercises that can help control anxiety. Some surgical nurses are applying their knowledge of complementary therapies to promote relaxation (see Chapter 32). In particular the appropriate use of massage and aromatherapy have been found to be beneficial. Music as relaxation therapy has also been advocated by Moss (1988).

The nurse should ask if family members, partners or friends can provide support. The patient/client may want someone else present when the nurse provides instructions or explanations. They may also wish a friend, relative or partner to accompany them to the operating theatre.

## Expressing Sexuality

Sexual health care is a relatively new domain for the nurse and he or she needs to be comfortable with his or her own sexuality, feelings, values and attitudes regarding a variety of sexual activities and behaviours before he or she can advise patients. Salter (1988) asserts that if nursing is about caring for the whole person then body image and sexuality must be included in the care plan.

## Body image

Surgical removal of a diseased body part may leave permanent disfigurement or alteration in body function. Concern over mutilation, loss of a body part or physical attraction compounds an individual's fears. The nurse assesses for the **body image alterations** that patients/clients perceive will result from surgery. Individuals will react differently, depending on occupation, self-concept, and degree of self-esteem (Price, 1990a,b; Price, 1992; Price, 1993).

## SEXUAL FUNCTIONING

Often, surgery changes the physical or psychological aspects of patients'/clients' sexuality. Excision of breast tissue, colostomies or ureterostomies, or removal of prostate glands may affect sexuality. Surgery, such as hernia repair or cataract extraction, forces people to refrain from sexual intercourse until they return to normal physical activity.

### Mental Health Nursing
### Preparing a mental health patient/client for surgery

When preparing a person with a mental illness or someone who has a history of mental distress for surgery, there must be the same care and attention to providing appropriate information which is understandable. Where there are other carers involved, there needs to be liaison and clear communication requesting their support in preparing the patient/client.

Like any other person, the individual with a mental illness may be anxious about the nature of the surgery he or she will undergo. However, the way this individual articulates his or her fears may sometimes seem bizarre or incomprehensible. This does not mean that the need for comfort and reassurance is any less real compared to any other patient/client receiving surgery.

Today, all student nurses will have the advantageous opportunity to work in mental health care settings. Students should maximize the opportunities such placements will offer in enabling them to develop appropriate communication skills with those who are mentally ill or who are mentally distressed.

The nurse should provide the opportunity for patients/clients to express concerns about sexuality. The patient/client facing even temporary sexual dysfunction requires understanding and support. Discussions about the person's sexuality should be held with his or her sexual partner so that they can gain a shared understanding of how to cope with limitations in sexual function (McCracken, 1988).

## Communicating Pain Relief Information

One of the surgical patient's/client's greatest fears is pain (see Chapter 27). The family is also concerned about the person's comfort. Pain is subjective and individualistic therefore no two people will have the same pain experience. Past pain experiences and coping methods need to be identified by the patient/client.

Inform the individual and family of therapies available for pain relief, for example, analgesics, positioning and relaxation exercises. The individual should be encouraged to inform the nurses as soon as pain becomes a constant discomfort and should also know the length of time that it takes for a drug to act and that all discomfort is rarely eliminated.

Encourage the patient/client to use analgesics as required. Unless the pain is controlled, it will be difficult for the person to participate in postoperative rehabilitation. Surgical patients/clients may delay asking for pain relief because they think that they may be a bother to the nurse. They may also avoid taking pain-relief drugs for fear of becoming dependent. Both these myths need to be dispelled.

Most drug doses and the required intervals between administration are not sufficient to cause dependence. During assessment, the nurse should ascertain the person's drug history including any history of abuse or dependence, and prescribed analgesics. Hospitalized patients/clients usually receive intramuscular analgesia injections, depending on the nature of surgery. As they become able to tolerate food, oral analgesics can be given.

For many patients/clients a more appropriate and effective form of pain relief is patient-controlled analgesia (PCA). The nurse assess the person's ability and willingness to understand and perform PCA. Clark (1992) discusses the pros and cons of this strategy for surgical patients/clients. Patient controlled analgesia enables patients/clients to have control over their pain and promotes earlier independence.

## Working and Playing

Preparation for discharge must commence on admission. Surgery may result in physical alterations, for example, that hinder or prevent an individual from returning to paid work or housework and/or as a carer of chidren, elderly partner or parent. The nurse assesses his or her occupational history to anticipate the possible effects of surgery on rehabilitation and eventual work performance. When an individual is unable to return to a job, the nurse often confers with a social worker to refer the person to a job-retraining programme. Economic assistance in the form of grants or benefits may also be provided. Child care provision and social services, such as meals on wheels, may also have to be arranged.

**Adult Nursing**
**Physiological factors that place an older adult at risk for surgery**

With advancing age, an individual's physical capacity to adapt to the stress of surgery is hampered because of deterioration in certain body functions. Despite the risk, most patients/clients undergoing surgery are older adults.

| Alterations | Risks | Nursing Implications |
|---|---|---|
| **CARDIOVASCULAR SYSTEM** | | |
| Degenerative change in myocardium and valves. | Change reduces cardiac reserve. | Assess baseline vital signs. |
| Rigidity of arterial walls and reduction in sympathetic and parasympathetic innervation to heart. | Alterations predispose patient/client to postoperative haemorrhage and rise in systolic and diastolic blood pressure. Increase in calcium and cholesterol deposits within small arteries; thickened arterial walls. Problems predispose patient/client to clot formation in lower extremities. | Teach patient/client techniques for performing leg exercises and proper turning. |
| **PULMONARY SYSTEM** | | |
| Rib cage stiffened and reduced in size. | Complication reduces vital capacity. | Teach patient/client proper technique for coughing and deep-breathing exercises. |
| Reduced range of movement in diaphragm. | Greater residual capacity of volume of air is left in lung after normal breath increases, reducing amount of new air brought into lungs with each inspiration. | |
| Stiffened lung tissue and enlarged airspaces. | Alteration reduces blood oxygenation. | May require 28% oxygen at 2L/min following surgery. |
| **RENAL SYSTEM** | | |
| Reduced blood flow to kidneys. | Reduced flow increases danger of shock when blood loss occurs. | For patients/clients hospitalized before surgery, determine baseline urinary output for 24 hr. |
| Reduced glomerular filtration rate and excretory times. | Problem limits ability to remove drugs or toxic substances. | |
| Reduced bladder capacity. | Voiding frequency increases, and larger amount of urine stays in bladder after voiding. | Teach patient/client to notify nurse immediately when sensation of bladder fullness develops. |
| | Sensation of need to void may not occur until bladder is filled. | Keep call bell and bedpan within easy reach. |
| **NEUROLOGICAL SYSTEM** | | |
| Sensory losses, including reduced tactile sense and increased pain tolerance. | Patient/client is less able to respond to early warning signs of surgical complications. | Orient patient/client to surrounding environment. Observe for nonverbal signs of pain. |
| Decreased reaction time. | Patient/client becomes easily confused after anaesthesia. | Promote a safe environment and protect the patient/client from harm. |
| **METABOLIC SYSTEM** | | |
| Lower basal metabolic rate. | Lower rate reduces total oxygen consumption. | |
| Reduced number of red blood cells and haemoglobin levels. | Ability to carry adequate oxygen to tissues is reduced. | Administer necessary blood products. |
| Change in total amounts of body potassium and water volume. | Greater risk for fluid and electrolyte imbalance occurs. | Monitor electrolyte levels. |

## Physical Factors

The nurse observes the patient's/client's general appearance. Gestures and body movements may reflect weakness caused by illness. The person may appear malnourished. Height and body weight are important indicators of nutritional status.

Preoperative assessment of vital signs, including blood pressure, provides important baseline data with which to compare alterations that occur during and after surgery. Anxiety and fear commonly cause elevations in heart rate and blood pressure. Anaesthetic agents typically depress all vital functions. As the effects of the anaesthesia diminish after surgery, the nurse closely monitors vital signs and compares findings with **preoperative baselines**.

An elevated temperature before surgery is a cause for concern. If the patient/client has an underlying infection, the surgeon may choose to postpone surgery until the infection has been treated.

## PHYSICAL FACTORS ASSOCIATED WITH AGE

Very young and old patients/clients are at risk during surgery because of immature or declining physiological status. During surgery, an infant has difficulty maintaining a normal circulatory blood volume. The total blood volume of an infant is considerably less than that of an older child or adult. Even a small amount of blood loss can be serious. A reduced circulatory volume makes it difficult for the infant to respond to the need for increased oxygen during surgery. Thus, the infant is highly susceptible to **dehydration**. However, if blood or fluids are replaced too quickly, **overhydration** may occur. The physiological factors that place an older adult at risk are listed in the previous box.

## PERSONAL CLEANSING AND DRESSING

Assess the skin overlying all body parts. Give particular attention to bony prominences, such as the elbows, sacrum, and scapula. During surgery, a patient/client must lie in a fixed position, often for several hours. Thus, the individual is susceptible to pressure sores (see Chapter 30), especially if the skin is thin and dry. The overall condition of the skin also reveals the person's level of hydration.

## BREATHING

Assessment of the person's breathing pattern will help the nurse to determine respiratory function. When a person is under general anaesthesia, the lungs do not ventilate fully. After surgery, the patient/client has a reduced lung volume and needs greater effort to breathe.

Patients/clients are encouraged to deep breathe and cough postoperatively. A decline in ventilatory function may place the person at risk of developing respiratory complications. For example, a person who has high abdominal surgery will have difficulty breathing deeply because of a painful abdominal incision.

**Diaphragmatic breathing** improves lung expansion and oxygen delivery without using excess energy. The patient/client learns to use the diaphragm during deep breathing to take slow, deep, and relaxed breaths. Eventually the person's lung volume improves. Deep breathing also helps clear out anaesthetic gases remaining in the airways.

An individual who smokes is at a greater risk of postoperative pulmonary complications than a person who does not. The chronic smoker already has an increased amount and thickness of mucous secretions in the lungs. General anaesthetics increase airway irritation and stimulate pulmonary secretions, which are retained as a result of reduction in ciliary activity during anaesthesia. After surgery an individual who smokes has greater difficulty clearing the airways of mucous secretions and is more susceptible to postoperative chest infection.

## MOBILIZING

Encouraging patients/clients to remain mobile in the preoperative period will improve blood flow to the extremities and thus reduce stasis. Contraction of lower leg muscles promotes venous return, making it difficult for clots to form. Patients/clients are taught leg exercises and the nurse should encourage the person to perform these at least every two hours while awake. During surgery, venous blood flow to the legs slows. Stasis of circulation may lead to clot formation in the deep veins of the legs. A clot (thrombus) can become dislodged from the wall of the vein, and travel in the venous system to the lungs where it causes a pulmonary embolism, a potentially fatal complication.

To reduce the risk of a deep vein thrombosis many doctors prefer patients/clients to wear **antiembolism stockings** for the perioperative period. These are designed to support the lower extremities and to maintain compression of small veins and capillaries. The constant compression forces blood into larger vessels, thus promoting venous return and preventing circulatory stasis. When correctly sized and properly applied, antiembolism stockings can reduce the risk of thrombi (see Chapter 24).

## ELIMINATING

Establish the patient's/client's routine bladder and bowel performance (see Chapters 22 and 23). Routine urinalysis is performed to detect any abnormality in the urine. Analysis of a urine specimen consists of screening for urinary infection, renal disease, and diabetes mellitus. The nurse collects a clean-voided specimen. The urinalysis measures urine colour, pH, and specific gravity. It also determines the presence of protein, glucose, ketones, and blood.

Determine whether the person has regular bowel movements. Bowel preparation (for example, an aperient or enema, rectal washout) is sometimes undertaken especially when surgery involves the gastrointestinal system. Manipulation of portions of the gastrointestinal tract during surgery results in absence of peristalsis for 24 hours and sometimes longer. Bowel preparation helps to cleanse the gastrointestinal tract, to prevent intraoperative incontinence and postoperative constipation. An empty bowel reduces risk of injury to the intestines and prevents contamination of the operative wound when a portion of the bowel is incised or opened.

## EATING AND DRINKING

**Food intake** Assess the patient's/client's regular eating and drinking habits. Normal tissue repair and resistance to infection depend on adequate nutrients. Surgery intensifies this need.

After surgery, a person requires at least 1500 kcal/day to maintain energy reserves (Keithley, 1982). A malnourished person is prone to improper wound healing, reduced energy stores, and infection after surgery. If a patient/client has elective surgery, nutrient imbalances can be corrected before surgery, often with the provision of parenteral nutrition (Torrance, 1991). However, if a malnourished person has to undergo an emergency procedure, efforts to restore nutrients occur after surgery.

**Obesity increases surgical risk**  The obese patient/client may have reduced ventilatory and cardiac function and has difficulty resuming normal physical activity after surgery. An obese person is susceptible to poor wound healing and wound infection because of the structure of fatty tissue, which contains a poor blood supply. This slows delivery of essential nutrients, antibodies, and enzymes needed for wound healing. It is often difficult to close the surgical wound of an obese person because of the thick adipose layer. An obese person is also at risk of **dehiscence** (opening of the suture line).

**Fluid intake**  The importance of tactfully eliciting information regarding drinking habits is required, because habitual use of alcohol predisposes the person to adverse reactions to anaesthetic drugs. In addition, the doctor may need to increase postoperative dosages of analgesics. Excessive alcohol ingestion can also lead to malnutrition, which may contribute to delayed wound healing.

**Fluid and electrolyte balance**  The body responds to surgery as a form of trauma. As a result of the adrenocortical stress response, hormonal reactions cause sodium and water retention and potassium loss within the first 2 to 5 days after surgery. Severe protein breakdown causes a negative nitrogen balance. The severity of the stress response influences the degree of fluid and electrolyte imbalance. The more extensive the surgery, the more severe the stress. A person who is hypovolaemic or who has serious preoperative electrolyte alterations is at significant risk during and after surgery. For example, an excess or depletion of potassium increases the chance of dysrhythmias during or after surgery. If the person has pre-existing renal, gastrointestinal, or cardiovascular abnormalities, the risk of fluid and electrolyte alterations is even greater.

### Medical History

A review of the patient's/client's medical notes should include past illnesses and the primary reason for seeking medical care. The person's medical record can be a valuable source of data.

### Safeguarding Valuables

If a person has any valuables, the nurse should turn them over to family members or secure them for safekeeping. Many hospitals require patients/clients to sign a disclaimer form to free the institution of responsibility for lost valuables. Valuables can usually be stored and locked in a designated location. A wedding ring can be taped in place prior to surgery.

### Diagnostic Screening

Patients/clients are screened prior to surgery to determine normal bodily functioning and to detect any abnormalities. Many individuals are tested on an outpatient basis before surgery or the day before or the morning of surgery. However, a person may also enter the hospital several days in advance to complete all the necessary tests. If diagnostic tests reveal severe problems, the surgeon may postpone surgery until the condition stabilizes.

Routine screening tests may include a full blood count (FBC) and haemoglobin concentration, serum electrolyte analysis, coagulation studies, serum creatinine tests, a chest x-ray, an electrocardiogram (ECG). The nurse may undertake the blood tests and ECG. He or she should review the diagnostic results as they become available.

### FULL BLOOD COUNT

A FBC is the analysis of a peripheral venous blood specimen that measures erythrocyte count, leucocyte count, haemoglobin concentration, and haematocrit (packed erythrocyte volume). An abnormal FBC may indicate a number of alterations (for example, dietary deficiency and chronic blood loss), placing the person at risk for cardiovascular and pulmonary complications. In such a case the patient/client may undergo a blood transfusion prior to surgery.

### SERUM ELECTROLYTE ANALYSIS

Analysis of **serum electrolyte** levels also requires a peripheral venous blood sample. Because of the potential for fluid and electrolyte imbalances after surgery, the surgeon screens preoperative electrolyte levels to determine whether electrolyte replacement is necessary before surgery.

### COAGULATION STUDIES

The ability of blood to clot or coagulate is essential for minimizing the risk of haemorrhaging. The prothrombin time (PT), partial thromboplastin time (PTT), and platelet count are routine tests for the clotting ability of blood. **Coagulation** studies allow identification of patients/clients at risk for bleeding tendencies and thrombus formation.

### SERUM CREATININE TEST

A **serum creatinine test** assesses renal function. Creatinine is the by-product of muscle metabolism. The body excretes a constant amount through the kidneys, which serves as an excellent measure of the glomerular filtration rate. The creatinine level can be an indicator of renal failure when the value rises.

### CHEST X-RAY STUDY

A **chest x-ray** allows the doctor to examine the condition of the heart and lungs before surgery. Although the x-ray study does not always detect subtle pathological changes, it can reveal the overall size and shape of the heart, lung lesions and chest wall abnormalities, and position of the diaphragm and aorta. If the doctor detects lung abnormalities, a different type and dosage of sedatives or anaesthetic agents may be used. Before sending a female patient/client for an x-ray examination, the nurse should be sure that she is not pregnant, because exposure of the fetus to radiation may cause injury.

## ADDITIONAL SCREENING TESTS

If an individual is over the age of 40 or has heart disease, the doctor may order an ECG to measure the heart's electrical activity to determine whether the heart rate, rhythm, and other factors are normal. The procedure takes less than 5 minutes and requires the patient/client simply to lie flat and relax.

Depending on the type of surgery the person will undergo, there are several diagnostic tests for specific anatomical structures and physiological functions. If the person is likely to lose a large amount of blood during surgery, the doctor orders a blood specimen for type and crossmatching. This enables the laboratory to determine the proper blood type and Rh factor. The surgeon usually designates the number of blood units to have available during and following surgery.

 **PLANNING**

Planning preoperative care also includes **discharge planning**: this is especially relevent for the patient/client undergoing day surgery. Malby (1992) provides a standard plan for discharge.

It is essential to include any patient/client, especially the surgical patient/client, in health care planning. Involving the individual early when developing the surgical care plan can help minimize surgical risks and postoperative complications. A person who has been informed about the surgical experience is less likely to be fearful and can prepare for expected outcomes.

Broad goals of care for the preoperative patient/client include:

- understanding physiological and psychological responses to surgery
- understanding intraoperative and postoperative events
- remaining safe from harm during surgery
- achieving physical and psychological comfort and rest
- achieving independent physiological, psychological and social functioning after surgery
- remaining free of postoperative complications.

 **IMPLEMENTATION**

Preoperative nursing interventions aim to provide the patient/client with a complete understanding of the surgery and to prepare him or her physically and psychologically for surgical intervention and recovery.

### Informed Consent

A surgeon cannot legally perform surgery until a person has given his or her **informed consent**. In order to give this, the person has to understand the need for the procedure, the steps involved, risks, expected results, and alternative treatments. The primary responsibility for informing the person rests with the surgeon. Consent is not informed if the person is unclear about the nature of the operation, confused, unconscious, mentally incompetent,

or under the influence of sedatives. Tschudin (1989) illustrates the concept of informed consent in relation to a surgical patient/client with cancer of the ovary.

The legal age of consent is 16 years. A patient's/client's signature on a consent form implies that the person has been thoroughly informed about the procedure; however, the nurse should reinforce this knowledge to ensure that the appropriate information has been understood.

After the patient's/client's consent form has been completed, it is placed with his or her notes. The form accompanys the individual to the operating theatre.

### Preoperative Teaching

Educating patients/clients influences recovery positively, by promoting feelings of independence (Toms, 1993), collaboration, participation and control (Breemhaar and van den Borne, 1991). Earlier patient/client discharge and reduced use of postoperative medication are other cited benefits (Sutherland, 1980).

The nurse needs to determine what the person already knows and any gaps in knowledge. Acknowledging past learning can inspire self-confidence and self-esteem in patients/clients and negates the risk of patronizing the patient/client.

Patient/client participation in setting realistic goals for learning will augment a positive outcome. Physical and psychological factors need to be considered as these can affect a person's attention span and the ability to retain information. Anxiety and fear are barriers to learning, and both emotions are heightened as surgery approaches. The physical environment of a busy surgical ward may also inhibit concentration due to noise and constant distractions. Consequently, a 5 to 10 minute interaction may be sufficient and as effective as a more lengthy teaching session. Guiding principles which facilitate retention and recall in patients/clients are provided by Ewles and Simnett (1992).

It is preferable whenever possible to begin preoperative teaching well in advance of scheduled surgery to provide time for reinforcement of information. The nurse assesses the surgical

**Learning Disabilities Nursing**
**Providing information before surgery**

People with learning disabilities must be thoroughly prepared for each step of surgery. This is of greatest importance when the patient/client is profoundly handicapped. The nurse must ensure that the patient/client is informed about the procedure. Avoid long explanations and use visual aids to reinforce the most important aspects of the explanation. You can assess the effectiveness of your explanation and information by asking yourself, "What have I explained and what do I think my patient/client has understood?"

An effective way to reduce preoperative trauma for people with learning disabilities is to ensure that all preoperative care is carried out by the same nurse. Remember to include the individual's family in the process, because it will help them, will enhance your partnership with them, and will benefit the patient/client.

## PROCEDURE 29-1  Demonstrating Postoperative Exercises

| SEQUENCE OF ACTIONS | RATIONALE |
|---|---|
| **Controlled Coughing** | |
| 1. Explain importance of maintaining upright position. | Position facilitates diaphragm excursion and enhances thorax expansion. |
| 2. Demonstrate coughing. Take two slow, deep breaths, inhaling through nose and exhaling through mouth. | Deep breaths expand lungs fully so that air moves behind mucus and facilitates effects of coughing. |
| 3. Inhale deeply the third time and hold breath to count of 3. Cough fully for two or three consecutive coughs without inhaling between coughs. (Tell patient/client to push all air out of lungs.) | Consecutive coughs help remove mucus more effectively and completely than does one forceful cough. |
| 4. Caution patient/client against just clearing throat instead of coughing. | Clearing throat does not remove mucus from deep in airways. |
| 5. If surgical incision will be abdominal or thoracic, teach patient/client to place one hand over incisional area and other hand on top of first. During breathing and coughing exercises, patient/client presses gently against incisional area to splint or support it. Pillow over incision is optional (see photograph). | Surgical incision cuts through muscles, tissues, and nerve endings. Deep breathing and coughing exercises place additional stress on suture line and cause discomfort. Splinting incision with hands provides firm support and reduces incisional pulling. (Some patients/clients prefer to have a pillow to place over incision.) |

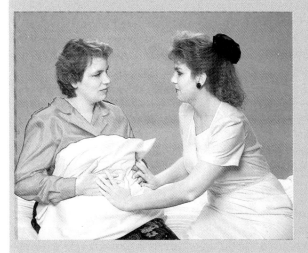

Step 5, Controlled coughing

| | |
|---|---|
| 6. Patient/client continues to practise coughing exercises, splinting imaginary incision. Instruct patient/client to cough two to three times every 2 hours while awake. | Value of deep coughing with splinting is stressed to effectively expectorate mucus with minimal discomfort. |
| 7. Instruct patient/client to examine sputum for consistency, amount, and colour changes. | Sputum consistency, amount, and colour changes may indicate presence of pulmonary complication, such as pneumonia. |
| **Leg Exercises** | |
| 1. Have patient/client assume supine position in bed. Demonstrate leg exercises by performing passive range of motion exercises and simultaneously explaining exercise. | Provides normal anatomical position of lower extremities. |
| 2. Rotate each ankle in complete circle. Instruct patient/client to draw imaginary circles with big toe. Repeat five times. | Leg exercises maintain joint mobility and promote venous return. |
| 3. Alternate dorsiflexion and plantar flexion of both feet. Direct patient/client to feel calf muscles contract and relax alternately (see photograph overleaf). Repeat five times. | Stretches and contracts gastrocnemius muscles. |

(Cont'd)

## PROCEDURE 29-1   Demonstrating Postoperative Exercises (Cont'd)

| STEPS | RATIONALE |
|---|---|
| Leg Exercises | |
| 4. Have patient/client continue leg exercises by alternately flexing and extending knees.  Repeat 5 times (see photograph). | Contracts muscles of upper legs and maintains knee mobility. |
| 5. Have patient/client alternately raise each leg straight up from bed surface, keeping legs straight. Repeat five times. | Promotes contraction and relaxation of quadriceps muscles. |
| 6. Have patient/client practise exercises at least every 2 hours while awake.  Instruct patient/client to coordinate leg exercises with diaphragmatic breathing, and coughing exercises. | Repetition of sequence reinforces learning. Establishes routine for exercises that develops habit for performance. |
| 7. Observe patient's/client's ability to perform all exercises independently. | Ensures that patient/client has learned correct technique. |
| 8. Record exercises demonstrated and patient's/client's ability to perform them independently. | Documents patient's/client's education and provides data for instructional follow-up. |

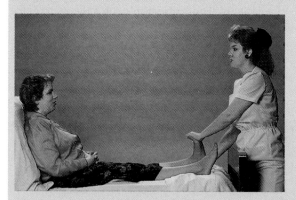

Step 3, Leg exercises

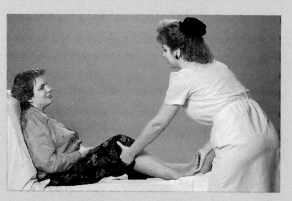

Step 4, Leg exercises

patient's/client's readiness and ability to learn. Specific learning goals should be documented in the nursing care plan. Most patients/clients, however, will need to be taught, often in conjunction with the physiotherapist, deep breathing and leg exercises (see Procedure 29-1).

### Eating and Drinking

Surgical procedures may cause extensive loss of blood and other body fluids. The nurse should ensure that the person eats and drinks sufficient amounts before fasting. This prevents fluid and electrolyte imbalances and reduces the risk of infection. The patient's/client's diet should include foods high in protein, with sufficient carbohydrates, fat, and vitamins. If a person cannot eat because of gastrointestinal alterations or impairments in consciousness, an intravenous route for fluid replacement is commenced. The doctor relies on serum electrolyte levels to determine the type of intravenous fluids and electrolyte additives to administer.

Patients receiving a general anaesthetic are required to refrain from eating and drinking for several hours prior to surgery, to allow the patient's/client's gastrointestinal tract to empty, so the risks of inhalation of stomach contents during surgery are minimal. A person who is at home the evening before surgery must understand the importance of not taking food or fluids, and must be willing to follow restrictions.

Ritualistic approaches to starving patients/clients are identified by Walsh and Ford (1989); typically patients/clients are starved from midnight for surgery the next morning. A minimum period of 6 hours was considered to be policy by many of the nurses and anaesthetists in a study undertaken by Smith (1972). A minimum of 4 hours is advocated by Torrance (1991). Despite the lack of consensus, research studies (Thomas, 1987; Smith, 1972) have demonstrated that many patients/clients are starved for much longer periods. An individualized approach should negate the potential risk of prolonged starvation, especially in the older adult. If the person eats or drinks during the fasting period the nurse should notify the surgeon immediately.

### Cleansing and Dressing

The risk of developing a surgical wound infection is determined by the amount and type of microorganisms contaminating a wound, susceptibility of the host, and condition of the wound at the end of the operation (largely determined by the surgeon's operative technique). All three factors may interact to cause infection.

The skin is a favourite site for microorganisms to grow and multiply. An antimicrobial bathing solution may be prescribed, however, most surgeons advocate a general bath or shower the evening before surgery. Some doctors may order patients/clients to bathe or shower more than once, whereas others may have them give special attention to cleansing the proposed operative site. Depending on the surgical procedure, a person may repeat skin preparation the morning of surgery.

If the surgical procedure involves the head, neck, or upper chest area, the patient/client may also be required to shampoo the hair. Cleansing and trimming of fingernails and toenails may be necessary, as well as ensuring that the person undergoing abdominal surgery has a clean umbilicus.

In the past, a surgical patient's/client's skin was routinely shaved to remove hair around the incision site. The rationale for the procedure was to remove microorganisms residing in body hair. However, it has been found that shaving the surgical site can cause superficial cuts and nicks in the skin that allow entry for microorganisms (Winfield, 1986). Some hospitals and clinics still perform shaving. The nurse should question the necessity of this procedure. If hair removal is advocated, a depilatory cream is recommended which has been associated with lower postoperative infection rates (*Lancet* editorial, 1983).

Another way to reduce the risk of a postoperative wound infection is to keep the person's preoperative hospital stay short. A number of researchers have shown that a short stay is associated with low wound infection rates (Cruse, 1980). Thus, patients/clients have less opportunity to acquire pathogens from the hospital.

### Resting and Sleeping

Rest is essential for normal healing. Anxiety about surgery can easily interfere with the ability to relax or sleep. The underlying condition requiring surgery may be painful, further impairing rest.

The nurse should attempt to make the patient's/client's environment quiet and comfortable. Night sedation will usually be prescribed by the doctor, however, McMahon (1990a) suggests that nurses have many other interventions they can turn to before resorting to a pharmacological solution (McMahon, 1990 b). Nevertheless, it may be preferable for an individual to take sleeping tablets rather than to lie awake in the early hours worrying about the impending operation.

An advantage of day surgery is that the person is able to sleep at home the night before surgery. The person is likely to get more rest in a familiar environment.

### Day of Surgery
### PROMOTING A SAFE ENVIRONMENT

Before the patient/client goes to theatre, the nurse checks the medical notes to ensure that pertinent laboratory results are present. Check that the consent form has been signed and that the patient/client is wearing identification bracelets. A preoperative checklist (Fig. 29-2) provides guidelines for ensuring completion of nursing interventions.

**Preoperative Checklist**

Patient's Name: _____

| | |
|---|---|
| • Identity bands (2) correctly labelled are in place | YES/NO |
| • Consent form is signed | YES/NO |
| • Wedding ring is taped, all other jewellery/hair grips, etc, removed | YES/NO |
| • Dentures are removed; caps and crowns, loose teeth noted | YES/NO |
| • Other prostheses are removed (specify) e.g. contact lenses and hearing aid | YES/NO |
| • Site is marked (specify) | YES/NO |
| • Patient/client has voided urine | YES/NO |
| • Internal tampon removed (as appropriate) | YES/NO |
| • Did theatre staff visit? | YES/NO |
| • X-rays to accompany patient to theatre | YES/NO |
| • Positioned correctly on canvas | YES/NO |
| • Notes to accompany patient | YES/NO |
| • Baseline observations | YES/NO |
| • Allergies noted | YES/NO |
| • Blood results (cross match, haemoglobin) | YES/NO |
| • Fluid chart to accompany patient | YES/NO |

**Fig. 29-2** Preoperative check list. Courtesy of Joyce Green Hospital, Dartford, Kent.

**Documenting Vital Signs** Ensure preoperative assessment of vital signs has been documented. The anaesthetist uses these values as baselines for intraoperative vital signs. If preoperative vital signs are abnormal, surgery may need to be postponed. For example, an elevated temperature increases the person's surgical risk. Notify the doctor of abnormalities before sending the person to surgery.

**Personal cleansing and dressing** Once basic hygiene measures have been undertaken the patient/client is required to remove all clothing and to wear a theatre gown; some hospitals provide a paper cap as well. The nurse must be sensitive to the feelings of some individuals who may feel embarrassed or whose cultural and religious practices may be compromised at having to remove their undergarments.

During surgery under general anaesthesia, the anaesthetist positions the person's head to introduce an endotracheal tube into the airway **(intubation)**. To avoid injury, ask the patient/client to remove hairpins or clips before leaving for surgery. Hairpieces or wigs should also be removed.

During and after surgery, the anaesthetist and nurses assess skin, mucous membranes and nail beds to determine the patient's/client's level of oxygenation and circulation. Therefore, all makeup (lipstick, powder, blush, nail polish) must be removed to expose normal skin and nail colouring. The nurse ensures that the patient/client lies correctly on a theatre canvas and clean bedlinen prior to surgery.

**Removal of prostheses** It is easy for any type of prosthetic device to become lost or damaged during surgery, or to cause injury while the patient/client is anaesthetized. The person must remove all prostheses, including partial or complete dentures, artificial limbs, artificial eyes, and contact lenses. Hearing aids, false eyelashes, and spectacles must also be removed.

For many, it is embarrassing to remove dentures or other devices that enhance appearance. Thus, privacy should be offered as the dentures are removed. Dentures must be placed in special containers for safekeeping to prevent loss or breakage, and the person is assessed for any loose teeth, crowns or caps. These can become damaged during intubation or become dislodged and lead to obstruction of the airway.

**Eliminating** The patient/client may require bowel preparation on the morning of surgery. If so, this should be undertaken as early in the day as possible to enable the person to recover and freshen up.

The patient/client should empty his or her bladder prior to the operation. An empty bladder prevents a person from being incontinent during surgery. This is important during abdominal surgery, when it may become necessary for the surgeon to manipulate the bladder. An empty bladder also makes abdominal organs more accessible during surgery. A Foley catheter is often inserted in theatre to maintain an empty bladder.

**Administering premedication** The anaesthetist or doctor, unless contraindicated, routinely orders a **premedication** to alleviate the patient's/client's fear and anxiety, nowadays usually administered via the oral route. Tranquillizers, for example, temezepan, reduce anxiety and cause drowsiness. Narcotic analgesics, such as pethedine or morphine, provide sedation and reduce pain and anxiety. An antiemetic, for example, metaclopramide hydrochloride (maxolon) is also commonly prescribed.

Typically the intramuscular premedication is administered approximately 1 hour before the patient/client leaves for the operating theatre. As the drugs cause sedation, the person is advised to remain in bed. The patient/client should be warned to anticipate drowsiness. The 'nurse call button' should be easily accessible and the person left comfortable. The nurse should, however, regularly check on the patient/client to evaluate the effectiveness of the premedication and any adverse reactions.

**Children's Nursing**
**The infant undergoing surgery**

During surgery, nurses and doctors are especially concerned with maintaining an infant's normal body temperature. The infant's shivering reflex is underdeveloped, and often wide temperature variations occur. Anaesthesia adds to the risk because anaesthetics can cause vasodilation and heat loss.

 **EVALUATION**

It is essential to evaluate the effectiveness of preoperative preparation and care. Occasionally, there is limited time to evaluate the outcomes of the preoperative care plan. This is especially so with an emergency admission. However, evaluation of care should be undertaken at the change of each shift, i.e. two to three times a day. Bedside handovers are advocated whenever possible, enabling the patient/client to participate in the evaluation of his or her care.

### Transport to the Operating Theatre

The patient/client is transported to the operating theatre in his or her bed or on a trolley. Safety checks include ensuring that the person's head is correctly positioned on the theatre canvas and that his or her arms are placed by his or her side to avoid injury en route to theatre. The medical notes, x-rays, prescription charts and nursing care plan should accompany the person. The ward nurse and if wished a family member, friend or partner will escort the patient/client to provide reassurance and emotional comfort. In the theatre receiving area the patient's/client's identification bracelets, consent form and removal of prosthesis are re-checked.

When the person has been safely left in theatre the nurse should, as soon as possible on return to the ward, prepare the bed area ready for the patient's/client's return. As a general rule, routine **postoperative equipment** to be placed at the bedside includes:

* suction and oxygen equipment
* sphygmomanometer, stethoscope, and thermometer
* postoperative observation and pain assessment chart (see Fig. 29-3)
* receiver and tissues
* intravenous infusion (IVI) and fluid balance chart
* clean bed linen folded into a special pack to cover the patient/client, to prevent heat loss, on his or her immediate return from theatre
* mouthwash.

Other specific equipment will also be required depending on the type of surgery performed.

### INTRAOPERATIVE PHASE

Care of the patient/client during surgery requires careful preparation and knowledge of the events that occur during the surgical procedure.

### Admission to the Operating Theatre

Once the patient/client has been anaesthetized he or she is transferred to the theatre and correctly and securely positioned on the operating table. The choice of position is usually determined by the surgical approach. Ideally, the person's position provides good access to the operative site and sustains adequate circulatory and respiratory function. It should not impair neuromuscular structures. The patient's/client's safety and comfort must not be

# Postoperative Nursing Observation Chart

Name _____ Ward _____ Unit No. _____

Returned from Theatre at: _____

Pre-op B/P: _____

Date: _____

Time: _____

Blood Pressure

170
160
150
140
130
120
110
100
90

Pulse

80
70
60
50
40

Respiration

30
20
10
0

Temperature   °C

## Pain assessment

Analgesia _____

Dose _____

Route _____

Time

Severity

Severe
Moderate
Slight
None/Asleep

## Analgesia evaluation

Amount of Relief

Complete
Almost Complete
Moderate
Slight
None

**Fig. 29-3** Postoperative observation chart. Adapted from Hosking J, Welchew E: *Postoperative pain*, London, 1985, Faber & Faber.

compromised. Many day surgery patients/clients remain awake during the procedure because only local anaesthetic is used. The nurse supports the person by explaining procedures and encouraging the person to ask questions, as sights and sounds in the surgical suite can be alarming.

It is sometimes difficult for surgical ward nurses to appreciate the discomfort a person may feel after surgery (for example, discomfort of the left arm or side of a patient/client whose right kidney was removed). Normal range of joint motion is maintained in an alert person by pain and pressure receptors. If a joint is extended too far, pain stimuli provide a warning that muscle and joint strain are too great. In a person who is anaesthetized, normal defence mechanisms cannot guard against joint damage, muscle stretch, and strain. The muscles are so relaxed that it is relatively easy to place the patient/client in a position that the individual normally could not assume while awake.

The person may remain in a given position for several hours. Although it may be necessary to place a patient/client in an unusual position, the nurse should attempt to maintain correct alignment and protect the person from pressure, abrasion, and other injuries. Attachments to the operating table allow protection and padding of extremities and bony prominences. Positioning should not impede normal movement of the diaphragm or interfere with circulation to body parts.

## Introduction of Anaesthesia

Patients/clients undergoing surgical procedures receive anaesthesia in one of three ways: general, regional or local.

## General Anaesthesia

Under **general anaesthesia**, a patient/client loses all sensation and consciousness. Muscles relax to ease manipulation of body parts. The person also experiences amnesia of all surgical events.

An anaesthetist gives general anaesthetics by intravenous and inhalation routes. There are four stages of anaesthesia. Stage 1 begins with the person awake. The patient/client gradually becomes drowsy and loses consciousness, and a state of analgesia begins. Stage 2 is the stage of excitement. The person's muscles are often tense and almost spasmodic. Swallowing and vomiting reflexes remain intact, and the patient/client may have an irregular breathing pattern. Stage 3 begins with the onset of regular rhythmical breathing. Vital functions are depressed, reflexes are depressed or temporarily lost, and the surgeon begins the operation during this phase. Stage 4 is the stage of complete respiratory depression, which can be fatal.

To move the patient/client quickly to stage 3 of general anaesthesia, the anaesthetist usually gives an intravenous dose of a barbiturate. To prevent possible aspiration and other respiratory complications, the anaesthetist inserts an endotracheal tube into the patient's/client's airway. Succinylcholine is administered to cause temporary paralysis of vocal cords and respiratory muscles while the tube is being positioned. The anaesthetist then provides artificial ventilation until succinylcholine's effects wear off and the person again breathes spontaneously. From that point, anaesthetic gases or vapours are usually delivered by inhalation

through the endotracheal tube. The person also receives a continuous supply of oxygen.

The duration of anaesthesia depends on the length of surgery. The greatest risks from general anaesthesia are the side effects of anaesthetic agents, including cardiovascular depression or irritability, respiratory depression, and liver and kidney damage.

## Regional Anaesthesia

Induction of **regional anaesthesia** results in loss of sensation in an area of the body. The method of induction influences the portion of sensory pathways that is anaesthetized. The anaesthetist gives regional anaesthetics by infiltration and local application. Infiltration of anaesthetic agents may involve one of the following induction methods:

- **nerve block** — local anaesthetic is injected into a nerve (for example, brachial plexus in the arm), blocking the nerve supply to the operative site.
- **spinal anaesthesia** — the anaesthetist performs a lumbar puncture and introduces local anaesthetic into the cerebrospinal fluid in the spinal subarachnoid space. Anaesthesia can extend from the tip of the xiphoid process down to the feet. Positioning of the patient/client influences movement of the anaesthetic agent up or down the spinal cord.
- **epidural anaesthesia** — this is a safer procedure than spinal anaesthesia because the anaesthetic agent is injected into the epidural space outside the dura mater and the level of anaesthesia is not as great as spinal anaesthesia. Because epidural anaesthesia provides an effective loss of sensation in the vaginal and perineal areas, it is the best anaesthetic for obstetrical procedures.
- **caudal anaesthesia** — this is a form of epidural anaesthesia achieved by giving the local anaesthetic at the base of the spine. The extent of anaesthesia affects only the pelvic region and legs.

There are risks involved with all types of infiltrative anaesthetics, so the nurse ensures careful monitoring of the patient/client during and immediately after surgery. A person under regional anaesthesia is awake throughout the surgery unless the doctor prescribes a tranquillizer that promotes sleep. Nurses must remember, however, that burns and other trauma can occur on the anaesthetized part of the body without the person being aware of the injury. It is therefore necessary to frequently observe the position of extremities and the condition of the skin.

## Local Anaesthesia

**Local anaesthesia** involves loss of sensation at the desired site (for example, a growth on the skin or the cornea of the eye). The anaesthetic agent, for example, lignocaine, inhibits nerve conduction until the drug diffuses into the circulation. The patient/client experiences a loss in pain sensation and touch. Local anaesthesia is commonly used for minor procedures performed in day surgery and outpatient departments.

## Nurse's Role During Surgery

Usually the nurse assumes one of two roles during the surgical procedure:

- **scrub nurse** — provides the surgeon with instruments and supplies, which requires strict asepsis and familiarity with surgical instruments. Each instrument is designed for a specific purpose during a phase or step in surgery. It needs knowledge and skill to anticipate which instrument the surgeon requires and to pass it quickly and smoothly. The scrub nurse also disposes of soiled gauze sponges and accounts for sponges, needles, and instruments on the surgical field and in body cavities.

- **circulating nurse** — an assistant to the scrub nurse and surgeon. When the patient/client first enters the operating room, the circulator may help to position the patient/client and apply necessary equipment and surgical drapes. During surgery, the circulator provides the scrub nurse with supplies, disposes of soiled equipment and sponges, and keeps a count of instruments, needles, and sponges used.

At the end of each surgical procedure, the scrub and circulating nurses count the number of used instruments, needles, and gauze sponges. This procedure prevents the accidental loss of such items within the patient's/client's surgical wound. It is not difficult for a sponge saturated with blood to be overlooked within a wound. Careful monitoring of items is essential for the patient's/client's safety.

## POSTOPERATIVE PHASE

After surgery, a patient's/client's care can become complex as a result of physiological changes that may occur. Individuals who have undergone general anaesthesia are more likely to face complications than those who have had local anaesthesia. A day surgery or outpatient/client who has had local anaesthesia with no sedation and has stable vital signs will usually be discharged soon after the procedure.

To assess a person's postoperative condition the nurse relies on information from the preoperative nursing assessment and on knowledge regarding the surgical procedure performed and events occurring during surgery. The nurse must be able to detect change. A variation from the norm may indicate onset of surgically related complications.

A patient's/client's postoperative course involves two phases: the immediate recovery period and postoperative convalescence. For a day surgery patient/client, recovery normally lasts only 1 to 2 hours, and convalescence takes place at home. For a hospitalized patient/client, recovery may last a few hours, and convalescence takes 1 or more days, depending on the extent of surgery and the person's response.

### Immediate Postoperative Recovery

The patient/client is admitted to the recovery area after surgery. After reviewing events in the operating room, the recovery room nurse makes a complete assessment of the patient's/client's status. Until stabilized, the person remains in the recovery unit.

After the initial assessment of the patient/client in recovery, the nurse records vital signs, oxygen administration and other key observations at least every 15 minutes and remains with the person until he or she has regained consciousness.

The patient/client often has an oral (or nasal airway) inserted in order to maintain a patent airway. As respiratory function and consciousness return, the nurse should ask the person to cough out the airway. The ability to do so signifies the return of a normal cough reflex.

Airway obstruction can be caused by aspiration of vomit, accumulation of mucus secretions in the pharynx, or swelling or spasm of the larynx. Airway patency can be maintained by positioning the patient/client in the recovery position, on one side with the face down and the neck slightly extended. Neck extension prevents occlusion of the airway at the pharynx. When the face is kept turned downward, the tongue moves forward and mucus secretions flow out of the mouth instead of accumulating in the pharynx. If the nature of the surgery prevents turning the person on one side, the head of the bed or trolley is slightly elevated and the patient's/client's neck slightly extended, with the head turned to the side. Suction is initiated as required to remove secretions.

The nurse rouses the person by calling the name in a moderate tone of voice and notes whether he or she responds appropriately or seems confused and disorientated. If the patient/client remains asleep or unresponsive, the nurse attempts arousal through touch or by gently moving a body part.

**Orientation** to the recovery room environment is important in maintaining the patient's/client's alertness. The nurse explains that surgery is completed and describes procedures and nursing measures within the recovery area. The patient/client who was properly prepared before surgery is less likely to be as anxious when recovery nurses begin their care.

### Communicating Pain

As patients/clients awaken from general anaesthesia, the sensation of pain becomes prominent. Pain can be perceived before full consciousness is regained. Acute incisional pain causes patients/clients to become restless and may be responsible for changes in vital signs. Unless contraindicated it should be common practice in the operating theatre to initiate patient/client controlled analgesia or to administer narcotic analgesics immediately after surgery, or to give epidural analgesia to expedite pain relief and minimize respiratory depression. The patient/client who had regional or local anaesthesia usually does not experience pain initially because the incisional area is still anaesthetized.

### Discharge from the Recovery Room

Once the patient's/client's condition stabilizes, the ward nurse will be asked to collect him or her from theatre. If the patient/client received a general anaesthetic the nurse must check that he or she is in possession of postanaesthetic instruments and a receiver, and that there is oxygen and suction equipment to hand. **Postanaesthetic instruments** include tongue holding forceps, sponge holding forceps and gauze swabs and a tongue depressor. This emergency equipment must be available to the ward nurse should the patient's/client's airway become obstructed while being transported back to the ward.

The recovery room nurse evaluates the person's readiness for return to the ward on the basis of vital sign stability, body temperature control, good ventilatory function, orientation to surroundings, absence of complications, minimal pain and nausea, controlled wound drainage, adequate urine output, and fluid and electrolyte balance. The ward nurse must be satisfied that the person's condition is stable before he or she agrees to escort the patient/client back to the ward. Allin (1991) describes the key elements in ensuring a safe and individualized comprehensive handover.

 ## ASSESSMENT

The same measurements and observations performed in the recovery room are continued in the ward, as a patient's/client's postoperative condition can change rapidly. The postoperative ward care plan (see Fig. 29-4) identifies the importance of continuously assessing vital signs and the need for the early detection of postoperative complications particularly shock and haemorrhage, respiratory depression, nausea and vomiting, retention of urine. Pain assessment is ongoing.

The speed of recovery depends on the type or extent of surgery, potential risk factors, postoperative complications, and the nurse's knowledge and skill in implementing the nursing care plan.

 ## PLANNING

The nurse considers the effects of the stress of surgery and limitations it produces when establishing goals of care for the patient/client.

Throughout the postoperative rehabilitation period the nurse promotes the individual's independence and active participation in care. When a patient/client is in pain or suffers from complications, there is little motive for self-care. The nurse must maintain a balance between providing for patients'/clients' needs when they are physically and psychologically dependent and promoting more involvement when their conditions allow.

The goals a nurse sets for an individual's involvement in care must be realistic. Surgery may limit the ability to participate effectively. It is inappropriate for the nurse to involve the person if movement is highly restricted or if participation increases discomfort.

The nurse should keep the patient/client and family informed of recovery progress. Many patients/clients become depressed if they think recovery is slow. The nurse should explain that it can take many days or weeks to feel fully recovered. Surgery may also cause permanent physical limitations that require time for acceptance.

The nurse and patient/client, whenever possible, plan the care together, focusing on the goals to be achieved for recovery and

rehabilitation. From the moment that the person enters the hospital, through surgery, and during the postoperative phase, the nurse anticipates the person's return home.

Family mambers may need support throughout the perioperative period, and nurses should try to be sensitive to how worried they may be at this time. They should be given full information on when they can telephone to enquire about progress and, when they do telephone, should be given a considerate reply. It can be reassuring to hear that their relative has awoken, taken sips of water, or been able to sit up in bed. Before they visit, the nurse can warn them that their relative may look pale, or may have an intravenous line, but that this is all usual. When they visit the nurse can offer them the opportunity to share concerns, or to see the surgeon when he/she is available.

Involvement of family members in the patient's/client's care plan can facilitate recovery. If the person requires additional care at home, such as dressing changes, assistance with ambulation, or drug administration, the nurse advises family members on proper care techniques. When there are problems or no family member, partner or friend, the social support services may be utilized.

Specialist nurses, for example the stoma therapist, breast care nurse, or incontinence adviser, should be accessed to provide ongoing support and information for patients/clients, family and staff. Kelly (1985) cites his stoma therapist as a 'major source of strength'. Support groups such as the Mastectomy Association and Ileostomy Association should also be utilized. These groups provide written guidance and personal contact as required.

 ## IMPLEMENTATION

### Body Temperature

On return to the ward the specially prepared pack of bedlinen is placed over the patient/client to restore body temperature. Increasing body warmth causes the person's metabolism to rise and circulatory and respiratory functions to improve. Shivering may not be a sign of hypothermia but rather a side effect of certain anaesthetic agents. Closs (1992) discusses the thermoregulation and the implications of postoperative fluctuations in temperature.

### Communicating Pain

Pain can significantly slow recovery. The person becomes reluctant to cough, breathe deeply, turn, mobilize, or perform necessary exercises. The nurse assesses and records the patient's/client's pain (see Fig. 29-3). The nurse should provide analgesics as often as allowed the first 24 to 48 hours after surgery to improve pain control. The PCA system allows patients/clients to administer their own analgesia. If patients/clients gain a sense of control over their pain, they usually have fewer postoperative problems, mobilize quicker and are able to rest and sleep more easily.

Epidural infusion of narcotics, such as morphine, is also a popular method of postoperative analgesia. Epidural narcotics relieve severe pain, often without the central nervous system depression that often occurs with systemic narcotics.

| DATE | ACTIVITIES OF LIVING: (A) ACTUAL (P) POTENTIAL PROBLEMS | PATIENT'S PROBLEMS | AIM/EXPECTED OUTCOME | POSTOPERATIVE NURSING CARE PLAN FOR 24-48 HOURS FOLLOWING SURGERY | SIGNED |
|---|---|---|---|---|---|
| | 3(P) | (i) Respiratory depression following anaesthesia | Early detection of hypoventilation | Maintain clear airway. Record respiratory rate (specify). | |
| | | | | Position patient (specify) O₂ prescribed | |
| | | (ii) Chest infection/fear of coughing | Patient will expectorate independently | Suction prn. Teach wound support when coughing/deep breathing/expectorating. | |
| | | | | Notify physiotherapist. Note colour, consistency, amount of sputum. | |
| | 1(P) | Unable to maintain safe environment due to post-operative shock-haemorrhage | Early detection of shock/haemorrhage | Record and interpret pulse, blood pressure 1/2 hourly, gradually increase length of time as observations stabilize. | |
| | | | | Investigate restlessness. | |
| | | | | Report changes in colour, peripheral perfusion, responsiveness; breathlessness. | |
| | | | | Check wound and drains. Monitor and record amount of leakage/drainage. | |
| | 2(A) | Pain/anxiety due to surgery | Pain to be of an acceptable level. | Perform pain assessment on return to ward and at regular intervals. | |
| | | | Anxiety to be relieved, minimal disturbance of rest and sleep | Interpret and respond to verbal and nonverbal signs of anxiety/discomfort | |
| | | | | Administer prescribed analgesia and monitor effect or monitor patient-controlled analgesia. | |
| | | | | Assist patient/client into a more comfortable position. | |
| | 4(P ) | (i) Nausea/vomiting due to anaesthetic | Patient will not feel nauseated | Administer prescribed antiemetic and monitor effect. | |
| | | (ii) Nil by mouth (to decrease risk of ileus) | Reduce risk of oral infection | Provide mouthwashes/oral hygiene – frequency: | |
| | | | Early detection of paralytic ileus | Aspirate nasogastric tube           Hourly. Note appearance/amount aspirate. | |
| | | (iii) Risk of dehydration following surgery | Intake of 2-3 litres in 24 hours | Monitor intravenous infusion as per regimen | |
| | | | To remain hydrated | Oral fluids commence: Amount: | |
| | 5(P) | Retention of urine following surgery | Patient will have passed urine within 12 hours | Offer urinal/bedpan within 6 hours. Time of voiding:          Amount: | |
| | | | If catheterized output 30 ml/hour minimum | Catheter in situ. YES/NO Empty drainage bag (specify) | |
| | | | Reduced risk of urinary tract infection | Catheter care (specify) | |
| | 1(P) | Wound infection due to surgical incision | Promote wound healing | Dressing to remain undisturbed until | |
| | | Risk of haematoma formation | | Dressing to be performed. | |
| | | | | Record temperature and pulse 4 hourly. Observe wound for signs of infection/necrosis. | |
| | | | | Drain/s (specify) | |
| | | | | Specific care | |
| | | | | Suture/s YES/NO Deep tension YES/NO Clips YES/NO | |

**Fig. 29-4** Section of postoperative care plan. Courtesy of Joyce Green Hospital, Dartford, Kent.                    (Cont'd)

| DATE | ACTIVITIES OF LIVING (A) ACTUAL (P) POTENTIAL PROBLEMS | PATIENT'S PROBLEMS | AIM/EXPECTED OUTCOME | POSTOPERATIVE NURSING CARE PLAN FOR 24-48 HOURS FOLLOWING SURGERY | SIGNED |
|---|---|---|---|---|---|
| | 8(A) | Reduced mobility due to effects of surgery | Increasing mobilization lessening risks of immobility | Encourage leg exercises. TED stockings YES/NO | |
| | | Pressure sore risk assessment score: | | Change patient's/client's position/observe pressure area (specify) | |
| | | | | Gradually mobilize. Aids to comfort (specify) | |
| | 6(A) | Unable to independently perform personal hygiene | Patient/client will achieve increasing independence in performing personal hygiene | Ensure patient/client is pain free. Maintain patient's/client's dignity. | |
| | | | | Personal hygiene needs (specify) | |

**Fig. 29-4 (Cont'd)** Postoperative care plan. Courtesy of Joyce Green Hospital, Dartford, Kent.

## Breathing and Circulation

The patient/client is at risk of cardiovascular complications resulting from actual or potential blood loss from the surgical site, side effects of anaesthesia, electrolyte imbalances, and depression of normal circulatory regulating mechanisms. Careful assessment of heart rate and rhythm along with blood pressure reveals the person's cardiovascular status. The values are monitored and recorded (see Fig. 29-3) at least every 30 minutes until they have stabilized and then decreased accordingly until 4 hourly. The nurse compares preoperative vital signs with postoperative values.

The nurse assesses circulatory perfusion by noting the colour of nail beds and skin. If the person has had vascular surgery or has a plaster cast or bandages that may impair circulation, the nurse assesses peripheral pulses distal to the site of surgery. Warmth of skin, sensation and movement of the limb are also important observations.

There is a potential risk of haemorrhage. Blood loss may occur externally through a drain or incision, or internally within the surgical wound. Either type of haemorrhage may manifest itself by a fall in blood pressure; elevated heart and respiratory rate; thready pulse; cool, clammy, pale skin; and restlessness. If haemorrhage is external, the nurse notes increased blood on dressings or in drainage bottles. An alert nurse always checks under the bedclothes for signs of external haemorrhage. The first signs of suspected haemorrhage should be reported to the doctor immediately.

Coughing assists in removing retained mucus in the airways. A deep, productive cough is more beneficial than merely clearing the throat. Postoperative incisional pain makes coughing difficult. The person must anticipate the pain and understand the importance of coughing. The nurse encourages coughing and deep breathing exercises every 2 hours while patients/clients are awake and maintains pain control to promote a full productive cough.

## Safe Environment

After surgery, most surgical wounds are covered with a dressing that protects the wound site and collects drainage. The nurse observes the amount, colour, odour, and consistency of drainage on dressings. The nurse estimates the amount of drainage by noting the number of saturated dressings.

Different approaches to wound care have been researched by Webster (1991) who identified ritualistic practices. There is no need to disturb a wound dressing until the sutures are due to be removed, unless there are signs of infection (Walsh and Ford, 1989).

A wound may undergo considerable physical stress. Strain on sutures from coughing, vomiting, distention, and movement of body parts can disrupt the wound layers. A critical time for wound healing is 24 to 72 hours after surgery. If a wound becomes infected, it usually occurs 3 to 6 days after surgery. A clean surgical wound usually does not regain strength against normal stress for 15 to 20 days after surgery. If wounds require re-dressing, an aseptic technique using either sterile forceps or gloves is required to minimize the risk of infection.

## Eliminating

A number of elimination problems may occur after surgery. A person may not pass urine for up to 10-12 hours following anaesthesia. Retention of urine may occur. An epidural or spinal anaesthetic may prevent the person from feeling bladder fullness or distention.

When the patient/client does urinate, the time, amount, colour and odour of urine is noted. Haematuria will often be present when surgery has been performed on the urinary tract or prostate gland. The nurse or the patient/client may measure fluid intake and output after surgery until normal fluid intake and urinary output are achieved.

If a person does not void within 10-12 hours of surgery, it may be necessary to insert a urinary catheter. When a Foley catheter is *in situ*, there should be a continuous flow of urine of 30 ml/hour in adults. Specific meatal cleansing is advocated by some health authorities. There is, however, no evidence to support the value of this intervention in reducing infection (Walsh and Ford, 1990). A high fluid intake, when permissible, will prevent urinary stasis in the bladder and reduce the risk of developing a urinary tract infection.

## Mobilizing

Early measures directed at preventing circulatory complications will reduce the risk of circulatory stasis. Some individuals are at greater risk of venous stasis because of the nature of their surgery. Venous return and circulatory blood flow can be promoted by encouraging the person to perform leg exercises, every 1 to 2 hours while awake. Antiembolism stockings should be in place except when contraindicated.

Early mobilization is encouraged whenever possible. When vital signs have stabilized and pain is controlled, the nurse first assists the person to slowly sit on the side of the bed. Too-rapid movements may lead to dizziness. At first the person may be seated at their bedside but planned care should identify when the person is able to walk down the ward and to the toilet. This promotes physical, psychological and social feelings of regaining independence (see box).

---

### Benefits of early postoperative mobility

**Physiological**
- Increased rate and depth of breathing
- Increased circulation
- Increased micturition
- Increased metabolism
- Increased appetite
- Increased peristalsis
- Improved muscle tone
- Improved healing

**Psychological**
- Increased mental alertness
- Raised morale

**Social**
- Greater social interaction

Adapted from Long B, Phipps W: *Medical-surgical nursing: a nursing process approach*, St Louis, 1989, CV Mosby.

---

When the patient/client sits in a chair, his or her legs should be elevated on a footstool to promote venous return. Always discourage patients/clients from sitting or lying with crossed legs. Further guidelines for promoting mobility are discussed by Pugh and Millar (1989).

Anticoagulant drugs, such as heparin, are sometimes prescribed for individuals at greatest risk of thrombus formation. Some patients/clients receive aspirin for anticoagulation.

The nurse promotes adequate fluid intake orally or intravenously. Adequate hydration prevents concentrated build up of formed blood elements, such as platelets and red blood cells. When the plasma volume is low, these elements may gather to form small clots within blood vessels.

## Eating and Drinking

General anaesthetics slow gastrointestinal motility and can induce nausea and vomiting. Antiemetic drugs are often prescribed. For the first few hours after surgery many patients/clients receive only intravenous fluids. The nurse provides frequent oral hygiene. Adequate hydration and cleansing of the oral cavity eliminate dryness and bad tastes. Frequent observations of the intravenous infusion and the cannula site are essential to ensure the patency of the giving set and accurate assessment and maintenance of fluid intake.

Oral fluids are gradually introduced. If the person tolerates liquids without nausea, a light diet is introduced. The nurse encourages a gradual progression in dietary intake providing nutritional guidance as appropriate. Protein, vitamin C and zinc are essential nutrients for wound healing.

A person may lose interest in eating if meal times have been preceded by exhausting activities, such as mobilization, coughing and deep breathing exercises, or extensive dressing changes. When a patient/client has pain, the associated nausea often causes a loss of appetite.

If the person has a nasogastric (NG) tube *in situ*, the nurse keeps it patent and removes gastric juices by regular aspirations. The nurse must ensure that the tube is firmly secured, preferably at the point of entry.

It takes several days for a person who has had surgery on gastrointestinal structures (for example, a bowel resection) to resume a normal dietary intake. Normal peristalsis may not return for 2 to 3 days. The nurse assesses for return of peristalsis by inquiring if the person is passing flatus. This is an important sign indicating the return of normal bowel function.

Patients/clients who have had abdominal surgery are usually nil by mouth (nbm) for the first 24 to 48 hours. As peristalsis returns, the nurse provides clear liquids, followed by full liquids, a light diet of solid foods, and finally a normal diet.

Physical activity stimulates a return of peristalsis as well as reducing abdominal distention and flatulence. Mobilization also often helps to prevent constipation. A high fluid intake should be encouraged; fresh orange juice and warm liquids are especially effective.

## Personal Identity

The appearance of wounds, bulky dressings, and extruding drains and tubes threatens a patient's/client's self-concept. The effects of surgery, such as disfiguring scars, may create permanent changes in the patient's/client's body image. If surgery leads to impairment in body function, the person's role within the family can change significantly.

---

 **Learning Disabilities Nursing Motivation and rehabilitation after surgery**

The following principles underly effective postoperative rehabilitation for people with learning disabilties:
- encourage patients/clients to do as much as possible for themselves, as quickly as is safely possible (to return them to their 'normal' preoperative state as soon as possible)
- consider early discharge from hospital, in appropriate cases, so rehabilitation can occur in the patient's/client's familiar surroundings
- coordinate the patient's/client's postoperative recovery with a therapist skilled in working with people who have learning disabilties

---

| DISCHARGE PLAN | | | PROPOSED DATE | | |
|---|---|---|---|---|---|
| Agency | Yes/No | Date arranged by whom | Information/ equipment | Yes/No | Date arranged by whom |
| District nurse | | | Outpatient appointment | | |
| Social worker | | | Door keys | | |
| Home help | | | Tablets/medicine | | |
| Do relatives know? | | | Certificate | | |
| Meals-on-wheels | | | Transport home | | |
| Occupational therapy | | | Diet sheet | | |
| Physiotherapy | | | Other (specify) | | |
| Aids arranged (specify) | | | | | |
| | | | | | |
| | | | | | |
| | | | | | |

**Fig. 29-5** Discharge planning checklist. Courtesy of Joyce Green Hospital, Dartford, Kent.

The nurse observes patients/clients for alterations in self-concept. Patients/clients may show a revulsion towards their appearance by refusing to look at incisions, carefully covering dressings with bedclothes, or refusing to get out of bed because of tubes and devices. The fear of not being able to return to a functional role in their families may even cause individuals to avoid participating in the nursing care plan.

The family becomes an important part of the nurse's efforts to improve the person's self-concept. The family needs to be accepting of the person's needs and still encourage the patient's/client's independence.

The nurse provides the family with opportunities to discuss ways to promote the patient's/client's self-concept. Encouraging independence can be difficult for a family member who has a strong desire to assist the person in any way.

Personal Cleansing and Dressing The nurse assists the person with his or her personal hygiene, gradually promoting independence. Night clothes should be changed daily or more frequently if they become soiled through wound drainage. Care of the hair and oral hygiene will also enable the patient to feel refreshed. Gradual rehabilitation measures by the nurse should encourage patients/clients to shower or bathe and to wear their day clothes around the ward whenever possible.

Traditional nursing practices that require all patients/clients to bathe before lunch are outmoded and inappropriate in promoting independence. The person should decide, whenever possible, when he or she wishes to bathe. Many patients/clients may choose to bathe or shower in the evening before retiring.

 **EVALUATION**

In an acute care setting the evaluation of a surgical patient/client is ongoing. If a person fails to progress as expected, the nurse revises the care plan based on the priorities of the patient's/client's needs. Every effort is made to assist the person to return to as healthy and functional a state as possible.

Part of the nurse's evaluation is determining the extent to which the patient/client and family have learned self-care measures. A person may have to continue wound care, follow activity restrictions, continue medication therapy, and observe for signs and symptoms of complications on returning home. A discharge planning checklist is shown in Fig. 29-5. The person should be discharged only when their specific needs have been met.

## SUMMARY

Care for the patient/client during all phases of the surgical experience needs to be continuous and integrated. Before the operation the nurse prepares the person and family for the surgical experience and assesses the patient/client in preparation for the operation. During surgery the nurse assists the surgeon and other operating room personnel to ensure that the person receives optimal care. After surgery, the nurse assists the patient/client in physical, psychological and social rehabilitation. Through all phases of care, the nurse involves the patient/client and family as much as possible in the care plan and helps maintain the person's dignity. Caring for surgical patients/clients is a rewarding and highly skilled area of nursing practice.

## CHAPTER 29 REVIEW

### Key Concepts
- Perioperative nursing is professional nursing care provided for the surgical patient/client before, during, and after surgery.
- In addition to the nature of nursing care provided, previous illnesses and past surgeries influence the person's ability to tolerate surgery.
- The duration of the preoperative period may be several days or only a few hours.
- Family members are important in assisting patients/clients with any physical limitations and in providing emotional support.
- Preoperative assessment of vital signs and physical and psychological findings provides an important baseline with which to compare postoperative assessment data.
- A patient's/client's feelings about surgery can have a significant impact on relationships with the nursing staff and the person's ability to participate in care.
- Surgical removal of a body part may permanently alter a person's body image, as well as the individual's sexuality.
- Informed consent cannot be obtained if a patient/client is confused, unconscious, mentally incompetent, or under the influence of sedatives.
- Structured preoperative teaching has a positive influence on postoperative recovery.
- Basic to preoperative teaching is explanation of all preoperative and postoperative routines and demonstration of postoperative exercises.
- A routine preoperative checklist is a guide for final preparation of the patient/client before surgery.
- Many responsibilities of nurses within the operating theatre focus on protecting the person from potential harm.
- The recovery unit nurse reports to the ward nurse on the patient's/client's current physical and psychological status and pain relief requirements.
- Assessment of the postoperative patient/client centres on the body systems most likely to be affected by anaesthesia, immobilization, and surgical trauma.
- The speed of recovery depends on the type or extent of surgery, potential risk factors, postoperative complications, and the nurse's knowledge and skill in implementing the nursing care plan.
- Throughout the postoperative rehabilitation period, the nurse promotes the individual's independence and participation in care.
- From the time of admission the nurse plans for the surgical patient's/client's discharge.

## CRITICAL THINKING EXERCISES

1. Mrs Williams is a 52-year-old patient/client who is going to have abdominal surgery in the morning. She has a history of smoking one pack of cigarettes per day for 30 years. What areas would you concentrate on during Mrs William's preoperative teaching?

2. Your patient/client has undergone abdominal surgery to remove a cancerous growth. Describe the postoperative measures you would use to promote rest and comfort.

3. Mrs Aswar is 39 years old and has undergone a right mastectomy. You notice that she refuses to look at her incision and has been staying in bed even though she has been advised to increase her activity as tolerated. How can you encourage Mrs Aswar's independence and maintain her self-concept?

4. Mr Esterfez, an 84-year-old man is being admitted for a cataract extraction under a general anaesthetic. Name three of the physiological changes that occur in older adults that would place your patient/client at risk of surgery.

### Key Terms

Anaesthesia (general, local, epidural), p.608
Antiembolism stockings, p. 600
Body image alterations, p. 598
Continuity of care, p. 594
Dehydration/overhydration, p. 600
Diaphragmatic breathing, p. 600
Discharge planning, p. 602
Informed consent, p. 602
Intubation, p. 605
Orientation, p. 609
Perioperative nursing, p. 594
Postanaesthetic instruments, p. 610
Premedication, p. 606
Preoperative baselines/baseline data, p. 600
Postoperative equipment, p .606

## REFERENCES

Allin K: Post-operative handover, *Surg Nurs* 4(3):23, 1991.

Biley F: Nurses' perceptions of stress in preoperative surgical patients, *J Advance Nurs* 14:575, 1989.

Breemhaar B, van den Borne: Effects of education and support for surgical patients: the role of perceived control, *Patient Education Counselling* 18:199, 1991.

Burnard P: *Learning human skills*, Oxford, 1985, Heinemann.

Clark EC: Post-operative patient controlled analgesia, *Surg Nurs* 5(3):20, 1992.

Closs J: Monitoring the body temperature of surgical patients, *Surg Nurs* 5(1):12, 1992.

Cruse PJE, Foord R: The epidemiology of wound infection: a ten-year prospective study of 62,939 wounds, *Surg Clin North Am* 60(1): 1980.

Ewles L, Simnett J: *Promoting health: a practical guide*, London, 1992, Scutari.

Fraser M: *Using conceptual nursing in practice*, London, 1990, Lippincott Nursing Series, Harper and Row.

Fulbrook P: Assessing needs and planning actions, *Senior Nurs* 12(1):42, 1992.

Hayward J: *Information — a prescription against pain*, London, 1975, Royal College of Nursing.

Holmes TH, Rahe RH: The social readjustment rating scale, *J Psychosomatic Res* 11:213, 1967.

Keithley JK: Wound healing in malnourished patients, *AORN J* 35:1094, 1982.

Kelly M: Loss and grief reactions as responses to surgery, *J Advanced Nurs* 10:517, 1985.

*Lancet* editorial: *Lancet* 8337:1311, 1983.

McCall J: Ethnic minorities, *Surg Nurs* 4(4):20, 1991.

McMahon R: Sleep management, *Surg Nurs* 3(4):25,1990a.

McMahon R: Sleep therapies, *Surg Nurs* 3(5):17, 1990b.

McRobb A: Ann's last lesson, *Nurs Standard* 8(10), 1993.

Malby R: Discharge planning, *Senior Nurs* 5(1):4, 1992.

Manley K: Ethical problems and the care of the surgical patient, *Surg Nurs* 3(6):408, 1990.

Marr J: Meeting the needs of ethnic patients, *Nurs Standard* 8(3): 31, 1993.

Moss VA: Music and the surgical patient, the effect of music on anxiety, *AORN J* 48(1):64, 1988.

Pape KE: Cost containment and the short-stay needs of surgical patients, *Nurs Management* 12(3): 61, 1990.

Pellett J: General anaesthesia, *Surg Nurs* 3(5):21, 1990.

Price B: *Body image: nursing concepts and care*, New York, 1990a, Prentice Hall.

Price B: A model for body image care, *J Adv Nurs* 15: 58 5-593, 1990b.

Price B: Living with altered body image: the cancer experience, *Br J Nurs* i(13) 641-645,1992.

Price B: Profiling the high risk body image patient, *Senior Nurs* 13 (4), 1993.

Pugh J, Millar B: Mobility in the post-operative phase of care, *Surg Nurs*, 2(5):15, 1989.

Roper N, Logan W and Tierney A: *The elements of nursing*, ed 3, Edinburgh, 1990, Churchill Livingstone.

Salter M: *Altered body image*, New York, 1988, John Wiley & Sons.

Sims C: *Spiritual care as part of holistic nursing*, NSMA/Imprint, 34(4), November 1987.

Smith SH: *Nil by mouth?*, London, 1972, Royal College of Nursing.

Sutherland MS: Education in the medical care setting, *Health Education* 39:25, 1980.

Taylor AG, Skelton JA and Czakowski RW: Do patients understand patient-education brochures?, *Nurs Health Care* 3:305, 1982.

Thomas EA: Pre-operative fasting — a question of routine, *Nurs Times* 83(49):46, 1987.

Thompson F: Management of terminally ill patients on an acute surgical ward, *Surg Nurs* 5(3):16, 1992.

Torrance C: Preoperative nutrition, fasting and the surgical patient, *Surg Nurs* 4(4):4, 1991.

Toms E: Patient teaching, a neglected area of nurse practice? *Senior Nurs* 13(1):37, 1993.

Tschudin V: Informed consent, *Surg Nurs* l2(6):15, 1989.

Visitainer M, Wolfer J: Pediatric surgical patients' and parents' stress responses and adjustment, *Nurs Res* 24(4):244, 1975.

Walsh M, Ford P: *Nursing rituals, research and rational actions*, Oxford, 1989, Heinemann.

Webster R: Use of research in wound care, *Nurs Times* 87(33):48, 1991.

Winfield U: Too close a shave, *Nurs Times* 82(10):64, 1986.

## Further Reading

### Adult Nursing

Barasi S: The physiology of pain, *Surg Nurs* 4(5):14, 1991.

Chalmer H: Nursing models: enhancing or inhibiting practice? *Nursing Standard* 5(11):1990.

Hosking J, Welchew E: *Postoperative pain — understanding its nature and how to treat it*, London, 1985, Faber & Faber.

Latter S *et al*: Perceptions and practice of health education and health promotion in acute ward settings, *Nurs Times* 89:51, 1993.

Morrison P: Psychology of pain, *Surg Nurs* 4(6):18, 1991.

Redman BK: *The process of patient education*, St Louis, 1993, Mosby.

Tilley JD: The nurse's role in patient education: incongruent perceptions among nurses and patients, *J Adv Nurs* 12:291, 1987.

Webb C: A study of nurses' knowledge and attitudes about sexuality in health care, *Int J Nurs Stud* 25(3):235, 1988.

### Children's Nursing

Brykczynska F: Informed consent, *Paed Nurs* 1(5), 1989.

Colliss V: Pre and postoperative management, *Paed Nurs* 2 (5) 1989.

Glasper A: Parents in the anaesthetic room: a blessing or a curse? *Prof Nurs* 3(4), 1989.

Radford P: Physical and emotional care, *Paed Nurs* 2(5), June, 1990.

Sherwood P: Why can't my mummy stay until I'm asleep? *Paed Nurs* 2(3), 1990.

Turner L: Creating the right atmosphere, *Nurs Times* 85(32):34, 1989.

Wattley LA, Muller DJ: *Investigating psychology — a practical approach for nursing*, 1984,London, Harper & Row.

# Tissue Viability and Wound Care

## CHAPTER OUTLINE

**Normal Integument**

**Wound Classifications**
*Acute wounds*
*Chronic wounds*

**Wound Healing Process**
*Healing by primary intention*
*Healing by secondary intention*

**Factors Influencing Wound Healing**
*Intrinsic factors*
*Extrinsic factors*
*Additional factors*

**Complications of Wound Healing**
*Haemorrhage*
*Infection*
*Dehiscence*
*Evisceration*
*Fistulas*
*Delayed wound closure*

**Psychosocial Impact of Wounds**

**Nursing Process, Tissue Viability**
*Assessment*
*Planning*
*Implementation*
*Evaluation*

## LEARNING OUTCOMES

After studying this chapter, you should be able to:

- *Define the key terms listed.*
- *Discuss normal skin structure and function, different types of wounds, and wound classifications.*
- *Explain the two wound healing processes and discuss the factors that impair or promote wound healing.*
- *Describe complications of wound healing, manifestations, and their usual time of occurence.*
- *Assess patients/clients for risk of pressure ulcer development.*
- *Assess closed, open, acute, and chronic wounds.*
- *Correctly cleanse and dress a wound site or drain, and obtain a wound culture specimen.*
- *Discuss the principles of first aid in wound care.*
- *Discuss the impact of positioning techniques.*
- *Discuss the impact of correct dressing selection on wound healing and pressure ulcer prevention.*
- *Apply a dressing, using sterile technique.*
- *Understand the qualities of the 'ideal' dressing.*
- *Discuss the purpose of bandages and their correct usage.*

The body's integument is a protective barrier against disease-causing organisms and is a sensory organ for pain, temperature, and touch. A major aspect of nursing care is the maintenance of **skin integrity**. Consistent, planned skin-care interventions are critical to ensuring quality and cost-effective care (Hoff, 1989). Nurses are able to constantly observe patients'/clients' skin for breaks or impairment in skin integrity. Impaired skin integrity can result from:

- prolonged pressure, irritation of the skin, or immobility (leading to the development of pressure ulcers)
- local tissue changes (for example, those leading to leg ulcers)
- wounds resulting from trauma or surgery.

Failure to recognize and treat impaired skin integrity can lead to the development of chronic open wounds, such as pressure ulcers and leg ulcers. It is imperative, therefore, to recognize alterations in skin integrity and to implement appropriate interventions.

Injury to the integument triggers a complex healing response. Knowing the normal healing pattern helps you recognize alterations that require intervention. The nurse's main responsibilities are to prevent invasion of microorganisms into wounds, to support the body's defences in achieving wound repair, and to educate the patient/client in preventing and caring for wounds. When choosing interventions, it is important to consider the type of wound, the pain associated with it, conditions that affect healing, and the patient's/client's psychological well-being.

## NORMAL INTEGUMENT

In relation to wound healing, the integument has two principal layers: the epidermis and the dermis (Fig. 30-1). Understanding the structure of the integument layers will help you understand and promote wound healing.

The **epidermis** is the outer layer of the integument, and is composed of two layers. The *stratum corneum* is the thin, outermost layer of the epidermis. It consists of flattened, dead cells. The cells originate from the second epidermal layer, the *stratum malpighii*. Cells in the stratum malpighii divide, proliferate, and migrate towards the epidermal surface. After cells reach the stratum corneum, they flatten and die. This constant movement ensures replacement of surface cells sloughed off during normal **desquamation**. The thin stratum corneum protects underlying cells and tissues from dehydration and prevents entrance of certain chemical agents. However, it also allows evaporation of water from the skin and permits absorption of certain topically applied medications. **The function of the epidermis is to resurface wounds and restore the barrier against invading organisms**.

The **dermis** differs from the epidermis in that it contains no skin cells. It is composed of collagen (a tough, fibrous protein), and contains blood vessels and nerves. *Fibroblasts*, which are responsible for collagen formation, are the only distinctive cell type within the dermis. **The function of the dermis is to restore the structural integrity and the physical properties of the skin**.

Even though a wound may close in the upper epidermal layer, the patient/client is at risk for infection, circulatory impairment, and tissue breakdown if the underlying dermis fails to heal.

## WOUND CLASSIFICATIONS

There are many ways to classify wounds. Wound classification systems describe the cause, severity of tissue injury, status of skin integrity, cleanliness, or descriptive qualities of the wound. These classifications overlap. For example, a penetrating knife wound is also an open wound, and a contused wound is also a closed wound. Wound classifications enable you to understand the risks associated with a wound and the implications for its care. An open wound, for example, presents a greater risk of infection than a closed wound. Wounds that have been present for some time, such as leg ulcers or pressure sores, are classified according to their appearance; for example, necrotic, sloughy, granulating, epithelializing. (For a detailed description of wounds and wound

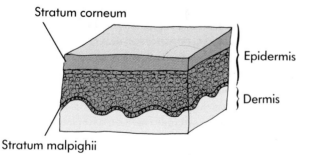

Stratum corneum

Epidermis

Dermis

Stratum malpighii

**Fig. 30-1** Layers of the integument.

---

### Causes of Leg Ulcers

Principal causes:
- chronic venous hypertension, usually due to incompetent valves in the deep and perforating veins.
- arterial disease, e.g. atherosclerotic occlusion of large vessels leading to tissue ischaemia.
- combined chronic venous hypertension and arterial disease

Unusual causes (2-5% of cases)
- neuropathy, e.g. associated with diabetes mellitus, spina bifida, leprosy
- vasculities, e.g. associated with rheumatoid arthritis, polyarteritis nodosum
- malignancy, e.g. squamous cell carcinoma, melanoma, basal cell carcinomal, Kaposi's sarcoma
- infection, e.g. tuberculosis, leprosy, syphilis, fungal infections
- blood disorders, e.g. polycythaemia, sickle cell disease, thalassaemia
- metabolic diorder, e.g. pyoderma gangrenosum, pretibial myxoedema
- lymphoedema
- trauma, e.g. lacerations, burns, irradiation injuries
- iatrogenic, e.g. over-tight bandaging, ill-fitting plaster case
- self-inflicted

Adapted from Morison M, Moffatt C: *A colour guide to the assessment and management of leg ulcers, ed 2* London, 1994, Mosby.

---

management, refer to Morison, M: *A Colour Guide to the Nursing Management of Wounds*, London, 1992, Mosby–Wolfe.)

### Acute Wounds

**Acute wounds** are caused by a single incident, such as surgery or trauma to the skin. Once the skin has been repaired, the goal is to promote wound healing as fast as possible, as comfortably as possible, and with minimum scarring. The majority of uncomplicated acute wounds heal satisfactorily.

### Chronic Wounds

**Chronic wounds** are complicated by factors such as impaired blood supply, changes in the tissues surrounding the wound, or general systemic changes (such as diabetes or inadequate nutrition). They may take longer to develop than acute wounds, and usually heal more slowly. Pressure ulcers and leg ulcers are the most commonly encountered chronic open wounds in the United Kingdom (Morison, 1994).

### Leg Ulcers

Approximately 1–2% of the population in the United Kingdom will develop a **leg ulcer** at some point in their lives (Laing, 1992). The problem of leg ulcers increases with age and presents major health and economic implications. In the UK, for example, the cost of managing leg ulcers is estimated to range from £150–600 million per year (Morison and Moffatt, 1994). More than 80% of all leg ulcers are treated in the community by district and practice nurses (Cornwall *et al*, 1986).

Ulceration of the leg may be caused by venous disease, arterial disease, neuropathic changes, trauma, haematological disease,

**Adult Nursing**
**Economic consequences of pressure ulcers**

When a pressure ulcer occurs, the length of stay in hospital may be increased and the overall cost of health care rises. The actual cost of treatment is difficult to approximate. Estimates suggest that £755 million is being spent annually by the NHS to treat pressure sores (West and Priestly, 1994) and that the cost per patient/client might be around £26,000 (Hibbs, 1988). However, these figures do not allow for delays in rehabilitation or for other costs which may not be immediately apparent. For example, the lengthened hospital stay of affected clients results in admission opportunities lost to other patients. Although treatment of pressure ulcers is more costly than prevention, the preventive measures themselves are expensive. Extra equipment such as special beds and mattresses and increased nursing time are needed to administer these measures. When an ulcer develops, the cost of increased nursing care alone is estimated at 50% (Maklebust, 1987). Some equipment available for pressure relief has not been validated by research. It is important to choose equipment which is validated by controlled clinical trials (Bliss and Thomas, 1992).

**Children's Nursing**
**Pressure ulcers in infants**

Infants and children are also prone to pressure ulcers. Neonates have very fragile skin which can easily break down if the neonate's position is not changed regularly. Tape stronger than Micropore should not be used, because the adhesive may tear the infant's skin.

Children who are immobilized move around in their beds more than immobilized adults, and thus are less prone to pressure ulcers. However, children who are malnourished, unconscious, or immobilized on one area for a long period are at risk and should be assessed for pressure ulcers.

Prevention and treatment for pressure ulcers in children is the same as for adults.

patients/clients, and is not limited to those with restrictions in mobility. Impaired skin integrity is a serious and potentially devastating problem in the ill or debilitated patient/client (USDHHS, 1992; Gröer and Shekleton, 1989; Shekleton and Litwack, 1991).

## PATHOGENESIS OF PRESSURE ULCERS

Tissues receive oxygen and nutrients and eliminate metabolic wastes via the blood. Any factor that interferes with this affects cellular metabolism and the function or life of the cell. Pressure affects cellular metabolism by decreasing or obliterating tissue circulation, resulting in tissue ischaemia.

A pressure ulcer occurs as a result of a time–pressure relationship (Stotts, 1988). The greater the force and the duration of the pressure, the greater the incidence of ulcer formation. The skin and subcutaneous tissue can tolerate some pressure; however, externally applied pressure greater than the pressure in the capillary bed decreases or obliterates blood flow to adjacent tissues. These tissues become hypoxic, and ischaemic injury results.

**Tissue ischaemia** is the localized absence of blood or a major reduction of blood flow resulting from mechanical obstruction (Pires and Muller, 1991). The reduction in blood flow causes blanching. **Blanching** is seen when the normal red tones of the skin are absent. Tissue damage occurs when the capillary closing pressure exceeds the normal range of 16 to 32 mmHg (Gröer and Shekleton, 1989; Maklebust, 1987). If the pressure is greater than 32 mmHg and remains unrelieved to the point of hypoxia, the vessels collapse and thrombose (develop a clot) (Maklebust, 1987). If the pressure is relieved before the critical point, circulation to the affected tissues is restored through the physiological mechanism of **reactive hyperaemia**. It has been demonstrated that 32 mmHg is the pressure at which arterial capillaries close in young healthy volunteers. Individuals at risk of pressure sores will have a much lower capillary closing pressure. The exact pressure is individual to each patient.

The effect of pressure can be increased by unequal distribution of body weight. Because of gravity, a person is

bacterial infections, autoimmune disease, inflammatory disease, or tumours. Ulcers may cause considerable discomfort to the patient/client, as well as changes in body image and restriction in activity.

In order to treat leg ulcers appropriately, nurses need to recognize the differing causes (see box) and manifestations. Recent studies indicate that dramatic improvements in healing rates can be achieved when leg ulcer management services are rationalized and research-based protocols are implemented consistently (Moffatt *et al*, 1992).

### Pressure Ulcers

The frequency of pressure ulcers ranges from 8.8% (Barbenel *et al*, 1977) to 66% (Versluysen, 1986) of all patients in hospital. Barbenel identified 8.8% of clients on the district nurses' list as having pressure ulcers, although an accurate presence of clients in the community is not known. People with pressure ulcers account for between 3.8% and 10.82% of all district nurses' workload, depending upon the grade of staff (NHS, 1992). Due to their important health care and economic implications, specific information about the prevention and treatment of pressure ulcers is presented throughout this chapter.

*Pressure sore*, *pressure ulcer*, *decubitus ulcer*, and *bedsore* are terms used to describe impaired skin integrity. The most current terminology is pressure ulcer. An ill person experiencing decreased mobility (see Chapter 24), impaired neurological functioning, decreased sensory perception, or decreased circulation is at risk for pressure ulcer development. Prevention and treatment of pressure ulcers are major nursing priorities and the ability to identify patients/clients at risk helps contain health care costs (Gosnell, 1973; Norton *et al*, 1962). Preventing pressure ulcers is a priority in caring for all

**Learning Disabilities Nursing**
**Pressure area care**

People with learning disabilities who are confined to bed may have a higher risk of pressure-induced ulcers, due to factors such as heavy sedation, or a lack of motivation to move independently.

If the individual is being nursed in a general surgical ward without the assistance of a learning disabilities nurse, he or she may receive only rudimentary care, because misconceptions about learning disabilities can result in a failure to recognize basic needs, such as assistance with feeding, the patient's/client's ability to comprehend instructions, or the patient's/client's ability to communicate physical discomfort or the need to eliminate.

subjected to constant pressures of the body against any surface on which it rests (Berecek, 1975). If the pressure is unevenly distributed on the body, a pressure gradient is increased on tissues receiving the pressure. The cellular metabolism of the skin is altered at the point of pressure.

The compensatory response of the tissues to ischaemia, reactive hyperaemia, permits ischaemic tissue to be flooded with blood when pressure is removed. Increased blood flow increases delivery of oxygen and nutrients to tissue. The metabolic debt resulting from pressure can then be met. Healthy equilibrium is restored, and necrosis of the compressed tissue is avoided (Berecek, 1975; Maklebust, 1991a, 1991b; Pires and Muller, 1991). Reactive hyperaemia is effective only if pressure is removed before damage occurs. Some researchers believe that the interval before damage occurs can be between one or two hours. However, this is a subjective time interval, and it is not based on patient/client assessment data.

## WOUND HEALING PROCESS

Wound healing involves integrated physiological processes. The nature of healing is the same for all wounds with variations, depending on the location, severity, and extent of injury. The ability of cells and tissues to regenerate or return to normal structure by cell growth also affects healing. Cells of the liver, renal tubules, and neurons of the central nervous system typically regenerate slowly or not at all.

There are two types of wounds: those with tissue loss and those without. A clean surgical incision is an example of a wound with little tissue loss. The surgical wound heals by **primary intention**. The skin edges **approximate**, or close together, and the risk of infection is lower. In contrast a wound involving loss of tissue, such as a burn, pressure ulcer, or severe laceration, heals by **secondary intention**. The wound edges do not approximate. The wound is left open until it becomes filled by new tissue. It takes longer for a wound to heal by secondary intention, and thus the chance of infection is greater. If scarring from secondary intention is severe, there may be permanent loss of tissue function. Healing by secondary intention, the method of healing in chronic wounds, is similar to primary intention, apart from time-scale.

### Healing by Primary Intention

An example of the normal healing process is repair of a clean surgical wound. Healing occurs in four stages as described by Westaby (1986): inflammatory, destructive, proliferative, and maturation.

### Inflammatory Phase

Inflammation begins within minutes of injury and lasts about 3 days. Reparative processes control bleeding **(haemostasis)**, deliver blood and cells to the injured area (inflammation), and form epithelial cells at the injury site **(epithelization)**. During haemostasis, injured blood vessels constrict and platelets gather to stop bleeding. Clots form a **fibrin** matrix that later provides a framework for cellular repair. Damaged tissue and mast cells secrete histamine, resulting in vasodilatation of surrounding capillaries and exudation of serum and leucocytes into damaged tissues. This results in localized redness, oedema, warmth, and throbbing. The inflammatory response is beneficial, and there is no value in attempting to cool the area or reduce the swelling unless the swelling occurs within a closed compartment (for example, fascial compartment or neck).

Leucocytes reach the wound within a few hours. The primary acting leucocyte is the neutrophil, which begins to ingest bacteria and small debris. The neutrophils die in a few days and leave behind an enzyme **exudate** that attacks bacteria or interferes with tissue repair. In chronic inflammation the dying neutrophils create pus. The second important leucocyte is the monocyte, which transforms into macrophages. The macrophages (engulfing and digesting) clean a wound of bacteria, dead cells, and debris by **phagocytosis**. The macrophages also digest and recycle substances, such as amino acids and sugars, that aid in wound repair.

After the macrophages clean the wound and make it ready for tissue repair, epithelial cells move from the wound margins under the base of the clot or scab. Epithelial cells continue to gather under the wound space for about 48 hours. Eventually a thin layer of epithelial tissue forms over the wound as a barrier against infectious organisms and toxic materials.

The inflammatory phase is prolonged and repair processes are slowed if too little inflammation occurs, as in debilitating disease or after administration of steroids. Too much inflammation also prolongs healing because arriving cells compete for available nutrients.

### Destructive Phase

The **destructive phase** (2 to 5 days) begins before inflammation ends. Macrophages continue the process of clearing the wound of debris, attracting further macrophages, and stimulating formation of **fibroblasts**, the cells that synthesize collagen. Collagen can be found as early as the second day and is the main component of scar tissue. Fibroblasts require vitamins B and C, oxygen, and amino acids to function properly. Collagen provides strength and structural integrity to a wound.

### Proliferative Phase

With the appearance of new blood vessels as reconstruction progresses, the **proliferative phase** begins and lasts from 3 to 24 days. During this period, the wound begins to close with new tissue.

As reconstruction progresses, the tensile strength of the wound increases, and the risk of wound separation or rupture is less likely. The degree of stress on a wound influences the amount of scar tissue formed. For example, more scar tissue forms in an extremity wound than in a less mobile area such as the scalp or chest. Impairment of healing during this stage usually results from systemic factors such as age, anaemia, hypoproteinaemia, and zinc deficiency.

## Maturation

**Maturation**, the final stage of healing, may take more than a year, depending on the depth and extent of the wound. The collagen scar continues to gain strength for several months. However, a healed wound usually does not have the strength of the tissue it replaces. Collagen fibres undergo remodelling or organization before assuming their normal appearance. Usually, scar tissue contains fewer pigmented cells (melanocytes) and has a lighter colour than normal skin.

## Healing by Secondary Intention

When tissue loss in a wound is extensive, wound healing takes longer. A large open wound typically drains more fluid than a closed wound. Inflammation is often chronic, and tissue defects become filled with fragile granulation tissue rather than collagen. **Granulation tissue** is a form of connective tissue that has a more abundant blood supply than collagen. Because the wound is larger, the amount of connective tissue scarring is larger.

When epithelial and connective tissue cells are unable to close a wound defect, contraction may occur. **Wound contraction** involves movement of the dermis and epidermis on each side of the wound. The mechanism of contracture is not completely understood. It is known, however, that collagen is not essential and any event that interferes with cell viability at the wound margin inhibits contraction. Wound contraction begins on about the fourth day and occurs simultaneously with epithelization. The cell that provides the motive force is the myofibroblast. Wound contraction results in thinning of surrounding tissues, and the size and shape of the final scar corresponds to tension lines in the damaged area. For example, a square wound in the abdomen assumes the shape of two Y's, end to end. There are areas of the body where contraction gives poor results, such as wounds on the face, sternum, and anterior lower leg. Wound contraction is not the same as a contracture or deformity resulting from muscle shortening and joint fixation.

## FACTORS INFLUENCING WOUND HEALING

A number of factors influence the rate of wound healing. A patient/client with any factors listed in Table 30-1 is at risk for wound complications. The nurse's knowledge of factors influencing healing helps in providing preventive care and selecting appropriate wound care therapies.

Factors that affect wound healing can be *intrinsic* (such as adverse conditions at the wound site, or an underlying medical condition) or *extrinsic* (such as adverse effects of other therapies, or inappropriate wound management) (Morison, 1992).

## Intrinsic Factors
## Nutrition

Normal wound healing requires proper nutrition (McLaren, 1992; Pinchofsky-Devin, 1993). Physiological processes of wound healing depend on the ready availability of protein, vitamins (especially A and C), and the trace minerals zinc and copper. Collagen is a protein formed from amino acids acquired by fibroblasts from protein ingested in food. Vitamin C is needed for synthesis of collagen. Vitamin A reduces the negative effects of steroids on wound healing (see Table 30-1). Trace elements are needed for epithelization (zinc), collagen synthesis (zinc), and collagen fibre linking (copper).

Malnutrition is second only to excessive pressure in the aetiology, pathogenesis, and nonhealing of pressure ulcers (Hanan and Scheele, 1991; NPUAP, 1989). Poor nutrition often leads to serious muscle atrophy, oedema and/or anaemia, all of which increase a person's risk for pressure ulcers. Moderate-to-severe obesity can also increase the risk of pressure ulcers, because the adipose and underlying tissues are poorly vascularized and are more susceptible to ischaemic damage.

**The nutritional status of the patient/client should be a primary consideration, even if the patient/client has a weight equal to or above the ideal body weight (IBW).** For individuals weakened or debilitated by illness, nutritional therapy is especially important. A person who has undergone surgery (see Chapter 29) and is well nourished still requires at least 1500 kcal/day for nutritional maintenance. Enteral feedings (see Chapter 21) and parenteral nutrition (see Chapter 18) are alternatives for people who are unable to maintain normal food intake.

## Blood and Oxygen Supply

Wounds with poor blood supply heal slowly (Morison, 1992), because blood transports essential healing factors, such as oxygen and nutrients.

Patients/clients who have impaired peripheral circulation due to peripheral vascular disease, shock, or vasopressor-type medications have impaired wound healing and have a higher risk of pressure ulcers. Smoking has been shown to increase the risk of pressure ulcer development by a factor of 3 (Guralnik et al, 1988). This effect is enhanced in people with spinal cord impairment (Lamid and Ghatit, 1983).

Anaemia (decreased levels of haemoglobin) also alters cellular metabolism and impairs wound healing, because the oxygen-carrying capacity of the blood and the amount of oxygen available to tissues is reduced.

## Pathophysiological Factors

Underlying physiological conditions can delay wound healing and can increase the risk of pressure ulcers. These conditions include respiratory and cardiovascular disorders, immune disorders, nutritional disorders, and other chronic conditions such as diabetes and rheumatoid arthritis. There are many mechanisms by which these conditions can affect wound healing. These include reduction of oxygen, vitamins or minerals at the wound site; decreased resistance to infection; or through adverse effects of therapies, such as cytotoxic drugs or radiotherapy.

## TABLE 30-1 Factors that Impair Wound Healing

| PHYSIOLOGICAL EFFECTS | NURSING IMPLICATIONS |
|---|---|
| **Age** | |
| Ageing alters all phases of wound healing. | Teach patient/client on safety precautions to avoid injuries. |
| Vascular changes impair circulation to wound site. | Be prepared to provide wound care for longer time period. |
| Reduced liver function alters synthesis of clotting factors. | Teach wound care techniques to patients/clients. |
| Inflammatory response is slowed. | |
| Reduced formation of antibodies and lymphocytes occurs. | |
| Collagen tissue is less pliable. | |
| Scar tissue is less elastic. | |
| **Malnutrition** | |
| All phases of wound healing are impaired. | Provide balanced diet rich in protein, carbohydrates, lipids, vitamins A and C, and minerals (e.g. zinc, copper) |
| Stress from burns or severe trauma increases nutritional requirements. | |
| **Obesity** | |
| Fatty tissue lacks adequate blood supply to resist bacterial infection and deliver nutrients and cellular elements for healing. | Observe obese patients/clients for signs of wound infection and evisceration. |
| **Impaired Oxygenation** | |
| Low arterial oxygen tension alters synthesis of collagen and formation of epithelial cells. | Provide diet adequate in iron. |
| If local circulating blood flow is poor, tissues fail to receive needed oxygen. | Monitor haematocrit and haemoglobin levels of patients/clients with wounds. |
| Decreased haemoglobin in blood (anaemia) reduces arterial oxygen levels in capillaries and interferes with tissue repair. | |
| **Smoking** | |
| Smoking reduces amount of functional haemoglobin in blood, thus decreasing tissue oxygenation. | Discourage patient/client from smoking by explaining its effects on wound healing. |
| Smoking may increase platelet aggregation and cause hypercoagulability. | |
| Smoking interferes with normal cellular mechanisms that promote release of oxygen to tissues. | |
| **Drugs** | |
| Steroids reduce inflammatory response and slow collagen synthesis. | Carefully observe patients/clients receiving these drugs, because signs of inflammation may not be obvious. |
| Anti-inflammatory drugs suppress protein synthesis, wound contraction, epithelization, and inflammation. | Prolonged antibiotic use may increase risk of superinfection. |
| Chemotherapeutic drugs can depress bone marrow function, lower number of leucocytes, and impair inflammatory response. | |
| **Diabetes** | |
| Chronic disease causes small blood vessel disease that impairs tissue perfusion. | Teach diabetic patients/clients to take preventive measures to avoid cuts or breaks in skin. |
| Diabetes causes haemoglobin to have greater affinity for oxygen, so it fails to release oxygen to tissues. | Provide preventive foot care. |

(Cont'd)

**TABLE 30-1 Factors that Impair Wound Healing (Cont'd)**

| PHYSIOLOGICAL EFFECTS | NURSING IMPLICATIONS |
|---|---|
| **Diabetes (Cont'd)**<br>Hyperglycaemia alters ability of leucocytes to perform phagocytosis and also supports overgrowth of fungal and yeast infection. | Control blood sugar to reduce the physiological changes associated with diabetes. |
| **Radiation**<br>Fibrosis and vascular scarring eventually develop in irradiated skin layers.<br>Tissues become fragile and poorly oxygenated. | Closely observe patients/clients who have surgery after radiation for wound complications. |
| **Wound Stress**<br>Vomiting, abdominal distension, and respiratory effort may stress suture line and disrupt wound layer.<br>Sudden, unexpected tension on incision inhibits formation of endothelial cell and collagen networks. | Control nausea with ordered antiemetics.<br>Keep nasogastric tubes patent and drain to avoid accumulation of secretions.<br>Teach and assist patient/client to support abdominal wound during coughing. |

**Cachexia** (generalized ill health and malnutrition, marked by weakness and emaciation) is usually associated with severe diseases such as cancer and end-stage cardiopulmonary diseases. This condition increases the risk of pressure ulcers, because the cachexic person has lost the adipose tissue necessary to protect bony prominences from pressure.

### Dehydration and Moisture

Dehydration can delay wound healing, because the epithelial cells at the wound margins migrate below the skin surface in search of moist conditions that promote healing. Over the long-term, dehydration increases tissue loss and scarring. (In some cases, however, such as facial burns, exposure of the wound is a favourable solution.)

*Excess* moisture on the skin increases the risk of ulcer formation because it reduces the skin's resistance to other physical factors such as pressure or shearing force. The presence of moisture increases the risk of pressure ulcer formation fivefold (Reuler and Cooney, 1981). Moisture on the skin can originate from wound drainage, perspiration, condensation from humidified oxygen-delivery systems, vomitus, and incontinence. Certain body fluids (for example, urine, diarrhoea, and wound drainage) cause skin erosion, and with pressure the patient's/client's risk increases. Research has shown a strong association between faecal incontinence and pressure ulcer development (St Claire, 1992; Allman *et al*, 1986).

### Temperature

A decrease in temperature at the wound site can arrest leucocyte activity and delay wound healing. The temperature of a wound can drop to as low as 12°C during lengthy dressing changes or while waiting for the doctor's round (Morison, 1992).

Fever, on the other hand, increases the metabolic needs of the body, making an already hypoxic (decreased oxygen) tissue more susceptible to ischaemic injury (Shekleton and Litwack, 1991) and pressure ulcers. Fever also creates diaphoresis (sweating) and increased skin moisture, which further predispose the patient/client to skin breakdown (maceration).

### Ageing

Although the rates for the stages of healing among older patients/clients may be slowed, the physiological aspects of healing are unchanged from the younger adult. Problems that arise during healing are difficult to assign to the ageing process or to other possible causes, such as poor nutrition, environment, or individual response to stress. Before surgery, it is important to assess any factors that may influence or alter the wound healing in older patients/clients (see Table 30-1).

Pressure ulcers occur more frequently in older adults. Studies by Barbenel *et al*, (1977), Versluysen (1986) and Norton *et al*, (1962) note a greater incidence of ulcer development in people over 70 years of age. In Barbenel's study, 71% of patients with ulcers were 70 years or older. Versluysen found that only 10% of her sample group were below 70 years of age.

### Extrinsic Factors
### Physical Forces

Recurrent mechanical trauma can damage the newly formed tissue of a healing wound, thus delaying the healing process. **Shearing force**, another type of mechanical trauma, is the third major factor contributing to the development of pressure ulcers. Shearing force is the pressure exerted against the skin when a patient/client is moved or repositioned in bed by being pulled or being allowed to slide down in bed (Fig. 30-2). When a shearing force is present, the skin and subcutaneous layers adhere to the surface of the bed, and the layers of muscle and even the bones

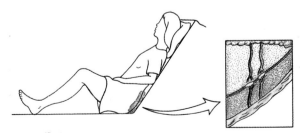

**Fig. 30-2** Diagrammatic sketch of shearing force exerted against sacral area.

slide in the direction of body movement. The underlying tissue capillaries are compressed and severed by the pressure (Knight, 1988; Bennett and Lee, 1988). The sacral areas and heels are the most susceptible (Maklebust, 1987).

## Additional Factors

Other factors may increase the risk of pressure ulcers. These include:

- **impaired sensory input** — people with altered sensory perception for pain and pressure are at greater risk for impaired skin integrity, because their body cannot sense when there is too much pressure or pain.
- **impaired motor function** — people who have impaired motor function can perceive the pressure, but are unable to independently change positions to relieve it. The incidence of pressure ulcers in people with spinal cord injuries is estimated to be as high as 85%, and ulcers or ulcer-related complications are the cause of death in 8% of this population (Reuler and Cooney, 1981). A patient/client with a cast also has an increased risk of pressure ulcer development because of the mechanical external force of friction from the surface of the cast rubbing against the skin.
- **alterations in level of consciousness** — patients/clients who are confused or disoriented or have changing levels of consciousness may be able to feel external pressure, but may not be able to relieve it. Sedative drugs that impair consciousness may create similar effects. People who are in a coma may not perceive pressure and are unable to voluntarily move into a more protective position.

## COMPLICATIONS OF WOUND HEALING

### Haemorrhage

Haemorrhage, or bleeding from a wound site, is normal during and immediately after the initial trauma. **Primary haemorrhage** occurs at the time of the injury and is normally controlled by the contraction of the blood vessel, the formation of a clot, pressure, ligature or diathermy. **Secondary haemorrhage** occurs a few hours after the injury or operation and is caused by the increase of the blood pressure to its usual level. Secondary haemorrhage usually occurs about seven days after injury or operation and is caused when infection erodes the clots which have formed to seal the wound. Haemostasis occurs within several minutes unless large blood vessels are involved or the patient/client has poor clotting function. Haemorrhage occurring after haemostasis indicates a slipped surgical suture, a dislodged clot, infection, or erosion of a blood vessel by a foreign object (for example, a drain). Haemorrhage may occur externally or internally. For example, if a surgical suture slips off a blood vessel, bleeding occurs within the tissues, and there are no visible signs of blood unless a surgical drain is present. (The surgeon often inserts a drain into tissues beneath a wound to remove fluid that collects in underlying tissues.) Internal bleeding can be detected by looking for distension or swelling of the affected body part, a change in the type and amount of drainage from a surgical drain, or signs of **hypovolaemic shock** (for example, fall in blood pressure,

increased thready pulse, increased respirations, restlessness, and diaphoresis). A **haematoma** is a localized collection of blood underneath the tissues. It appears as a swelling or mass that often takes on a bluish discolouration. A haematoma near a major artery or vein is dangerous because pressure from the expanding haematoma may obstruct blood flow.

External haemorrhaging is more obvious. Observe dressings covering the wound for bloody drainage. If bleeding is extensive, the dressing soon becomes saturated, and frequently blood escapes along the sides of the dressing and pools beneath the patient/client. Observe all wounds closely, particularly surgical wounds in which the risk of haemorrhage is great during the first 24 to 48 hours after surgery.

### Infection

Wound infection is the second most common **nosocomial** (hospital-related) **infection**. A wound may be infected if purulent material drains from it, even if a culture is not taken or has negative results. A sample of drainage from an infected wound may not reveal bacteria in a culture because of poor culture technique or because the patient/client has already received antibiotics. Positive culture findings do not always indicate an infection because many wounds contain colonies of noninfective resident bacteria. The chances of wound infection are greater when the wound contains dead or necrotic tissue, when there are foreign bodies in or near the wound, and when blood supply and local tissue defences are reduced. Bacterial wound infection inhibits wound healing.

A contaminated or traumatic wound may show signs of infection early, within 2 to 3 days. A surgical wound infection usually does not develop until the fourth or fifth day. The patient/client has a fever, tenderness and pain at the wound site, and an elevated leucocyte count. The edges of the wound may appear inflamed. If drainage is present, it is purulent, odourous, and has a yellow, green, or brown colour, depending on the causative organism.

### Dehiscence

When a wound fails to heal properly, the layers of skin and tissue may separate. This most commonly occurs before collagen formation (3 to 11 days after injury). **Dehiscence** is the partial or total separation of wound layers. A person with poor wound healing is at risk for dehiscence. However, obese people have a high risk because of the constant strain placed on their wounds and the poor healing qualities of fatty tissue. Dehiscence often involves abdominal surgical wounds and occurs after a sudden strain, such as coughing, vomiting, or sitting up in bed. Patients/clients often report feeling as though something has given way. When there is an increase in serosanguineous drainage from a wound, the nurse should be alert for dehiscence.

### Evisceration

With total separation of wound layers, **evisceration** (protrusion of visceral organs through a wound opening) may occur. Although rare, this condition is an emergency that requires surgical repair. When evisceration occurs, place sterile towels soaked in sterile saline over the extruding tissues to reduce chances of bacterial invasion and drying. If the organs protrude through the wound, blood supply to the tissues is compromised.

### Fistulas

A **fistula** is an abnormal passage between two organs or between an organ and the outside of the body. A surgeon may create a fistula for therapeutic purposes (for example, making an opening between the stomach and the outer abdominal wall to insert a gastrostomy tube for feeding). Most fistulas, however, form as a result of poor wound healing. Trauma, infection, radiation exposure, and diseases such as cancer prevent tissue layers from closing properly and allow the fistula tract to form. Fistulas increase the risk of infection and increase the risk of fluid and electrolyte imbalances from fluid loss. Chronic drainage of fluids through a fistula can also predispose a person to skin breakdown.

### Delayed Wound Closure

Sometimes referred to as *third-intention wound healing*, delayed wound closure is a deliberate attempt by the surgeon to allow effective drainage of a clean-contaminated or contaminated wound. The wound is not closed until all evidence of oedema and wound debris has been removed, usually several days, occasionally weeks. An occlusive dressing is used to prevent bacterial contamination of the wound. Then the wound is closed as in primary closure, or first intention. Experimentally, it has been demonstrated that scarring or delayed healing does not significantly increase when this technique is used (Cooper, 1992).

### PSYCHOSOCIAL IMPACT OF WOUNDS

Although not always considered along with the physiological process of healing, a person's psychological response is an important contributing factor in how he or she adapts to a wound. Body-image changes may impose a great stress on the patient's/client's adaptive mechanisms. In addition, body-image changes influence self-concept (Price, 1990). The patient's/client's personal and social resources for adaptation should also be a part of the nursing assessment. Factors that may affect the individual's perception of the wound include the

presence of scars, drains, odour, bandages, and temporary or permanent prosthetic devices.

## NURSING PROCESS, TISSUE VIABILITY AND WOUND HEALING

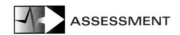 ASSESSMENT

### Assessing Risk of Pressure Ulcer Development

Baseline and continual assessment data provide critical information about the individual's skin integrity and the increased risk for pressure ulcer development. Assessment for pressure ulcers is not limited to the skin, because pressure ulcers have multiple aetiological factors.

Many risk assessment scores have been devised to identify patients/clients with the highest risk of pressure ulcers. Therefore, preventive measures should be targeted only to these high-risk people. Patients/clients with little risk for pressure ulcer development are spared the unnecessary preventive treatments and the risk of complications (Stotts, 1988). Commonly used risk assessment tools include:

- the **Norton Scale** (Table 30-2), designed to score five risk factors — physical condition, mental condition, activity, mobility, and continence. The range is 5 to 20, with a lower score indicating a higher risk for pressure ulcer development. This tool also offers descriptive information regarding potential risk factors (Hoff, 1989).
- the **Waterlow Score** (Fig. 30-3), a popular alternative to the Norton Score in the United Kingdom. The Waterlow Score addresses important factors which are omitted by the Norton, such as nutrition and smoking. In a comparison of the Norton and Waterlow tools (Dealey, 1989), the Waterlow Score was more sensitive but less specific.
- the **Braden Scale**, a 23-point instrument composed of six subscales: sensory perception, moisture, activity, mobility, nutrition, friction, and shear. A hospitalized adult with a score of 16 or below is considered at risk. In older clients, a

## TABLE 30-2 Norton Scale

| Physical Condition | | Mental Condition | | Activity | | Mobility | | Incontinence (bowel and/or bladder) | |
|---|---|---|---|---|---|---|---|---|---|
| Good | 4 | Alert | 4 | Ambulant | 4 | Full | 4 | Never | 4 |
| Fair | 3 | Apathetic | 3 | Walk/help | 3 | Slightly limited | 3 | Occasional | 3 |
| Poor | 2 | Confused | 2 | Chairbound | 2 | Very limited | 2 | (< 2 per 24 hr) Usually | 2 |
| Very bad | 1 | Stuporous | 1 | Bedfast | 1 | Immobile | 1 | (> 2 per 24 hr) Always | 1 |

Maximum score = 20 (good physical condition); minimum score = 5; high risk for pressure ulcers = 12 or below
From Trelease CC: *Ostomy/Wound Manage* 20: 46, 1988.

| Build/ weight for height | | Skin type and visual risk areas | | Sex and age | | Special risks | |
|---|---|---|---|---|---|---|---|
| | | | | | | **Tissue malnutrition** | |
| Average | 0 | Healthy | 0 | Male | 1 | e.g. Terminal cachexia | 8 |
| Above average | 1 | Tissue paper | 1 | Female | 2 | Cardiac failure | 5 |
| Obese | 2 | Dry | 1 | 14-49 | 1 | Peripheral vascular disease | 5 |
| Below average | 3 | Oedematous | 1 | 50-64 | 2 | Anaemia | 2 |
| | | Clammy (Temp Δ) | 1 | 65-74 | 3 | Smoking | 1 |
| | | Discoloured | 2 | 75-80 | 4 | | |
| | | Broken/spot | 3 | 81+ | 5 | | |
| **Continence** | | **Mobility** | | **Appetite** | | **Neurological deficit** | |
| Complete/ catheterized | 0 | Fully | 0 | Average | 0 | e.g. Diabetes, MS, CVA, motor/sensory, paraplegia | 4-6 |
| Occasional incontinent | 1 | Restless/fidgety | 1 | Poor | 1 | | |
| | | Apathetic | 2 | Nasal gastric | | **Major surgery/trauma** | |
| Cath/incont of faeces | 2 | Restricted | 3 | tube/ fluids only | 2 | Orthopaedic | |
| Doubly incontinent | 3 | Inert/traction | 4 | NBM/anorexic | 3 | Below waist, spinal | 5 |
| | | Chairbound | 5 | | | On table >2 hours | 5 |
| | | | | | | **Medication** | |
| | | | | | | Steroids, cytotoxics High dose Anti-inflammatory | 4 |

| **Score** | 10+ At risk | 15+ High risk | 20+ Very high risk |
|---|---|---|---|

**Fig. 30-3** Waterlow risk assessment scale. From Waterlow J: A risk assessment card, *Nurs Times* 81(48):49, 1985.

score of 17 or 18 may be a more efficient prediction of risk (Bryant *et al*, 1992). This instrument is highly reliable in identifying patients/clients at greatest risk of pressure ulcers (Bergstrom *et al*, 1987a).

Although the Norton and Braden scales are valid and reliable, tests have shown that the Norton Scale overpredicts by 64% and the Braden scale overpredicts by 36% (Bergstrom *et al*, 1987). It is important to correctly identify people at risk without overprediction, because a majority of the preventive measures are costly and can cause the cost of care to rise unnecessarily.

Risk assessment scores should *never* be used as a substitute for clinical judgement (Barrat, 1987). Clark (1991) points out that there are no published accounts of prospective comparisons of the predictive power of different risk evaluators.

## SKIN

Continually assess the patient's/client's skin for signs of ulcer development, especially those with high risk as described earlier in this chapter. Assessment for tissue pressure indicators includes:

- Visual and tactile inspection of the skin (Pires and Muller, 1991).
- Baseline assessment to determine the client's normal skin characteristics and any actual or potential areas of breakdown, with particular attention given to areas exposed to casts, traction, or splints. The frequency of pressure checks depends on the schedule of appliance application and the skin's response to the external pressure.

When **hyperaemia** (an increased blood flow to part of the body) is noted, it is important to:

- Document it, noting location, size, and colour, and to reassess the area after 1 hour.
- Outline the affected area with a marker to facilitate reassessment, if you suspect abnormal reactive hyperaemia
- Observe for early warning signs, such as a blister or pimple over the weight-bearing area with possible hyperaemia. Pires and Muller (1991) report that a frequently overlooked sign of early pressure is a scabbing over of the weight-bearing areas in the absence of trauma.

All of these signs are very early indicators of impaired skin integrity, but damage to the underlying tissue may be more progressive. Tactile assessment (using palpation) enables you to acquire further data about induration, and damage to the skin and underlying tissues.

Include *visual* and *tactile* inspection over the body areas most frequently at risk for pressure ulcer development (Fig. 30-4). When a patient/client lays in bed or sits in a chair, body weight is heavily placed on certain bony prominences. Body surfaces subjected to the greatest weight or pressure are at greatest risk for decubitus ulcer formation.

## MOBILITY

Documenting the level of mobility and the potential effects of impaired mobility on skin integrity (see Chapter 24) is an important factor in assessment for pressure ulcers. Assessment of mobility should also include obtaining data on the quality of muscle tone and strength. For example, determine whether the individual can lift his or her weight off the ischial tuberosities and can roll to a side-lying position. The patient/client may have adequate range of motion (ROM) to independently move into a more protective position. Also, note the person's activity tolerance (see Chapter 24). The frequency of position changes is based on ongoing skin assessment and is revised as data change.

## NUTRITIONAL STATUS

Assessment of the patient's/client's nutritional status is an integral part of the initial assessment. Albumin assessment is often used to evaluate the individual's protein status. A person with a serum albumin level below 3 g/100 ml is at greater risk of pressure ulcers than someone with a higher albumin level. In addition, low albumin levels are associated with poor wound healing (Hanan and Scheele, 1991; Pinchcofsky-Devin and Kaminski, 1989; Natlow, 1983). Although serum albumin levels are slow to reflect changes in visceral proteins, they are the best predictors of malnutrition in all age groups (Hanan and Scheele, 1991).

The patient's/client's percentage of ideal body weight is also obtained. A person who is malnourished or cachexic and whose body weight is less than 90% of IBW, or a person whose body weight is greater than 110% of IBW, has an increased risk for the development of pressure ulcers (Hanan and Scheele 1991). Percentage of IBW alone is not a good predictor. However, when used with a low serum albumin or total protein level, the patient's/client's percentage of IBW can have an impact on the occurrence of pressure ulcers.

## Assessing Wounds

You will often assess wounds under two conditions: at the time of injury (before treatment) and after therapy when the wound is relatively stable. A chronic wound may be assessed at *any* stage in its history; therefore, **each condition requires you to make different observations and to take different actions.**

You may see wounds in any setting, including a clinic, patient's/client's home, hospital ward, or accident and emergency department. The type of wound determines the criteria for inspection. For example, you need not inspect for signs of internal bleeding after an abrasion but should do so in the event of a puncture wound.

## EMERGENCY SETTING

In an emergency setting, wound assessment begins when the patient's/client's condition is judged to be stable, as indicated by the presence of spontaneous breathing, a clear airway, and a strong carotid pulse (see Chapter 18). To begin the assessment, inspect the wound for bleeding. An **abrasion** is usually superficial with little bleeding. The wound may appear 'weepy' because of plasma leakage from damaged capillaries. A **laceration** may bleed more profusely, depending on the wound's depth and location. For example, minor scalp lacerations tend to bleed profusely because of the rich blood supply to the scalp. Lacerations greater than 5 cm long or 2.5 cm deep can cause serious bleeding. **Puncture** wounds bleed in relation to the depth and size of the wound. The primary dangers of puncture wounds are internal bleeding and infection.

Next, inspect the wound for foreign bodies or contaminant material. Most traumatic wounds are dirty. Soil, broken glass,

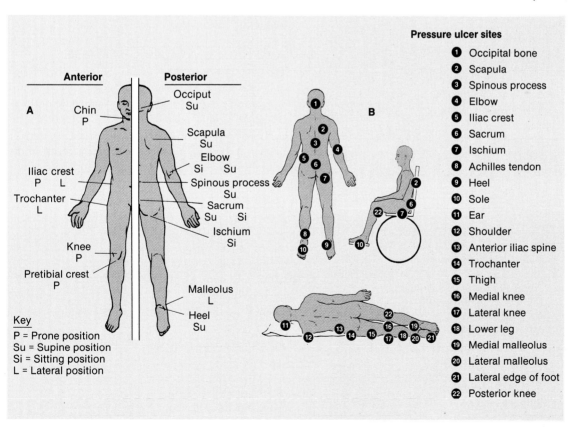

**Fig. 30-4 A,** Bony prominence most frequently underlying pressure ulcer. **B,** Pressure ulcer sites. From Trelease CC: *Ostomy/Wound Manage* 20:46, 1988.

shreds of cloth, and foreign substances clinging to penetrating objects can become embedded in the wound.

The size of the wound is the next criterion for inspection. A deep laceration requires suturing by a doctor. A large open wound may expose bone or tissue that should be protected.

When the injury is the result of trauma from a dirty penetrating object, determine when the patient/client last received a tetanus toxoid injection. Tetanus bacteria reside in soil and in the gut of humans and animals. A tetanus antitoxin injection is necessary if the patient/client has not had one within 5 years.

## STABLE SETTING

In a stable setting (for example, after surgery or in the client's home) assess the wound to determine its progress towards healing. If the patient/client has a high risk of pressure ulcers (especially if he or she is immobilized), the skin integrity should also be assessed.

## WOUND APPEARANCE

Note whether wound edges are closed. A surgical incision should have clean, well-approximated edges. Crusts often form along the wound edges from exudate. A puncture wound is usually a small, circular wound with the edges coming together towards the

centre. If a wound is open, the wound edges are separated, and the condition of underlying tissue such as adipose and connective tissue should be inspected. Also look for complications such as dehiscence and evisceration. The outer edges of a wound normally appear inflamed for the first 2 to 3 days, but this slowly disappears. Within 7 to 10 days a normally healing wound fills with epithelial cells, and edges close. If infection develops, the wound edges become brightly inflamed and swollen.

Skin discolouration usually results from bruising of interstitial tissues or possibly haematoma formation. Blood collecting beneath the skin first takes on a bluish or purplish appearance. Gradually, as the clotted blood is broken down, shades of brown and yellow appear. If the wound becomes chronic it should be assessed according to its appearance: necrotic, sloughy, granulating, epithelizing or infected.

- **necrotic** wounds have a leathery, black appearance, due to the dehydrated dead tissue
- **sloughy** wounds have a yellow or green appearance, often associated with odour and exudate; slough is dead fat colonized heavily with bacteria
- **granulating** wounds are healthy and healing well; new tissue has an irregular, shiny, red appearance
- **epithelizing** wounds are filled will new tissue to skin level; they have smooth edges and the epithelial tissue is pink in colour
- infected wounds may be tender and painful with purulent material draining from it.

An example of a nursing protocol for the care of sloughly wounds is outlined in the box below.

## CHARACTER OF WOUND DRAINAGE

It is important to note the amount, colour, odour, and consistency of drainage. The amount of drainage depends on the location and extent of the wound. For example, drainage is minimal after a simple appendectomy. In contrast, wound drainage is moderate for 1 to 2 days after resection of a portion of the small bowel. If you need an accurate measurement of the amount of drainage within a dressing, the dressing can be weighed and compared with the weight of the same dressing when clean and dry. A rule of thumb is 1 g of drainage equals 1 ml. The colour and consistency of drainage vary depending on the components. Types of drainage include:

- **serous**, a clear, watery plasma
- **sanguineous**, which indicates fresh bleeding
- **serosanguineous**, a pale, more watery drainage than sanguineous drainage
- **purulent**, a thick, yellow, green, or brown drainage.

If the drainage has a pungent or strong odour, an infection should be suspected.

## WOUND MEASURING

It is important to calculate wound size at each dressing change so that healing can be assessed. Accurate measurement of depth is difficult, especially if the wound base is uneven. Suggested ideas for promoting accurate assessment are the use of a quill to

| Protocol 3: Sloughy Wounds | |
|---|---|
| EXAMPLE: | Common in chronic wounds — pressure sores, ulcers, abscess cavity. |
| PROBLEM: | Exudate. Odour, due to bacteria and necrotic tissue. Slough and necrotic tissue may encourage the growth of bacteria and this may delay healing (Haury, 1989). |
| GOAL: | Removal of sloughy and necrotic tissue. |
| CARE PLAN: | If unsure whether wound infection is present take a wound swab and send for microscopy and culture. |
| Cleaning: | Sodium chloride 0.9% (seek advice from nurse specialist if an antiseptic cleanser is being considered). |
| Dressing: | *Non-cavity, sloughy wound* Minimal/moderate exudate --> hydrocolloid sheet Moderate/heavy exudate --> alginate sheet *Sloughy, cavity wound* Minimal/moderate exudate --> hydrogel occluded with film Moderate/heavy exudate --> alginate rope or desloughing agent |

From James H (editor): *The Royal Hospitals NHS Trust wound management guidelines,* London, 1993, The Royal Hospitals NHS Trust.

measure the deepest point, and aligning the quill against a ruler. Surface area can be assessed by tracing the wound outline on a sterile plastic sheet. This can then be measured using a centimetre squared grid.

Record the wound integrity, size and drainage character. Describe the wound's appearance according to characteristics observed. An example of accurate recording is:

*Pressure ulcer on sacrum measures 5 cm x 6 cm and is Grade 4, depth 5 cm at deepest point. It is 50% sloughy, 50% granulating. Exudate is purulent green/yellow and has saturated outer dressing within 10 hours.*

## DRAINS

The doctor inserts a drain into or close to a surgical wound if a large amount of drainage is expected and if keeping wound layers closed is especially important. If fluid is allowed to accumulate under tissues, the inner wound edges may never close.

Assess drain placement, character of drainage, and condition of collecting apparatus. First, observe the security of the drain and its location with respect to the wound. Next, note the character of drainage. If there is a collecting device, measure the drainage volume. Because a drainage system must be patent, look for drainage flow through the tubing. A sudden decrease may indicate a blocked drain, and the doctor should be notified. When a drain is connected to suction, assess the system to be sure that the pressure ordered is being exerted. Evacuator units, such as a Minivac™ or Redivac™ pump, exert a constant low negative pressure as long as the suction bladder or bag is fully compressed (Fig. 30-5). When the evacuator device is unable to maintain a vacuum on its own, the nurse notifies the surgeon, who will then order a secondary vacuum system. If fluid is allowed to accumulate within the tissues, wound healing will not progress at an optimal rate, and the risk of infection is increased.

## WOUND CLOSURES

Surgical wounds are closed with staples, sutures, or wound closures. Look for irritation around staple or suture sites and note whether closures are intact. Normally for the first 2 to 3 days after surgery the skin around sutures or staples is swollen. Continued swelling may indicate that the closures are too tight. The skin can be cut by overly tight suture material, leading to wound separation. Sutures that are too tight are a common cause of wound dehiscence. Early suture removal reduces formation of defects along the suture line and minimizes chances of scar malformation.

## PALPATION OF WOUND

When inspecting a wound, you may observe swelling or separation of wound edges. Light palpation on wound edges enables you to detect localized areas of tenderness, drainage collection or infection. Apply sterile gloves before palpating any wound. Gently apply the fingertips along the wound edges. If pressure causes fluid to be expressed, note the character of the drainage. It may be necessary to collect the drainage for culture. The patient/client is normally sensitive to palpation of wound edges. Extreme tenderness may indicate infection.

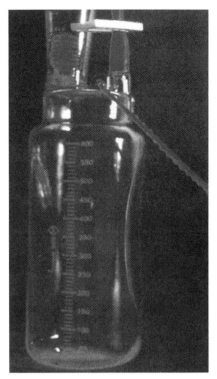

**Fig. 30-5** A disposable pre-vacuumed lightweight drainage system with vacuum indicator and Luer lock safety feature for disconnecting bottles, System 600 (Summit Medical). From: Morrison: *A Colour guide the nursing management of wounds*, 1992, Mosby.

## PAIN

Pain assessment is an important part of wound assessment in terms of detecting complications and planning for future wound care. If the patient/client experiences serious discomfort while you inspect or palpate the wound, look for underlying problems. If the wound is extensive and discomfort seems to be related to dressing removal or application, plan to administer analgesics before future dressing changes.

## Wound Cultures

If you detect purulent or suspicious-looking drainage, collecting a specimen for culture may be necessary. Never collect a wound culture sample from old drainage. Resident colonies of bacteria from the skin grow within exudate and may not be the true causative organisms of a wound infection. Clean the wound first to remove skin flora. Aerobic organisms grow in superficial wounds exposed to the air, and anaerobic organisms tend to grow within body cavities.

To collect an aerobic specimen use a sterile swab and a culturette tube (Fig. 30-6). If wound edges are separated, slowly and gently insert the tip of the swab into the wound to collect deeper secretions. After collecting the specimen place the swab in the tube and cap the tube. The medium must moisten and coat the swab tip. Send the labelled specimen to the laboratory immediately. Swabs to identify anaerobic bacteria are taken in the same way but treated in a different manner on reaching the laboratory.

Gram's stains are often performed, as well. This test allows earlier broad identification of the microorganism type involved.

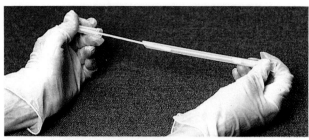

**Fig. 30-6** Wound culturette tube.

The doctor can then order appropriate treatment before culture results are ready. No additional specimens are usually required. The microbiology laboratory needs only to be notified to perform the additional test. In every case, the doctors in the laboratory need a clinical history of the patient/client to enable correct diagnosis of the microorganisms cultured.

After completing an assessment of the patient's/client's wound, identify nursing actions that will direct supportive and preventive care. Existence of a wound clearly indicates action to treat actual impaired skin integrity and to initiate interventions that promote the healing process, such as ensuring adequate nutrition.

 **PLANNING**

After assessing the wound and identifying interventions, develop a care plan for the patient/client. The plan is based on the patient's/client's identified needs and priorities. Goals are established which enable you to plan therapies according to severity and type of wound; the presence of any complicating conditions (for example, infection, poor nutrition, immunosupression, and pathophysiological conditions) that may affect wound healing; and interventions for patients/clients with actual or potential risks to skin integrity.

Because patients are often discharged from hospital earlier than in the past, it is important to consider the patient's/client's home when planning therapies to promote wound healing. Patients/clients, their families, and community nurses may need to continue the objectives of wound management after discharge. Whether the patient/client is in hospital or at home, it is important to involve him or her in the nursing care to promote wound healing.

The nurse's priorities in wound care depend on whether the patient's/client's condition is *stable*, *emergent* or *chronic*. The type of wound care administered depends on the type of wound, its size and location, and complications. Nursing interventions will be both *dependent* and *independent*. Goals of care for people with any type of wound include the following:
- promoting wound haemostasis and healing
- preventing infection
- maintaining skin integrity and vitality through hygiene and topical care
- reducing and preventing injuries to the skin and musculoskeletal system from mechanical trauma, pressure, and shearing force

- improving nutritional intake
- regaining normal function (including improving mobility)
- gaining comfort
- addressing the cause (e.g. relieving pressure, promoting venous return)
- educating the patient/client about health promotion and wound healing.

 **IMPLEMENTATION**

In an emergency setting, the nurse uses first aid measures for wound care. Under more stable conditions, the nurse uses a variety of interventions to ensure wound healing. For chronic wounds, nursing interventions focus on prevention or treatment.

### Cleansing

Gentle cleansing of a wound removes contaminants that might serve as sources of infection. However, vigorous cleaning can cause bleeding or further injury. For abrasions, minor lacerations, and small puncture wounds, rinse the wound in running water. When a laceration is bleeding profusely, brush away surface contaminants and concentrate on haemostasis until the patient/client can be cared for in a clinic or hospital. Pressure sores should be gently irrigated with warmed normal saline at each dressing change.

On reaching the accident and emergency department a wound which is contaminated with gravel should be irrigated thoroughly to prevent a 'tattoo' effect. Irrigation is usually performed with saline. Occasionally Savlon™, a combination of cetrimide and chlorhexidine, is used. The detergent effect of the centrimide helps to remove the gravel.

To prevent chronic open wounds (pressure ulcers), the patient's/client's skin must be kept clean and dry (see Guidelines for Treating Pressure Ulcers). The types of products available for skin care are numerous, and their uses need to be matched to the specific needs of the individual (Maklebust, 1991a, 1991b).

#### TOPICAL AGENTS FOR CLEANSING WOUNDS

Topical antiseptics (such as hypochlorite, hydrogen peroxide, and povidone-iodine) are rarely used in the United Kingdom to clean wounds, as they have been found to be too irritant. Gentle cleansing with normal saline is the preferred method for most wounds. It is isotonic and does not cause chemical damage to cells. If a large surface area is to be irrigated the solution should be warmed, as a drop in temperature at the wound face is known to decrease the rate of cell division (Lock, 1980).

Avoid soaps when cleaning the skin. Soaps and alcohol-based lotions cause drying and leave an alkaline residue. The alkaline residue discourages the growth of normal skin bacteria, thus promoting an overgrowth of opportunistic bacteria, which can then enter an open wound (Barnes, 1987).

The use of prophylactic creams to prevent pressure ulcers has largely been discontinued in the UK due to lack of research validation proving their effectiveness. Creams and sprays do not prevent pressure sores and some may even be harmful (Norton *et*

## Guidelines for Treating Pressure Ulcers

| SEQUENCE OF ACTIONS | RATIONALE |
|---|---|
| 1. Assess pressure ulcer and surrounding skin: | |
|   a. Note and document colour and appearance of skin around ulcer. | Skin condition may indicate progressive tissue damage. |
|   b. Measure diameter of pressure ulcer with ruler or transparency film. | Provides objective measure of wound size. May determine type of dressing chosen. |
|   c. Measure depth of ulcer using sterile, cotton-tipped applicator or other device that will allow measurement of wound depth. | Depth measure is important for staging ulcer. Kundin scale is a three-dimensional (length, width, and depth) tool for wound volume calculations (Cooper, 1992). |
|   d. Measure depth of undermining skin by lateral tissue necrosis. Use cotton-tipped applicator and gently probe under skin edges. | Undermining may indicate progressive tissue necrosis. |
| 2. Wash skin around ulcer gently with warm water. | Reduces number of resident bacteria. |
| 3. Rinse area thoroughly with water. | |
| 4. Gently dry skin thoroughly by patting lightly with towel. | Retained moisture causes maceration of skin layers. |
| 5. Cleanse ulcer thoroughly with normal saline or cleansing agent: | Removes debris from wound from digested material. Previously applied enzymes may require soaking for removal. |
|   a. Use irrigating syringe for deep ulcers. | |
|   b. Use shower with hand-held shower head. | |
|   c. Use whirlpool treatments to assist with wound cleansing and debridement. | |
| 6. Apply topical agents or dressings, if prescribed: | |
|   a. Enzymes | |
|     (1) Reconstitute enzyme in sterile solution as per manufacturer's instructions. | |
|     (2) Cover with light dressing and film. | Stops enzyme drying out and maintains function. |
|   b. Hydrogels: | |
|     (1) Apply hydrogel onto wound cavity up to skin level. | Maintains moist wound healing environment. |
|     (2) Cover in light dressing and film. | Prevents dehydration and holds hydrogel in place. |
|   c. Hydrocolloid beads/paste: | |
|     (1) Fill wound to approximately half of total depth with hydrocolloid beads or paste. | Assists in absorbing wound drainage. Highly draining wounds are best treated with hydrocolloid beads or granules. |
|     (2) Cover with hydrocolloid dressing; extend dressing 2.5–4 cm beyond edges of wound. | Dressing maintains wound humidity. May be left in place up to 7 days. |
|   d. Dextranomer beads: | |
|     (1) Hold container of beads approximately 2.5 cm above site and lightly sprinkle 5 mm diameter layer over wound. | Absorbs wound exudate. |
|     (2) Apply gauze dressing over ulcer. | |
|   e. Hydrogel agents: | |
|     (1) Cover surface of ulcer with hydrogel using sterile applicator or gloved hand. | Provides maintenance of wound humidity while absorbing excess drainage. May be used as carrier for topical agents. |
|     (2) Apply dry, fluffy gauze over gel to completely cover ulcer. | Holds hydrogel against wound surface. Used as absorbent. |

## TABLE 30-3 Devices Used to Prevent or Treat Pressure Ulcers

### DEVICES TO REDUCE PRESSURE

- These aids are thought to reduce interface pressures, that is, the pressure encountered by the patient's/client's skin on the supporting surface.
- Examples are silicone fibre pads, replacement pressure relieving mattresses, contoured foam overlays.

### DEVICES TO AID IN TURNING

- A CircOletric™ bed is electronically controlled and can be rotated vertically 210 degrees to rotate patient/client from prone to supine position.
- A Guttman™ bed rotates the patient/client from prone to supine positions and from side to side.
- A Rotokinetic™ treatment table continuously rotates the patient/client 270 degrees every 3 min.
- A Stryker™ wedge turning frame rotates the patient/client horizontally from the prone to the supine position.

### DEVICES TO MINIMIZE AND RELIEVE PRESSURE

- Alternating pressure mattresses are made of polyvinyl cells attached to a motor which inflates and deflates them alternately on a 7 to 12 minute cycle. This emulates patient movement and thus relieves pressure points regularly. Alternating pressure mattresses can be used instead of a mattress or above the mattress, depending on its depth. They are considerably cheaper than the others in this group and their efficacy has been proven in controlled trials (Bliss and Thomas, 1992).
- An air-fluidized bed decreases pressure and reduces shearing friction, and distributes the patient's/client's weight through a gentle flow of temperature controlled air forced through a mass of fine ceramic microspheres. The air flow is particularly good for patients/clients with extensive skin loss and maceration.
- Low air-loss therapy places the patient/client on a layer of air-controlled cells which conform to their shape by low air loss. This therapy is given as a replacement mattress or can be incorporated into a total replacement bed.

al, 1967). When using any water-repellent ointment, clean the area completely on a routine basis. If left in place too long, ointment can be a medium for bacteria and can cause further skin problems, such as maceration and infection.

### PROTECTION

Regardless of whether bleeding has stopped, protect the wound from further injury by applying sterile or clean dressings and immobilizing the body part. A light dressing applied over minor wounds prevents entrance of microorganisms.

The more extensive the wound, the larger the bandage required in the first aid situation. In the home a clean tea towel may be the best dressing. A bulky dressing applied with pressure minimizes movement of underlying tissues and helps immobilize the entire body part. If applied with pressure it can also help to assuage bleeding during transfer to Accident and Emergency. A bandage or cloth wrapped around a penetrating object should immobilize it adequately. A penetrating object such as a knife or piece of glass should not be removed in the first aid setting as further trauma may ensue.

When patients/clients are incontinent, the area should be cleansed, and a skin barrier containing petrolatum or zinc oxide applied. These barriers protect the skin from excessive moisture and toxins from urine or stool (Maklebust, 1991b). Absorptive underpads, such as incontinence pads, can be used to drain moisture away from the person's skin (USDHHS, 1992). The absorptive garments have a quilted lining and contain a polymer filling. Do not place disposable, plastic-lined underpads directly under the patient's/client's skin because the pads do not drain moisture away from the skin. These products protect the bed, not the patient/client. The plastic also causes diaphoresis, which can lead to skin maceration. Moist, macerated skin is more susceptible to pressure, friction, and the shearing force, so tissue breakdown occurs more rapidly.

### POSITIONING

Positioning interventions are designed to reduce pressure and shearing force to the skin. The immobilized patient's/client's position should be changed according to activity level, perceptual ability, and daily routines (Pajk et al, 1986; Bergstrom et al, 1987a). Therefore a standard turning interval of 1.5 to 2 hours may not prevent pressure sore development in some people.

People who sit out of bed in chairs are at equal or greater risk of sustaining sores than those who remain in bed (Bliss, 1990). More than 50% of people who are confined to a wheelchair will eventually develop a pressure sore (Mawson *et al*, 1993). The patient's/client's time spent in the chair should be limited to 2 hours or less. Do not allow the person to sit for a period longer than the recommended interval calculated during the assessment. Teach patients/clients who sit in chairs to shift their weight every 15 minutes. Foam, gel, or air cushions can help redistribute the individual's weight, but do not completely remove pressure from the ischial tuberosities. Rigid and ring-shaped cushions are contraindicated, because they reduce blood supply to the area, resulting in wider areas of ischaemia (Maklebust, 1991a).

After the patient/client is repositioned, reassess the skin and observe for normal reactive hyperaemia and blanching. The reddened areas should *never* be massaged. This change in practice is a result of nursing research (Maklebust, 1991a; USDHHS, 1992). Massaging the reddened areas increases breaks in the capillaries in the underlying tissues and increases the risk of pressure ulcer formation.

### Therapeutic Beds and Mattresses

A variety of special beds and mattresses are available that help reduce the incidence of pressure ulcers in high-risk patients/clients. However, no single mattress entirely eliminates the effects of pressure on the skin.

When selecting speciality beds, thoroughly assess the

patients'/clients' needs. Patients/clients and families should be taught the reason for and proper use of the beds or mattresses.

## Dressings

The use of dressings requires an understanding of wound healing. A variety of dressing materials is commercially available. Unless a dressing is suited to the characteristics of a wound, the dressing can hinder wound repair:

- For **surgical wounds** that heal by primary intention, it is common to remove dressings as soon as drainage stops. Patients/clients with surgical wounds have had similar infection rates whether the wound is covered or not. This implies that the wound is sealed to microorganisms at an early stage (Chrnitz *et al*, 1989). Wounds healing by secondary intention require dressings which are biointeractive with the wound face and thus promote a faster rate of healing.

- For reddened areas or areas of **superficial broken skin integrity**, a semipermeable film dressing may promote healing. However, there is little research surrounding the efficacy of dressing application to these superficial sores. It is most important to concentrate efforts towards improving pressure relief. When the ulcer is pink with granulation tissue throughout, a dressing is indicated to promote healing. A clean, moist environment promotes migration of epithelial cells across the ulcer surface (Fowler, 1982).

The choice of dressings and the method of dressing a wound influence the progress of wound healing. The proper dressing should not allow a draining wound to become overly dry with extensive scab formation. When this occurs, the dermis dehydrates and crusts. As a result, a barrier forms against normal epidermal cell growth, leaving a depression or defect in the new epidermal surface. Furthermore, dryness of the wound may increase the patient's/client's discomfort. Ideally a dressing leaves a wound slightly moist to promote epithelial cell migration. The dressing should also absorb drainage to prevent pooling of exudate that may promote bacterial growth.

## PURPOSES OF DRESSINGS

A dressing may serve several purposes:

- Aiding haemostasis — pressure dressings promote haemostatis. Applied with elastic bandages, a pressure dressing exerts localized downward pressure over an actual or potential bleeding site. A pressure dressing eliminates dead space in underlying tissues so that wound healing progresses normally. Check pressure dressings to be sure that they do not interfere with circulation of a body part. Assess skin colour, pulses in distal extremities, the patient's/client's comfort, and changes in sensation. Pressure dressings are not routinely removed.

- Supporting or splinting the wound site — a firmly taped or wrapped dressing supports or immobilizes a body part, minimizing movement of the underlying incision and injured tissues.

- Protecting the patient/client from seeing the wound (if perceived as unpleasant).

- Providing conditions which promote wound healing.

The characteristics of the ideal dressing for this purpose have been outlined (see Table 30–4).

## TYPES OF DRESSINGS

There are many different types of dressings and this can be confusing when choosing a dressing for a particular wound type. The nurse should group dressings into major types, according to their effect upon the wound. Before instituting treatment measures for chronic wounds, assess the wound thoroughly and determine the correct dressing based on the stage of ulcer development. Types of dressing are described in many sources such as the British National Formulary. (*Pharmaceutical Press, 1994*).

## CHANGING DRESSINGS

To prepare for changing a dressing, you must know the type of dressing, the presence of underlying drains or tubing, and the type of supplies needed for wound care. Poor preparation may cause a break in aseptic technique (see Chapter 28) or an accidental dislodging of a drain. Your judgement in modifying a dressing change procedure is important during wound care, particularly if the character of a wound changes. Notifying the doctor of any change is essential.

## Cleansing Skin and Drain Sites

Although a moderate amount of wound exudate promotes epithelial cell growth, the doctor may order cleansing of a wound or drain site if a dressing does not properly absorb drainage or if an open drain deposits drainage onto the skin. An ulcer that has necrotic tissue or eschar or shows signs of sloughing must be debrided. **Eschar** is the scab or dry crust that results from excoriation of the skin. **Sloughing** is the shedding of dead tissue as the result of skin ulceration. **Debridement** is the removal of necrotic tissue so that healthy tissue can regenerate.

Wound cleansing requires good handwashing and aseptic techniques (see Chapter 28). The nurse may apply normal saline solution locally or may use irrigation to remove debris.

## BASIC SKIN CLEANSING

Clean surgical or traumatic wounds by applying saline solution with sterile gauze or by irrigation. The following three principles are important when cleaning an incision or the area surrounding a drain:

1. Cleanse in a direction from the least contaminated area, such as from the wound or incision to the surrounding skin (Fig. 30-7) or from an isolated drain site to the surrounding skin (Fig. 30-8).
2. Use gentle friction when applying saline locally to the skin.
3. When irrigating, allow the solution to flow from the least to most contaminated area.

A wound is thought to be less contaminated than the surrounding skin; therefore it is important to clean *away* from the wound. Never use the same piece of gauze to cleanse across an incision or wound twice.

## TABLE 30-4 Characteristics of the 'Ideal' Dressing

The characteristics of the ideal dressing have been outlined by Morgan (1990). Many of these recommendations are based upon research. Although they are not all essential, all have valuable applications for various wound types.

**Morgan's Ideal Dressing Characteristics**

1. *Provide the optimum environment for wound healing*
   This has been defined as moist but not macerated, free of infection, free of toxins, optimum temperature, infrequent temperature, optimum pH value (Thomas, 1991).
2. *Maintain a moist wound environment at the wound dressing interface*
   If dry conditions exist under a dressing, the wound dehydrates and a scab forms which acts as a barrier to epidermal migration across the wound (Winter, 1962).
3. *Allow gaseous exchange of oxygen, carbon dioxide and water vapour*
   This is an area of ongoing research. Because oxygen is metabolized by leucocytes, it was previously thought that gaseous permeability was an essential quality for a dressing. However, recent research with hydrocolloid dressings has cast some doubt on this theory (Thomas, 1991).
4. *Provide thermal insulation*
   Research has shown that cell division and replication takes several hours to return to pre-wound dressing levels following the drop in wound temperature at cleansing (Myers, 1982).
5. *Impermeable to microorganisms*
   Microorganisms, especially motile bacteria such as pseudomonas sp, will pass quickly across a wet dressing. This can be prevented by certain properties, such as the semipermeable film backings of most hydrocolloidal dressings. Even so, once the dressing is wet on the outside, bacteria will quickly pass through and increase the risk of infection.
6. *Free from particulate contaminants*
   Traditional dressings, such as gauze, have been shown to shed fibres into the wound which have histological changes several months after wound occurrence (Wood, 1976).
7. Nonadherent
   Many dressings describe themselves as non-adherent, and this is strictly incorrect. Because serum in exudate is inherently sticky, all dressings will adhere to a certain extent. However, some wound coverings possess low adherent qualities which prevent disruption of cells at the wound surface.
8. *Safe in use*
   Presently, many wound coverings do not pass through the five stages associated with pharmaceutical trials, and many are not product licensed. Many, however, are supported by extensive clinical trials, which are an essential consideration when deciding to use a product.
9. *Acceptable to the patient/client*
   This is of particular importance in community care, where patient/client compliance is of paramount importance to ensure effective treatment. Before any dressing is implemented, the patient's/client's consent must be sought and an explanation given.
10. *High absorption characteristics*
    Many wounds exude large quantities of serum, plasma proteins and bacterial debris. If the dressing is to prevent cross infection, absorptive qualities are essential for this type of wound.
11. *Cost effective*
    Many of the modern dressings require less frequent changing, thus providing a cost effective saving of nursing time.
12. *Carrier for medicaments*
    This is a rarely used property at present, but may become more frequently used as growth factors are used in clinical practice.
13. *Capable for standardization and evaluation*
    All dressings should be subject to ongoing clinical trials.
14. *Allow monitoring of wound*
    Not an essential characteristic, but useful in semipermeable film dressing and sheet hydrogels.
15. *Provide mechanical protection*
    A dressing should protect the wound from mechanical damage. When a wound is granulating, the tissue is more vascular, will bleed, and will be more susceptible to damage.
16. *Properties must remain constant*
    Dressings are not medications; however, their properties must remain consistent and predictable whenever they are used.
17. *Non-inflammable*
18. *Sterilization*
19. *Available (hospital and community)*
    Unfortunately the community tariff means that many dressings available in hospital are not obtainable in the community. When a patient/client is discharged, therefore, it is important that the hospital team considers the availability of the prescribed product in the community.
20. *Require infrequent changing*
    All dressings must be changed when wound exudate strikes through the outer dressing. However, if the qualities of the dressing give a greater time before this occurs, there is a cost saving in terms of nursing time. This property also reduces disturbance at the wound face and promotes a faster healing rate.
21. *Conformable*
    To increase wear time and promote patient/client comfort it is important that a dressing is able to conform to body contours. This presents a particular challenge when the wound is on a heel.

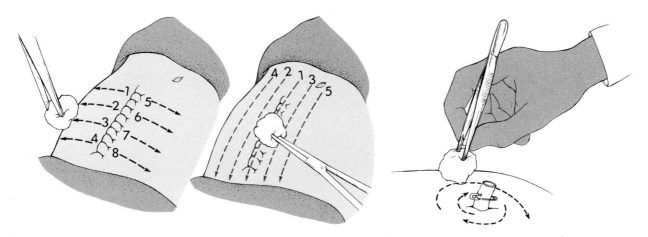

**Fig.30-7** Methods for cleansing a wound site.

**Fig. 30-8** Cleansing a drain site.

A drain site is highly contaminated because the moist drainage harbours microorganisms. If a wound has a dry incisional area and a moist drain site, cleansing moves from the incisional area towards the drain.

## Suture Care

A surgeon closes a wound by bringing the wound edges as close together as possible to reduce scar formation. Proper wound closure involves minimal trauma and tension to tissues with control of bleeding.

**Sutures** are threads of a variety of materials used to sew body tissues together. The patient's/client's history of wound healing, site of surgery, tissues involved, and purpose of the sutures determine the suture material to be used. For example, if the person has had repeated surgery for an abdominal hernia, the surgeon might choose proline sutures to provide greater strength for wound closure. In contrast a small laceration of the face calls for the use of very fine Dacron™ (polyester) sutures to minimize scar formation.

Sutures are available in a variety of materials, including silk, steel, cotton, linen, wire, nylon, and Dacron™. Commonly seen are steel staples, a type of outer skin closure that causes less trauma to tissues than sutures, yet provides extra strength. It is also common to see wounds closed with Steri-Strips™. A Steri-Strip™ is a sterile butterfly tape, applied along both sides of a wound to keep the edges closed.

Sutures are placed within tissue layers in deep wounds and superficially as the final means for wound closure. The deeper sutures are usually an absorbable material that disappears in several days. Sutures are foreign bodies and thus are capable of causing local inflammation. The surgeon can minimize tissue injury by using the finest suture possible and the smallest number necessary.

In general, nurses remove sutures following doctors' orders, and instructions and policies vary within institutions as to who may remove sutures.

To remove staples, simply insert the tips of the staple remover under each wire staple. While slowly closing the ends of the staple remover together, squeeze the centre of the staple with the tips, freeing the staple from the skin.

To remove sutures, first check the type of suturing used (Fig. 30-9). With **interrupted suturing**, the surgeon ties each individual suture made in the skin. **Continuous suturing**, as the name implies, is a series of sutures with only two knots, one at the beginning and one at the end of the suture line. **Retention sutures** are placed more deeply than skin sutures. The manner in which the suture crosses and penetrates the skin determines the method for removal. The most important principle in suture removal is to *never* pull the visible portion of a suture through underlying tissue. Sutures on the skin's surface harbour microorganisms and debris. The portion of the suture beneath the skin is sterile. Pulling the contaminated portion of the suture through tissues may lead to infection. Clip suture materials as close to the skin edge on one side as possible and then pull the suture through from the other side (Fig. 30-10).

## Bandages and Binders

A simple dressing is often not enough to immobilize or provide support to a wound. **Binders** and bandages applied over or around dressings can provide extra protection and therapeutic benefits by:

- creating pressure over a body part (for example, an elastic pressure bandage applied over an arterial puncture site)
- immobilizing a body part (for example, an elastic bandage applied around a sprained ankle)
- supporting a wound (for example, an abdominal binder applied over a large abdominal incision and dressing)
- reducing or preventing oedema (for example, to reduce the effects of venous stasis which results in leg ulceration)
- securing a splint (for example, a bandage applied around hand splints for correction of deformities)
- securing dressings (for example, a retention bandage used to secure a dressing to a laceration on the ankle).

Bandages have been classified by Thomas (1991) according to their characteristics:

- **Nonextensible** bandages are now rarely used, due to their lack of conformability, which made them difficult to apply.
- **Extensible** bandages are the most common group and range from conforming cotton (such as Slinky™) to high

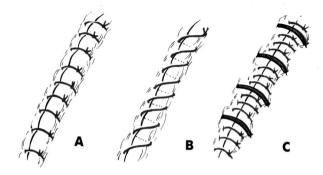

**Fig. 30-9** Examples of suturing methods. **A,** Intermittent. **B,** Continuous. **C,** Retention.

compression (such as Setopress™) and are used to promote venous return. Crepe bandages also fall into this category, although any pressure they apply is drastically reduced within 20 minutes of application.

- **Adhesive** bandages were previously used to apply compression; for example, to support fractured ribs. An example of an adhesive bandage would be Elastoplast™.
- Some **tubular** bandages, such as Tubigrip™, apply gentle support. Others, such as Surginet™, are fixing bandages to hold dressings in place.
- **Medicated** bandages or **paste** bandages have been used to treat leg ulceration for many years. However, they provide little support, do not provide venous return, and can promote skin sensitivity.

## PRINCIPLES FOR APPLYING BANDAGES

Correctly applied bandages do not cause injury to underlying and nearby body parts or create discomfort for the patient/client (Procedure 30-1). Before a bandage is applied, the nurse's responsibilities include the following:

- inspecting the skin for abrasions, oedema, discolouration, or exposed wound edges
- covering exposed wounds or open abrasions with a sterile dressing
- assessing the condition of underlying dressings and changing them if soiled
- assessing the skin of underlying body parts and parts that will be distal to the bandage for signs of circulatory impairment (coolness, pallor or cyanosis, diminished or absent pulses, swelling, numbness, and tingling) to provide a means for comparing changes in circulation after bandage application
- if a bandage is to be used on a leg that is ulcerative the cause of that pathology must be assessed. Before compression is applied measurement of Doppler pressure (usually done by a doctor) is essential. This involves measuring the blood pressure in the patient's/client's arm and leg to establish that circulatory supply to the leg is adequate to support compression without skin damage.

After a bandage is applied, assess, document, and immediately report changes in circulation, skin integrity, comfort level, and body function such as movement. Loosen or readjust the bandage as necessary.

## Nutritional Status

Maintaining adequate protein intake and haemoglobin levels are important in treatment of all wounds. Clients with a potential for, or decreased serum albumin levels, or poor protein intake need a nutritional evaluation to ensure proper caloric intake (Maklebust, 1991a). A person can lose as much as 50 g of protein per day from

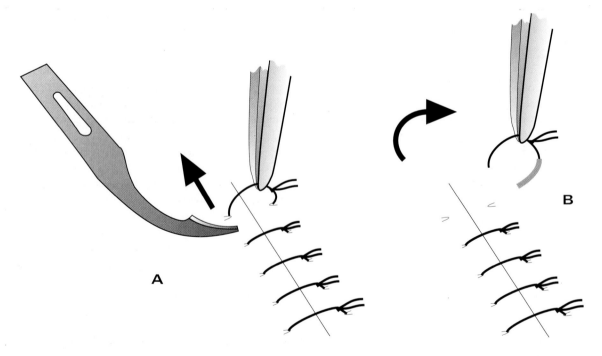

**Fig. 30-10** Removal of intermittent suture. **A,** Cut the suture as close to the skin as possible, away from the knot. **B,** Remove the suture. Never pull the contaminated stitch through tissues.

## PROCEDURE 30-1 Applying a Compression Bandage to the Lower Leg

| SEQUENCE OF ACTIONS | RATIONALE |
|---|---|
| 1. Inspect skin for alterations in integrity as indicated by abrasions, discolouration, chafing, or oedema. (Look carefully at bony prominences, e.g. malleoli.) | Altered skin integrity contraindicates the use of compression bandage. Pressure drainage most commonly occurs on the shins and ankles. |
| 2. Observe adequacy of circulation by noting surface temperature, skin colour, state of toenails, and sensation of body parts to be wrapped. | Comparison of area before and after application of bandage is necessary to ensure continued adequate circulation. Impairment of circulation may result in coolness to touch when compared with opposite side of body, cyanosis or pallor of skin, diminished or absent pulses, oedema or localized pooling, and numbness or tingling of body parts. |
| 3. Review medical record for specific orders related to application of elastic bandage. Note area to be covered, type of bandage required, frequency of change, and previous response to treatment. Note any Doppler pressure readings. | Specific prescription may direct procedure, including duration of treatment. Doppler readings should indicate a higher blood pressure in the lower limbs than the arms. Compression should not be applied if a lower pressure is found. |
| 4. Obtain necessary equipment and supplies (determine if present bandage will be reused or replacement be obtained): | |
|   a. Correct widths and number of bandages. | Increasingly wider bandages are used (e.g. 7.5-, 10-, and 15-cm bandages may be used to cover foot, calf, thigh) as circumferences increase. Manufacturers will indicate the subcutaneous pressure for each bandage size and type. |
|   b. Orthopaedic wool padding. | Wool padding protects bony prominences from excess pressure. |
|   c. Safety pins, tape. | Secures bandage in place. |
| 5. Explain procedure to patient/client. Reinforce teaching that smooth, even, light pressure will be applied to improve venous circulation and promote healing of venous leg ulcers. | Promotes cooperation and reduces anxiety. Improves knowledge level regarding need for compression bandages. |
| 6. Wash hands. | Reduces transmission of infection. |
| 7. Close room door or curtains. Assist patient/client to assume comfortable, anatomically correct position. | Maintains comfort and dignity. Maintains alignment. Prevents musculoskeletal deformity. |
| 8. Hold roll of elastic bandage in dominant hand and use other hand to lightly hold beginning of bandage at distal body part. Continue transferring roll to dominant hand as bandage is wrapped. | Maintains appropriate and consistent bandage tension. Manufacturers will state correct amount of bandage extension (e.g. 50%) required, or overlap (usually 50%) and method of application (usually spiral). |
| 9. Apply bandage evenly from toes to knees | Bandage is applied in manner that conforms evenly to body part and promotes venous return. |
| 10. Unroll and very slightly stretch bandage. Overlap turns. | Maintains uniform bandage tension. Prevents uneven bandage tension and circulatory impairment. |
| 11. Secure first bandage before applying additional rolls. | Prevents wrinkling or loose ends. |
| 12. Wash hands. | Reduces transmission of microorganisms. |
| 13. Evaluate distal circulation as application is completed and at least twice during 8-hr period (note colour, warmth, pulses, and numbness). | Early detection of circulatory difficulties ensures healthy neuromuscular status. |
| 14. Record bandage application and patient's/client's response in nurses' notes. | Documents procedures and ensures continuity of care. |
| 15. If the bandage is applied to a community client, supply client with a contact number in case pain develops. | Pain can indicate pressure damage and the client will require treatment review. |

an open, weeping pressure ulcer. This is a sizeable amount of the daily recommended requirement of 60 g for women and 70 g for men (Kavchak-Keyes, 1977).

Increased protein intake, 2 to 4 times above the daily recommended requirement, helps rebuild epidermal tissue. Increased caloric intake, at least 1.5 times the recommended amount, helps replace subcutaneous tissue. Increased intake of vitamin C promotes protein synthesis and tissue repair (Shekleton and Litwack, 1991; Kavchak-Keyes, 1977).

A low haemoglobin level decreases delivery of oxygen to the tissues and leads to further ischaemia. When possible, haemoglobin should be maintained at 12 g/100 ml.

 **EVALUATION**

Evaluate wound healing on an ongoing basis; for example, during dressing changes, when therapies are administered, and as a patient/client attempts to perform self-care in the presence of a nurse. Teach patients/clients and family members how to evaluate wound healing after discharge from a health care setting. For example, patients/clients should be told to notify the GP or community nurse if signs of infection develop.

Evaluate each intervention designed to promote wound healing, or to prevent or treat pressure ulcers, and compare the status of the wound with the assessment data. Review with the patient/client any teaching plans designed to enable him or her and their family to care for the wound. Modify the nursing care and teaching plans based on evaluation data. Also evaluate specific interventions designed to promote skin integrity and to teach the client and family to reduce future threats to skin integrity. Lastly, investigate the patient's/client's and family's need for additional support services (for example, home health care, physiotherapy, and counselling) and initiate the referral process.

## SUMMARY

The nurse delivers various forms of therapy to patients/clients with acute or chronic wounds. The type of wound determines the types of dressing used, their methods of application, the manner of caring for drains and sutures, and observations to make for monitoring wound repair. Patients/clients most at risk for impaired wound healing require close observation.

Principles to promote wound healing include use of aseptic technique, protection of the wound from further injury, and promotion of the stages of healing.

Pressure ulcers adversely affect the patient/client in all dimensions. Although in some cases immobilization is necessary to promote wound healing, proper skeletal alignment, or rest after an illness, it involves risks. Nursing care prevents the adverse effects of reduced mobility on skin integrity. Using the nursing process, assess the risk for pressure ulcers, determine actual or potential problems related to impaired skin integrity, and plan and deliver nursing care to meet the client's needs. Because of the cost, increased nursing time, and prolonged hospital stay to treat

pressure ulcers, nursing care aims first to prevent pressure ulcers and then to minimize the effects of pressure ulcers after they develop. As more people are cared for in the community, due to NHS reforms and a shift from acute to community care, it is increasingly important that nurses involve carers actively in pressure area care, prevention and management.

## CHAPTER 30 REVIEW
### Key Concepts

- In normal wound healing the epidermal skin layer resurfaces wounds, and the dermis restores the structural integrity and physical properties of the skin.
- Healing by primary intention proceeds through four stages: inflammation, destruction, proliferation, and maturation.
- Haemorrhaging often occurs during the destructive stage of wound healing.
- When there is extensive tissue loss, a wound heals by the slower process of secondary intention.
- The chances of wound infection are greater when the wound contains dead or necrotic tissue, when foreign bodies lie on or near the wound, and when blood supply and tissue defences are reduced.
- Any factor that lowers a patient's/client's immune response impairs wound healing.
- Alterations in mobility, sensory perception, level of consciousness, and nutrition; the use of casts; and the presence of severe infection or other debilitating diseases increase the risk for pressure ulcer development.
- External pressure, shearing force, moisture, impaired peripheral circulation, oedema, and obesity are also contributing factors to the development of pressure ulcers.
- Pressure ulcers increase length of stay in hospitals and extended care settings, as well as the overall cost of nursing care needed to manage the wound.
- Wound assessment requires a description of the appearance of the wound, palpation of the area, and information regarding character of drainage, drains and wound closures, and pain.
- Meticulous assessment of the skin and underlying tissue and identification of risk factors are important in decreasing the opportunity for pressure ulcer development.
- In addition to assessing the reactive hyperaemia, the nurse must also palpate adjacent tissue for signs of induration.
- Wound drains remove secretions within tissue layers to promote wound closure.
- Wounds should be cleaned from the least to most contaminated area.
- The type of suture securing a wound influences the method of suture removal. Correct removal is vital in the prevention of infection.
- Modern wound dressings create a moist environment which promotes wound healing and hastens epithelial migration.
- Decreased circulation to the tissues results in tissue hypoxia; if untreated, tissue necrosis results.
- Preventative skin care is aimed at controlling external pressure on bony prominences and keeping the skin clean,

well lubricated and hydrated, and free of excess moisture.

- Plastic-lined pads protect the bed, not the patient's/client's skin, because they do not remove moisture away from the individual's skin.
- Proper positioning should reduce the effects of pressure and guard against the shearing force.
- Therapeutic beds and mattresses reduce the effects of pressure; however, selection is based on assessment data to identify the best bed for individual needs.
- Nutritional interventions are directed at improving wound healing.

## CRITICAL THINKING EXERCISES

1. You are caring for a client with a spinal cord injury. What are your priorities for reducing the risk for pressure ulcers a) in a hospital setting and b) in the client's home.
2. While changing your patient's/client's dressing, you note a foul odour and observe serous yellow drainage from the suture line. What doctor's order would you anticipate?
3. You are working with an elderly, physically frail person who has Alzheimer's Disease. How would you perform an assessment on this person in order to obtain sufficient information regarding pressure ulcer risk?
4. List the characteristics of an ideal wound dressing.

### Key Terms

Acute wound, p. 618
Chronic wound, p. 618
Debridement, p. 633
Dehiscence, p. 624
Desquamation, p. 618
Epithelization, p. 620
Evisceration, p. 624
Exudate, p. 620
Granulating (wounds), p. 621
Haematoma, p. 624
Haemostasis, p. 620
Hyperaemia, p. 619
Inflammation (phase of healing), p. 620
Leg ulcer, p. 618
Necrotic (wounds), p. 618
Pressure ulcer, p. 619
Shearing force, p. 623
Sloughing, p. 618
Sutures, p. 635
Tissue ischaemia, p. 619

## REFERENCES

Allman *et al:* Pressure sores amongst hospitalised patients, *Ann Intern Med* 105(3):337, 1986.

Barbenel JC *et al:* Incidence of pressure sore in the greater Glasgow health board area, *Lancet* 2:548, 1977.

Barnes SH: Patient/family education for the patient with a pressure necrosis, *Nurs Clin North Am* 22:463, 1987.

Barrat E: Putting risk calculators in their place, *Nurs Times,* Feb. 19, 1987.

Bennett L, Lee BY: Vertical shear existence in animal pressure threshold experiments, *Decubitus* 1(1):18, 1988.

Berecek KH: Etiology of decubitus ulcers, *Nurs Clin North Am* 10:157, 1975.

Bergstrom N *et al:* The Braden Scale for predicting pressure sore risk, *Nur Res* 36:205, 1987a.

Bergstrom N, Demuth PJ, Braden, B: A clinical trial of the Braden Scale for predicting pressure sore risk, *Nurs Clin North Am* 22(2):417, 1987b.

Bliss MR: Medical implications of the sedentary posture, *Care Science Practice* 8(3):104, 1990.

Bliss MR, Thomas J: Clinical trials with budgetary implications, *Prof Nurs* 8(5):292, 1992.

Bryant RA *et al:* Pressure ulcer. In Bryant RA, editor: *Acute and chronic wounds: nursing management,* St Louis, 1992, Mosby.

Chrnitz H *et al:* Need for surgical wound dressings, *BJS* 76:204, 1989.

Clark M, Farrar S: *Comparisons of pressure sore risk assessment calculators,* London, 1991, Macmillan.

Cooper DM: Acute surgical wounds. In Bryant RA (editor): *Acute and chronic wounds: nursing management,* St Louis, 1992, Mosby.

Cornwall J, Dore CJ, Lewis JD: Leg ulcers: epidemiology and aetiology, *Br J Surg* 73:693, 1986.

Dealey C: Risk assessment scores: a comparative study of Norton and Waterlow, *Care Science Practice* 7(1):5, 1989.

Department of Health: *Your guide to pressure sores.* London, 1994, HMSO.

Fowler E: Pressure sores: a deadly nuisance, *J Gerontol Nurs* 12:6809, 1982.

Gosnell DJ: An assessment tool to identify pressure sores, *Nurs Res* 22(1):55 1973.

Gröer MW, Shekleton ME: *Basic pathophysiology: a conceptual approach,* ed 3, St Louis, 1989, Mosby.

Guralnik JM et al: Occurrence and prediction of pressure sores in the national health and nutritional survey, *J Am Geriatr Soc* 36:807, 1988.

Hanan K, Scheele L: Albumin vs. weight as a predictor of nutritional status and pressure ulcer development, *Ostomy/Wound Manage* 33:22, 1991.

Haury B, Debridement; an essential component of traumatic wound care in wound healing. In Hunt TK (editor): *Wound healing.* New York, 1989, Appleton Century Crofts.

Hibbs P: *City and Hackney pressure sore prevention policy,* ed 1, London , 1988, City and Hackney Provider Unit.

Hoff J: Effecting a change in nursing practice: pressure ulcer prevention, *J Nurs Qual Assur* 3(4):56, 1989.

Kavchak-Keyes MA: Four proven steps for preventing decubitus ulcers, *Nurs 77* 7:58, 1977.

Knight AL: Medical management of pressure sores, *J Fam Pract* 27(1):95, 1988.

Laing W: *Chronic venous diseases of the leg.* London, 1992, Office of Health Economics.

Lamid S, Ghatit AZ: Smoking, spacticity and pressure sores in spinal cord injured patients, *Am J Psysical Med* 62:300, 1983.

Lock PM: The effect of temperature on mitotic activity at the edge of experimental wounds. In Lundgren A, Soner A: Symposium of wound healing, *Plast Surg Dermatol Aspects,* Sweden, 1980, Molndal.

Maklebust J: Impact of AHCPR pressure ulcer guidelines on nursing practice, *Decubitus* 4(2):46, 1991a.

Maklebust J: Pressure ulcer update, *RN* 41(12):56, 1991b.

Maklebust J: Pressure ulcers: etiology and intervention, *Nurs Clin North Am* 22(2):359, 1987.

Mawson A *et al:* A literature review: Enhancing host resistance to pressure ulcer formation — a new approach to prevention, *Preventative Med* 22:433, 1993.

McLaren SMG: Nutrition and wound healing, *J Wound Care* 1(3):45, 1992.

Moffatt CJ *et al*: Community clinics for leg ulcers and impact on healing, *BMJ* 305:1389, 1992.

Morgan D: *Formulary of wound management products: a guide for health care staff* (ed 5), Chichester, 1992, Media Medica Publications Ltd.

Morison M: *A colour guide to the nursing management of wounds*. London, 1992, Mosby-Wolfe.

Morison M, Moffatt C: *A colour guide to the assessment and management of leg ulcers* ed 2. London, 1994, Mosby.

Myers J: Modern plastic surgical dressing, *J Health Soc Serv* 18 March:336, 1982.

National Pressure Ulcer Advisory Panel (NPUAP): Pressure ulcers: incidence, economics, risk assessment. Consensus Development Conference Statement, *Decubitus* 2(2):24, 1989.

National Pressure Ulcer Advisory Panel (NPUAP): Pressure ulcers, incidence, economics, risk assessment, Consensus Development Conference Statement, *Decubitis* 2(2):24, 1989.

Natlow AB: Nutrition in prevention and treatment of decubitus ulcers, *Top Clin Nurs* 5(2):39, 1983.

NHS 1992

Norton D, McLaren R, Exton-Smith AN: *An investigation of geriatric nursing problems in a hospital*, London, 1962, National Corporation for the Care of Old People.

Pajk M *et al*: Investigating the problem of pressure sores, *J Gerontol Nurs* 12(7):11, 1986.

Pinchcofsky-Devin GD, Kaminski MV: Correlation of pressure sores and nutritional status, *J Am Geriatr Soc* 34:435, 1989.

Pinchcofsky-Devin GD: *Proceedings of the third European conference in wound management*. London, 1993, Macmillan.

Pires M, Muller A: Detection and management of early tissue pressure indicators: a pictorial essay, *Progressions* 3(3):3, 1991.

Price B: *Body image: nursing concepts and care*. New York, 1990, Prentice Hall.

Reuler JB, Cooney TG: The pressure sore: pathophysiology and principles of management, *Ann Int Med* 94(5):661, 1981.

Shekleton ME, Litwack K: *Critical care nursing of the surgical patient*, Philadelphia, 1991, Saunders.

St Claire M: Survey of use of Pegasus airwave mattress, *J Tissue Viability* 2(1):9, 1992.

Stotts NA: Predicting pressure ulcer development in surgical patients, *Heart Lung* 17(6):641, 1988.

Thomas S: Evidence fails to justify the use of hypochlorites, *J Tissue Viability* 1(1), 1991.

US Department of Health and Human Services Agency for Health Care Policy & Research: *Pressure ulcers in adults, prediction and prevention*, Roshville, Maryland, 1992, USDHHS.

Versluysen M: Pressure sores in elderly patients: the epidemiology related to hip operations, *J Bone Joint Surg* 67(1):10, 1985.

Versluysen M: Elderly patients with femoral fractures develop pressure sores whilst in hospital, *BMJ* 292, 1986.

Waterlow J: A risk assessment card, *Nurs Times* 81(29):45, 1985.

West P, Priestley J: Money under the mattress, *Health Serv J* 14 April:20, 1994.

Westaby S: *Wound care*, St Loius, 1986, Mosby.

Winter GD: Formation of scab and the rate of epithelialisation in the wounds of a young domestic pig, *Nature* 193:293 1962.

Wood R: Disintegration of cellulose dressings in open granulating wounds, *BMJ* 1:1444, 1976.

## FURTHER READING

### Adult Nursing

Bale S, Harding KG: Using modern dressings to effect debridement, *Prof Nurs* 5:244, 1990.

Department of Health: *Your guide to pressure sores*, London, 1994, HMSO.

Hess CT, Miller P: The management of open wounds: acute and chronic, *Ostomy/Wound Manage* 31:58, 1990.

Hunt TK: Basic principles of wound healing, *J Trauma* 30:S122, 1990.

Jones PL, Millman A: Wound healing and the aged patient, *Nurs Clin North Am*, 25:263, 1990.

Kloth LC, McCulloch JM, Feedar JA, editors: *Wound healing: alternatives in management*, Philadelphia, 1990, Davis.

LaVan FB, Hunt TK: Oxygen and wound healing, *Clin Plast Surg* 17:463, 1990.

Nightengale K: Making sense of wound closure, *Nurs Times* 86:35, 1990.

North A: The effect of sleep on wound healing, *Ostomy/Wound Manage* 27:56, 1990.

Pinchcofsky DG: Why won't this wound heal? *Ostomy/Wound Manage* 27:56, 1990.

Rosenberg CS: Wound healing in the patient with diabetes mellitus, *Nurs Clin North Am* 25:247, 1990.

Thomas AC, Wysocki AB: The healing wound: a comparison of three clinically useful methods of measurement, *Decubitus* 3:18, 1990.

Turner V: Standardization of wound care, *Nurs Stand* 5:25, 1991.

Young J, Cotter D: Pressure sores — do mattresses work? *Lancet* 336:183, 1990.

### Children's Nursing

Bale S *et al*: Wound management in children, Paediatric Nursing 6(1) Feb p12-14. 1994.

Garvin G: *Wound healing in pediatrics*, Nursing Clinics of North America 25(1) Mar p181-192. 1990.

Turril S: Supported positioning in intensive care, *Paed Nurs* 4(4), 1992.

Wong D: *Nursing care of infants and children* ed 5 St Louis, 1995, Mosby.

# Administering Medicines

## CHAPTER OUTLINE

## LEARNING OUTCOMES

After studying this chapter, you should be able to:

■ *Define the key terms listed.*
■ *Differentiate between the clinical, generic, official and trade names of drugs.*
■ *Discuss the nurse's legal responsibilities in drug prescription and administration.*
■ *Describe the physiological mechanisms of drug action, including absorption, distribution, metabolism, and excretion.*
■ *Differentiate between toxic, idiosyncratic, allergic, and side effects of drugs.*
■ *Discuss factors that influence drug pharmacokinetics and factors that influence drug actions.*
■ *Describe the different routes of administration available and*

*factors to consider in choosing the correct method.*
■ *Correctly calculate a prescribed drug dosage.*
■ *List four common types of drug order, and describe the roles of the pharmacist, doctor, and nurse in drug administration.*
■ *Assess the patient's/client's response to drug therapy, ensuring that safe administration techniques are used.*
■ *List and discuss the 'five rights' of drug administration.*
■ *Discuss methods of educating a patient/client about medications.*
■ *Describe special considerations for patients clients from different developmental age groups.*
■ *Correctly prepare and administer (under supervision) subcutaneous, intramuscular and oral medicines; topical skin preparations; eye, ear, and nose drops; vaginal instillations; rectal suppositories; and inhalants.*

**S**afe and accurate administration of medications is one of the nurse's important responsibilities. Drugs may be a primary means of therapy for patients/clients with health problems, but any drug can cause harmful effects when administered incorrectly. The nurse is responsible for understanding a drug's action and its side effects, administering it correctly, monitoring the patient's/client's response, and helping the patient/client to self-administer drugs correctly and knowledgeably.

In addition to knowing about a specific drug's action, the nurse must also understand the patient's/client's previous and current health problems to ascertain whether a particular medication is safe to give. The nurse's judgement is critical for proper and safe drug administration.

## DRUG NOMENCLATURE AND FORMS

A drug is a substance used in the diagnosis, treatment, cure, relief, or prevention of disease.

### Names

A single medication may have as many as four different names. See Table 31-1 for a description of these names. As you will encounter drugs under a variety of different names, it is extremely important to obtain the exact name and spelling for a particular drug.

### Classification

Drugs with similar characteristics are categorized by **functional class**. This classification indicates the effect on a body system, the symptoms relieved, or the desired effect. Each class contains drugs prescribed for similar types of health problems. The physical and chemical composition of drugs within a class is not necessarily the same. A drug may also belong to more than one functional class. For example, aspirin is an analgesic, an antipyretic, and an anti-inflammatory drug.

Nurses should know the general characteristics of drugs in each class. Each class has nursing implications for proper administration and monitoring. Nursing implications for all drugs within a class provide guidelines for safe and effective care.

### Drug Forms

Drugs are available in a variety of forms or preparations. The form of the drug determines its route of administration. For example, a capsule is usually taken orally, and a solution may be given intravenously. The composition of a drug is designed to enhance its absorption and metabolism within the body. Many drugs are available in several forms such as tablets, capsules, elixirs, and suppositories. When administering a medication, you must be certain to give it in the proper form (Table 31-2).

## DRUG LEGISLATION AND STANDARDS

### Legislation and Control

Legislation of medicines has developed in a piecemeal fashion throughout the years, often in response to specific problems. There were no restrictions in the UK on the sale of drugs or poisons until the middle of the nineteenth century. The first controls were established in 1851 for the sale of arsenic. The following year, regulations were established to regulate pharmacists, and later legislation developed to control poisons. The rapid development of medicines during the Second World War highlighted the need for new controls over medicines. As a result, the Medicines Act 1968 was developed to replace all previous legislation relating to medicines. The Poisons Act 1972 deals with nonmedicinal poisons and the Misuse of Drugs Act 1971 deals with the misuse of amphetamines and other psychotropic drugs. Recently, the manufacture and distribution of medicines and recognition of pharmaceutical qualifications in the UK have been influenced by EC legislation.

The Medicines Act 1968 regulates the manufacture, distribution and importation of medicines for human use (as well as medicines for animals). The Medicines Control Agency of the Department of Health controls the licensing system according to these regulations and the Medicines Inspectorate enforces the regulations. Health care institutions establish policies that conform to legislation, and local regulations. The size of an institution, the types of services it

---

### Table 31-1 Medication Names, Using Aspirin as an Example

| Name | Description | Example |
|------|-------------|---------|
| Chemical name | Provides an exact description of the drug's composition. | acetylsalicylic acid |
| Generic name | Given by the manufacturer who first develops the drug before it receives official approval. | aspirin |
| Official name | The name under which the drug is listed in official publications such as the *British National Formulary*. A drug's generic name often becomes its official name. | aspirin |
| Trade name, brand name, or proprietary name | The name under which a manufacturer markets a drug. A generic drug may have many different trade names. The trade name has the symbol ® at the upper right of the name, indicating that the drug has been registered. Manufacturers try to choose trade names that are easier to pronounce and spell to help the lay person recognize and remember the medications more readily. Since many companies may produce the same drug, similarities in trade names can be confusing. | Disprin® |

## TABLE 31-2 Forms of Medication

| Form | Description |
|------|-------------|
| Capsule | Solid dosage form for oral use; medication in powder, liquid, or oil form and encased by gelatine shell; capsule coloured to aid in product identification. |
| Elixir | Clear fluid containing water and/or alcohol; designed for oral use. |
| Enteric-coated tablet | Tablet for oral use coated with materials that do not dissolve in stomach; coatings dissolve in intestine, where medication is absorbed. |
| Extract | Concentrated drug form made by removing active portion of drug from its other components (e.g. fluid extract is drug made into solution from vegetable source). |
| Liniment | Preparation usually containing alcohol, oil, or soapy emollient that is applied to the skin. |
| Lotion | Drug in liquid suspension applied externally to protect skin. |
| Lozenge | Flat, round dosage form containing drug, flavouring, sugar, and mucilage; dissolves in mouth to release drug. |
| Ointment | Semisolid, externally applied preparation, usually containing one or more drugs. |
| Paste | Semisolid preparation, thicker and stiffer than ointment; absorbed through skin more slowly than ointment. |
| Solution | Liquid preparation that may be used orally, parenterally, or externally; can also be instilled into body organ or cavity (e.g. bladder irrigations); contains water with one or more dissolved compounds; must be sterile for parenteral use. |
| Suppository | Solid dosage form mixed with gelatine and shaped in form of pellet for insertion into body cavity (rectum or vagina); melts when it reaches body temperature, releasing drug for absorption. |
| Suspension | Finely divided particles dispersed in liquid medium; when suspension is left standing, particles settle to bottom of container; commonly oral medication and not given intravenously. |
| Syrup | Medication dissolved in concentrated sugar solution; may contain flavouring to make drug more palatable. |
| Tablet | Powdered dosage form compressed into hard disks or cylinders; in addition to primary drug, contains binders (adhesive to allow powder to stick together), disintegraters (to promote tablet dissolution), lubricants (for ease of manufacturing), and fillers (for convenient tablet size). |
| Transdermal patch | Medication contained within semipermeable patch, which allows medications to be absorbed through skin slowly over long period. |
| Tincture | Alcohol or water–alcohol drug solution. |

provides, and the types of professional personnel it employs influence policies for drug control, distribution, and administration. Institutional policies are often more restrictive than government controls. Legislation and local policy governs nursing practice, including the administration of medicines. In addition, standards for nurses regarding the administration of medicines are published by the UKCC in *Standards for the Administration of Medicines*, 1992.

Doctors and dentists prescribe the majority of drugs in the UK. However, limited prescribing for community nurses who hold recognized community health care qualifications (currently DN and HV) is on the statute book, with the legislation permitting nurse prescribing receiving Royal Assent in March, 1992. The main purposes behind this plan are to help elderly and chronically ill people to obtain dressings, lotions and creams they need without visiting their GP, and eventually to save health care costs.

Nurses must know the regulations affecting drug administration in their practice areas. When moving from one hospital or area to another, nurses may discover significant differences in the policies governing drug administration. For example, policies vary concerning the prescription and administration of intravenous (IV) drugs and single nurse administration.

The nurse is responsible for following legal provisions when administering a **controlled drug**. This is a prescrption drug which is subject to specific prescribing, dispensing and storage requirements under the Misuse of Drugs Act 1971. The purpose of these requirements is to monitor the usage of such drugs in order to prevent drug dependence or misuse. Hospitals and other health care institutions have policies for the ordering, correct storage and distribution of controlled drugs (including checking stock levels).

## Drug Standards

Standards for drug strength, quality, purity, packaging, safety, labelling, and dosage form are published in the *European Pharmacopoeia* and in the *British Pharmacopoeia*. The standards set in the *European Pharmacopoeia* take precedence over standards in other publications. Doctors, nurses, and pharmacists depend on these standards to ensure that patients/clients receive pure drugs in safe and effective dosages. Accepted standards must be met in the following areas:

- purity — manufacturers must meet purity standards for the type and concentration of substances allowed in drug products
- potency — the concentration of active drug in the preparation affects strength or potency
- bioavailability — the ability of a drug to be released from its dosage form and dissolved, absorbed, and transported by the body to its site of action is its **bioavailability**
- efficacy — detailed laboratory studies can help determine a drug's effectiveness
- safety — all drugs should be continually evaluated to determine their side effects.

Other publications, such as the *Monthly Index of Medical Specialties* (MIMS) and the *British National Formulary* (BNF) publish complete information about most drugs currently available in the United Kingdom.

## Nontherapeutic Drug Use

Despite legislative controls, some people use drugs for purposes other than their proper purpose. Nontherapeutic drug use poses serious health problems for the user, family, and community. In the past, the misuse or **abuse of drugs** was related to use for therapeutic qualities, such as the relief of pain or reduction in anxiety. Today, factors such as peer pressure, curiosity, and the pursuit of pleasure are motivators for drug use. Problems with drug use are not limited to heroin, cocaine, and other 'hard' drugs. Our society is drug conscious, as shown by the frequent advertisements for pain relievers, decongestants, and antacids on television.

Nurses have ethical and legal responsibilities to understand the problems of people using drugs improperly. When caring for patients/clients with suspected drug misuse or drug dependence, nurses must be aware of their own values and attitudes about the use of potentially harmful substances.

A problem involving the misuse of drugs by health professionals also exists. Stress in the work place, personal problems, and the strong desire to perform well are some of the factors that may cause nurses to rely on drugs. Misuse of drugs by a nurse contravenes the UKCC Code of Professional Conduct.

### Mother and Child Nursing
### Supply and administration of medicines

Under the Medicines Act 1968, certain classes of people are exempt from the conditions or restrictions on the retail sale and/or supply of medicines on the general sale list, pharmacy medicines, and prescription only medicines. According to the Act, registered midwives may administer parenterally (in the course of professional practice) certain Prescription Only Medicines that contain a specific list of substances (see Medicines Act 1968, SI 1983 No. 1212). Midwives may also administer two local anaesthetics (lignocaine and lignocaine hydrochloride) and the antipsychotic drug, promazine hydrochloride, while attending a woman in childbirth. Midwives may also supply any medicinal product that is not a prescription only medicine.

Adapted from: Appelbe G, Wingfield J: *Dale and Appelbe's Pharmacy Law and Ethics*, ed 5, London, 1993, The Pharmaceutical Press.

## NATURE OF DRUG ACTIONS

Drugs act to produce therapeutically useful effects. A drug does not create a function in a tissue or organ but rather alters physiological functions. Drugs may protect cells from the influence of other chemical agents, promote cell function, or accelerate or slow cell processes. A drug may replace a substance that is missing; for example, insulin, thyroxine, or oestrogen.

### Mechanisms of Action

Drugs produce actions by:

- altering body fluids — for example, the drug aluminium hydroxide gel exerts its effect by altering the chemical properties of a body fluid (specifically, neutralizing the stomach's acid contents).
- altering cell membranes — for example, drugs such as general anaesthetic gases interact with cell membranes. After properties of the cells become altered, the drug exerts its effects.
- interacting with cell receptor sites — this is the most common mechanism of drug action. Receptors localize drug effects. Sites on the receptors interact with drugs because of similar chemical shapes. The drug and receptor bind together like a lock-and-key fit. When receptors and drugs lock together, the therapeutic effects are realized.

### Pharmacokinetics

**Pharmacokinetics** is the study of how drugs enter the body, reach their site of action, are metabolized, and exit the body. The doctor and nurse use the knowledge of pharmacokinetics when timing drug administration, selecting the route of administration, judging the risk for alterations in drug action, and observing the patient/client response. The pharmacokinetics of individual drugs are described in the manufacturer's literature as well as in publications, such as *MIMS* and the *BNF*.

## Absorption

**Absorption** is the passage of drug molecules into the blood. Most drugs, except those applied topically for local effects, must enter the systemic circulation to exert therapeutic effect. Factors influencing absorption include route of administration, ability of the drug to dissolve, and conditions at the site of absorption.

Each route has a different influence on drug absorption, depending on the physical structure of the tissues. The skin is relatively impermeable to chemicals, making absorption slow. The mucous membranes and respiratory airways allow quick drug absorption because of the high vascularity of mucosal and alveolar-capillary surfaces. Because orally administered drugs must pass through the gastrointestinal tract to be absorbed, the overall rate of absorption may be slowed. Intravenous injection produces the most rapid absorption because this route provides immediate access to the systemic circulation.

The ability of an oral medication to dissolve after ingestion depends largely on its form or preparation. Solutions and suspensions already in a liquid state are absorbed more readily than tablets or capsules. Solid dosage forms must first disintegrate to expose the chemical to gastric and intestinal secretions. Acidic drugs pass through the gastric mucosa rapidly. Drugs that are basic are not absorbed before reaching the small intestine.

Conditions at the site of absorption influence the ease with which medications enter the systemic circulation. Topical substances normally prescribed for local effect can cause serious reactions when absorbed through the skin's layers. The formation of oedema in mucous membranes slows drug absorption because drugs take longer to diffuse to blood vessels. The absorption of parenterally administered medications depends on the blood supply of the tissues. Before administering a drug by injection,

assess the patient/client for local factors, such as oedema, bruising, or scarring, which might impair the absorption of the medication. Since muscles have a richer blood supply than subcutaneous tissues, a drug given intramuscularly (IM) is absorbed more quickly than one injected subcutaneously (SC). In some instances a delayed subcutaneous absorption is preferable as it produces longer-lasting drug effects. If an individual's tissue perfusion is poor, as in the case of circulatory shock, the intravenous route is more effective. Intravenous (IV) administration provides the most rapid and dependable absorption (Fig. 31-1).

Oral drugs are absorbed more easily when administered between meals. When the stomach is filled with food, the contents are emptied slowly into the duodenum, thus slowing drug absorption. Certain foods and antacids cause drugs to bind into complexes that cannot pass through the gastrointestinal tract lining. For example, milk interferes with the absorption of iron and tetracycline. Some drugs are destroyed by the increased acidity of gastric contents and protein digestion during a meal. Enteric coatings on certain tablets resist dissolution in gastric juices and prevent certain medications from being digested in the upper gastrointestinal tract. The coating also protects the stomach lining from irritation by the medication.

The route of drug administration is prescribed by the doctor. Nurses may need to request a medication be given by an

**Children's Nursing
Administering medications to neonates**

Drugs are usually administered via the intravenous route in neonates because their rate of absorption via the oral route is very erratic. The rectal route of administration is rarely used because of its fast absorption rate.

alternative route or in a different form, based on physical assessments of the patient/client. For example, an individual may not be able to swallow tablets; therefore the nurse would request the medication as an elixir or syrup. Knowledge of factors that alter or impair drug absorption helps the nurse administer drugs correctly. It is important to be aware of the nursing implications for each medication given. For example, drugs such as aspirin, iron, and phenytoin sodium irritate the gastrointestinal tract and should be administered with or immediately after a meal. However, food may interfere with the absorption of drugs such as cloxacillin and penicillin; therefore they should be given 1 to 2 hours before meals or 2 to 3 hours afterwards.

## Distribution

After a drug is absorbed, it is distributed within the body to tissues and organs and ultimately to its specific site of action. The rate and extent of distribution depend on the physical and chemical properties of the drug and the physiological make-up of the person taking the drug.

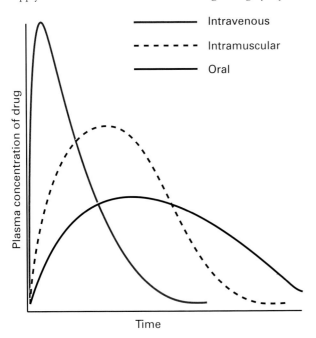

Fig. 31-1 The effect of the route of administration of a drug on the plasma concentration. Redrawn from Trounce JR: *Clinical pharmacology for nurses*, ed 9, Edinburgh, 1981, Churchill Livingstone.

**Children's Nursing**
**Considerations when**
**administering drugs to children**

Children require very careful prescriptions and nurses need to be extremely vigilant for the effects and side effects of medication on children. A brief overview of the reasons includes: smaller body weight; children are generally more sensitive; renal tubules are smaller, indicating a prolonged glomerular filtration rate and tubular absorption; and the liver is inadequate in detoxifying drugs.

## BODY SIZE

A direct relationship exists between the amount of drug administered and the amount of body tissue in which it is distributed. Most medications are distributed to body fat or water (Simonson, 1984). An increase in the percentage of body fat may cause a longer duration of drug action because of slower distribution throughout the body. In an obese patient/client a lower concentration accumulates in the body tissues, thus reducing the targets for drug action. The older adult experiences a change in fat/protein/tissue ratio and height, and often requires a lower drug dosage than a younger person.

## CIRCULATORY DYNAMICS

Drugs pass more easily from interstitial to intravascular spaces than between body compartments. Blood vessels are permeable to most dissolved substances unless drug particles are large or bound to serum proteins. The **concentration** of a drug at a specific site depends on the number of blood vessels in tissues, the degree of local vasodilatation or vasoconstriction, and the rate of blood flow to a tissue site. Exercise, warming, and chilling alter local circulation. For example, if an individual applies a warm compress to an intramuscular injection site, the resultant vasodilatation increases drug distribution.

## PROTEIN BINDING

The degree to which drugs **bind** to the protein albumin in the bloodstream affects drug distribution. Most medications bind to this protein to some extent. When drug molecules are bound to albumin, they cannot exert any pharmacological activity. **Unbound** or 'free' drug is the active form of the drug. Older adults have a decreased albumin level in the bloodstream, probably caused by a change in liver function. The same is true for individuals with liver disease or malnutrition. Because of this, older adults may be at risk for an increase in drug activity, toxicity, or both.

### Metabolism

After a drug reaches its site of action, it is metabolized into an inactive form that is more easily excreted. This **biotransformation** occurs under the influence of enzymes that detoxify, degrade (break down), and remove biologically active chemicals. Most biotransformation occurs within the liver, although the lungs, kidneys, blood, and intestines also metabolize drugs.

The liver is especially important because its specialized structure oxidizes and transforms many toxic substances. The liver degrades many harmful chemicals before they are distributed to the tissues. The decrease in liver function that occurs with ageing or with liver disease influences the rate at which a drug is eliminated from the body. The resultant slowing of metabolism causes the drug to accumulate in the body. Thus, a patient/client would be at greater risk for drug toxicity. If any of the organs that participate in drug metabolism are altered, a patient/client is at risk for drug toxicity.

### Excretion

After drugs are metabolized, they exit the body through the kidneys, liver, bowel, lungs, and exocrine glands. The chemical make-up of a drug determines the organ of excretion. Gaseous and volatile compounds such as ether, nitrous oxide, and alcohol exit through the lungs. Deep breathing and coughing help the postoperative patient/client eliminate anaesthetic gases more rapidly.

The exocrine glands excrete lipid-soluble medications. When drugs exit through sweat glands, the skin may become irritated. If a drug exits through the mammary glands, a breast-fed baby may absorb the chemicals. Nurses should be aware of a drug's contraindications for breast-feeding or pregnant patients/clients, and should advise these individuals accordingly. The nurse must carefully consider the balance between the risk to the infant receiving the drug and the risk to the mother *not* taking the drug.

The gastrointestinal tract is another route for drug excretion. Many drugs enter the hepatic circulation to be broken down by the liver and excreted into the bile. After chemicals enter the intestines through the biliary tract, they may be reabsorbed by the intestines. Factors increasing peristalsis, such as laxatives and enemas, accelerate drug excretion through the faeces, whereas factors slowing peristalsis, such as inactivity and improper diet, may prolong a drug's effects.

The kidneys are the main organs for drug excretion. Some drugs escape extensive metabolism and exit relatively unchanged in the urine. Others undergo biotransformation in the liver before they are excreted by the kidney. If renal function declines, a common change in ageing, the risk for drug toxicity increases. If the kidneys cannot adequately excrete a drug, it may be necessary to reduce the dosage. Maintenance of a normal fluid intake promotes proper elimination of drugs.

### Types of Drug Actions

Because of its chemical make-up and physiological action, a drug may produce more than one effect.

### Therapeutic Effects

The **therapeutic effect** is the intended or predicted physiological response that a drug causes. Each drug has a desired or therapeutic effect for which it is prescribed; for example, codeine phosphate is administered to create analgesia. A single medication may have many therapeutic effects. For example, aspirin is an analgesic, antipyretic, and anti-inflammatory, and it reduces platelet aggregation (clumping) if the dose is reduced to 75 mg a day.

## Side Effects

Predictably a drug will cause unintended, secondary effects. These **side effects** may be harmless or injurious. For example, with codeine phosphate, a person may also experience constipation, and this side effect may be considered harmless. However, digoxin may cause cardiac dysrhythmias that could be lethal. If the side effects are serious enough to negate the beneficial effects of a drug's therapeutic action, the doctor may discontinue it. Patients/clients often stop taking drugs without consulting their doctors because of side effects.

## Toxic Effects

Generally, **toxic effects** develop after prolonged intake of high doses of medication, or after a drug accumulates in the blood because of impaired metabolism or excretion. *One* dose of medication can have toxic effects for some individuals. Excess amounts of a drug within the body may have lethal effects, depending on the drug's action. For example, morphine relieves pain by depressing the central nervous system. However, toxic levels of morphine cause severe respiratory depression and death.

## Allergic Reactions

An **allergic reaction** is an unpredictable response to a drug; allergic reactions compose 5 to 10% of all drug reactions. Exposure to an initial dose of a medication may cause an immunological response; the person has then been sensitized. With repeated administration the patient/client will also develop an allergic response to the drug, its chemical preservatives, or a metabolite. In this case the drug or chemical acts as an antigen, triggering the release of antibodies, and a faster and often more severe reaction.

A drug allergy may be mild or severe. Allergic symptoms vary, depending on the individual and the drug; for example, antibiotics cause many allergic reactions. Common allergy symptoms are summarized in Table 31-3. Severe or **anaphylactic reactions** are characterized by sudden constriction of bronchiolar muscles, oedema of the pharynx and larynx, and severe wheezing and shortness of breath. The person may also become severely hypotensive, necessitating emergency resuscitation. An individual with a known history of an allergy to a medication should wear an identification bracelet that alerts nurses and doctors to the allergy should the person be unconscious.

## Drug Tolerance

Some people have unusually low metabolisms in response to a drug. An increase in dosage may be required to cause a therapeutic effect. Patients/clients that are taking various drugs for pain may develop a tolerance over time. Frequently, patients/clients require increasing dosages of morphine over time to relieve pain.

## Drug Interaction

When one drug modifies the action of another, a **drug interaction** occurs. Drug interactions are common in individuals taking several medications. A drug may potentiate or diminish the action of other drugs and may alter the way in which another drug is absorbed, metabolized, or eliminated from the body.

When two drugs are given simultaneously, they can have a synergistic or addictive effect. With a **synergistic effect** the physiological action of the two drugs in combination is greater than the effect of the drugs when given separately. Alcohol is a central nervous system depressant that has a synergistic effect on antihistamines, antidepressants, and opioid analgesics.

## Drug Dose Responses

After the drug is administered, it undergoes absorption, distribution, metabolism, and excretion. Except when administered intravenously, drugs take time to enter the bloodstream. The quantity and distribution of a drug in different body compartments changes constantly.

When a medication is prescribed, the goal is to achieve a constant blood level within a safe therapeutic range. Repeated doses are required to achieve a **constant therapeutic concentration** of a medication because a portion of a drug is always being excreted. When absorption ceases, only metabolism, excretion, and distribution continue. The highest **plasma concentration** (peak concentration) of the drug usually occurs just before the last of the drug is absorbed. After peaking, the plasma concentration falls progressively. With intravenous drug infusions, the peak concentration occurs quickly, but the plasma level also begins to fall immediately.

All drugs have a **plasma half-life**, or the time it takes for excretion processes to lower the plasma concentration by half. To maintain a therapeutic level, the patient/client must receive regular, fixed doses or a continuous infusion. After an initial dose

### TABLE 31-3 Allergic Reactions

| Symptom | Description |
|---|---|
| Urticaria | Raised, irregularly sized and shaped skin eruptions with reddened margins and pale centres |
| Eczema (rash) | Small, raised vesicles that are usually reddened; often distributed over entire body |
| Pruritus | Itching of skin; accompanies most rashes |
| Rhinitis | Inflammation of mucous membranes lining nose; causes swelling and clear, watery discharge |

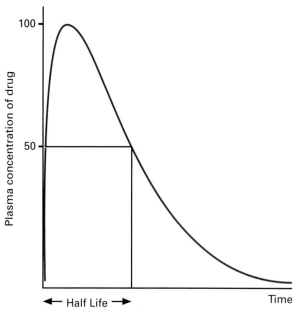

**Fig. 31-2** The plasma levels of a drug after a single intravenous injection. The plasma half-life of a drug is the time taken for the plasma concentration to drop by 50%. From Trounce JR: *Clinical pharmacology for nurses,* ed 9, Edinburgh, 1981, Churchill Livingstone.

the person receives each successive dose when the previous dose reaches its half-life (Fig. 31-2). In this way an almost constant therapeutic drug concentration is maintained.

Knowledge of the following time intervals of drug action also helps to anticipate a drug's effect:

1. Onset of drug action, or period of time it takes after a drug is administered for it to produce a response.
2. Peak action, time it takes for a drug to reach its highest effective concentration.
3. Duration of action, or length of time during which the drug is present in a concentration great enough to produce a response.
4. Plateau, blood serum concentration reached and maintained after repeated, fixed doses of the medication.

The ideal way to achieve a constant therapeutic drug level is continuous IV infusions, which eliminate the fluctuating effects of intermittent dosages.

## FACTORS INFLUENCING DRUG ACTION

Due to differences in the manner in which medications act and their types of action, responses to drugs vary considerably. Factors other than characteristics of the medication also influence its actions. A patient/client may not respond in the same way to each successive dose of a medication. Similarly, the same drug dosage may cause very different responses in different individuals. It is essential for nurses to monitor the effects.

### Genetic Differences
Genetic make-up affects the manner in which biotransformation of drugs occurs. Metabolic patterns are often similar within

families. Genetic factors determine whether naturally occurring enzymes are present to assist in medication degradation. As a result, members of a family may share a sensitivity to a drug.

### Physiological Variables
Hormonal differences between men and women alter the metabolism of certain drugs. Hormones and drugs compete with each other in biotransformation because they are degraded by the same metabolic processes. Diurnal variations in oestrogen secretion may be responsible for cyclic fluctuations in drug reactions experienced by women.

Age has a direct effect on drug action. Infants lack many of the enzymes necessary for normal drug metabolism. A number of physiological changes accompanying the ageing process influence the response to drug therapy (see box opposite).

If a person's nutritional status is poor, proper cell function for biotransformation cannot occur. Like all body functions, drug metabolism relies on adequate nutrition for enzyme and protein formation. Most drugs bind with proteins before being distributed to their sites of action.

Any disease state that impairs the function of organs responsible for normal pharmacokinetics also impairs drug action. Altered skin integrity, reduced gastrointestinal absorption or motility, and impaired renal or hepatic function are just some of the disease-related conditions that can reduce a drug's efficacy or place a person at risk for drug toxicity.

### Environmental Conditions
A patient's/client's exposure to severe physical and emotional stress triggers a hormonal response that eventually may interfere with drug metabolism. Ionizing radiation creates a similar effect by altering the rate of enzyme activity. Use of alcohol can also affect drug action.

Exposure to heat and cold can affect responses to drugs. Vasodilators are used to control the blood pressure of hypertensive patients/clients. In hot weather, it may be necessary to reduce vasodilator dosages because the temperature adds to the medication's effects. Cold weather tends to promote vasoconstriction, necessitating an increase in vasodilator dosage.

A reaction to a medication may vary, depending on the setting in which it is taken, and who administers the medication.

### Psychological Factors
A number of psychological factors influence the use of drugs and the response to them. A person's attitude about drugs may stem from early experiences or family influences.

The meaning or significance that a drug or taking a drug has for patients/clients influences the response to therapy. A drug may serve as a means for overcoming feelings of insecurity. In this situation, patients/clients depend on drugs as a means of coping with life. In contrast, if patients/clients resent their physical conditions, anger and hostility may result in adverse reactions to medications. Medications often provide a sense of security. The regular use of nonprescription medications, or **over-the-counter drugs**, such as vitamins, laxatives, and aspirin, gives many people a sense of control over their health. The colour and shape of

## Adult Nursing
### Influence of drug actions in older adults

| Physiological Change | Drug Action/Patient/Client Response | Nursing Interventions |
| --- | --- | --- |
| **GASTROINTESTINAL TRACT** | | |
| **Oral cavity**<br>Loss of elasticity in oral mucosa, which becomes dry and easily cracks. | Difficulty in swallowing tablets or capsules; sensitivity to drugs that cause dryness of mouth; susceptibility to gum disease and dental caries. | Rinse patient's/client's oral cavity frequently with tepid clear water or an antiseptic mouthwash. Brush teeth and gums gently. |
| **Oesophagus**<br>Delayed oesophageal clearance because of weakened contractions and failure of lower oesophageal sphincter to relax. | Difficulty in swallowing large tablets or capsules; tissue erosion caused by drugs such as aspirin and uncoated potassium chloride. | Position patient/client upright. Administer full glass of liquid with drug. Crush tablets and mix with food but do not empty capsules. Obtain elixirs. |
| **Stomach**<br>Decrease in gastric acidity and peristalsis. | Potentiation of irritating effects of highly acidic drugs (e.g. aspirin); alteration of solubility of certain drugs. | Have patient/client drink full glass of water/milk and take medication with food to reduce gastric irritation. |
| **Large intestine**<br>Reduced colon muscle tone; loss of defaecation reflex; decreased intestinal blood flow. | Slowing of drug excretion; overuse and abuse of laxatives by patient/client; delayed drug absorption. | Provide normal fluid intake. Instruct patient/client to eat bulk-forming foods and avoid use of constipating drugs. |
| **SKIN AND VASCULAR SYSTEM**<br>Reduced skin fold thickness in extremities (less body fat); reduced elasticity in skin and vascular system. | Fragile blood vessels; patient/client prone to bleeding after injection. | Apply pressure to injection sites after administration. Observe injection sites for bleeding. |
| **LIVER**<br>Reduced liver size; decrease in hepatic blood flow. | Longer biotransformation time; longer-than-normal duration of drug action; greater risk for drug sensitivity and toxicity. | Monitor for signs of liver impairment (jaundice, pruritus, dark urine). Question dosages for patients/clients. |
| **KIDNEYS**<br>Reduced glomerular filtration; decreased tubular function and renal blood flow. | Risk of drug accumulation and toxicity. | Prevent urinary retention (keep catheters free flowing and observe frequency of micturition). Monitor for signs of renal impairment (reduced output and difficulty in urinating). Question dosages for patients/clients with renal disease. |

tablets and capsules is very significant and drug companies invest great resources in this area.

The nurse's behaviour when administering a medication can have a significant impact on the person's response. If you convey a sense that the medication can be helpful, it is more likely that it will have a positive effect. If you seem uncaring when the patient/client experiences discomfort, the medication administered may prove relatively ineffective. The information given by the nurse, for example about the type of drug and possible side effects is also important in compliance. Some side effects are short lived if the patient/client perseveres with taking the medication, but he or she needs to be informed.

### Diet
Drug and nutrient interactions can alter a drug's action or the effect of a nutrient. For example, vitamin K is a nutrient that antagonizes the effect of warfarin, decreasing its effect on clotting mechanisms. Mineral oil decreases the absorption of fat-soluble vitamins. Patients/clients may be required to take nutritional supplements when taking drugs that reduce a nutrient's effect.

**Mental Health Nursing
Oral medications**

When administering oral medication, particularly in tablet form, to patients/clients in the mental health setting, it is essential to follow all local safety procedures and to ensure that the patient/client has actually swallowed the medication. Vigilance in this area can prevent accidental or deliberate self harm by the patient/client. It is not unusual for certain people in the mental health setting to 'hoard' tablets with the intention of harming themselves.

Similarly, withholding certain nutrients may ensure a drug's therapeutic effect.

## ROUTES OF ADMINISTRATION

The route chosen for administering a drug depends on its properties, and the desired effect and the person's physical and mental condition (Table 31-4). The nurse is frequently involved in judging the best route for a medication, as in the following hypothetical situation:

*Mr Bush's physical condition has progressively deteriorated. His temperature is 39.2° C. He complains of nausea and is unable to tolerate oral fluids. The nurse checks Mr Bush's drug chart, which reads, 'Aspirin 600 mg orally for temperature above 38.5°C.' On the basis of the assessment, the nurse believes that Mr Bush will be unable to tolerate an oral dose of aspirin. By consulting the doctor, a rectal suppository is prescribed instead.*

### Oral Routes
The oral route is the easiest and the most commonly used. Medications are given by mouth and swallowed. Orally administered medications are less expensive than many other preparations. They have a slower onset of action and a more prolonged effect. Patients/clients generally prefer the oral route.

### Sublingual Administration
**Sublingual** drugs are designed to be readily absorbed after being placed under the tongue to dissolve. A drug given sublingually should not be swallowed, because the desired effect will not be achieved. The patient/client should not drink any fluid until the drug is completely dissolved.

### Parenteral Routes
**Parenteral** administration involves giving a drug via an injection into body tissues. Parenteral administration of a medication involves four major types of injections:

1. **Subcutaneous (SC)**, or injection into tissues just below the dermis of the skin.
2. **Intradermal (ID)**, injection into the dermis just under the epidermis.
3. **Intramuscular (IM)**, injection into a muscle.
4. **Intravenous (IV)**, injection into a vein.

A doctor may use additional routes for parenteral injections, including intrathecal or epidural, intracardiac, intrapleural, intra-arterial, and intra-articular.

A strict sterile technique should be used when preparing drugs for parenteral injection. Contamination of the medication solution, syringe needle, or the syringe itself can lead to infection.

### Topical Administration
Drugs applied to the skin and mucous membranes principally have local effects. The **topical** medication preparation is applied to the skin by painting or spreading it over an area, applying moist dressings, soaking body parts in a solution, or giving medicated baths. Systemic effects can occur if a patient's/client's skin is thin, if the drug concentration is high, or if skin contact is prolonged.

Some drugs (for example, nitroglycerin and oestrogens) are applied topically by a transdermal patch. The patch secures the ointment to the skin. These topical applications may be applied for as little as 24 hours or up to 7 days. Drugs delivered by this route have systemic effects.

Drugs can also be applied to mucous membranes. They are quickly absorbed. If the drug concentration is high enough or applied in great quantities, systemic effects may occur.

Mucous membranes differ in their sensitivity to drugs. The cornea of the eye and nasal mucous membranes are particularly sensitive. The person may complain of a burning sensation when eye drops or nose drops are administered. Drugs are generally less irritating to vaginal or rectal mucosa. The following methods can be used to apply drugs to mucous membranes:

- **direct** application of liquid (for example, applying eye drops, having the person gargle, swabbing the throat)
- **insertion** of the drug into a body cavity (for example, placing a suppository in the rectum or a pessary in the vagina)
- **instillation** of fluid into a body cavity (for example, instilling ear drops, nose drops, and bladder and rectal fluids)
- **irrigation** (washing out) of body cavity (for example, flushing the eye, ear, vagina, bladder, or rectum with medicated fluid)
- **spraying** (for example, instilling medication into nose and throat)

### Inhalation
The deeper passages of the respiratory tract provide a large surface area for drug absorption. The vascular alveolar-capillary network readily absorbs gases and mists introduced through the airways. Medications introduced into the lung's airways must not interfere with normal gas exchange such as constricting bronchioles. Inhaled medications may have local effects. Drugs such as oxygen and general anaesthetics create general systemic effects. Some medications given by inhalation are designed to produce local effects but have potentially dangerous systemic side effects. Oxygen must be administered with the appropriate oxygen delivery equipment (see Chapter 17). Nurses must teach patients/clients how to administer local-acting medications with a hand-operated inhaler.

### Nebulizers
The drug is introduced into the lungs as a mist when oxygen or air is bubbled through the drug chamber on the oxygen mask.

**TABLE 31-4 Factors Influencing Choice of Administration Routes**

| Advantages | Disadvantages or Contraindications |
|---|---|
| **ORAL, BUCCAL, SUBLINGUAL ROUTES** | |
| Routes are convenient and comfortable for patient/client. | These routes are avoided when patient/client has alterations in gastrointestinal function (e.g. nausea, vomiting), reduced motility (after general anaesthesia or bowel inflammation and surgical resection of portion of gastrointestinal tract. |
| Routes are economical. | |
| Medications may produce local or systemic effects. | |
| Routes rarely cause anxiety for patient/client. | Some drugs are destroyed by gastric secretions. Oral administration is contraindicated in patients/clients unable to swallow (e.g. patients/clients with neuromuscular disorders, oesophageal strictures, mouth lesions). |
| | Oral medications cannot be given when patient/client has gastric suction and are contraindicated in patients/clients before some tests or surgery. |
| | Unconscious or confused patient/client is unable or unwilling to swallow or hold medication under tongue. |
| | Oral medications may irritate lining of gastrointestinal tract, discolour teeth, or have unpleasant taste. |
| **SC, IM, IV INJECTIONS** | |
| Routes provide means of administration when oral drugs are contraindicated. | There is risk of introducing infection, drugs are expensive, and these routes are avoided in patients/clients with bleeding tendencies. |
| More rapid absorption occurs than with topical or oral routes. | There is a risk of tissue damage with SC injections. |
| Intravenous infusion provides drug delivery when patient/client is critically ill. If peripheral perfusion is poor, IV route is preferred over injections. | IM and IV routes are potentially dangerous because of rapid absorption. |
| | These routes cause considerable anxiety in many patients/clients, especially children. |
| **SKIN** | |
| **Topical** | |
| Topical skin applications primarily provide local effect. | Extensive applications may be bulky and cause difficulty in manoeuvring. |
| Route is painless. | |
| Limited side effects occur. | Patients/clients with skin abrasions are at risk for rapid drug absorption and systemic effects. |
| **Transdermal** | |
| Transdermal applications provide prolonged systemic effects, with limited side effects. | Application leaves oily or pasty substance on skin and may soil clothing. |
| **MUCOUS MEMBRANES *** | |
| Therapeutic effects are provided by local application to involved sites. | Mucous membranes are highly sensitive to some drug concentrations. |
| Aqueous solutions are readily absorbed and capable of causing systemic effects. | Insertion of rectal and vaginal medication often causes embarrassment. |
| Mucous membranes provide route of administration when oral drugs are contraindicated. | Patient/client with ruptured eardrum cannot receive irrigations. |
| | Rectal suppositories are contraindicated if patient/client has had rectal surgery or if active rectal bleeding is present. |
| **INHALATION** | |
| Inhalation provides rapid relief for local respiratory problems. | Some local agents can cause serious systemic effects. |
| Route provides easy access for introduction of general anaesthetic gases. | |

* Includes eyes, ears, nose, vagina, rectum, buccal, sublingual routes.

## SYSTEMS OF DRUG MEASUREMENT

The proper administration of medications depends on the nurse's ability to compute drug dosages accurately and measure medications correctly. The nurse is responsible for checking the dose before giving a drug and teaching patients/clients about prescribed doses. The metric system of measurement is used in drug therapy.

### Metric System

Because it is a decimal system, the **metric system** is the most logically organized of the measurement systems. Metric units can easily be converted and computed through simple multiplication and division. Each basic unit of measurement is organized into units of 10. Multiplying or dividing by 10 forms secondary units. In multiplication, the decimal point moves to the right; in division, the decimal moves to the left. For example:

$10.0$ mg $\times$ 10 = 100. mg

$10.0$ mg $\div$ 10 = 1.00 mg

The basic units of measurement in the metric system are the metre (length), litre (volume), and gram (weight). For drug calculations, use primarily volume and weight units. In the metric system, small and large letters are used to designate the basic units (for example, gram = g and litre = l or L). Small letters are abbreviations for subdivisions of major units (for example, milligram = mg and millilitre = ml).

A system of Latin prefixes designates subdivision of the basic units: *deci-* ( 1/10 or 0.1), *centi-* ( 1/100 or 0.01), *milli-* ( 1/1,000 or 0.001), and *micro-* (1/1000,000 or 0.000001). Greek prefixes designate multiples of the basic units: *deca-* (10), *hecto-* (100), and *kilo-* (1000).

### Solutions

In clinical practice, nurses use solutions of various concentrations for injections, irrigations, and infusions. It is important to understand the terms that describe concentrations of solutions. A **solution** is a given mass of solid substance dissolved in a known volume of fluid or a given volume of liquid dissolved in a known volume of another fluid. When a solid is dissolved in fluid, the **concentration** is in units of mass per units of volume (for example, g/ml, g/L, mg/ml). A concentration may also be expressed as a percentage. A 10% solution, for example, is 10 g of solid dissolved in 100 ml of solution. A **proportion** also expresses concentrations. A 1:1000 solution is a solution containing 1 g of solid in 1000 ml of liquid or 1 ml of liquid with 1000 ml of another liquid.

## DOSAGE CALCULATIONS

The following simple formula can be used for many types of dosage calculations. The formula can be applied when preparing solid or liquid forms of drugs:

$$\frac{\text{Prescribed dose}}{\text{Available form}} \times \text{Volume available} = \text{Amount to administer}$$

The **prescribed dose** ordered is the amount of pure drug that the doctor prescribes for a patient/client. The **available form** is the weight or volume of drug available in units supplied by the pharmacy; it may be expressed on the drug label as the contents of a tablet or capsule or the amount of drug dissolved per unit volume of liquid. The **volume available** is the basic unit or quantity of the drug containing the available form. For solid drugs, the amount on hand may be one tablet or capsule; the amount of liquid on hand may be a millilitre or litre. The amount to administer is always expressed in the same unit as the volume available.

The following example illustrates how to apply the formula. The doctor prescribes the patient/client to receive ampicillin 250 mg IM. Thus, the *prescribed dose* is 250 mg. The medication is available only in ampoules containing 500 mg per 2 ml. Thus, the *available form* is 500 mg in an *volume available* of 2 ml. The formula is applied as follows:

$$\frac{250}{500} \times 2 \text{ ml} = \text{Volume to administer in millilitres}$$

To simplify the fraction, divide the numerator and denominator by 250:

$$\frac{1}{2} \times 2 \text{ ml} = 1 \text{ ml to administer}$$

Another example demonstrates how the formula is applied to solid dosage forms. The doctor orders 125 micrograms of digoxin orally (125 µg = 0.125 mg). The drug is available in tablets containing 0.25 mg or 250 µg.

$$\frac{0.125 \text{ mg}}{0.250 \text{ mg}} \times 1 \text{ tablet} = \text{Number of tablets to administer}$$

The fraction 0.125/0.250 equals 1/2 or 0.5. Therefore

$$0.5 \times 1 \text{ tablet} = 0.5 \text{ or } 1/2 \text{ tablet to be administered}$$

Many tablets come with scores or indentations across the centre. A scored tablet is easy to break for divided dosages. Never attempt to estimate the amount of medication in a broken, unscored tablet. The potential for giving a dangerously low or high dosage of medication is likely if you attempt to estimate dosage by breaking unscored tablets.

Liquid medications often come prepared in volumes greater than 1 ml. In this situation the formula still applies. For example, the medication order is, 'Erythromycin suspension 250 mg po by mouth'. The pharmacy delivers 100-ml bottles with the labels stating, '5 ml contains 125 mg of erythromycin'.

$$\frac{250}{125} \times 5 \text{ ml} = \text{Volume to administer}$$

The fraction 250/125 equals 2. Therefore

$$2 \times 5 \text{ ml} = 10 \text{ ml to administer}$$

In this situation, ignore the total volume of medication available and instead use the dosage values noted on the label.

## Paediatric Dosages

Calculating a child's drug dosages requires caution. A child is unable to metabolize many drugs as readily as an adult. The child's body size also necessitates smaller dosages. Doctors calculate the safe dosage for a child before ordering the medication. However, nurses should be aware of the formula used to calculate paediatric dosages and should recheck all dosages before administration. Most drug references list the normal ranges for paediatric dosages.

The most accurate method of calculating paediatric dosages is based on body surface area. **Body surface area** is estimated on the basis of weight. Standard nomograms, or charts, list body surface area by weight and approximate age. The formula is a ratio of the child's body surface area compared with the body surface area of an average adult (1.7 square metres, or 1.7 m$^2$).

$$\text{Child's dose} = \frac{\text{Surface area of child}}{1.7 \text{ m}^2} \times \text{Normal adult dose}$$

For example, a doctor orders ampicillin for a child weighing 12 kg, but the normal single adult dose is 250 mg. The nomogram chart shows that a child weighing 12 kg has a surface area of 0.54 m$^2$.

$$\text{Child's dose} = \frac{0.54 \text{ m}^2}{1.7 \text{ m}^2} \times 250 \text{ mg}$$

The m$^2$ units cancel out and can be ignored.

$$\text{Child's dose} = \frac{0.54}{1.7} \times 250 \text{ mg}$$

$$\frac{0.54}{1.7} = 0.3$$

$$\text{Child's dose} = 0.3 \times 250 \text{ mg} = 75 \text{ mg}$$

Extra care should be taken when calculating the amount of drug to administer. Smaller doses necessitate the use of decimal points and micrograms which are not often required when dealing with adult doses.

## ADMINISTERING MEDICATIONS

The nurse does not bear sole responsibility for drug administration. The doctor and pharmacist play key roles in ensuring that the right medication gets to the right patient/client. However, the nurse giving the medications bears responsibility and accountability for the accuracy of the 'five rights' of drug administration (see p. 657).

### Doctor's Role

The doctor prescribes drugs on the patient's/client's drug chart, or on the outpatient drug form or on a FP10 prescription pad in the community. In some situations a doctor may also order a medication by telephone or by giving the nurse a verbal order. This will be countered by local policy. Hospital and community policies vary as to which personnel can take verbal or telephone orders and the nurse must adhere to these. *No* medication may be given without an order.

Common abbreviations (see box) are used when writing orders. The abbreviations indicate dosage frequencies or times, routes of administration, and special information to follow in giving the drug.

### Types of Orders

The four common types of medication orders are based on the frequency of drug administration.

### REGULAR PRESCRIPTIONS

A regularly prescribed drug is administered until the doctor cancels it or until a prescribed number of days elapse. A regular prescription may have a final date. Local policy will determine when the drug chart needs to be rewritten by the doctor.

### 'AS REQUIRED' PRESCRIPTIONS (PRN)

The doctor may order a drug to be given as the patient requires it (prn). The nurse uses discretion in determining the patient's/client's need. Often the doctor sets minimal intervals for the time of administration. The nurse may decide to lengthen the interval if the patient/client does not need the drug, for example, aspirin 600 mg orally 4 hourly, metoclopramide 10 mg orally 6 hourly prn.

### SINGLE (ONE-TIME) ORDERS

A doctor may order a drug to be given only once at a specified time. This is common for preoperative drugs or drugs given before diagnostic examinations.

| Abbreviation | Latin term | Meaning |
| --- | --- | --- |
| bd | *bis die* | twice a day |
| om | *omni mane* | every morning |
| on | *omni nocte* | every night |
| po | *per os* | by mouth |
| prn | *Pro re nata* | as occasion arises (repeat when necessary) |
| qds | *quater die sumendum* | to be taken four times a day |
| stat | *statim* | immediately |
| tds | *ter die sumendum* | to be taken three times a day |

## 'STRAIGHT AWAY' SINGLE DOSE PRESCRIPTIONS

This order signifies that a single dose of a medication is to be given immediately and only once (stat). Prescriptions are written for emergencies when a patient's/client's condition changes suddenly.

### Pharmacist's Role

The pharmacist prepares and distributes prescribed drugs. The pharmacist is responsible for ensuring that prescriptions are valid and accurate. The pharmacist calls the doctor if an ordered dose seems outside the safe therapeutic range. In some hospitals, pharmacists can write on the drug card, usually in green, for example to put the drug name if the doctor has used the proprietary one.

Most drug companies deliver drugs in a form ready for administration. Dispensing the correct drug, in the correct dosage and amount, with an accurate label is the pharmacist's chief responsibility. The pharmacist can also provide information about drug side effects, toxicity, interactions, and incompatibilities. Ward pharmacists are a valuable resource and nurses should not hesitate to seek advice.

### Distribution Systems

Systems for the storage and distribution of medications vary according to the care setting. Special drug and lotion cupboards, portable locked trolleys, and individual storage units for patient self administration are some of the facilities used. Nurses are responsible for the supply and ordering of medications, making sure that storage areas are locked when unattended and that drugs are stored correctly.

## STOCK SUPPLY

With a ward stock system, medications are available in quantity in stock containers. Nurses prepare individual doses from a large stock supply container. Many areas now have a 'top up' system in

---

conjunction with the pharmacy. Patients/clients requiring 'non stock' drugs will have a designated supply from the pharmacy, kept on the ward trolley.

### Nurse's Role

The nurse's role extends beyond simply giving drugs to a patient/client. The nurse must determine whether a patient/client should receive a drug at a given time, provide medications at the proper time, and monitor the effects of prescribed medications. Patient/client and family education about correct drug administration and monitoring is also the nurse's role. It is important to use the nursing process to integrate drug therapy into care.

## NURSING PROCESS AND DRUG ADMINISTRATION

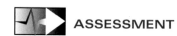 ASSESSMENT

To determine the need for and potential response to drug therapy, it is important to assess many factors.

### Medical History

A medical history provides indications or contraindications for drug therapy. Disease or illness may place patients/clients at risk for adverse drug effects. For example, if a person has a gastric ulcer or bleeding tendency, compounds containing aspirin or anticoagulants will increase the probability of bleeding. Long-term health problems such as diabetes mellitus or arthritis, which require medications, suggest to the nurse the type of drugs a patient/client is taking. A patient's/client's surgical history may indicate use of medications, for example, after a thyroidectomy a patient/client may require hormone replacement.

### History of Allergies

Inform other members of the health care team if the patient/client has a history of allergies to medications. Food allergies should also be carefully documented because many drugs have ingredients found in food sources, for example shellfish. If patients/clients are allergic to shellfish, they may be sensitive to any product containing iodine. All allergies should be noted on the nurse's admission notes, drug chart, and doctor's history. If the 'known allergy' box on the drug chart is empty, it must not be assumed that the patient/client has no allergies. It may be that they have not been asked. If a patient/client has no known allergies, the chart should say this.

### Drug Data

Assess information about each drug, including action, purpose, normal dosages, routes, side effects, and nursing implications for administration and monitoring. Common questions to ask include the following: 'Is this the smallest possible dose ordered?' (a question pertinent to older adults), 'Can a certain drug interact with other drugs being used?' and 'Are there special instructions for administering the drug?'.

---

> **Learning Disabilities Nursing Self-medication**
>
> For people with learning disabilities, it is important to encourage the highest level of personal independence possible, that is compatible with an acceptable level of risk. Achieving a balance between independence and risk is frequently difficult when encouraging patients/clients to take responsibility for their own medication.
>
> Before establishing a self-medication programme, the nurse must carefully assess the patient's/client's ability to comply with self-administration requirements, such as the ability to identify the medicine, dispense an accurate dosage, and take it at the appropriate times. Deficits in any of these areas must be addressed through systematic training and supervised self-administration. Regular monitoring of patients/clients who are handling their own medications is also important.
>
> In addition to the self-medication skills listed above, it is also important to teach patients/clients to recognize the side effects of the medication and to have their medication reviewed regularly.

Often, several resources have to be consulted in order to gather the necessary information. Pharmacology textbooks, nursing journals, the *British National Formulary*, drug package inserts, and the pharmacist are valuable resources. You are responsible for knowing as much as possible about each drug given.

### Diet History

A diet history reveals the patient's/client's usual eating patterns. The nurse can then plan the dosage schedule more effectively.

### Patient's/Client's Current Condition

The ongoing physical or mental status of a patient/client may affect whether a drug is given or how it is administered. Assess the patient/client carefully before giving any drug; for example, check blood pressure before giving an antihypertensive. If the person is nauseated, it is unlikely that a tablet can be swallowed. Assessment findings can also serve as a baseline in evaluating the effects of drug therapy.

### Patient's/Client's Perceptual or Coordination Problems

For a person with perceptual or coordination limitations, self-administration may be difficult on discharge home. During pre-discharge assessment, it is important to assess the person's ability to prepare dosages and take medications correctly. If the individual is unable to self-administer drugs, find out whether family members or friends are available to assist. The community nursing service and Social Services can assist individuals who live alone.

### Patient's/Client's Knowledge and Understanding of Drug Therapy

The patient's/client's knowledge and understanding of drug therapy influences his or her willingness or ability to follow a drug regimen. Unless a patient/client understands a drug's purpose, the importance of regular dosage schedules and proper administration methods, and the possible side effects, compliance is unlikely. When assessing knowledge of a drug, ask the person the following questions:

1. What is it for?
2. How and when is it taken?
3. Have there been any side effects?
4. Have you ever stopped taking doses?
5. Is there anything else that you do not understand or would like to know about the drug?

### Patient's/Client's Learning Needs

By assessing the patient's/client's level of knowledge about a medication, you can determine the need for teaching. It may be necessary to explain the action and purpose of the drug, expected side effects, correct administration techniques, and ways to remember the drug regimen. If a person has been placed on a newly prescribed drug, instruction may need to be more comprehensive. It is useful to provide written guidelines that the person can take home. Many drug companies produce patient information leaflets, under recent EC directives. It is important to ensure any written information given to the patient/client

corresponds with verbal information given, that the information is appropriate in style and language for the patient/client, and that it addresses the specific needs of the patient/client (for example, ethnic minority considerations).

### Cultural or Religious Considerations

It is important to be aware of the origins of drug preparations in order that cultural beliefs and practices are not infringed.

Jewish or Muslim people may be unwilling to accept drugs derived from pigs, such as porcine insulin, and Hindus may be unwilling to accept drugs derived from cows. Catholics may be unwilling to accept drugs which have been prepared from aborted fetal tissue.

Some people, for example Christian Scientists, may refuse to accept all drugs.

 **PLANNING**

Organize care activities to ensure that safe administrative techniques are used. Giving patients/clients medications in a hurry can lead to errors. Also utilize the time during administration to teach patients/clients about their medications.

In situations in which individuals learn to self-administer medications, for example insulin, plan to use all available teaching resources. Inclusion of family members or friends in teaching is very important. Patients/clients may be unable to consistently self-administer drugs. There may be other non-health-related reasons. When there is little time for teaching, brochures or pamphlets describing drug therapy are available. Whether a patient/client attempts self-administration or the nurse assumes responsibility for administering drugs, the following goals should be met:

- absence of complications related to the route of administration
- achievement of the therapeutic effect of the prescribed drugs safely while maintaining the person's comfort
- understanding on the part of the patient/client and family members regarding drug therapy
- safe self-administration of medication.

 **IMPLEMENTATION**

### ACCURATE DOSAGE CALCULATION AND MEASUREMENT

The nurse who gives the wrong medication or an incorrect dosage is legally responsible for the error. The procedure for drug measurement is systematic to lessen the chance of error. Calculate each dose when preparing the drug, pay close attention to calculation, and avoid interference from other activities.

When measuring liquid drugs, use standard cups or syringes.

### CORRECT ADMINISTRATION

Use aseptic technique and correct procedures when handling and giving medications. Certain drugs require you to perform assessments at the time of administration, such as assessing heart rate before giving antidysrhythmics.

| ADDRESSOGRAPH | | WARD | | HOUSE OFFICERS | |
|---|---|---|---|---|---|
| | | CONSULTANT | | | |
| WEIGHT | STEROID HISTORY | | | | |

| Date | Time | Once only and Pre-Med Drugs | Dose | Route | Signature | Given | W'ness | Pharm. | DIET | OXYGEN |
|---|---|---|---|---|---|---|---|---|---|---|
| | | | | | | | | | | |
| | | | | | | | | | | |
| | | | | | | | | | | |
| | | | | | | | | | | |
| | | | | | | | | | DRUG IDIOSYNCRASY | |
| | | | | | | | | | | |
| | | | | | | | | | | |
| | | | | | | | | | | |
| | | | | | | | | | Yellow Card Sent | |
| | | | | | | | | | | |

| AS REQUIRED PRESCRIPTIONS | | | Date | Time | Dose | Given | W'ness | Date | Time | Dose | Given | W'ness | Date | Time | Dose | Given | W'ness |
|---|---|---|---|---|---|---|---|---|---|---|---|---|---|---|---|---|---|
| Drug (approved name) | | Dose | | | | | | | | | | | | | | | |
| Route | Maximum Frequency | Start Date | Signature | Pharm. | | | | | | | | | | | | | |
| Drug (approved name) | | Dose | | | | | | | | | | | | | | | |
| Route | Maximum Frequency | Start Date | Signature | Pharm. | | | | | | | | | | | | | |

**Fig. 31-3** Example of medication record. Courtesy of St. Bartholomew's Hospital, London.

## RECORDING DRUG ADMINISTRATION

To prevent another nurse giving a medication without knowing that the patient/client has already received a dose, document medications at the time of administration (Fig. 31-3). If the medication is not given due to patient/client refusal or physical assessment findings **contraindicating** drug use, the drug chart must be completed according to local policy and the doctor informed.

### Patient/Client and Family Teaching

Unless patients/clients are properly informed about drugs, they may take them incorrectly or not at all. It is important to provide information about the purpose of medications and their actions and effects. Patients/clients must know the way to take drugs properly and the effects if they fail to do so, for example, a patient/client receiving a prescription for an antibiotic must understand the importance of taking the full course. Failure to do this can lead to a worsening of the condition, as well as the development of bacterial resistance to the drug.

Patients/clients must be aware of the symptoms of drug side effects or toxicity, for example, patients/clients taking anticoagulants learn to notify the doctor immediately when signs of bleeding or frequent bruising develop. Family members should be informed of drug side effects, such as changes in behaviour, because they are often the first people to recognize such effects. Patients/clients are better able to cope with problems caused by drugs if they understand how and when to act. All patients/clients should learn the following basic guidelines for drug safety in the home:

1. Keep each drug in its original, labelled container.
2. Be sure labels are legible.
3. Discard any outdated medications by returning them to the pharmacy/chemist.
4. Always finish a prescribed drug unless otherwise instructed. Never save a drug for future illnesses.
5. Do not give a family member or friend a drug prescribed for another.
6. Store medicines according to manufacturers recommendations, for example out of bright light or below 50° C.
7. Read labels carefully and follow all instructions
8. If side effects occur, contact GP.
9. If buying 'over the counter' medicines, inform pharmacist of prescribed drugs.
10. Carry a medications identification card or wear an ID bracelet if you have any drug allergies (e.g. penicillin) or take particular drugs, such as insulin or steroids.

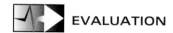 **EVALUATION**

Monitor the patient's/client's response to medications on an ongoing basis. In order to do this, you must know the therapeutic action and common side effects of each medication. A change in a patient's/client's condition can be physiologically related to health status, may result from medications, or both. It is important to be alert for reactions, particularly when a person is taking several medications.

The goal of safe and effective drug administration involves a careful evaluation of technique, the person's response to therapy and ability to assume responsibility for self-care. To evaluate the effectiveness of nursing interventions when meeting established goals of care, use evaluative measures to identify actual outcomes:

- **observe** injection sites for bruises, inflammation, localized pain, or bleeding
- **question** the patient/client about localized numbness or tingling at injection sites
- **assess** the person for gastrointestinal disturbances, including nausea, vomiting, and diarrhoea
- **inspect** IV sites for phlebitis, including fever, swelling, and localized tenderness.

Examples of evaluative measures for determining whether the therapeutic effect of prescribed medication has been achieved safely include the following:

1. Questioning the patient/client for expected response to the drug (for example, pain relief, or reduction in symptoms).
2. Monitoring patient's/client's physical response to medication (e.g. antidysrhythmic medication, regular heart rhythm; hypertension medication, lowered blood pressure; diuretics, increased urine output).

Examples of evaluative measures for maintaining the person's safety and comfort include the following:

1. Monitoring the patient/client for potential side or toxic effects, allergic reactions, or interactions.
2. Assessing the patient/client up to 30 minutes after administration of medications for symptoms of discomfort.

Examples of evaluative measures for understanding drug therapy include the following:

1. Asking the person to explain the drug's purpose, action, dosage, schedule of administration, and possible side effects.
2. Asking the person to describe when each medication is taken during the day.

Examples of evaluative measures for determining the patient's/client's ability to self-administer medications safely include the following:

1. Observing the person preparing an ordered dose of medication.
2. Observing the patient/client administering the ordered dose of medication.

## MEDICATION DELIVERY

Preparing and administering drugs requires accuracy by the nurse. Use the following guidelines, the 'five rights' of drug administration, to ensure safe drug administration:

1. The *right* drug.
2. The *right* dose.
3. The *right* patient/client.
4. The *right* route.
5. The *right* time.

### Right Drug

When administering drugs, compare the label of the drug container with the drug chart. Nurses administer *only* the drugs they prepare. If an error occurs, the nurse administering the drug is responsible for its effects.

If an individual questions the medication, do not ignore these concerns. An alert person will know whether a drug is different from those received before. In most cases the prescription has been changed. However, the patient's/client's questions might reveal an error. The nurse should withhold the drug and the preparation should be rechecked. Patients/clients who self-administer drugs should keep them in their original labelled containers, separate from other drugs, to avoid confusion.

Never prepare medications from unmarked containers or containers with illegible labels. If a patient/client refuses a drug, never return it to the original container or transfer it to another container.

### Right Dose

When a medication has to be prepared from a larger or smaller volume or strength than needed, the chance of error increases.

After calculating dosages, prepare the medication by using standard measurement devices, for example, many liquid paediatric medications come with a scaled dropper. Graduated cups, syringes, and specially designed spoons can be used to measure medications accurately. In the home, medicine cups and special spoons supplied with the medicine should be used. Household teaspoons may vary in volume.

To break a scored tablet, make sure that the break is even. A tablet may be cut in half by using a knife edge or by folding a tissue over the tablet and breaking it with the fingers. Any tablets that do not break evenly are discarded. After a tablet is split, the two halves may be given in successive doses, but only if the second half has been repackaged and labelled.

A tablet may be prepared by crushing it in a mortar with a pestle or in a special tablet crusher so that it can be mixed in food or jam, especially when a person has difficulty with swallowing and an injection is unnecessary or undesirable. The mortar should always be cleaned out completely before the tablet is crushed. Remnants of previously crushed drugs may increase a drug's concentration or result in the person receiving a portion of an unprescribed drug. Crushing the tablet in a small container avoids loss of any substance. Crushed medications should be mixed with very small amounts of jam or liquid. Foods and liquids that patients/clients are taking well or especially like should not be used, because the medication may decrease the person's desire for the food after it has been altered with 'bitter' or 'bad-tasting' medications. Some suggestions are jelly, syrup, and chocolate syrup or other ice cream toppings. Capsules should never be broken to mix contents with food. The gelatin capsule is designed to survive its journey through the hydrochloric acid in the stomach.

## Right Patient/Client

It is important when administering drugs to ensure that the medication is given to the right patient/client. The nurse working in a hospital, community, or extended care setting is frequently responsible for administering drugs to several patients/clients. Patients/clients may have similar last names, and it is difficult to remember every name and face, especially if a nurse has been off duty for several days. To identify patients/clients correctly, check the drug chart against the person's identification bracelet and ask him or her to state his or her name. This is vital even if you have been caring for a person for several days. To avoid making the patient/client feel uneasy, simply explain that the safety checks for giving a medication requires identification by name. If an identification bracelet becomes smudged or illegible, replace it with a new one. In some areas, photographs may be used to identify patients/clients. Photographs must show an accurate and clear likeness of the person.

## Right Route

If a drug prescription does not designate a route of administration, consult the doctor. Similarly, if the specified route is not the recommended route, you should alert the doctor immediately.

When administering injections (see the section on parenteral routes), ensure that medications are given correctly. It is also important to prepare injections only from preparations designed for parenteral use. The injection of a liquid designed for oral use can produce local complications such as a sterile abscess or fatal systemic effects. Drug companies label parenteral drugs for 'injection only'.

## Right Time

The nurse must understand why a drug is ordered for certain times of the day and know whether the time schedule can be altered. Each care area has a recommended time schedule for medications ordered at frequent intervals.

The doctor often gives specific instructions about when to administer a medication. A preoperative medication is to be given when the operating theatre notifies the ward.

When a nurse is responsible for administering several medications, those that must act at certain times are given priority, for example, insulin should be administered at a precise interval before a meal. All routinely ordered medications should be given within 30 minutes of the times ordered, if possible, although some variation is acceptable.

Some drugs require the nurse's clinical judgement in determining the proper time for administration. A sleeping medication should be administered when the person is prepared for sleep. Many hospitalized patients prefer to go to sleep earlier than they might normally at home. However, if you are aware that a procedure might interrupt the person's sleep, it is appropriate to withhold the drug until a time when the patient/client can gain full benefit from it. Also use your judgement in administering analgesics. When a patient's/client's prescription reads '4 hourly', then the medication may be given as often as every 4 hours. However, first assess the individual's level

## Community Nursing
## Administering medications in the community

### Community practice

- Nurses must be familiar with the local drugs policy.
- Managers must ensure that all nurses authorized to administer medicines read and understand the drugs policy and are updated regularly on the policy.
- Nurses must read and understand the policy and follow the UKCC Code of Conduct.
- Nurses must act within the boundaries of their role/grade.
- Nurses act within their level of competence, with reference to grade and UKCC Code of Conduct.
- Advice can be obtained from managers, colleagues, community pharmacy.
- Community nurses usually do not need to carry drugs.
- Adrenaline and chlorpheniramine may be carried if the nurse is performing a procedure which may result in anaphylaxis, e.g. immunization at home.

### Stock, storage of drugs and related equipment in clinic

- Stocked by pharmacy.
- Labelled by pharmacy.
- Locked, designated cupboard.
- Injectable and systemic drugs kept separately from topical drugs.
- Needles and syringes in a locked cupboard.
- Anaphylactic shock packs should be sealed prior to use and stored in secure accessible place.
- If drugs should be stored in a refrigerator, it should be locked and the temperature checked daily.

### Drugs at home

- Client's responsibility.
- Nurses advise regarding storage and safety.
- If the nurse is concerned regarding storage, the nurse should notify the manager.

of pain to determine the degree of discomfort. If the person is made to wait until the pain becomes severe, the analgesic effect may not be sufficient (see Chapter 27).

## Avoiding Errors

Most drug administration errors occur when a nurse fails to follow agreed procedures (Table 31-5).

An error should be acknowledged immediately. The nurse has an ethical and professional responsibility for reporting the error to the doctor and the nurse manager (see Chapter 12). Measures to counteract the effects of the error, such as administering an antidote when the wrong drug is given, withholding a dose when a previous medication has been given too soon, or monitoring the effects when an unusually high dosage is given, may be necessary. A note is made in the nursing records or case notes.

The nurse is also responsible for completing an **incident form** describing the nature of the incident. The report is not an

## TABLE 31-5 Ways to Prevent Drug Administration Errors

| Precaution | Rationale | Precaution | Rationale |
|---|---|---|---|
| Read drug labels carefully | Many products come in similar containers, colours, and shapes. | When new or unfamiliar drug is ordered, consult BNF or pharmacist. | If doctor is also unfamiliar with drug, there is greater risk of inaccurate dosages being ordered. |
| Question administration of multiple tablets or vials for single dose | Most doses are one or two tablets or capsules or one single-dose vial. Incorrect interpretation of order may result in excessively high dose. | Do not administer drug ordered by unofficial abbreviation. | Many doctors refer to commonly ordered medications by unofficial abbreviations. If nurse or pharmacist is unfamiliar with name, wrong drug may be dispensed and administered. |
| Be aware of drugs with similar names | Many drug names sound alike. | Do not attempt to decipher illegible writing. | When in doubt, ask doctor. Unless nurse questions order that is difficult to read, chance of misinterpretation is great. |
| Check decimal point | Some drugs come in quantities that are multiples of one another. | Know patients/clients with same last names. Also have patients/clients state their full names. Check name bands carefully. | It is common to have two or more patients/clients with same or similar last names. Special labels on Kardex or drug chart can warn of potential problem. |
| Question abrupt and excessive increases in dosages | Most dosages are made gradually so that doctor can monitor therapeutic effect and response. | Do not confuse equivalents. | When in a hurry, it may be easy to misread equivalents (e.g. milligram instead of millilitre). |

**IF IN DOUBT, DO NOT GIVE DRUG AND CONSULT DOCTOR AND/OR PHARMACIST**

admission of guilt or the basis for punishment and is not a part of the patient's/client's legal medical record. The report provides an objective analysis of what went wrong and is a means for the hospitals' or community unit's Clinical Practice Committee and Medicine Committee (or other mechanism) to monitor such occurrences. Incident reports assist in identifying errors and solving recurrent problems affecting care.

## Special Considerations for Age Groups

A patient's/client's developmental level is a factor in the way in which nurses administer drugs. Knowledge of a person's developmental needs helps you anticipate responses to drug therapy.

## Infants and Children

Children vary in age, weight, body surface area, and the ability to absorb, metabolize, and excrete drugs. Children's dosages are lower than those of adults, so special caution is needed in preparing drugs for them.

A child's parents are valuable resources for learning the best way to give a child medications. Sometimes it is less traumatic for the child if a parent gives the drug and the nurse supervises.

All children require special psychological preparation before receiving medications. Supportive care is needed if a child is expected to cooperate. Explain the procedure to the child, using short words and simple language appropriate to the child's level of comprehension. Long explanations may increase anxiety, especially for painful procedures such as an injection. Approach the child with confidence and act as though the child is expected to cooperate (Wong, 1995). Giving medication may be more successful if it is possible to involve the child; for example, saying "It's time to take your tablet now. Do you want it with water or juice?" allows the child to make a choice. *Never* give a child the option of *not* taking a medication. After a drug is given, praise the child and offer a simple reward such as a star or token. Depending on the route of administration, there are several tips for administering drugs to children (see left box overleaf).

## Older Adults

Older adults also require special consideration during drug administration. Age has an effect on the absorption, distribution, metabolism, and excretion of drugs (see earlier section). In addition to the physiological changes of ageing, behavioural and economic factors influence older peoples' use of drugs.

**Noncompliance** with drug therapy is the failure of patients/clients to follow instructions regarding the use of

**Children's Nursing**
**Tips for administering medications to children**

ORAL MEDICATIONS
- Liquid forms are safer to swallow to avoid aspiration.
- Juice, or a soft drink, is offered after a drug is swallowed.
- When mixing drugs with palatable flavourings, such as syrup and honey, use only a small amount. The child may refuse to take all of a larger mixture. Avoid mixing a drug with foods or liquids that the child is taking well, because the child may in turn refuse them.
- A plastic, disposable syringe is the most accurate device for preparing liquid dosages, especially those less than 10 ml. (Cups, teaspoons, and droppers are inaccurate.)
- Special syringe droppers are now used for administration.

INJECTIONS
- Be very careful when selecting IM injection sites. Infants and small children have underdeveloped muscles.
- Children can be unpredictable and uncooperative. Someone should always be available to hold a child.
- Always awaken a sleeping child before giving an injection, and prepare the child, e.g. 'This will be a little hurt to take away a big hurt'.
- Distract the child with conversation or a toy to help reduce pain perception.
- Give the injection quickly and do not fight with the child.

ENEMAS
- Never give a retention enema to a child younger than 6 years of age. He or she will not be able to retain it. The amount of solution is important and smaller children require smaller amounts.

**Adult Nursing**
**Medications and older adults**

The medications given to older people have been under scrutiny for some years, as they potentially have widespread implications in both human and financial terms.

In 1988, the total cost of drugs dispensed to older people was estimated at £782 million. The average number of prescriptions dispensed per person over retirement age was 17.4, compared to 5.6 prescriptions per person below retirement age (London and Thames Valley Pharmaceutical Group, 1989).

Older people are prescribed more drugs than younger people for many reasons, such as multiple illnesses. However, older people also experience more medication-related problems, such as increased sensitivity to side effects (Bliss, 1981).

Older people are not always able to take their drugs as prescribed. One report suggested that 75% of older people make errors in their compliance with prescriptions, and that 25% of these errors could cause serious problems (Royal College of Physicians, 1984).

Nurses play a key role in helping older people to reduce medication consumption (for example, in promoting sleep or avoiding constipation rather than taking medications for these problems). When drugs are prescribed, nurses should ensure that the regimen is as straightforward as possible, and that it is consistent with the older person's lifestyle and available support. Other considerations for older adults include:
- being able to open the drug packaging
- knowing who to contact in case of difficulties
- understanding the purpose of the medication, dosage instructions, side effects, and action to take in case of problems (Quilligan, 1990)
- knowing how to dispose of unused medications
- checking with the pharmacist before taking any over-the-counter preparations.

Special considerations may also be necessary for older people with hearing-impairment.

medication. Noncompliance may involve failure to take a medication by choice, intentional reduction in drug dosage, failure to take a drug at the right time, increasing the frequency or dosage of medication, or discontinuing use of a drug prematurely. Older adults may also deny the presence of an illness and therefore choose not to take a medication.

Although noncompliance may occur in any age group, it is a special problem for older adults. Older people are more prone to suffer serious physical effects from particular diseases when medications are not taken. Simonson (1984) summarizes the following patient/client-related factors that may cause non-compliance with drug therapy in older adults:

- Lack of understanding of drug therapy. People who are prescribed several medications can easily become confused about when, how and why they have been prescribed.
- Poor self-medication practices. Patients may consume more nonprescription drugs than needed. These drugs can interfere with the action of prescription drugs.
- Lack of social supervision. People living alone are less likely to comply with prescribed medication therapy than those living with another person.

- Feeling too ill or tired to take the medication. These feelings may be complicated by older peoples' difficulty with ambulating and adverse effects of certain drugs.
- Sensory losses. Visual alterations make it difficult to read prescriptions. Hearing problems may alter the ability to understand oral instructions.
- Keeping old medicines and self-dosing. Old medications may be *inappropriate* or have little therapeutic effect.

Compliance can be improved by offering patients/clients simple, realistic plans for drug therapy. The least possible number of medications should be prescribed and complement daily habits (for example, meals and bedtime). Eliopoulos (1987) makes the following recommendations for teaching and assisting older adults with drug regimens:
1. Provide detailed written and oral descriptions to patients/clients and care givers. Outline the drug's name, dosage schedule, route of administration, action, special

### Mental Health Nursing
### Noncompliance

There are occasions in mental health nursing when individuals may not readily accept medication as it is prescribed. It requires considerable interpersonal skills on the part of the nurse to explain to the patient/client the necessity of medication at that particular point of the treatment programme. The Mental Health Act 1983 has particular legal provisions for enforcing treatment, and medication is included in its provision. However, the enactment of the law requires that the nurse be aware of his or her own motives in exercising control and the skilful assessment of the patient's/client's mental health status at any given time.

It is important to be sensitive to and receptive to the patient's/client's concern about his or her medication. However, the issue of safety is paramount. At no time should the nurse take his or her eyes off the patient/client when the patient/client is taking oral medication. If in doubt, adopt a direct approach by politely asking the patient/client to open the palm of his or her hands and his or her mouth to allow you to check that the medication has been swallowed. If the patient/client refuses, seek guidance from a qualified nursing practitioner promptly.

Medication not swallowed and not returned to the staff may subsequently be collected and used with the intention of self-harm. Also, medication collected by one patient/client may contribute to self-harm by another patient/client. Any concerns about medication must be discussed with qualified nursing staff.

precautions, incompatible foods or drugs, and adverse reactions.

2. Offer a colour-coded dosage schedule for people who have visual deficits or cannot read.
3. Be sure that all medication labels are typed in large print.
4. Provide medicine containers with easy-to-remove caps for weak or arthritic hands.
5. Offer memory aids to remind patients/clients of medication schedules (for example, a partitioned plastic box containing prescribed doses for 1 week, labelled plastic bags holding each timed dose, or a colour-coded chart describing each drug and time to be taken).

## ADMINISTERING ORAL MEDICATIONS

The most desirable way to administer medications is by mouth. Unless the person has impaired gastrointestinal functioning or is unable to swallow, an oral medication is the safest and most straightforward.

Most tablets and capsules should be swallowed and administered with an adequate amount of fluid, providing an opportunity for you to increase the patient's/client's fluid intake. For individuals with nasogastric feeding tubes, liquid preparations are preferred, but some tablets can be crushed (see box).

When administering medications orally, it is important to protect the person against possible aspiration. Positioning the patient/client in a sitting or side-lying position will prevent accumulation of a liquid or a solid medication in the back of the throat. A patient/client who swallows slowly should not be forced to take a large amount of liquid with each swallow. Similarly, most patients/clients should swallow only one pill or capsule at a time. If a person begins to cough while taking a medication, withhold the remaining portion of the drug until he or she can breathe more easily. If the patient/client has difficulty with swallowing tablets, other forms of the medications should be considered.

## ADMINISTERING INJECTIONS

Administering an injection is an invasive procedure that must be performed using aseptic techniques (see box overleaf). After a needle pierces the skin, the risk of infection exists. Drugs are administered parenterally by the SC, IM and IV routes. Each type of injection requires certain skills to ensure that the drug reaches the proper location. The effects of a parenterally administered drug can develop rapidly, depending on the rate of drug absorption. It is important to closely observe the person's response.

### Equipment

A variety of syringes and needles are available; each is designed to deliver a certain volume of a drug to a specific type of tissue. Use your judgement to decide which syringe or needle will be the most effective.

### Syringes

Syringes consist of a cylindrical barrel with a tip designed to fit the hub of a hypodermic needle and a close-fitting plunger (Fig. 31-4). Disposable, single-use plastic syringes that are inexpensive and easy to manipulate are used. The syringes are packaged separately, with or without a sterile needle, in a paper wrapper or rigid, plastic container. Glass syringes are also available, although they are reserved for specific drugs and not commonly used.

Fill the syringe by aspiration, pulling the piston outward while keeping the needle tip immersed in the prepared solution. You may handle the outside of the syringe barrel and the handle

### Guidelines for Giving Drugs Through a Nasogastric Tube, J-Tube, G-Tube, or Small-Bore Feeding Tube

- Administer medications in a liquid form (suspension, elixir, or solution) when possible, to prevent tube obstruction
- Read medication labels carefully before crushing a tablet
- Do not crush buccal or sublingual tablets
- Do not crush enteric-coated or sustained-action medications
- Dissolve crushed tablets and powders in warm water
- Irrigate the tube before and after all medication is given with 50–150 ml of water
- Avoid giving syrups or medications with a pH of less than 4
- Do not attempt to give whole or undissolved medications

Adapted from Petrosin BM et al: Crit Care Nurs Q 12:1, 1989.

of the plunger. To maintain sterility, avoid letting any unsterile object touch the tip or inside of the barrel, the shaft of the plunger, or the needle.

Syringes come in a number of sizes, from 0.5 to 60 ml. It is unusual to use a syringe larger than 5 ml for a SC or IM injection. A 2–3-ml syringe is adequate. A larger volume creates discomfort. Larger syringes are used to prepare IV drugs. However, you may change needle sizes. The hypodermic has a scale on the barrel, divided into millilitres and tenths of a millilitre.

Insulin syringes hold 0.5 to 1 ml and are calibrated in units. Insulin syringes are U-100s, designed for use with U-100 strength insulin. Each millilitre of solution contains 100 units of insulin.

---

### Patient's/Client's Perceptual or Coordination Problems
### Preventing Infection During an Injection

- To prevent contamination of solution, draw medication from ampoule quickly. Do not allow it to stand open.
- To prevent needle contamination, avoid letting needle touch contaminated surface (e.g. outer edges of ampoule or vial, outer surface of needle cap, nurse's hands, table surface).
- To prevent syringe contamination, avoid touching length of plunger or inner part of barrel. Keep tip of syringe covered with cap or needle while preparing.
- To prepare skin, wash skin soiled with dirt, drainage, or faeces with soap and water and dry.

---

### Needles

Needles come packaged in individual sheaths to allow flexibility in choosing the right needle. Some needles are pre-attached to standard-size syringes. Most are made of stainless steel and are disposable.

The needle has three parts: the hub, which fits onto the tip of a syringe; the shaft, which connects to the hub; and the bevel or slanted tip (see Fig. 31-4). You may handle the needle hub to ensure a tight fit on the syringe; however, the shaft and bevel must remain sterile.

Each needle has three characteristic features: the slant of the bevel, the length of the shaft, and the needle gauge or diameter. Long bevels are sharper, which minimizes discomfort caused by SC and IM injections. Needles vary in length. Choose needle length according to patient/client size and weight and the type of

tissue into which the drug is to be injected. A child or a very slender adult generally requires a shorter (blue) needle. Use a longer (green) needle for IM injections and a shorter (orange) needle for SC injections.

The smaller the gauge, the larger the needle diameter. The selection of a gauge depends on the viscosity of the fluid to be injected or infused. An IM injection usually requires a 19- to 23-gauge needle, depending on the viscosity of the medication. Subcutaneous injections require smaller-diameter needles, such as a 25-gauge needle.

### Disposable Injection Units

Disposable, single-dose, prefilled syringes are available for many medications. When using these, be careful to check the medication and concentration, because all prefilled syringes appear very similar.

### Preparing an Injection from an Ampoule

Ampoules contain single doses of medication in a liquid and are available in several sizes, from 1 ml to 10 ml or more. An ampoule is made of glass with a constricted neck that must be snapped off to allow access to the medication. A coloured ring around the neck indicates where the ampoule is prescored to break easily. Aspiration of the drug into a syringe should be done with an orange, blue or green needle, to avoid picking up minute pieces of glass which could occur if a syringe is used without a needle, or indeed with a quill or a smaller gauge white needle.

### Preparing an Injection from a Vial

A vial is a single-dose or multidose glass container with a rubber seal at the top. A metal cap protects the seal until it is ready for use. Vials contain liquid and/or dry forms of medications. Drugs that are unstable in solution are packaged dry. The vial label specifies the solution (solvent) used to dissolve the drug and the amount needed to prepare a desired drug concentration. Normal saline and sterile water are solutions commonly used to dissolve drugs.

Unlike the ampoule, the vial is a closed system, and air must be injected into it to permit easy withdrawal of the solution. Failure to inject air before withdrawing the solution leaves a vacuum within the vial that makes withdrawal difficult. The amount of air injected should equal the amount of fluid to be withdrawn.

To prepare a powdered drug, draw up the amount of solvent recommended on the vial's label, then inject the solvent into the vial in the same manner as injecting air into the vial. Clear the top of the bottle (but let the spirit evaporate). Most powdered drugs dissolve easily, but it may be necessary to withdraw the needle to mix the contents thoroughly. Gently shaking or rolling the vial between the hands will dissolve the powdered drug. The needle is reinserted to draw up the dissolved medication.

### Insulin

Insulin is the hormone used to treat insulin-dependent (Type I) diabetes mellitus. It is also sometimes used to treat non-insulin-dependent (Type II) diabetes mellitus. Insulin must be

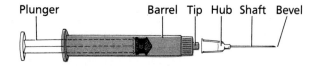

**Fig. 31-4** Parts of a syringe and hypodermic needle.

administered by injection because it is a protein and therefore would be digested and destroyed in the gastrointestinal tract. Most patients/clients with insulin-dependent diabetes mellitus learn to self-administer injections, and children from about the age of seven can do this successfully.

Until the last few years there were different types of insulin available (for example, short-acting and long-acting) and patients/clients would mix these together for use. However, there were problems with mixing. Consequently, most patients/clients now use premixed insulins. Specialists suggest that blood sugar control is improved with premixed insulins, particularly in children. If blood sugar should prove difficult to control for a period of time, a prescribed amount of soluble insulin may be added.

### Insulin Syringes and Injection Devices
Insulin is provided in 100 units per millilitre of solution. When preparing insulin, a scaled syringe is used. Special insulin syringes are manufactured so that there is virtually no 'dead-gap' (the amount of insulin remaining in a syringe after injection is minimal). Insulin syringes are also manufactured with the correct-sized needle attached. Insulin needles are microfine and are of the correct size to inject into the subcutaneous tissues.

Insulin 'pens' are now very common injection devices, and many different pens are available. In some areas, newly-diagnosed children are given insulin pen devices from the start, although this decision depends on the doctor.

### Insulin Preparation and Storage
When preparing medium-acting, long-acting, or premixed insulin for injection, the bottle should be gently rotated. Insulin should not be shaken, as this breaks down the crystals and alters the action time. If the insulin looks cloudy because the crystals have clogged, it should not be used. It is preferable to inject air into the insulin bottle before drawing up. The same amount of air as insulin should be injected into the bottle, particularly if the

person is mixing insulins.

It is not absolutely necessary to keep insulin vials currently being used in the refrigerator, only the stock. In fact, cold insulin can sting. The fridge should be set on a low temperature and the insulin stored well away from the freezer. Insulin pen devices should not be kept in the refrigerator.

### Insulin Injections
Insulin injections should be given at an angle of 90 degrees to the skin surface. The British Diabetic Association now recommends that it is not necessary to withdraw the plunger to check for blood in the syringe, as this tends to cause additional trauma to the area.

Selecting and alternating the injection site is very important. If the same site is used too many times, lipohypertrophy (building of subcutaneous fat tissue) will develop, which may cause erratic insulin absorption and unstable blood sugar control. An injection diagram allows nurses and patients/clients to record daily injections to ensure that sites are rotated (Fig. 31-5).

### Administering Injections
Each injection route is unique in regard to the type of tissues into which the medication is injected. The characteristics of the tissues influence the rate of drug absorption and thus the onset of drug action. Before injecting a drug, you should know the volume of the drug to administer, the drug's characteristics and viscosity, and the location of anatomical structures underlying injection sites (Procedure 31-1).

Serious consequences may occur if an injection is administered incorrectly. Failure to select an injection site in relation to anatomical landmarks can result in nerve or bone damage during needle insertion. Failure to aspirate the syringe (withdraw fluid) before injecting a drug, may result in the drug being accidentally injected directly into an artery or vein. Injecting too large a volume of medication for the site selected can cause extreme pain and may result in local tissue damage.

Many patients/clients, particularly children, fear injections. Patients/clients with serious or chronic illness often are given multiple injections daily. You can attempt to minimize discomfort in the following ways:

- use a new, bevelled needle in the smallest suitable length and gauge
- position the person as comfortably as possible to reduce muscular tension
- select the appropriate injection site, using anatomical landmarks
- apply EMLA (eutetic mixture of local anaesthetic) cream if prescribed to numb skin, particularly useful for children
- divert the patient's/client's attention from the injection through conversation
- spread the tissue out firmly and insert the needle smoothly and quickly to minimize tissue pulling
- hold the syringe steady while the needle remains in tissues, and withdraw the plunger to check that there is no blood (this would indicate that a blood vessel had been punctured)
- massage the injected area very gently for several seconds unless contraindicated.

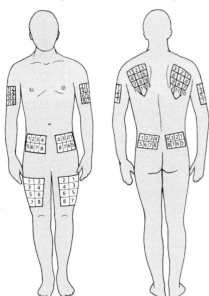

**Fig. 31-5** Common sites for SC injections. Note how sites might be rotated.

## PROCEDURE 31-1 Administering Injections

| SEQUENCE OF ACTIONS | RATIONALE |
|---|---|
| 1. Assess indications for proper route for medication. | Ensures proper drug absorption and distribution through tissues to enhance drug action. Ensures proper route appropriate for patient/client as per doctor's orders. |
| 2. Assess patient's/client's medical history and history of allergies. | May influence certain drugs. Parenteral medications often create sensitivities in form of allergies. |
| 3. Observe verbal and nonverbal responses to receiving injection. Maximize opportunities for communication. | Injections can be painful. Patients/clients may experience considerable anxiety, which can increase pain. Communication may alleviate some anxiety. |
| 4. Wash hands. | Reduces transmission of microorganisms. |
| 5. Prepare needed equipment and supplies:<br>  a. Proper-size syringe: | Volume injected should be compatible with tissue type. |
|   b. Proper-size needle: | Prevents injury to patient/client and ensures distribution of drug. |
|   c. Disposable gloves.<br>  d. Medication ampoule or vial.<br>  e. Drug card. | Identifies medication, dose ordered and patient's/client's name. |
| 6. Check drug card. | Checks prescription. |
| 7. Prepare correct medication dose from ampoule or vial. (Procedure 31-1). Check carefully. Be sure all air is expelled. | Ensures that medication is sterile. Preparation techniques differ for ampoule and vial. |
| 8. For IM injection, change needle if medication is irritating to SC tissue. | Prevents tracking of irritating substance through tissues as needle passes into muscle. |
| 9. Apply disposable gloves. | Injections could cause mild seepage of blood at injection site. Gloves reduce risk of exposure. |
| 10. Identify patient/client by checking identification armband and asking name. | Ensures that correct patient/client is receiving prescribed medication. |
| 11. Explain procedure to patient/client and proceed in calm, confident manner. | Helps patient/client anticipate actions. Calm approach minimizes anxiety. |
| 12. Draw curtains around bed, or close door. | Provides privacy. |
| 13. Keep sheet or gown draped over body parts not requiring exposure. | Proper selection of injection site may require exposure of body parts. |
| 14. Select appropriate injection site. Inspect skin surface over sites for bruises, inflammation, or oedema:<br>  a. SC: palpate sites for masses of tenderness.<br>  b. IM: note integrity and size of muscle and palpate for tenderness. | Injection sites should be free of abnormalities that may interfere with drug absorption.<br><br>Site used repeatedly can become hardened from lipohypertrophy (increased growth in fatty tissue). |
| 15. If injections are given frequently, rotate sites. | |
| 16. Assist patient/client to comfortable position: | Relaxation of site minimizes discomfort. |

(Cont'd)

## PROCEDURE 31-1 Administering Injections (Cont'd)

| SEQUENCE OF ACTIONS | RATIONALE |
|---|---|
| 17. Relocate site using anatomical landmarks. | Accurate injection requires insertion in correct site to avoid injury to underlying tissues, blood vessels, nerves, or bone. |
| 18. Remove cap from needle by pulling it straight off. | Prevents contamination. |
| 19. Hold syringe correctly between thumb and forefinger of dominant hand:<br>  a. SC: hold as dart (see Fig.19a) - or at 90-degree angle.<br>  b. IM: hold as dart. | Quick, smooth injection requires proper manipulation of syringe parts. |
| 20. Administer injection:<br><br>  a. SC:<br>    (i) For average-size patient/client, spread skin tightly across injection site or pinch skin with nondominant hand. | Needle penetrates tight skin easier than loose skin. Pinching skin elevates SC tissue. |
|     (ii) Inject needle quickly and firmly at 90-degree angle (see Fig. 20a). (Then release skin, if pinched.) | Quick, firm insertion minimizes discomfort. (Injecting medication into compressed tissue irritates nerve fibres.) |
|     (iii) For obese patient/client, pinch skin at site and inject needle below tissue fold. | Obese patients/clients have fatty layer of tissue above SC layer. |
|   b. IM:<br>    (i) Position nondominant hand at proper anatomical landmarks and spread skin tightly. Inject needle quickly at 90-degree angle into muscle. | Speeds insertion and reduces discomfort. |
|     (ii) If patient's/client's muscle mass is small, grasp body of muscle between thumb and other fingers. | Ensures that medication reaches muscle mass. |
|     (iii) If medication is irritating, use the track method (see section on the track method). | Used to prevent tracking of drug through SC tissue. |

(Cont'd)

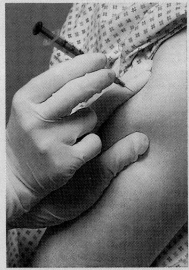

19a

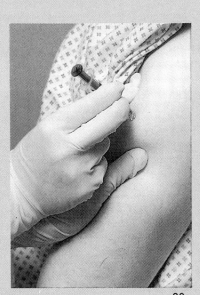

20a

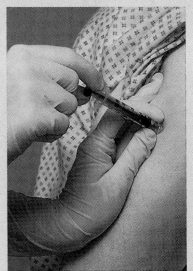

21

## PROCEDURE 31-1 Administering Injections (Cont'd)

| SEQUENCE OF ACTIONS | RATIONALE |
|---|---|
| 21. After needle enters site of IM injections, grasp lower end of syringe barrel with nondominant hand. Move dominant hand to end of plunger. Avoid moving syringe, while slowly pulling back on plunger to aspirate drug (see Fig. 21). If blood appears in syringe, remove needle, discard medication and syringe and repeat procedure. | Aspiration of blood into syringe indicates IV placement of needle. IM injections are not for IV use. |
| 22. Inject medication slowly. | Minimizes discomfort and trauma at site. |
| 23. Withdraw needle while applying alcohol swab gently above or over injection site. | Supports tissues around injection site to minimize discomfort during needle withdrawal. |
| 24. Assist patient/client to comfortable position. | Gives patient/client a sense of well-being. |
| 25. Discard unsheathed needle and attached syringe into appropriately labelled receptacles. | Prevents injury to patients/clients and health care personnel. |
| 26. Remove disposable gloves. Wash hands. | Reduces transmission of microorganisms. |
| 27. Return to ask if patient/client feels acute pain, burning, numbness, or tingling at injection site. | Continued discomfort may indicate injury to underlying bones or nerves. |
| 28. Return to evaluate response to medication in 10 to 30 min. | IM medications absorb quickly; undesired effects may also develop rapidly. Observations determine efficacy of drug action. |
| 29. Chart medication dose, route, and site and time and date given in medication record. Correctly sign according to local policy. | Timely documentation prevents administration errors. |

### Subcutaneous (SC) Injections

SC injections involve placing medication into the loose connective tissue under the dermis (Procedure 31-2). Since SC tissue is not as richly supplied with blood as the muscles, drug absorption is somewhat slower than with IM injections. However, drugs are absorbed completely if circulatory status is normal. As SC tissue contain pain receptors, the person may experience some discomfort.

The optimum sites for SC injections include vascular areas around the outer aspect of the upper arms, the abdomen from below the costal margins to the iliac crests, and the anterior aspect of the thighs. These areas are easily accessible, especially for patients/clients with diabetes who self-administer insulin. The site most frequently recommended for heparin injections is the abdomen. The injection site chosen should be free of infection, skin lesions, scars, bony prominences, and large underlying muscles or nerves.

Only small doses (0.5–1 ml) of water-soluble medication should be given by the SC route. Subcutaneous tissue is sensitive to irritating solutions and large volumes of medication. Collecting of medication within the tissues can cause sterile abscesses, which appear as hardened, painful lumps under the skin.

Generally a 25-gauge needle inserted at a 90-degree angle (Fig. 31-6) deposits medication into the SC tissue of a normal-sized patient/client (Watson, 1988). If the individual is obese, pinch the tissue and use a needle long enough to insert through fatty tissue at the base of the skinfold.

A thin, cachectic individual may have insufficient tissue for SC injections; in this case the upper abdomen is the optimum site for injection.

### Intramuscular (IM) Injections

The IM route provides faster drug absorption than the SC route because of a muscle's greater vascularity. The danger of causing tissue damage is less when drugs enter deep muscle, but there is the risk of inadvertently injecting drugs directly into blood vessels. Use a longer and heavier-gauge needle to pass through SC tissue and penetrate deep muscle tissue (Procedure 31-2), but also consider the patient's/client's weight when selecting the needle size (blue or green). The angle of insertion for an IM injection is 90 degrees (see Fig. 31-6). Muscle is less sensitive to irritating and viscous drugs. A normal, well-developed person can safely tolerate as much as 3 ml of medication in larger-developed muscles such as the gluteal quadriceps or deltoids. Smaller muscles can tolerate only smaller amounts of medication without severe muscle discomfort. Children, older adults, and thin individuals tolerate less than 2 ml of medication. Wong (1995) recommends giving no more than 1 ml to small children and older infants.

Assess the integrity of the muscle before giving an injection. The muscle should be free of tenderness. Repeated injections in the same muscle cause considerable discomfort. By asking the person to relax, you can palpate the muscle to rule out the presence of hardened lesions. Normally a muscle feels soft when relaxed and firm when tense. You can minimize discomfort during an injection by helping the person assume a position that will help reduce the strain on the muscle.

## SITES

When selecting an IM site, consider the following questions:

- is the area free of infection or necrosis?
- are there local areas of bruising or abrasions?
- what is the location of underlying bones, nerves, and major blood vessels?
- what volume of medication is to be administered?

Each site has certain advantages and disadvantages (see box).

## TRACK METHOD

When irritating preparations (for example, iron) are given intramuscularly, the **track method** of injection minimizes tissue irritation by sealing the drug within the muscle tissues. Select the IM site, preferably in larger, deeper muscles such as the dorsogluteal muscle. A new needle must be applied to the syringe after preparing the drug so that no solution remains on the outside needle shaft. Pull the overlying skin and SC tissues approximately 2.5–3.5 cm laterally to the side. Holding the skin taut with the nondominant hand, inject the needle deep into the muscle. With practice you will learn to hold the syringe and aspirate with one hand. Inject the drug and air slowly, if there is no blood return on aspiration. The needle remains inserted for 10 seconds to allow the medication to disperse evenly. Release the skin after withdrawing the needle. This leaves a zigzag path that seals the needle track wherever tissue planes slide across each other (Fig. 31-7). The drug cannot escape from the muscle tissue.

## Intradermal (ID) Injections

Specially trained nurses can give ID injections for skin testing (for example, tuberculin screening and allergy tests) and for immunizations. These substances are potent. They are injected into the dermis, where the blood supply is reduced and drug absorption occurs slowly. A patient/client may have a severe anaphylactic reaction if the medications enter the circulation too rapidly. IV cortisone should be available in case of this.

## Intravenous (IV) Administration

Nurses with advanced training can administer drugs intravenously by the following methods:

- as mixtures within large volumes of IV fluids
- by injection of a bolus, or small volume, of medication through an existing IV infusion line or heparin lock
- by 'piggyback' **infusion** of a solution containing the prescribed drug and a small volume of IV fluid through an existing IV line.

In all three methods the person has an existing IV infusion line or an IV access site such as a heparin lock. In most institutions, policies and procedures list personnel who may give IV medications and the situations in which these may be given. These policies are based on the drug, capability and availability of staff, and the type of monitoring equipment available.

Administering drugs by the IV route has advantages. In

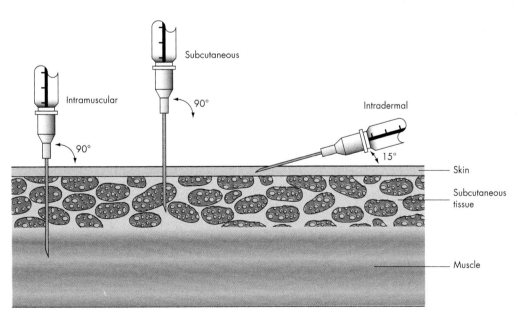

**Fig. 31-6** Comparison of the angles of insertion for IM (90 degrees), SC (90 degrees), and ID (15 degrees) injections.

## Characteristics of IM Sites

Vastus Lateralis Muscle
- This large, developed muscle lacks major nerves and blood vessels
- Rapid drug absorption occurs
  Dorsogluteal Muscle
- A deep site
- The nurse runs the risk of striking the underlying sciatic nerve, greater trochanter, or major blood vessels
- This site is not used with infants or children under 3 years of age due to underdeveloped muscle
- This site must be clean to avoid contamination
  Deltoid Muscle
- This site is easily accessible, but the muscle is not well developed in most patients/clients
- Nurses use this site for small amounts of medications
- The nurse avoids using the deltoid muscle in infants or children with underdeveloped muscles
- There is potential for injury to radial and ulnar nerves or brachial artery
- Less discomfort is felt in the deltoid, and this site is less likely to impair circulation

emergencies when a fast-acting drug must be delivered quickly, the IV route is the most desirable. The IV route is also the best when constant therapeutic blood levels must be established. Some medications are highly alkaline and irritating to muscle and SC tissue. Therefore giving these drugs intravenously causes less discomfort.

## LARGE-VOLUME INFUSIONS

Of the three methods of administering IV medications, mixing drugs in large volumes of fluids is the safest and easiest. Drugs are diluted in large volumes (500 ml or 1000 ml) of compatible IV fluids such as normal saline or Ringer-Lactate solution. In most institutions the pharmacist adds drugs to the primary container of IV solution to ensure asepsis. Because the drug is not in a concentrated form, the risk of side effects or fatal reactions is minimal. Vitamins and potassium chloride are two types of drugs commonly added to IV fluids. The danger with continuous infusion is that the person may suffer circulatory fluid overload if the IV fluid is infused too rapidly (see Chapter 18).

### Disposal of Equipment

After administering injections, it is imperative to properly dispose of used equipment. A stray needle can injure the patient/client, nurse, or other health care personnel. A needlestick injury can be the source of hepatitis or human immunodeficiency virus.

Infection control policy strongly recommends that needles

### Mental Health Nursing
### Self-medication

Many patients/clients in the mental health setting are not reliable with self-medication. Therefore, these individuals are given a slow-release drug which is suspended in an oily base and which is injected deep into muscle tissue. The medication can be given on a three-weekly to monthly basis.

should not be re-sheathed before disposal. Covering a needle may predispose the nurse to a needlestick injury. Discard the needle and syringe intact into clearly marked, appropriate containers (Fig. 31-8). Containers should be puncture- and leak-proof. Needles and plungers should *not* be broken. Never force a needle into a full needle disposal receptacle.

## APPLYING TOPICAL APPLICATIONS

### Skin Applications

Since many locally applied drugs such as lotions, pastes, transdermal patches, and ointments can create systemic and local effects, these drugs should be applied using gloves and applicators.

Skin encrustations and dead tissues harbour microorganisms and block contact of medications with the tissues to be treated. Simply applying new medications over previously applied drugs does little to prevent infection or offer therapeutic benefit. Before applying medications, clean the skin thoroughly by washing the area gently with soap and water.

When applying ointments or pastes, spread the medication on evenly, but not excessively, over the involved surface. Opaque ointments prevent visualization of underlying skin.

Each type of application, for example, ointment, lotion or powder should be applied as directed by the manufacturer to ensure proper penetration and absorption. During any skin application, first assess the skin thoroughly. Apply lotions and creams by smearing them lightly onto the skin's surface. Rubbing may cause irritation. A liniment is applied by rubbing it gently but firmly into the skin. A powder is dusted lightly to cover the affected area with a thin layer. To record administration, note the area applied, name of the medication, and condition of skin.

### Eye Applications

Many people receive prescribed ophthalmic drugs for eye conditions such as glaucoma and for treatment after procedures such as cataract extraction. A large percentage of patients/clients receiving eye medication are older adults. Age-related problems, including poor vision, hand tremors, and difficulty in grasping or manipulating containers, affect the ease with which older adults can self-administer eye medications. It is important to teach patients/clients and family members about the following proper techniques for administering eye medications:

1. The cornea of the eye is richly supplied with pain fibres and thus is very sensitive to anything applied to it; therefore, avoid instilling any form of eye medication directly onto the cornea.
2. The risk of transmitting infection from one eye to the other is high; therefore, avoid touching the eyelids or other eye structures with eye droppers or ointment tubes.
3. Use eye medication only for the affected eye.
4. Never allow a person to use another person's eye medications.

### Ear Instillations

Internal ear structures are very sensitive to temperature extremes. Failure to instil ear drops or irrigating fluid at room temperature may cause vertigo (severe dizziness) or nausea. Although the structures of the outer ear are not sterile, it is wise to use sterile

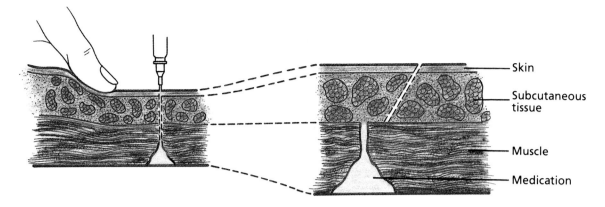

Skin
Subcutaneous tissue
Muscle
Medication

**Fig. 31-7** The track method of injection prevents the deposit of medication through sensitive tissues.

drops and solutions in case the eardrum is ruptured. Entrance of nonsterile solutions into middle ear structures could result in infection. With ear drainage, check with the doctor to ensure that the patient/client does not have a ruptured eardrum. Never occlude the ear canal with the dropper or irrigating syringe. Forcing medication into an occluded ear canal creates pressure that may injure the eardrum.

The external ear structures of children are different from those of adults. When instilling drops or irrigating the canal, straighten the ear canal. In infants and young children straighten the cartilaginous canal by grasping the pinna of the ear and pulling it gently *down* and backward. In adults the ear canal is longer and composed of underlying bone and is straightened by pulling the auricle *upward* and backward. Failure to straighten the canal properly may prevent medicinal solutions from reaching the deeper external ear structures.

## Nasal Instillations

Individuals with nasal sinus alterations may receive drugs by spray, drops, or gauze packs. The most commonly administered form of nasal instillation is decongestant spray or drops, which are used to relieve symptoms of sinus congestion and colds. Patients/clients must be cautioned to avoid overuse because it can lead to a rebound effect in which the nasal congestion worsens. When excess decongestant solution is swallowed, serious systemic effects may also develop, especially in children. Saline drops are safer as a decongestant for children than nasal preparations.

It is easier to have the patient/client self-administer sprays. With the head tilted back, the patient/client holds the tip of the container just inside the nares. The person inhales as the spray enters the nasal passages. For patients/clients who use nasal sprays repeatedly, check the nares for irritation. In children, nasal sprays should be given with the head in an upright position so that excess spray will drip anteriorly from the nostrils and not be swallowed.

## Vaginal Instillations

Vaginal medications are available as pessaries, foam, jellies, or creams. Pessaries come individually packaged in foil wrappers. Storage in a refrigerator prevents the solid, oval-shaped pessaries from melting. After a pessary is inserted into the vaginal cavity, body temperature causes it to melt and be distributed and absorbed. Foam, jellies, and creams are administered with an inserter or applicator. A pessary is given with a gloved hand. Patients/clients often prefer administering their own vaginal medications and should be given privacy. After instillation, patients/clients may wish to wear sanitary pads to collect excess drainage. Because vaginal medications are frequently given to treat infection, any discharge may be foul smelling. An aseptic technique should be followed, and patients/clients should be offered frequent opportunities to maintain perineal hygiene (see Chapter 25).

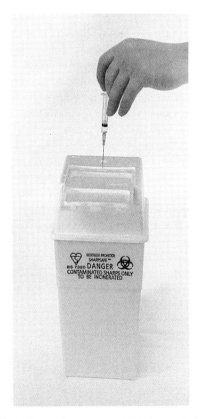

**Fig. 31-8** Special containers are available in nursing units for the disposal of contaminated syringes. *Photograph © Bruce Bailey, Select Photos London.*

### Rectal Instillations

Rectal suppositories differ in shape from vaginal pessaries; they are thinner and bullet shaped (Procedure 31-3). The rounded end prevents anal trauma during insertion. Rectal suppositories contain medications that exert local effects, such as promoting defaecation, or systemic effects, such as reducing nausea.

During administration, place the suppository past the internal anal sphincter and against the rectal mucosa, otherwise the suppository may be expelled before it can melt and be absorbed into the mucosa. With practice, you will learn to recognize the sensation of the sphincter relaxing around the finger. The suppository should not be forced into a mass of faecal material. It may be necessary to clear the rectum with a disposable cleansing enema before a suppository can be inserted. Some drugs may be given in a retention enema, for example prednisolone.

## ADMINISTERING DRUGS BY INHALATION

Drugs administered with hand-held inhalers are dispersed through an aerosol spray, mist, or powder that penetrates lung airways (see guidelines overleaf). The alveolar-capillary network absorbs medications rapidly. Metered-dose inhalers (MDIs) are usually designed to deliver medications that produce local effects such as bronchodilation. The advantage of MDIs is that drugs can be delivered into the airways in high concentrations and systemic side effects are usually avoided. The major disadvantage of MDI therapy is that training and skill are required to coordinate activation of the metered-dose inhaler with inhalation of the drug (Mellins, 1989).

Patients/clients who receive drugs by inhalation frequently suffer chronic respiratory disease such as chronic asthma, emphysema, or bronchitis. Drugs given by inhalation provide these patients/clients with control of airway obstruction, and because these clients depend on medications for disease control, they must learn about them and their safe administration (see guidelines).

### Nebulizers

A nebulizer relies on the power of compressed gas through a liquid solution of drug to spray it as a mist. Prescribed oxygen or air are the gases used. The drug will travel from the nebulizer chamber on a face mask to the patients/clients mouth and nose, from where it is inhaled. This method of inhalation is particularly effective for individuals who have difficulty in using metered inhalers due to severe dyspnoea, such as that experienced in an acute asthma attack. It is very useful in infants and small children.

## IRRIGATIONS

Medications may be used to irrigate or wash out a body cavity and are delivered through a stream of solution. Irrigations are most commonly performed with sterile water, saline, or antiseptic solutions on the eye, ear, throat, vagina, and urinary tract. When there is a break in the skin or mucosa, use aseptic technique to perform an irrigation. When the cavity to be irrigated is not sterile, as in the case with the ear canal, vagina, or eye, clean technique is acceptable. Sterile solutions may be used. An irrigation can be used to cleanse an area or apply a medication or heat or cold to injured tissue. When performing irrigations, follow these principles:

- avoid further injury to tissue
- prevent the transmission of infection
- maintain the patient's/client's comfort.

## SUMMARY

The nurse is responsible for safely and effectively ordering, storing and administering medications, which requires understanding of legal guidelines affecting drug prescription and administration. The nurse's care of patients/clients also involves making decisions about the need for drug therapy.

The nurse must have detailed knowledge about a drug being used and the patient/client receiving it. A thorough assessment of the patient's/client's physical condition, medical history, allergies, diet, and medication history ensures that accurate judgements are made about drug therapy.

Preparation of medication requires accurate calculation and a methodical approach. Application of physiological, anatomical, and aseptic principles ensures safe administration of drugs. When monitoring a response to medications, the nurse uses physical assessment skills and knowledge of expected drug effects. The nurse also teaches patients/clients and families to administer drugs safely and to follow schedules for drug therapy. A patient's/client's well-being depends on the nurse's application of all the principles of drug administration.

## CHAPTER 31 REVIEW

### Key Concepts

- Learning drug classifications improves the understanding of nursing implications for administering drugs with similar characteristics.
- Nurse practice acts define and set limits on the scope of a nurse's professional functions and responsibilities in giving medications.
- All controlled substances are handled according to strict procedures that account for each drug.
- Apply understanding of the physiological action of drug action when timing administration, selecting routes, initiating actions to promote drug efficacy, and observing responses to drugs.
- Patients/clients with alterations in organs that metabolize or excrete drugs are at risk for drug toxicity.
- The older adult's body undergoes structural and functional changes that alter drug actions and influence the manner in which nurses provide drug therapy.
- Children's drug dosages are calculated on the basis of body surface area.
- Repeated doses or intravenous infusion of a drug are required to achieve constant therapeutic blood levels.

## PROCEDURE 31-2 Giving Rectal Suppositories

| SEQUENCE OF ACTIONS | RATIONALE |
|---|---|
| 1. Inform the patient/client of the intended activity and explain the procedure. | To obtain consent and cooperation and reduce anxiety of patient/client during the procedure (Wilson-Barnett 1978). |
| 2. Offer the patient/client the opportunity to empty bladder. | A full bladder can cause discomfort during the procedure. |
| 3. Collect appropriate equipment: | |
| (i) one or two suppositories as prescribed | |
| (ii) lubricating jelly | Eases introduction of suppository by reducing friction. |
| (iii) waterproof incontinence pad | To protect bedclothes and prevent soiling. |
| (iv) toilet tissue and gauze squares | To maintain patient's/client's personal hygiene. |
| (v) disposable gloves. | Prevents transmission of microorganisms from faeces and reduces risk of cross-infection. |
| 4. Pull curtains around the patient's/client's bed or close the door. | To provide privacy and reduce embarrassment. |
| 5. With the patient/client on the bed, arrange clothing so that hips and buttocks are exposed. Place an incontinence pad under the patient/client then cover with a blanket so that only rectal area is exposed. | Provides warmth, prevents embarrassment, demonstrates concern for dignity and helps reduce anxiety. Prevents faecal soiling of clothing and bedlinen. |
| 6. Position the patient/client on the left side with the buttocks near the edge of the bed and the right knee well flexed. | Flexing the knee permits easier insertion |
| 7. Wash hands thoroughly, dry, and put on disposable gloves. | Reduces risk of cross infection through faecal contamination. |
| 8. Squeeze lubricating jelly onto gauze swab and lubricate blunt end of the suppository. | Eases insertion into the anus and prevents trauma to the rectal mucosa (NB systemic effect suppositories should be inserted blunt end first to maximize effect) (Walker, 1982). |
| 9. Ask the patient/client to breathe slowly and deeply through the mouth while suppositories are inserted. | Promotes relaxation of external anal sphincter and facilitates introduction. |
| 10. Administer suppositories by separating buttocks and introducing them one at a time, inserting at least 4 cm. | Suppositories are inserted beyond anal canal into rectum. |
| 11. Gently wipe dry the patient's/client's anus with gauze or toilet tissue. | Prevents irritation/excoriation of the perianal area and promotes patient/client comfort and cleanliness. |
| 12. a. Ask patient/client to remain in bed and retain suppository for 10–15 minutes. b. If suppositories with a systemic action are given, alter instructions for retention time according to prescription. | Longer retention promotes more effective stimulation of peristalsis and defaecation as suppository will melt. Retention for the appropriate time will ensure systemic effects are maximized. |
| 13. Discard used gloves into the appropriate disposable bag | To prevent accidental cross-infection through faecal contamination. |
| 14. Provide call bell for patient/client. Check that toilet is available or bring a bedpan/commode to bedside. If necessary, assist patient/client to use toilet facilities. | Access to appropriate facilities prevents accidental soiling and decreases anxiety. |
| 15. Note and record in nursing notes character of stool passed. | Communicates relevant information to other health team members and provides a record of bowel function. |
| 16. Assist patient/client to meet personal hygiene needs and rearrange clothing if required. | Faeces are irritant to the skin. Promotes feelings of cleanliness and maintainance of dignity. |

**Guidelines for helping and teaching patients/clients to use metered dose inhalers.**

• Check the person's name (and identification number), drug, dosage and times of administration with the medical prescription.

• Explain and demonstrate how the canister fits into the inhaler.

• Assess the person's ability to comfortably hold and manipulate the inhaler (see illustration A).

• Ask the patient/client to sit as upright as possible, to breathe out, then place the mouthpiece of the inhaler into the mouth (see illustration B). Then, while inhaling slowly, to press down on the top of the inhaler thus releasing the medication.

• Ask the patient/client to hold his or her breath for approximately 10 seconds, or to breathe slowly, as recommended for the individual person, drug or inhaler.

• Ensure that the patient/client understands any special precautions (for example, waiting time between the inhalation of different drugs) and any medication side effects.

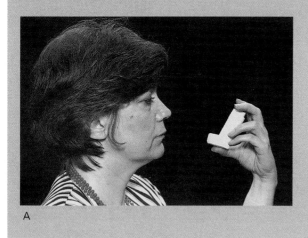

A

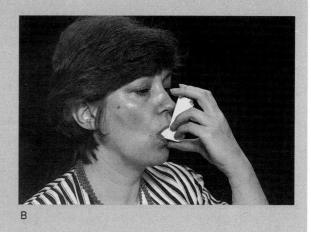

B

• Drugs given parenterally are absorbed more quickly than drugs administered by other routes.
• Each drug order should include the patient's/client's name, order date, drug name, dosage, route and frequency of administration, and doctor's signature.
• A teaching plan for drug therapy should include guidelines for drug safety.
• The 'five rights' of drug administration ensure accurate preparation and administration of drug dosages.
• Nurses administer only those medications they prepare.
• Never administer a drug without accurately identifying a patient/client.
• Drugs should be charted and signed for immediately after administration.
• Report a drug error immediately.
• When preparing medications, check the drug container label against the drug prescription.
• Never leave a prepared medication unattended.
• Rotate injection sites when giving repeated parenteral administrations.
• Failure to select injection sites by anatomical landmarks may lead to tissue, bone, or nerve damage.

## CRITICAL THINKING EXERCISES

1. During your placement in a mental health setting what aspects of intra- and interpersonal skills did you observe in a nurse who persuaded a patient/client who was refusing to accept his or her medication?

2. You are preparing to give a parenteral injection of preoperative atropine. You check the prescription and calculate the dose. You note that your calculations result in a 3-ml dose. You recognize that this is an excessive dose, and you recalculate the dose and obtain the same answer. You check the dose information against the doctor's order and confirm that the order is excessive. You verify this information with the nurse in charge, who says 'The prescription is correct'. What action do you take at this point?

3. When preparing to give a controlled drug to your patient/client you observe that the number remaining indicated for that particular drug is wrong. What do you do?

4. You need to give an injectable pain medication to a

patient/client with metastatic cancer. The patient's/client's pain increases with change of position, the person is cachexic, and is receiving multiple injections. What information do you need to prepare the medication, the syringe, and the needle and to determine the site of injection?

## Key Terms

Absorption, p. 645
Allergic reaction, p. 647
Anaphylactic reaction, p. 647
Bioavailability, p. 644
Biotransformation, p. 646
Constant therapeutic concentration, p. 647
Contraindication, p. 656
Controlled drugs, p. 643
Drug interaction, p. 647
Drug misuse/abuse, p. 644
Generic name, p. 654
Non-compliance, p. 659
Pharmacokinetics, p. 644
Plasma concentration, p. 647
Plasma half-life, p.647
Prescribed dose, p. 652
Side effects, p. 645
Synergistic effect, p. 647
Therapeutic effect, p. 646
Toxic (effects), p. 647

## REFERENCES

Bliss MR: Prescribing for the elderly, *BMJ* 283:203, 1981.

Eliopoulos C: Geriatric pharmacology. In Eliopoulos C: *Gerontological Nurs,* ed 2, Philadelphia, 1987, Lippincott.

London and Thames Valley Pharmaceutical Group: *Focus on Medicines,* newsletter in conference, *Can We Afford the Elderly?* London, December, 1989.

Mellins RB: Patient education is key to successful management of asthma, *J Respir Dis* 10:8 S47 (suppl), 1989.

Petrosin BM et al: Implications of selected problems with nasoenteral tube feedings, *Crit Care Nurs Q* 12:1, 1989.

Quilligan S: Tablets to take away: why some old people fail to comply with their medication, *Prof Nurs* Aug, 1990.

Ractoo S, Bamber J: Testing times, *Nurs Mirror* 153(24):26, 1983.

Royal College of Physicians: Medication for the elderly: a report by the Royal College of Physicians, *J of RCP Lond,* 18:7, 1984.

Simonson W: *Medications and the elderly: a guide for promoting proper use,* Rockville, Md, 1984, Aspen.

Trounce JR: *Clinical pharmacology for nurses,* Edinburgh, 1988, Churchill Livingstone.

United Kingdom Central Council for Nursing, Midwifery and Health Visiting: *Standards for the administration of medicines,* London, 1992, UKCC.

Walker R: Suppository insertion, *World Med* 18:58, 1982.

Watson JE, Royle JA: *Watson's medical–surgical nursing and related physiology,* ed 3, London, 1988, Balliére Tindall.

Wilson-Barnett J: Patients' emotional responses to barium x-rays *J Adv Nurs* 3(1):37, 1978.

Wong DL: *Nursing care of infants and children,* ed 5, St Louis, 1995, Mosby.

## FURTHER READING

### Adult Nursing

Hawkins: *Drugs and pregnancy,* Edinburgh, 1987, Churchill Livingstone.

Heenan A: Side effects of drugs: monitoring adverse reactions, *Nurs Times* 85(39):25, 1989.

Joshua A, King T (eds): *Guy's hospital 1995–96 nursing drug reference,* London, 1994, Mosby.

Kolcaba K, Miller CA: Geropharmacology treatment, *J Gerontol Nurs* 15:29, 1989.

Laurence: *Clinical pharmacology,* Edinburgh, 1992, Churchill Livingstone.

McPherson ML: Medicating the elderly in home health care, *Home Health Care Pract* 2:16, 1989.

Neal MJ: *Medical pharmacology at a glance,* Oxford, 1992, Blackwell Scientific Publishers.

Smith F, Ross F: Principles of drug therapy, *Commun Outlook* February:25, 1992.

Smith F, Ross F: Prescribing topical agents, *Commun Outlook* July:29, 1992.

### Children's Nursing

Beecroft PC, Redick S: Possible complications of intramuscular injections on the paediatric unit, *Pediatr Nurs* 15:333, 1989.

Glasper A, Oliver RW: A simple guide to infant drug calculations, *Nurs* 22:649, 1984.

Holmes, A, Davidson LF: Sugar-free medicine: a lost opportunity? *Br Dental J* 163:240, 1987.

Hurrel F: Choosing inhaler devices for children with asthma, *Paed Nurs* 5(7):22, 1993.

Insley J: *A paediatric vade mecum,* Birmingham, 1990, Edward Arnold.

Jerrett M: Taking the ouch out of injections, *Can Nurs* 79(1):24, 1983.

Kendrick R: Giving intravenous therapy at home, *Paed Nurs* 5(1):22, 1993.

Mason G: Medicine round, *Paed Nurs* 3(3):1, 1993.

Royal College of Nursing: *Drug administration : a nursing responsibility,* London, 1987, RCN.

Webb C et al: Patient controlled analgesia as post operative pain treatment for children, *J Paed Nurs* 4(3):163, 1989.

### Learning Disabilities Nursing

Manley G, Sheiham A, Eadsforth W: Sugar-coated care? *Nurs Times,* 90(7):34, 1994.

Society of Mental Handicap Nursing: *Medication and people with a mental handicap,* London, 1988, Royal College of Nursing.

### Mental Health Nursing

Healy D: *Psychiatric drugs explained,* London, 1993, Mosby.

Ritter SAH: *Bethlem Royal and Maudsley Hospital manual of clinical psychiatric nursing principles and procedures,* London, 1989, Harper and Row, Chapter 35 and 37.

# Complementary Therapies

## CHAPTER OUTLINE

## LEARNING OUTCOMES

After studying this chapter, you should be able to:
- *Define the key terms listed.*
- *Discuss the availability of complementary therapy and describe the extent to which it is currently integrated with orthodox nursing care.*
- *Describe 10 of the most commonly used therapies, using correct terminology to express the central concepts of each.*
- *Relate the major therapies currently used to legal and political issues surrounding their use.*
- *Discuss the cultural philosophies which underpin particular therapies.*
- *Discuss the ways in which nursing care is supported by the use of therapeutic interventions.*
- *Relate costs of complementary therapies to other interventions.*
- *Discuss the disadvantages of using a variety of therapeutic interventions.*
- *Identify the nurse's role as patient/client advocate in his or her choice of complementary therapy.*
- *Apply the UKCC Code of Conduct to the concept of accountability in the use of complementary therapies.*

Hardly a day passes without a health care professional suggesting that either a patient/client or, more interestingly, a member of the clinical team would benefit from some method of relaxation, such as massage, acupressure, or aromatherapy. This reflects the present shift away from the orthodox system of medical diagnosis and cure, to a system of individual choice. Several theorists have discussed possible reasons for society's change in attitude and the revision of practices by the medical and nursing professions (Pietroni, 1990; Fulder, 1989; Lewith and Aldridge, 1990). According to a 1990 Mori & Mintel Public Opinion Poll, 75% of the respondents wished to see complementary therapies freely available on the NHS. In response to public and professional interest in complementary therapies, the government established the Special Health Committee to determine ways in which the National Health Service is supporting the integration of complementary and supplementary therapies into its daily services.

Several studies have demonstrated nurses' increased interest in complementary therapies and the additional training they have undertaken in order to expand their clinical role and integrate the therapies into nursing care (Rankin-Box, 1989; Rankin-Box, 1992). As more nurses adopt these practices, there is a greater need for standardization in courses training complementary therapists. Any nurse practising complementary therapies must adhere to the UKCC Code of Professional Conduct. There are many professional, political and ethical issues to be considered when offering these therapies as a part of daily nursing care. Also there is a need to explore the issues of accountability and advocacy that concern the health care professional and patient/client in receipt of care.

## Useful Addresses

### Aromatherapy

Aromatherapy Organisations Council, 3 Latymer Close, Braybrooke, Market Harborough, Leicester LE16 8LN.

International Federation of Aromatherapists, c/o Department of Continuing Education, The Royal Masonic Hospital, London W6 0TN.

The International Society of Professional Aromatherapists, 41 Leicester Road, Hinckley, Leicester LE10 1LW.

### Chiropractic

British Chiropractic Association, 29 Whitley Street, Reading, Berkshire RG2 0EG.

### Herbalism

National Institute of Medical Herbalists, 9 Palace Gate, Exeter, Devon EX1 1JA.

British Herbal Medicine Association, PO Box 304, Bournemouth, Dorset BH7 6JZ.

### Homeopathy

The Society of Homeopaths, 2 Artizan Road, Northampton NN1 4HU.

The British Homeopathic Association, 27a Devonshire Street, London W1N 1RJ.

The British Institute of Homeopathy, Victor House, Norris Road, Staines, Middlesex TW18 4DS.

The Faculty of Homeopathy, The Royal London Homeopathic Hospital, Great Ormond Street, London WC1N 3HR.

The Register and Council of Homeopathy and UK Homeopathic Medical Association, 243 The Broadway, Southall, Middlesex UB1 3AN.

### Hypnosis

The Institute of Complementary Medicine, PO Box 194, London SE16 1QZ.

### Naturopathy

The British Naturopathic Association, Frazer House, London NW3 5RR

### Osteopathy

The British and European Osteopathic Association, c/o 15 Station Road, Sidcup, Kent DA15 7EN.

British Osteopathic Association, 8–10 Boston Place, London NW1 6QH.

### Reflexology

The British Reflexology Association, 12 Pond Road, London SE3 9JL.

Association of Reflexologists, 27 Old Gloucester Street, London WC1 3XX.

### Therapeutic Massage

The British Massage Therapy Council, c/o 9 Elm Road, Worthing, West Sussex.

### Therapeutic Touch

The Didsbury Trust, Sherbourne Cottage, Litton, near Bath, Avon BA3 4PS.

Because complementary or alternative therapies developed from the basis of different belief systems, individuals who do not subscribe to these beliefs may find these approaches unacceptable. Beliefs that may be particularly offensive to some people might be the life force to others and how this influences health. Nurses should never assume that patients/clients will automatically welcome complementary practices. It is vital to ensure fully informed consent as described in Chapter 13.

Many schools, colleges, registration councils and referral agencies can provide information about complementary therapies to professionals and to patients/clients (see box).

## EVOLUTION OF COMPLEMENTARY THERAPIES

What factors have influenced this renewed interest in complementary therapies? The economic and political influences of the last few decades have changed health care service and delivery. Although economic pressures have created a health care system that now provides a more organized approach to health care and its delivery, this system sometimes also neglects the importance of the needs of the individual seeking health care. Thus, some people seek an individualized approach to health care through complementary therapies. In addition, improved standards of living and improved health education have enabled individuals to become health care 'consumers' who can be informed about their health and health care. Some of these consumers have begun to seek alternative treatments to those provided by conventional health care; for example, as an alternative to conventional medical care which may have failed, or to avoid taking conventional medications which may cause undesirable side effects. Thirdly, the increasing number of people from various cultures and economic environments living in the UK have varying health care attitudes and needs (see Chapter 8) which are not always met by the current medical system (Pietroni, 1990).

### The Development of Holism and Holistic Caregiving

The nursing profession in the UK has historically embraced holistic caregiving in the definition of nursing care. The mind-body-spirit potential of holistic caring has been an overriding feature of the evolving nursing culture in the UK and in many other countries (Orem, 1991; Riehl and Roy, 1980). The modern nurse's role in the management of care, including involving the patient/client in his or her own health and well-being, has been extensively developed in a variety of nursing theories (Reihl and Roy, 1980; Henderson, 1966; Orem, 1991; McFarlane, 1986). Florence Nightingale supported the following philosophy of nursing care:

> Pathology teaches the harm that disease has done. But it teaches nothing more. We know nothing of the principle of health, the positive of which pathology is the negative, except from observation and experience. And nothing but observation and experience will teach us the ways to maintain or to bring back the state of health. It is often thought that medicine is the curative process. There is no such thing; medicine is the surgery of functions, as surgery proper is that of limbs and organs. Neither can do anything but remove obstructions; neither can cure; nature alone cures .... And what nursing has to do in either case, is to put the patient in the best condition for nature to act upon him (Nightingale, 1860).

Several studies have been undertaken in which a duality of treatments and care initiatives have been developed for patients/clients. For example, the Hoxton Health Group (Kettle, 1993), a care provider for an inner city area of East London, provides a combination of acupuncture, chiropractic, herbal medicine, osteopathy, massage and shiatsu. In an effort to meet the needs of the local community, the therapy clinics have become part of a successful group development of interdisciplinary collaboration and direct management. They have close links with local health services and are included in health service audits and quality evaluations. This type of interdisciplinary therapeutic care is considered to be the way forward in health-care delivery. Since there has not been significant time for complementary therapies to be tested and developed in conjunction with, or separately to, orthodox medical treatments, it is difficult to assess the effectiveness of these collaborative efforts.

## AVAILABILITY OF COMPLEMENTARY THERAPIES

Approximately 5% of the population seeks treatment from a complementary therapist each year; but despite the availability of such therapies, few people receive this treatment within the NHS (Lewith and Aldridge, 1990; NAHAT, 1993).

Presently, the main therapies require regulation and formal incorporation into the NHS. Homeopathy (see p. 681) is presently available in six NHS hospitals, and several hospitals have incorporated acupuncture as one of a variety of therapies available to patients/clients in pain clinics. The Royal Marsden Hospital, for example, employs a specialist nurse to provide therapeutic massage and aromatherapy. This has been incorporated into care services, since research has demonstrated that stress combined with a learned personal response may be involved in the induction and progress of cancer (Conference:'Cancer and the Mind' London, February, 1990). In 1993, the National Association of Health Authorities and Trusts recommended a critical review of the effectiveness and appropriate use of complementary therapies in the NHS be undertaken (NAHAT, 1993). A research and development strategy is still to be developed as a result of this review.

There is a demand for approved educational courses on complementary therapies, to provide objective information about the nature of different therapies, their effectiveness, appropriate

**Mental Health Nursing**
**Use of complementary therapies**

**Dance and body movement** is not a new phenomenon and its healing properties have been recognized for centuries. Dance/movement therapy is the psychotherapeutic use of movement to enhance the emotional and physical integration of the individual. The dance therapist focuses on movement, positive breathing and interaction, and thereby complements the therapeutic flow of words with a more immediate flow of movement.
**Transcendental meditation** is concerned with the development and maintenance of perfect mental and physical health. In transcendental meditation, the meditator allows his or her attention to turn within, enabling the mind to sink to a resting state and the emotional state to become quieter.

uses, potential complications, training standards and legal implications. Yet, there are major difficulties in researching complementary therapies because appropriate research methods have not been developed and associated quality of care criteria have not yet been established.

The Institute of Complementary Medicine has established the British Register of Complementary Practitioners — a statutory body that will define the training criteria which conform to EC directives, and which will establish qualification criteria for membership on the British Register.

## Use of Therapies in the United Kingdom and European Community

Although statutory requirements for education and training in all therapies are mandatory, the UK has yet to implement its interpretation of EC education and training directives (see p. 686). The suggested duration of training for complementary health practitioners is three years. This is to facilitate the establishment of a European standard that can also be interpreted locally, so complementary practitioners can travel and trade within the EC, as do nurses, doctors and midwives (Lewith and Aldridge, 1990; Buchan, 1992; Fulder, 1989).

Currently, all complementary therapy practitioners in the UK can practise if they have qualifications obtained from any course. Some of these practitioners may not have a sufficient level of skill or competence, since there is little national vocational qualification (NVQ) work available in these areas. Osteopaths are the exception; in 1993, Parliament passed a bill to regulate their training and practice, implemented in 1995 (The Osteopath's Bill, 1993).

## PHILOSOPHICAL AND PHYSIOLOGICAL BASIS OF THERAPEUTIC INTERVENTIONS

To attempt an exact definition of complementary therapies would be unrealistic. Several types of therapies are available:
* **ancient**, such as acupuncture
* **modern**, such as biofeedback
* **curative**, such as naturopathy
* **allopathic symptomatology**, such as homeopathy and medical herbalism
* those that avoid all artificial aid, such as nature cure.

It is possible to distinguish the pathways of conventional medicine and complementary medicine based upon their philosophical focuses. For example, conventional medicine has developed through a theoretical and practical model that uses a dynamic interventionist approach to alleviate suffering by controlling *symptoms* of disease processes diagnosed through pathology. Complementary, or *alternative* or *supplementary* therapeutic medicines, view symptoms as having accumulated over time and through mismanagement of health-related behaviour or lifestyle. These therapies therefore recruit the *self-healing* capacities of the body by amplifying the natural recuperative processes and by augmenting the energies upon which the individual's health depends. They relate 'directly to an

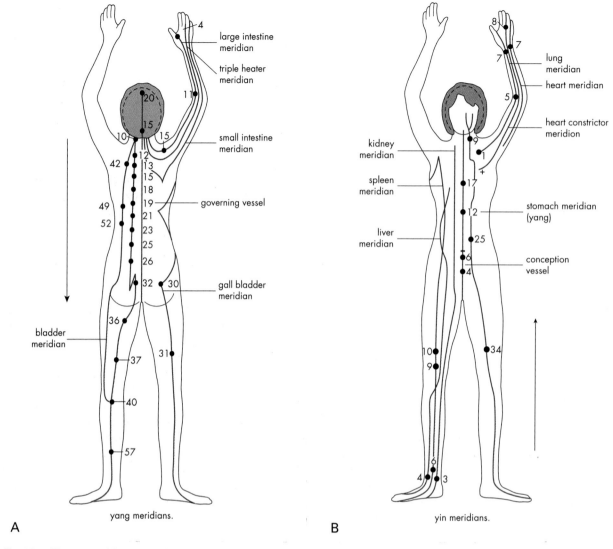

**Fig. 32-1** There are 12 basic meridians which are named after the organs or function to which they are attached. A, Six are predominatly Yin: heart, heart protector, spleen, lungs, kidney and liver (understood as organs of storage); B, six are predominantly Yang: small intestine, triple heater, stomach, colon, bladder and gall bladder (organs of activity).

adaptation process to promote a harmony with that person's surroundings' (Fulder, 1989).

## The Influence of Ancient Philosophies and Systems of Medicine

Most of the complementary therapies discussed in this chapter have evolved from the philosophies and systems of medicines in ancient cultures. One of the most influential is the traditional Chinese system of medicine. Traditional Chinese medicine uses herbs, diet and exercise, and acupuncture to prevent and treat disease. The philosophy underlying this system is opposite to that of the West. It is derived from the 'Law of Nature' and in particular the 'Rules of the Universe', in which life is activated by **Chi**, or a vital life, or energy, force. Chi pervades all things and, in humans, this energy is derived partly from heredity and partly from the environment. As long as the Chi is flowing freely through the body, then health is maintained in balance with

nature. Many Chinese practise **T'ai-chi**, a set of exercises designed to promote the free flow of Chi and thus prevent disease.

One of the main tenets of traditional Chinese medicine is that humans are regarded as 'whole beings'; that is, as an indivisible combination of mind, body and spirit, in which it is impossible to treat one aspect without affecting the others. The person is also seen as being an inextricable part of the environment. Disease is interpreted as originating within the individual (internal) or as being derived from the environment (external). Since emotions are part of the holistic view of the individual, emotional problems can be traced to a physical origin and physical symptoms can be traced to emotional origins. The process of diagnosis emphasizes the individual's ability to cope with internal and external factors, and the quality of the person's Chi is vital for the prognosis.

When diagnosing illness, the Chinese consider the impact of *natural* forces on the individual, and the balance that is achieved between **Yin** and **Yang**, the opposing forces in each person (Fig.

32-1). Yin represents a person's 'female' aspects, which the ancient Chinese believed to be coldness, darkness, passivity, inwardness, and negativity. Yang represents a person's 'male' aspects. Traditionally, these are warmth, light, activity, expressivity, and positivity. The organs of the body are accorded yin and yang features; for example, empty/full; hot/cold; excess/deficiency and interior/exterior. These are used to define signs that are discovered by using the four stages of diagnosis (also called the *Four Examinations* ) — looking; listening and smelling (together as they are the same word in Chinese); asking; and palpating.

## THE MOST COMMONLY PRACTISED THERAPIES

The following descriptions provide a general overview of some of the most commonly practised complementary therapies in the UK.

### Acupuncture

**Background**: The ancient Chinese practice of **acupuncture** is based on a series of **meridians** (pathways of energy) in the body which are mapped to 'flow' from the head towards the feet or hands, and return to the head. They connect with the inner organs (see Fig. 32-1) and constitute channels through which energy can pass. In 3000 BC, the Chinese noticed that soldiers wounded by arrows sometimes recovered from diseases that had been troubling them for years. The Chinese thus developed a system of medicine which cured some diseases by penetrating the skin at specific points. This system is based on the principle that in all diseases (physical and psychological) there are tender areas at certain points of the body **(acupuncture points)**, which disappear when the disease is cured. The Chinese believed that any reversible disease could be cured with acupuncture.

Acupuncture can be applied in two ways — to *stimulate* energy release or to *gather* energy from the meridians. To **tonify** (stimulate the acupuncture points), needles are inserted into the recognized points on a pathway for approximately 30 seconds. To disperse the energy, needles are then inserted for between 10 and 60 minutes. There is normally no blood loss. Some special needles may be left in place under a plaster for up to three weeks, according to requirements. Treatment is often followed by dietary and lifestyle advice for the individual. The treatment may be repeated until relief is obtained.

**Physiological basis for action**: Therapeutic acupuncture utilizes processes (meridians and the flow of energy) which have so far defied measurement by modern scientific instruments. However, there has been investigation into the nature of the meridians and acupuncture points. These points are known to be areas of low electrical resistance on the skin, and this resistance can now be measured (Bergsman and Woolley-Hart, 1973; Voll, 1975; Vincent and Mole, 1989). Research reveals that acupuncture stimulates the release of **endorphins** (the body's own analgesic) in the brain and provides long-term pain relief (Stanway, 1982). Other chemical messengers in the brain, such as serotonin, which have a profound effect on well-being, are also known to be involved. **Kirlian electrophotography** (a system of high energy photography that records the 'vitality' of living things, including the energy fields of the meridian lines) reveals the meridians clearly, and also the changes that occur after acupuncture treatment. There is extensive research literature on therapeutic acupuncture. Successful treatment with acupuncture has been reported frequently in China and the Far East and occasionally in the West. However, additional trials need to be conducted under strictly controlled, double-blind conditions (Weigant *et al*, 1991).

**Contraindications:** Acupuncture should not be used to treat undiagnosed pain, any type of infection, cancer, or conditions requiring emergency treatment. This treatment should not be used to treat pregnant women (except as an anaesthetic during delivery) because stimulating energy flow may induce premature labour.

**Current uses**: Traditional, Chinese-trained practitioners often use acupuncture in conjunction with herbal treatment to treat a variety of disorders, including infectious diseases, forms of paralysis, migraine, shingles, hypertension, insomnia, hay fever, and irritable bowel syndrome. Today, sterilization of acupuncture needles is mandatory, to prevent hepatitis and AIDS. The needles may be destroyed after use unless each patient/client prefers to use the same needles until the end of his or her course of treatment (Grange, 1990).

**Training requirements**: Training to administer acupuncture can take many years. Course lengths vary. Individuals who have medical or nursing qualifications can obtain a licentiate to practise, using Western Diagnosis, after one year of study. A higher qualification may be obtained after three years of study.

Individuals who have no previous medical qualifications may obtain a licentiate after three years of study. They may obtain a higher qualification after two years of part-time study while practising acupuncture.

### Acupressure

**Background: Acupressure** also follows the philosophy of Oriental diagnosis and treatment. It is an ancient Japanese therapy which arose spontaneously with, but independently from, acupuncture. For nurses, acupressure may be a more easily adaptable form of helping the patient/client, who may not appreciate the connotations of 'needles' in a clinical setting.

**Physiological basis for action**: Acupressure works on the same basis as acupuncture, but without the needles. Its purpose is to stimulate the body's own recuperative powers. During treatment, pressure is applied with the fingers to sensitive areas on the body, along the energy meridians. The pressure is sustained for an interval of 3 seconds to 5 minutes. It is believed that this procedure removes energy blockages and fatigue by diffusing the lactic acid and carbon monoxide that accumulates in muscle tissue. When all pathways (meridians) are open and energy flow is unhindered, the body's energy is balanced, thus promoting good health.

**Contraindications**: There have been no reported adverse effects of acupressure. However, the treatment should be used with caution in pregnant women, to avoid inducing premature labour or abortion. It should also be used cautiously on people who have a skin condition or an acute infectious disease.

Acupressure experts do not recommend working in areas of tumour, especially malignant tumours where there is a danger of haemorrhaging. However, acupressure can be useful to relieve stress and aid relaxation in people undergoing chemotherapy.

**Current uses**: These include asthma, constipation, insomnia, sciatica, dizziness, fatigue, sore throat, impotence, ulcers, gastrointestinal disorders, arthritis, back pain, migraines, muscle cramps and hypoglycaemia. Acupressure is also used as a first aid treatment for nose bleeds, sprains, contusions, fractures and vomiting. Treatments have been used effectively by nurses in chemotherapy units (Price *et al*, 1991) as well as in other situations.

**Required training**: A minimum of 86 days of practical tuition is required to qualify. Therefore, course lengths vary from 12 months to 3 years, depending on time available for study. After two years of study, a student can practise as a supervised student practitioner before becoming a qualified practitioner.

## Aromatherapy

**Background**: **Aromatherapy** is an ancient healing practice and religious ritual which uses **essential oils** extracted from plants to provide psychological and physiological healing. Humans have been extracting chemical substances from plants for thousands of years; for example, digitalis (now used as a beta blocker) is extracted from the foxglove plant, *digitalis, digitalis*. The use of plants in Indian medicine reflects the religious and philosophical view of man as part of the continually changing process of nature; the scientific basis of their use forms the basis of Ayurvedic medicine today. Chinese herbal medicine is another ancient practice that uses essential oils. The classic text of this practice is *Pen ts/ao kang-mou*, a formulary that lists 8,160 different formulae including minerals such as sulphur, iron and mercury. According to archaeological evidence and ancient records, this book was in use before 1000 BC.

The use of oils from plants was revived by Rene Gattefosse during the 1920s. He found that the essential oils used in his firm's products were better antiseptics than the chemical antiseptics being added to the same products. His interest in this area began when he burnt his hand in an explosion, and plunged it into lavender oil to cool it down. The wound healed in only a few hours, did not become infected and left no scar. Thus, he began to research the dermatological use of essential oils.

**Physiological basis for action**: Stanway (1982) defines aromatherapy as "a combination of body and face massage using essential oils extracted from plants." Some of the oils may be taken internally as well. Essential oils vary in their properties and their effects; some may stimulate, others sedate. The oils are extracted from various parts of plants, trees and shrubs, and are distilled into concentrated chemicals with complex organic structures. Chemical analogues of essential oils can be produced in the laboratory, but they do not have the same properties as those extracted from the plants (Stanway, 1982).

Essential oils used in aromatherapy act directly on the **limbic system** (pleasure centre) of the brain via the olfactory nerve. The aromas are sensed at the olfactory bulb, which then sends a nerve impulse to the brain to stimulate the release of endorphins. The

**Learning Disabilities Nursing**
**Aromatherapy for relaxation**

When working with adults who have a learning disability, it is easy to underestimate the need for, and effect of, physical contact. People with learning disabilities sometimes express their need for physical contact by approaching other people, including strangers, in an overly intimate way. The use of aromatherapy oils with massage (particularly hand and foot massage) enables these people to have their physical contact needs met in a socially acceptable and age-appropriate way. Massage enables these individuals to enjoy the undivided attention of their carer and to exert some control over their own life by participating in decisions, such as choice of essential oil, and determining the time, place and duration of the massage.

essential oils used in massage permeate the skin and enter the circulating venous blood in the capillaries.

**Contraindications:** Most people find essential oils relaxing; however, they should be used with caution, because some people may be sensitized to some aromas and may find that particular smells evoke bad memories rather than pleasant ones. Some aromas may cause nausea. At the Royal Marsden Hospital, strong aromatic oils are not used in conjunction with chemotherapy and other treatments that cause violent nausea and vomiting. Because it is difficult to control the drift of the aroma, sufficient ventilation should be provided in public places where aromatherapy is used, such as in critical care units, wards, and outpatient clinics.

Undiluted essential oils should never be used directly on the skin or where the skin is broken or bruised. Massage with essential oils is contraindicated in patients/clients who have a high risk of thrombosis due to bed rest.

**Current uses:** Today, specially trained nurses use essential oils for research purposes in cardiothoracic units, paediatric intensive care units, labour wards (Burns and Blamey, 1994) and cancer treatment centres, as well as in the community setting for venous ulcer treatments, stress reduction and terminal care in the home (Swaffield, 1992; Wright, 1990; Rankin-Box, 1989; Marshall, 1991; Crowther, 1991; Faulkner, 1990; Smith, 1991; Swinnerton, 1991). Some nurses use essential oils with massage for people with learning disabilities in order to facilitate communication, as this is sometimes the only channel of communication for people with severe or profound disabilities. This therapy is also used to empower the disabled individual: by enabling him or her to choose oils; become aware of his or her body; and to help him or her to relax (Sanderson and Carter, 1994). Common oils used include lavender, lemon balm, rosemary and marjoram. When used in massage, the oils are often mixed in a low dilution with a *carrier* or base oil — often a light vegetable oil.

**Training requirements:** Training in aromatherapy is offered by a variety of nursing colleges, as well as by unclassified organizations. Nurses should ensure the course they undertake is of a sufficient academic level and provides a sufficient research base to provide the skills and knowledge particular to nursing needs. The European Community requires all practitioner courses to be at least three years in duration. This cost requirement will limit nurse practitioners unless managers consider aromatherapy skills an integral part of the care offered for particular situations.

## Chiropractic

**Background:** Chiropractic is a manipulative therapy designed to maintain the spinal column and nervous system in good health without the use of surgery or medications. **Chiropractic** is derived from the Greek words *cheir* (hands) and *practikos* (done by). Ancient Egyptian manuscripts describe chiropractic techniques and ancient Hindu, Babylonian and Assyrian physicians used a similar manipulative treatment.

Chiropractic was revived by Dr Daniel Palmer who manipulated the vertebrae in the neck of his caretaker, thus curing his long-standing deafness. After further successes, Palmer researched the anatomy and physiology of his methods, thus providing the philosophy for the treatment now called *chiropractic*. Further research supported the therapy and a science developed from this in America.

**Physiological basis for action:** Chiropractors manipulate a person's joints by hand to re-balance the body's function. The principle theory is that modern life produces stresses which cause abnormalities in the joints and subsequent deformities in the muscles. Diet, rest and exercise also form a part of the advice given in the treatment.

**Current uses:** Chiropractic is used as an aid to conventional medicine. It is used to correct distortions of posture, to restore function to spinal and pelvic joints, to remove nerve irritation which might be causing pain or disturbed function (such as low back pain or migraine), to treat asthma, or to treat arthritis or other musculoskeletal pain.

**Contraindications:** This treatment may be therapeutic for a variety of conditions when administered by a qualified practitioner. It is contraindicated for people with carcinomatous lesions or in people who may benefit more from conventional medicine.

**Training requirements:** Training for chiropractic consists of four years of full-time study. The main focus of study is on the spine and nervous system, but much of the supporting education in anatomy and physiology is similar to that provided in medical training. Chiropractic is therefore singularly physiological in defining disease and in providing an alternative to medical cure. Of all the alternative therapies, it is the most widely recognized by the medical profession.

## Herbalism

**Background: Herbalism** or **herbal medicine** is an ancient system of medicine that uses plants to prevent and cure disease. To the medical herbalist, a herb is any plant of medicinal value. There are at least 350,000 known species of plants, but only 10,000 have been examined for medicinal purposes. Plants almost exclusively contain three of the fatty acids essential to life; linoleic, linolenic and arachidonic acids.

**Physiological basis for action:** Naturally occurring medicinal substances are modified by other natural substances that occur in the plant. Research has shown that plants contain *secondary substances* which enhance other substances or medications, or which eliminate side effects. For example, digitalis, as used originally from the foxglove plant, cures the accumulation of body fluids secondary to heart failure with few side effects. However, when the active agent was isolated, it was found to be more potent and to produce more side effects than the natural whole leaf in the right dose.

**Contraindications:** Herbal remedies should be administered only by a qualified medical herbalist, because the remedies may either enhance or reduce the effects of conventional medications, or may cause allergic reactions.

**Current uses:** Thousands of pounds are invested annually in screening for potential anti-cancer properties of plants, but only 20 or 30 have shown any opportunities for use. For example, vincristine, extracted from the periwinkle plant, is used to treat leukaemia. Vinblastine, also extracted from periwinkle, is used to treat Hodgkin's disease. Other herbal remedies are used to treat Raynaud's disease, rheumatoid arthritis, sinus problems, sciatica, thrush, toothache, vertigo, colitis, and viral infections.

**Training requirements:** Training to become a medical herbalist takes several years. This does not include a medical education. The National Institute of Medical Herbalists offers a four-year course. Doctors can take a one-year course at the School of Herbal Medicine.

## Homeopathy

**Background: Homeopathy** is a system of medicine based on the principle that agents which produce certain signs and symptoms in health also cure those signs and symptoms in disease. This therapy is also based on the principle that the more a remedy is diluted, the more powerful it becomes. The principle is, for example, that of heat curing the effect of heat. In homeopathy, it is the patient/client who is treated and not the disease, as in **allopathic medicine**. The philosophy is that the body has a 'vital force' which is re-established to gain the natural balance, eliminating symptoms and preventing them in the future.

**Physiological basis for action:** Samuel Hahnemann (1775-1843) believed **miasms**, the inherited effect of a disease that has been suppressed, to be at the root of all disease. He maintained that the miasm is the 'residue' left by the disease and passed on to generations, and that many of today's diseases are the aftermath of these miasms. In homeopathy, the sets of behaviours and traits in the illness experience are classified into groups that share characteristics. Homeopaths have found that in the course of true healing, symptoms and suppressed manifestations of a miasm always reappear in the reverse order of their original development. Hering, a nineteenth century American homeopath, encapsulated this principle in his 'Law of Cure'. This states that the disease will leave the body:

- from the top downwards
- from the mind to the body
- from inside outwards
- from the main organs to those of lesser importance.

**Homeopathic remedies** are made from a variety of substances, such as plants, animals, insects, reptiles, minerals, and metals. More than 2000 remedies are now in use, and are available in forms such as tablets, tinctures and powders. Most remedies are available over-the-counter in a 6c or 30c potency ('c' refers to the dilution of the remedy). The remedies can be diluted in water and sipped, placed under the tongue, or placed on a lactose tablet and dissolved in the mouth (Trevelyan, 1994a).

**Contraindications:** Although some remedies may not be useful for some conditions, they are generally considered to be safe. Some remedies can be used to supplement orthodox treatment.

**Current uses:** In the nineteenthth century, homeopathic hospitals were successful in treating cholera. Today, homeopathy is available on the NHS and in at least six homeopathic hospitals in the UK. Research has found homeopathy to be effective in treating rheumatoid arthritis (Gibson, 1980) and hay fever (Taylor Reilly, 1986). The remedies are also popular for children, for use during childbirth, and are available in first aid kits. Nurses should not use the remedies, however, unless permission has been obtained from the patient's/client's doctor, or the employing hospital, trust, health authority or board (Trevelyan, 1994b).

**Training requirements:** There are now more than 2000 GPs in the UK who use homeopathic remedies or who refer patients to homeopathic hospitals (Trevelyan, 1994a). Training in homeopathy should take place at a recognized college or institute. Completion of a three-year, intensive full-time course allows membership of the British Homeopathic Association. Many medically trained doctors are also homeopaths who incorporate homeopathic remedies into orthodox treatments. Currently, nurses who are trained homeopaths cannot prescribe the remedies as a part of their nursing role. They have to practise homeopathy outside the NHS unless they are employed as a homeopath within the NHS and not as a nurse.

## Hypnosis

**Background: Hypnosis** is used in certain circumstances to induce a trance-like state of compliance and suggestibility in an individual. Almost everybody is susceptible to hypnosis and it has been proven that the more intelligent the person, the more easily he or she can be hypnotized (Stanway, 1982). Historically, hypnosis dates back to the Greeks who used it as a form of therapy for anxiety and hysterical states. These conditions are effectively treated with hypnosis today. Sigmund Freud used hypnosis in his early work, because it was one of the only ways to relax patients/clients for surgery, other than the use of ether which was introduced in 1846 (Stanway, 1982).

**Physiological basis for action:** Hypnosis is an altered state of mind, but is not sleep. Studies using electroencephalography to investigate cerebral impulse patterns have demonstrated that a person under hypnosis is neither awake nor asleep. The induction process of hypnosis usually occurs as the subject is closing his or her eyes, and the hypnotist verbalizes positive phrases that are familiar to the person. There is a critical area of the consciousness which has to be bypassed by both the subject and the hypnotist before being able to access the subject's unconscious mind where control over all the body functions is achieved. **Age regression** is a technique which enables the hypnotist to allow the subject to 'experience childhood' again, and even experience his or her birth.

**Mother and Child Nursing**
**Use of complementary therapies in midwifery**

Complementary and supplementary therapies are accepted as part of the midwife's strategy for care. For example, relaxation techniques have been in use for a few decades. Aromatherapy, acupuncture, massage, and hypnosis are among the complementary methods practised by midwives, but prior to their acceptance there is a need to consider both the altered physiology of the mother and the well-being of the fetus. Midwives are therefore advised to become knowledgeable and competent before putting complementary therapies into practice and to ensure that these are acceptable to the mothers. Bennett and Brown (1989) state: "Midwives who are interested in alternative forms of pain relief should be prepared to make a thorough study of the remedies available, their uses and mode of action and the possible side effects".

**Contraindications:** Hypnosis should not be used with patients/clients who have severe depression or who are in a psychotic state. Their problems can be made worse by trying to induce a hypnotic trance. Initial hypnotherapy sessions should focus on establishing a sound relationship with the patient/client. Creating a therapeutic relationship will enhance further sessions and enable a positive outcome. Some counselling techniques are used, and the hypnotherapist should use a nonjudgemental approach. Carl Rogers' practice of unconditional positive regard for the patient/client is beneficial because the person will become relaxed enough to become induced into a trance state.

**Current uses:** Today, hypnosis is used for pain control, for example when anaesthetics are dangerous to use. Physical conditions in patients/clients that may have a psychological element (particularly stress) will benefit from the therapy. Caesarean sections without the use of any drugs have been performed on prepared subjects who were hypnotized. Migraine, skin problems such as psoriasis, and problems with the gastrointestinal tract, such as colitis and constipation, can be helped using hypnosis (Tamin, 1988; Whorwell *et al*, 1992). Some dentists use hypnosis for pain control during surgery (Conway, 1989; Hartland, 1971). Self-hypnosis is also useful. A randomized trial of analgesia during labour demonstrated that women who used self-hypnosis were more satisfied with their delivery than those who did not use hypnosis (Freeman *et al*, 1986).

Hypnosis is also used to help people stop smoking or to break other habits; to help resolve stress-related conditions; and to help change self-image perceptions, for instance following mastectomy. Nurses whose work involves counselling and guided imagery therapy may be trained to use hypnosis. Some research studies suggests that nurses who work in Accident and Emergency departments may find the application of hypnosis useful for patients/clients who are anxious or in pain (Puskar, 1990).

**Training requirements:** Training in hypnosis is provided by several colleges. An accredited course for nurses is available at Manchester University in conjunction with the Institute for Complementary Medicine and the Royal College of Nursing. Training can range from four months to one year.

## Osteopathy

**Background:** Osteopathy is a manipulative therapy which is similar to chiropractic, although the practice of osteopathy is 20 years older. **Osteopathy** uses the philosophy of the structure and mechanical function of the body to diagnose problems and alleviate dysfunctions. The spine is the main area of treatment and the biomechanical principle of 'structure governs function' supports the theory that, after alleviating the stress of dysfunction, the body will be able to heal and resolve the health problems that caused the presenting difficulties. The whole person is considered when planning the treatment.

**Physiological basis for action:** Andrew Taylor Still, a doctor in the US, began to research the therapeutic concepts of osteopathy. He considered the spine to be important in maintaining health because of its protective structure for the nerves and cerebrospinal fluid. The process of **manipulation** was developed by Still to reverse damage to the muscles, and thus enable the body to cure itself.

The governing principles of osteopathy are:

*   a holistic perception of the body's functioning
*   the body has the mechanisms of defence and repair to regulate and treat itself
*   the maintenance of the circulation of all the body's fluids will help restore the imbalances of ill-health which are the result of disturbances to the normal state of equilibrium.

This 'circulatory' theory supports the notion that nerves are involved with the genesis of many medical problems and the correction of lesions in mechanical joints will resolve health imbalances. Often, osteopaths counsel patients/clients in genetic, environmental, developmental, dietary, psychological, bacteriological and toxicological features and characteristics. Although many of these problems are not treatable through osteopathy, there may be a positive understanding of self-regulation for the individual through health education. This may be regarded as part of the treatment, along with a drug-free way to resolve some of the problems.

### Children's Nursing
### Use of hypnosis and relaxation in children

Hypnosis can be used effectively with children aged 4–5 years (Lansdown, 1987) and can be used to control pain, irritation and anxiety. The more imaginative the child, and the more used he or she is to being immersed in stories, the more successful it will be. Lansdowne used guided imagination, such as 'a magic room', to induce sleep and relieve pain. Learning the technique can take as little as three sessions, as children are more susceptible than adults. However, the child will need sufficient powers of concentration in order to attend to a story. If the child is motivated and the parents supportive, this technique can be effective.

Relaxation is also useful for relieving pain in children. Asking children to take a deep breath and to "go as limp as a rag doll" while exhaling slowly, followed by yawning, is very effective (Wong, 1995). This is particularly effective in younger children.

**Contraindications:** Osteopathy should not be used in people who have osteoporosis or inflamed joints from arthritis, or in pregnant women (because of the increased risk of miscarriage in the first trimester — due to the potentially stressful alterations to the mother's circulatory system).

**Current uses:** Osteopathy is used to restore structure and function to the back, neck, and any other abnormal joint. It is also used in the treatment of bronchitis, asthma, trigeminal neuralgia, and menstrual problems. **Cranial osteopathy** (manipulation of the skull bones) is used to treat migraine.

**Training requirements:** In 1874, osteopathy was officially recognized as a therapeutic treatment in the United Kingdom. There are now degree programmes which are often taught alongside degrees for physiotherapy in universities. The degree course and other nonuniversity courses range from three to four years, depending on the institute, and incorporate theoretical and practical instruction.

Nurses should not use osteopathic treatments unless they have been trained and have qualified from a reputable school. Training is governed by statutes outlined in the Osteopath's Bill (1993). From 1995, there will be regulation of osteopaths similar to that for nursing, midwifery, medicine and dentistry.

## Reflexology

**Background:** The principles of **reflexology** are based on the belief that the body's natural healing can be enhanced by applying pressure to certain areas of the feet and hands. These areas are said to be connected by a flow of energy. The word *reflex* refers to the areas or zones of the feet that are said to be connected to specific organs of the body which can be mapped out (Fig. 32-2). The reflexive effect of treatment is explained through present knowledge about neurology. There are areas on the surface of the body that represent internal organs, due to the close and sequential development during embryonic and fetal growth.

Therapies that used pressure for healing were in use some 5,000 years ago. William Fitzgerald, an American ear, nose and throat specialist practising in the early 1900s, first revived the treatment in its present form by discovering the analgesic effects of pressure upon certain parts of his patients'/clients' nose, mouth and throat. Since then, Eunice Ingham, an American physiotherapist, has defined specific areas of the foot where therapeutic effects are produced when pressure is applied to a specific distal area of the body. In the 1960s, a student of Miss Ingham's, Doreen Bayley, began the first training school for reflexology therapists based in the UK.

**Physiological basis for action:** The philosophy of reflexology is loosely associated with the theories of meridians and energy flows of the body, as mapped by the Chinese for their acupressure techniques. However, there is a more evenly defined zoning of areas in reflexology and it is therefore more easily understood and practised. Illness is seen as energy which is misdirected through 'energy zones'. The therapist identifies crystalline deposits in certain areas of the feet (which relate to an organ) that are impeding the flow of energy. Treatment consists of gently dispersing these deposits with firm massage of the area on the foot.

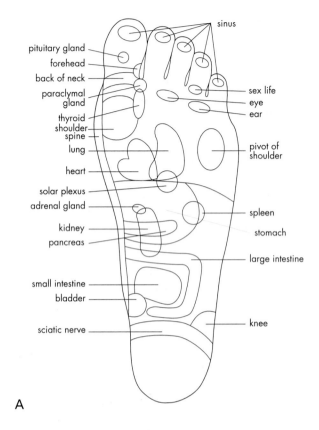

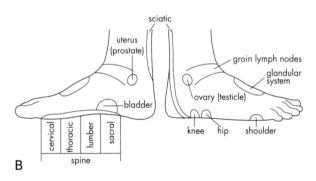

**Fig. 32-2** An example of selected reflex zones charted on the right foot. A, Dorsal view B, lateral view.

The zones of the body are aligned vertically with zones on each foot. The soles of each foot are mapped in accordance with the main structures of the body; that is, the head area is related to the toes, the chest area to the ball of the foot and the waistline may be compared to the narrowest part of the foot. The zones also relate to areas on the upper surface of the foot where, for instance, there may be a relationship between the ankle area and the organs in the pelvic region of the body.

**Contraindications:** Although reflexology is considered to be a safe procedure, contraindications for this therapy include:

- deep vein thrombosis
- leg ulcers
- pronounced varicose veins
- viral infections, such as verrucas
- fungal diseases, such as athlete's foot
- phlebitis or other circulatory disorders of the lower limbs.

Reflexology should be used with caution in pregnant women and in patients/clients who have gallstones, kidney stones, a pacemaker, or liver problems.

**Current uses:** Few, if any, clinical trials have been conducted to test the effectiveness of reflexology. However, the treatment is promoted as being beneficial for gastrointestinal disorders (such as heartburn, constipation and diarrhoea); skin problems (such as acne, eczema, and psoriasis); arthritis; menstrual problems; asthma; and migraines (Trevelayan and Booth, 1994). Some beneficial effects from the procedure have been noted in recent case histories. The treatment was considered beneficial, for example, to mothers and babies in a post-natal ward (Evans, 1990), for new mothers (Sofroniou, 1993), and for oncology patients/clients (Burke, 1992).

**Training requirements:** Training in reflexology requires six to nine months. The Association of Reflexologists provides training standards, a code of ethics, a professional register and continuing education. The British Reflexology Association provides a professional register, insurance coverage, and publications (see box on p. 676).

## Therapeutic Massage

**Background: Therapeutic massage** uses a variety of manual tactile movements that involve applying pressure on specific areas of the body. Through this movement and use of pressure, internal muscles and soft tissue are manipulated externally from the skin surface. The principle philosophy of therapeutic massage is that the manipulation stimulates circulation of blood and lymph, thereby cleansing the body of potential deposits of toxins. Therapeutic massage works on the same principle as acupuncture. The object is to strengthen and relax the muscles, and to release blockages in the flow of the body's energy, or *chi*.

Historically, the writings in the *Ayur Veda*, an Indian text from 1800 BC, formally describe the effective use of massage as a treatment. The theories of Hippocrates (d. 370 BC) advocate the use of massage as a valuable treatment for preventing illness and for maintaining health. It was also a known treatment of Galen, a Greek physician in the second century.

**Physiological basis for action:** The theories of the use of 'touch' as a therapy may be easily combined with those of massage; massage should be considered as directed contact with an aim or goal. Social touching may be directional but not necessarily therapeutic, and therefore can be misconstrued by patients/clients. Massage is a natural remedy for localized pain.

Work by Melzac and Wall (1988) has helped to define three sensory systems in the skin: pressure, heat and pain. When stimulated, these systems stimulate the nervous system, which integrates with spinal response mechanisms as well as the cerebral pathways. Systematic reaction from 'gates' which close on a prolonged pain stimulus (see Gate Control Theory of Pain, Chapter 27) enable the brain to produce endorphins and other pain reducing substances as a normal reaction to chronic pain. Massage also aids relaxation and may be used to treat stress-related problems such as shoulder stiffness, insomnia, and headaches. Subjective data indicate massage may be effective as a complementary therapy to orthodox treatment of oncology patients/clients and people who have AIDS. It may also be beneficial in treating people with hypertension, asthma, constipation, depression, tension and anxiety, as well as secondary psychological symptoms of lack of self-esteem, and low self-confidence (Sanderson and Carter, 1994). It is used as a supporting treatment for athletes, both pre- and postactivities, to prevent sports-related injuries and problems.

**Contraindications:** Therapeutic massage should not be used in people with skin lesions from infections or inflammation or in people receiving anticoagulation therapy, due to the high risk of subcutaneous haemorrhage. It should not be used on any area of the body that has undergone recent trauma, and should not be used to treat pregnant women in their first trimester, although gentler forms of effleurage may be used if the abdominal and pelvic areas, and the ankles, are avoided.

**Current uses:** Nurses have found that the use of massage, as part of planned interventions, enhances the therapeutic relationship with patients/clients (Sanderson and Carter; 1994). The process of touch and care by nurses for patients'/clients' physical and psychological (emotional) pain has been appropriately mastered in the professional setting and is supported by nursing theory for practice (Benner and Wrubel, 1989; Rogers, 1970). Massage is used frequently as an adjunct to other therapies, such as osteopathy and chiropractic, reflexology, aromatherapy; and by several professions allied to medicine, such as physiotherapy. Massage is also practised by Indian parents on their newborn and young infants to promote bonding. This is being practised increasingly by health visitors as a way of supporting parents. Massage is also used as a complementary treatment for sports injuries.

Therapeutic massage should be given in a suitable environment. If the masseur is also a nurse and a formal massage room is available, then all the rules of maintaining dignity and provision of privacy are applied. Inform the patient/client that a full body massage may take one hour. In some circumstances, the relaxation induced by the massage may also cause patients/clients to release their emotions; therefore, additional time should be allocated for this. Nurses and health visitors who use massage in the patient's/client's home should use a similar professional approach.

---

 **Children's Nursing**
**Use of massage in infants**

It has been recognized recently that neonates benefit greatly from massage (Russell, 1993). The need for human contact is consistent from the time the fetus leaves the uterus and becomes physically separated from the mother. Montague (1986), states that denial or deprivation of primary tactile experiences may be revealed as crucial in the development of personalities and character structure. It is very important for neonates in special care units to be exposed to tactile stimulation; however, for the very immature infant minimal handling is required. Massaging these infants also benefits the mother, who may feel her baby belongs to nursing and medical staff. Encouraging the mother to massage her infant gently, under supervision, will stimulate emotional contact and bonding.

---

**Training requirements:** Training for massage is often combined with training for other therapies. Courses vary in time and in the intensity of learning; counselling is almost never included as a part of the course. Considering the personal and intimate nature of the treatment, a caring professional will appreciate the potential situations promoted by the therapy and enhance the time spent with the patient/client by utilizing other skills, such as active listening.

### Therapeutic Touch

**Background: Therapeutic touch** is an ancient healing art and science. It is based on the philosophy that living beings are 'energy fields' and an integral part of a universal life force that extends beyond the physical body and interacts with the environment. Health is seen as a manifestation of this 'vital' energy and therefore ill health results from problems with the energy flow. The therapist draws energy from the environment through his or her body, or from other areas in the patient/client where there is congestion, and directs it into the area where it is lacking. Symmetry is then restored to the field, which allows the body to regenerate its wholeness. It is not essential to have skin-to-skin contact in this therapy, since the energy exists in contact fields beyond the skin surface (Sayre-Adams, 1993).

**Physiological basis for action:** Martha Rogers provided a nursing model for therapeutic touch in the US called the 'Science of Unitary Human Beings', and this has been propounded by Jean Sayre-Adams in the UK (Sayre-Adams, 1993). The Kreiger-Kuntz method of therapeutic touch is the harnessing of healing power that is believed to be latent in everyone. Many experiments have been undertaken to prove the efficacy of therapeutic touch. One experiment demonstrated that therapeutic touch increased haemoglobin levels in volunteers (Krieger, 1975). As a result of this research, the technique is widely used by nurses in the US. Research has also been conducted in using therapeutic touch to relieve tension headaches and stress in children and adults (Sayre-Adams, 1994). Therapeutic touch has been used beneficially in mental health nursing (Hill and Oliver, 1993).

**Contraindications**: There are no contraindications for the use of therapeutic touch. Individuals who hold particular religious beliefs where 'laying on of hands' may be offensive, and where spiritual or psychic healing may cause offence, will not wish to undertake this therapy.

**Training requirements:** In the UK, the Didsbury Trust offers courses in therapeutic touch, from introductory to practitioner level (see box on p. 676).

## THE NURSE AS PRACTITIONER OF COMPLEMENTARY THERAPIES

The United Kingdom Central Council allows nurses to train for and practise complementary therapies, but does not validate or approve courses. The Royal College of Nursing has issued guidelines to assist in course selection, and the RCN indemnity insurance scheme covers the majority of complementary therapies (up to £1,000, plus legal costs), except herbalism and homeopathy. The RCN Complementary Therapies in Nursing Special Interest

Group issues a regular newsletter to keep its 2,000 members up-to-date on UK activities, and plans to initiate annual conferences in this area.

Many medical professionals are now attending courses in nonmedical therapies; however, educational standards for most of the therapies have yet to be established. Nurses who successfully complete a full course in a particular therapy, will be able to use their skills within and without the nursing profession. However, unlike doctors or other professionals allied to medicine, nurses are *not* able to advertise as nurses if they are using their therapeutic skills as a part of their practice repertoire. In 1993, the International Council for Nursing proposed that nurses should be allowed to practice their profession outside the NHS as independent practitioners; however, this issue has not yet been resolved.

### Training and Education for Practioners

Training and education for complementary therapies is described in a publication by the Institute of Complementary Medicine (see box on p. 676), who also hold a register of qualified practitioners. However, since January 1993, the European Community has declared that training courses should be of at least three years in length for all therapies. Many colleges have already acted on this requirement and provide courses for osteopathy, chiropractic, homeopathy and acupuncture to comply with the degree status which will become the norm. In addition, some nursing schools provide university accreditation in complementary therapies courses; such courses do not train nurses to practise the therapies, but do enable them to respond to patients'/clients' questions and needs, and to evaluate the effectiveness and appropriateness of various therapies (Trevelyan, 1994b). All EC member states will have to realize a level of comparability in training programmes. There are now plans in the UK to provide competency standards under the National Vocational Qualifications scheme. Nurses, midwives and health visitors who hold qualifications in a variety of therapies will be required to register according to their training received in each therapy. This will support the accountability and professional practice of nurses.

This committee also reviews the training and education of complementary therapies practitioners, who are considered to be at a different level of expertise to practitioners in other European Community countries (Gaier, 1990).

### SUMMARY

Interest in the use of complementary therapies has recently increased in both health care professionals and consumers, mirroring the move towards a more holistic attitude to nursing care and the maintenance of good health. This rediscovery of the potential of complementary therapies represents a shift from the straightforward medical diagnosis–cure approach. Instead, these traditional remedies concentrate on a mind-body spirit approach, enlisting the self-healing capacity of the body and treating symptoms in a broader context, encompassing the health-related behaviour and lifestyle considerations of each individual.

Demand for these therapies is growing, and the wide range of treatments available can provide the patient/client with an individualized programme consisting of a specific therapy or combination of therapies. Therapies are based on the use of sensory stimulation, the manipulation of body parts, and promotion of relaxation techniques. Stemming from ancient philosophies, knowledge of plant properties, and understanding of the healing properties of touch, therapies have much to offer patients/clients, especially when planned in conjunction with orthodox treatments. The health care profession has recognized this, and current demand for an improved system of formal training and registration reflects this move.

### CHAPTER 32 REVIEW
### Key Concepts

- An increasing number of nurses are including complementary therapies in their practice and are undertaking additional training in this field.
- A variety of social, economic and medical factors are influencing an increasing number of patients/clients to utilize complementary therapies.
- The philosophy of holism and holistic caregiving underlies the historical basis for delivering nursing care, and is the historical basis for the development of complementary therapies.
- The UK is developing training and education requirements to comply with EC directives for education and training in complementary therapies.
- Most complementary therapies have evolved from ancient philosophies and systems of medicine.
- Acupuncture uses needles to stimulate energy release or to gather energy from the energy meridians of the body.
- Pressure applied with the fingers to pressure points along the meridians is used to stimulate energy release in acupressure treatment.
- Aromatherapy uses essential oils extracted from plants either to stimulate or relax the patient/client.
- Chiropractic is a manipulative therapy designed to maintain the spinal column and nervous system in good health without the use of surgery or medications.
- Qualified medical herbalists use a variety of plant extracts to treat conditions such as rheumatoid arthritis, sinus problems, colitis, and toothache.
- Homeopathic remedies are made from substances such as plants, animals, and minerals, and are used in diluted form, sometimes as an adjunct to orthodox medical treatment.
- Hypnosis is used for pain control and to treat physical conditions that may have a psychological element, such as migraine, psoriasis, or colitis.
- Osteopathy is a manipulative therapy that operates on the basis that alleviating the stress of mechanical dysfunction will enable the body to heal and resolve health problems.
- The principles of reflexology are based on the belief that the body's natural healing can be enhanced by applying pressure to certain areas of the feet and hands.
- The principle of therapeutic massage is that applying pressure to specific areas of the body stimulates circulation of blood and lymph, thereby cleansing the body of potential toxins.

- Therapeutic touch is based on the philosophy that redirecting a person's energy fields helps restore wholeness and health.
- The UKCC allows nurses to train for and practise complementary therapies, but does not validate or approve courses.

## Key Terms

Acupressure, p. 679
Acupuncture, p. 679
Allopathic medicine, p. 681
Aromatherapy, p. 680
Chi, p. 678
Chiropractic, p. 681
Endorphin(s), p. 679
Essential oil(s), p. 680
Herbalism/herbal medicine, p. 681
Homeopathy, p. 681
Hypnosis, p. 682
Life force, p. 676
Meridians, p. 679
Osteopathy, p. 683
Reflexology, p. 683
T'ai-chi, p. 678
Therapeutic massage, p. 685
Therapeutic touch, p. 685
Yin and Yang, p. 678

## CRITICAL THINKING EXERCISES

1. In which way does the professional nurse make best use of his or her skills in practising holistic nursing within the complementary therapy field?
2. What aspects of assessment of a patient/client would you ensure you included now, as a result of reading this chapter?
3. How may nurses relate to their professional accountability when using skills associated with complementary therapies?
4. Should nurses not use these therapies formally at all, and bring non-nurse therapists in from the private sector to provide these services?

## REFERENCES

Benner P, Wrubel J: *The primacy of caring,* Reading MA, 1989, Addison-Wesley Publishing Co., Inc.

Bennett VR, Brown LK: *Myles textbook for midwives,* ed 11, Edinburgh, 1989, Churchill Livingstone.

Bergsman O, Woolley-Hart A: Differences in electrical skin conductivity between acupuncture points and adjacent skin areas, *Am J Acupuncture* 1:27, 1973.

Buchan J et al: *International mobility of nurses: a UK perspective,* IMS report no 230, London, 1992, Institute of Manpower Studies/Royal College of Nursing.

Burke C, Sikora K: Cancer: the dual approach, *Nurs Times* 88(38):62, 1992.

Burns E, Blamey C: Using aromatherapy in childbirth, *Nurs Times* 90(9):54, 1994.

Conway A: Hypnosis and research into mind/body relationships, *Complement Med Res* 3(2):9, 1989.

Crowther D: Complementary therapy in practice, *Nurs Standard* 5(23):25, 1991.

Evans M: Reflex zone therapy for mothers, *Nurs Times* 86(4):29, 1990.

Faulkner A: Autogenics-neighborhood venture, *Nurs Times* 86(16):50, 1990.

Freeman RM et al: Randomised trial of self hypnosis for analgesia in labour, *BMJ* 292:657, 1986.

Fulder S: *The handbook of complementary medicine,* London, 1989, Hodder & Stoughton.

Gaier H: Reveille for biocentric medicine. In Lewith G, Aldridge D, editors: *Complementary medicine and the European community,* London, 1990, CW Daniel.

Gibson RG et al: Homeopathy therapy in rheumatoid arthritis: evaluation by double blind clinical therapeutic trials, Br J Clin Pharm, 9(5): 413-419, 1980.

Grange JM: Infectious hazards of acupuncture and their prevention, *Complement Med Res* 4(2):39, 1990.

Hartland J: *Medical and dental hypnosis,* London, 1971, Bailliere Tindall.

Henderson V: *The nature of nursing,* New York, 1966, Macmillan.

Hill L, Oliver N: Therapeutic touch and theory-based mental health nursing, *J Psychosoc Nurs* 31(2):19, 1993.

Kettle C: Hoxton Health Group: a central resource for complementary health care. In *Complement Therapies Med* 1(3):148, 1993.

Krieger D: *The therapeutic touch: how to use your hands to help all heal.* New York, 1979, Prentice Hal.l

Lansdown R: A child's magic world where pain melts away, The Independent, 13:17.2.1987.

Lewith G, Aldridge D, editors: *Complementary medicine and the European community,* London, 1990, CW Daniel.

Marshall M: Stress management in dermatology patients, *Nurs Standard* 5(24):29, 1991.

McFarlane J: The value of models for care. In Kershaw B, Salvage J, editors: *Models for nursing,* Chichester, 1986, John Wiley & Sons.

Melzack R, Wall PD: *The challange of pain,* ed 2, Harmondsworth, 1988, Penguin Books.

Montague A: *Touching: the human significance of the skin,* New York, 1986, Harper & Row.

National Association of Health Authorities and Trusts: Survey Paper no.10, London, 1993, DOH.

Nightingale F: *Notes on nursing; what it is and what it is not,* Ontario, 1969, Dover Publications.

Orem DE: *Nursing, concepts of practice,* ed 4, St Louis, 1991, Mosby.

Pietroni P: *The greening of medicine,* London, 1990, Victor Gollancz.

Price H, Lewith G, Williams C: Acupressure as an anti-emetic in cancer chemotherapy, *Complement Med Res* 5(2):93, 1991.

Puskar K, Mumford K: The healing power, *Nurs Times* 86(33):50, 1990.

Rankin-Box DF: *Complementary health therapies: a guide for nurses and the caring professions,* London, 1988, Chapman and Hall.

Rankin-Box DF: European developments in complementary medicine, *Br J Nurs* 1(2):103, 1992.

Reihl JP, Roy C, editors: *Conceptual models for nursing practice,* ed 2, Conn, 1980, Appleton-Century Crofts.

Rogers ME: *The theoretical basis for nursing,* Philadelphia, 1970, FA Davis.

Russell J: Touch and infant massage, *Paediatr Nurs* 5(3):1993.

Sanderson H, Carter A: Healing hands, *Nurs Times* 90(11):46, 1994.

Sayre-Adams J: Therapeutic touch-principles and practice, *Complement Therapies Med* 1(2):96, 1993.

Sayre-Adams J: Therapeutic touch: a nursing function, *Nurs Standard* 8, 1994.

Smith M: Complementary support, *Nurs Times* 87(32):36, 1991.

Sofroniou P: Reflexology: the practitioner's story. In: Booth B: *Complementary Therapy,* London, 1993, Macmillan.

Stanway A: *Alternative medicine,* Harmondsorth, 1982, Penguin Books.

Swaffield L: New age nursing, *Nurs Times* 88(27):19, 1992.

Swinnerton T: Alternative remedies during labour, *Nurs Times* 87(9):64, 1991.

Taylor Reilly D *et al*: Is homeopathy a placebo response?, *Lancet*, 2, (8152):881-885, 1986.

Tamin J: Hypnosis. In Rankin-Box, editor: *Complementary health therapies: a guide for nurses and the caring professions*, London, 1988, Chapman and Hall.

Trevelyan J: Homeopathy, *Nurs Times* 90(4):56, 1994a.

Trevelyan J: Courses of action, *Nurs Times* 90(7):21, 1994b.

Trevelyan J, Booth B: Complimentary medicine for nurses, midwifes and health visitors, London, 1994, Macmillan Publishers.

Vincent C, Mole P: Acupuncturists and research, *Complementary Med Res* 3(3):25, 1989.

Voll R: Twenty years of acupuncture diagnosis, *Am J Acupuncture* 3:7, 1975.

Weigant FAC, Kramers CW, van Wijk R: Clinical research in complementary medicine: the importance of patient selection, *Complement Med Res* 5(2):110, 1991.

Whorwell PJ, Houghton LA, Taylor EE *et al*: Physiological effects of emotion: assessment via hypnosis, *Lancet* 340(8811):69, 1992.

Wong D: *Nursing care of infants and children*, ed 5 St Louis, 1995, Mosby.

Wright S: Editorial, *Nursing Practice* 4(3):1, 1990.

## FURTHER READING

### Adult Nursing

Body Shop Team: *Mamatoto — a celebration of birth*, London, 1991, Virago Press.

de Aloysio D, Renaccioni P: Morning sickness control in early pregnancy by Neiguan acupressure, *Obstet Gynaecol* 80(5):852, 1992.

Fisher P: Research into homeopathic treatment of rheumatological disease: why and how? *Complement Med Res* 4(3):34, 1990.

Furnham A: Attitudes to alternative medicine: a study of the perceptions of those studying orthodox medicine. In *Complement Therapies Med* 1(3):120, 1993.

Jarmey C, Tindall J: *Acupressure for common ailments*, London, 1991, Gaia Books.

Jenkins MW, Prichard MH: Hypnosis: practical applications and theoretical considerations in normal labour, *Br J Obstet Gynaecol* 110(3):221, 1993.

Kaptchuk TJ: *The web that has no weaver: understanding Chinese medicine*, New York, 1983, Congdon and Weed.

Leigh S: Aromatherapy: making good scents, *MIDIRS Midwifery Digest* 1(3):305, 1991, Institute of Child Health, Bristol.

Smith M: Healing through touch, *Nurs Times* 86(4):31, 1990.

Taylor Reilly D: Homeopathy in focus: the modern state of the discussion, *Complmentary Medical Research*, 4(2): 41-54, 1990.

### Children's Nursing

Atherton D: Chinese herbs for eczema, *Lancet* 336(8725):1250, 1990.

David T: False allergic reactions in children with atopic eczema, *Eur J Clin Nutr* 45(suppl) 1:4751, 1991.

Kachyoeanos M, Friedhoff M: Cognitive and behavioural strategies to reduce children's pain, *MNC* 18:14, 1993.

McCaffery M: Pain relief for the child: problem areas and selected non-pharmacological methods, *Paediatr Nurs* 3:11, 1977.

Skinner S: Asthma treatment must consider the whole person, *Nurse Pract* 17(4):8, 1992.

### Learning Disabilities Nursing

Sanderson H, Harrison J, Price S: *Aromatherapy and massage for people who have learning difficulties*, Birmingham, 1991, Hands-on Publishing.

### Mental Health Nursing

Davis M: Movement characteristics of hospitalized psychiatric patients. In *American Dance Therapy Association proceedings* 25, (5th annual conference) Columbia, 1970.

Laban R: *The mastery of movement*, London, 1950, MacDonald & Evans.

Otis LS: The facts on transcendental meditation: if well integrated but anxious, try TM, *Psychol Today* 7:45, 1974.

Turnbull M, Norris H: Effects of transcendental meditation on self identity indices and personality, *Br J Psychol* 73:57, 1982.

# Index

# Index